# A **PRACTICAL** GUIDE TO OBSTETRICS & GYNECOLOGY

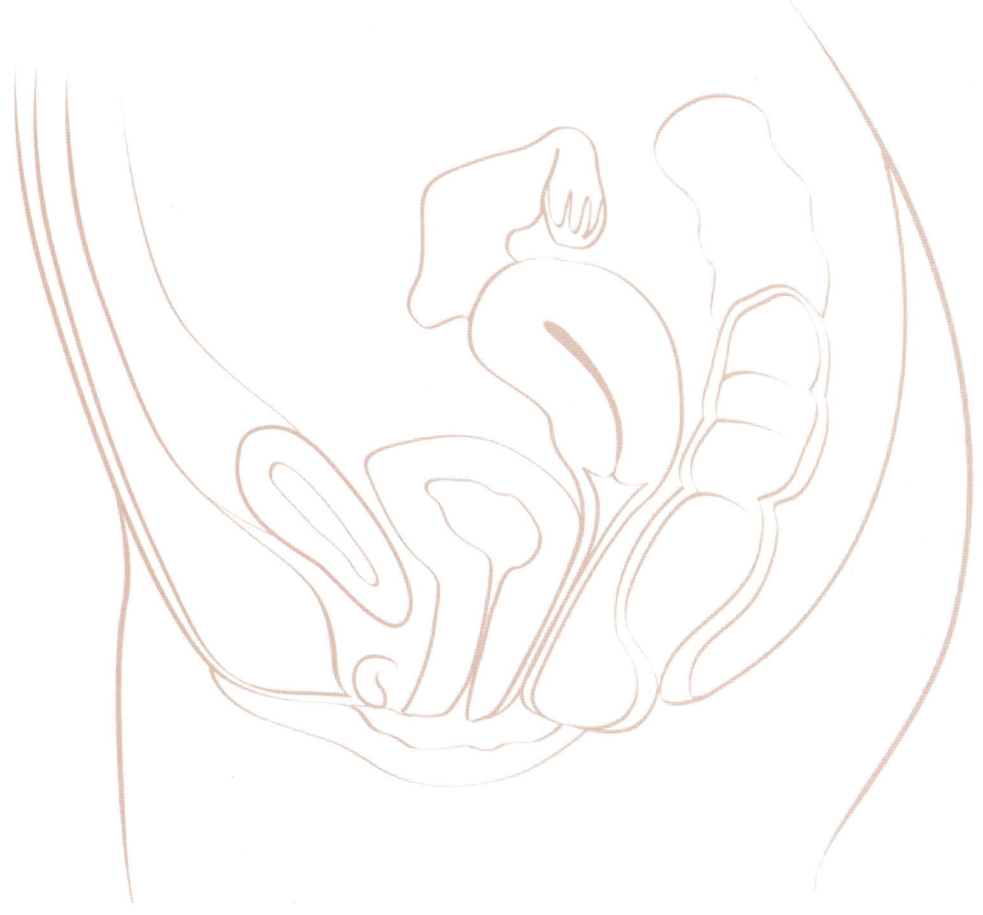

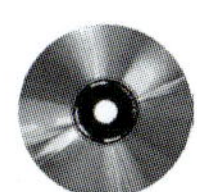

**System requirements:**
- Operating System—Windows Vista or above
- Web Browser—Google Chrome, Mozilla Firefox, Internet Explorer 9 and above
- Essential plugins—Java and Flash player
  - Facing problems in viewing content—it may be your system does not have java enabled.
  - If Videos don't show up—it may be the system requires Flash player or need to manage flash setting. To learn more about flash setting click on the link in the help section.
  - You can test java and flash by using the links from the help section of the CD/DVD.

**Accompanying CD/DVD-ROM is playable only in Computer and not in DVD player.**
The CD/DVD has Autorun function—it may take few seconds to load on your computer. If it does not works for you then follow the steps below to access the contents manually:
- Click on my computer
- Select the CD/DVD drive and click open/explore—this will show list of files in the CD/DVD
- Find and double click file—"launch.html"

For more information about troubleshoot of Autorun click on: http://support.microsoft.com/kb/330135

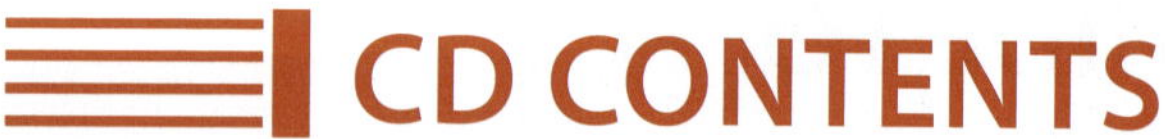# CD CONTENTS

**Video 1**: Fetal Skull: The Passenger

**Video 2**: Maternal Pelvis: The Passage

**Video 3**: Mechanism of Labor: The Journey

# A PRACTICAL GUIDE TO OBSTETRICS & GYNECOLOGY


**Richa Saxena**
MBBS MD (Obstetrics and Gynecology)
PG Diploma in Clinical Research
Obstetrician and Gynecologist
New Delhi, India


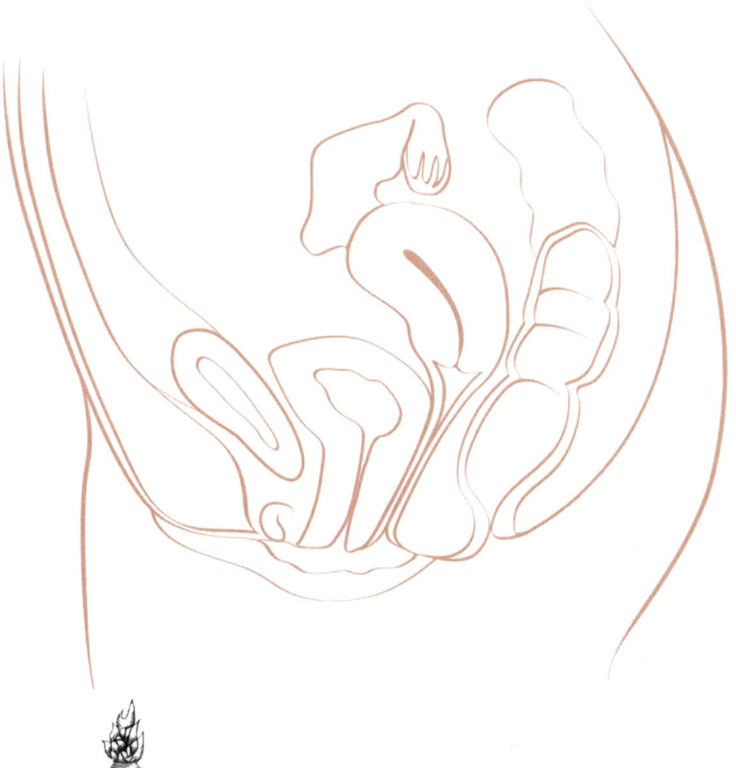


JAYPEE *The Health Sciences Publisher*

New Delhi | London | Philadelphia | Panama

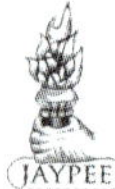 **Jaypee Brothers Medical Publishers (P) Ltd.**

**Headquarters**
Jaypee Brothers Medical Publishers (P) Ltd.
4838/24, Ansari Road, Daryaganj
New Delhi 110 002, India
Phone: +91-11-43574357
Fax: +91-11-43574314
E-mail: jaypee@jaypeebrothers.com

**Overseas Offices**

J.P. Medical Ltd.
83, Victoria Street, London
SW1H 0HW (UK)
Phone: +44-20 3170 8910
Fax: +44(0)20 3008 6180
E-mail: info@jpmedpub.com

Jaypee-Highlights Medical Publishers Inc.
City of Knowledge, Bld. 237, Clayton
Panama City, Panama
Phone: +1 507-301-0496
Fax: +1 507-301-0499
E-mail: cservice@jphmedical.com

Jaypee Medical Inc.
The Bourse
111, South Independence Mall East
Suite 835, Philadelphia, PA 19106, USA
Phone: +1 267-519-9789
E-mail: jpmed.us@gmail.com

Jaypee Brothers Medical Publishers (P) Ltd.
17/1-B, Babar Road, Block-B, Shaymali
Mohammadpur, Dhaka-1207
Bangladesh
Mobile: +08801912003485
E-mail: jaypeedhaka@gmail.com

Jaypee Brothers Medical Publishers (P) Ltd.
Bhotahity, Kathmandu, Nepal
Phone: +977-9741283608
E-mail: kathmandu@jaypeebrothers.com

Website: www.jaypeebrothers.com
Website: www.jaypeedigital.com



**Inquiries for bulk sales may be solicited at:** jaypee@jaypeebrothers.com

*A Practical Guide to Obstetrics & Gynecology*

*First Edition:* **2015**

ISBN: 978-93-5152-479-3

*Printed at* Replika Press Pvt. Ltd.

# Dedication

Dedicated to all the women, especially to the woman
whom I admire the most, my mother, "Mrs Bharati Saxena"

"A woman is the full circle. Within her is the power to create, nurture and transform."

**—Diane Mariechild**

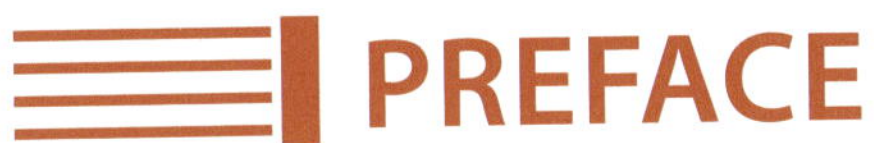

# PREFACE

*"If you don't believe in miracles, perhaps you have forgotten that you are one."*

—**God**

Childbirth can be considered as one of the most miraculous and mesmerizing processes of nature. While being extremely glorious and magnificent, it is equally intricate and complex. When undergraduate students first encounter a childbirth in the labor room, they are likely to get awestruck; even I was. To visualize how the baby's head negotiates through the delicate narrow maternal passage after undergoing a series of pre-decided movements is indeed marvellous. An undergraduate student who for the first time enters the labor room must understand that childbirth is not as difficult as may appear at the first glance, but a series of clever maneuvers which the passenger (the baby) undertakes while passing through the slender maternal passage (maternal pelvis) to complete its journey (childbirth).

Childbirth can be considered as a story illustrating the journey (process of childbirth) of a passenger (the baby), traveling via maternal passage. This is what the book, *"A Practical Guide to Obstetrics & Gynecology"* aims to offer by providing the complete coverage of all practical aspects of obstetrics and gynecology from both examination and viva point of view. This is not a quick-read handbook just before examinations, but a complete manual, which would serve as a comprehensive guide for undergraduate students. The book would not only be extremely useful for the undergraduates preparing for the practical/viva examination, but will also aid the postgraduate and DNB students for brushing up their basics. The book covers all important topics encountered by a student at the time of practical viva examination: history taking and examination in both obstetrics and gynecology; important clinical cases in obstetrics and gynecology; normal labor room and operation theater (OT) procedures; important drugs used in obstetrics and gynecology; contraception; imaging; instruments and specimens in obstetrics and gynecology. The book also features an appendix at the end covering useful topics such as nutritional values, biochemistry and hematological parameters. The process of childbirth has been well illustrated by an accompanying CD-ROM covering basics related to obstetrics such as: bony pelvis, fetal skull, and mechanism of normal vaginal delivery.

Writing a book is a colossal task. It can never be completed without divine intervention and approval. Therefore, I have decided to end this preface with a small prayer of thanks to the Almighty, which I was taught in my childhood.

*"Father, lead me day by day, ever in thy own sweet way.*
*Teach me to be pure and good and tell me what I ought to do."*

—**Amen**

Simultaneously, I would like to extend my thanks and appreciation to all the related authors and publishers whose references have been used in this book. Book creation is teamwork, and I acknowledge the way the entire staff of M/s Jaypee Brothers Medical Publishers (P) Ltd., New Delhi, India, worked hard on this manuscript to give it a final shape. I would like to thank Shri Jitendar P Vij (Group Chairman), Jaypee Brothers Medical Publishers, for being the guiding beacon, and source of inspiration and motivation behind this book. I would also like to thank Mr Ankit Vij (President) and Mr Tarun Duneja (Director-Publishing). Last but not the least, I would also like to thank the entire staff of Jaypee Brothers, especially, Mr Nitish Kumar Dubey, Mr Amit Rai, and Mr Syed Amir Haider (Medical Editors) for editing the manuscript and coordinating the process of publication; Mr Vinod Kumar Sharma (DTP Operator) for typesetting the book; Mr Manoj Pahuja (Senior Graphic Designer) and Mr Vijay Singh (Graphic Designer) for making beautiful illustrations. May God bless them all!

I believe that writing a book involves a continuous learning process. Though extreme care has been taken to maintain accuracy while writing this book, constructive criticism would be greatly appreciated. Please e-mail me your comments at the email address: *richa@drrichasaxena.com*. Also, please feel free to visit my website *www.drrichasaxena.com* for obtaining information related to various other books written by me and to make use of the free resources available for the medical students.

**Richa Saxena**
*(richa@drrichasaxena.com)*
*www.drrichasaxena.com*

# SPECIAL ACKNOWLEDGMENTS

**Saunitra Inamdar** MD
Professor
Department of Obstetrics and Gynecology
Jawaharlal Nehru Medical College, Wardha, Maharshtra, India
For providing pictures for Chapter 14 (Specimens in Obstetrics and Gynecology)


**Kiran Agarwal** MD FICOG
Associate Professor, Rohilkhand Medical College and Hospital
Pilibhit Bypass Road, Bareilly, India
Vice President, Rohilkhand Medical College and Hospital
Institute of Dental Sciences
Rohilkhand College of Nursing, Bareilly, India
For providing pictures for Chapter 13 (Instruments in Obstetrics and Gynecology)

# ≡ CONTENTS

Section 2:  Gynecology

## Section 3: Imaging, Instruments, Specimens and Drugs

### 12. Imaging in Obstetrics and Gynecology　　377



### 13. Instruments in Obstetrics and Gynecology　　403

## Section 4:  Appendices

# ABBREVIATIONS

| | | |
|---|---|---|
| ACE | : | Angiotensin-Converting-Enzyme |
| ACOG | : | The American Congress of Obstetricians and Gynecologists |
| AHA | : | American Heart Association |
| AIDS | : | Acquired Immunodeficiency Syndrome |
| ALT | : | Alanine Aminotransferase |
| APGAR | : | Activity, Pulse, Grimace, Appearance and Respiration |
| APH | : | Antepartum Hemorrhage |
| ART | : | Assisted Reproductive Technology |
| ASRM | : | American Society for Reproductive Medicine |
| AST | : | Aspartate Aminotransferase |
| AUB | : | Abnormal Uterine Bleeding |
| BMI | : | Body Mass Index |
| BP | : | Blood Pressure |
| BPP | : | Biophysical Profile |
| CBC | : | Complete Blood Count |
| CDC | : | Centers for Disease Control and Prevention |
| CNS | : | Central Nervous System |
| COCP | : | Combined Oral Contraceptive Pill |
| COPD | : | Chronic Obstructive Pulmonary Disease |
| D&C | : | Dilatation and Curettage |
| DLC | : | Differential Leukocyte Count |
| DUB | : | Dysfunctional Uterine Bleeding |
| EB | : | Endometrial Biopsy |
| EDD | : | Expected Date of Delivery |
| ESHRE | : | European Society of Human Reproduction and Embryology |
| ESR | : | Erythrocyte Sedimentation Rate |
| FGR | : | Fetal Growth Restriction |
| FSH | : | Follicle-Stimulating Hormone |
| GA | : | General Anesthesia |
| GnRH | : | Gonadotropin-Releasing Hormone |
| GPE | : | General Physical Examination |
| hCG | : | Human Chorionic Gonadotropin |
| HIV | : | Human Immunodeficiency Virus |
| HPV | : | Human Papillomavirus |
| HRT | : | Hormone-Replacement Therapy |
| HSG | : | Hysterosalpingography |
| IDA | : | Iron-Deficiency Anemia |
| IM | : | Intramuscular |
| ISSHP | : | International Society for the Study of Hypertension in Pregnancy |
| IUCD | : | Intrauterine Contraceptive Device |
| IUD | : | Intrauterine Death |
| IUGR | : | Intrauterine Growth Restriction |
| IV | : | Intravenous |
| IVF | : | In Vitro Fertilization |
| IVP | : | Intravenous Pyelography |
| KFT | : | Kidney Function Test |
| LA | : | Local Anesthesia |
| LDH | : | Lactate Dehydrogenase |
| LFT | : | Liver Function Test |
| LH | : | Luteinizing Hormone |
| LMP | : | Last Menstrual Period |
| LOA | : | Left Occiput Anterior |
| LOP | : | Left Occiput Posterior |
| LOT | : | Left Occiput Transverse |
| LSA | : | Left Sacrum Anterior |
| LSP | : | Left Sacrum Posterior |
| MCH | : | Mean Corpuscular Hemoglobin |
| MCHC | : | Mean Cell Hemoglobin Concentration |
| MCV | : | Mean Corpuscular Volume |
| MTP | : | Medical Termination of Pregnancy |
| NHBPEP | : | National High Blood Pressure Education Program |
| NPO | : | Nil Per Os |
| NSAIDs | : | Nonsteroidal Anti-Inflammatory Drugs |
| NST | : | Nonstress Test |
| OCP | : | Oral Contraceptive Pill |
| OPD | : | Outpatient Department |
| Pap smear | : | Papanicolaou smear |
| PCOD | : | Polycystic Ovarian Disease |
| PCR | : | Polymerase Chain Reaction |
| PCV | : | Packed Cell Volume |
| PGE2 | : | Prostaglandin E2 |
| PID | : | Pelvic Inflammatory Disease |
| PMS | : | Premenstrual Syndrome |
| PPH | : | Postpartum Hemorrhage |
| PPROM | : | Preterm Premature Rupture of Membranes |
| PROM | : | Premature Rupture of Membranes |
| PUBS | : | Percutaneous Umbilical Cord Blood Sampling |
| RCOG | : | Royal College of Obstetricians and Gynaecologists |
| ROA | : | Right Occiput Anterior |
| ROM | : | Rupture of Membranes |
| ROP | : | Right Occiput Posterior |
| ROT | : | Right Occiput Transverse |
| RSA | : | Right Sacrum Anterior |
| RSP | : | Right Sacrum Posterior |
| SC | : | Subcutaneous |
| STDs | : | Sexually Transmitted Diseases |
| TAH | : | Total Abdominal Hysterectomy |
| TAS | : | Transabdominal Sonography |
| TIBC | : | Total Iron-Binding Capacity |
| TLC | : | Total Leukocyte Count |
| TOLAC | : | Trial of Labor after Cesarean |
| TVS | : | Transvaginal Sonography |
| VBAC | : | Vaginal Birth after Cesarean Delivery |
| WHO | : | World Health Organization |
| WNL | : | Within Normal Limits |

# Obstetrics

# History Taking and Examination in Obstetrics

## CHAPTER OUTLINE

- Introduction
- History
- Clinical Presentation
- Clinical Examination

## Introduction

The duration of pregnancy has been traditionally considered to be 10 lunar months or 40 weeks or 280 days. It is customary to divide the entire period of gestation into three trimesters: first trimester (until 14 weeks); second trimester (15–28 weeks); third trimester (29–42 weeks). The gestational age is usually calculated from the first day of LMP. During the antenatal period, planned antenatal care is given to a pregnant woman in order to ensure good maternal and neonatal outcome.

## History

### History at the Time of First Antenatal Visit

The aim of history taking is to determine the period of gestation and thereby EDD. History taking also helps in determining if the pregnancy is associated with any high risk factors. Taking appropriate history helps the clinician to determine the further management and mode of delivery. Components of complete history elicitation and physical examination are tabulated in Table 1.1.

### History of Presenting Complaints

The various complaints with which the woman presents are listed in a chronological order from the time of their onset. These complaints need to be described detailing their mode of onset, severity, aggravating or relieving factors. Regarding the present pregnancy, the following points need to be considered:

- The first day of the LMP must be determined as accurately as possible. The clinician must ask the patient how long she had been married or has been in relationship with the present partner. The clinician must also ask the woman if she had previously received any treatment for infertility. The patient must be asked if the present pregnancy is a planned one and since how long she had been planning this pregnancy. The patient must be enquired if she ever used any contraceptive agents in the past.

**Table 1.1:** Components of complete history elicitation and physical examination

| Components of history taking | Components of clinical examination |
|---|---|
| • History of presenting complaints<br>• Menstrual history<br>• Previous obstetric history<br>• Medical history<br>• Treatment history<br>• Surgical history<br>• Family history<br>• Social history<br>• Personal history<br>• Family planning/contraceptive history<br>• Nutritional history<br>• Gynecological history | • General physical examination<br>• Obstetric examination (done using Leopold's maneuvers)<br>  – Fundal height<br>  – Fetal lie, position<br>  – Fetal presentation, weight and viability<br>  – Assessment of the amount of liquor<br>• Vaginal examination (done only if required) |

- The clinician needs to take the history of any medical or obstetric problems, which the patient has had since the start of this pregnancy, for example, pyrexial illnesses (such as influenza) with or without skin rashes; symptoms suggestive of a urinary tract infection and history of any vaginal bleeding.

Enquiry must be also made regarding normal symptoms related to pregnancy, which the patient may be experiencing, e.g. nausea and vomiting, heartburn, constipation, etc. Some symptoms, which may be both due to physiological or pathological changes in pregnancy, include abdominal pain (Table 1.2), shortness of breath (Table 1.3), back pain (Table 1.4), etc.

### Menstrual History

It is important to elicit the proper history regarding the last (normal) menstrual period. It is also important for the clinician to find out if the previous cycles were normal and regular or not. In absence of regular, predictable, cyclic, spontaneous menstrual cycles, accurate dating of pregnancy based solely on history and clinical examination is impossible. The clinician must also enquire about the length of periods and amount of bleeding. Excessive amount of menstrual blood loss in previous cycles may be associated with anemia.

Last menstrual period can be used for calculating the EDD. To calculate the EDD, 7 days are added to the first day of LMP and then 9 months are added to this date. For example, if the LMP was on February 2, 2014, the EDD will be on November 9, 2014. If the LMP was on October 27, 2013, the EDD will be on August 3, 2014. This method of estimating EDD is known as the Naegele's rule. This rule can also be applied by adding

| **Table 1.2:** Causes of abdominal pain during pregnancy |
| --- |
| • Stretching of uterus and ligaments due to uterine enlargement during pregnancy<br>• Gastritis, hepatitis, pancreatitis<br>• Abruptio placentae<br>• Fibroid uterus<br>• Ovarian cysts |

| **Table 1.3:** Causes of shortness of breath during pregnancy |
| --- |
| • Normal physiological changes of pregnancy<br>• Anemia, heart disease during pregnancy<br>• Chest infection, asthma |

| **Table 1.4:** Causes of back pain during pregnancy |
| --- |
| • Calcium deficiency, osteoporosis<br>• Lumbar lordosis, lumbar subluxation<br>• Occipitoposterior position<br>• Abruptio placentae |

7 days to the first day of LMP, subtracting 3 months and then adding 1 year to this. The rule should be used to measure the duration of pregnancy, only if the patient had been having regular menstrual cycles previously. Naegele's rule is based on the assumption that pregnancy had begun approximately 2 weeks before ovulation. In clinical practice, this gestational age is used for marking the temporal events occurring during pregnancy. In contrast, ovulatory or fertilization age which is typically 2 weeks lesser is utilized by the embryologists and other reproductive biologists.

The history of using steroidal contraception prior to conception is important as in this case EDD may not be accurately determined with help of Naegele's rule. This is so as ovulation may not immediately resume following withdrawal bleeding; there may be a delay of 2–3 weeks.

### Previous Obstetric History

Details regarding the past obstetric history are important because many complications, which had occurred in the previous pregnancy, are likely to recur again. Each previous pregnancy must be described in a chronological manner with details such as place of delivery, mode of delivery, type of labor, use of any anesthesia or interventions during the labor, presence of any complications at the time of labor or delivery. Details of each delivered baby such as birthweight, APGAR score at birth, sex, time of birth, any complications, immunizations, history of breastfeeding, etc. must be recorded.

The woman's past obstetric history must be denoted by the acronym GPAL, where G stands for gravida, P for parity, A for number of abortions and L for number of live births. It is also important to ask the woman, how long she has been married.

*Gravida:* This refers to the number of pregnancies, including the present pregnancy, the woman has ever had. This is irrespective of the fact whether the pregnancies were viable at the time of birth or not.

*Nulligravida:* This implies a woman who has never been pregnant.

*Primigravida:* This stands for a woman who is pregnant for the first time (Gravida 1).

*Multigravida:* This stands for a woman who has had at least one previous pregnancy, irrespective of whether it was viable or not (depending on the number of previous pregnancies, she could be gravida 2, 3, or more). For example, a woman who has had three previous pregnancies and is now pregnant for the fourth time will be gravida 4.

*Abortions:* Number of the pregnancies, which have terminated before reaching the point of viability (20 weeks). The clinician must note their exact gestational period and also mention whether they were spontaneous or induced abortions; the reason for the induced abortion also needs to be asked.

*Viability:* This refers to the ability of the fetus to live outside the uterus after birth.

*Parity:* This refers to the number of previous viable pregnancies (including infants who were either stillborn or born alive). Parity is determined by the number of viable pregnancies and not by the number of fetuses delivered. Thus, parity does not change even if twins or triplets are born instead of a singleton fetus or if woman gives birth to a live or stillborn infant.

*Nullipara:* A woman who has never carried a previous pregnancy to a point of viability (para 0).

*Primipara:* Woman who has had one previous viable pregnancy (para 1). For example, if the woman is gravida 4 and only two of the previous pregnancies of this woman were viable, she would be gravida 4, para 2.

*Multipara:* Woman who has had two or more previous viable pregnancies (para 2, 3, or more).

*Grand multipara:* Woman who has had five or more previous viable pregnancies (para 5, 6 or more).

*Elderly primigravida:* Woman having her first pregnancy at the age of 30 years or above.

A woman is considered as a high-risk mother, if she is either a primigravida or nullipara over the age of 30 or if she is a young teenaged primigravida or if she is a grand multipara.

It is important to take the history of previous pregnancies including history of previous abortions (period of gestation < 20 weeks), precipitate labor, preterm pregnancies (period of gestation < 37 completed weeks), abnormal presentations, preeclampsia or eclampsia, cesarean section, retained placenta, postpartum hemorrhage, stillbirths, history of episiotomies, perineal tears, and history of receiving epidural anesthesia during the previous pregnancies. History about any episodes of hospitalization during previous pregnancies can be helpful. History of complications during previous pregnancy, such as preeclampsia, placenta previa, abruptio placentae, IUGR, polyhydramnios or oligohydramnios is important because many complications in previous pregnancies tend to recur in subsequent pregnancies (e.g. patients with a previous history of perinatal death or spontaneous preterm labor or preeclampsia or multifetal gestation are likely to experience the recurrence of these complications in their subsequent pregnancies). It is also important to take the history of previous pregnancy losses. A history of three or more successive first trimester miscarriages suggests a possible genetic abnormality in the father or mother. Previous midtrimester miscarriages could be associated with cervical incompetence. Patient may often forget to give the history about previous miscarriages and ectopic pregnancies. Therefore, the clinician needs to ask specifically about the history of previous miscarriages and ectopic pregnancies. Approximate birthweight of previous children and the approximate period of gestation, especially if the infant was low birthweight or preterm, are useful. Low birthweight at the time of birth is indicative of either IUGR or preterm delivery.

It is important to know if the woman has experienced a prolonged labor during her previous pregnancy, as this may indicate cephalopelvic disproportion. History of previous birth in form of assisted delivery, including forceps delivery, vacuum application and cesarean section, suggest that there may have been cephalopelvic disproportion. In case of previous cesarean delivery, a detailed history of the previous surgery needs to be taken (*See* chapter 5). The patient should always be asked if she knows the reason for having had a cesarean delivery. She should be asked to show the hospital notes related to the surgery, if available. This may help to provide some information regarding the type of incision made in the uterus, any complications encountered during the surgery, etc. Detailed history of the previous live births as well as of previous perinatal deaths is important. The following points need to be elicited:

*Birthweight of each infant born previously:* This is important as previous low birthweight infants or spontaneous preterm labors tend to recur during future pregnancies. Also, history of delivering a large-sized baby in the past is suggestive of maternal diabetes mellitus or gestational diabetes, which may recur during subsequent pregnancies.

*Method of delivery of each previous infant:* The type of previous delivery is also important because a forceps delivery or vacuum extraction may suggest that some degree of cephalopelvic disproportion may have been present. If the patient had a previous cesarean section, the indication for that cesarean section must be determined.

*History of previous perinatal deaths:* Previous history of having one or more perinatal deaths in the past places the patient at high risk of further perinatal deaths. Therefore, every effort must be made to find out the cause of any previous deaths. If no cause can be found, then the risk of a recurrence of perinatal death is even higher.

### Medical History

Patients must be specifically asked about the previous medical history of diabetes, epilepsy, hypertension, renal disease, rheumatic disease, heart valve disease, epilepsy, asthma, tuberculosis, psychiatric illness or any other significant illness that she may have had in the past.

History regarding any previous hospital admission, surgery, blood transfusion, etc. also needs to be taken. It is important to elicit the patient's medical history as some medical conditions may become worse during pregnancy, e.g. a patient with heart valve disease may go into cardiac failure, while a hypertensive patient is at a high risk of developing preeclampsia.

### Treatment History

The woman must be asked if she has previous history of allergy to any drugs (specifically allergy to penicillin), history of receiving immunization against tetanus or administration of Rhesus (Rh) immunoglobulins during her previous pregnancies. The patient must be asked if she had received any treatment in the past (e.g. hypoglycemic drugs, antihypertensive drugs, etc.). Certain drugs may be teratogenic to the fetus during the first trimester of pregnancy, e.g. retinoids, which are used for acne and anticoagulant drugs like warfarin. Also certain drugs, which the women may be regularly taking prior to pregnancy, are relatively contraindicated during pregnancy, e.g. antihypertensive drugs like ACE inhibitors, β-blockers, etc.

### Surgical History

The woman must be enquired if she ever underwent any surgery in the past such as cardiac surgery, e.g. heart valve replacement; operations on the urogenital tract, e.g. cesarean section, myomectomy, cone biopsy of the cervix, operations for stress incontinence and vesicovaginal fistula repair, etc.

### Family History

Family history of medical conditions, such as diabetes, multiple pregnancy, bleeding tendencies or mental retardation, etc. increases the risk for development of these conditions in the patient and her unborn infant. Since some birth defects are inherited, it is important to take the history of any genetic disorder, which may be prevalent in the family.

### Social History

It is important to elicit information regarding the patient's social circumstances. The mother should be asked if she has social or family support to help her bring up the baby, for example, a working mother may require assistance to help her plan the care of her infant. Social problems, like unemployment, poor housing and overcrowding increase the risk of mother developing medical complications like tuberculosis, malnutrition and IUGR. Patients living in poor social conditions need special support and help. Sometimes it may become difficult to ask the patient directly regarding her socioeconomic status. In these cases, taking the history regarding the occupation of the husband or partner is likely to give clues regarding the patient's socioeconomic history. Classification of the women based on their socioeconomic status is usually done using the Kuppuswamy Prasad's classification system* (revised for 2013), which is based on the per capita monthly income (Table 1.5).

### Personal History

History of behavioral factors (smoking or tobacco usage, alcohol usage, utilization of prenatal care services, etc.) needs to be taken. The patient should be specifically asked if she has been smoking or consuming alcohol. Smoking and alcohol both may cause IUGR. Additionally, alcohol may also cause congenital malformations.

### Family Planning/Contraceptive History

The patient's family planning needs and wishes should be discussed at the time of her first antenatal visit. If she is a multipara having at least two live babies, she should be counseled and encouraged for postpartum sterilization. In case the woman is not willing to undergo permanent sterilization procedure, the patient's wishes should be respected; she can be offered temporary methods of contraception like oral contraceptive pills, Cu-T, etc.

Previous history of use of various contraception methods with details such as type of contraceptive devices used, duration of their use, patient satisfaction, associated problems and complications, etc. also need to be mentioned.

### Nutritional History

A record of patient's daily food intake is documented to calculate the daily calorie intake. Caloric values of some commonly used food stuffs have been described in Appendix 1. Dietary history may be particularly important in some pregnancy-related complications where dietary modifications are suggested, e.g.

| Social class | Original classification of the per capita income in (Rs/month), 1961 | Revised classification for 2013 (in Rs/month) |
|---|---|---|
| I | 100 and above | 5,113 and above |
| II | 50–99 | 2,557–5,112 |
| III | 30–49 | 1,533–2,556 |
| IV | 15–29 | 767–1,532 |
| V | Below 15 | Below 767 |

**Table 1.5:** Revision of the Kuppuswamy Prasad's social classification* for the year 2013

* Kuppuswamy Prasad's classification system is applicable only for Indian population. Per capita income is calculated by dividing total income of the household by the number of individuals.

diabetic diet in case of gestational diabetes, iron and protein-rich diet in case of anemia in pregnancy, etc.

### Gynecological History

The clinician must record the history of previous gynecological problems, such as recurrent vaginal discharge, pelvic pain, fibroids, ovarian cysts, previous infertility, etc. The clinician also needs to enquire if some treatment (both medical and surgical) was instituted for any of these problems.

## Summary of History

Once the history is complete, a summary is made along with the possible diagnosis or differential diagnosis. This should include the woman's name, age, time since marriage, gravida, parity, any previous miscarriages, number of live children, weeks of gestation and any associated medical or surgical disease along with any other possible complications. This allows differentiation between normal pregnancy and a high-risk pregnancy.

# Clinical Presentation

Clinical presentation during various trimesters of pregnancy is as follows:

## First Trimester of Pregnancy

- *Cessation of menstruation:* Cessation of menstrual cycles in a woman belonging to the reproductive age group, who had previously experienced spontaneous, cyclical, predictable periods, is the first most frequent symptom of pregnancy. Since there may be considerable variation in the length of ovarian and thus menstrual cycle amongst women, amenorrhea is not a reliable indicator of pregnancy.
- *Nausea and vomiting:* Also known as morning sickness, these symptoms appear 1 or 2 weeks after the period is missed and last until 10–12th week. Its severity may vary from mild nausea to persistent vomiting, e.g. hyperemesis gravidarum.
- *Urinary symptoms:* Increased frequency of urination during the early months of pregnancy is due to relaxant effect of progesterone on the bladder, in combination with the pressure exerted by the gradually enlarged uterus on the bladder.
- *Mastodynia:* Mastodynia or breast discomfort may be present in early pregnancy and ranges in severity from a tingling sensation to frank pain in the breasts.
- *Cervical mucus:* High levels of progesterone during pregnancy helps in lowering the concentration of NaCl in cervical mucus, which prevents the formation of ferning pattern; instead the cervical mucus shows an ellipsoid pattern.

## Second Trimester of Pregnancy

There is disappearance of subjective symptoms of pregnancy such as nausea, vomiting and frequency of micturition. Other symptoms, which may appear include the following:

- *Abdominal enlargement:* Progressive enlargement of the lower abdomen occurs due to the growing uterus.
- *Fetal movements*: Fetal movements generally occur after 18–20th week of gestation.
- *Quickening:* Fetal movements (quickening) can usually be seen or felt between 16 to 18 weeks of gestation in a multigravida. A primigravida, on the other hand, is capable of appreciating fetal movements after approximately 2 weeks (i.e. 18–20 weeks).
- *Fetal heart sounds:* This is the most definitive clinical sign of pregnancy and can be detected between 18 to 20 weeks of gestation. The rate usually varies from 120 beats/minute to 160 beats/minute.
- *Palpation of fetal body parts:* The fetal body can usually be palpated by the 18–20 weeks of gestation unless the patient is obese; there is abdominal tenderness or there is an excessive amount of amniotic fluid.
- *External ballottement:* This can be elicited as early as 20th week of gestation because the size of fetus is relatively smaller in comparison to the amniotic fluid. In this method, repercussion is felt by the examiner's hand placed on the woman's abdomen when the fetus is given a push externally.
- *Internal ballottement:* This can be elicited between 16 to 28 weeks of gestation. This is an obsolete method for diagnosing pregnancy. Tip of forefinger of the right hand is placed in the anterior fornix and a sharp tap is made against the lower segment of uterus where the fetus, if present, gets tossed upwards. It is felt by the examiner's finger to strike against the uterine wall as it falls back.
- *Skin changes:* There is appearance of pigmentation over the forehead and cheeks by 24th week of gestation. There is appearance of linea nigra and stria gravidarum over the abdomen.

## Changes in the Third Trimester

- *Abdominal enlargement:* There occurs progressive enlargement of the abdomen, which can result in development of symptoms of mechanical discomfort such as palpitations and dyspnea. Lightening is another phenomenon, which occurs at approximately 38 weeks of gestation especially in the primigravida. This results in a slight reduction in fundal height, which provides relief against pressure symptoms.

- *Frequency of micturition:* There is an increased frequency of micturition, which had previously disappeared in the second trimester.
- *Fetal movements become more pronounced:* The fetal movements become more pronounced and palpation of fetal parts becomes easier.
- Braxton Hicks contractions become more evident.
- Fetal lie, presentation and period of gestation can be determined.

## Changes in Genital Organs

The changes in genital organs occurring at the time of pregnancy are described as follows:

### Vagina

- *Chadwick's or Jacquemier's sign:* The vaginal walls show a bluish discoloration as the pelvic blood vessels become congested. This sign can be observed by 8–10 weeks of gestation.
- *Osiander's sign:* There is increased pulsation in the vagina felt through the lateral fornix at 8 weeks of gestation.

### Uterus

- Enlargement of the uterus occurs due to hypertrophy and hyperplasia of the individual muscle fibers under the influence of hormones such as estrogen and progestogens.
- For the first few weeks of pregnancy, the uterus maintains its original pear shape, but becomes almost spherical by 12 weeks of gestation. Thereafter, it increases more rapidly in length, than in width becoming ovoid in shape. Until 12 weeks, the uterus remains a pelvic organ after which it can be palpated per abdominally.
- The uterus increases in weight from pre-pregnant 70 g to approximately 1,100 g at term.
- Due to uterine enlargement, the normal anteverted position gets exaggerated up to 8 weeks. Since the enlarged uterus lies on the bladder making it incapable of filling, the frequency of micturition increases. However, after 8 weeks the uterus more or less conforms to the axis of the inlet.
- *Hegar's sign:* At 6–8 weeks of gestation, the cervix is firm in contrast to the soft isthmus. Due to the marked softness of uterine isthmus, cervix and body of uterus may appear as separate organs. As a result, the isthmus of the uterus can be compressed between the fingers palpating vagina and abdomen, which is known as Hegar's sign (Fig. 1.1).
- *Palmer's sign:* Regular rhythmic uterine contractions, which can be elicited during the bimanual examination can be felt as early as 4–8 weeks of gestation.
- *Braxton Hicks contractions:* In the early months of pregnancy, uterus undergoes contractions known as

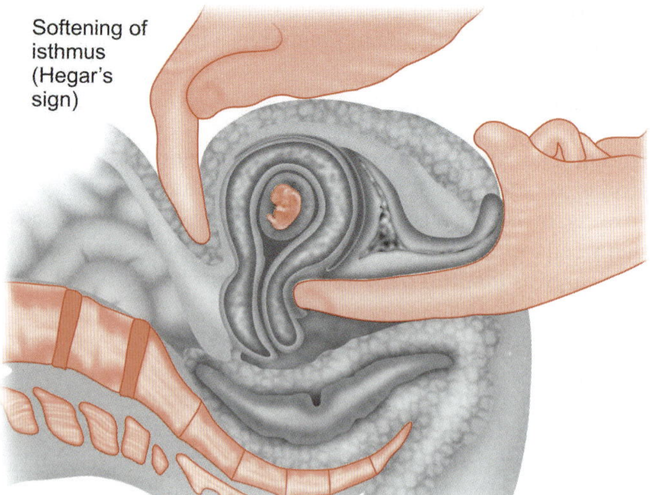


**Fig. 1.1:** Hegar's sign

Braxton Hicks contractions, which may be irregular, infrequent and painless without any effect on the cervical dilatation and effacement. Towards the last weeks of pregnancy, these contractions increase in intensity, resulting in pain and discomfort for the patient and may occur after every 10–20 minutes, thereby assuming some form of rhythmicity. Eventually, these contractions merge with the contractions of labor.

- There is hypertrophy of the uterine isthmus to about three times its original size during the first trimester of pregnancy.
- *Formation of lower uterine segment:* After 12 weeks of pregnancy, the uterine isthmus unfolds from above downwards to get incorporated into the uterine cavity and also takes part in the formation of lower uterine segment.
- There is an increase in the uteroplacental blood flow ranging between 450 mL/minute to 650 mL/minute near term. This increase is principally due to vasodilatation.
- *Uterine soufflé:* This is a soft blowing sound synchronous with the maternal pulse. It is caused by rush of blood through the dilated uterine arteries. On the other hand, fetal soufflé is a sharp whistling sound synchronous with the fetal pulse. It is caused by the rush of blood through the fetal umbilical arteries.

### Cervix

- There occurs hypertrophy and hyperplasia of the elastic and connective tissue fibers and increase in vascularity within the cervical stroma. This is likely to result in cervical softening (known as Goodell's sign), which becomes evident by 6 weeks of pregnancy. Increased vascularity is likely to result in bluish discoloration beneath the squamous epithelium of portio vaginalis resulting in a positive Chadwick's sign.

- With the advancement of pregnancy, there is marked proliferation of endocervical mucosa with downward extension of the squamocolumnar junction. There is copious production of cervical secretions resulting in the formation of a thick mucus plug, which seals the cervical canal.
- When the cervical mucus (secreted during pregnancy) is spread over the glass slide and dried, it shows a characteristic crystallization or beading pattern due to presence of progesterone.

If the history and examination suggest that the patient is pregnant, the diagnosis is usually confirmed by urine pregnancy test or a urine hCG assay. The test becomes positive by the time the first menstrual period is missed. A transvaginal or abdominal scan helps in providing 100% confirmation of pregnancy.

# Clinical Examination

## GENERAL PHYSICAL EXAMINATION

The general appearance of the patient is of great importance as it can indicate whether or not she is in good health. A woman's height and weight may reflect her past and present nutritional status.

The signs which must be carefully looked for in a pregnant woman include the following:
- Pallor (lower palpebral conjunctiva, palms of the hand, nail beds, tongue, lips).
- Edema [foot (Table 1.6), face, vulva, sacral region]. Simple strategies, which can be used for the alleviation of physiological pedal edema in pregnancy, are reduction of salt and carbohydrate intake in the diet; foot elevation; and use of elastic stockings.
- Jaundice (sclera, nail beds).
- Enlarged lymph nodes (neck, axillae and inguinal areas).
- *Thyroid gland:* The clinician must look for an obviously enlarged thyroid gland (goiter). In case, there is obvious enlargement of the thyroid gland or it feels nodular, the patient must be referred for further investigations.
- *Skin changes:* There may be increased skin pigmentation due to increased production of melanotropin. This may manifest as the following:
  - *Face:* Melasma, a frequently encountered skin change during pregnancy
  - *Breasts:* Darkening of areolas
  - *Abdomen:* Linea nigra.

| Table 1.6: Causes of pedal edema in pregnancy |
| --- |
| • Normal, physiological changes of pregnancy |
| • Anemia, malnutrition, hypoproteinemia |
| • Renal failure/disease |
| • Hypertension |
| • Hepatic or cardiac disease |
| • Varicose veins and varicose ulcers |

- Signs of past pregnancy such as breast pigmentation, striae gravidarum, abdominal laxity, perineal or vulval damage, perineal repair, any stress incontinence, etc. may be present.

## Examination of the Breasts

There is pronounced pigmentation of the areola and nipples during pregnancy. There is also appearance of secondary areola, Montgomery's tubercles and presence of increased vascularity. Routine breast examination during antenatal examination is not recommended for the promotion of postnatal breastfeeding. The breasts should be examined with the patient both sitting and lying on her back, with her hands above her head. Changes in the breasts are best evident in the primigravida in comparison to multigravida. Presence of secretions from the breasts of a primigravida who has never lactated is an important sign of pregnancy.

## SPECIFIC SYSTEMIC EXAMINATION

During pregnancy a detailed abdominal and vaginal examination may be required. Besides this, the other body systems like the respiratory system and the cardiovascular system must also be briefly examined. In case any pathological sign is observed, a detailed examination of the respective body system must be carried out.

## ABDOMINAL EXAMINATION

Even in the present time of technological advancements, the clinicians must not underestimate the importance of clinical abdominal examination. The abdominal examination in the antenatal period usually comprises of the following:
- Inspection
- Estimation of height of uterine fundus
- Obstetric grips (Leopold's maneuvers)
- Evaluation of uterine contractions
- Estimation of fetal descent
- Auscultation of fetal heart.

Each of these is described next in detail.

## Preparation of the Patient for Examination

- Before starting the abdominal examination, the clinician should ensure that the patient's bladder is empty; she should be asked to empty her bladder in case it is not empty.
- The patient must lie comfortably on her back with a pillow under her head and her abdomen must be fully exposed. She should not lie in a left lateral position.
- Verbal consent must be taken from the patient before beginning the examination. A female chaperone must be preferably present, especially if the examining clinician is a male.

## Inspection of the Abdomen

The following should be specifically looked for at the time of abdominal inspection:

*Shape and size of the distended abdomen*
- In case of a singleton pregnancy and a longitudinal lie, the shape of the uterus is usually oval.
- The shape of the uterus may be round with a multiple pregnancy or polyhydramnios.
- The flattening of the lower part of the abdomen suggests a vertex presentation with an occipitoposterior position (ROP or LOP).
- A suprapubic bulge may be suggestive of a full bladder.

*Presence or absence of scars:* In case scar marks as a result of previous surgery are visible, a detailed history must be taken. This should include the reasons of having the surgery and the type of surgery performed [myomectomy or previous lower segment cesarean section (LSCS)]. In case the scar is related to previous LSCS, detailed history as described in Chapter 5 needs to be taken.

*Presence of stria gravidarum and linea nigra:* In many pregnant women, a black-brownish colored line may sometimes develop in the midline of the abdomen. This is known as linea nigra (Fig. 1.2). In many women, in later months of pregnancy, stretch marks called stria gravidarum (Fig. 1.2) may develop over the skin of abdomen, breast or thighs.

## Abdominal Palpation

Besides the fetal and uterine palpation, other abdominal organs like the liver, spleen and kidneys must also be specifically palpated. Presence of any other abdominal mass should also be noted.

The presence of an enlarged organ, or a mass, should be appropriately followed up.

### Examination of the Uterus and the Fetus

- The clinician must firstly check whether the uterus is lying in the midline of the abdomen or it is dextrorototated either to the right or the left. In case the uterus is dextrorotated, it needs to be centralized.
- The wall of the uterus must be palpated for the presence of any irregularities. An irregular uterine wall may be suggestive of either the presence of myomas or a congenital abnormality such as a bicornuate uterus. Uterine myomas may enlarge during pregnancy and become painful.

### Determining the Fundal Height

In the first few weeks of pregnancy, there is primarily an increase in the anterior posterior diameter of the uterus. By 12 weeks, the uterus becomes globular and attains a size of approximately 8 cm. On the bimanual examination, the uterus appears soft, doughy and elastic. In the initial stages of pregnancy the cervix may appear firm. However with increasing period of gestation, the cervix becomes increasingly softer in consistency. From the second trimester onwards, the uterine height starts corresponding to the period of gestation. The rough estimation of fundal height with increasing period of gestation is shown in Figure 1.3.

*Determining size of the uterus through estimation of fundal height:* After centralizing the dextrorotated uterus with right

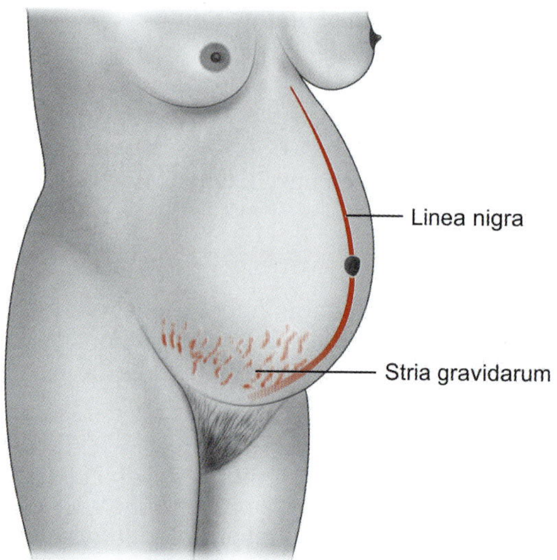


**Fig. 1.2:** Linea nigra and stria gravidarum

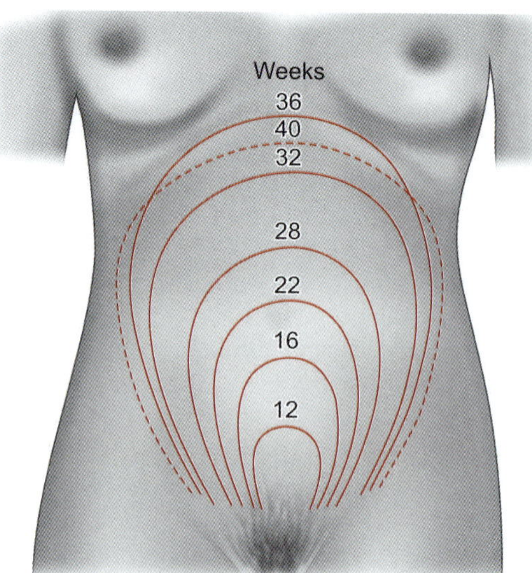


**Fig. 1.3:** Estimation of fundal height with increasing period of gestation

hand, the upper border of the uterus is estimated with the ulnar border of the left hand. Anatomical landmarks used for determining the size of uterus through estimation of fundal height mainly include the symphysis pubis and the umbilicus:

- If the fundus is palpable just above the symphysis pubis, the gestational age is probably 12 weeks.
- If the fundus reaches half way between the symphysis and the umbilicus, the gestational age is probably 16 weeks.
- If the fundus is at the same height as the umbilicus, the gestational age is probably 22 weeks (one finger under the umbilicus = 20 weeks and one finger above the umbilicus = 24 weeks).
- The distance between the xiphisternum and umbilicus is divided into three equal parts. Upper one-third corresponds to 28 weeks; upper two-thirds corresponds to 32 weeks whereas the tip of xiphisternum corresponds to 36 weeks. At 40 weeks, due to the engagement of fetal head, the height of the uterus reduces slightly and corresponds to the level of 32 weeks. As a result even though the fundal height is same at 32 weeks and 40 weeks of gestation, at 32 weeks the fetal head is free floating, while it is engaged at 40 weeks of gestation.
- At every antenatal visit from 28 weeks of gestation onwards, the wellbeing of the fetus must be assessed. Having determined the height of the fundus, the clinician needs to assess whether the height of the fundus corresponds to the patient's dates and to the size of the fetus.

*Measurement of symphysisfundus (S-F) height:* Method of measuring the S-F height is shown in Figure 1.4. After centralizing the dextrorotated uterus, the upper border of the fundus is located by the ulnar border of left hand and this point is marked by placing one finger there. The distance between the upper border of the symphysis and the marked point is measured in centimeter with help of a measuring tape. After 24 weeks, the S-F height, measured in centimeters corresponds to the period of gestation up to 36 weeks. Though a variation of 2 cm (more or less) is regarded as normal, there are numerous conditions where the height of uterus may not correspond to the period of gestation (Table 1.7). If the fundus is palpable just above the symphysis pubis, the gestational age is probably 12 weeks.

## Palpation of the Fetus

The lie and presenting part of the fetus only becomes important when the gestational age reaches 34 weeks. The following must be determined:

### Fetal Lie

Fetal lie refers to the relationship of cephalocaudal axis or long axis (spinal column) of fetus to the long axis of the centralized uterus or maternal spine. The lie may be longitudinal, transverse or oblique (Figs 1.5A to D).

- *Longitudinal lie:* The fetal lie can be described as longitudinal when the maternal and fetal long axes are parallel to each other.
- *Transverse lie:* The fetal lie can be described as transverse when the maternal and fetal long axes are perpendicular to each other.
- *Oblique lie:* The fetal lie can be described as oblique when the maternal and fetal long axes cross each other obliquely or at an angle of 45°. The oblique lie is usually unstable and becomes longitudinal or transverse during the course of labor.

### Fetal Presentation

Fetal presentation can be described as the fetal body part, which occupies the lower pole of the uterus and thereby first enters the pelvic passage. Fetal presentation is determined by fetal lie and may be of three types: cephalic (head), podalic (breech), or shoulder (Figs 1.6A to E).

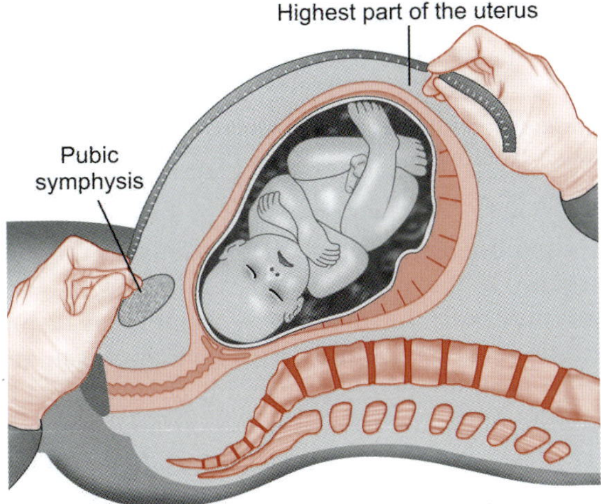


**Fig. 1.4:** Method of measuring the symphysisfundus height

| **Table 1.7:** Conditions where the height of uterus may not correspond to the period of gestation ||
|---|---|
| *Fundal height is greater than the period of gestation* | *Fundal height is lesser than the period of gestation* |
| • Multifetal gestation | • Oligohydramnios |
| • Polyhydramnios | • IUGR baby |
| • Wrong dates | • Wrong dates |
| • Macrosomic baby | • Intrauterine death |
| • Pelvic tumor (uterine fibroid or ovarian cyst) | • IUGR |
| • Hydatidiform mole | • Missed abortion |
| • Concealed abruptio placentae | • Transverse lie |

*Abbreviation:* IUGR, intrauterine growth restriction

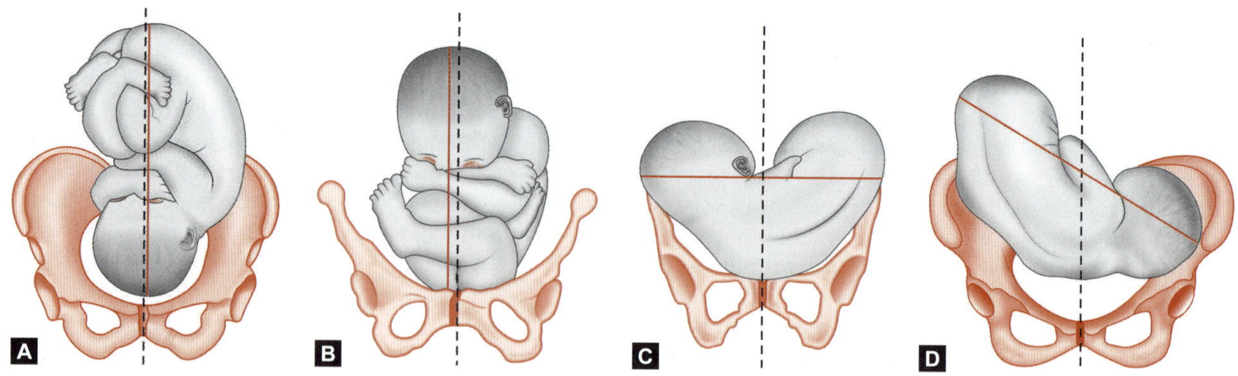

**Figs 1.5A to D:** Fetal lie. (A) Longitudinal lie (vertex presentation); (B) Longitudinal lie (breech presentation); (C) Transverse lie (shoulder presentation); (D) Oblique lie

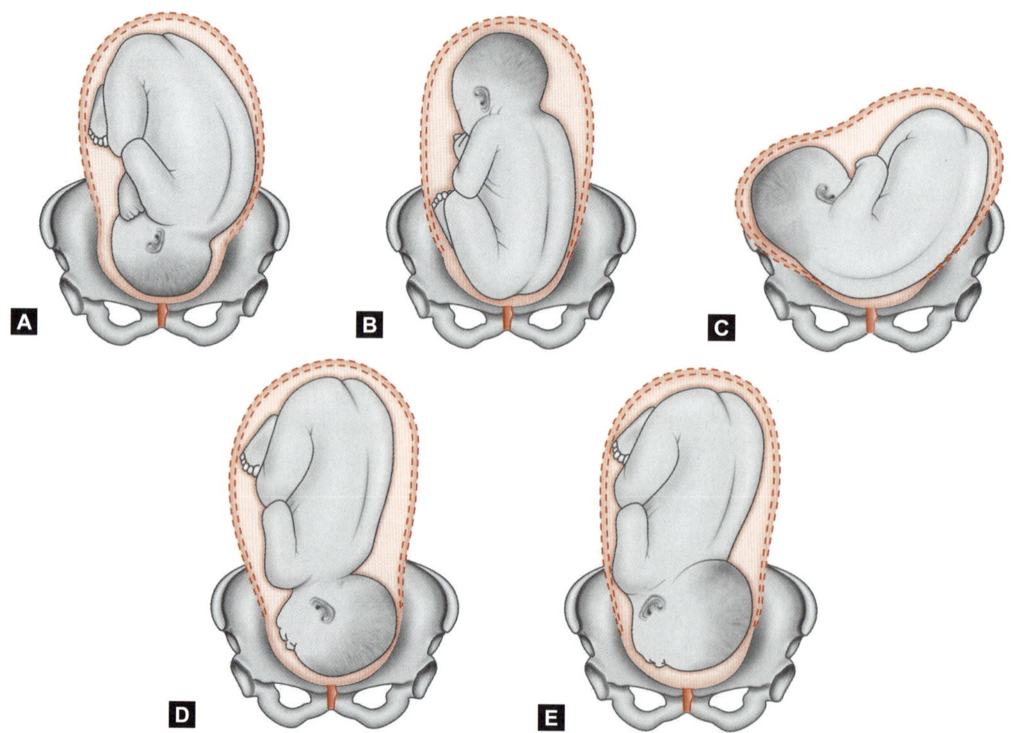

**Figs 1.6A to E:** Type of fetal presentation. (A) Vertex presentation; (B) Breech presentation; (C) Shoulder presentation; (D) Brow presentation; (E) Face presentation

Cephalic or the head presentation is the most common and occurs in about 97% of fetuses. Breech and shoulder presentations are less common and may pose difficulty for normal vaginal delivery. Thus, these two presentations are also known as malpresentations. As described previously, in cephalic presentation, the fetal head presents first. Depending on the part of fetal head presenting first, cephalic presentation can be divided as follows:

*Vertex or occiput presentation:* When the head is completely flexed onto chest, the smallest diameter of the fetal head (suboccipitobregmatic diameter) presents. In these cases, the occiput is the presenting part. Usually the occiput presents anteriorly. In some cases, occiput may be present posteriorly (Figs 1.7A and B). This type of presentation is known as occipitoposterior position. Though most of the cases with occipitoposterior position undergo normal vaginal delivery, labor is usually prolonged in these cases. In some cases with occipitoposterior presentation, cesarean delivery may be required.

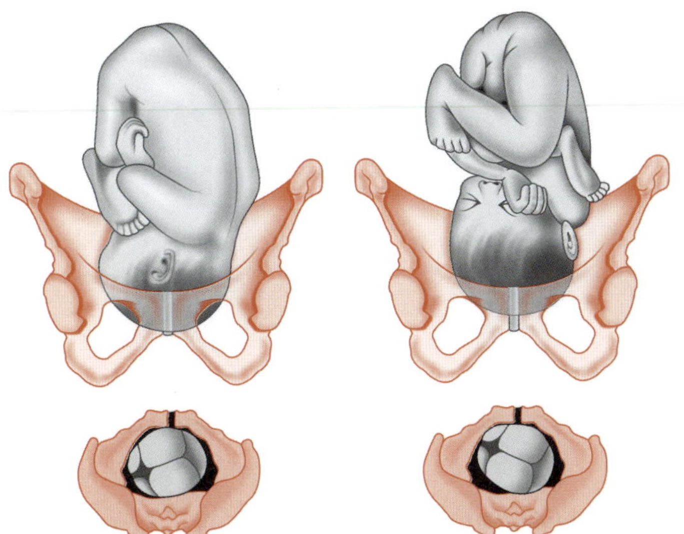

**Figs 1.7A and B:** Different positions of the occiput.
(A) Occipitoanterior; (B) Occipitoposterior

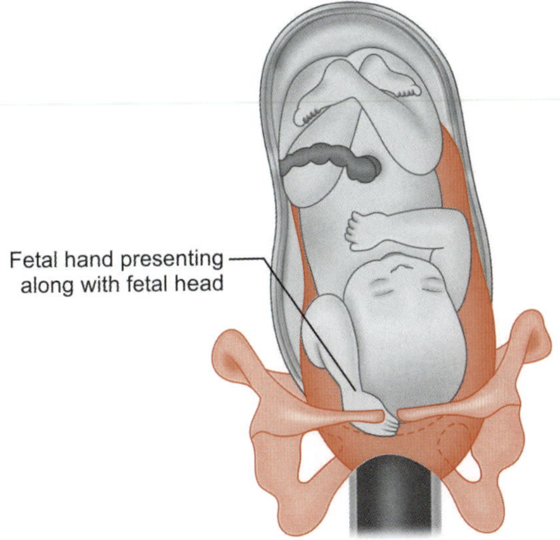



**Fig. 1.8:** Compound presentation

*Face presentation:* When the fetal head is sharply extended, occiput and the back are in contact with one another. In these cases, face is the foremost part of fetal head inside the birth canal and it presents first.

*Brow presentation:* When the fetal head is only partially extended, fetal brows are the foremost part of fetal head inside the birth canal and they present first. Brow presentation is usually transient because with the progress of labor, as further extension of neck takes place, brow presentation almost invariably gets converted into face presentation. If the brow presentation remains persistent, the labor gets arrested and a cesarean section is almost always required.

*Sinciput presentation:* When the fetal head is only partially flexed, the anterior fontanel or bregma is the foremost inside the birth canal and it presents. With progress of labor, as the flexion of neck takes place, sinciput presentation invariably gets converted into vertex presentation.

*Compound presentation:* Compound presentation is a term used when more than one part of the fetus presents (Fig. 1.8). For example, presence of fetal limbs alongside the head in case of a cephalic presentation or one or both arms in case of breech presentation. This can commonly occur in case of preterm infants.

Since fetal presentation can undergo a change in the early weeks of gestation, fetal presentation should be reassessed by abdominal palpation at 36 weeks or later, when fetal presentation is unlikely to change by itself and it is likely to influence the plans for the birth. In case of suspected fetal malpresentation, an ultrasound examination must be performed to confirm the presentation.

### Presenting Part

This can be defined as the part of fetal presentation which is foremost within the birth canal and is therefore first felt by the clinician's examining fingers:
- *Cephalic:* In case of cephalic presentation, the fetal presenting parts are as follows:
  - Completely flexed fetal head: Vertex
  - Deflexed fetal head: Sinciput
  - Partially extended fetal head: Brow
  - Completely extended fetal head: Face
- *Breech presentation:* In case of breech presentation, the fetal presenting part is the sacrum.
- *Shoulder presentation:* In case of shoulder presentation, fetal presenting part is the back.

### Fetal Attitude

Fetal attitude refers to the relationship of fetal parts to each other (Figs 1.9A to D). The most common fetal attitude is that of flexion in which the fetal head is flexed over the fetal neck; fetal arms are flexed unto chest and the fetal legs are flexed over the abdomen.

### Denominator

Denominator can be described as an arbitrary fixed bony point on the fetal presenting part (Table 1.8).

### Fetal Position

Fetal position can be defined as the relationship of the denominator to the different quadrants of maternal pelvis

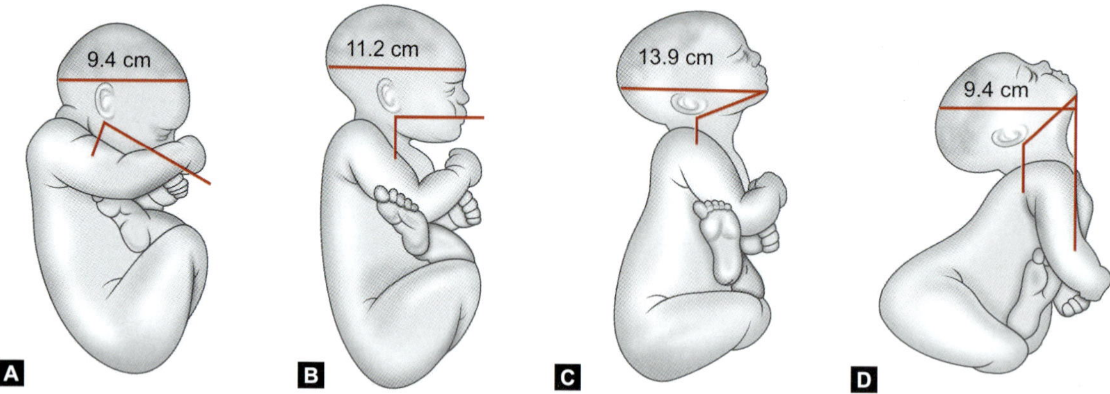



**Figs 1.9A to D:** Different types of fetal attitudes. (A) Complete flexion; (B) Marked deflexion; (C) Partial extension; (D) Complete extension

| **Table 1.8:** Fetal denominator in relation to fetal presenting parts | |
|---|---|
| *Fetal presenting part* | *Denominator* |
| Vertex | Occiput |
| Face | Mentum |
| Brow | Frontal eminence |
| Breech | Sacrum |
| Shoulder | Acromion |

(anterior, transverse and posterior). Since the presenting part would be either directed to the left or right side of maternal pelvis, six positions would be possible for each of the fetal presentation. For example, with vertex presentation, the six positions that would be possible are LOA, ROA, LOT, ROT, LOP and ROP (Figs 1.10A and B). The fetal position gives an idea regarding whether the presenting part is directed towards the front, back, left or right of the birth passage.

## Diagnosis of Fetal Presentation and Position

It is most important for the clinician to correctly identify the fetal presentation and position. This is usually done by performing Leopold's maneuvers on abdominal examination or via vaginal examination.

## Obstetric Grips or Leopold's Maneuvers of Abdominal Palpation

Obstetric grips which help in determining fetal lie and presentation are also known as Leopold's maneuvers. Leopold's maneuvers basically include four steps and must be performed while the woman is lying comfortably on her back. The examiner faces the patient for the first three maneuvers and faces towards her feet for the fourth. Obstetric grips must be conducted when the uterus is relaxed and not when the woman is experiencing contractions (Figs 1.11A to D).

### Maternal Position

The mother should be comfortable lying in supine position and her abdomen is to be bared. She should be asked to semiflex her thighs in order to relax the abdominal muscles.

These maneuvers can be performed throughout the third trimester and between the contractions, when the patient is in labor. These grips help in determining fetal lie and presentation. The fetal head feels hard and round, and is easily movable and ballotable. The breech feels soft, broad and irregular and is continuous with the body. Besides estimating the fetal lie and presentation, many experienced clinicians are also able to estimate fetal size and weight through these maneuvers. The following obstetric grips/ Leopold's maneuvers are carried out:

### Fundal Grip (Leopold's First Maneuver)

This is conducted while facing the patient's face. This grip helps the clinician to identify which of the fetal poles (head or breech) is present at the fundus. The fundal area is palpated by placing both the hands over the fundal area. Palpation of broad, soft, irregular mass is suggestive of fetal legs and/ or buttocks, thereby pointing towards cephalic presentation. Palpation of a smooth, hard, globular, ballotable mass at the fundus is suggestive of fetal head and points towards breech presentation.

### Lateral Grip (Leopold's Second Maneuver)

This grip is also conducted while facing the patient's face. The hands are placed flat over the abdomen on the either side of the umbilicus. Lateral grip helps the clinician in identifying the position of fetal back, limbs and shoulder in case of vertex or breech presentation. The orientation of the fetus can be determined by noting whether the back is directed vertically (anteriorly, posteriorly) or transversely. In case of transverse lie, hard, round, globular mass suggestive

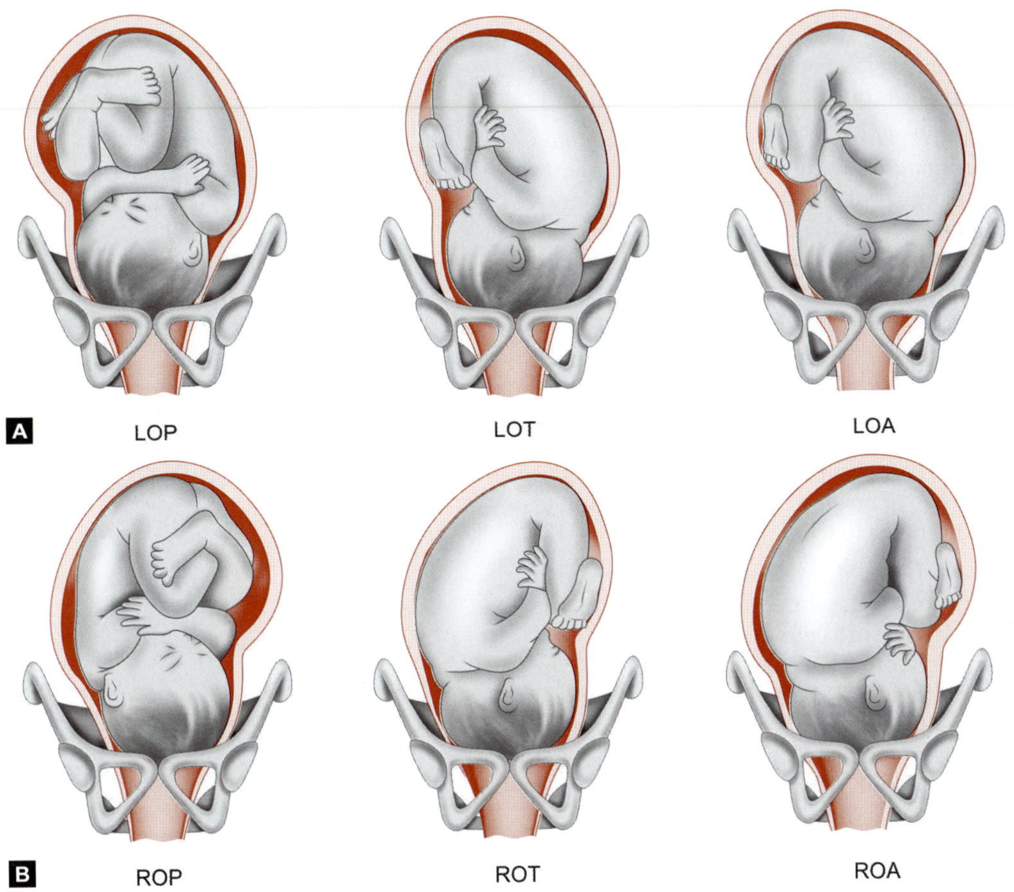

**Figs 1.10A and B:** Different positions with occipitoanterior position
*Abbreviations:* LOA, left occiput anterior; LOP, left occiput posterior; LOT, left occiput transverse; ROA, right occiput anterior; ROP, right occiput posterior; ROT, right occiput transverse

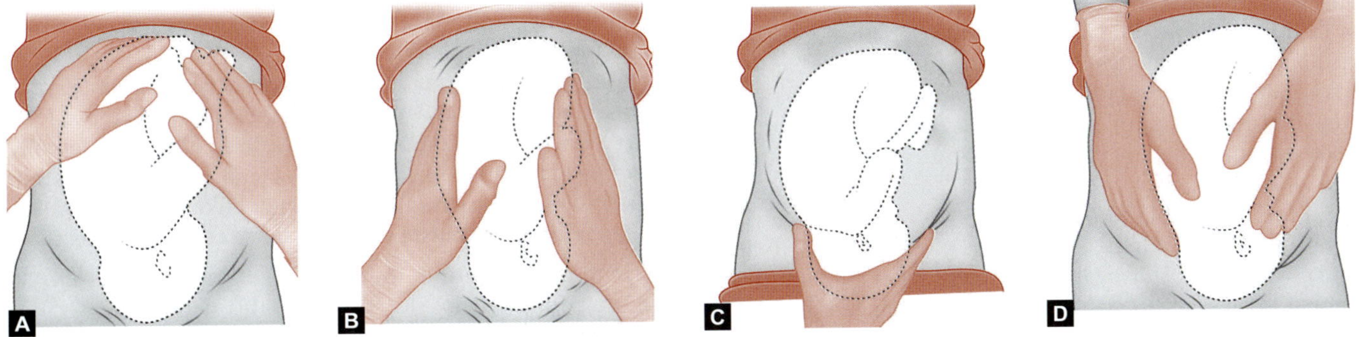

**Figs 1.11A to D:** Obstetric grips. (A) First Leopold's maneuver; (B) Second Leopold's maneuver; (C) Third Leopold's maneuver; (D) Fourth Leopold's maneuver

of fetal head can be identified horizontally across the maternal abdomen. The fetal back can be identified as a smooth curved structure with a resistant feel. The position of the fetal back on the left or right side of the uterus would help in determining the position of the presenting part. The fetal limbs would be present on the side opposite to the fetal back and present as small, round, knob-like structures. After identifying the back, the clinician should try to identify the anterior shoulder, which forms a well-marked prominence just above the fetal head.

*Pelvic Grips*

These include two maneuvers: first pelvic grip (Leopold's fourth maneuver) and second pelvic grip (Leopold's third maneuver)

*Second pelvic grip (Pawlik's grip) or third Leopold's maneuver:* This examination is done while facing the patient's face. The clinician places the outstretched thumb and index finger of the right hand keeping the ulnar border of the palm on the upper border of the patient's pubic symphysis. If a hard globular mass is gripped, it implies vertex presentation. A soft broad part is suggestive of fetal breech. If the presenting part is not engaged, it would be freely ballotable between the two fingers. If the presenting part is deeply engaged, the findings of this maneuver simply indicate that the lower fetal pole is in the pelvis. Further details would be revealed by the next maneuver. In case of transverse presentation the pelvic grip is empty. Normally, the size of head in a baby at term would fit in the hand of the examining clinician.

*First pelvic grip (Fourth Leopold's maneuver):* The objective of this step is to determine the amount of head palpable above the pelvic brim in case of a cephalic presentation. First pelvic grip is performed while facing the patient's feet. Tips of three fingers of each hand are placed on the either side of the midline in downwards and backwards direction in order to deeply palpate the fetal parts present in the lower pole of the uterus. The fingers of both the hands should be placed parallel to the inguinal ligaments and the thumbs should be pointing towards the umbilicus on both the sides. In case of vertex presentation, a hard, smooth, globular mass suggestive of fetal head can be palpated on pelvic grip. In case of breech presentation, broad, soft, irregular mass is palpated.

In case of cephalic presentation, the following need to be assessed: precise presenting part; fetal attitude and engagement of the fetal head. The fetal attitude or the amount of flexion of the fetal head can be evaluated by assessing the relative position between the sinciput and occiput (Fig. 1.12). In case of a fully flexed fetal head the sinciput can be palpated way above the occiput. As the amount of flexion of the fetal head reduces, the sinciput and occiput can be palpated at almost equal levels.

If the fingers of the palpating hands appear to converge below the fetal head, the fetal head is most likely free floating and not engaged. However, if the fingers of the palpating hand appear to diverge, the head is most likely engaged (Figs 1.13A and B).

## Auscultation of Fetal Heart

The fetal wellbeing is usually assessed by listening to the fetal heart. The auscultation of fetal heart will also give some idea regarding the fetal presentation and position. The region of maternal abdomen where the heart sounds are most clearly heard would vary with the presentation and extent of descent of the presenting part (Fig. 1.14). The fetal heart is

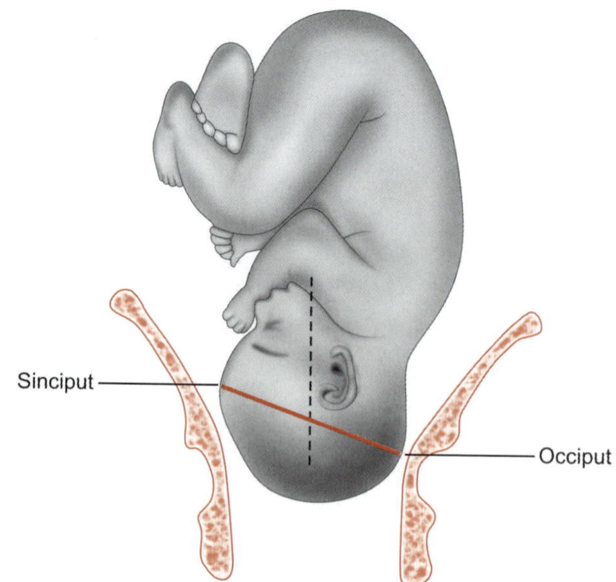


**Fig. 1.12:** Position of the fetal occiput and sinciput in a fully flexed fetal attitude

most easily heard by listening over the back of the fetus. The fetal heart rate can be monitored either through electronic fetal monitoring, using an external fetal monitor or through intermittent auscultation, using a Doppler instrument or Pinard's fetoscope or even an ordinary stethoscope. Instruments utilizing Doppler instruments can be commonly used for detecting fetal heart sounds by 10 weeks. Cardiac activity can be visualized as early as five menstrual weeks using real-time ultrasound with a vaginal transducer. Normal fetal heart rate varies from 110 beats/minute to 160 beats/minute with the average rate being about 140 beats/minute. The fetal heart sounds appear as the ticking of a watch when heard from under the pillow.

Auscultation of fetal heart rate is particularly important in cases whether the woman is unable to perceive the fetal movements. To make sure that the clinician is not accidentally listening to mother's heart instead of fetal heart, the maternal pulse must also be simultaneously palpated. In normal cases, the fetal heart rate must be auscultated as described next.

*Normal cases:* During the first stage of labor; every 30 minutes, followed by every 15 minutes during the second stage of labor.

*High-risk cases:* In high-risk cases (e.g. preeclampsia), the fetal heart rate must be auscultated every 15 minutes during first stage and every 5 minutes during the second stage of labor.

## VAGINAL EXAMINATION

Routine vaginal examination is not required in the antenatal period. Vaginal examination may be required for confirmation of the signs of pregnancy such as Hegar's sign, Chadwick's and

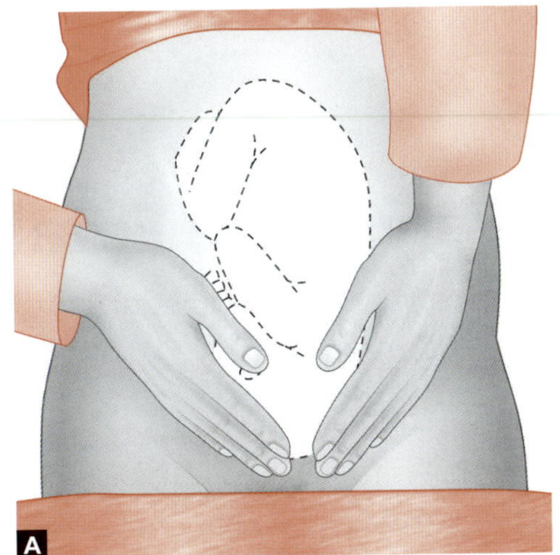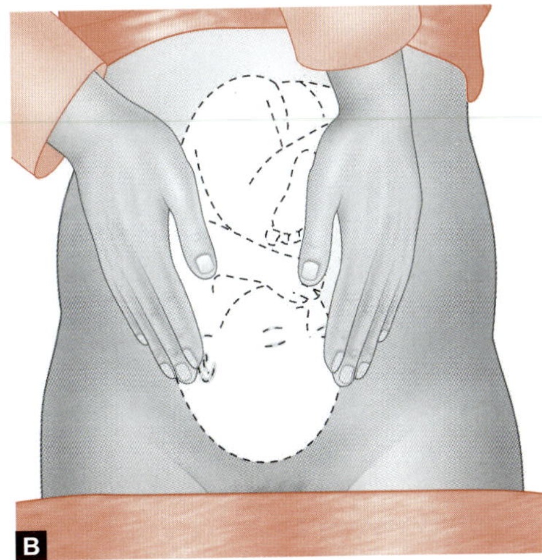

**Figs 1.13A and B:** Checking the engagement of fetal head on fourth Leopold's maneuver. (A) Unengaged fetal head; (B) Engaged fetal head

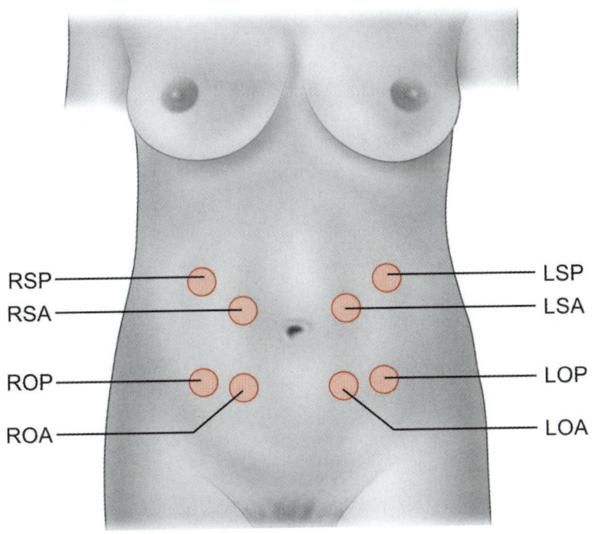


**Fig. 1.14:** Auscultation of fetal heart
*Abbreviations:* LOA, left occiput anterior; LOP, left occiput posterior; LSA, left sacrum anterior; LSP, left sacrum posterior; ROA, right occiput anterior; ROP, right occiput posterior; RSA, right sacrum anterior; RSP, right sacrum posterior

Jacquemier's sign. Vaginal examination may also be required in cases of recurrent vaginal discharge, pelvic pain, suspected labor or ectopic pregnancy. Vaginal examination assumes importance in labor where the palpation of sagittal sutures and fontanels through the open cervix helps in evaluation of the baby's position and the amount of descent of the fetal presenting part. Vaginal examination has been described in details in Chapter 3.

## Per Speculum Examination

Per speculum examination can help in evaluation of the following parameters: checking the presence of any discharge or lesions; to note the color and consistency of cervix; and to obtain cervical samples for testing.

## Pelvic Examination

Since the routine antenatal pelvic examination does not accurately assess gestational age, nor does it accurately predict preterm birth or cephalopelvic disproportion, it is not recommended in routine clinical practice.

## FURTHER READINGS

1. American College of Obstetricians and Gynecologists Committee on Gynecologic Practice. ACOG Committee Opinion No. 483: Primary and preventive care: periodic assessments. Obstet Gynecol. 2011;117(4):1008-15.
2. Committee on Nutritional Status during Pregnancy and Lactation, Institute of Medicine, National Academy of Science. "Dietary intake during pregnancy". Nutrition during pregnancy: Part I: Weight gain, Part II: Nutrient supplements. Washington DC: National Academy Press; 1990.
3. National Institute for Clinical Excellence. (NICE, 2008). Antenatal care: Routine care for the healthy pregnant woman. [online] Available from www.nice.org.uk/nicemedia/pdf/CG062NICEguideline.pdf [Accessed November, 2014].
4. Sharma R Revision of Prasad's social classification and provision of an online tool for real-time updating. [online] Available from: www.prasadscaleupdate.weebly.com [Accessed November, 2014].

# Bony Pelvis and Fetal Skull



## Introduction

Five important factors are responsible for the normal progress of labor. These include the passage (i.e. the maternal pelvis), the fetus, the relationship between the passage and the fetus, the force of labor and psychosocial considerations. This can be remembered by the mnemonic called the five "Ps" of labor: **P**assageway (maternal pelvis), **P**assenger (fetus), **P**ower (uterine contractions), **P**osition and **P**sychologic responses.

## The Maternal Pelvis: Passageway

The birth passage comprises of three parts, namely the pelvic inlet, pelvic cavity and the pelvic outlet (Video 2). The bony pelvis can be classified into four types: gynecoid, android, anthropoid and platypelloid (Figs 2.1A to D and Table 2.1). Of these, the gynecoid type of pelvis is the most common, with its diameters being most favorable for vaginal delivery. The anterior view of maternal gynecoid pelvis is shown in Figure 2.2. Gynecoid pelvis is an ideal type of pelvis and is characterized by the presence of the following features:

- The pelvic brim is almost round in shape, but slightly oval transversely.
- Anteroposterior (AP) diameter is the shortest in a gynecoid pelvis.
- Ischial spines are not prominent.
- Subpubic arch is rounded and measures at least 90° in size.
- Obturator foramen is triangular in shape.
- Sacrum is wide with average concavity and inclination.
- Sacrosciatic notch is wide.

The pelvic brim (Fig. 2.3) anatomically divides the pelvis into false pelvis and true pelvis. The boundaries of the pelvic brim or inlet include the following: sacral promontory,

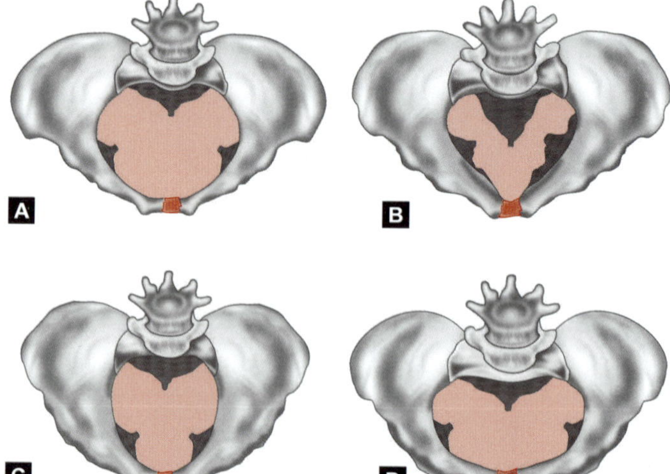

**Figs 2.1A to D:** Different types of pelvis. (A) Gynecoid pelvis; (B) Android pelvis; (C) Anthropoid pelvis; (D) Platypelloid pelvis

sacral alae, sacroiliac joints, iliopectineal lines, iliopectineal eminence, upper border of superior pubic rami, pubic tubercles, pubic crest and upper borders of pubic symphysis.

- *False pelvis:* False pelvis lies above the pelvic brim and has no obstetric significance.
- *True pelvis:* True pelvis lies below the pelvic brim and plays an important role in the childbirth and delivery. The true pelvis forms a bony canal through which the fetus passes at the time of labor. It is formed by the symphysis pubis anteriorly and sacrum and coccyx posteriorly. The true pelvis can be divided into three parts: pelvic inlet, cavity and outlet.

**Table 2.1:** Various pelvic dimensions in different types of pelvis

| Part of pelvis | Dimension | Gynecoid | Anthropoid | Android | Platypelloid |
|---|---|---|---|---|---|
| Pelvic inlet | The widest diameter of pelvic inlet | 12 cm | < 12 cm | 12 cm | 12 cm |
| | Shape of the pelvic inlet | Oval at the inlet with anteroposterior diameter being just slightly less than the transverse diameter | Oval, long and narrow; the anteroposterior diameter of the inlet exceeds the transverse diameter giving it an oval shape | Heart-shaped/triangular with the base towards the sacrum. As a result, posterior segment is short, and anterior segment is narrow | Pelvic brim is flat and transverse kidney-shaped. Transverse diameter is much larger than the anteroposterior diameter |
| | Anteroposterior diameter of inlet | 11 cm | > 12 cm | 11 cm | 10 cm |
| | Forepelvis | Wide | Divergent | Narrow | Straight |
| Pelvic midcavity | Sidewalls | Straight | Narrow | Convergent (widest posteriorly) | Wide (diverge downwards) |
| | Sacrosciatic notch | Wide and shallow | Wider and more shallow | Narrow and deep | Slightly narrow and small |
| | Inclination of sacrum | Sacrum is well-curved, and sacral angle exceeds 90° | Sacrum is long and narrow with usual curve; sacral angle is > 90° | Sacrum is inclined forward and straight; sacral angle is < 90° | The sacrum is prominent and the sacral promontory tends to encroach upon the area of the hind pelvis; sacral angle is > 90° |
| | Ischial spines | Not prominent | Not prominent | Prominent | Not prominent |
| Pelvic outlet | Subpubic arch | Wide and curved subpubic arch (subpubic angle is not < 85°) | Subpubic arch is long and narrow; subpubic angle may be slightly narrowed | Long and straight subpubic arch; narrow subpubic angle | The subpubic arch is generally wide, and the subpubic angle is in the excess of 90° |
| | Transverse diameter of the outlet | 10 cm | 10 cm | < 10 cm | 10 cm |

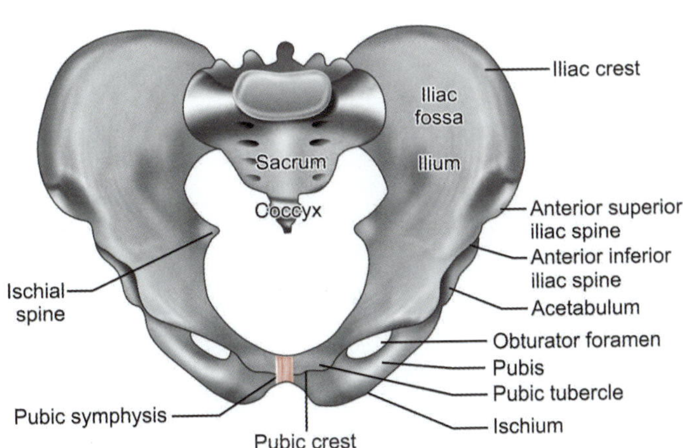


**Fig. 2.2:** Anterior view of maternal pelvis

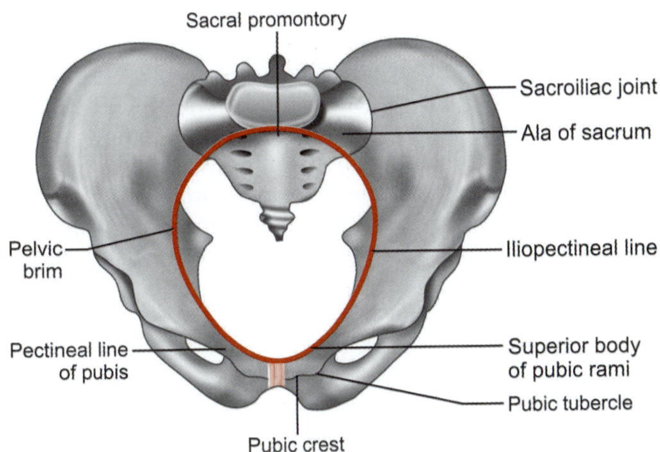


**Fig. 2.3:** Boundaries of the pelvic brim

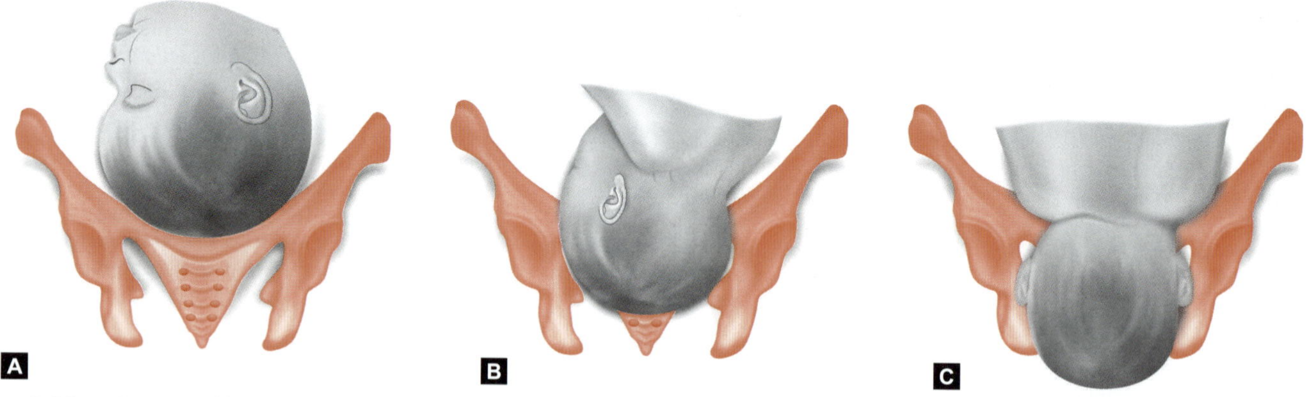

**Figs 2.4 A to C:** Entry of fetal head into the maternal pelvis. (A) The engaging anteroposterior diameter of fetal head engages in the transverse diameter of the inlet; (B and C) The fetal head undergoes internal rotation by 90° inside the pelvic cavity so that the longest diameter of fetal head engages in anteroposterior diameter of the outlet, which is its largest diameter

## PELVIC INLET

Pelvic inlet is round in shape and is the narrowest in anteroposterior dimension and the widest in transverse diameter. The fetal head enters the pelvic inlet with the longest diameter of the fetal head (AP diameter) in the widest part of the pelvic inlet (transverse diameter) (Figs 2.4A to C). The plane of the pelvic inlet (also known as superior strait) is not horizontal, but is tilted forwards. It makes an angle of 55° with the horizontal. This angle is known as the angle of inclination. Radiographically, this angle can be measured by measuring the angle between the front of the vertebra L5 and plane of inlet and subtracting this from 180°. Increase in the angle of inclination (also known as the high inclination) has obstetric significance because this may result in delayed engagement of the fetal head and delay in descent of fetal head. Increase in the angle of inclination also favors occipitoposterior position. On the other hand, reduction in the angle of inclination (also known as low inclination) may not have any obstetric significance.

The axis of the pelvic inlet is a line drawn perpendicular to the plane of inlet in the midline (Fig. 2.5). It is in downwards and backwards direction. Upon extension, this line passes through the umbilicus anteriorly and through the coccyx posteriorly. For the proper descent and engagement of fetal head, it is important that the uterine axis coincides with the axis of inlet.

### Diameters of the Pelvic Inlet

#### Anteroposterior Diameter (Fig. 2.6)

- *Anteroposterior diameter (true conjugate or anatomical conjugate = 11 cm):* This is measured from the midpoint of sacral promontory to the upper border of pubic symphysis.
- *Obstetric conjugate (10.5 cm):* The obstetric conjugate is measured from the midpoint of sacral promontory to the

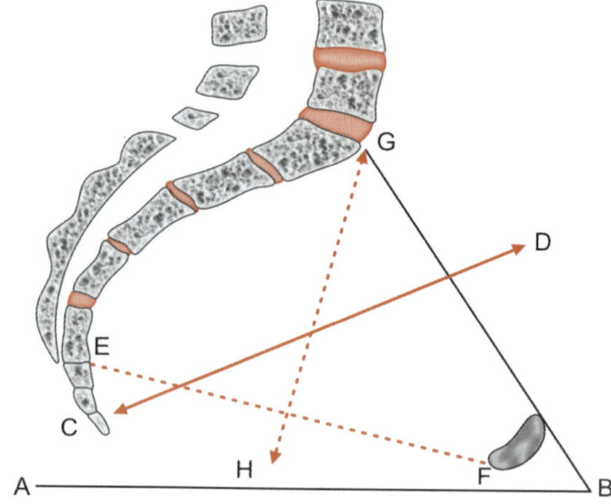

**Fig. 2.5:** Different planes and axes of the pelvis. AB—Horizontal line; GB—Plane of inlet; FE—Plane of obstetric outlet; DC—Axis of the inlet; GH—Axis of obstetric outlet

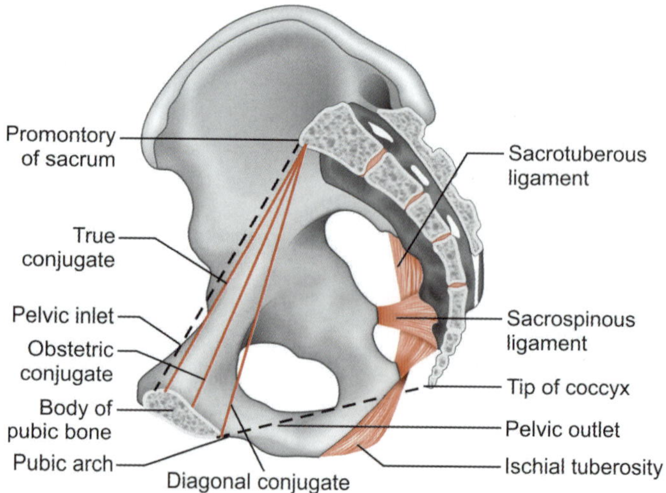


**Fig. 2.6:** Medial view of maternal pelvis (from left)

most bulging point on the back of pubic symphysis. This is the shortest AP diameter of the pelvic inlet and measures about 10.5 cm.

- *Diagonal conjugate (12.5 cm):* It is measured from the tip of sacral promontory to the lower border of pubic symphysis.

Out of three AP diameters of pelvic inlet, only diagonal conjugate can be assessed clinically during the late pregnancy or at the time of the labor. Obstetric conjugate can be calculated by subtracting 1.5–2 cm from the diagonal conjugate. Also the true conjugate can be inferred by subtracting 1.2 cm from the diagonal conjugate.

### Measurement of the Diagonal Conjugate

After placing the patient in dorsal position and taking all aseptic precautions, two fingers are introduced into vagina. The clinician tries to feel the anterior sacral curvature with these fingers (Fig. 2.7). In normal cases it will be difficult to feel the sacral promontory. The clinician may be required to depress the elbow and wrist while mobilizing the fingers upwards in order to reach the promontory. The point at which the bone recedes from the finger is sacral promontory. A marking is placed over the gloved index finger by the index finger of the other hand. After removing the fingers from the vagina, the distance between the marking and the tip of the middle finger is measured in order to obtain the measurement of diagonal conjugate. In clinical situations it may not always be feasible to measure the diagonal conjugate. In these cases, if the middle finger fails to reach the sacral promontory or reaches it with difficulty, the diagonal conjugate can be considered as adequate. Under normal circumstances, an adequate pelvis would be able to allow an average-sized fetal head to pass through.

### Transverse Diameter of Pelvic Inlet

- *Anatomical transverse diameter (13 cm):* It is the distance between the farthest two points on the iliopectineal line (Fig. 2.8). It is the largest diameter of the pelvic inlet and lies 4 cm anterior to the promontory and 7 cm behind the symphysis.
- *Obstetric transverse diameter:* This diameter passes through the midpoint of true conjugate and is therefore slightly shorter than the anatomical transverse diameter.

### Oblique Diameters of Pelvic Inlet

There are two oblique diameters, right and left (12 cm). The right oblique diameter passes from right sacroiliac joint to the left iliopubic eminence, whereas the left diameter passes from left sacroiliac joint to the right iliopubic eminence.

## Pelvic Cavity

The pelvic cavity is almost round in shape and is bounded above by the pelvic brim and below by the plane of least pelvic dimension, anteriorly by the symphysis pubis and posteriorly by sacrum. The plane of least pelvic dimension extends from the lower border of pubic symphysis to the tip of ischial spines laterally and to the tip of fifth sacral vertebra posteriorly.

### Plane of Cavity (Plane of Greatest Pelvic Dimensions)

This plane passes between the middle of the posterior surface of the symphysis pubis and the junction between second and the third sacral vertebra. Laterally, it passes through the center of acetabulum and the upper part of greater sciatic notch. Since this is the roomiest plane of pelvis, it is also known as the plane of greatest pelvic dimensions. This is almost round in shape. Internal rotation of the fetal head occurs when the biparietal diameter of the fetal skull occupies this wide pelvic plane while the occiput is on the pelvic floor, i.e. at the plane of least pelvic dimensions.

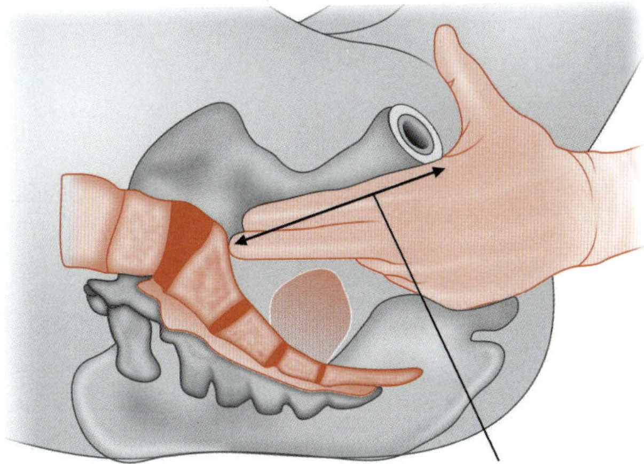


**Fig. 2.7:** Measurement of diagonal conjugate

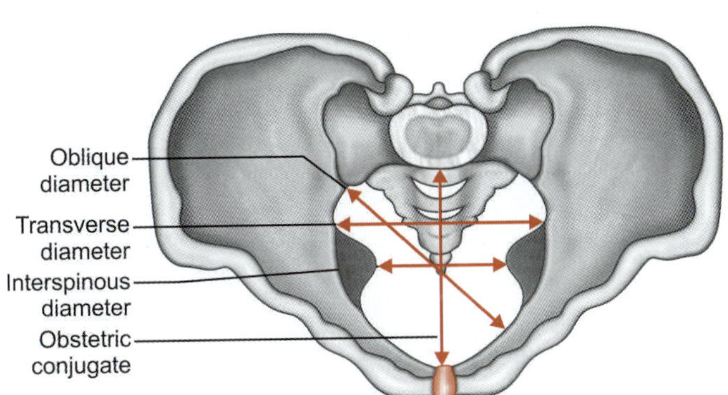


**Fig. 2.8:** Superior view of pelvic inlet

### Diameters of Pelvic Cavity

- *Anteroposterior diameter (12 cm):* It measures from the midpoint on the posterior surface of pubis symphysis to the junction of second and third sacral vertebra.
- *Transverse diameter (12 cm):* It is the distance between two farthest points laterally. Since there are no bony landmarks, the diameter cannot be exactly measured and can be roughly estimated to be about 12 cm.

## Pelvic Outlet

- *Anatomical outlet:* It is a lozenge-shaped cavity bounded by anterior border of symphysis pubis, pubic arch, ischial tuberosities, sacrotuberous ligaments, sacrospinous ligaments and tip of coccyx.
- *Plane of anatomical outlet:* It passes along with the boundaries of the anatomical outlet and consists of two triangular planes with a common base, which is the bituberous diameter (Fig. 2.9A).
- *Anterior sagittal plane:* Its apex is at the lower border of the symphysis pubis.
- *Anterior sagittal diameter (6–7 cm):* It extends from the lower border of the pubic symphysis to the center of bituberous diameter.
- *Posterior sagittal plane:* Its apex lies at the tip of the coccyx.
- *Posterior sagittal diameter (7.5–10 cm):* It extends from the tip of the sacrum to the center of bituberous diameter.
- *Obstetric outlet:* It is bounded above by the plane of least pelvic dimensions, below by the anatomical outlet, anteriorly by the lower border of symphysis pubis, posteriorly by the coccyx and laterally by the ischial spines.

### Diameters of Pelvic Outlet

- Anteroposterior diameters of pelvic outlet include the following:
    - *Anatomical AP diameter (11 cm):* It extends from tip of the coccyx to the lower border of symphysis pubis.
    - *Obstetric AP diameter (13 cm):* It extends from the lower border of symphysis pubis to the tip of coccyx (as it moves backwards during the second stage of labor).
- Transverse diameter of the pelvic outlet includes the following:
    - *Bituberous diameter (11 cm):* This is the transverse diameter of the anatomical outlet and extends between the inner aspects of ischial tuberosities. The bituberous diameter is measured with the knuckles of the closed fist of the hand placed between the two ischial tuberosities (Figs 2.9A and B). If the pelvis is adequate, the intertuberous diameter allows four knuckles.
    - *Bispinous diameter (10.5 cm):* This is the transverse diameter of the obstetric outlet and extends between the tips of ischial spines.

Measurement of various pelvic diameters is summarized in Table 2.2.

**Table 2.2:** Summary of the measurement of the diameters of the pelvis

| Diameter | Pelvic brim | Pelvic cavity | Pelvic outlet |
|---|---|---|---|
| Anteroposterior | 11 cm | 12 cm | 13 cm |
| Oblique | 12 cm | 12 cm | – |
| Transverse | 13 cm | 12 cm | 11 cm |

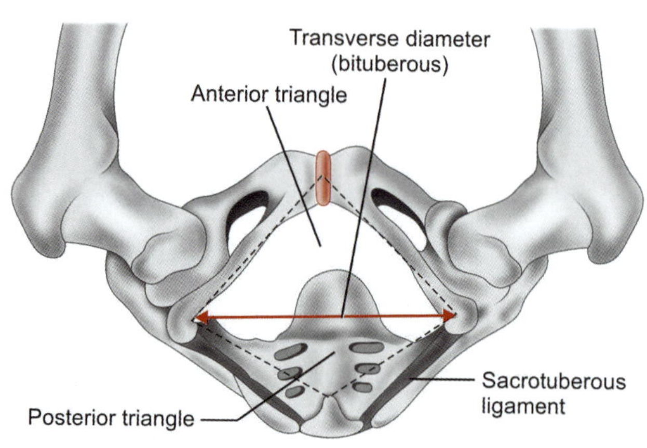


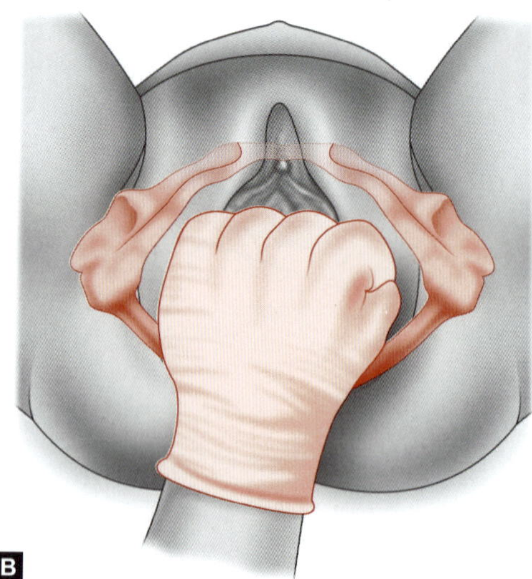


**Figs 2.9A and B:** Measurement of transverse diameter of the outlet

## Pelvic Axis

*Anatomical axis (Curve of Carus):* This is an imaginary line joining the central points of the planes of inlet, cavity and outlet. This axis is C-shaped with concavity directed forwards. It has no obstetric significance.

*Obstetric axis:* It is an imaginary line, which represents the direction in which the fetal head passes during the labor. It is J-shaped and passes downwards and backwards along the axis of the inlet till the ischial spines are reached after which it passes downwards and forwards along the axis of pelvic outlet (Fig. 2.10).

## Midpelvis

This is the part of pelvis which is bounded above by the plane of greatest pelvic dimensions and below by the plane known as the midpelvic plane.

*Midpelvic plane:* This plane is bounded anteriorly by the lower margin of symphysis pubis. It extends through the ischial spines to the junction of S4 and S5 or the tip of fifth sacral piece, depending upon the structure of the sacrum. If this plane meets at the tip of the S5 sacral piece, this plane becomes same as that of the plane of least pelvic dimensions; otherwise it forms a wedge posteriorly.

### Diameters of Midpelvis

- *Anteroposterior diameter (11.5 cm):* It is measured from the lower border of the symphysis pubis to the junction of S4 and S5 or the tip of S5, whichever is applicable.
- *Bispinous or transverse diameter (10.5 cm):* It is the distance between two ischial spines. Ischial spines are palpated for the assessment of midpelvis. After assessing

the sacrum, the clinician must move his/her fingers lateral to the midsacrum where the sacrospinous ligaments can be felt. If these ligaments are followed laterally, the ischial spines can be palpated (Fig. 2.11).

- *Subpubic angle:* It is the angle between two pubic rami. It varies from 85 ± 5°.

## Waste Space of Morris

Normally, the width of the pubic arch is such that a round disk of 9.4 cm (diameter of a well-flexed head) can pass through the pubic arch at a distance of 1 cm from the midpoint of the inferior border of the symphysis pubis. This distance is known as the "waste space of Morris" (Fig. 2.12). In case of an inadequate pelvis with narrow pubic arch, the fetal head would be pushed backwards and the waste space of Morris would increase. As a result, reduced space would be available for fetal head to pass through, due to which the fetal head would be forced to pass through a smaller diameter termed as the "available AP diameter". This is likely to injure the perineum or sometimes cause the arrest of fetal head.

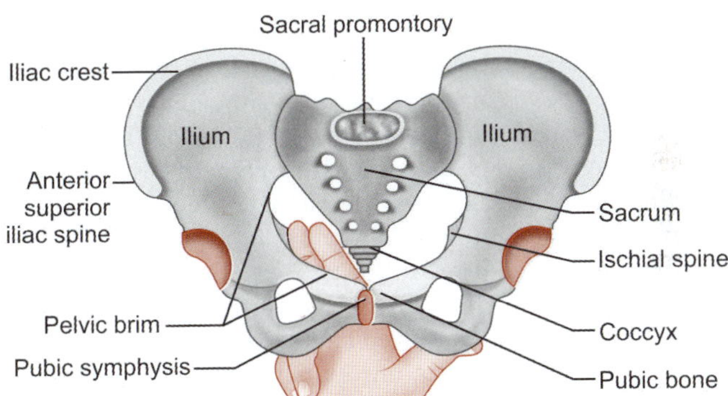


**Fig. 2.11:** Assessment of ischial spines

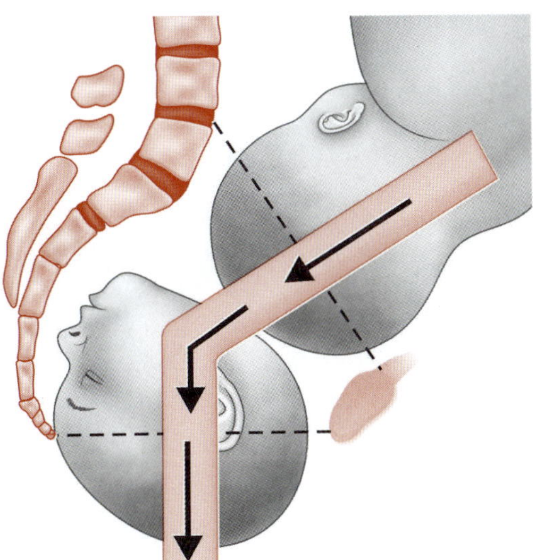

**Fig. 2.10:** Obstetric axis

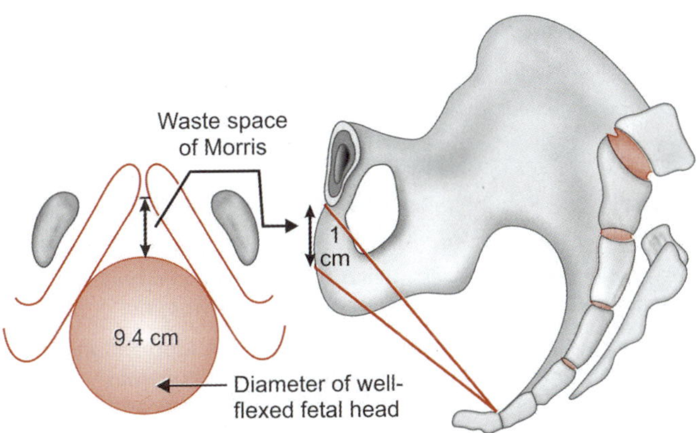


**Fig. 2.12:** Waste space of Morris

### Pelvic Joints

There are four joints in the pelvis, namely the symphysis pubis, sacroiliac joints (left and right) and the sacrococcygeal joint (Table 2.3).

## Pelvic Assessment

While assessing the pelvis, it is important to adopt a step-by-step method to assess the pelvis, i.e. first assessing the size and shape of the pelvic inlet, then the midpelvis and lastly the pelvic outlet. The parameters described in Table 2.4 need to be assessed.

The clinician must begin the pelvic assessment by starting with the sacral promontory and then following the curve of the sacrum down the midline. In an adequate pelvis, the promontory cannot be easily palpated, the sacrum is well curved and the coccyx cannot be felt. In case of an inadequate pelvis, the sacral promontory is easily palpated and prominent, the sacrum is straight and the coccyx is prominent and/or fixed. After assessing the sacrum, the clinician must move his/her fingers lateral to the midsacrum where the sacrospinous ligaments can be felt. If these ligaments are followed laterally, the ischial spines can be palpated. In an adequate pelvis, the sacrospinous ligaments are 3 cm or longer, i.e. at least two of the clinician's fingers can be placed over the sacrospinous ligaments. In case of an inadequate pelvis, it may not be possible to place two fingers over the sacrospinous ligaments; the ligaments usually allow less than two fingers. Also, the ischial spines may appear sharp and prominent. Next, the retropubic area is palpated. For this the clinician must put two examining fingers with the palm of the hand facing upwards, behind the symphysis pubis. The hand is then moved laterally to both sides. In case of an adequate pelvis, the retropubic area is flat. In case of an inadequate pelvis, the retropubic area is angulated. To measure the subpubic angle, the examining fingers are turned so that the palm of the hand faces downwards. At the same time, the third finger is also held out at the vaginal introitus and the angle under the pubis is felt. If three fingers can be placed under the pubis, the subpubic angle is approximately 90°, which can be considered as adequate (Fig. 2.13). If the subpubic angle allows only two fingers, the subpubic angle is about 60° which is indicative of an inadequate pelvis. Finally, as the clinician's hand is withdrawn from the vaginal introitus, the intertuberous diameter is measured with the knuckles of the closed fist of the hand placed between the ischial tuberosities. If the pelvis is adequate, the intertuberous diameter allows four knuckles. In case of an inadequate pelvis the intertuberous diameter allows less than four knuckles.

## Passenger: Fetus

Obstetrically, the head of fetus is the most important part, since an essential feature of labor is an adaptation between the fetal head and the maternal bony pelvis (Video 1). Only a comparatively small part of the head of the fetus at term is represented by the face; the rest is composed of the firm skull, which is made up of two frontal, two parietal and two temporal bones, along with the upper portion of the occipital bone and the wings of the sphenoid. The bones are not united rigidly but are separated by membranous spaces, the sutures. The fetal skull has four main sutures (Figs 2.14 and 2.15A and B), which are as follows:

- *Sagittal or longitudinal suture:* This suture lies longitudinally across the vault of the skull in midline. It lies between the two parietal bones. The obstetric significance of sagittal suture is described in Table 2.5.
- *Coronal suture:* These sutures are present between the parietal and frontal bones, and extend transversely on either side from the anterior fontanel.

| Table 2.3: Joints in the pelvis | |
|---|---|
| *Joint* | *Type* |
| Symphysis pubis | Fibrocartilaginous joint |
| Sacroiliac joint | Synovial joint |
| Sacrococcygeal joint | Synovial hinge joint |

| Table 2.4: Parameters to be evaluated at the time of pelvic assessment | | |
|---|---|---|
| *Assessment of pelvic inlet* | *Assessment of midpelvis* | *Assessment of the pelvic outlet* |
| The sacral promontory is palpated | The curve of sacrum, the sacrospinous ligaments and the ischial spines are palpated | The subpubic angle, intertuberous diameter and mobility of the coccyx are determined |

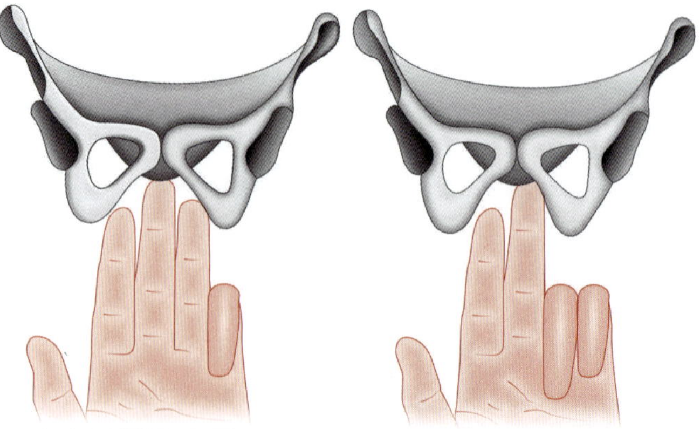

**Fig. 2.13:** Assessment of subpubic angle

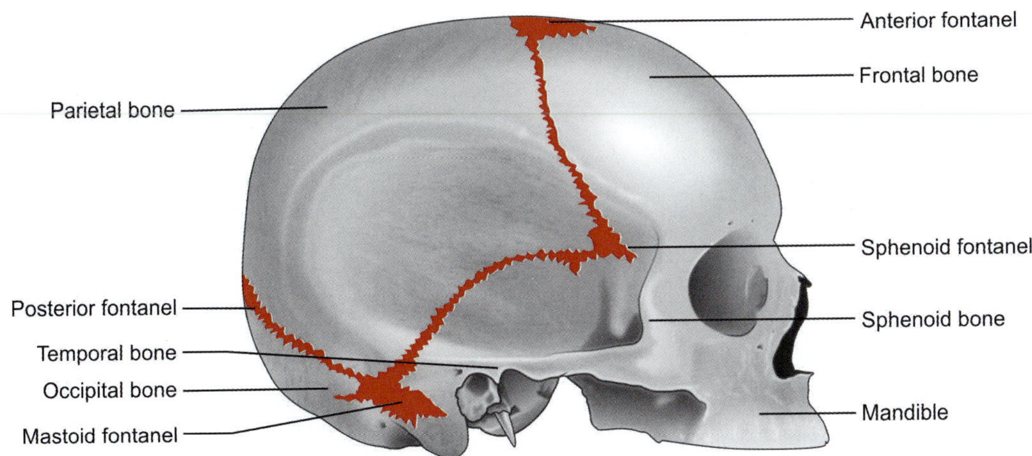



**Fig. 2.14:** Important sutures and bones of fetal skull

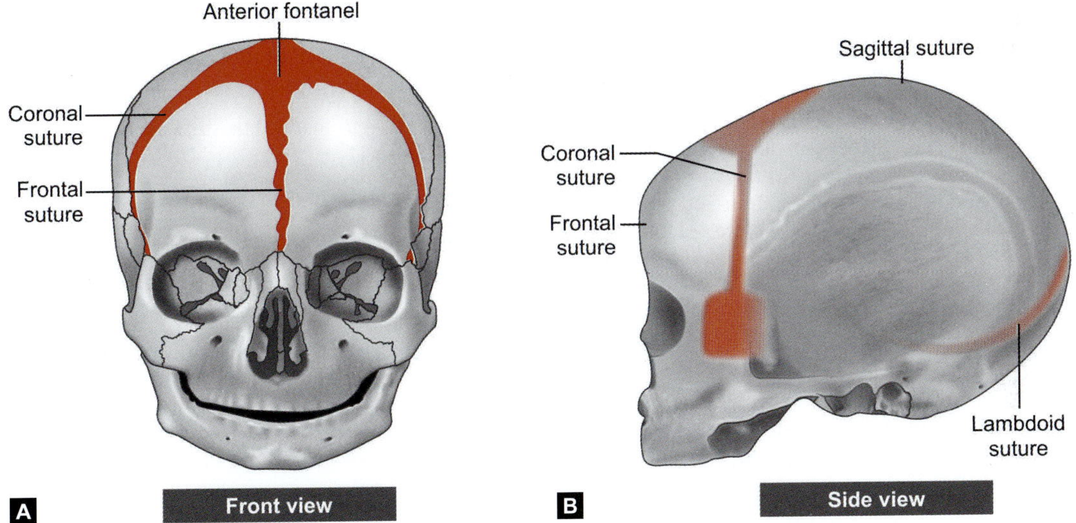



**Figs 2.15A and B:** Important sutures and fontanels in the fetal skull

| Table 2.5: Obstetric significance of sagittal suture |
| --- |
| • Allows gliding movement of the skull bones over one another, thereby permitting the molding of fetal head<br>• Gives an idea about the degree of synclitism and asynclitism of fetal head<br>• Gives an idea regarding the degree of internal rotation and molding of fetal head |

- *Lambdoid suture:* This suture separates the occipital bone from the two parietal bones and extends transversely both on the right and left side from the posterior fontanel.
- *Frontal suture:* This suture is present between the two halves of the frontal bone in the skull of infants and children and usually disappears by the age of 6 years.

Where several sutures meet, an irregular space is formed, which is enclosed by a membrane and is designated as a fontanel. The greater or anterior fontanel is a lozenge-shaped space situated at the junction of the sagittal and coronal sutures (Fig. 2.16). The lesser, or posterior fontanel is represented by a small triangular area at the intersection of the sagittal and lambdoid sutures. Both may be felt readily during labor, and their recognition gives important information concerning the presentation and position of the fetus. The two main fontanels having obstetric significance in the fetal head are: anterior fontanel (bregma) and posterior fontanel (lambda). Anterior fontanel is formed by joining of four sutures: frontal suture (anteriorly); sagittal suture (posteriorly) and coronal sutures on the two sides (laterally). The

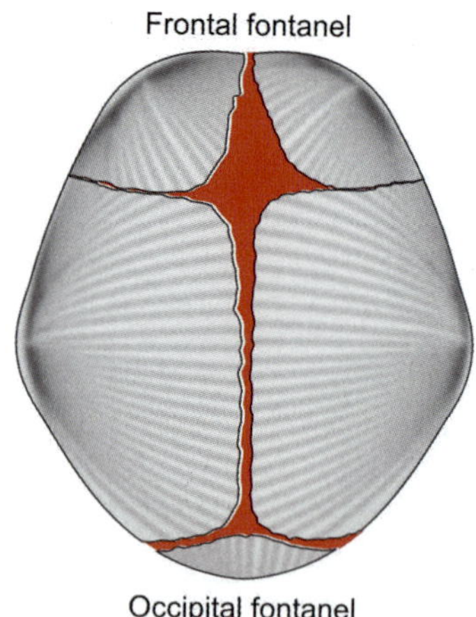



**Fig. 2.16:** Anterior and posterior fontanels in fetal head

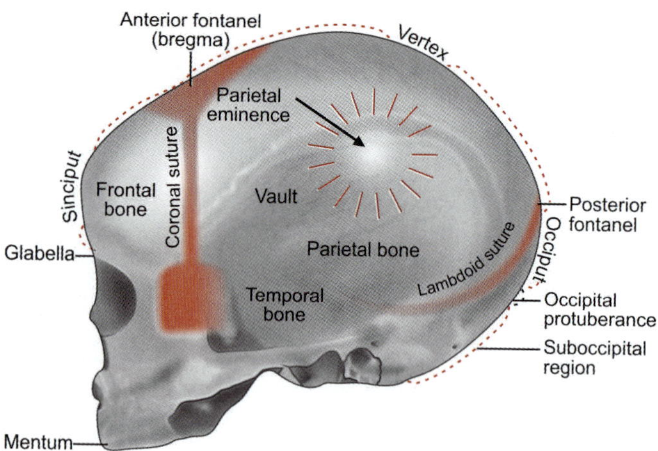



**Fig. 2.17:** Important landmarks of fetal skull

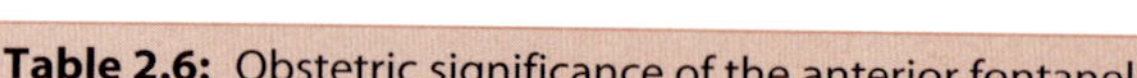

| **Table 2.6:** Obstetric significance of the anterior fontanel |
| --- |
| • Palpation of anterior fontanel indicates degree of flexion of fetal head<br>• It facilitates molding of fetal head<br>• The membranous nature of anterior fontanel helps in accommodating the rapid growth of brain during neonatal period<br>• Floor of the anterior fontanel reflects the intracranial status. The floor may be depressed in case of dehydration and elevated in case of hydrocephalus or other conditions with raised intracranial tension |

palpation of anterior fontanel on vaginal examination is of great obstetric significance (Table 2.6). Both AP and transverse diameters of the anterior fontanel measure about 3 cm. It usually becomes ossified by one and a half years of age. On the other hand, posterior fontanel is triangular in shape and measures 0.5 inch × 0.5 inch.

## Presenting Parts of Fetal Skull (Fig. 2.17)

These include the following:

*Vertex:* This is a quadrangular area bounded anteriorly by bregma (anterior fontanel) and coronal sutures; posteriorly by lambda (posterior fontanel) and lambdoid sutures; and laterally by arbitrary lines passing through the parietal eminences. When vertex is the presenting part, fetal head lies in complete flexion.

*Face:* This is an area bounded by the root of the nose along with the supraorbital ridges and the junction of the chin or floor of mouth with the neck. Fetal head is fully extended during this presentation.

*Brow:* This is an area of forehead extending from the root of nose and supraorbital ridges to the bregma and coronal sutures. The fetal head lies midway between full flexion and full extension in this presentation.

Some other parts of fetal skull, which are of significance, include the following:

*Sinciput:* Area in front of the anterior fontanel corresponding to the forehead.

*Occiput:* Area limited to occipital bone.

*Mentum:* Chin of the fetus.

*Parietal eminences:* Prominent eminences on each of the parietal bones.

*Subocciput:* This is the junction of fetal neck and occiput, sometimes also known as the nape of the neck.

*Submentum:* This is the junction between the neck and chin.

## Important Diameters of Fetal Skull

### Anteroposterior Diameters

The important AP diameters of the fetal skull are: suboccipitobregmatic (9.4 cm); suboccipitofrontal (10 cm); occipitofrontal (11.2 cm); mentovertical (13.9 cm); submentovertical (11.3 cm) and submentobregmatic (9.4 cm). These diameters are described in Table 2.7 and Figure 2.18.

### Transverse Diameters

- *Biparietal diameter (9.5 cm):* It extends between the two parietal eminences. This diameter nearly always engages.
- *Supersubparietal diameter (8.5 cm):* It extends from a point placed below one parietal eminence to a point placed above the other parietal eminence of the opposite side.
- *Bitemporal diameter (8 cm):* Distance between the anteroinferior ends of the coronal sutures.

**Table 2.7:** Anteroposterior diameters of the fetal head which may engage

| Diameter | Extent | Length | Attitude of head | Presentation |
|---|---|---|---|---|
| Suboccipitobregmatic | Extends from the nape of the neck to the center of bregma | 9.4 cm | Complete flexion | Vertex |
| Suboccipitofrontal | Extends from the nape of the neck to the anterior end of anterior fontanel or center of sinciput | 10 cm | Incomplete flexion | Vertex |
| Occipitofrontal | Extends from the occipital eminence to the root of nose (glabella) | 11.2 cm | Marked deflexion | Vertex |
| Mentovertical | Extends from midpoint of the chin to the highest point on sagittal suture | 13.9 cm | Partial extension | Brow |
| Submentovertical | Extends from the junction of the floor of the mouth and neck to the highest point on sagittal suture | 11.3 cm | Incomplete extension | Face |
| Submentobregmatic | Extends from the junction of the floor of the mouth and neck to the center of bregma | 9.4 cm | Complete extension | Face |

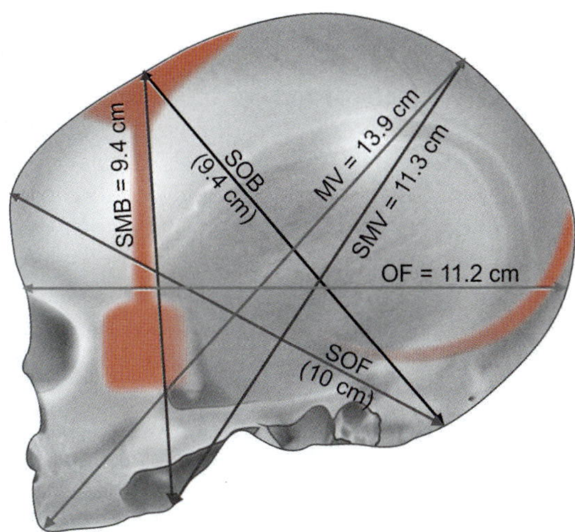


**Fig. 2.18:** Diameters of fetal skull
*Abbreviations:* SMB, submentobregmatic; SOB, suboccipitobregmatic; OF, occipitofrontal; MV, mentovertical; SMV, submentovertical; SOF, suboccipitofrontal

- *Bimastoid diameter (7.5 cm):* Distance between the tips of the mastoid process. This diameter is nearly incompressible.

The fetal head is said to be engaged when maximum transverse diameter of fetal head can pass through the pelvic brim. The shape and the diameter of the circumference of the fetal skull varies with the degree of flexion and hence the presentation. A normal pelvis would be easily able to permit the

**Table 2.8:** Plane of engagement of fetal head depending upon its attitude

| Attitude of head | Plane of shape | Engagement |
|---|---|---|
| Complete flexion | Biparietal-suboccipitobregmatic | Almost round |
| Deflexion | Biparietal-occipitofrontal | Oval |
| Incomplete extension | Biparietal-mentovertical | Bigger oval |
| Complete extension | Biparietal-submentobregmatic | Almost round |

engagement of the fetal skull in vertex and face presentations. This is so as in case of vertex and face presentations, the engaging AP diameters of fetal skull are respectively suboccipitobregmatic (9.4 cm) and submentobregmatic (9.4 cm) (Table 2.8). However, the passage of the fetal head in brow presentation would not be able to take place in a normal pelvis as the engaging AP diameter of fetal skull is mentovertical (13.9 cm) in this case. Therefore, arrest of labor occurs when the fetal head is in brow presentation.

## FURTHER READINGS


1. Moore KL, Agur AM, Dalley AF. Clinically Oriented Anatomy. 7th edition. Philadelphia: Lippincott Williams and Wilkins; 2013.
2. Snells RS. Clinical Anatomy by Regions, 9th edition. Philadelphia: Lippincott Williams and Wilkins; 2011.

# Normal Pregnancy and Labor



## Antenatal Care

### Antenatal Schedule

The antenatal schedule as devised by WHO is shown in Figure 3.1. The antenatal visits should be at every 4 weeks up to 28 weeks; at every 2 weeks up to 36 weeks and thereafter weekly till the EDD. A minimum of four visits are recommended by the WHO—first at 16th week; second at 24–28 weeks; third at 32 weeks and fourth at 36 weeks. The various antenatal visits would now be described in detail.

#### First Antenatal Visit

The woman must be called for the first antenatal visit preferably before 12 weeks of gestation. Since detailed history including previous medical and obstetric history needs to be taken, this visit takes about 30–40 minutes. The woman should be given an opportunity to discuss issues and ask questions. The presence of pregnancy needs to be confirmed during this visit. The accurate period of gestation can be established by first trimester ultrasound examination. A complete general physical and systemic examination as described in Chapter 1 must be performed. Advice regarding diet, exercise and folic acid intake must be given. She should be offered verbal information supported by written information (leaflets, brochures, etc.) on topics such as diet and lifestyle considerations. She should be advised to stop smoking and consuming alcohol, if previously doing so. High-risk women who may require additional care need to be identified and pattern of care for the pregnancy needs to be planned. The

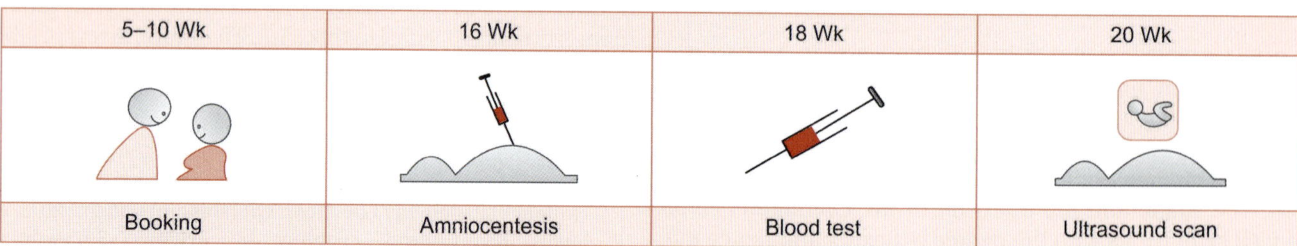



**Fig. 3.1:** Antenatal schedule

**Table 3.1:** Routine investigations to be done during the first antenatal visit

- Determination of the patient's blood group (ABO and Rh)
- Hemoglobin estimation
- Blood sugar (random)
- Urine test for proteins, glucose and pus cells
- Serological screening test for syphilis (VDRL)
- A rapid HIV screening test after pretest counseling and written consent
- Screening for HbsAg and hepatitis C virus
- Wet smear of any symptomatic vaginal discharge (i.e. itching, burning or offensive) must be examined under a microscope
- Screening for asymptomatic bacteriuria
- Screening for Down syndrome, if available (nuchal translucency at 11–14 weeks or serum screening at 14–20 weeks)
- First trimester ultrasound scan for gestational age assessment
- Ultrasound screening for structural anomalies (20 weeks)

*Abbreviation:* VDRL, venereal disease research laboratory

investigations, which need to be performed during first antenatal visit, are listed in Table 3.1.

### Second Antenatal Visit

Second antenatal visit must be scheduled at about 26 weeks of gestation. This visit is much shorter and lasts for about 20 minutes. At 18–20 weeks, an ultrasound scan should be performed for the detection of structural anomalies. For a woman whose placenta is found to be extending across the internal cervical os during this time should be offered another scan in third trimester and the results of this scan reviewed at the next appointment. Anti-D immunoglobulins must be offered to the Rh-negative women where available and indicated (at 28 weeks of gestation).

### Third Antenatal Visit (30–36 Weeks)

The clinician needs to review, discuss and document the results of screening tests undertaken during previous visits. Planned pattern of care for the pregnancy needs to be reassessed and the women who require additional care need to be identified.

### Fourth Antenatal Visit (36–40 Weeks)

During this last visit, the position of baby needs to be checked. In case of suspected malpresentation, ultrasound examination must be performed to confirm the fetal position. For women whose babies are in the breech presentation, external cephalic version can be considered after 37 completed weeks of gestation. Ultrasound scans may be required to confirm the placental position if the placenta had extended over the internal cervical os during the previous ultrasound scans. She should be asked to revisit her clinician in case she does not deliver until 41 weeks. Fetal heart rate monitoring needs to

be done in these cases. Induction may be considered, if the cervix is inducible and favorable.

## ROUTINE ANTENATAL CARE

### Nutrition

- Pregnant women require 15% more kilocalories than nonpregnant women, usually 100–300 kcal more per day, depending on the patient's weight and activity.
- Supplementation with iron, folic acid, protein and calcium is required during pregnancy.
- One tablet of fersolate ($FeSO_4$) containing 60 mg of elemental iron is prescribed daily from 16 weeks onwards or even earlier, if possible (WHO, 2012). Iron supplementation is recommended throughout the pregnancy.
- During second half of pregnancy, extra protein intake of 5–6 g/day is recommended.
- The woman should be informed that dietary supplementation with folic acid, before conception and up to 12 weeks of gestation, helps in reducing the risk of having a baby with neural tube defects (anencephaly, spina bifida, etc.). The recommended dose is 400 µg/day (WHO, 2012).
- The recommended dose of calcium supplementation in pregnancy is 1.5–2.0 g elemental calcium/day (WHO, 2013). Calcium supplementation is recommended for all pregnant women, particularly those at higher risk of gestational hypertension.

### Weight Gain

The total weight gain recommended during pregnancy based on the prepregnancy body mass index is described in Table 3.2. Presently the focus is on lower weight gain during pregnancy because of concerns regarding the epidemic of obesity. The physiological average weight gain in a healthy primigravid woman eating without restriction is expected to be about 12.5 kg, of which 1 kg is gained during the first trimester. Approximately 3.2 kg (7 lbs) is gained at 10–20 weeks and approximately 4.6 kg (10 lbs) at 20–30 weeks. It has been found that the woman who gained less than 15 lbs during

**Table 3.2:** Recommended weight gain in pregnancy by the IOM (1990), endorsed by ACOG (2007)

| Category | BMI | Recommended weight gain |
| --- | --- | --- |
| Low | <19.8 | 12.5–18 kg (28–40 lbs) |
| Normal | 19.8–26 | 11.5–16 kg (25–35 lbs) |
| High | 26–29 | 7–11.5 kg (15–25 lbs) |
| Obese | >29 | ≤7 kg (<15 lbs) |

*Abbreviations:* ACOG, american college of obstetricians and gynecologists; BMI, body mass index; IOM, institute of medicine

pregnancy are associated with lower rate of preeclampsia, large for gestational age infants and cesarean delivery.

## Exercise and Employment

In the absence of obstetric or medical complications, most pregnant women are able to work throughout the pregnancy. Heavy weight lifting and excessive physical activity should be avoided. Pregnant women should also be informed that beginning or continuing a moderate course of exercise during pregnancy is not associated with adverse outcomes.

## Prescribed Medicines

Use of prescribed medicines during pregnancy should be limited to circumstances where the benefits outweigh the risks. Pregnant women should be informed that only a few over-the-counter (OTC) medicines have been established as being safe during pregnancy. OTC medicines should be therefore used as less as possible during pregnancy.

## Immunizations

- All women of childbearing age should be immune to measles, rubella, mumps, tetanus, diphtheria, poliomyelitis and varicella through natural or vaccine-conferred immunization.
- All pregnant women should be screened for hepatitis B surface antigen. Pregnancy is not a contraindication to the administration of hepatitis B virus (HBV) vaccine for hepatitis B.
- All vaccines with a live virus, e.g. rubella, yellow fever, etc., should be avoided during pregnancy.
- *Tetanus toxoid:* According to recent recommendations by the WHO, all pregnant women should be immunized against tetanus and diphtheria. Places where DT (diphtheria, tetanus toxoid) is not available, immunization should be with TT (tetanus toxoid). For unimmunized women, TT or DT must be administered intramuscularly in the dosage of 0.5 mL at 6 weeks interval with the first dose being administered at 16–24 weeks. For women who have been immunized in the past, a booster dose of 0.5 mL may be administered in the third trimester.
- Varicella zoster immunoglobulin should be administered to any newborn whose mother has developed chickenpox within 5 days before or 2 days after delivery.

## Sexual Intercourse

No restriction of sexual activity is necessary for pregnant women. Avoidance of sexual activity must be recommended for women at risk of preterm labor, placenta previa or women with previous history of pregnancy loss.

## Counseling and Screening for Down Syndrome, Thalassemia, Etc.

*Noninvasive Prenatal Screening Tests for Down Syndrome*

These mainly include assessment of biochemical parameters in the form of triple test or quadruple test. Addition of nuchal translucency to the biochemical markers helps in improving the accuracy of detection rate by 80%. The maternal triple test, performed at 15–20 weeks of pregnancy, involves measurement of the following in maternal serum: maternal serum alpha-fetoprotein (MSAFP); hCG and unconjugated estriol levels. Low maternal levels of MSAFP and unconjugated estriol and high maternal levels of hCG are associated with an increased risk of Down syndrome. Quadruple test includes the same parameters as described with triple test along with measurement of serum inhibin A levels. High levels of inhibin A are indicative of Down syndrome.

If the woman is found to be at a high risk (>1 in 250) for Down syndrome based on the results of these tests and maternal age over 35 years, then they are offered a diagnostic test—either amniocentesis or chorionic villus sampling.

Women belonging to ethnic groups at high risk for thalassemia must be offered screening tests for identification of affected fetuses.

## Ultrasound Examination

Pregnant women should be offered an early ultrasound scan to determine gestational age, especially if the woman is not sure about her LMP. Pregnant women should be offered an ultrasound scan to screen for structural anomalies, preferably between 18 to 20 weeks of gestation.

## Education Regarding Breastfeeding, Birth Spacing and Contraception

During the antenatal classes, the pregnant women should be taught about how to breastfeed their babies and to take care of their own hygiene. The importance of birth spacing should be stressed and they should be informed about all the methods of contraception that can be safely used during the postpartum period when they are breastfeeding their babies.

## Alcohol and Tobacco Use during Pregnancy

Due to increased fetal risks, it is suggested that women should avoid or limit their alcohol consumption to no more than one standard unit per day when pregnant. One "unit" of alcohol is constituted by the following: a single measure of spirits, one small glass of wine, or a half pint of ordinary strength beer, lager or cider.

Pregnant women should be informed about the specific risks related to smoking/tobacco use during pregnancy (e.g. risk of having a baby with low birthweight, IUGR or preterm birth) and therefore they should be encouraged to quit.

### Screening for Infections

Pregnant women should be offered routine screening for asymptomatic bacteriuria by midstream urine culture early in pregnancy. Identification and treatment of asymptomatic bacteriuria reduce the risk of preterm birth. Serological screening for HBV and HIV infection should be offered to pregnant women so that effective postnatal interventions can reduce the risk of mother-to-child transmission. Screening for syphilis should be offered to all pregnant women at an early stage in antenatal care because treatment of syphilis is beneficial to the mother as well as the fetus. Rubella-susceptibility screening should also be offered early in pregnancy to identify women at risk of contracting rubella infection.

### Psychiatric Screening

History of any previous psychiatric illnesses in the past must be taken from the women. Women having had a past history of serious psychiatric disorder should be referred for a psychiatric assessment during the antenatal period.

### Abdominal Examination

Abdominal examination has been described in details in Chapter 1.

# Normal Labor

## INTRODUCTION

Labor comprises of a series of events taking place in the genital organs, which help to expel the fetus and other products of conception outside the uterine cavity into the outer world. It can be defined as the onset of painful uterine contractions accompanied by any one of the following: rupture of membranes (ROM), bloody show, cervical dilatation and/or effacement. Two to three weeks prior to the onset of true labor in a primigravida and a few days in a multigravida, a premonitory stage called prelabor may sometimes occur.

## PRELABOR

Prelabor is associated with the following features:
- *Lightening:* The fetal presenting part may sink into the pelvis due to the formation of lower uterine segment during this phase. This causes a reduction in the fundal height and also reduces pressure on the diaphragm. As a result, it provides relief from cardiorespiratory embarrassment. However, at the same time, there may be an increase in the frequency of micturition or constipation due to the pressure exerted by the engaged presenting part. Lightening is a welcome sign because it helps in excluding cephalopelvic disproportion.
- *Cervical change:* Few days prior to the onset of labor, the cervix may become ripe (i.e. soft) and may begin to dilate and efface. It is able to admit a finger and is less than 1.5 cm in length.
- *False labor:* There may be appearance of false labor pain (described later in the text).

## TRUE LABOR

True labor, which may be sometimes preceded by a premonitory stage (prelabor), is associated with the following features:
- *Labor pains/uterine contractions:* Described later in the text.
- *Show:* There is expulsion of cervical secretions mixed with blood, released due to the rupture of capillary vessels caused by the separation of membranes from the lower uterine segment.
- *Dilatation of internal os:* Dilatation begins in the upper part of the cervix and is accompanied by the corresponding stretching of the lower uterine segment.
- *Formation of the bags of membranes (BOM):* As the lower uterine segment is stretched, fetal membranes get detached from the decidua. With the progressive cervical dilatation, the membranes tend to become unsupported and bulge into the cervical canal. Due to the rise of intra-amniotic pressure at the time of uterine contractions, these membranes tend to become tense and convex resulting in the formation of bag of membranes. This bulging of membranes usually disappears as the contraction passes off. Formation of bag of membranes is a certain sign of labor.

## STAGES OF LABOR

Labor can be either spontaneous or induced and normally comprises of three stages—first stage, second stage and third stage. Since the most common fetal position is occipitolateral (transverse) position (Fig. 3.2), the mechanism of labor in context to this position comprises of the following cardinal movements: engagement, flexion, descent, internal rotation, extension and external rotation of fetal head (Flow chart 3.1). Various stages of labor are described in Table 3.3 and depicted in Figures 3.3A and B.

## First Stage of Labor

The first stage of labor begins with the onset of regular uterine contractions and ends with complete dilatation and effacement of cervix. It is divided into two phases:

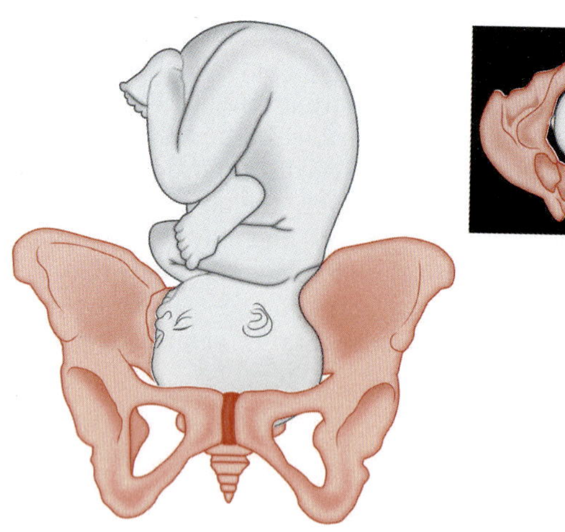
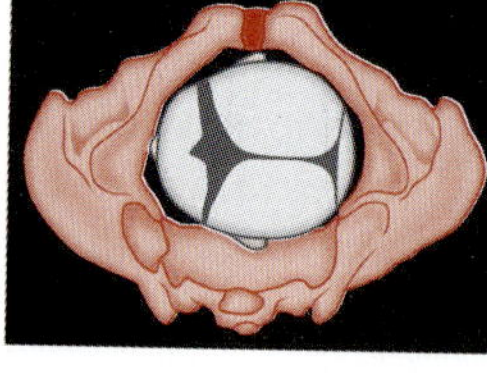

**Fig. 3.2:** Occipitolateral (transverse) position

*Latent Phase (Preparatory Phase)*

Latent phase begins with onset of regular contractions, with contractions occurring after every 15–20 minutes, lasting for 20–30 seconds. Gradually the frequency of contractions increases and they can occur after every 5–7 minutes, lasting for 30–40 seconds. This phase ends when cervix becomes about 3–5 cm dilated. The latent phase lasts for approximately 8–9 hours in the primigravida, and less than 6 hours in multigravida. Prolonged latent phase can be defined as greater than 20 hours in primigravida and greater than 14 hours in multigravida.

*Active Phase*

Active phase begins when the cervix is about 4 cm dilated and ends when it becomes fully dilated. The normal rate of cervical dilatation during this stage is approximately 1–1.5 cm/hour. The intensity of contractions increases with the contractions occurring after every 2–3 minutes and lasting for about 40–60 seconds. This stage lasts for an average of 4.6 hours in a primigravida and approximately 2.4 hours in multigravida.

## Second Stage of Labor

The second stage of labor begins when the cervical dilatation and effacement is complete and ends with the delivery of the fetus. Its mean duration is 50 minutes for nullipara and 20 minutes for multipara. During this stage, the woman begins to bear down. The abdominal muscles contract, which help in the descent of fetal head. When the crowing of fetal head has occurred at vulvar opening, birth of the baby is imminent.

## Third Stage of Labor

Third stage of labor begins after expulsion of the fetus and is associated with expulsion of placenta and membranes.

## CLINICAL EXAMINATION IN LABOR

### History and Clinical Presentation

If detailed history had not been taken during the time of antenatal check-up, it must be taken now, at the time of admission. The details, which need to be elicited at the time of taking history, are described in Chapter 1.

### General Physical Examination

This involves assessment of patient's vital signs, similar to that done during the time of antenatal examination (Chapter 1).

### Specific Systemic Examination

Findings of specific systemic examination are summarized in Table 3.4.

## ABDOMINAL EXAMINATION

The abdominal examination forms an important part of every complete physical examination in labor. The abdominal examination must be done at the time of admission and each time before a vaginal examination is performed. The parameters to be assessed at the time of abdominal examination of a patient who is in labor are similar to those observed at the time of antenatal examination and have been described before in Chapter 1. Additionally, descent and engagement of the fetal presenting part, assessment of fetal position and uterine contractions are especially important when the patient is in labor. The amount of descent and engagement of the presenting part is assessed by feeling how many fifths of the head are palpable above the brim of the pelvis.

Various parameters on abdominal examination, such as estimation of fundal height, detection of fetal lie, presentation, position, conducting the four Leopold's maneuvers and auscultation of fetal heart rate, have been described in details in Chapter 1. Besides this, other parameters, which need to be assessed at the time of abdominal examination during labor, are as follows:

### Assessment of Fetal Size

While palpating the fetus, the clinician must try to assess the size of the fetus itself. A note should be made regarding the expected fetal weight. A fetus, which feels smaller than expected, could be indicative of IUGR or oligohydramnios or wrong dates. A fetus, which feels larger than expected, could be indicative of fetal macrosomia (particularly in association with gestational diabetes); polyhydramnios or multifetal gestation. In multifetal gestation, though the uterine size is larger than the period of gestation, the size of individual fetuses per se is small.

**Flow chart 3.1:** Mechanism of labor

**Engagement**
Biparietal diameter is able to negotiate through the pelvic inlet

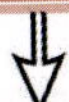

**Flexion**
Flexion of the fetal head permits the smallest diameter of the fetal head (suboccipitobregmatic) to enter the pelvis

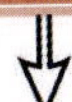

**Descent**
This is a continuous process which continues occurring throughout labor

**Internal rotation**
Internal rotation of the fetal head occurs by 2/8 of the circle, resulting in the development of similar amount of torsion on fetal neck. Simultaneous rotation of fetal shoulders occurs by 1/8 of the circle so that the torsion on the fetal neck is reduced to 1/8 of the circle. Shoulders would now be placed in the oblique diameter: right oblique with right occipitolateral position and left oblique with left occipitolateral position

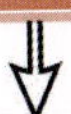

**Crowning**
This occurs with increasing descent of fetal head. In this stage, the biparietal diameter of fetal head stretches the vaginal introitus

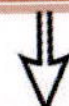

**Extension**
Delivery of fetal head occurs by extension. Head delivers first, followed by the occiput, face and chin

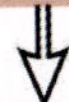

**Restitution**
The neck comes back to its original position and aligns along the long axis of the fetus

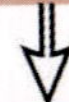

**External rotation of the fetal head**
As the shoulders rotate through 1/8 of the circle to engage in the anterior-posterior diameter of the pelvis, external rotation of the head occurs by 1/8 of the circle

**Delivery of shoulders**
Following the external rotation of the head, the anterior shoulder delivers first, followed by the posterior one

**Lateral flexion of the trunk**
Rest of the body delivers via the lateral flexion of the trunk

| Stages of labor | Description | Characteristics | Duration in primigravida | Duration in multigravida |
|---|---|---|---|---|
| Stage I | Starts from the onset of true labor pain and ends with complete dilatation of cervix | Can be divided into:<br>• Latent phase: Slow and gradual cervical effacement and dilatation (up to 3 cm)<br>• Active phase: Active cervical dilatation (3–10 cm) and fetal descent. It comprises of:<br>– Acceleration phase:<br>- Phase of maximum slope<br>- Deceleration phase | 8–20 hours<br><br>6–12 hours | 6–14 hours<br><br>3–6 hours |
| Stage II | Starts from full dilatation of cervix and ends with expulsion of the fetus from birth canal | — | 50–180 minutes | 30–50 minutes |
| Stage III | It begins after expulsion of the fetus and is associated with expulsion of placenta and membranes | — | 15 minutes | 15 minutes |
| Stage IV | Stage of observation which lasts for at least 1 hour after the expulsion of afterbirths | — | 60 minutes | 60 minutes |

*Table 3.3:* Various stages of labor

If the clinician feels that the size of the head appears to be smaller in relation to the period of gestation, he/she must try to assess the size as well as hardness of the fetal head. The fetal head feels harder as the pregnancy reaches closer to term. A relatively small fetal head with a hard feel is suggestive of IUGR rather than prematurity.

## Engagement

With the progress of second stage of labor, there is progressive downwards movement of the fetal presenting part in relation to the pelvic cavity. Engagement is said to have occurred when largest diameter of the presenting part passes through the pelvic inlet. Engagement of fetal presenting part is evident from abdominal and vaginal examination. The indicators of engagement of fetal head on abdominal/vaginal examination are as follows:

- Both the fetal poles, occiput and sinciput cannot be felt on per abdominal examination.
- There is divergence of the examining fingers when trying to palpate the fetal head using fingers of both the hands on the Leopold's fourth maneuver.
- Vaginal examination reveals the descent of fetal head in relation to the ischial spines (would be described in details with the vaginal examination). In case of an engaged head, lower pole of the unmolded head is at or below the ischial spines.

Engagement of the fetal presenting part is of great importance as it helps in ruling out fetopelvic disproportion. In a primigravida, engagement occurs by 38–42 weeks of gestation. However, in a multigravida, engagement occurs late in the first stage of labor. Some of the causes for nonengagement of the fetal head are listed in Table 3.5.

## Abdominal Assessment of Fetal Descent (Figs 3.4A and B)

The assessment of fetal descent through the abdominal examination is done by using the Fifth's formula. In this method, number of fifths of fetal head above the pelvic brim is estimated. The amount of fetal head that can be palpated per abdominally is estimated in terms of finger breadth which is assessed by placing the radial margin of the index finger above the symphysis pubis successively. Depending upon the amount of fetal head palpated per abdominally, other fingers of the hand can be placed in succession, until all the five fingers cover the fetal head.

A free-floating head would be completely palpable per abdomen. This head accommodates full width of all the five fingers above the pubic symphysis and can be described as 5/5. A head which is fixing but not yet engaged may be three-fifths palpable per abdominally and is known as 3/5. A recently engaged fetal head may be two-fifths palpable per abdominally and is known as 2/5, while a deeply engaged fetal head may not be palpable at all per abdominally and may be described as 0/5.

## Assessment of the Amount of Liquor Present

Under normal circumstances, the amount of liquor decreases as the pregnancy approaches term. The amount of liquor can be clinically assessed by feel the way that the fetus can

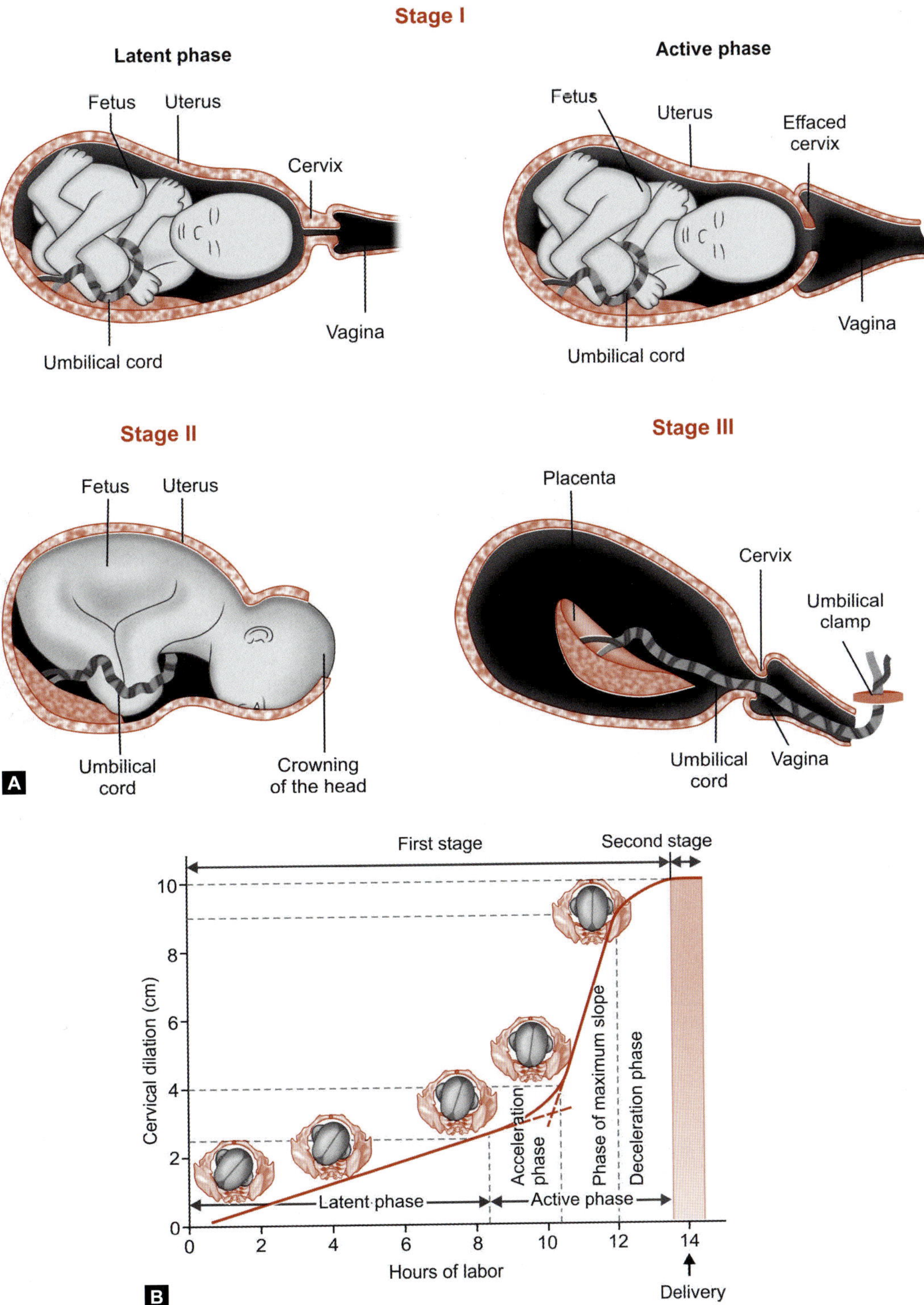


**Figs 3.3A and B:** (A) Stages of normal labor; (B) Graphical representation of normal labor

| **Table 3.4:** Findings of specific systemic examination | | |
|---|---|---|
| *Abdominal examination* | *Per speculum examination* | *Per vaginal examination* |
| • Estimation of height of uterine fundus<br>• The fetal lie may be longitudinal, transverse or oblique<br>• Fetal presentation may be cephalic, podalic (breech) or shoulder<br>• Obstetric grips (Leopold's maneuvers)<br>• Uterine contractions<br>• Estimation of fetal descent<br>• Assessing the engagement of fetal presenting part<br>• Auscultation of fetal heart rate<br>• Assessment of the fetal size<br>• Assessment of the amount of liquor present |   Indicators of ruptured membranes are as follows:<br>• Gross vaginal pooling of fluid<br>• Positive results on Nitrazine paper test and fern testing of vaginal secretions<br>• Evidence of meconium | • Cervical dilatation<br>• Cervical consistency and effacement<br>• Fetal presentation and position<br>• Assessment of fetal membranes and amount of liquor<br>• Fetal descent (Station of fetal head)<br>• Molding of fetal skull<br>• Pelvic assessment |

| **Table 3.5:** Causes for nonengagement of the fetal head |
|---|
| • Deflexed fetal head<br>• Cephalopelvic disproportion<br>• Hydrocephalus<br>• Pelvic tumors (fibroids, ovarian cysts, etc.)<br>• Poor formation of the lower uterine segment |

be balloted at the time of abdominal examination. Reduced degree of fetal ballottement at the time of abdominal palpation is indicative of reduced amount of amniotic fluid or oligohydramnios. On the other hand, increased degree of fetal ballottement at the time of abdominal palpation is suggestive of increased amount of amniotic fluid or polyhydramnios.

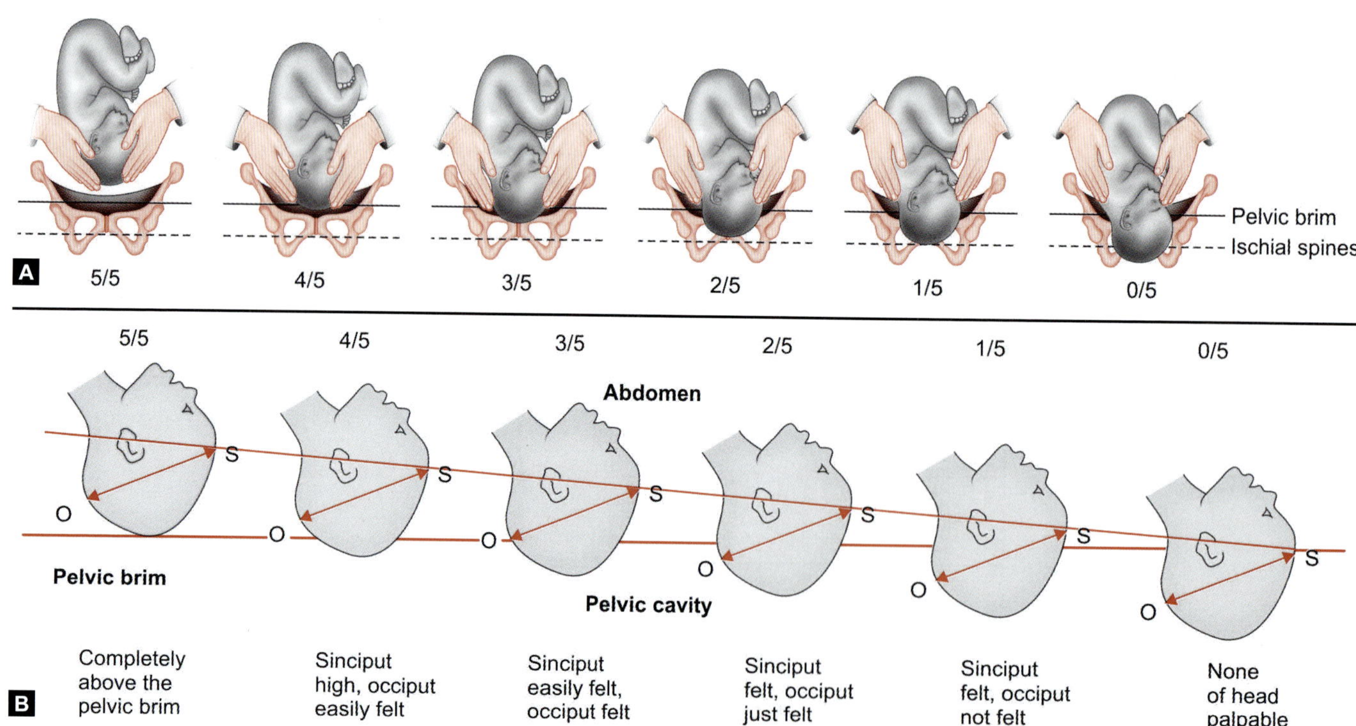


**Figs 3.4A and B:** Estimation of the descent of fetal head using the Fifth's formula. (A) Abdominal examination for fetal descent (B) Stages of fetal descent through the pelvic cavity

## Uterine Contractions

The clinician will get an idea regarding the woman's uterine contractions by typically placing hands on the patient's abdomen and feeling her uterus contract. The parameters to be assessed at the time of abdominal examination include, number of uterine contractions in a 10-minute period, duration of contractions, regularity of contractions and intensity of contractions. Another important parameter to assess is whether the contractions result in simultaneous dilatation of the cervix. One way to determine the intensity of a contraction is by comparing the firmness of the uterus to areas on the clinician's face. For example, the cheek could be considered as mild, the tip of the nose as moderate and forehead as strong. In the early stages of labor, the frequency of the uterine contractions may be after every 15–20 minutes, lasting for about 20–30 seconds. However, as the labor progresses, the frequency and duration of uterine contractions greatly increase with contractions occurring after every 1–2 minutes and lasting for about 60–120 seconds. Some of the features of uterine contractions, which need to be assessed, are:

### Duration of Uterine Contractions

Placing a hand on the abdomen and feeling when the uterus becomes hard and when it relaxes helps in assessing the duration of the uterine contractions. Depending upon the time duration for which the contractions last, they can be classified as strong, moderate and weak contractions. Grading of the duration of uterine contractions is described in Table 3.6.

### Strength of Contractions

Measuring the degree of hardness, which the uterus undergoes at the time of contraction, helps in assessing the strength of contractions or their intensity. Experienced clinician can estimate the intensity of uterine contractions by palpating the uterine fundus during the contractions. During a mild contraction, the uterine wall can be indented, whereas during a strong contraction, it cannot be indented.

### Frequency of Uterine Contractions

This measures the number of times the uterine contractions occur in a period of 10 minutes.

## True/False Labor Pains

During the first stage of labor, the clinician needs to determine whether the woman is having true or false uterine contractions. False labor pains can occur prior to the onset of true labor pains. They occur more frequently in a primigravida where they may occur 1–2 weeks prior to the onset of true labor pains. In multigravida, they may precede the true labor pains by a few days.

The false labor pain is usually dull in nature and is confined to the lower abdominal and groin region. They occur at irregular intervals, with their intensity remaining same over a period of time. They tend to become shorter in duration over time and do not cause any effect on cervical dilatation and effacement. This pain is usually relieved by enema and administration of sedatives. False labor pain is related to the formation of lower uterine segment and taking up of cervix, which may cause cervical stretching and irritation of the surrounding ganglia.

On the other hand, true labor pain comprises of painful uterine contractions at regular intervals; these contractions tend to increase in intensity and duration with the progression of labor; they are usually experienced at lower back and radiate to abdomen, and tend to become more intense with walking, cervical changes, and with fetus moving into the lower pelvis. True labor pain is accompanied with the appearance of show (expulsion of cervical mucus plug mixed with blood) and progressive cervical dilatation and effacement. True labor pain is not relieved by sedation. There may be the formation of bag of membranes. There may also be an accompanying "show".

True uterine contractions usually follow a rhythmic pattern with periods of contractions followed by periods of relaxation in between, which would allow the woman to rest. During the phase of relaxation, restoration of placental circulation occurs, which is important for the baby's oxygenation. The uterus appears to be hard during the strong uterine contractions and it may be difficult to palpate the fetal parts. Abnormal uterine hardness and tenderness could be due to causes such as abruption placenta or a ruptured uterus.

## VAGINAL EXAMINATION

Vaginal examination must be performed at the time of admission of the pregnant patient in labor. It is carried out at least once every 4 hours during first stage of labor or if there is ROM or if any intervention is needed. Preparations for delivery are made as the cervical dilatation and effacement

| **Table 3.6:** Grading the duration of contractions | |
|---|---|
| **Duration of contraction** | **Grading of contractions** |
| Contraction lasting less than 20 seconds | Weak |
| Contractions lasting for 20–40 seconds | Moderate |
| Contractions lasting more than 40 seconds | Strong |

approaches completion and/or crowning of the fetal presenting part becomes evident at the vaginal introitus. Pelvic assessment is best done before the onset of labor or just before the induction of labor. Any history of vaginal bleeding is a contraindication for vaginal examination.

### Prerequisites for a Vaginal Examination

Following are the prerequisites for vaginal examination:
- The patient must be carefully explained about the method of examination, prior to performing the examination.
- Adequate permission must be taken from the patient.
- There should be a valid reason for performing the examination.
- A vaginal examination must always be preceded by an abdominal examination.

### Indications for a Vaginal Examination

Indications for performing a vaginal examination during the various stages of labor are as follows:
- Assessment of the ripeness of the cervix prior to induction of labor.
- Performance of artificial rupture of the membranes to induce labor.
- Detection of cervical effacement and/or dilatation (Figs 3.5A to D).
- Identification of the fetal presenting part.
- Performance of pelvic assessment.
- To note progress of labor.
- Following rupture of membranes to rule out cord prolapse.
- Whenever interference is contemplated.
- To confirm the second stage of labor.

### Contraindications for Vaginal Examination

Antepartum hemorrhage and preterm ROM without contractions are conditions in which the vaginal examination is contraindicated. In these cases a sterile speculum examination can be done to confirm or exclude ROM.

### Preparation for Vaginal Examination

- The patient's bladder must be empty.
- The procedure must be carefully explained to the patient.
- The patient must be placed in either the dorsal or lithotomy position. In clinical practice, dorsal position is most commonly used because it is more comfortable and less embarrassing than the lithotomy position.
- If the membranes have not ruptured or are not going to be ruptured during the examination, an ordinary surgical glove can be used and there is no need to swab the patient with antiseptic solution. However, if the membranes

Cervical effacement and dilatation during labor

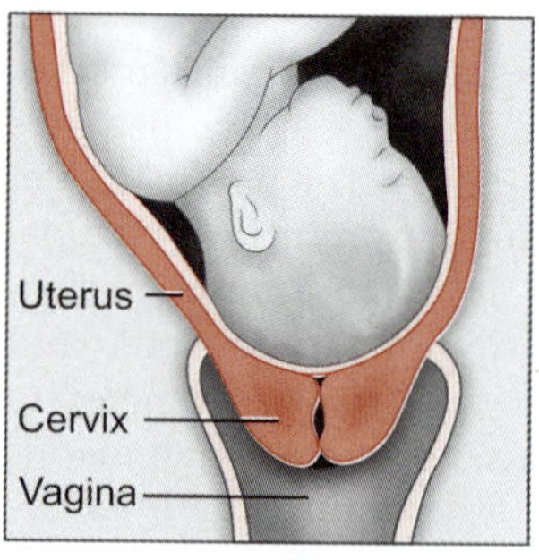

Cervix not effaced or dilated
**A**

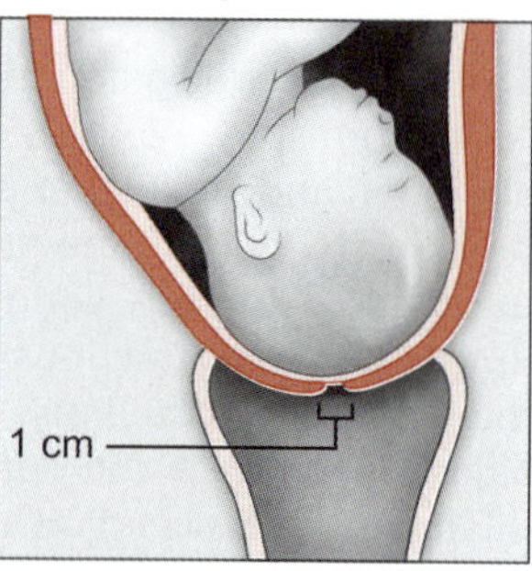

Cervix is fully effaced and dilated to 1 cm
**B**

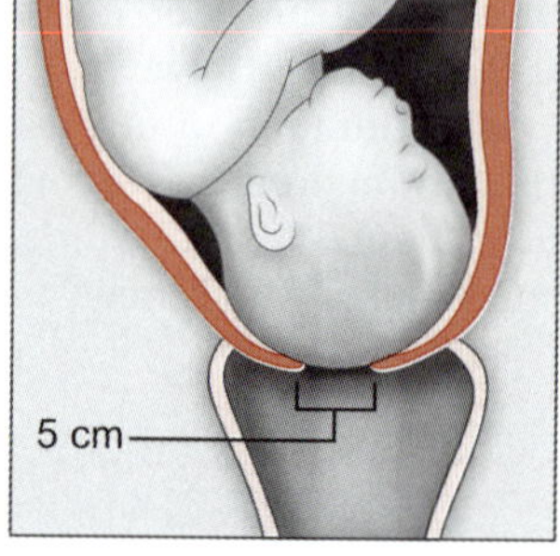

Cervix is dilated to 5 cm
**C**

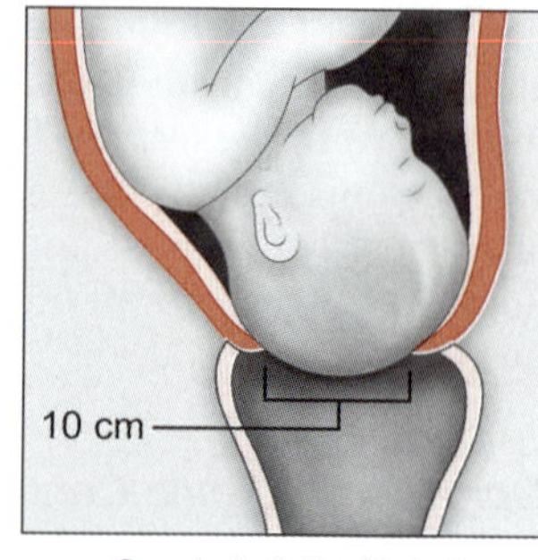

Cervix is fully dilated to 10 cm
**D**

**Figs 3.5A to D:** Cervical dilatation and effacement

have ruptured or are going to be ruptured during the examination, vaginal examination in labor should be performed as a sterile procedure.
- In case of ruptured membranes or if an ARM is planned, the clinicians before performing the vaginal examination must either scrub or thoroughly wash their hands and wear sterile gloves. The patient's vulva and perineum must be swabbed with savlon or betadine solution. This is done by first swabbing the labia majora and groin on both sides and then swabbing the introitus while keeping the labia majora apart with the thumb and forefinger.
- A vaginal examination must be preceded by the inspection of the external and internal genitalia for signs of sexually transmitted diseases such as presence of single or multiple ulcers, a purulent discharge or enlarged inguinal lymph nodes. The vulva must also be carefully inspected for any abnormalities, e.g. scars, warts, varicosities, congenital abnormalities, ulcers or discharge. Vagina and cervix can be inspected by performing a per speculum examination. The vagina must be assessed for the presence or absence of the following features: vaginal discharge; a fully loaded rectum, vaginal stricture or septum or prolapse of the umbilical cord through the vaginal introitus.
- Presence of a wart-like growth or an ulcer on the cervix may be suggestive of cervical carcinoma. The cervical

surface can also be assessed while performing a vaginal examination. A bimanual examination helps in assessing the cervical dilatation and effacement, the size of the uterus and masses in the adnexa (ovaries and Fallopian tubes).

- Lastly, the fornices are palpated to exclude any masses, the most common of which is an ovarian cyst or tumor.

In the first trimester of pregnancy, a bimanual examination helps in assessment of the uterine size in comparison with the period of amenorrhea. After the first trimester, the uterine size is primarily assessed on abdominal examination.

Special care must be taken, when performing a vaginal examination late in pregnancy, especially in the presence of a high presenting part. The nonengagement of the presenting part could be due to an undiagnosed placenta previa. If this is suspected, the finger must not be inserted into the cervical canal. Instead, the presenting part is gently palpated through all the fornices. If any bogginess is noted between the fingers of the examining hand and the presenting part, the examination must be immediately abandoned and the patient must be referred urgently for an ultrasound examination. Preparations for an emergency cesarean delivery must also be begun.

## Parameters to Be Observed during Vaginal Examination

The parameters to be observed while performing a vaginal examination are described in Table 3.7.

| **Table 3.7:** Parameters to be observed while performing a vaginal examination |
|---|
| • Consistency and position of cervix<br>• Cervical dilatation<br>• Cervical effacement<br>• Fetal presentation<br>• Position<br>• Assessment of fetal membranes<br>• Assessment of liquor<br>• Fetal descent (station of the fetal presenting part)<br>• Molding of fetal skull<br>• Pelvic assessment (to rule out cephalopelvic disproportion) |

### Cervical Dilatation and Effacement

Dilatation of cervix refers to the opening up of cervical os (both internal and external). Cervical dilatation must be assessed in centimeters and is best measured by assessing the degree of separation of the fingers on vaginal examination. Initial cervical dilatation is sometimes described in terms of fingers (one-finger dilated, two-fingers dilated or three-fingers dilated). Cervical dilatation is also described in terms of centimeters. When fully dilated, cervical os measures about 10 cm.

Cervical effacement is a process in which the muscular fibers of cervix are pulled upwards and merge with the lower uterine segment. Cervical effacement is described in terms of the length of endocervical canal in the vagina. Cervical effacement refers to the distance between the internal os and the external os on digital examination. In an uneffaced cervix, the endocervical canal is approximately 3 cm. Cervical effacement is usually measured in terms of a percentage (10%, 25%, 50%, 75%, etc.). The cervix becomes paper thin when it is 100% effaced. In primigravida, effacement usually occurs before dilatation of cervix, whereas in case of multigravida, both of them occur simultaneously. Anterior lip of the cervix is usually the last cervical structure to become effaced.

### Evaluation of State of Cervix

This is done by calculation of the Bishop's score (Table 3.8). A maximum score of 13 is possible with this scoring system. Labor is most likely to commence spontaneously with a score of 9 or more, whereas lower scores (especially those <5) may require cervical ripening and/or augmentation with oxytocin.

### Fetal Presentation

An abdominal examination performed earlier helps in determining the fetal lie and the presenting part. The presenting part of the fetus can be confirmed on vaginal examination. The presenting part could be head, breech or shoulder. If the head is presenting, the exact fetal presenting part, e.g. vertex, brow or face needs to be determined.

*Features of a vertex presentation:* The posterior fontanel is normally felt. It is a small triangular space. In contrast,

| **Table 3.8:** Bishop's score (modified) | | | | | |
|---|---|---|---|---|---|
| *Score* | *Dilation (cm)* | *Effacement (%)* | *Station of the presenting part* | *Cervical consistency* | *Position of cervix* |
| 0 | Closed | 0–30 | – 3 | Firm | Posterior |
| 1 | 1–2 | 40–50 | –2 | Medium | Mid position |
| 2 | 3–4 | 60–70 | –1,0 | Soft | Anterior |
| 3 | >5 | >80 | +1, +2 | — | — |

the anterior fontanel is diamond-shaped. If the head is well flexed, the anterior fontanel will not be felt. If the anterior fontanel can be easily felt, the head is deflexed.

*Features of a face presentation:* On abdominal examination the presenting part is the head. However, on vaginal examination the following features are observed:
- Instead of a firm skull, something soft is felt
- The gum margins distinguish the mouth from the anus
- The cheek bones and the mouth form a triangle
- The orbital ridges above the eyes can be felt
- The ears may be felt.

*Features of a brow presentation:* The presenting part is high. The anterior fontanel is felt on one side of the pelvis, the root of the nose on the other side and the orbital ridges may be felt laterally.

*Features of a breech presentation:* On abdominal examination the presenting part is the breech (soft and triangular). On vaginal examination, instead of a firm skull, something soft is felt; the anus does not have gum margins; the anus and the ischial tuberosities form a straight line.

*Features of a shoulder presentation:* On abdominal examination the lie will be transverse or oblique. Features of a shoulder presentation on vaginal examination will be quite easy if the arm has prolapsed. The shoulder is not always that easy to identify, unless the arm can be felt. The presenting part is usually high.

### Fetal Position

Fetal position refers to relationship of the designated landmark on the fetal presenting part with the left or right side of the maternal pelvis. Fetal position has been described in details previously in Chapter 1.

### Assessment of the Membranes

Drainage of liquor indicates that membranes have ruptured. However, even if the liquor is obviously draining, the clinician must always try to feel for the presence of membranes overlying the presenting part. If the presenting part is high, it is usually quite easy to feel the intact membranes. However, it may be difficult to feel the membranes, if the presenting part is well applied to the cervix. In this case, one should wait for a contraction, when some liquor often comes in front of the presenting part, allowing the membranes to be felt. If the membranes are intact, and the patient is in the active phase of labor, the membranes should be ruptured.

### Condition of the Liquor When the Membranes Rupture

An important parameter, which must be assessed at the time of assessing the membranes, is the condition of liquor following ROM. Clear colored liquor following ROM is indicative of a normal healthy fetus. Greenish colored liquor is suggestive of presence of meconium. The presence of meconium may change the management of the patient as it indicates the presence of fetal distress. In these cases, it may be required to expedite the delivery.

### Determining the Descent and Engagement of the Head

The engagement of the fetal head is assessed on abdominal and not on vaginal examination. However, the vaginal examination does help in assessing the descent of fetal presenting part. The level of the fetal presenting part is usually described in relation to the ischial spines, which is halfway between the pelvic inlet and pelvic outlet. When the lower most portion of the fetal presenting part is at the level of ischial spines, it is designated as "zero" station. The ACOG has devised a classification system that divides the pelvis above and below the spines into fifths. This division represents the distance in centimeters above and below the ischial spine. Thus, as the presenting fetal part descends from the inlet towards the ischial spine, the designation is –5, –4, –3, –2, –1, then 0 station. Below the ischial spines, the fetal head passes through +1, +2, +3, +4 and + 5 stations till delivery (Fig. 3.6). +5 Station represents that the fetal head is visible at the introitus. If the leading part of the fetal head is at the zero station or below, the fetal head is said to be engaged. This implies that the biparietal plane of the fetal head has passed through the pelvic inlet. However, in the presence of excessive molding or caput formation, engagement may not have taken place even if the head appears to be at zero station.

### Molding

Molding is the overlapping of the fetal skull bones at the regions of sutures, which may occur during labor due to the

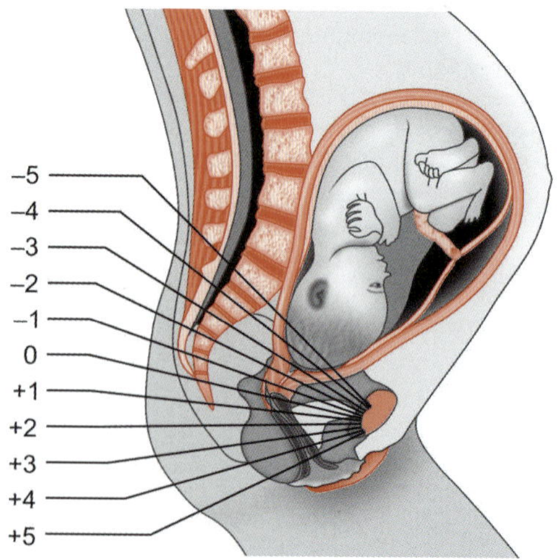


**Fig. 3.6:** Fetal descent

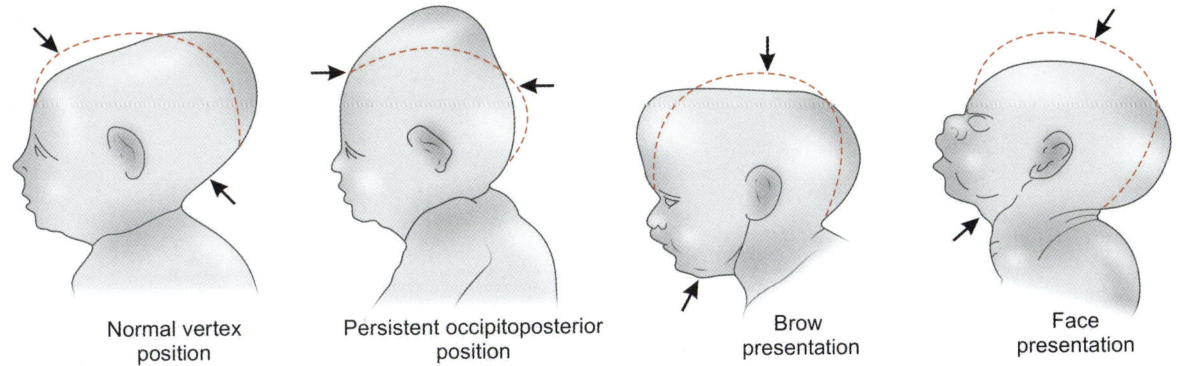



**Fig. 3.7:** Pattern of molding in different types of cephalic presentations

head being compressed as it passes through the pelvis of the mother. Molding results in the compression of the engaging diameter of the fetal head with the corresponding elongation of the diameter at right angles to it (Fig. 3.7). For example, if the fully flexed fetal head engages in the suboccipitobregmatic diameter, this diameter gets compressed. At the same time, the mentovertical diameter (which is at right angles to the suboccipitobregmatic diameter) gets elongated.

*Diagnosis of molding:* In a cephalic presentation, molding is diagnosed by feeling overlapping of the sutures of the skull on vaginal examination and assessing whether or not the overlap can be reduced (corrected) by pressing gently with the examining finger.

The presence of caput succedaneum (soft tissue edema of fetal scalp) can also be felt as a soft, boggy swelling, which may make it difficult to identify the presenting part of the fetal head clearly. With severe caput, the sutures may be impossible to feel. For grading the degree of molding, the occipitoparietal and the sagittal sutures are palpated and the relationship or closeness of the two adjacent bones is assessed. The degree of molding is assessed according to the scale described in Table 3.9 and is also described in Figures 3.8A to D.

### Pelvic Assessment

For details related to pelvic assessment kindly refer to Chapter 2.

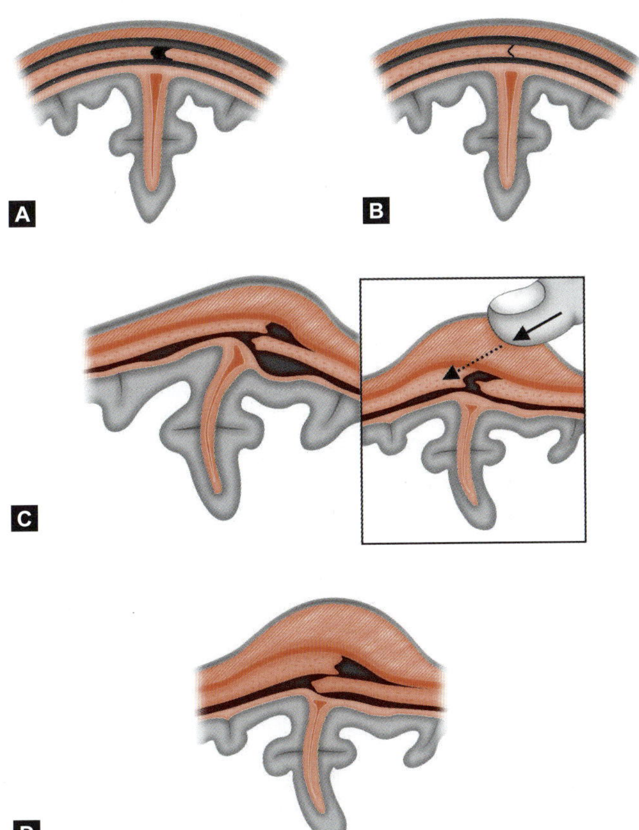

**Figs 3.8A to D:** Grading of molding of fetal skull: (A) Minimal molding; (B) Mild molding; (C) Moderate molding; (D) Marked molding and caput succedaneum

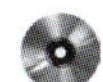 **MECHANISM OF NORMAL LABOR**

Figure 3.9 and Video 3 illustrate the mechanism of normal labor in occipitolateral position. In normal labor the fetal head enters the pelvic brim most commonly through the available transverse diameter of the pelvic inlet. This is so because the most common fetal position is occipitolateral

**Table 3.9:** Degree of molding of fetal skull

| Degree of molding | Description |
| --- | --- |
| 0 (normal) | Normal separation of the bones with open sutures |
| 1+ (mild molding) | Bones touching each other |
| 2+ (moderate molding) | Bones overlapping, but can be separated with gentle digital pressure |
| 3+ (severe molding) | Bones overlapping, but cannot be separated with gentle digital pressure |

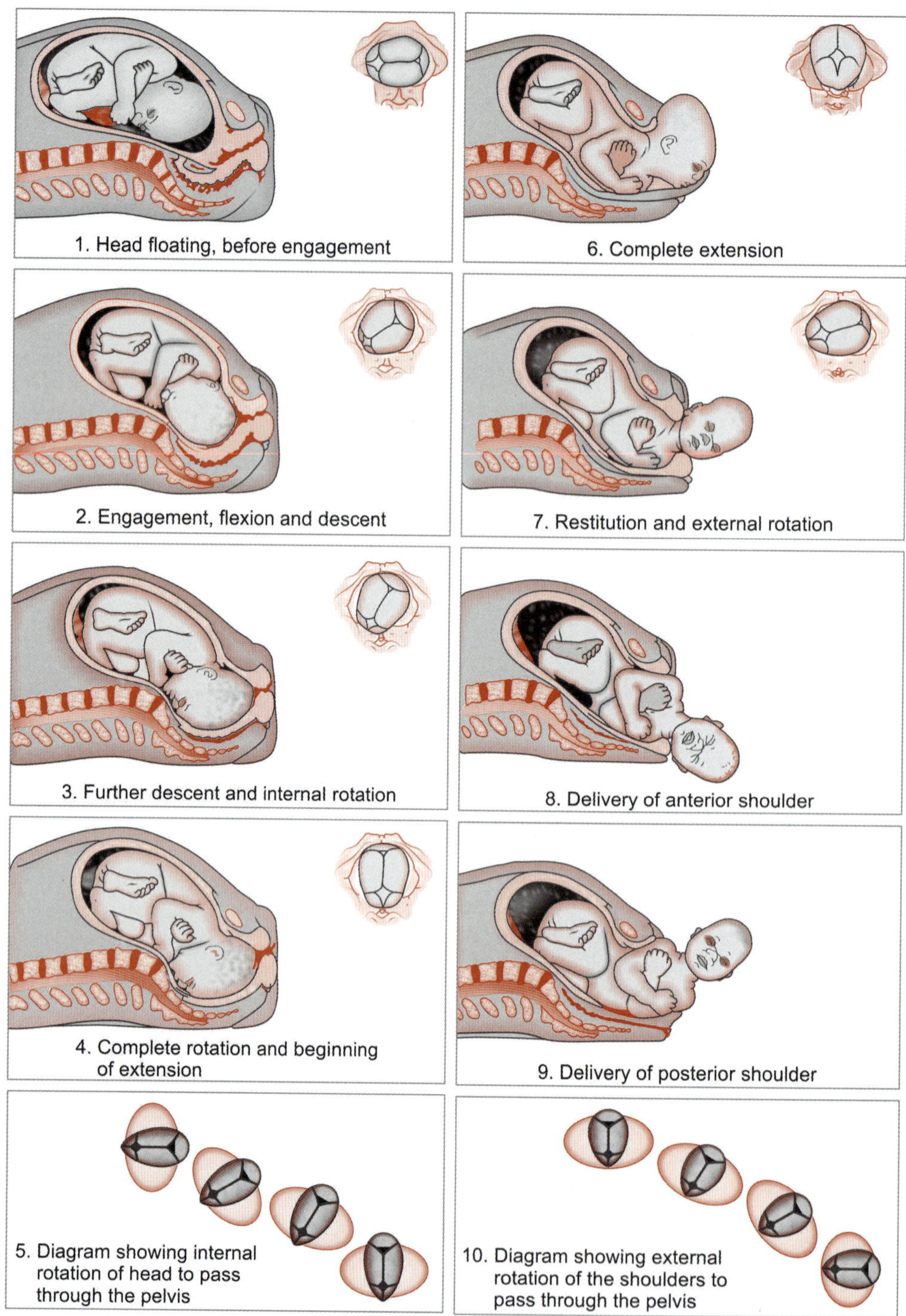



**Fig. 3.9:** Mechanism of normal labor in occipitolateral position

(transverse position). In some cases the fetal head may enter through one of the oblique diameters. The fetal head with left occipitoanterior position (Figs 3.10A to C) enters through right oblique diameter, whereas that with right occipitoanterior position enters through left oblique diameter of the pelvic inlet. Left occipitoanterior position is slightly more common than the right occipitoanterior position as the left oblique diameter is encroached by the rectum. The engaging AP diameter of the fetal head is suboccipitobregmatic (9.4 cm) in position of complete flexion. The engaging transverse diameter of the fetal head is biparietal diameter (9.5 cm). As the occipitolateral position of the fetal head is the most common, the mechanism of labor in this position would be discussed. The cardinal fetal movements during the occipitolateral position comprise of the following: engagement, flexion, descent, internal rotation, crowning, extension, restitution, external rotation of the head and expulsion of the trunk.

## Engagement

In primigravida, the engagement of fetal head usually occurs before the onset of labor, while in multigravida, it may occur only during the first stage of labor, following ROM.

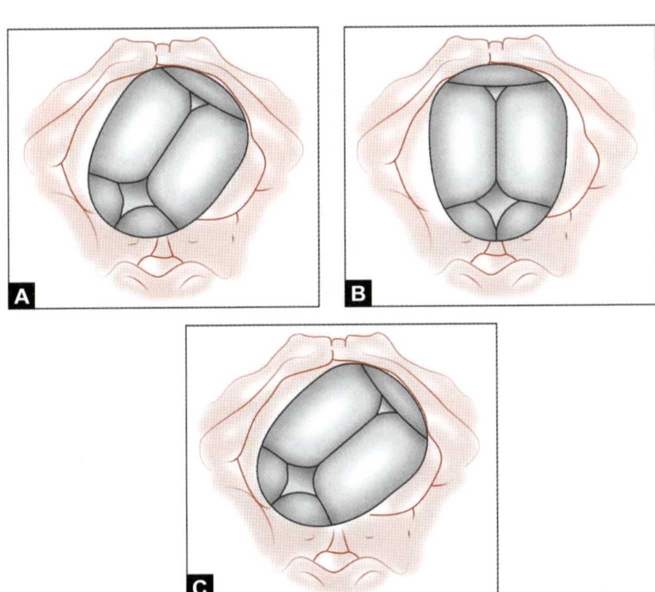

**Figs 3.10A to C:** Position of sagittal suture in case of occipitoanterior position (A) At the time of engagement; (B) Completion of internal rotation; (C) External rotation of fetal head

### Asynclitism of the Fetal Head

At the time of engagement, the head may have a lateral inclination due to which the sagittal sutures may not strictly correspond with the available transverse diameter of the pelvic inlet. As a result, the head may be either deflected anteriorly towards the pubic symphysis or posteriorly towards the sacral promontory. This lateral deflection of the fetal head in relation to the pelvis is known as asynclitism (Figs 3.11A to C). When the sagittal sutures lie anteriorly, the posterior parietal bone becomes the leading presenting part, and this is known as posterior asynclitism or posterior parietal presentation or Litzmann's obliquity. This is commonly encountered in the primigravida due to the good tone of the abdominal muscles and the uterus. If the sagittal sutures lie posteriorly, the anterior parietal bone becomes the leading part, and this is known as anterior parietal presentation or anterior asynclitism or Naegele's obliquity. This is more common amongst the multigravida. While mild degrees of asynclitism are common, severe degrees indicate cephalopelvic disproportion. In case of posterior parietal presentation, the posterior lateral flexion of the head occurs to glide the anterior parietal bone past the pubic symphysis. In the anterior parietal presentation, lateral flexion of the head occurs in opposite direction. Following this movement, synclitism occurs. In nearly one-fourth of the cases, the head on its own enters the brim in synclitism, i.e. sagittal sutures correspond with the diameter of engagement.

## Descent

Descent of the fetal head is a continuous process that occurs throughout the second stage of labor in such a way that towards the end of second stage, crowning of fetal head occurs.

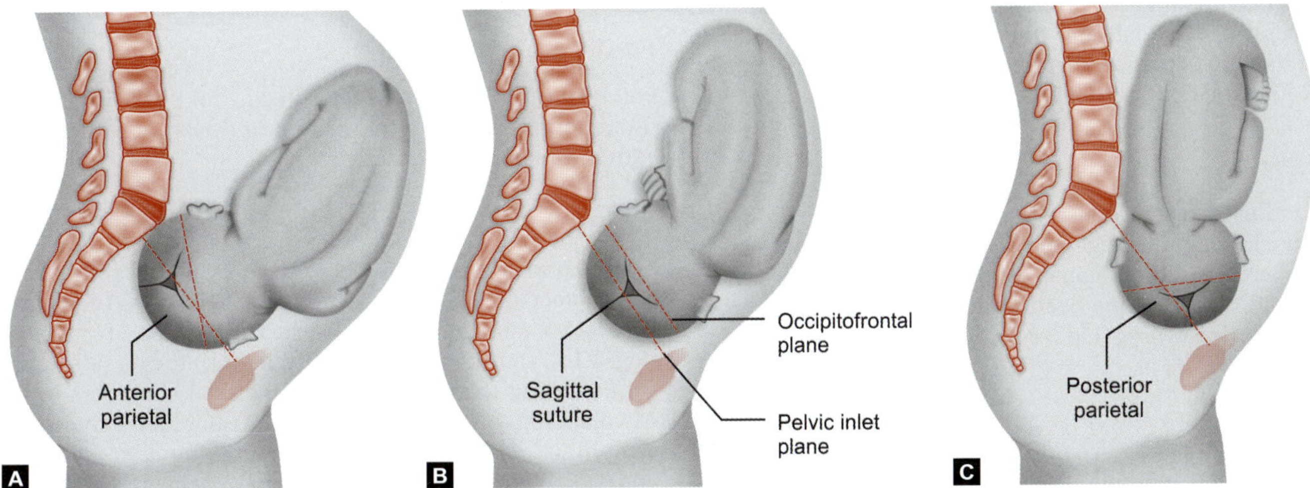


**Figs 3.11A to C:** (A) Anterior asynclitism (Naegele's obliquity); (B) Normal synclitism; (C) Posterior asynclitism (Litzmann's obliquity) ear presentation

## Flexion

In normal cases, increased flexion of fetal chin against the chest helps in presenting the smallest fetal diameter. Flexion of the head occurs as it descends and meets the pelvic floor, bringing the chin into contact with the fetal thorax. Adequate flexion of the fetal head produces the smallest diameter of presentation, i.e. the suboccipitobregmatic diameter, which may change to the larger occipitofrontal diameter, when the fetal head is deflexed. With increasing descent, lever action produces increasing flexion of the fetal head; converting from occipitofrontal to suboccipitobregmatic diameter, which typically reduces the AP diameter from nearly 12 cm to 9.5 cm.

## Internal Rotation

Fetal head must rotate to accommodate the pelvis. The head rotates as it reaches the pelvic floor. In the occipitolateral position, there is anterior rotation of the fetal head by two-eighths of the circle in such a way that the occiput rotates anteriorly from the lateral position towards the pubic symphysis. In case of anterior oblique position, rotation will be by one-eighth of the circle placing the occiput behind the pubic symphysis. There always occurs some descent with internal rotation. Torsion of fetal neck is a phenomenon, which will inevitably occur during internal rotation of the fetal head. In case of occipitolateral position, the internal rotation of the fetal head by two-eighths of the circle is likely to cause the torsion of fetal neck by two-eighths of the circle. Since the neck would not be able to sustain this much amount of torsion, there would be simultaneous rotation of the fetal shoulders in the same direction by one-eighth of the circle. This would cause the torsion on the fetal neck to get reduced to one-eighth of the circle and would place the shoulders in an oblique diameter, i.e. right oblique with right occipitolateral and left oblique with left occipitolateral.

In occipitoanterior position, the neck is able to sustain a torsion of one-eighth of the circle. Therefore, there is no simultaneous rotation of the shoulders which are already placed in the oblique diameter of the pelvis.

## Crowning

With the increasing descent of the fetal head, crowning occurs. During this stage, the biparietal diameter of the fetal head stretches the vaginal introitus. Even as the uterine contractions cease, the head would not recede back during the stage of crowning (Fig. 3.12).

## Extension

Fetal head pivots under symphysis pubis and emerges out through extension, followed by occiput, then the face, and finally the chin (Fig. 3.13).

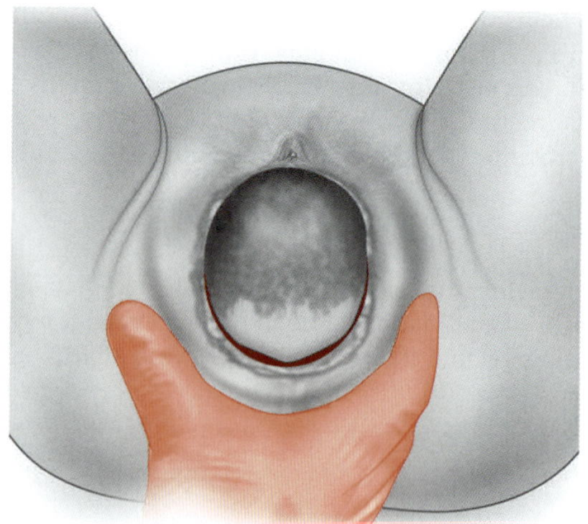

**Fig. 3.12:** Crowning of the fetal head

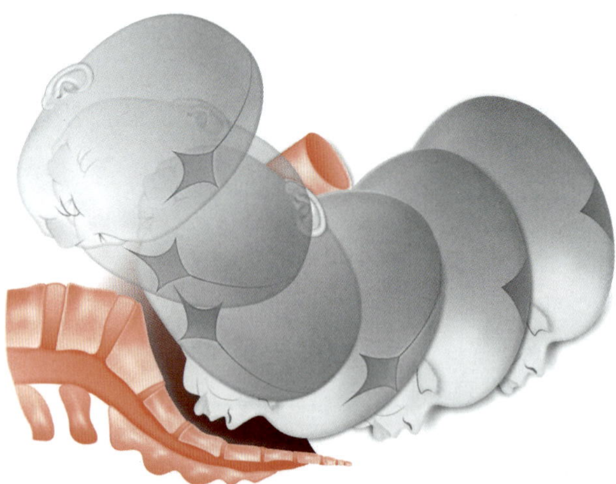

**Fig. 3.13:** Delivery of the fetal head by extension

## Restitution

Following the delivery of fetal head, the neck, which had undergone torsion, previously, now untwists and aligns along with the long axis of the fetus.

## External Rotation of the Head

As the undelivered shoulders rotate by one-eighth of the circle to occupy the AP diameter of the pelvis, this movement is visible outside in form of the external rotation of fetal head (Fig. 3.14), causing the head to further turn to one side.

Following the engagement of the fetal shoulders in the AP diameter of the pelvis, anterior shoulder slips under symphysis pubis, followed by posterior shoulder (Figs 3.15 and 3.16). Once both the shoulders have delivered, rest of the trunk is delivered by lateral flexion.

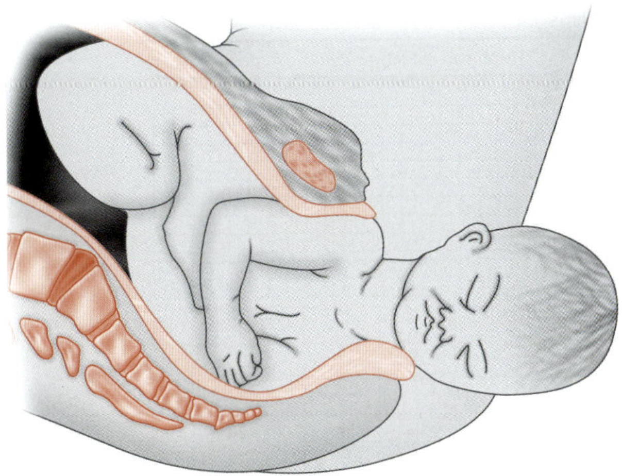

**Fig. 3.14:** External rotation of head allowing delivery of shoulders

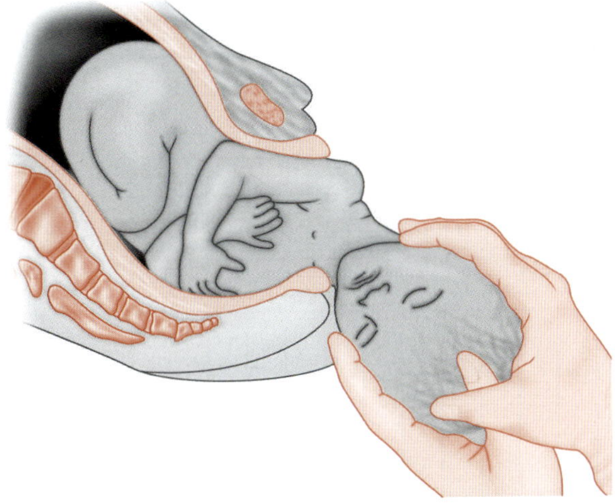

**Fig. 3.15:** Delivery of anterior shoulder

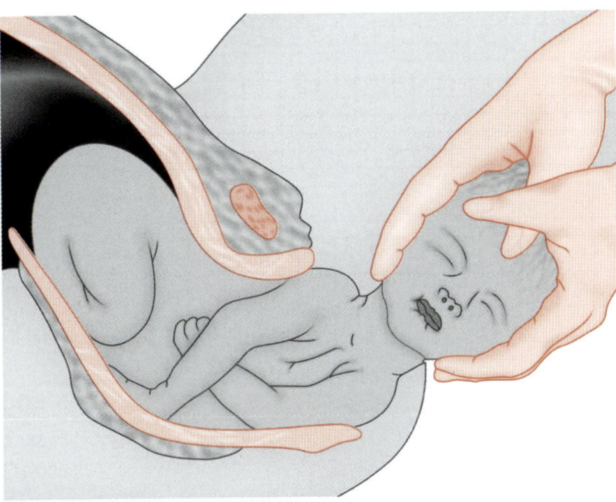

**Fig. 3.16:** Delivery of posterior shoulder

# Conducting Normal Vaginal Delivery

### Pre-delivery Preparation

- *Patient position:* The patient is commonly placed in the dorsal lithotomy position with left lateral tilt.
- *Cleaning and draping:* Vulvar and perineal cleaning and draping with antiseptic solution must be done. The sterile drapes must be placed in such a way that only the area immediately around the vulva and perineum is exposed.
- *Strict asepsis:* A complete aseptic technique must be adopted at the time of conducting the vaginal delivery.
- *Bladder to be emptied:* If at any time during the abdominal examination, the bladder is palpable, the patient must be encouraged to void. If despite of distended bladder the patient is unable to void, catheterization is indicated.
- *Patient monitoring:* Maternal blood pressure and pulse should be recorded every hour during the first stage of labor and every 10 minutes during the second stage of labor in a normal patient.
- *Fetal heart rate monitoring:* Continuous external electronic fetal monitoring must be preferably done throughout the active stage of labor in a high-risk patient. Intermittent auscultation can be done in low-risk patients. Parameters such as maternal-fetal conditions, patient preferences and health care resources must be taken into consideration before determining the auscultation intervals in these patients. Intermittent auscultation can be done after every 15–30 minutes during the first stage of labor and after every 5–15 minutes or following each contraction during the second stage of labor.
- *Induction of labor:* This is required to make the cervix soft and pliable and/or to induce uterine contractions.
- *Partogram:* Normal labor should be plotted graphically on a partograph (Fig. 3.17). The partograph is divided into a latent phase and an active phase. The latent phase ends, while the active phase begins when the cervix is 3 cm dilated. Cervical dilation and descent of the presenting part are plotted in relation to an alert line and an action line. Alert line starts at the end of latent phase and ends with the full dilation of the cervix (10 cm) within 7 hours (at the rate of 1 cm/hour). The action line is drawn 4 hours to the right of the alert line. Labor is considered to be abnormal when the cervicograph crosses the alert line and falls on zone II, and intervention is required when it crosses the action line and falls in the zone III.

### Conducting Normal Vaginal Delivery

Conducting a normal vaginal delivery involves the following steps:

- *Delivery of fetal head:* With increasing descent of the head, the perineum bulges and thins out considerably. As the largest diameter of the fetal head distends the vaginal introitus, the crowning (Fig. 3.12) is said to occur.

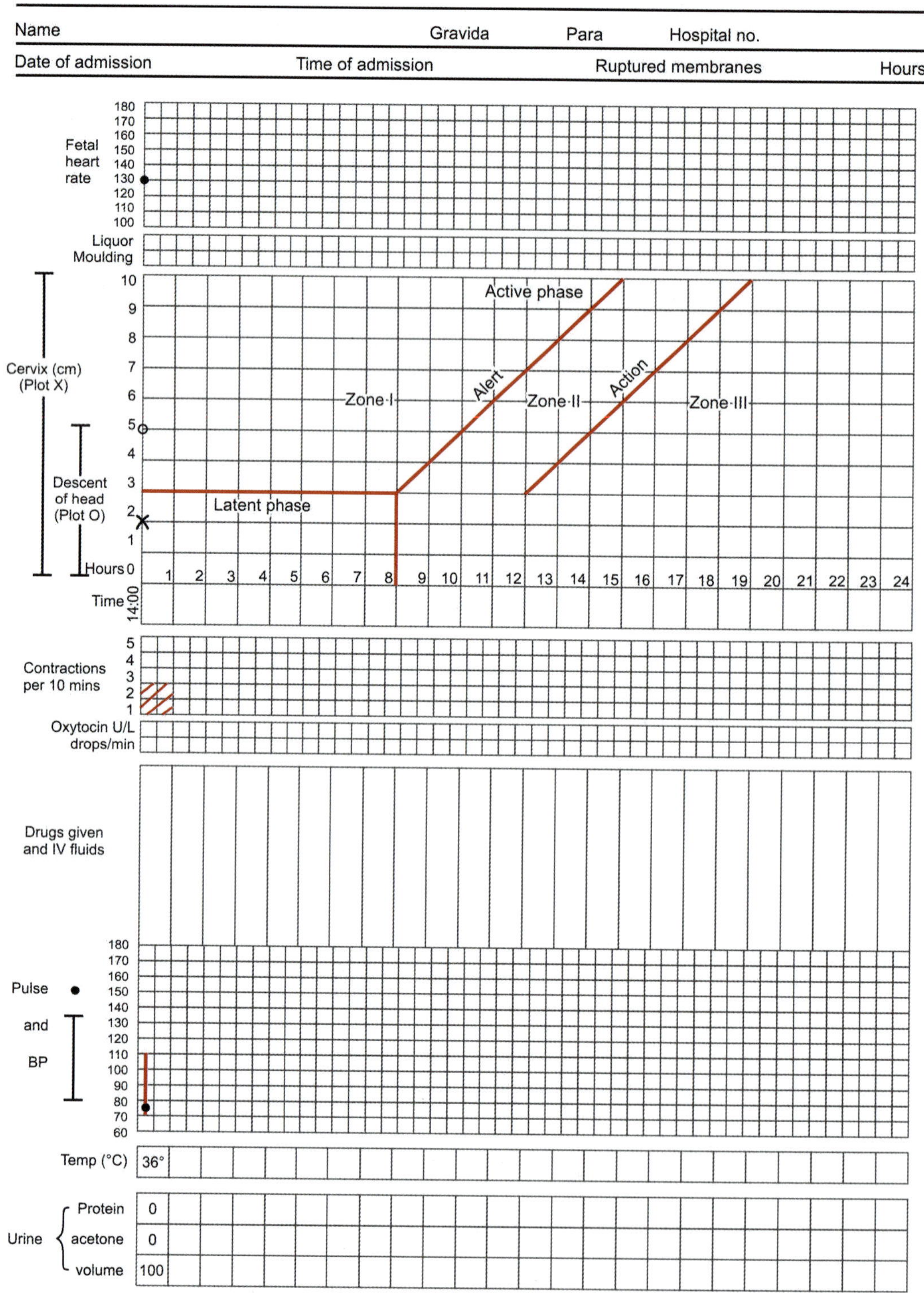


**Fig. 3.17:** Partograph

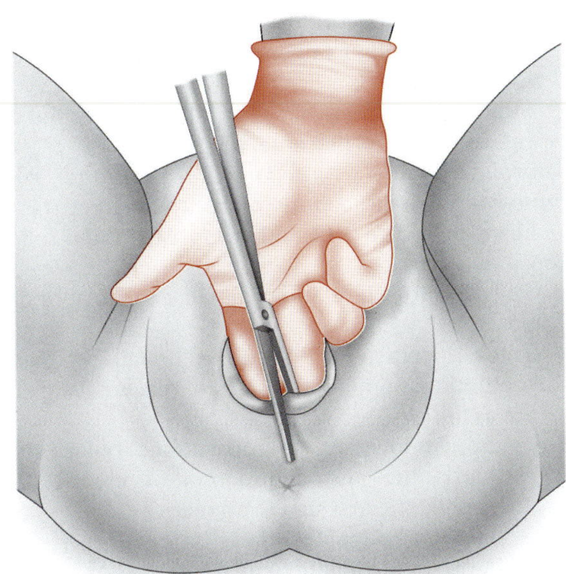

**Fig 3.18:** Administration of an episiotomy

- As the head distends the perineum and it appears that tears may occur in the area of vaginal introitus, mediolateral surgical incision called episiotomy may be given (Fig. 3.18). Episiotomy is no longer recommended as a routine procedure and is performed only if the clinician feels its requirement.
- As the fetal head progressively distends the vaginal introitus, the clinician in order to facilitate controlled birth of the head must place the fingers of one hand against the baby's head to keep it flexed and apply perineal support with the other hand. Increasing flexion of the fetal head would facilitate the delivery of the smallest diameter of fetal head. This can be achieved with help of Ritgen maneuver. In this maneuver, one of the clinician's gloved hands is used for exerting downwards and forwards pressure on the chin through the perineum, just in front of the coccyx. The other hand exerts pressure superiorly against the occiput. This helps in providing controlled delivery of the head and favors extension at the time of actual delivery so that the head is delivered with its smallest diameter passing through the introitus and minimal injury occurs to the pelvic musculature. Once the baby's head delivers, the woman must be encouraged not to push. The baby's mouth and nose must be suctioned. The clinician must then feel around the baby's neck in order to rule out the presence of cord around the fetal neck. If the cord is around the neck but is loose, it should be slipped over the baby's head. However, if the cord is tight around the neck, it should be doubly clamped and cut before proceeding with the delivery of fetal shoulders.
- *Delivery of the shoulders:* Following the delivery of fetal head, the fetal head falls posteriorly, while the face comes

in contact with the maternal anus. As the restitution or external rotation of the fetal head occurs, the occiput turns towards one of the maternal thighs and the head assumes a transverse position. This movement implies that bisacromial diameter has rotated and has occupied the AP diameter of the pelvis. Soon the anterior shoulder appears at the vaginal introitus. Following the delivery of the anterior shoulder, the posterior shoulder is born. The clinician must move the baby's head posteriorly to deliver the shoulder that is anterior.

Immediately following delivery of the thorax, the mouth and nasopharynx must be aspirated in order to reduce the fetal aspiration of amniotic fluid, particulate matter and blood.

- *Delivery of the rest of the body:* This is followed by delivery of the rest of the body. The rest of the baby's body must be supported with one hand as it slides out of the vaginal introitus.
- *Clamping the cord:* The umbilical cord must be clamped and cut if not done earlier. Two clamps must be placed on the umbilical cord and cord must be cut in between them with the help of scissors. Delayed clamping of the cord would help in transferring about 80 mL of blood from the placenta to the neonate which would help in supplying 50 mg of iron to the fetus. This strategy would help in preventing the development of anemia.
- The baby must be placed over the mother's abdomen and then handed over to the assisting nurse or the pediatrician. The baby's body must be thoroughly dried, the eyes be wiped and baby's breathing must be assessed.
- In order to minimize the chances of aspiration of amniotic fluid, soon after delivery of the thorax, the face must be wiped and the mouth and nostril must be aspirated.
- The baby must be covered with a soft, dry cloth, and a blanket to ensure that the baby remains warm and no heat loss occurs. Following the delivery of baby, the placenta needs to be delivered. The clinician must look for signs of placental separation following the delivery of the baby.
- The third stage of labor must be actively managed.

## MONITORING DURING LABOR

### Management during the First Stage of Labor

The following steps should be observed at the time of normal vaginal delivery:

- During normal labor, in absence of any complications, the following vital signs must be regularly monitored at every hourly interval: pulse, BP, temperature, frequency, duration and intensity of uterine contractions, fetal heart rate, fetal presentation, presence or absence of fetal membranes, and any vaginal bleeding.
- In normal pregnancy, there is no need to keep the patient confined to bed during the first stage of labor. She should

be encouraged to move about in the labor room or sit on a birthing ball. She can assume any position in which she is comfortable in the bed.

- Bladder distension must be avoided as it can hinder the normal progress of labor. This can subsequently lead to bladder hypotonia and infection.
- Spontaneous rupture of fetal membranes during labor is important to the following three reasons:
  - ROM is likely to fix the presenting part in the pelvis. If the presenting part is not fixed in the pelvis, there is a possibility of umbilical cord prolapse and cord compression
  - Labor is likely to begin soon following the ROM
  - If delivery is delayed for more than 24 hours following ROM, there is a high possibility of intrauterine infection. If membranes are ruptured for more than 18 hours, antimicrobial therapy must be administered in order to reduce the risk of infection.

## Management during the Second Stage of Labor

During the second stage of labor, the woman must be encouraged to push down with each uterine contraction and then relax at the time the contractions stop. During this period of active bearing down, the fetal heart rate must be auscultated following each uterine contraction. Though fetal heart sound (FHS) may be slow immediately following a contraction, it must normally recover in the time interval before the next contraction begins.

## Management during the Third Stage of Labor

The management during the third stage of labor is as follows:
- As previously mentioned, third stage of labor begins with the delivery of the fetus and ends following the completed delivery of the placenta and its attached membranes. Third stage of labor is particularly important because an important complication, postpartum hemorrhage, which is an important cause of maternal mortality and morbidity, can occur during this phase. The active management of the third stage of labor can help to prevent this. Active management comprises of the following steps:
  - Administering a uterotonic drug, usually 0.25 mg of methergine or ergometrine 0.2 mg (IM or IV) soon after the delivery of the anterior shoulder and/or oxytocin 5–10 IU (IV) within 1 minute of the birth of the baby.
  - Clamping the cord as soon as it stops pulsating.
  - Uterine massage (would be described later).
  - Controlled cord traction or Brandt-Andrews maneuver must be used.
  - Crede's method of placental expulsion must never be used. Crede's maneuver involves placing one hand

over the uterine fundus and squeezing it between the thumb and other fingers to aid placental separation and delivery.
  - Fundal pressure must not be applied over the atonic uterus to aid the placental delivery.
- *Controlled cord traction or Brandt-Andrews maneuver:* The procedure of controlled cord traction is shown in Figure 3.19 and comprises of the following steps:
  - The cord must be clamped as close to the perineum as possible.
  - The clinician must look for the signs of placental separation. Some of the signs of placental separation are as follows:
    - Appearance of a suprapubic bulge due to hardening and contraction of uterus. This is usually the first sign to appear.
    - Sudden gush of blood.
    - A rise in the height of the uterus (as observed over the abdomen) due to the passage of placenta to the lower uterine segment.
    - Irreversible cord lengthening.
- Once these above-mentioned signs occur, the clinician must hold the cord with the right hand and place the left hand over the mother's abdomen just above the pubic bone.
- The clinician must apply slight tension on the cord with right hand in downwards and backwards direction. At the same time the uterus must be stabilized by applying counter pressure in upwards and backwards direction while exerting controlled traction with the left hand.

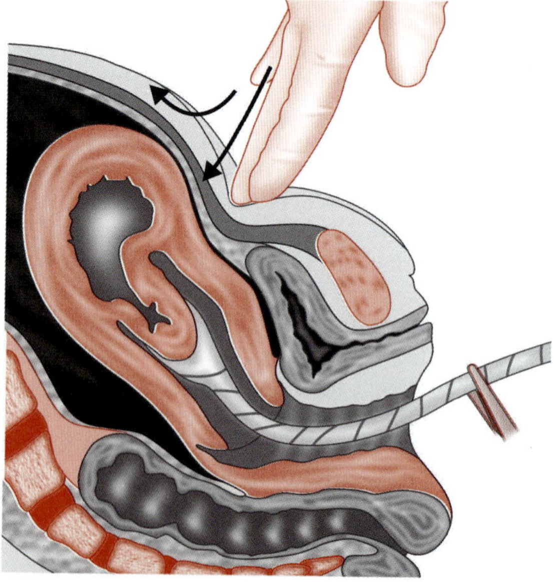

**Fig. 3.19:** Controlled cord traction

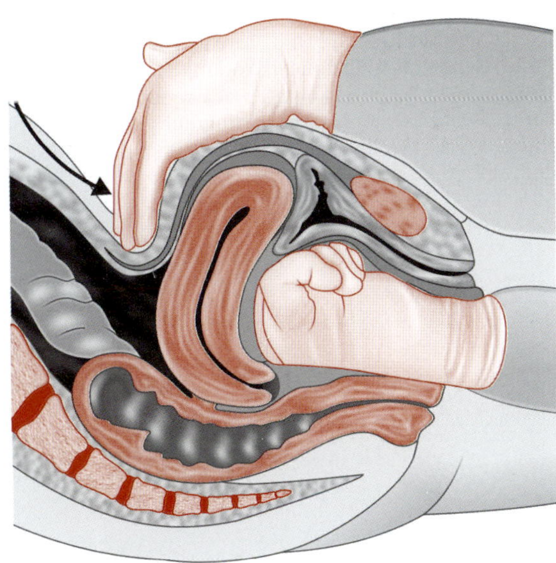

**Fig. 3.20:** Bimanual uterine compression

- The mother should be encouraged to push with the uterine contractions.
- The cord should never be pulled without applying counter traction above the pubic bone.
- As the placenta delivers, it should be held in two hands and gently turned, until the membranes are twisted and stripped off intact from the uterine wall.
- If the membranes tear, gentle examination of the upper vagina and cervix must be carried out to look for torn bits of membrane. These if present, can be removed with the help of a sponge forceps.
- *Bimanual uterine massage:* If the clinician finds the uterus to be soft upon bimanual examination, a bimanual uterine massage must be performed to contract the myometrial muscles. The maneuver involves the massage of the posterior aspect of the uterus with the abdominal hand and that of the anterior aspect of the uterus with the vaginal hand and comprises of the following steps (Fig. 3.20):
  - One of the clinician's hands is formed into a fist and placed inside the vagina, with the back of the hand directed posteriorly and knuckles in the anterior fornix so as to push against the body of the uterus.
  - The other hand compresses the fundus from above through the abdominal wall. The fundus of the uterus must be immediately massaged, until uterus is well contracted.
  - Uterus must be massaged every 15 minutes during the first 2 hours. If this maneuver controls bleeding, the clinician must maintain this compression for at least 30 minutes.

- Once the placenta and membranes have delivered, they should be carefully examined by the clinician. The maternal surface of the placenta is examined for its completeness to see that no cotyledon is missing, thereby ensuring that no placental remnants are left inside the uterine cavity. The fetal membranes, amnion and chorion must also be examined for completeness. The amnion is shiny in appearance, whereas the chorion is shaggy.
- The cut end of the umbilical cord is also observed for the number of blood vessels. Normally there are two umbilical arteries and one vein.
- The vulva and the perineum must be carefully inspected for any injuries and if present, they must be repaired. If an episiotomy had been administered, it is repaired during this stage.

## Fourth Stage

The mother should be monitored during this stage through assessment of her pulse, blood pressure, uterine tone, presence of any vaginal bleeding, etc. When the clinician is completely satisfied that the mother is stable, uterus is well contracted and there is no vaginal bleeding, she can be sent to the ward.

## FURTHER READINGS


1. American Academy of Pediatricians and American College of Obstetricians and Gynecologists. Guidelines for Perinatal Care, 6th edition. 2008;10(3):207.
2. American College of Obstetricians and Gynecologists. ACOG Practice Bulletin. Clinical Management Guidelines for Obstetrician-Gynecologists, Number 70, December 2005 (Replaces Practice Bulletin Number 62, May 2005). Intrapartum fetal heart rate monitoring. Obstet Gynecol. 2005;106(6):1453-60.
3. American College of Obstetricians-Gynecologists. ACOG Practice Bulletin. Episiotomy. Clinical Management Guidelines for Obstetrician-Gynecologists. Number 71, April 2006. Obstet Gynecol. 2006;107(4):957-62.
4. American College of Obstetricians and Gynecologists Practice Bulletin. Dystocia and Augmentation of Labor. Clinical Management Guidelines for Obstetricians Gynecologists. No 49. Washington, DC: American College of Obstetricians and Gynecologists; 2003.p.10.
5. Goetzl LM, ACOG Committee on Practice Bulletins-Obstetrics. ACOG Practice Bulletin. Clinical Management Guidelines for Obstetrician-Gynecologists Number 36, July 2002. Obstetric analgesia and anesthesia. Obstet Gynecol. 2002;100(1):177-91.
6. ACOG technical bulletin. Dystocia and the augmentation of labor. Number 218—December 1995 (replaces no. 137, December 1989, and no. 157, July 1991). American College of Obstetricians and Gynecologists. Int J Gynaecol Obstet. 1996;53(1):73-80.
7. Friedman EA. Labor. Clinical Evaluation and Management. New York: Appleton-Century-Crofts; 1978.p.34.

8. Neilson JP. Evidence-based intrapartum care: evidence from the Cochrane library. Int J Gynaecol Obstet. 1998;63 (Suppl 1): S97-102.

9. O'Driscoll K, Meagher D. Introduction. In: O'Driscoll K, Meagher D (Eds). Active Management of Labor, 2nd edition. Eastbourne, United Kingdom: Balliere Tindall; 1986.

10. World Health Organization (WHO), Maternal and Newborn Health/Safe Motherhood Unit. Care in Normal Birth: a Practical Guide. Report of a Technical Working Group. WHO: Geneva; 1996.pp.1-53.

11. World Health Organization partograph in management of labour. World Health Organization Maternal Health and Safe Motherhood Programme. Lancet. 1994;343 (8910):1399-404.

# 4

# Labor in Case of Malpresentations



## Breech Delivery

### Introduction

Breech presentation can be defined as a malpresentation in which the fetus lies longitudinally with its buttocks/feet/legs presenting in the lower pole of the uterus.

### Types of Breech Presentation

The different types of breech presentations are shown in Figure 4.1 and are described below in details.

### *Frank Breech*

This is the most common type of breech presentation (50–70% cases). Buttocks present first with flexed hips and legs extended on the abdomen. This position is also known as the pike position.

### *Complete Breech*

Also known as the cannonball position, this type of presentation is present in 5–10% of cases. In this, the buttocks present first with flexed hips and flexed knees. Feet are not below the buttocks.

### *Footling Breech*

One or both feet present in the lower pole of uterus as both hips and knees are in extended position. As a result, feet are palpated at a level lower than the buttocks.

The denominator of breech presentation is considered to be the sacrum. Depending on the relationship of the sacrum

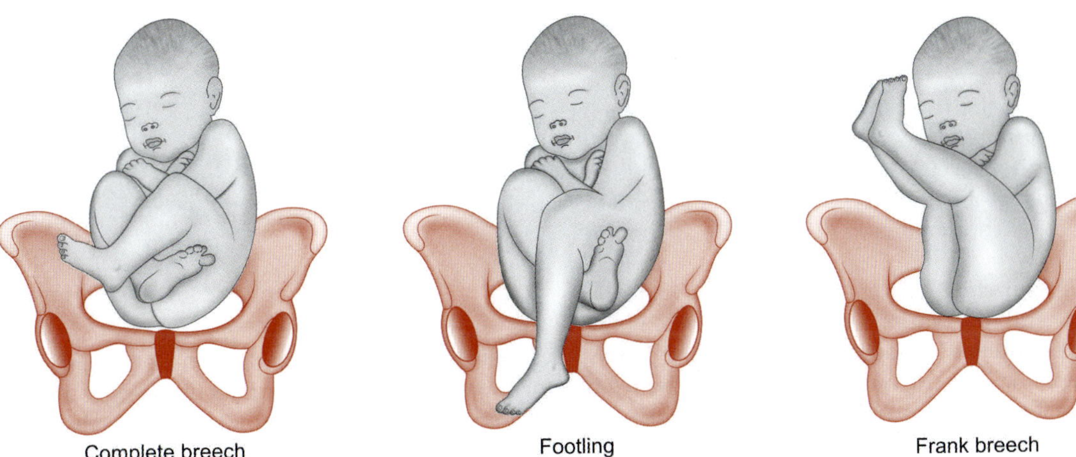



**Fig. 4.1:** Different types of breech presentation

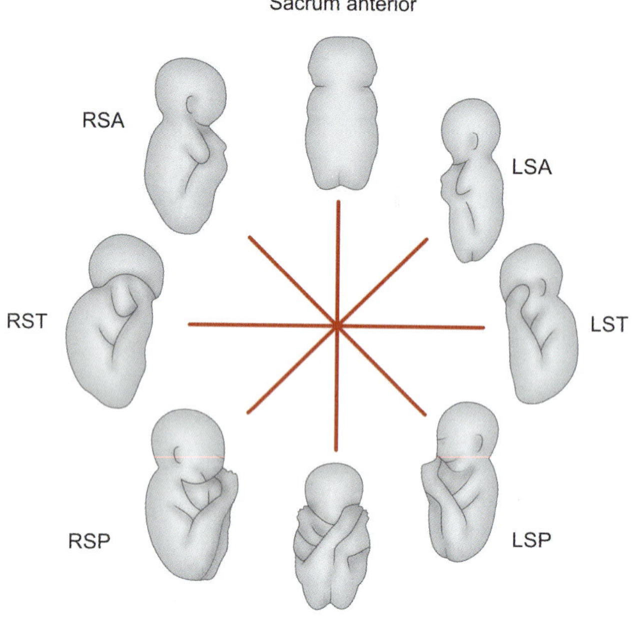



**Fig. 4.2:** Different positions of the breech

*Abbreviations:* LSA, left sacroanterior; LSP, left sacroposterior; LST, left sacrotransverse; RSA, right sacroanterior; RSP, right sacroposterior; RST, right sacrotransverse

with the sacroiliac joint, the following positions of the breech are possible (Fig. 4.2). These include the left sacroanterior (LSA) position; right sacroanterior (RSA) position; right sacroposterior (RSP) position and left sacroposterior (LSP) position. LSA position is the most common position.

## BREECH VAGINAL DELIVERY

Three types of vaginal breech deliveries are described:

1. *Spontaneous breech delivery:*  No traction or manipulation of the infant by the clinician is done. The fetus delivers spontaneously on its own. This occurs predominantly in very preterm deliveries.
2. *Assisted breech delivery:*  This is the most common mode of vaginal breech delivery. In this method a "no-touch technique" is adopted in which the infant is allowed to spontaneously deliver up to the umbilicus, and then certain maneuvers are initiated by the clinician to aid in the delivery of the remainder of the body, arms, and head.
3. *Total breech extraction:* In this method, the fetal feet are grasped, and the entire fetus is extracted by the clinician. Total breech extraction should be used only for a noncephalic second twin; it should not be used for singleton fetuses because the cervix may not be adequately dilated to allow passage of the fetal head.

## Indications

Certain indications for breech vaginal delivery are:
- Frank or complete breech (not footling)
- Estimated fetal weight between 1.5 kg and 3.5 kg
- Gestational age (36–42 weeks)
- Well-flexed fetal head (no evidence of hyperextension of the fetal head)
- Adequate pelvis (no fetopelvic disproportion)
- Normal progress of labor on partogram
- Uncomplicated pregnancy (No contraindications to vaginal birth, e.g. placenta previa, severe IUGR, etc.
- Multiparas
- No obstetric indication for cesarean section, e.g. placenta previa, etc.
- An experienced clinician
- Presence of severe fetal anomaly or fetal death
- Mother's preference for vaginal birth
- Delivery is imminent in case of breech presentation.

The major difference between the breech vaginal delivery and normal vaginal delivery in cephalic presentation is based on the fact that in cephalic presentation, the head which is the largest and least compressible structure of the fetus is delivered first followed by the rest of the body. Once the head has delivered in cases of cephalic presentation, the rest of the body follows without much difficulty. On the other hand in breech presentation, the buttocks which are compressible structures are delivered first followed by the head. This can result in the entrapment of fetal head. The maximum danger for entrapment of fetal head is in case of footling presentation. In these cases, the fetal leg and foot can deliver through partially dilated cervix followed by entrapment of fetal head. Also, breech presentation is a slow dilator of cervix. Due to an irregular-fitting presenting fetal part, the risk of PROM and cord prolapse is increased. Therefore, with breech vaginal delivery anytime during the course of vaginal delivery, a situation may arise when the clinician might have to resort to cesarean section for fetal or maternal sake. Thus, the vaginal breech birth should take place in a hospital with facilities for emergency cesarean section.

While in cephalic presentation, the head delivers gradually after undergoing molding, in breech presentation the fetal head delivers suddenly. As a result, sudden excessive pressure on the after-coming head of the breech is associated with a high risk of tentorial tears and intracranial hemorrhage in comparison to the fetuses in cephalic presentation.

## MECHANISM OF BREECH VAGINAL DELIVERY

The breech most commonly presents in LSA position, which causes the bitrochanteric diameter of the buttocks (9.5 cm) to enter through the pelvic inlet in the right oblique diameter of the pelvic brim (Fig. 4.3A). Once the bitrochanteric diameter has passed through the oblique diameter of pelvis,

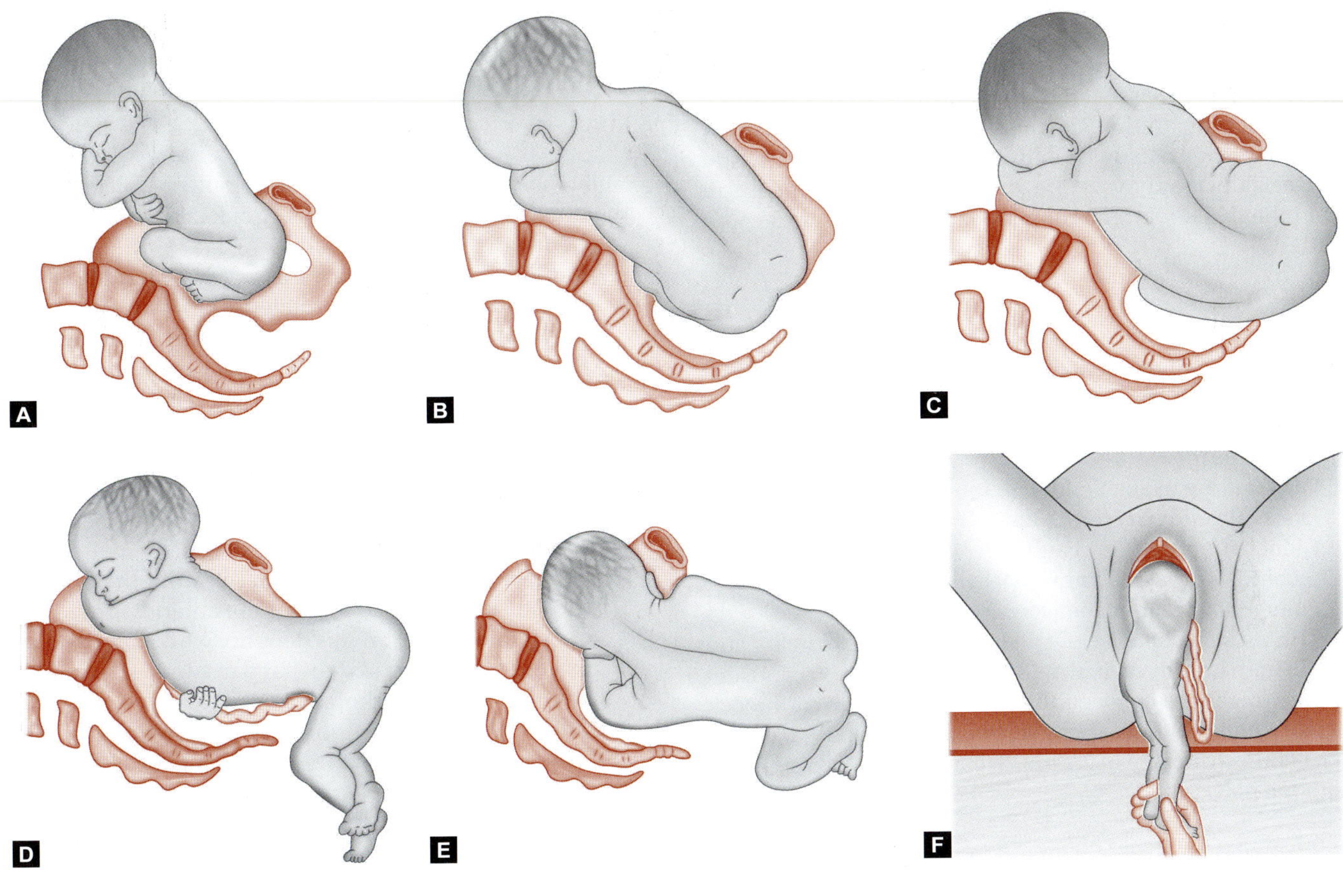

**Figs 4.3A to F:** Mechanism of breech vaginal delivery

engagement is said to occur (Fig. 4.3B). With full dilatation of the cervix, the buttocks descend deeply into the pelvis. The descent of remaining fetal parts is, however, slow. The descent of anterior hip is faster than that of the posterior hip.

When the buttocks reach the pelvic floor, the anterior hip which reaches the pelvic floor first, internally rotates through 45° so that the bitrochanteric diameter lies in the anteroposterior (AP) diameter of the pelvic outlet.

With continuing fetal descent, the anterior buttock appears at the vulva. With further uterine contractions, the buttocks distend the vaginal outlet. There is delivery of anterior hip followed by that of posterior hip by lateral flexion. The anterior hip slips out under the pubic symphysis followed by the lower limbs and feet (Fig. 4.3C).

Following the delivery of buttocks and legs, sacrum rotates by 45° in the direction opposite to the internal rotation, resulting in the external rotation of the breech. This causes the back to turn anteriorly (Fig. 4.3D). With continuing descent, the bisacromial diameter (12 cm) of the shoulders engages in right oblique diameter of the pelvis and descent continues (Fig. 4.3E). On touching the pelvic floor, the anterior shoulders undergo internal rotation by 45° so that the bisacromial diameter lies in the AP diameter of the outlet. Simultaneously, the buttocks and sacrum externally rotate anteriorly through 45°.

As the anterior shoulder impinges under the pubic symphysis, the posterior shoulders and arm are born over the perineum followed by the delivery of anterior shoulder. Following the delivery, anterior shoulders undergo restitution through 45° and assume a right oblique position. At the same time the neck undergoes torsion of 45°. As a result the engaging diameter of the head (suboccipitofrontal diameter, 10.5 cm) or suboccipitobregmatic diameter engages in the left oblique diameter of the pelvis (Fig. 4.3F). Descent into the pelvis occurs with flexion of the fetal head. The flexion of fetal head is often maintained by uterine contractions aided by suprapubic pressure applied by the delivery assistant at the time of delivery. When the head reaches the pelvic floor, it undergoes internal rotation by 45° so that the sagittal sutures lie in the AP diameter of the pelvis, with the occiput presenting anteriorly and brow in the hollow of the sacrum. As the nape of the neck impinges against the pubic symphysis, the chin, mouth, nose, forehead, bregma and occiput are born over the perineum by flexion.

## ASSISTED BREECH VAGINAL DELIVERY

In clinical practice, the most common mode of vaginal breech delivery is assisted breech delivery. In this method, a "no-touch technique" is adopted in which the infant is allowed to spontaneously deliver up to the umbilicus, and then certain maneuvers are initiated by the clinician to aid in the delivery of the remainder of the body, arms, and head.

### Prerequisites for a Vaginal Delivery

Prerequisites for breech vaginal delivery are as follows:
- Facilities for cesarean section are available.
- Anesthetist, operation theater staff and pediatrician have been informed.
- Facilities are available for continuous monitoring of fetal heart rate and ultrasonography.
- Clinician and other health care staff, well versed in the technique of vaginal breech delivery and facilities for safe emergency cesarean delivery are available.

The woman should be explained about the benefits and risks of both breech vaginal delivery and cesarean section and allowed to choose between the two. The decision for breech vaginal delivery or cesarean section is made based on the type of breech, degree of flexion of fetal head, fetal size, size of maternal pelvis, etc.

## STEPS FOR BREECH VAGINAL DELIVERY

- Once the buttocks have entered the vagina and the cervix is fully dilated, the woman must be advised to bear down with the contractions.
- Episiotomy may be performed, if the perineum appears very tight.

### Delivery of Buttocks and Lower Back

- A "no touch policy/hands off the breech policy" must be adopted by the clinician until the buttocks and lower back deliver till the level of umbilicus. At this point the baby's shoulder blades can be seen.
- Sometimes, the clinician may have to make use of maneuvers like Pinard's maneuver and groin traction (will be described later), if the legs have not delivered spontaneously.
- The clinician should be extremely careful and gently hold the baby by wrapping it in a clean cloth in such a way that the baby's trunk is present anteriorly. This will allow the fetal head to enter the pelvis in occipitoanterior (OA) position.
- The baby must be held by the hips and not by the flanks or abdomen as this may cause kidney or liver damage. At no point, must the clinician try to pull the baby out; rather the patient must be encouraged to push down.

- In order to avoid compression on the umbilical cord, it should be moved to one side, preferably in the sacral bay.

### Delivery of Fetal Shoulders and Arms

- Appearance of axilla at the vulval outlet indicates that the time has come for the delivery of fetal shoulders. Two methods can be used:
    - In the first method, once the scapula is visible at the vulval outlet, the trunk is rotated in clockwise direction by 90° in such a way that the anterior shoulder and arm appears at the vulva (Figs 4.4A to E). It can then be easily released and delivered. The body of the fetus is then rotated similarly in the reverse direction (anticlockwise) to deliver the other arm and shoulder.
    - Second method is employed if the first method is unsuccessful. In the second method, the posterior shoulder is delivered first (described later in the text). Following the delivery of posterior arm, the body of the fetus is depressed to allow the anterior arm to slip out spontaneously. If this does not work, the clinician can use two fingers of right hand to sweep the anterior arm down over the thorax.
- *Nuchal arms:* Sometimes, due to inappropriate traction and rotational maneuvers, the shoulder is extended and elbow is flexed. In these cases, the forearm gets trapped behind the occiput. If the clinician tries to hook down the trapped arm, there may occur fracture of the humerus. Therefore, in these cases, the following maneuver (Figs 4.5A and B) can be used—the fetus is rotated in the direction in which the baby's hand is pointing. This would cause the occiput to slip past the forearm. Friction of the rotation causes the shoulder to flex and become accessible for delivery.
- The clinician must wait to deliver the shoulders until axilla is visible. Attempts must not be made to release the arms immediately after the emergence of costal margins.
- The clinician must wait for the arms to deliver spontaneously. If arms are felt on chest, the clinician must allow the arms to disengage spontaneously one by one. Assistance should be provided only if necessary. After spontaneous delivery of the first arm, the buttocks must be lifted towards the mother's abdomen to enable the second arm to deliver spontaneously. If the arm does not spontaneously deliver, place one or two fingers in the elbow and bend the arm, bringing the hand down over the baby's face.
- If the arms still do not deliver, the clinician must reach into the vagina to determine their position. If they are flexed in front of the chest, gentle pressure must be applied to the crook of the elbow to straighten the arm and aid delivery.
- The same maneuver must be repeated with the other arm.
- The clinician needs to be aware that there are other maneuvers to deliver the arms and shoulders, if needed,

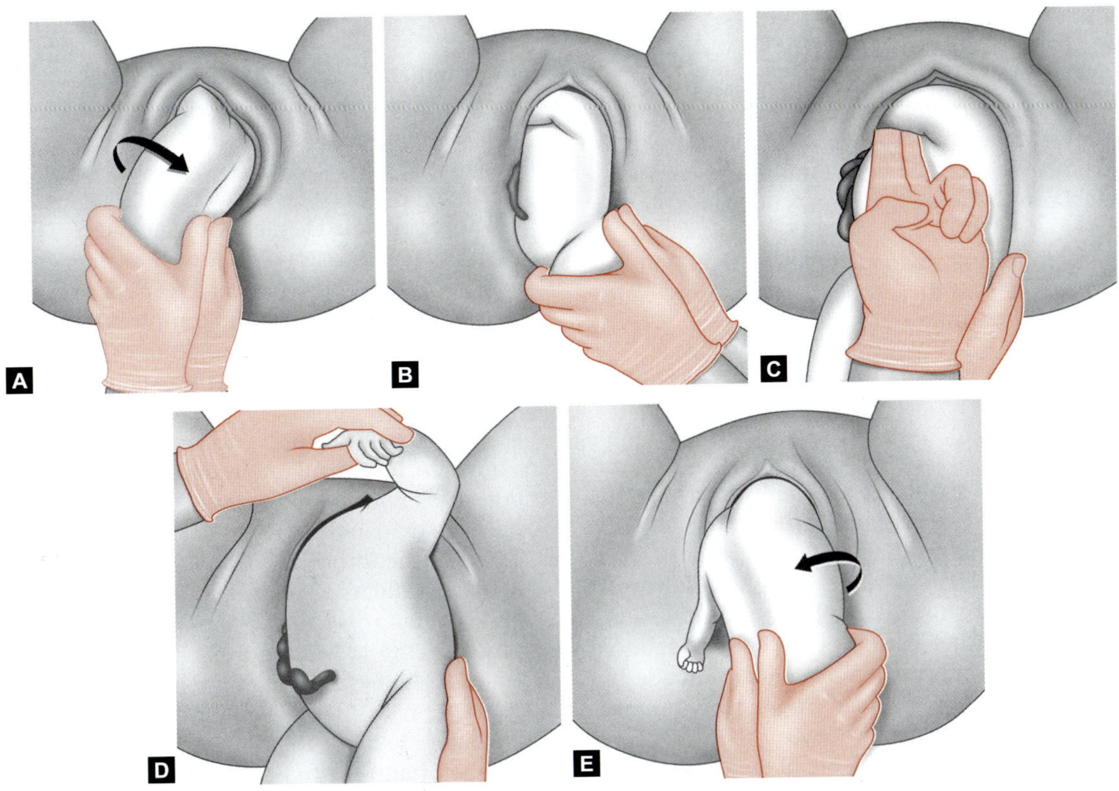

**Figs 4.4A to E:** Delivery of fetal shoulders and arms. (A) Rotation of fetal pelvis by 90° in clockwise direction; (B to D) Application of gentle traction to deliver the anterior shoulder, arm and forearm; (E) Rotation of the fetal pelvis in anticlockwise direction to deliver the posterior arm and forearm

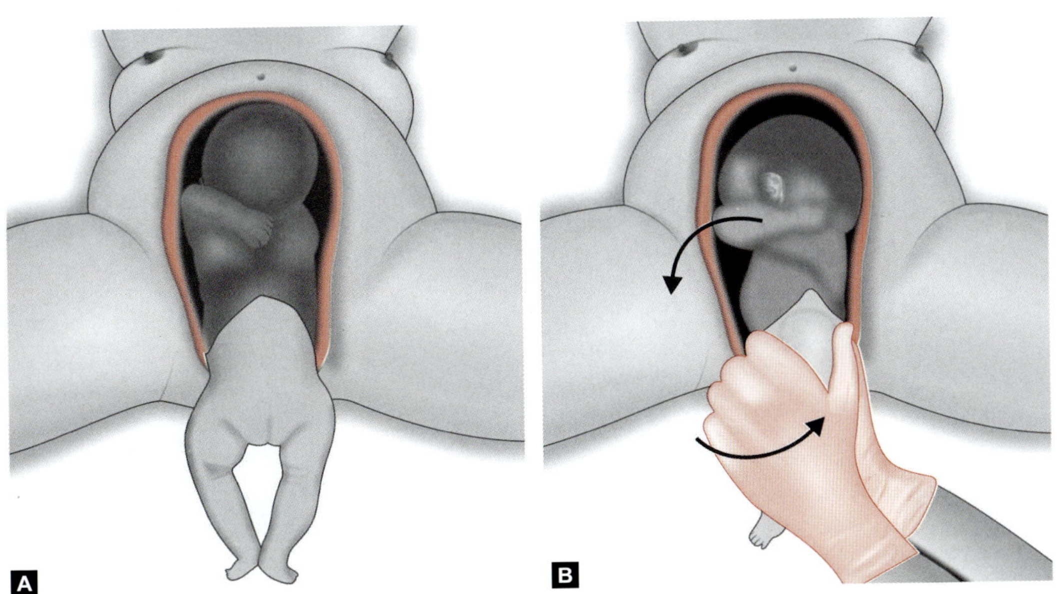

**Figs 4.5A and B:** Delivery of nuchal arm. (A) Forearm is trapped behind the occiput;
(B) Rotation of fetal body in the direction in which the baby's hand is pointing

including Løvset's maneuver (described later) to deliver the extended arms, which are stretched above the baby's head.

- Once the shoulders are delivered, the baby's body with the face down must be supported on the clinician's forearm. The clinician must be careful not to compress the umbilical cord between the infant's body and his/her arm.
- One of the following maneuvers, which would be described next, can be then used for delivery of after-coming head of the fetus.

### Maneuvers for Delivery of the After-Coming Head

#### Burns Marshall Technique

Following the delivery of shoulders and both the arms, the baby must be let to hang unsupported from the mother's vulva. This would help in encouraging flexion of fetal head (Fig. 4.6A). The nursing staff must be further advised to apply suprapubic pressure in downwards and backwards direction, in order to encourage further flexion of the baby's head. As the nape of baby's neck appears, efforts must be made by the clinician to deliver the baby's head by grasping the fetal ankles with the finger of right hand between the two. Then the trunk is swung up forming a wide arc of the circle, while maintaining continuous traction when doing this (Fig. 4.6B). The left hand is used to provide pelvic support and to clear the perineum off successively from the baby's face and brow as the baby's head emerges out.

#### Mauriceau–Smellie–Veit Maneuver

This is another commonly used maneuver for the delivery of after-coming fetal head and is named after the three clinicians who had described the method of using this grip. This maneuver comprises of the following steps:

- The baby is placed face down with the length of its body over the supinated left forearm and hand of the clinician.
- The clinician must then place the first finger (index finger) and second finger (middle finger) of this hand on the baby's cheek bones and the thumb over the baby's chin. This helps in facilitating flexion of the fetal head. In the method originally described by Mauriceau, Smellie and Veit, the index finger of the left hand was placed inside the baby's mouth. This is no longer advocated as placing a finger inside the infant's mouth is supposed to stimulate the vagal reflex. An assistant may provide suprapubic pressure to help the baby's head remain flexed.
- The right hand of the clinician is used for grasping the baby's shoulders. The little finger and the ring finger of the clinician's right hand is placed over the baby's right shoulder, the index finger over the baby's left shoulder and the middle finger over the baby's suboccipital region (Fig 4.7). With the fingers of right hand in this position, the baby's head is flexed towards the chest. At the same time left hand is used for applying downwards pressure on the jaw to bring the baby's head down until the hairline is visible.
- Thereafter the baby's trunk is carried in upwards and forwards direction towards the maternal abdomen, till the baby's mouth, nose and brow and lastly the vertex and occiput have been released.

In this maneuver, the clinician uses both the arms simultaneously, in synchronization to exert gentle downwards traction at the same time both on the fetal neck and maxilla.

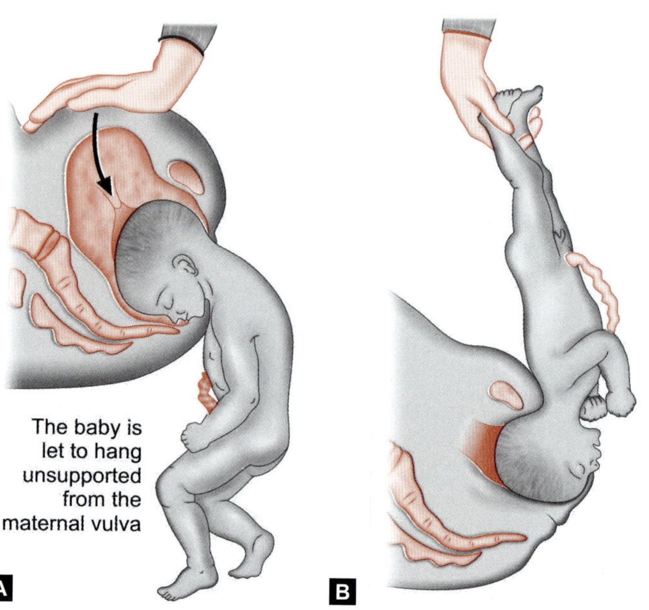


**Figs 4.6A and B:** Burns Marshall technique

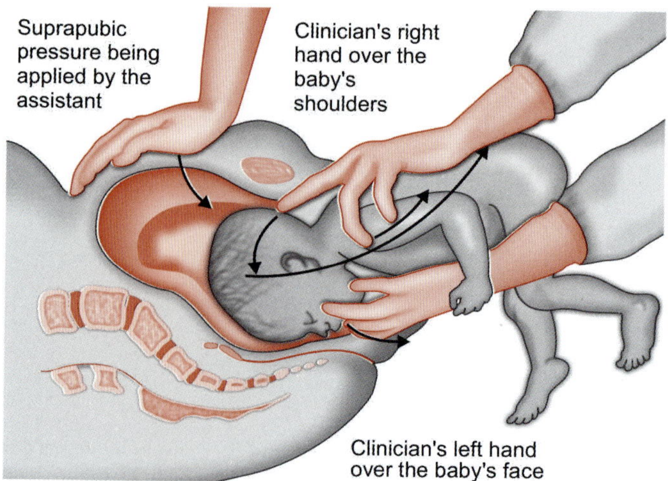


**Fig. 4.7:** Mauriceau–Smellie–Veit maneuver

*Delivery of After-Coming Head Using Forceps*

Application of forceps (Fig. 4.8) is the technique of choice to ensure safe delivery of baby's head because it provides protection to the fetal head from sudden forces of compression and decompression. Also, the use of forceps helps in better maintenance of flexion of fetal head and helps in transmitting the force to the fetal head rather than the neck. This helps in reducing the risk of fetal injuries. Furthermore, flexion of fetal head helps in reducing the diameter of fetal head, thereby aiding descent.

- Ordinary forceps or Piper's forceps (specially designed forceps with absent pelvic curve) or divergent Laufe's forceps can be used.
- While the clinician is applying forceps, the baby's body must be wrapped in a cloth or towel and held on one side by the assistant. Suspension of the baby in a towel prior to application of forceps helps in effectively holding the baby's body and keeping the arms out of the way. At the time of application of forceps, the assistant must hold the infant's body at or just above the horizontal plane. Assistant must be instructed not to hold the fetal body higher than this plane because hyperextension of fetal neck can cause injuries such as dislocation of cervical spine, bleeding in the venous plexus around the cervical spine and sometimes—even quadriplegia.
- Left blade of the forceps is applied first followed by the right blade and the handles are then locked.

  The forceps are used for both flexing and delivering the baby's head. During the initial descent of fetal head, fetal body must remain in horizontal plane. Once the chin and mouth are visible over the perineum, the forceps, body and legs of the fetus are raised to complete delivery.
- The head must be delivered slowly over 1 minute in order to avoid sudden compression or decompression of fetal head, which may be a cause for intracranial hemorrhage.

## Delivery of Baby's Shoulders

*Reverse Prague's Maneuver*

At times, the back of fetus may fail to rotate anteriorly. In these cases, stronger traction on fetal legs or bony pelvis may be applied to turn the back anterior. If the baby's back still remains posterior, head can be extracted using Mauriceau maneuver and delivering the baby with back down. Alternatively, modified Prague's maneuver can be used (Fig. 4.9). In this maneuver, two fingers of clinician's one hand grasp the shoulders of back down fetus from below and exert traction in downward and backward direction. Simultaneously, the other hand draws the feet up over the maternal abdomen to flex the infant and aid the delivery of occiput.

*Løvset's Maneuver*

If the baby's arms are stretched above the head, a maneuver called Løvset's maneuver is used for delivery of fetal arms. This maneuver is based on the principle that due to the curved shape of the birth canal, when the anterior shoulder is above the pubis symphysis, the posterior shoulder would be below the level of pubic symphysis. The maneuver should be initiated only when the fetal scapula becomes visible underneath the pubic arch and includes the following steps (Figs 4.10A to C):

- First the baby is lifted slightly to cause lateral flexion of the trunk.
- Then the baby which is held by pelvifemoral grip is turned by half a circle, keeping the back uppermost. Simultaneously, downwards traction is applied so that the arm that was initially posterior and below the level of pubic symphysis now becomes anterior and can be delivered under the pubic arch.

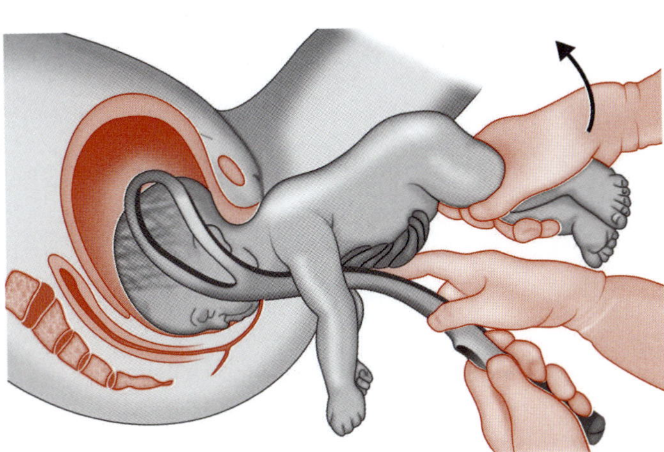

**Fig. 4.8:** Delivery of after-coming head of the breech using forceps

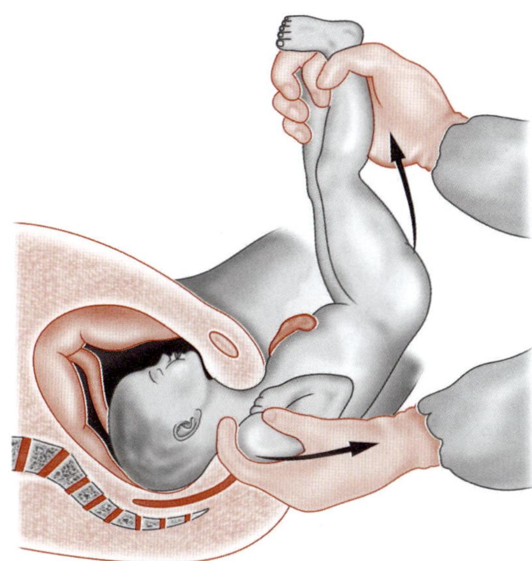

**Fig. 4.9:** Prague's maneuver

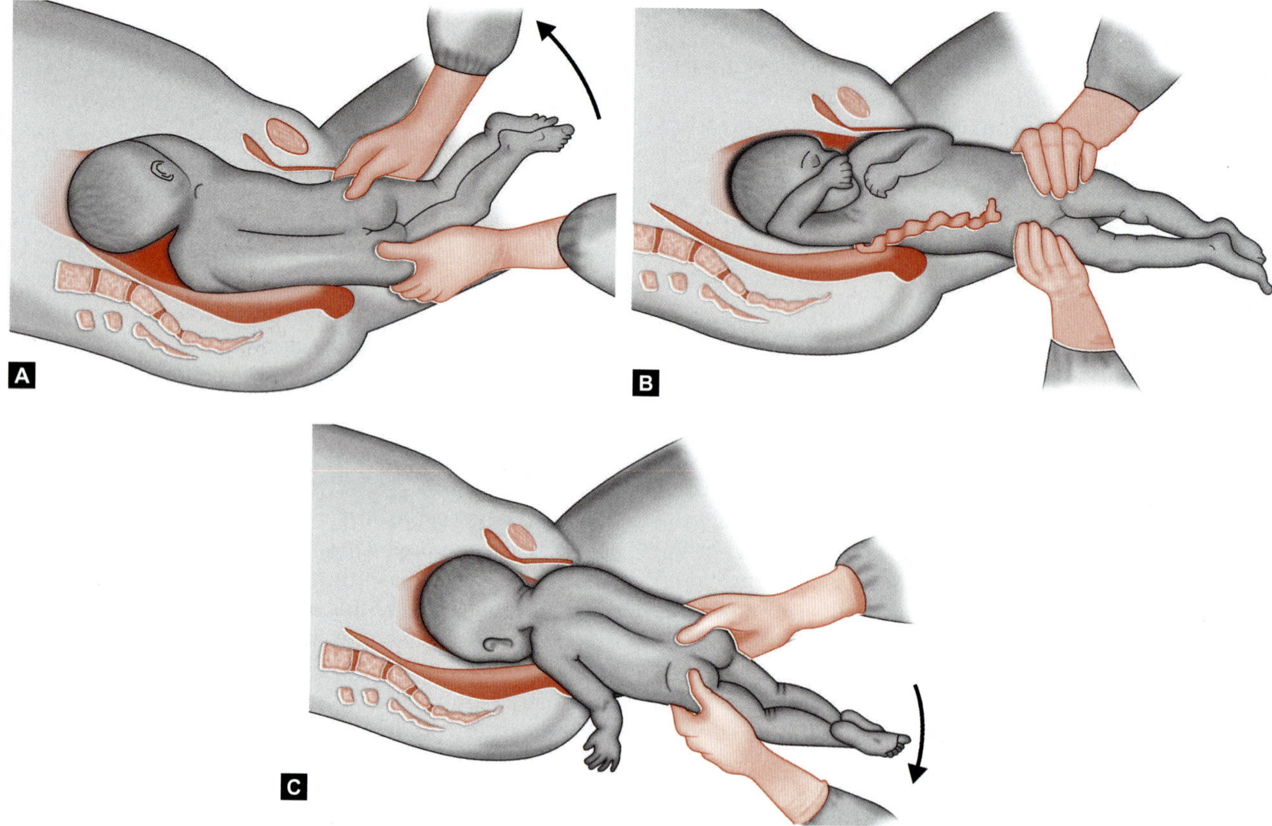

**Figs 4.10A to C:** Løvset's maneuver. (A) Trunk is rotated through 180° keeping the back anterior. This causes the posterior arm to emerge under the pubic arch; (B) Posterior arm is hooked out; (C) Trunk is rotated in reverse direction to deliver the anterior shoulder

Delivery of the arm can be assisted by placing one or two fingers on the upper part of the arm. Then the arm is gradually drawn down over the chest as the elbow is flexed, with the hand sweeping over the face.

- In order to deliver the second arm, the baby is again turned by 180° in the reverse direction, keeping the back uppermost and applying downward traction and then delivering the second arm in the same way under the pubic arch as the first arm was delivered.

### Delivery of the Posterior Shoulder

If the clinician is unable to turn the baby's body to deliver the arm that is anterior first, through Løvset's maneuver, then the clinician can deliver the shoulder that is posterior first (Fig. 4.11). Delivery of the posterior shoulder involves the following steps:

- The clinician must hold and lift the baby up by the ankles. At the same time, the baby's chest must be moved towards the woman's inner thighs. The clinician must then hook the baby's shoulder with fingers of his/her hand. This would help in delivering the shoulder that is posterior, followed by the delivery of arm and hand.

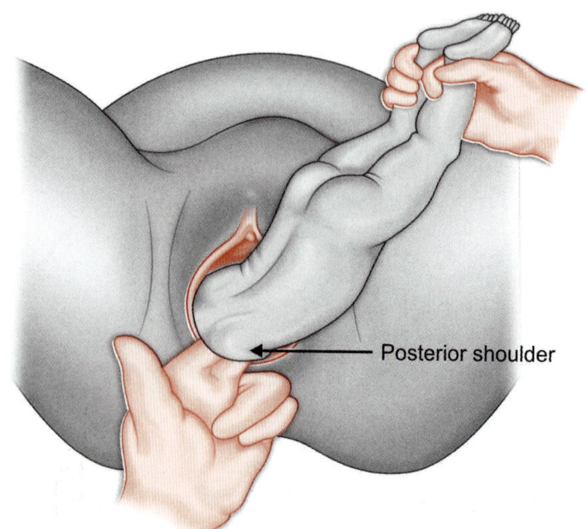


**Fig. 4.11:** Delivery of the shoulder that is posterior

- Then the baby's back should be lowered down, still holding it by ankles. This helps in the delivery of anterior shoulder followed by the arm and hand.

## Delivery of Baby's Legs

### Groin Traction

If the buttocks and hip do not deliver by themselves, the clinician can make use of simple maneuvers including groin traction or Pinard's maneuver to deliver the legs. Groin traction could be of two types: single or double groin traction. In single groin traction, the index finger of one hand is hooked in the groin fold and traction is exerted towards the fetal trunk rather than towards the fetal femur, in accordance with the uterine contractions. In double groin traction, the index fingers of both the hands are hooked in the groin folds and then traction is applied (Fig. 4.12).

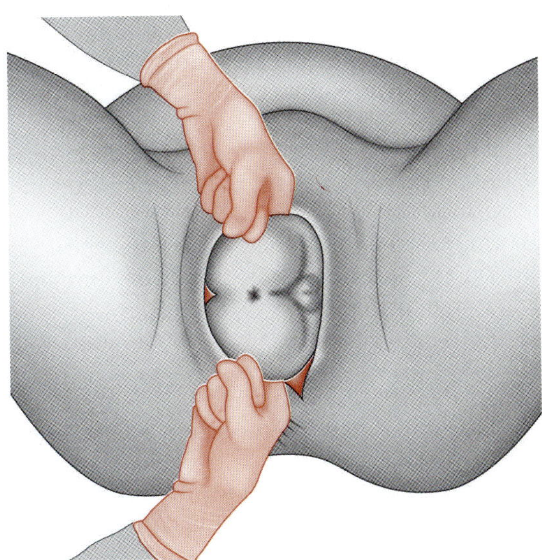

**Fig. 4.12:** Application of double groin traction

### Pinard's Maneuver

In this maneuver, pressure is exerted against the inner aspect of the knee (popliteal fossa), with help of the middle and index fingers of the clinician (Fig. 4.13A). As the pressure is applied, the knee gets flexed and abducted. This causes the lower leg to move downwards, which is then swept medially and gently pulled out of the vagina (Figs 4.13B and C).

## Post-Delivery Care

- The baby's mouth and nose must be suctioned
- The cord must be clamped and cut
- Active management of the third stage of labor needs to be done.

The cervix and vagina must be carefully examined for presence of any tears and the episiotomy must be repaired.

# Occipitoposterior Position

## Introduction

This is a type of abnormal position of the vertex where the occiput is placed over the left sacroiliac joint (LOP or 4th vertex) or right sacroiliac joint (ROP or 3rd vertex) (Figs 4.14A and B) or directly over the sacrum (direct occipitoposterior position). Occipitoposterior (OP) position can be considered as an abnormal position of the vertex rather than an abnormal presentation. ROP is more common than the LOP position as dextrorotation of the uterus favors ROP if the back is on right side. Also, the left oblique diameter is slightly reduced in size due to the presence of sigmoid colon due to which the right oblique diameter is slightly longer than the left oblique diameter.

Cesarean section is not indicated per se in the cases of OP position. Most of the fetuses in OP position before labor

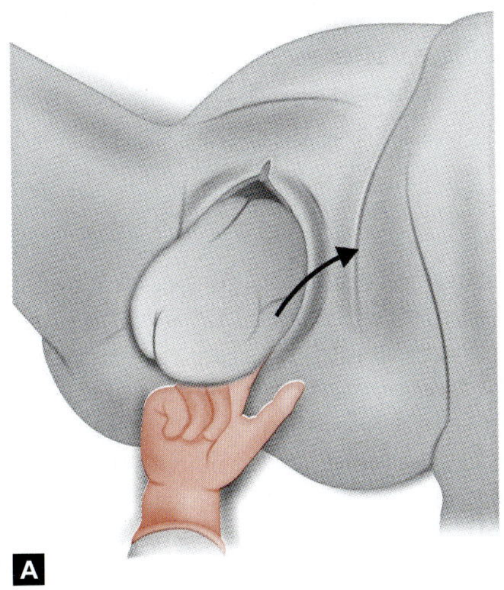



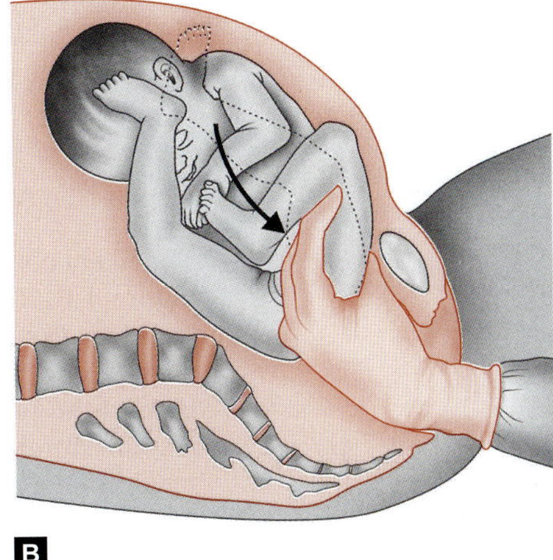



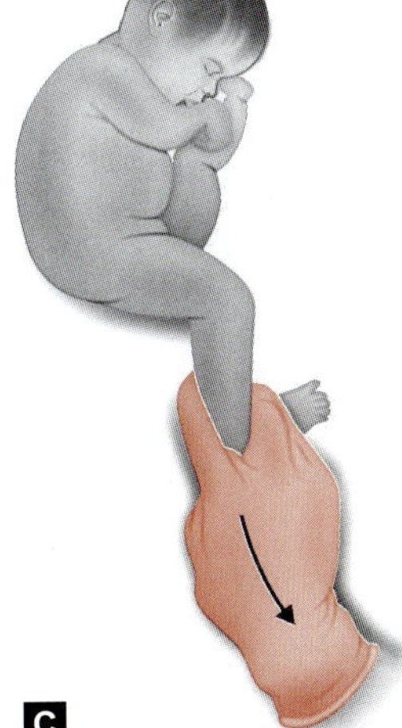



**Figs 4.13A to C:** Pinard's maneuver

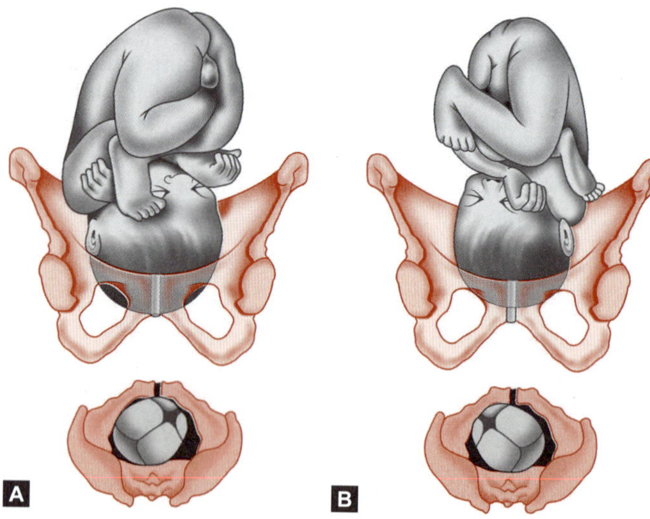

**Figs 4.14A and B:** (A) Right occipitoposterior position; and (B) Left occipitoposterior position

rotate back into OA position in the intrapartum period. Persistence of the OP position is important because it can be associated with labor abnormalities and numerous maternal and neonatal complications (e.g. birth trauma, neonatal acidosis, etc.). The likely outcomes in case of OP position are summarized in Flow chart 4.1.

## Etiology

Some risk factors for the development of OP position are as follows:

- Presence of an anthropoid or android pelvis.
- High pelvic inclination.
- Attachment of placenta on the anterior uterine wall.
- Brachycephaly of fetal head.
- Abnormal uterine contractions.
- Nulliparity.
- Maternal age over 35 years.
- Obesity.
- African-American race.
- Previous OP delivery.
- Decreased pelvic outlet capacity.
- Maternal kyphosis: The convexity of fetal back fits with the concavity of maternal spine (created due to maternal lumbar kyphosis).
- Gestational age greater than or equal to 41 weeks.
- Birthweight greater than or equal to 4,000 g.
- Prolonged first and/or second stage of labor.

## Diagnosis

### Abdominal Examination

- On abdominal inspection there is flattening of the abdomen below the umbilicus.

- Fetal limbs are palpated more easily nearly the midline on either side.
- Fetal back and anterior shoulders are far away from the midline.
- On pelvic grip, the head is not engaged. The cephalic prominence is not felt as prominently as felt in OA position (Figs 4.15A and B). The fetal heart sound (FHS) is difficult to locate and may be best heard in the flanks.

### Vaginal Examination

- Presence of an elongated bag of membranes.
- Posterior fontanel and lambdoid suture are felt near the sacroiliac joint.
- Anterior fontanel can be felt more easily due to the deflexed head and at times it may be at a lower level than the posterior one. Anterior fontanel would be felt anteriorly, while the posterior fontanel would be posterior and hence difficult to feel, especially if the head is deflexed.
- Sagittal sutures would be in one of the oblique diameters of maternal pelvis (e.g. right oblique diameter in case of ROP position).
- Cervix may not be well applied to the presenting part.
- With the progress of labor, posterior fontanel is felt laterally and then anteriorly.

In addition to the above, vaginal examination also shows the following:

- Degree of deflexion of fetal head.
- Degree of molding of fetal head (presence of caput succedaneum).
- Degree of cervical dilatation and effacement.
- Rupture of membranes (ROM) and cord prolapse.
- Direction of the occiput.
- Exclusion of contracted pelvis.

In late labor, diagnosis may be difficult due to considerable molding and formation of caput succedaneum over the presenting part which obliterates the sutures and the fontanels. In these cases, the occiput can be identified by the direction of the unfolded pinna, which points towards the occiput.

## Obstetric Management

The likely consequences related to OP position are shown in Figure 4.16. In majority of cases, good uterine contractions result in the flexion of fetal head. Descent occurs and the occiput undergoes rotation by three-eighths of the circle to lie behind the pubic symphysis, resulting in an OA position. In a small number of cases, the outcome may be unfavorable, resulting in short anterior rotation, nonrotation or short posterior rotation. In case of short anterior rotation, the occiput rotates through one-eighth of the circle anteriorly so that the sagittal sutures lie in the bispinous diameter.

**Flow chart 4.1:** Occipitoposterior position and its likely outcomes

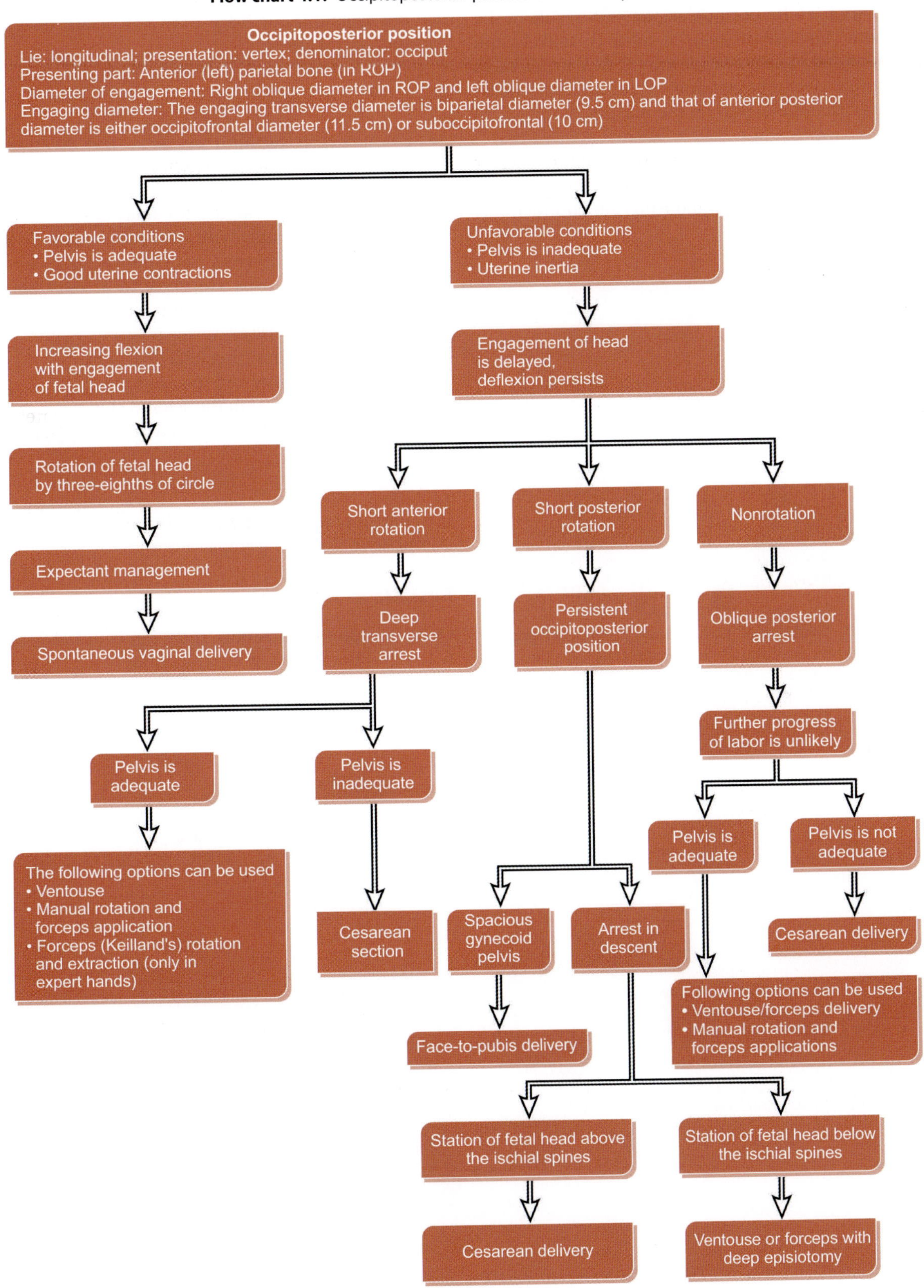

This position is known as the "deep transverse arrest". In case of nonrotation of the occiput, sagittal sutures lie in the oblique diameter. Further progress of labor is unlikely and this is known as "oblique posterior arrest". In case of short posterior rotation, posterior rotation of the sinciput occurs by one-eighth of the circle, putting the occiput in the sacral hollow.

This position is known as persistent occipitoposterior (POP) position. Under favorable conditions with an average-sized baby, spacious pelvis and good uterine contractions,

spontaneous face-to-pubis delivery can occur. If conditions are not favorable, delivery may not occur, resulting in an "occipitosacral arrest".

## Expectant Management

Occipitoposterior position per se is not an indication for cesarean delivery. The most common mode of management in the cases of occipitoposterior position comprises of watchful expectancy hoping for fetal descent and anterior rotation of the occiput. With expectant management, more than 50% multiparous women and more than 25% nulliparous women with OP fetuses are likely to achieve spontaneous vaginal delivery. Prerequisites for expectant management of OP position are described next:

- Presence of a reassuring fetal heart rate
- Average-sized baby and spacious pelvis
- Continued progress in the second stage
- Multiparous women with persistent OP fetuses.

## Intrapartum Management

Intrapartum management in the cases of OP position comprises of following steps:

### First Stage of Labor

Occipitoposterior position may be commonly associated with conditions such as contracted pelvis, cord presentation

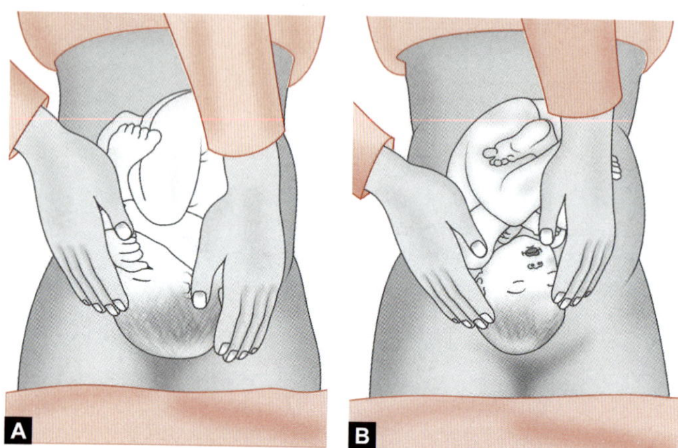

**Figs 4.15 A and B:** Palpation of the fetal head (third pelvic grip). (A) Occipitoanterior position; (B) Occipitoposterior position

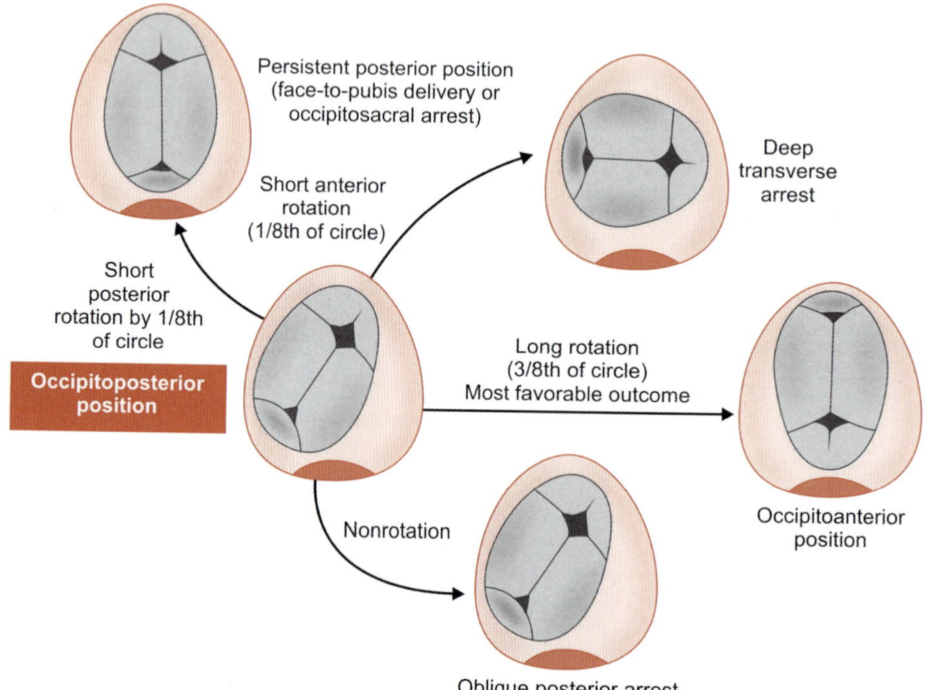



**Fig. 4.16:** Consequences related to occipitoposterior position

or cord prolapse. Therefore, pelvis must be assessed for adequacy and cord presentation or prolapse must be ruled out at the time of vaginal examination. Since cases of OP position are more liable to poor and abnormal progress of labor, PROM and abnormal and/or incoordinate uterine action, the following steps must be taken:

- Intravenous infusion of Ringer's lactate must be started in anticipation of prolonged labor.
- Due to high chances of PROM, the following steps must be observed to avoid early ROM:
  - Bed rest.
  - Maternal straining to be avoided even if there is a premature urge to bear down.
  - High enema must be avoided.
  - Vaginal examination must be minimized.
- There may be marked backache. Therefore, analgesic drugs in the form of pethidine or epidural analgesics may be administered.
- Since uterine inertia and prolonged labor are expected, oxytocin infusion must be started unless there is some contraindication present.
- Watchful expectancy must be observed for around 1 hour hoping for long anterior rotation of the occiput, which will result in normal delivery in 90% of the cases.

*Second Stage of Labor and Delivery of the Baby*

- During the second stage of labor, mother and fetus must be carefully assessed.
- Oxytocin can be used to combat inertia unless there is some contraindication to the use of oxytocin.
- Liberal episiotomy should be given to prevent perineal tears.
- Since in the majority of cases, long anterior rotation of head occurs, delivery occurs spontaneously or with application of low forceps or ventouse.
- In cases of occipitotransverse or oblique OP positions, ventouse application can be done. In cases of POP, under favorable conditions with an average-sized baby, spacious pelvis and good uterine contractions, spontaneous face-to-pubis delivery or vaginal delivery with the aid of forceps/ventouse can occur.
- Manual rotation of fetal head or rotation using Kielland's forceps, both of which were previously performed are no longer done nowadays.
- Nowadays, cesarean section is the most commonly used mode of delivery in cases of POP or occipitosacral arrest and deep transverse arrest.

## Complications

Complications related to occipitiposterior position are as follows:

- Prolonged duration of both first and second stages of labor (due to labor dystocia; delayed engagement of the fetal head and abnormal uterine contractions with slow dilatation of cervix.
- Early ROM.
- Extreme degree of molding of fetal skull can result in tentorial tears.
- Increased tendency for postpartum hemorrhage.
- High chances of perineal injuries and trauma including complete perineal tears: there are higher chances of perineal injuries with face-to-pubis delivery because the biparietal diameter stretches the perineum and occipitofrontal diameter emerges out of the introitus.
- High maternal morbidity due to an increased rate of operative delivery.
- Increased perinatal morbidity and mortality due to asphyxia or trauma.

# Deep Transverse Arrest

Deep transverse arrest can occur in cases of OP position where there is nonrotation of the occiput. As a result, in these cases, the occipitofrontal diameter is caught at the narrow bispinous diameter of the outlet. This occurs in about 1% of cases. The head is placed deep inside the pelvic cavity; sagittal suture is placed in the transverse bispinous diameter and there is no progress in the descent of fetal head even after half an hour to 1 hour of full cervical dilatation. Some likely causes for deep transverse arrest are as follows:

- Faulty pelvic architecture (prominent ischial spines, flat sacrum, convergent side walls, narrow pubic arch, etc.).
- Deflexed fetal head.
- Weak uterine contractions.
- Laxity of pelvic floor muscles.

### MANAGEMENT

Cesarean section may not be required in all cases with deep transverse arrest. In cases of even slight suspicion of cephalopelvic disproportion, cesarean delivery is the best option. In cases where there are no contraindications for vaginal delivery, the following methods of operative vaginal delivery can be employed:

- Ventouse application.
- Manual rotation and application of forceps.
- Forceps rotation and delivery with Kielland's forceps (refer to Chapter 6 for details).

Operative vaginal delivery in the form of manual/forceps rotation should only be performed in the hands of an expert who is conversant with these techniques. In absence of a skilled clinician, delivery via cesarean section is the best option.

### Manual Rotation

Manual rotation of fetal head must be avoided in the first stage of labor because this may disengage the fetal head, which could lead to prolapse of the umbilical cord. Rotation is more likely to be successful in the second stage of labor when the cervix has fully dilated. However, performing prophylactic manual rotation prior to the arrest of descent is likely to be more successful than the procedure performed after arrest of descent. When prophylactic rotation is performed, it must be performed at the beginning of the second stage, regardless of the station of the fetal head.

### Prerequisites

- The maternal bladder must be emptied prior to the procedure.
- The procedure is usually performed under general anesthesia.
- The patient must be placed in lithotomy position.
- Complete surgical asepsis must be maintained.
- Vaginal examination must be performed prior to the procedure to identify the direction of occiput.

### Procedure of Three-Finger Rotation

- In the procedure of three-finger rotation of fetal head (Figs 4.17A and B), the clinician uses tips of his/her index and middle fingers of the right hand to apply pressure on the fetal head at the level of the diameter of engagement. The pressure is applied on the side of fetal head or the parietal eminence.
- In right occipitotransverse (ROT) and ROP positions, the fingers are placed anterior to the head in the anterior segment of the lambdoidal suture near the posterior fontanel. Pressure is applied by the ulnar border of hand to perform digital rotation.
- In left occipitotransverse (LOT) and LOP positions, the fingers are placed posterior to the head and the pressure is applied by the radial border of the hand.

- After flexing and slightly dislodging the vertex, the clinician then rotates the fetal head to the OA position by rotating his/her hand and forearm.
- The fetal head may need to be held in place for a few contractions to prevent rotation back towards the posterior position.

### Full-Hand Method (Five-Finger Rotation)

- In this method (Figs 4.18A to F), the clinician's whole hand is used. The right hand is used for LOP and LOT) positions, whereas the left hand is used for ROP and ROT positions.
- After taking complete aseptic precautions, the clinician's corresponding supinated hand is introduced inside the vagina in a cone-shaped manner after separating the labia with two fingers of the other hand.
- In OT position, the clinician's four fingers are pushed in the sacral bay behind the posterior parietal bone with the palm up in such a way that the thumb is placed over the anterior parietal bone. The head is then grasped with the tips of the fingers and thumb. In oblique OP position, the four fingers of supinated hand are placed over the occiput and thumb over the sinciput.
- During a contraction, the patient is encouraged to push and the clinician attempts to flex and rotate the fetal head anteriorly by pronating his/her hand.
- Simultaneously, the back of fetus is rotated externally by the clinician's free hand or by an assistant in order to move the back from the flank into the midline.
- Manual rotation is more successful in multiparous women and women less than 35 years of age. The procedure of manual rotation may be unsuccessful due to the failure to grip the head because of lack of space or failure to dislodge the head from its impacted position. Sometimes, there

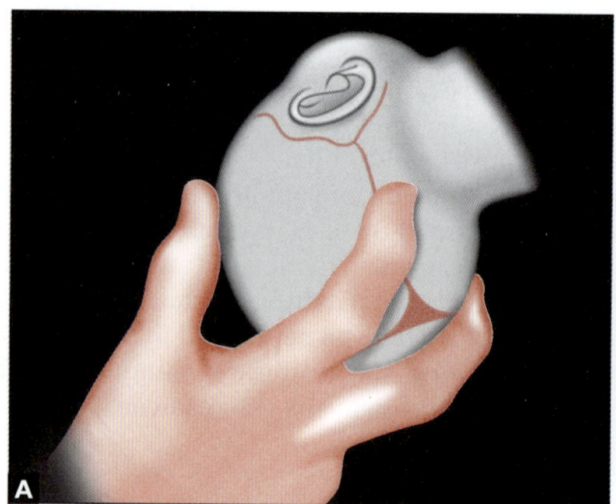 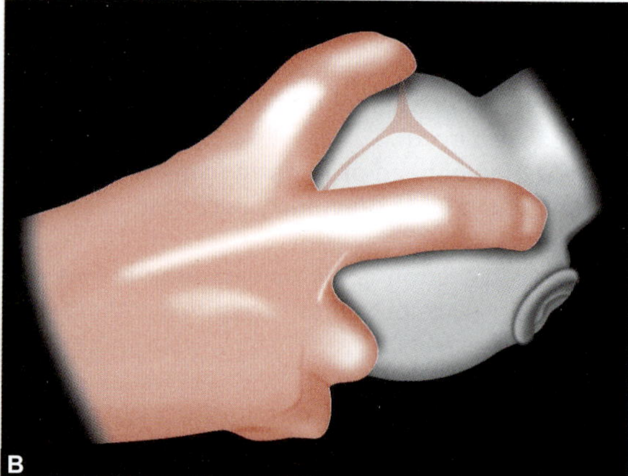

**Figs 4.17A and B:** Procedure of three-finger rotation of fetal head. The tips of the index and middle fingers are placed in the anterior segment of the lambdoidal suture near the posterior fontanels. The fingers are used for rotating the fetal head to the occipitoanterior position via rotation of the operator's hand and forearm

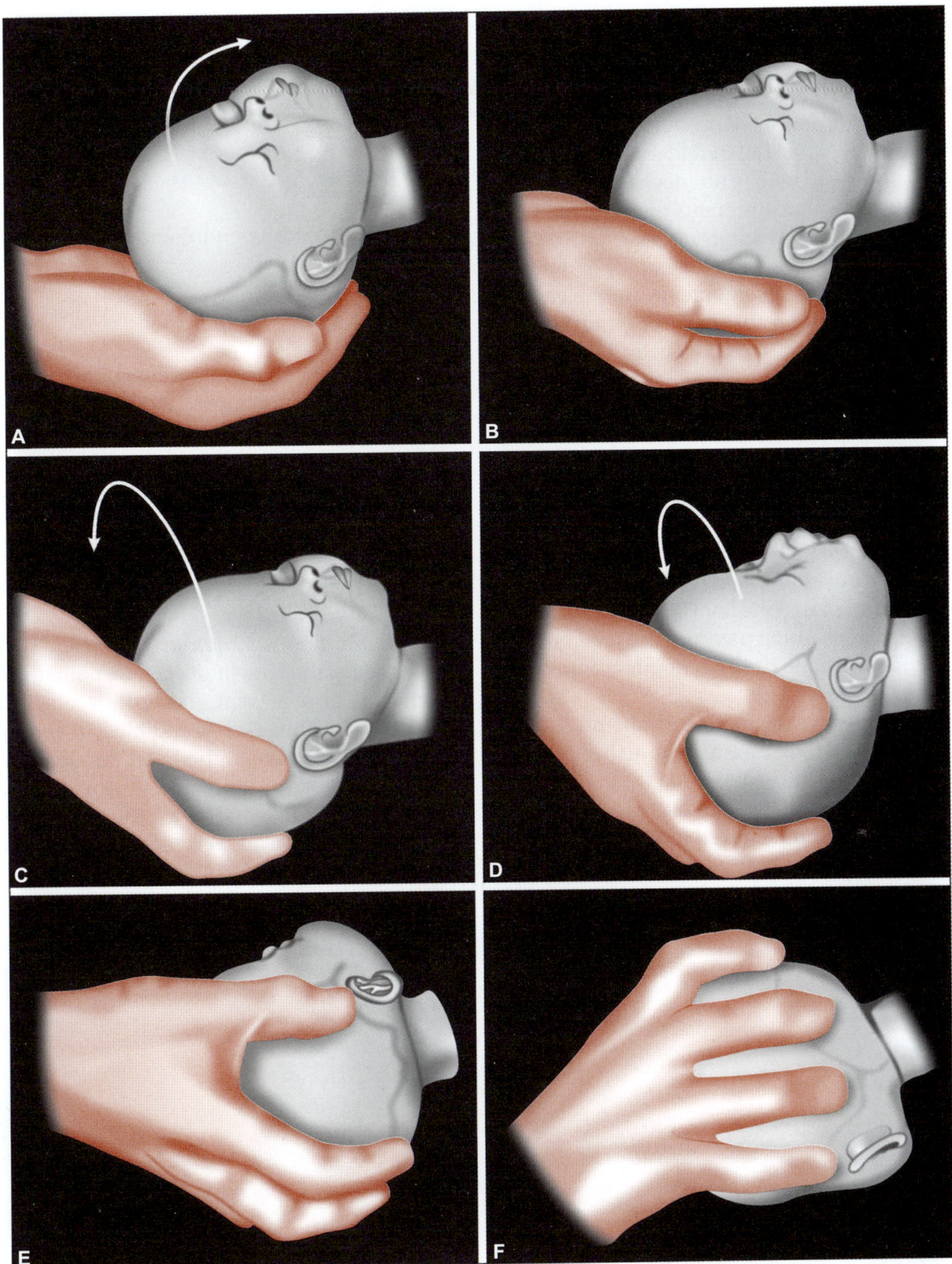

**Figs 4.18A to F:** The procedure of five-finger rotation of fetal head. (A) The operator places four fingers behind the posterior parietal bone with the palm up and the thumb over the anterior parietal bone. The head is grasped with the tips of the fingers and thumb; (B to F) During a contraction, the patient is encouraged to push and the operator attempts to flex and rotate the fetal head to the occipitoanterior position

may be accidental slipping of the head above the pelvic brim and resultant cord prolapse. Cesarean delivery is commonly performed after a failed manual rotation. However, if prompt delivery is indicated, failed manual rotation may be followed by vacuum or forceps delivery from the OP position in an appropriately assessed patient.

- The maneuvers of manual rotation must be performed only by skilled and experienced clinicians, fully conversant in this technique.

# Transverse Lie

## Introduction

Transverse lie is an abnormal fetal presentation in which the fetus lies transversely with the shoulders presenting in the lower pole of the uterus. There is no mechanism of labor for a fetus in transverse lie, which remains uncorrected until term. The management options for transverse lie include external cephalic version (ECV) during pregnancy or delivery by cesarean section (elective or an emergency). If the version is unsuccessful, the only option for delivering the fetus in transverse lie is performing a cesarean delivery. For details regarding the management of transverse lie, kindly refer to Chapter 5.

# Face Presentation

## Introduction

This is an abnormal fetal position characterized by an extreme extension of the fetal head so that the fetal face rather than the fetal head becomes the presenting part and the fetal occiput comes in direct contact with the back. Denominator in these cases is mentum or chin.

Four positions are possible depending on the position of the chin with left or right sacroiliac joints (Fig. 4.19):
- Right mentoposterior position (deflexed LOA)
- Left mentoposterior position (deflexed ROA)
- Left mentoanterior position (deflexed ROP)
- Right mentoanterior position (deflexed LOP).

The most common type of face presentation is left mentoanterior position.

## Etiology

### Maternal Causes

- Multiparity with pendulous abdomen.
- Contracted pelvis.

### Fetal Causes

- Congenital causes (anencephaly, congenital goiter, congenital bronchocele, etc.).
- Several twists of cord around fetal neck.
- Dolicocephalic head (with long AP diameter).
- Increased tone of extensor group of muscle.

## Diagnosis

### Clinical Examination

- *Abdominal examination:* In case of mentoanterior positions, the fetal limbs can be palpated anteriorly. Fetal chest is also present anteriorly against the uterine wall. The FHS is thus clearly audible. On abdominal palpation, the groove between the head and neck is not prominent and cephalic prominence lies on the same side as the fetal back. On abdominal examination in case of face presentation, head feels big and is often not engaged.

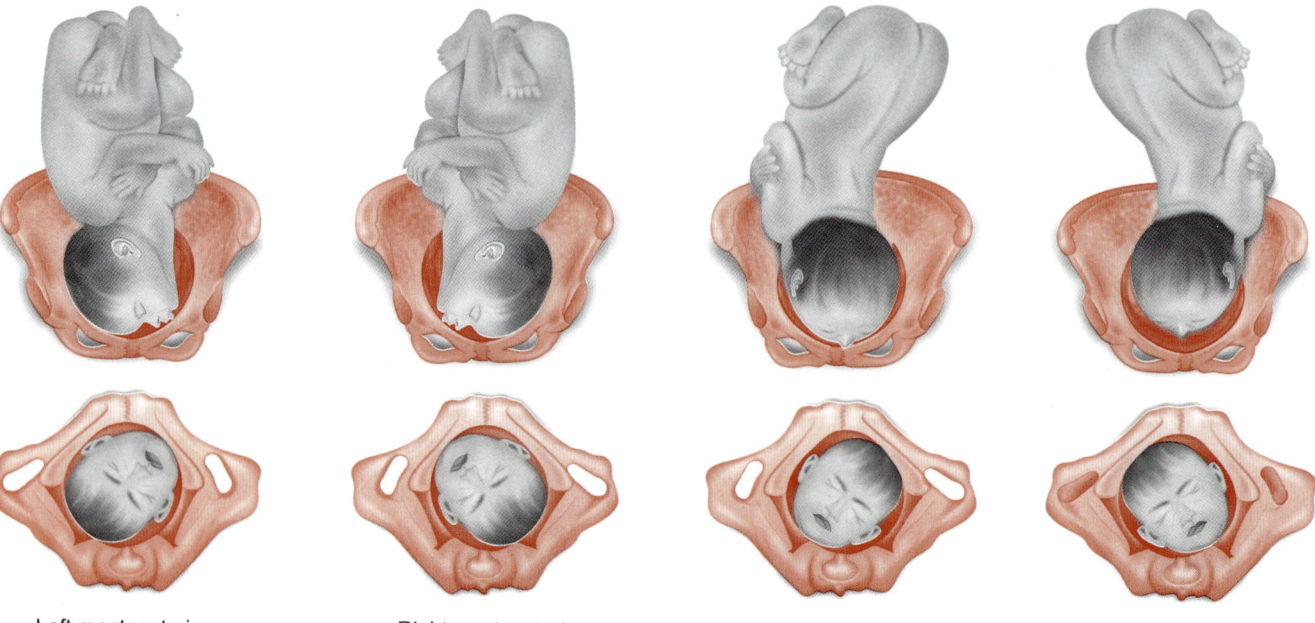



**Fig. 4.19:** Different positions in face presentation

- On pelvic grip, the head is not engaged. In case of mentoposterior positions, the back is better palpated towards the front.
- *Vaginal examination:* Diagnosis of face presentation is made on vaginal examination. On the vaginal examination, the following structures can be felt: alveolar margins of the mouth, nose, malar eminences, supraorbital ridges and the mentum (Fig. 4.20). There is absence of meconium staining on the examining fingers, unlike in breech presentation.

### Investigation

- *Ultrasonography:* Ultrasonography must be performed in order to assess fetal size and to rule out the presence of any bony congenital malformations.

### Differential Diagnosis

Diagnosis of face presentation can often be confused with that of breech presentation. This can be differentiated from breech presentation with the help of following two rules:
1. When the examining finger is inserted into the anus, it offers resistance due to the presence of anal sphincters.
2. Anus is present in line with the anal sphincters, whereas the mouth and malar prominences form a triangle.

### Obstetric Management

Delivery occurs spontaneously in most of the cases. In presence of normal cervical dilatation and descent, there is no need for the clinician to intervene. Labor will be longer, but if the pelvis is adequate and the head rotates to a mentoanterior position, a vaginal delivery can be expected.
- The mechanism of delivery and corresponding body movements in case of anterior face presentations are

similar to that of the corresponding OA positions. The only difference is that delivery of head occurs by flexion rather than extension. The engaging diameter is submentobregmatic in case of a fully extended head. If the head rotates backwards to a mentoposterior position, a cesarean section may be required. Although, the engaging diameter of the head in flexed vertex and face presentation is the same [submentobregmatic in face (9.5 cm) and suboccipitobregmatic in case of vertex (9.5 cm)], the clinical course of labor is significantly delayed. This could be due to the ill-fitting face in the lower uterine segment, which results in delayed engagement due to the absence of molding.
- While conducting a normal vaginal delivery, one should wait for spontaneous delivery. Liberal mediolateral episiotomy must be given to protect the perineum against injuries.
- Forceps may be applied in case of delay.
- Indications for an elective cesarean section in case of face presentation include co-existing conditions such as contracted pelvis, large sized baby or presence of associated complicating factors.
- In case of posterior face presentations, the mechanism of delivery is same as that of OP position except that the anterior rotation of the mentum occurs in only 20–30% of the cases. In the remaining 70–80% cases, there may be incomplete anterior rotation, no rotation or short posterior rotation of mentum. There is no possibility of spontaneous vaginal delivery in case of persistent mentoposterior positions. Cesarean section may be required in these cases.

### Complications

- Increased chances of cord prolapse.
- Delayed labor.
- Risk of perineal injuries.
- Postpartum hemorrhage.
- Caput formation and molding.
- Increased rate of operative deliveries.
- Fetal cerebral congestion due to poor venous return from head and neck.
- Neonatal infection.
- Increased maternal morbidity due to operative delivery and vaginal manipulation.
- Neglected cases of face presentation may result in obstructed labor and uterine rupture.
- Marked caput formation and molding may distort the entire face. This usually subsides within a few days.

## Brow Presentation

### Introduction

This is a type of cephalic presentation where the fetal head is incompletely flexed (Fig. 4.21). The head is short of complete

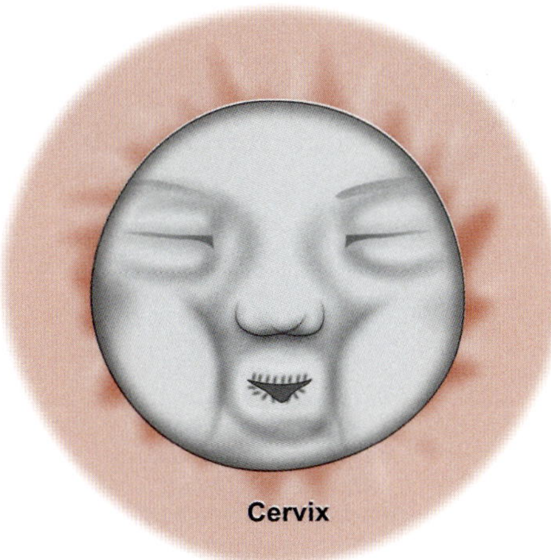


**Fig. 4.20:** Vaginal touch picture in case of face presentation

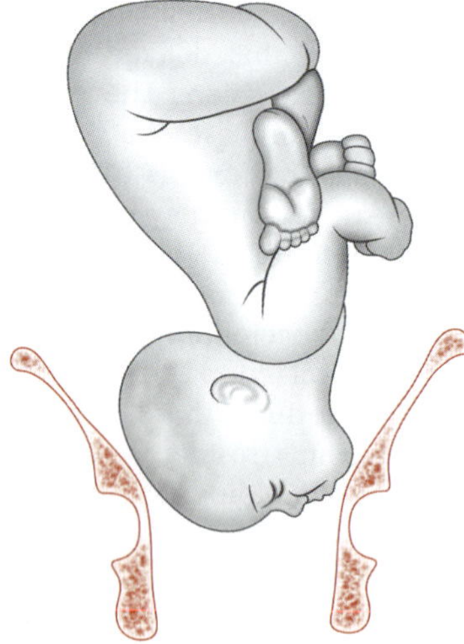

**Fig. 4.21:** Brow presentation

extension, which could have resulted in a face presentation. As a result, presenting part becomes the brow. Brow presentation may temporarily persist as it may get converted to either a vertex or face presentation with complete flexion or extension respectively. The predisposing factors for the brow presentation are similar to that for face presentation.

## Diagnosis

### Abdominal Examination

Findings on abdominal examination are similar to that of face presentation.

### Vaginal Examination

Brow presentation can be confirmed on vaginal examination due to the presence of supraorbital ridges and anterior fontanel.

### Investigations

*Ultrasonography:* This helps in ruling out the presence of any congenital malformations.

## Obstetric Management

Since the engaging diameter of the head is mentovertical (14 cm), there would be no mechanism of labor with an average-sized baby and a normal pelvis. Vaginal delivery may be the possible option only in cases where there is spontaneous conversion to face or vertex presentation. Therefore, after ruling out the cephalopelvic disproportion and fetal congenital anomalies, the clinician must await spontaneous delivery. In cases where this does not occur, cesarean section is the best method of treatment.

## Complications

- Obstructed labor and uterine rupture can occur in cases of neglected brow presentation.
- There can be considerable amount of molding and caput formation of the fetal skull.

# Cord Prolapse

## Introduction

Cord prolapse has been defined as descent of the umbilical cord through the cervix alongside the presenting part (occult presentation) or past it (overt presentation) in the presence of ruptured membranes. In occult prolapse, the cord cannot be felt by the examiner's fingers at the time of vaginal examination. In overt cord prolapse, the cord is found lying inside the vagina or outside the vulva following the ROM (Fig. 4.22). Cord presentation, on the other hand, is the presence of one or more loops of umbilical cord between the fetal presenting part and the cervix, with the membranes being intact (Fig. 4.23). Incidence of cord prolapse has greatly reduced due to the increased use of elective cesarean deliveries in cases of noncephalic presentation.

## Etiology

Various probable causes of cord prolapse are listed in the Table 4.1.

## Diagnosis

### Investigations

- *Cardiotocography:* There may be variable decelerations of heart rate pattern on continuous electronic fetal monitoring

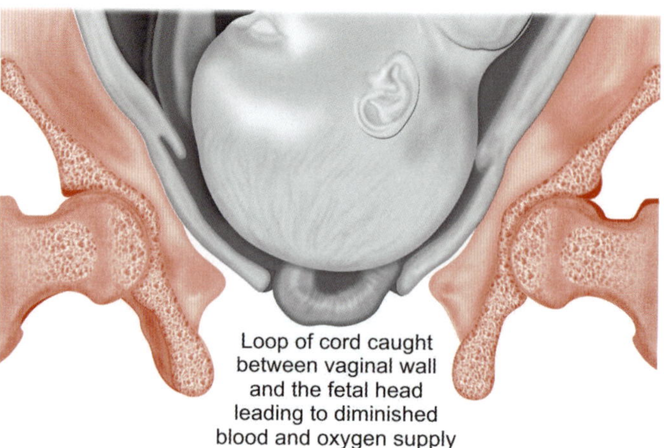


**Fig. 4.22:** Overt cord prolapse

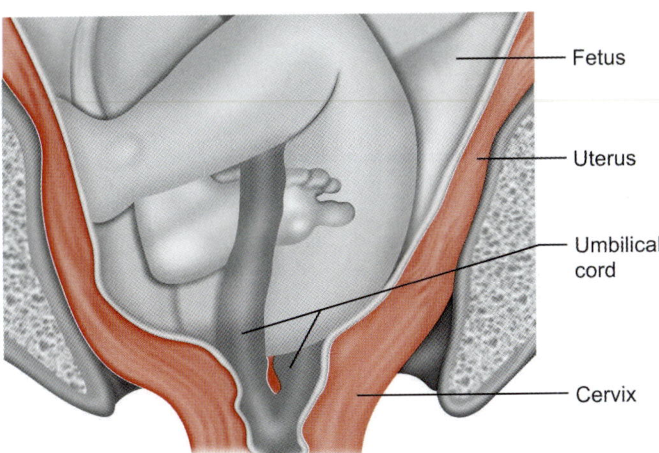



**Fig. 4.23:** Cord presentation

| **Table 4.1:** Causes of cord prolapse | |
| --- | --- |
| *General causes* | *Procedure related causes* |
| • Multiparity<br>• Low birthweight (< 2.5 kg)<br>• Prematurity (< 37 weeks)<br>• Fetal congenital anomalies<br>• Breech/shoulder presentation<br>• Second twin<br>• Polyhydramnios<br>• Unengaged presenting part<br>• Low placenta and other abnormal placentation<br>• Cord abnormalities (such as true knots or low content of Wharton's jelly) | • Artificial ROM (particularly with unengaged head)<br>• Vaginal manipulation of fetus with ruptured membranes<br>• External cephalic version<br>• Internal podalic version<br>• Stabilizing induction of labor<br>• Application of fetal scalp electrodes or placement of intrauterine catheters |

*Abbreviation:* ROM, rupture of membrane

- *Ultrasound examination:* Ultrasound, specifically Doppler ultrasound may help in identification of umbilical cord within the cervix.

## Management

Management of cases of cord prolapse has been described in Flow chart 4.2.

### Prevention and First Aid

- Artificial ROM should be avoided whenever possible if the presenting part has yet not engaged or is mobile. In cases where ROM becomes necessary even in such circumstances, this should be performed in an operation theater with facilities available for an immediate cesarean birth.

- In cases of cord prolapse where immediate vaginal delivery is not possible, assistance should be called immediately; venous access should be obtained, consent taken and immediate preparations be made for an urgent cesarean delivery. The following steps can be followed until facilities for cesarean section are made available:
  - To prevent vasospasm, there should be minimal handling of loops of cord lying outside the vagina, which can be covered with surgical packs soaked in warm saline.
  - To prevent cord compression, it is recommended that the presenting part be elevated either manually or by filling the urinary bladder with normal saline.
  - Cord compression can be further reduced by advising the mother to adopt knee-chest position or head-down tilt (preferably in left lateral position).
  - In order to prevent vasospasm of umbilical artery, there should be minimal handling of loops of cord lying outside the vagina.

### Definitive Management

Definitive management comprises of immediate delivery:

- In cases where vaginal delivery is possible, forceps can be applied in cases of cephalic presentation if the head has engaged. In case of breech presentation, breech extraction can be done.
- A cesarean section is the recommended mode of delivery in cases of cord prolapse when vaginal delivery is not imminent. A cesarean section should ideally be performed within 30 minutes or less (from the point of diagnosis to the delivery of the baby).

## Complications

*Maternal:* These is an increased maternal morbidity due to greater incidence of operative delivery.

*Fetal:* Cord compression and umbilical artery vasospasm may cause asphyxia, which may result in hypoxic-ischemic encephalopathy and cerebral palsy.

# Compound Presentation

## Introduction

In compound presentation, one or two of the fetal extremities enter the pelvis simultaneously with the presenting part. The most common combinations are head-hand (Fig. 4.24); breech-hand and head-arm-foot.

## Etiology

The predisposing factors for the development of compound presentation are described next:

**Flow chart 4.2:** Management of cases of cord prolapse

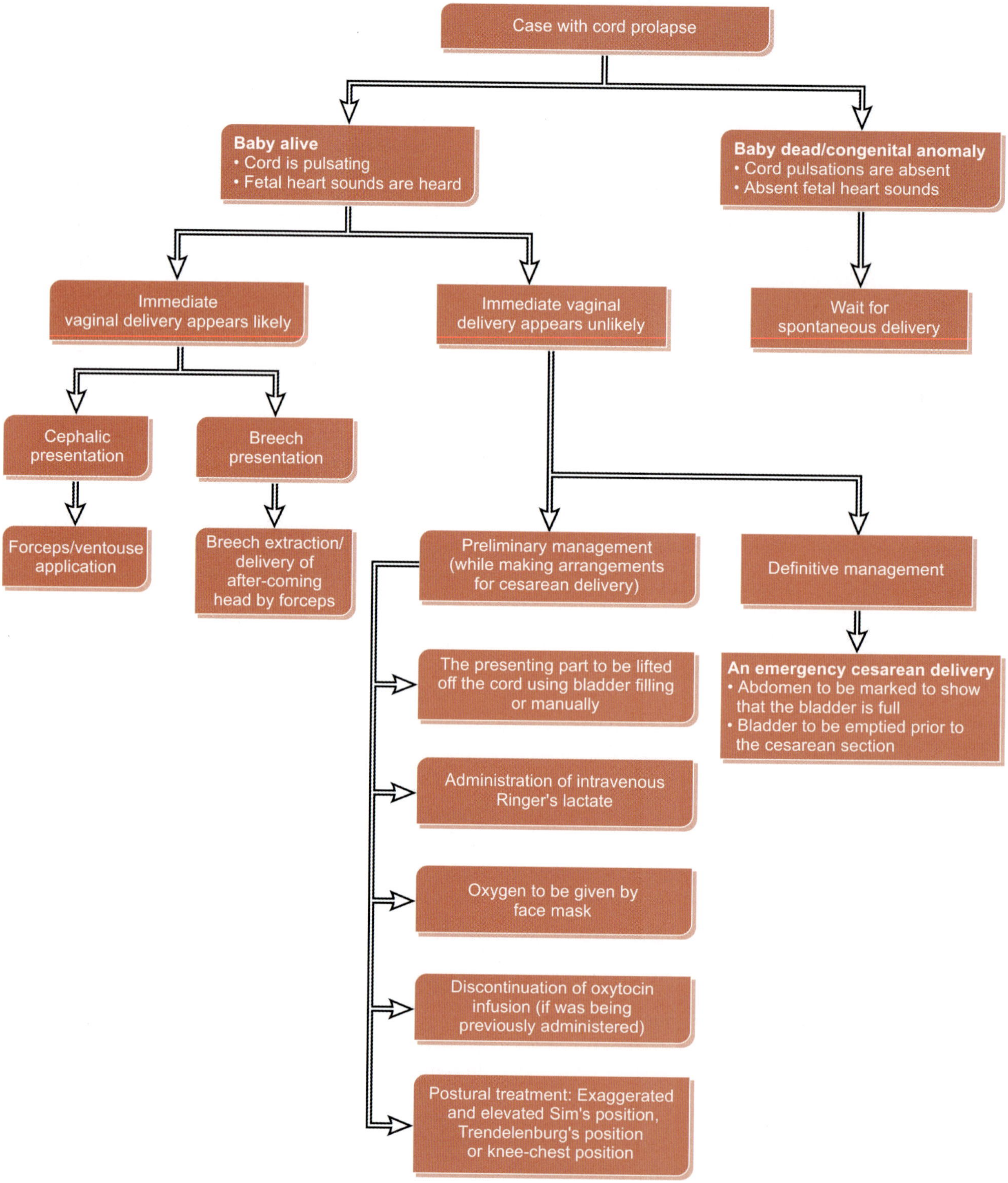

Case with cord prolapse

**Baby alive**
• Cord is pulsating
• Fetal heart sounds are heard

**Baby dead/congenital anomaly**
• Cord pulsations are absent
• Absent fetal heart sounds

Immediate vaginal delivery appears likely

Immediate vaginal delivery appears unlikely

Wait for spontaneous delivery

Cephalic presentation

Breech presentation

Forceps/ventouse application

Breech extraction/ delivery of after-coming head by forceps

Preliminary management (while making arrangements for cesarean delivery)

Definitive management

The presenting part to be lifted off the cord using bladder filling or manually

**An emergency cesarean delivery**
• Abdomen to be marked to show that the bladder is full
• Bladder to be emptied prior to the cesarean section

Administration of intravenous Ringer's lactate

Oxygen to be given by face mask

Discontinuation of oxytocin infusion (if was being previously administered)

Postural treatment: Exaggerated and elevated Sim's position, Trendelenburg's position or knee-chest position

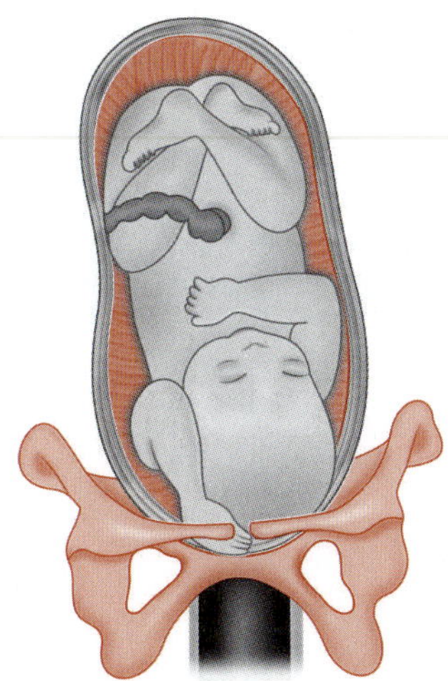

**Fig. 4.24:** Compound presentation where the fetal hand is seen to be entering the pelvis

- Prematurity
- Multiparity
- Twin/multiple gestation
- Pelvic tumors
- Cephalopelvic disproportion
- Macerated fetus.

## Diagnosis

*Clinical Presentation*

The diagnosis is confirmed on vaginal examination.

## Obstetric Management

In most cases, the prolapsed extremity does not cause any interference with the normal progress of labor and vaginal delivery. In most of the cases, the prolapsed limbs spontaneously rise up with the descent of the presenting part.

In presence of cephalopelvic disproportion and/or cord prolapse, cesarean section is required.

## Complications

- The most common complication associated with that of compound presentation is cord prolapse.
- Temptation to replace the limb early during labor is associated with an increased maternal and fetal mortality and morbidity.

## FURTHER READINGS


1. Committee on Obstetric Practice. ACOG committee opinion. Mode of term singleton breech delivery. Number 265, December 2001. American College of Obstetricians and Gynecologists. Int J Gynaecol Obstet. 2002;77(1):65-6.
2. ACOG Committee on Obstetric Practice. ACOG Committee Opinion No. 340. Mode of term singleton breech delivery. Obstet Gynecol. 2006;108(1):235-7.
3. Cruikshank DP, Cruikshank JE. Face and brow presentation: a review. Clin Obstet Gynecol. 1981;24:333-51.
4. Edwards RL, Nicholson HO. Management of the unstable lie in late pregnancy. J Obstet Gynaecol Br Commonw. 1969;76(8):713-5.
5. Løvset J. Vaginal operative delivery. Oslo: Scandinavian University Books; 1968.
6. Phelan JP, Boucher M, Mueller E, et al. The nonlaboring transverse lie. A management dilemma. J Reprod Med. 1986;31(3):184-6.
7. Posner AC, Friedman S, Posner LB. Modern trends in the management of the face and brow presentations. Surg Gynecol Obstet. 1957;104:485-90.
8. Royal College of Clinicians and Gynaecologists (RCOG). The management of breech presentation. London (UK): Royal College of Clinicians and Gynaecologists; 2006. p. 13 (Green-top guideline; no. 20b).

# 5

**C H A P T E R**

# Cases in Obstetrics

## CHAPTER OUTLINE

- Anemia in Pregnancy
- Hypertensive Disorders in Pregnancy
- Breech Presentation
- Previous Cesarean Delivery
- Multifetal Gestation
- Abnormalities of Liquor
- Polyhydramnios
- Transverse Lie
- Intrauterine Growth Restriction
- Antepartum Hemorrhage
- Intrauterine Death
- Preterm Labor, PROM
- Post-Term Pregnancy
- Bad Obstetric History/Recurrent Pregnancy Loss
- Rh Isoimmunization
- Cardiac Disease in Pregnancy
- Diabetes in Pregnancy

## Anemia in Pregnancy

### Case Study 1

Mrs XYZ, a 28-year-old woman, married for 8 years, resident of ABC, G4P3L3 with 28 weeks of gestation presents with complaints of easy fatigability and dyspnea since last 2 weeks. On general physical examination, pallor was observed on the lower palpebral conjunctiva, tongue and palmar surface of hands. Pedal edema of pitting type was present. No other significant finding was observed on systemic examination. Abdominal examination revealed presence of pregnancy corresponding to about 28 weeks of gestation with cephalic presentation.

#### Q. What is the likely diagnosis in the above-mentioned case study?

**Ans.** The above-mentioned case study most likely corresponds to anemia during pregnancy (to be confirmed by investigations). The questions to be asked at the time of taking history and the parameters to be assessed at the time of examination in such a case are described in Tables 5.1 and 5.2 respectively. The most likely diagnosis in this case is Mrs XYZ, 28-year-old woman, married for 8 years, resident of ABC, G4P3L3 with 7 months period of amenorrhea corresponding to 28 weeks period of gestation, with history and clinical examination suggestive of anemia in pregnancy. Diagnosis of anemia can only be confirmed only after the estimation of hemoglobin levels.

#### Q. What is anemia?

**Ans.** Anemia is one of the most common medical disorders present globally. It can be defined as reduction in circulating hemoglobin mass below the critical level. WHO defines anemia as presence of hemoglobin of less than 11 g/dL and hematocrit of less than 0.33 g/dL. CDC (1990) has defined anemia as hemoglobin levels below 11 g/dL in the pregnant woman in first and third trimester and less than 10.5 g/dL in second trimester. However, in India and most of the other developing countries, the lower limit is often accepted as 10 g percent. Depending on the levels of circulating hemoglobin in the body, WHO has graded anemia as mild (10–10.9), moderate (8–9.9), severe (7.9–7) and life-threatening (< 7.0).

#### Q. What are the causes for development of physiological anemia during pregnancy?

**Ans.** The two main reasons for development of physiological anemia due to pregnancy are:

1. Physiological hemodilution resulting in disproportionate increase in plasma volume.
2. Negative iron balance during pregnancy.

In developing countries, majority of women enter pregnancy in an already iron-depleted condition and may be consuming an iron-deficient diet. Iron depletion can be attributed to young age of childbearing and frequent occurrence of pregnancies in a woman without allowing the recovery of iron stores in the body. Moreover, in developing countries, most people consume vegetarian, low bioavailability diet which is low in ascorbic acid and

| **Table 5.1:** Symptoms to be elicited at the time of taking history in a case of anemia |
|---|
| *History of Presenting Complains* |
| • Vague complains of ill health, loss of appetite, digestive upset, breathlessness, palpitation, easy fatigability, fainting, lightheadedness, tinnitus, headache, restlessness, tiredness or exhaustion, nocturnal leg cramps, edema of the feet, hyperemesis in the first trimester, etc.<br>• The woman may also experience headache, paresthesias and numbness in the extremities, oral and nasopharyngeal symptoms (e.g. burning of tongue), dysphagia (due to mucosal atrophy in the laryngopharynx), hair loss, etc. |
| *Dietary History* |
| • A detailed dietary history is important. Vegetarians are more likely to develop iron deficiency. In developing countries due to poor socioeconomic conditions, patients may not be able to afford good nutritious diet rich in iron and proteins.<br>• History of pica: Pica can be the etiology of iron deficiency amongst people who habitually eat clay, dirt, paint or laundry starch. One-half of patients with moderate IDA may develop pagophagia, in which they develop strong craving to suck ice. |
| *History of Hemorrhage* |
| • Blood loss in any form from the body from any of the orifices (hematuria, hematemesis, hemoptysis, malena, excessive menstrual loss, etc.) needs to be elicited. Since occult bleeding from the gastrointestinal tract often goes unrecognized, the patient needs to be specifically asked if she ever had ulcers in the gastrointestinal tract. History of chronic ingestion of aspirin or other NSAIDs need to be elicited as this is commonly associated with occult gastric ulcerations.<br>• History of melanotic stools can be elicited by asking the patient if she has ever passed black-colored stools (provided that she is not taking iron). She should also be asked about the history of passing worms in the stool.<br>• History of excessive menstrual blood loss: The patient may not be able to give the correct estimate of menstrual blood loss, thus she should be specifically asked about the number of tampons or pads she needs to use in a day during the time of her periods and whether her menstrual flow is associated with passage of clots. Frequent pad changes and passage of clots signify greater blood loss. |
| *Obstetric History* |
| • Taking the history of obstetric factors such as gravidity, parity and history of previous preterm or small-for-gestational age deliveries and multifetal pregnancy is important.<br>• History of giving birth to babies at frequent intervals before the women has a chance to replenish her depleted iron stores is an important reason for development of anemia in women with low socioeconomic status, especially in developing countries.<br>• History of excessive blood loss at the time of delivery or during the antenatal period in her previous pregnancies.<br>• History of taking iron supplements during her previous pregnancies.<br>• Undernourished and anemic women are often observed to give birth to preterm or small-for-gestational age babies. |
| *Socioeconomic History* |
| • History regarding various social and demographic factors including age, level of formal education, marital status, area of residence (areas with hookworm infestation, malaria, etc.) needs to be elicited. |
| *Behavioral History* |
| • History related to smoking or tobacco usage, alcohol usage, utilization of prenatal care services, etc. should be asked. |
| *Medical History* |
| • History of medical conditions (diabetes, renal or cardiorespiratory diseases, chronic hypertension, etc.) can further aggravate the development of anemia during pregnancy. Cardiac disease must be ruled out by taking the history of chest pain, palpitations and cough with expectoration. |
| *Menstrual History* |
| • It is important to take a detailed history of previous menstrual cycles including the amount of blood loss and the number of days the blood loss occurs. Small amount of menstrual blood loss occurring over a long period of time can also result in the development of anemia. |
| *Treatment History* |
| History of taking iron supplements during pregnancy: An easy way of assessing whether the woman is speaking truth regarding the intake of iron tablets is to ask her the color of the stools. Due to continuous ingestion of iron tablets, the color of stools invariably turns black. |

*Abbreviations:* IDA, iron-deficiency anemia; NSAIDs, nonsteroidal anti-inflammatory drugs

high in biological proteins composed entirely of cereals (containing excessive iron inhibitors such as phytates), which further reduce iron absorption.

**Q. What are the probable causes of anemia during pregnancy?**
**Ans.** Anemia in pregnancy has a multifactorial etiology. Various factors responsible for aggravating anemia during pregnancy include the following:

• Prior history of menorrhagia (loss of more than 80 mL of blood per month)
• Multiparity, multiple gestations (multiple births at frequent intervals resulting in the depletion of iron stores)
• Low intake of dietary iron, vegetarian diet, low in heme iron
• Intake of a diet containing low amounts of vitamin C (which facilitates iron absorption) and high amount of phytates (which interfere with the absorption of iron)

**Table 5.2:** Various findings elicited at the time of clinical examination in a case of anemia

*General Physical Examination*

- *Pallor:* Reduced amount of oxygenated hemoglobin in anemic individuals results in development of nonspecific pallor of the mucous membranes. Paleness may be observed on the woman's face. Clinical examination may reveal pallor in lower palpebral conjunctiva, tongue, nail beds, palmar surface of hands, lips, vagina (on per speculum examination), etc.
- *Epithelial changes:* The epithelial tissues of nails, tongue, mouth, hypopharynx and stomach are affected resulting in development of brittle, fragile, spoon-shaped nails, glossitis, angular stomatitis, atrophic gastritis, etc.
- *Nail changes:* Thinning, flattening and development of concave "spoon-shaped nails", also known as koilonychias, occur.
- *Changes in the tongue or mouth:* There may be atrophy of lingual papilla accompanied by soreness or burning of the tongue. Glossitis and stomatitis can also develop. Angular stomatitis, characterized by development of ulcerations or fissures at the corners of the mouth is a less specific sign of anemia. It is commonly associated with deficiency of riboflavin or pyridoxine.
- *Jaundice:* Jaundice could be related to the presence of hemolytic anemia.
- *Pedal edema:* In severely anemic cases, there may be pedal edema.
- *Septic focus:* One must look for the presence of septic focus (suggestive of chronic infection) anywhere in the body (e.g. sore throat, dental caries, etc.).
- *Signs suggestive of congestive cardiac failure:* Raised jugular venous pressure (JVP), basal rales, liver tenderness and edema of the feet could be suggestive of congestive cardiac failure in cases with severe anemia.

*Specific Systemic Examination*

- *Cardiovascular system:* In cases of severe anemia increased blood flow to the heart results in the development of tachycardia and a soft systolic ejection murmur. In rapidly developing anemia (e.g. from hemorrhage), additional symptoms and signs may be noted, e.g. syncope on rising from bed, orthostatic hypotension (i.e. the blood pressure falls when the patient is raised from the supine to the sitting or standing positions) and orthostatic tachycardia.
- *Respiratory system:* Bilateral crepitations in the lungs could be related to the presence of congestion.
- *Abdominal examination:* Normal obstetric examination to be carried out (as described in Chapter 1).

- Inadequate iron absorption
- Chronic blood loss due to hookworm infestation, schistosomiasis, etc.
- Chronic infection (e.g. malaria)
- Chronic aspirin use.

### Q. What are the causes of microcytic anemia in pregnancy and how can one differentiate between them?

**Ans.** The three most common causes of microcytic anemia in pregnancy are iron deficiency anemia (IDA), thalassemia and anemia due to chronic infection.

- *Iron deficiency anemia:* IDA usually develops, when body iron stores become inadequate for normal erythropoiesis. Iron deficiency is the most common cause of anemia during pregnancy.
- *Thalassemia:* Thalassemia includes a group of genetically inherited disorders, which are characterized by impaired or defective production of one or more normal globin peptide chains. Abnormal synthesis of globin chains can result in ineffective erythropoiesis, hemolysis and varying degrees of anemia.
- *Chronic iron-deficiency anemia:* Anemia can be produced due to the diseases like chronic renal insufficiency, hypothyroidism, malignancies (hematologic malignancies, leukemia, lymphoma, myeloma, etc.). Anemia due to chronic disease is caused by a reduction in both the lifespan of existing RBCs and in the number of new RBCs produced to replace dying RBCs.

Iron deficiency anemia can be differentiated from other causes of hypochromic anemia including thalassemia and anemia due to chronic diseases (Table 5.3).

Anemia due to thalassemia can be differentiated on the basis of erythrocyte indices. Although MCV may be reduced in thalassemia to values as low as 60–70 fL, values this low are rarely encountered in cases with IDA. Serum iron concentration is usually normal or increased in thalassemic syndromes, while it is usually low in IDA. Bone marrow examination and hemoglobin electrophoresis also help in differentiating between IDA and thalassemia by respectively showing normal bone marrow iron stores and increased proportions of HbF and HbA2 in cases with thalassemia.

### Q. How should the cases of anemia be managed in pregnancy?

**Ans.** Treatment of the pregnant patient diagnosed with IDA basically depends on the period of gestation, severity of anemia and presence of any associated complications. If the period of gestation is less than 30 completed weeks, oral iron preparations (200 mg of ferrous sulfate containing 60 mg of elemental iron to be given thrice a day with or after meals) along with 500 µg of folic acid must be prescribed. This therapy must be continued until the peripheral smear becomes normal. After this, a maintenance dose of one tablet daily is continued for at least 100 days following delivery to replenish the iron stores.

If the patient is not compliant with oral therapy or other causes for ineffective oral treatment are present, parenteral therapy may be considered. Also, if period of gestation is between 30 to 36 weeks, parenteral therapy must be

**Table 5.3:** Differentiation between iron deficiency anemia and anemia due to chronic diseases

| Blood index | Iron-deficiency anemia | Anemia due to chronic diseases | Thalassemia |
| --- | --- | --- | --- |
| Peripheral smear | Microcytic hypochromic anemia | Microcytic hypochromic anemia (20–30%) | Microcytic hypochromic anemia |
| Serum iron | Reduced | Normal | Normal or high |
| TIBC | High | Reduced | Normal |
| Percentage saturation | Reduced (< 16%) | Reduced (> 16%) | Normal or high |
| Serum ferritin | Reduced | Normal | High |
| MCV, MCHC, MCH | All reduced proportionally to the severity of anemia | Low/normal | All reduced to very low levels in relation to the severity of anemia |
| HbF and HbA$_2$ | Normal | Normal | High |
| Bone marrow iron stores | Absent | Present | Present |

*Abbreviations:* TIBC, total iron binding capacity; HbF, fetal hemoglobin; HbA2, hemoglobin A consisting of two alpha and two delta chains; MCV, mean corpuscular volume; MCHC, mean corpuscular hemoglobin concentration; MCH, mean corpuscular hemoglobin

administered. The rise in hemoglobin levels by the parenteral route is same as that with oral route, but this route is preferred during 30–36 weeks of pregnancy as it guarantees certainty of administration. If the patient presents with severe anemia beyond 36 weeks and there is not enough time to achieve a reasonable hemoglobin level before delivery, blood transfusion may be required.

## Case Study 2

Mrs XYZ, a 28-year-old married for 6 years, resident of ABC, G5P3A1L3 woman with 6 months period of gestation presents with complaints of easy fatigability, dyspnea, weakness, poor appetite and chronic tiredness since past 6 months. On general physical examination, pallor was observed on the lower palpebral conjunctiva, tongue and palmar surface of hands. Pedal edema of pitting type was present. The vital signs were within normal limits (WNL), chest was clear bilaterally and the uterus was just palpable supraumbilically corresponding to 12 weeks of gestation. No other significant finding was observed on systemic examination. She also gave the history of using an intrauterine contraceptive device (IUCD) prior to this pregnancy due to which, she used to experience heavy menstrual bleeding. The device was eventually removed 6 weeks prior to the time of conception.

### Q. What investigations must be performed in the suspected cases of iron-deficiency anemia?

**Ans.** The following investigations need to be done in the suspected cases of IDA:

- *Hemoglobin and hematocrit:* Hemoglobin concentration reflects the capacity of blood to distribute oxygen from the lungs to tissues in the body. In IDA, the hemoglobin levels are typically less than 10 'g' percent. Hematocrit, on the other hand, reflects the measurement of the percentage of RBCs found in a specific volume of blood. Hematocrit is sometimes also known as packed cell volume (PCV).

Normal hematrocit value in women varies between 36.1% and 44.3%. In women with IDA, the hematocrit value may be less than 36.1%. Red cell count is also often measured and is less than 4 million/mm$^3$ in cases of anemia.

- *Blood cellular indices:* Some of these indices are mean corpuscular volume (MCV), mean corpuscular hemoglobin (MCH) and mean corpuscular hemoglobin concentration (MCHC). All these three indices are reduced in IDA. Each if these indices have been described below in details:
  - Mean corpuscular volume: This index indicates the morphology of the RBCs, which could be microcytic, normocytic or macrocytic. MCV is usually less than 76 fL in cases of IDA.

$$MCV = \frac{\text{Packed cell volume}}{\text{Red cell count per liter}} \times 10^{15}\ fL$$

  - Mean corpuscular hemoglobin: This index indicates average weight of hemoglobin in RBC. MCH is reduced in cases of microcytosis and hypochromia. MCH is less than 25 pg/cell in cases of IDA.

$$MCH = \frac{\text{Hb in g \%}}{\text{Red cell count per liter}} \times 10^{13}\ pg/cell$$

  - Mean corpuscular hemoglobin concentration: This index represents weight of hemoglobin/volume of cells. Since this index is independent of cell size, it is more useful than MCH in distinguishing between microcytosis and hypochromia. MCHC is typically less than 30% in cases of IDA. A low MCHC always indicates hypochromia, as a microcyte with a normal hemoglobin concentration will have a low MCH but a normal MCHC.

$$MCHC = \frac{MCH}{MCV} \text{ or } \frac{\text{Hb in g \%}}{\text{PCV}}$$

Out of the various indices used, MCV and MCHC are the two most sensitive indices of iron deficiency.

- *Red cell distribution width:* This indicates the variation in the size of RBCs. Thus, red cell distribution width is elevated in anemia resulting from iron deficiency.
- *Reticulocyte count:* This test helps in measuring the percentage of reticulocytes, which are slightly immature RBCs, in blood. Normally, about 1–2% of the RBCs in the blood are reticulocytes. The reticulocyte count may rise when there is an excessive blood loss or in certain diseases like hemolytic anemia in which RBCs are destroyed prematurely.
- *Peripheral smear:* Examination of the peripheral smear is an important part of the work-up of patients with anemia. The following findings are observed on the peripheral smear:
  - Peripheral blood smear in case of iron deficiency shows microcytic and hypochromic picture. There is presence of pale looking RBCs with large central vacuoles (hypochromic RBCs).
  - Anisocytosis (abnormal size of cells): The RBCs are small and deformed (microcytosis)
  - Poikilocytosis (abnormal shape of cells): Presence of pencil cells and target cells.
  - Presence of ring or pessary cells with central hypochromia (large central vacuoles).
- *Serum iron studies:* A low serum iron (< 60 µg/dL) and ferritin (< 20 ng/mL) with an elevated total iron binding capacity (TIBC) is diagnostic of iron deficiency. Transferrin delivers iron to bone marrow and storage sites. Circulating transferrin is normally only about 30% saturated with iron. The remaining 70% is unbound and represents the TIBC. Percentage saturation of transferrin is less than 10% and serum transferrin levels are more than 360 mg/dL in cases of IDA.
- *Stool examination:* Stool examination for ova and cysts (three consecutive samples) can help in determining if the cause of anemia can be attributed to parasitic infestation. Testing the stools for the presence of hemoglobin is useful in establishing gastrointestinal bleeding as the etiology of IDA.
- *Urine routine/microscopy:* Urine routine/microscopy helps in detecting the presence of pus cells, sugar, proteins/occult blood or schistosomes.
- *Hemoglobin electrophoresis:* Hemoglobin electrophoresis and measurement of HbA2 and fetal hemoglobin are useful in establishing either β-thalassemia or hemoglobin C or D as the etiology of microcytic anemia.
- *Bone marrow examination:* Bone marrow examination is not done as a routine in cases of IDA. While the performance of bone marrow examination for the diagnosis of iron deficiency has largely been displaced by the performance of serum iron, TIBC and serum ferritin, the absence of stainable iron in a bone marrow aspirate reflects absent iron stores.

**Q. Peripheral smear revealed presence of microcytic hypochromic type of anemia. What is the likely cause of anemia in the above-mentioned case study?**

**Ans.** Microcytic hypochromic picture on the peripheral smear examination is suggestive of IDA. In this case the history revealed that the patient had yet not started taking iron supplements and gave a history of menorrhagia related to IUCD use prior to conception. Moreover, she has three children, the oldest being 5 years old and the youngest just 1 year of age. She also had a miscarriage after the birth of her first child at 4 months of gestation. Frequent childbirths could be another cause for depleted iron stores. Also, she conceived the present pregnancy before the restoration of her already depleted iron stores. These could be the reasons for her to develop IDA.

**Q. What would be the first line of management in this case?**

**Ans.** Since in this case the period of gestation is less than 30 weeks, oral iron supplements were prescribed. Use of iron supplements helps in improving the iron status of the mother during pregnancy and during the postpartum period, even in women who enter pregnancy with reasonable iron stores. Since iron is absorbed in ferrous form, only ferrous salts must be used. Iron must be taken orally in 3–4 doses, 1 hour prior to meals. Oral iron therapy must be continued for at least 12 months after the anemia has been corrected in order to replenish the depleted iron stores.

**Q. What are the likely side effects of taking oral iron supplement?**

**Ans.** The main problems associated with the use of iron supplements is occurrence of side effects such as anorexia, diarrhea, epigastric discomfort, nausea, vomiting and constipation, passage of dark-greenish or black-colored stools, temporary staining of teeth, etc. Although associated with gastrointestinal side effects, oral iron supplements are not associated with the anaphylaxis that can occur with parenteral iron preparations.

**Q. What kind of response can be observed with iron therapy?**

**Ans.** Positive response to therapy is indicated by the sense of wellbeing, increased appetite and improved outlook of the patient. The earliest hematological response to iron therapy is reticulocytosis. Initially, there is an increase in reticulocytes by 4–6 days, which peaks by 9–12 days. Hemoglobin levels usually start rising at the rate of 2 g/dL after 3 weeks. The plasma iron will gradually increase and the initially elevated TIBC will return to normal in about 1 month. Blood ferritin levels return to normal in about 4–6 months. If the predictable rise in hemoglobin does not occur after oral iron therapy, the clinician must try to find out the possible reasons.

**Q. What are the methods of reducing side effects associated with oral iron therapy?**

**Ans.** The following steps can be taken for reducing the side effects associated with oral iron therapy:

- Starting with one tablet daily and slowly increasing the dosage every 3–5 days can sometimes help patients tolerate oral iron better than immediately starting with three times daily dosing.
- Avoiding the use of high-dose vitamin C supplements with iron tablets, as this may be associated with increased epigastric pain.
- Taking iron supplements with meals helps in reducing the frequency of side effects, even though this may be associated with reduced iron absorption.
- Administration of iron supplements at bed time.
- Use of iron formulations containing reduced amount of elemental iron.

**Q. What are the causes of failure of oral iron therapy?**

**Ans.** The causes of failure of oral iron therapy are as follows:

- Improper typing of anemia (e.g. presence of folate-deficiency anemia).
- Defective absorption of iron.
- Patient is noncompliant.
- Blood loss due to hookworm infestation or bleeding piles.
- Inhibition of erythropoiesis due to infection.

**Q. What are the factors which reduce the absorption of dietary iron?**

**Ans.** Factors for reducing the absorption of dietary iron are as follows:

- Phytates present in wholegrain cereals, legumes, nuts, seeds, etc.
- Calcium and phosphorus in milk.
- Tannins in tea (a cup of tea taken with meals can inhibit iron absorption by 11%).
- Polyphenols present in many vegetables.
- Increased gastric pH due to presence of antacids or reduced gastric acidity.
- High phenol content of some fruits, e.g. strawberries, melon, etc.
- Cow's milk with high content of calcium and casein inhibits iron absorption.

**Q. What are the methods for improving iron absorption in the diet?**

**Ans.** Methods for improving iron absorption in the diet are as follows:

- Adding lime juice, which is a good source of vitamin C, to one's food.
- Avoiding the intake of substances like tea, coffee and milk with the meals.
- Cooking food in iron vessels.
- Taking iron tablets with orange juice or water rather than with milk, tea or coffee.
- Avoiding the use of antacids with iron as lower gastric acidity reduces absorption of iron.
- Eating fermented food aids iron absorption by reducing the phytate content of diet.

- Increasing the intake of food containing ascorbic acid such as citrus food, broccoli and other dark-green vegetables.
- Increasing the intake of foods containing muscle protein (e.g. meat), which enhance iron absorption.
- Cereal milling to remove bran reduces its phytic acid content by 50%.

## Case Study 3

Mrs XYZ, a 26-year-old married for 4 years, resident of ABC, G3P2L2 woman at 34 completed weeks of gestation visited the ANC clinic with moderate pallor, weakness, poor appetite and easy fatigability. She was pale with vital signs within normal limits. The chest was bilaterally clear and the pregnancy corresponded to 32 weeks of gestation with a single live fetus in cephalic presentation. Minimal bilateral pedal edema was also present. Hemoglobin level was 7.5 g percent.

**Q. What should be the first line of management in this case?**

**Ans.** Since this case presented with severe anemia for the first time during 30–36 weeks of pregnancy, parenteral therapy in this case would be preferred over the oral route due to the certainty of its administration for correction of hemoglobin deficit. Since the response to parenteral iron is not observed before 4–9 weeks, this method is not suitable if at least 4 weeks time is not available to raise hemoglobin to a safe level of 10 g percent. The two main types of parenteral iron preparations, which can be used are iron dextran (Imferon), which can be used both intramuscularly and intravenously and iron sorbitol citrate, which can be used only by IV route. Besides these, another preparation of iron, which can be used via the intravenous route is iron (ferrous) sucrose.

**Q. What are the indications for the parenteral iron therapy?**

**Ans.** Indications for the parenteral iron therapy are as follows:

- Contraindications to the oral therapy (intolerance to oral iron, severe anemia).
- Patient is noncompliant to oral therapy.
- Patient presents for the first time between 30 and 36 weeks of pregnancy with severe anemia.

**Q. What are the risks associated with parenteral iron therapy?**

**Ans.** The main drawback of IM iron is the pain and staining of the skin at the site of injection, development of fever, chills, myalgia, arthralgia, injection abscess, etc. Both IM and IV injections can result in systemic reactions, which may be either immediate or delayed. Immediate side effects include hypotension, vascular collapse, tachycardia, dyspnea, cyanosis, vomiting, pyrexia, headache, malaise, urticaria, nausea and anaphylactic reactions, whereas delayed reactions include lymphadenopathy, myalgia, arthralgia, fever, etc.

The most serious side effects associated with the use of IV iron is the risk of anaphylactic reactions, which can occur in about 0.7% of patients taking IV iron dextran. Allergic reactions can be particularly more common in individuals with previous history of multiple drug allergies. Therefore, before administering parenteral iron, it is important to elicit history regarding allergies to any drugs in the past. Also, total dose of iron therapy by IV route should only be given in a hospital setting where facilities are available to manage severe anaphylactic reactions.

### Q. How is the total dose of iron, which is to be infused, calculated?

**Ans.** Since the symptoms of IDA do not appear until essentially all iron stores have been depleted, therapy should aim not only at the replenishment of hemoglobin iron but iron stores as well. Total dose for iron infusion is calculated through any of the following formulae:

Total dose of iron (mg) = whole blood hemoglobin deficit (g/dL) × body weight in pounds (lb)

or

Dose (mL) = 0.0442 [14 – patient's observed Hb (g/dL) × LBW + (0.26 × LBW)]

LBW = Lean body weight in kg.

or

Total dose (mL) = [patient's weight (kg) × 2.3 (14 – patient's observed hemoglobin (g/dL)] + 500 to 1,000 mg

or

Total dose (mg) = [15 – patient's Hb (g/dL)] × body weight (in kg) × 3

*For women:* lean body weight (LBW) = 45.5 kg + 2.3 kg for each inch of patient's height over 5 feet.

After the total dose of iron has been calculated, the infusion must be prepared by diluting each 5 mL of iron dextran with 100 mL of normal saline. The whole dose can be given in the form of a single infusion or may be divided into three parts to be administered intravenously over 3 consecutive days. The flow rate in the beginning must be kept at 20 drops/minute for the initial 5 minutes. If no side effects are observed, the flow rate may be eventually increased to 40–60 drops/minute. This way the IV infusion is given over 6–8 hours under constant observation.

### Q. What precautions must be observed prior to the administration of intravenous iron?

**Ans.** Precautions to be taken before administration of IV iron are listed next:

- Prior to receiving the therapeutic dose, all patients should be given an IV test dose of 0.5 mL.
- Severe/fatal anaphylactic reactions characterized by respiratory difficulty or cardiovascular collapse have been reported with the use of iron dextran injections. Therefore, the drug should be given only when resuscitation techniques and facilities for treatment of anaphylactic and anaphylactoid shock are readily available.
- Epinephrine should be immediately available in case there is development of acute hypersensitivity reactions. Usual adult dose of epinephrine is 0.5 mL of a 1:1,000 solution, administered through SC or IM route.

- Though most anaphylactic reactions, following IV iron administration, are usually evident within a few minutes, it is recommended that the patient must be observed for at least 1 hour before the administration of remainder of the therapeutic dose. If no adverse reactions are observed, iron can be administered until the calculated total amount of total iron has been administered.

### Q. What is the technique for administering intramuscular iron injections?

**Ans.** Intramuscular iron is administered in the form of daily injections or injections on every alternate day in the dosage of 2 mL intramuscularly. The technique of administration of IM iron injections is as follows:

- An IM test dose of 0.5 mL should be given before the administration of the total IM dose of iron.
- The maximum daily dose of undiluted iron dextran should not exceed 2 mL (100 mg). This dose may be given daily until anemia is corrected.
- Injection should be given into the muscle mass of the upper outer quadrant of the buttock.
- Deep injection with a 2 inch or 3 inch long 19 or 20 G needle is given.
- While giving the injection, the patient must be in a lateral position with the injection site being uppermost.
- A Z-track technique (displacement of the skin laterally prior to injection) is recommended to avoid tattooing of the skin.

### Q. What are the steps for management of anemic patients during intrapartum period?

**Ans.** Precautions to be taken at the time of first stage of labor are as follows:

- Patient's blood grouping and crossmatching needs to be done.
- Though ideally the patient must be placed in a propped up position, the woman can be placed in any position which is comfortable to her.
- Adequate pain relief must be provided.
- Oxygen inhalation through face mask must be provided.
- Digitalization may be required especially if the patient shows a potential to develop congestive heart failure.
- Antibiotic prophylaxis must be given, as the anemic women are prone to develop infections.
- Strict asepsis needs to be maintained at the time of delivery or while performing procedures like artificial rupture of membranes (ARM).
- In case of preterm labor, β-mimetics and steroids must be administered cautiously in order to prevent pulmonary edema.

The precautions, which must be observed during the second stage of labor, are as follows:

- In order to shorten the duration of second stage of labor, forceps or vacuum can be applied prophylactically.

The precautions, which must be taken during the third stage of labor, are as follows:

- Active management of third stage of labor
- Postpartum hemorrhage (PPH) is to be managed aggressively.
- Advice regarding contraception must be given (e.g. barrier contraception).
- Postpartum sterilization may be offered to these women if the family is complete.

### Q. What precautions must be observed to reduce the amount of blood loss at the time of labor and delivery?

**Ans.** The following precautions must be taken during the time of labor and delivery in order to reduce the amount of blood loss:

- Routine administration of oxytocics (methergine, oxytocin, etc.) during delivery in order to reduce the blood loss.
- Late clamping of cord at the time of delivery prevents anemia in infancy and should be employed as a routine practice in all babies. This simple practice helps in transferring 80 mL of blood with 50 mg of iron to the baby.
- Breastfeeding for first 6 months after delivery reduces maternal iron loss by producing amenorrhea. Maternal iron and folic acid supplementation should also be continued in postpartum period.

### Q. What are the adverse effects of anemia on the mother and the baby?

**Ans.** Adverse effects of anemia on the mother include the following:

- *High maternal mortality rate:* In India, 16% of maternal death is due to anemia.
- Cerebral anoxia, cardiac failure.
- Increased susceptibility to develop infection.
- Inability to withstand even slight blood loss during pregnancy or delivery.
- Abortions, preterm labor.
- *Maternal risk during antenatal period:* Poor weight gain, preterm labor, pregnancy-induced hypertension, placenta previa, accidental hemorrhage, eclampsia, premature rupture of membranes (PROM), preterm labor, intercurrent infection, heart failure (30–32 weeks of gestation), etc.
- *Maternal risk during intranatal period:* Dysfunctional labor, intranatal hemorrhage, shock, anesthesia risk, cardiac failure, etc.
- *Maternal risk during postnatal period:* Postpartum hemorrhage, puerperal sepsis, subinvolution, poor lactation, puerperal venous thrombosis, pulmonary embolism.

  Fetal adverse effects include the following:
- Preterm, low birthweight and intrauterine growth restricted babies.
- Fetal distress and neonatal distress requiring prolonged resuscitation and low APGAR scores at birth.
- Impaired neurological and mental development.

- Anemia can result in hypertrophy of placenta and cause increased placental: fetal ratio, which has been suggested to be a predictor for development of diabetes and cardiovascular diseases later in life.

Infants with anemia have higher prevalence of failure to thrive, poorer intellectual developmental milestones and higher rate of morbidity and neonatal mortality in comparison to the infants without anemia.

### Q. What are the periods of pregnancy during which the anemic mother is at an increased risk for mortality?

**Ans.** The periods during pregnancy when the mother is at an increased risk for mortality include the following:

- 30–32 weeks of pregnancy
- During labor
- Immediately following delivery
- Puerperium (pulmonary embolism/cardiac failure).

## Case Study 4

Mrs XYZ, a 32-year-old married for 10 years, resident of ABC, G6P4A1L4 woman was seen at 38 weeks of gestation. She presented with the complaints of difficulty in breathing, fainting spells and chronic tiredness since past few days. She did not use any contraception between her pregnancies and also did not take any iron supplements during her previous pregnancies. On physical examination, she was very pale, had pulse rate of 120 beats/minute, low-grade fever and normal blood pressure (BP). There was facial, abdominal, presacral and pedal edema.

### Q. What should be the first line of management in this case?

**Ans.** Women with severe anemia presenting late in pregnancy should ideally be managed in hospital settings. They may or may not present with heart failure. However, they all need urgent admission and require complete rest with sedation and oxygen. Packed red cells are the preferred choice for severe anemia in later part of pregnancy. In case of congestive cardiac failure, patients should be given digitalis, diuretics and packed red cells.

### Q. What are the indications for blood transfusion in a pregnant woman with anemia?

**Ans.** Indications of blood transfusion for correction of anemia during pregnancy are as follows:

- There is not enough time to achieve a reasonable hemoglobin level before delivery, e.g. patient presents with severe anemia beyond 36 weeks.
- There is acute blood loss or associated infections.
- Anemia is refractory to iron therapy.
- Micronormoblastic erythroid hyperplasia.
- Hemoglobin levels less than 6 g/dL.
- Moderate and severe anemia in patients with known heart disease or severe respiratory infections.

- Symptomatic anemia not responding to conventional therapy.
- Placenta previa with hemoglobin levels less than 10 g/dL.
- Patients developing side effects or showing no response to both oral or parenteral iron therapy.

### Q. What are the advantages of blood transfusion?

**Ans.** Blood transfusion is likely to result in the following:
- Improvement in the oxygen carrying capacity of blood.
- Hemoglobin from the hemolyzed cells in the blood can be used for the synthesis of new RBCs.
- Stimulation of erythropoiesis.
- Provision of natural blood constituents such as proteins, antibodies, etc.

### Q. What precautions must be observed at the time of blood transfusion?

**Ans.** Due to increased chances for development of circulatory overload, resulting in the development of pulmonary edema and cardiac failure in a severely anemic patient, the precautions which must be observed are described next:
- Intramuscular administration of injection phenergan in the dosage of 25 mg must be given prior to the transfusion.
- Diuretics (furosemide in the dosage of 20 mg is given intramuscularly 2 hours prior to the transfusion.
- Packed red cells must be slowly administered at the drip rate of about 10 drops per minute.
- Clinical parameters (pulse, respiratory rate and crepitations at the base of the lungs) must be regularly monitored.

### Q. What are the methods for prevention of iron-deficiency anemia?

**Ans.** Following steps can be taken for prevention of IDA:
- *Screening:* Routine determination of hemoglobin or hematocrit is required in women, starting from the time of adolescence. Hemoglobin or hematocrit should be routinely determined at the time of first prenatal visit in order to detect any preexisting anemia. Routine screening for anemia and provision of supplements to adolescent girls should also be done, starting right from the school days.
- *Dietary changes:* Improving nutritional status of women through dietary changes is one of the most important strategies for reducing the prevalence of IDA during pregnancy. A good-quality diet should not only be rich in iron and contain sufficient proteins for hemoglobin synthesis but must also contain various micronutrients, including vitamin A, zinc, calcium, riboflavin, vitamin B12, etc.
- *Examples of iron-rich foods:* Two types of iron are present in food, heme iron, which is principally found in animal products and nonheme iron, which is found mainly in the plant products. Heme iron is better absorbed (up to 35%) than nonheme iron, but heme iron forms smaller fraction of the diet. Nonheme iron is mostly in ferric form, and needs to be reduced to ferrous form for absorption. Sources of heme iron include animal flesh and viscera. Nonheme iron is present mainly in the plant products such as dried fruits, walnuts, cashew nuts, raisins, peanuts, green leafy vegetables, spinach, broccoli, kale, turnip greens and collard greens, pulses, cereals, jaggery, legumes, such as lima beans and green peas, dry beans and peas; yeast-leavened whole-wheat bread and rolls, iron-enriched white bread, pasta, rice and cereals.
- Since folate deficiency has been found to commonly coexist with that of iron deficiency, diet rich in both iron and folic acid must be encouraged. Milk is a poor source of iron.
- Heme iron is present in the following animal products red meat, beef, pork, lamb; poultry: chicken, duck, turkey; fish, shellfish (clams, mussels, sardines, anchovies and oysters); eggs [one large egg (70–80 mg) contains about 1 mg of iron].
- *Management of endemic infection:* Malaria and hookworm infections are the major factors responsible for causing anemia in pregnancy by causing hemolysis and chronic blood loss respectively. The preferred drug for treating malaria in pregnancy is chloroquine. Malaria prophylaxis should also be given to pregnant women in areas where malaria is endemic. Also, antihelminthic drugs like albendazole or mebendazole are recommended to all pregnant women after the first trimester of pregnancy to help treat hookworm infestation.
- *Fortification of food with iron:* Fortification of the food with iron and folic acid is being tried in some countries and has been found to be one of the most effective, inexpensive and simple strategy for ensuring adequate supply of iron to large segments of the population.
- *Exogenous iron supplementation:* Iron supplementation has presently become the most common strategy used for controlling iron deficiency in developing countries. The WHO recommends universal iron supplementation comprising of 60 mg elemental iron and 400 μg of folic acid once or twice daily for 6 months in pregnancy, in countries with prevalence of anemia less than 40% and an additional 3 months postpartum in countries where prevalence is greater than 40%.
- In developing countries, routine iron supplementation during pregnancy is practiced, regardless of the fact, whether the mother is anemic or not. In India, Ministry of Health and Family Welfare, Government of India (2013) has recently recommended that all pregnant ladies must be given iron and folic acid supplementation (amounting to 100 mg elemental iron and 500 μg of folic acid) every day for at least 100 days, starting after the first trimester, at 14–16 weeks of gestation. This must be followed by the same dose for 100 days in the postpartum period. In addition to this, all women in the reproductive age group in the preconception period and up to the first trimester

of the pregnancy must be prescribed 400 μg of folic acid tablets daily to reduce the incidence of neural tube defects in the fetus. In a woman seen late in pregnancy, 120 mg of elemental iron daily is recommended during pregnancy and puerperium.

## Case Study 5

Mrs XYZ, a 30-year-old married for 9 years, resident of ABC, G3P2L2 woman presented to the ANC with 24 weeks of gestation with the complaints of tiredness, weakness and poor appetite since last 2 months. There was moderate pallor and moderate pedal edema. The per abdominal examination corresponded to 24 weeks of gestation. There was no other significant finding on general physical or systemic examination. She had been taking iron supplements on her own since past 1 month. She, however, was not taking any folic acid supplements. The hemoglobin levels were 7.8 g/dL and the peripheral smear showed the presence of macrocytes.

### Q. What was the next step of management in the above-mentioned case study?

**Ans.** The findings of the peripheral smear are suggestive of macrocytic anemia in the above-mentioned case study. Detailed investigations (hemoglobin, hematocrit, blood cell indices, peripheral smear, etc.) need to be carried out to confirm the type of anemia and its likely cause. Since the most common cause of macrocytic anemia in pregnancy is the deficiency of folic acid, serum folate levels and the red cell folate levels also need to be carried out. The results of various investigations pointed towards anemia due to folate deficiency in this case.

In cases where anemia fails to show improvement with use of iron supplements only, addition of folic acid must be tried.

### Q. What is megaloblastic (macrocytic) anemia and why does it occur in pregnancy?

**Ans.** Megaloblastic anemia occurs as a result of derangement of red cell maturation due to impaired DNA synthesis, resulting in the production of abnormal precursors called megaloblasts in the bone marrow. The signs and symptoms in cases of megaloblastic anemia are similar to IDA. However, nail changes do not occur normally. Megaloblastic anemia commonly occurs in multiple pregnancies (20–28 weeks), in users of OCPs or those consuming antiepileptic drugs. It most commonly occurs due to folate deficiency during pregnancy. Deficiency of folate can also result in the development of neural tube defects, which can be prevented by periconceptional folic acid in the dosage of 0.4 mg/day in low-risk cases and in the dosage of 5 mg/day in high-risk women.

Megaloblastic anemia in nonpregnant women commonly occurs due to deficiency of vitamin B12 caused by the lack of intrinsic factor, resulting in the lack of absorption of vitamin B12. This, however, occurs rarely in pregnancy because deficiency of vitamin B12 may take months to manifest and usually causes infertility.

### Q. What are the various investigations, which must be done in cases of folate deficiency anemia?

**Ans.** The following investigations aid in the diagnosis of folate deficiency anemia:

- *Hemoglobin:* Less than 10 g/dL.
- *MCV:* Greater than 96 fL.
- *MCH:* Greater than 33 pg.
- *MCHC:* Within the normal range.
- *Serum folate:* Less than 3 mg/mL.
- *Red cell folate:* Less than 150 ng/mL is diagnostic of folic acid deficiency.
- *Peripheral smear:* At least two of the following criteria must be present on the peripheral smear to establish the diagnosis of megaloblastic anemia:
  - Presence of macrocytes and megaloblasts.
  - More than 4% of neutrophil polymorphs have five or more lobes (hypersegmented neutrophils).
  - Orthochromatic macrocytes having a diameter greater than 12 mm.
  - Howell-Jolly bodies must be demonstrated.
  - Presence of nucleated red cells.
  - Macropolycytes may be present.

### Q. What steps must be taken to prevent folate deficiency anemia during pregnancy?

**Ans.** In order to prevent folate deficiency, WHO recommends a daily folate intake of 800 μg in the antenatal period and 600 μg during lactation. Pregnant women must be advised to eat a diet rich in green vegetables (e.g. spinach and broccoli), offal (e.g. liver and kidney), etc. Treatment of folate deficiency comprises of administration of 5 mg folate/day, which must be continued for at least 4 weeks in the puerperium.

# Hypertensive Disorders in Pregnancy

## Case Study 1

Mrs XYZ, a 31-year-old married for 3 years, resident of ABC, primigravida patient with 39 completed weeks of gestation presented with the complaints of headache since last 10 days. Her BP was 144/95 mm Hg.

### Q. What is the likely diagnosis in the above-mentioned case study?

**Ans.** The above-mentioned case study most likely corresponds to hypertensive disorders during pregnancy (to be confirmed by estimation of proteinuria). The questions to be asked at the time of taking history and the parameters to be assured at the time of general physical examination in such a case are described in Tables 5.4 and 5.5 respectively. The most likely diagnosis in this case is 31-year-old married

**Table 5.4:** Symptoms to be elicited at the time of taking history in a case of hypertensive disorders of pregnancy

*History of Presenting Complains*

- *Edema:* Since edema is a universal finding in pregnancy, it is not considered as a criterion for diagnosing preeclampsia. The following parameters related to edema need to be elicited:
  - *Site of origin:* The body region which is affected by edema, is it face, legs, fingers, sacral region or vulva?
  - *Duration:* Since what time the edema has been present?
  - *Progress:* What are the relieving and aggravating factors of edema? Is edema aggravated by walking and relieved by rest?
  - *Type:* Whether the edema is of pitting or nonpitting type? Pitting edema implies that a pit (depression) is formed upon application of pressure in the region of edema.
- Symptoms suggestive of severe preeclampsia may include the following:
  - *Headache:* Dull, throbbing headache, often described as migraine-like, which would just not go away.
  - *Visual problems:* Vision changes include temporary loss of vision, sensations of flashing lights, sensitivity to light auras and blurry vision or spots. The problems related to vision are usually related to the spasm of retinal vessels.
  - *Epigastric or right upper quadrant abdominal pain:* Epigastric or the right upper quadrant pain is usually indicative of hepatocellular necrosis, ischemia, edema, hepatic dysfunction, etc. all of which are responsible for stretching the Glisson's capsule of the liver. There may be associated nausea and vomiting as well.
  - *Shortness of breath or dyspnea:* This could be reflective of pulmonary edema or acute respiratory distress syndrome.
  - *Oliguria:* Reduced urinary output of less than 300–400 mL in 24 hours could be indicative of reduced plasma volume or ischemic acute tubular necrosis.
- *Reduced fetal movements:* The patient may give a history of experiencing reduced fetal movements especially in association with IUGR and oligohydramnios.
- *History suggestive of multifetal gestation:* Ask for the history suggestive of excessive enlargement of the uterus or excessive fetal movements (which could be suggestive of multifetal gestation).

*History of the Likely Risk Factors*

- *Obesity:* A prepregnancy BMI of greater than or equal to 35 almost quadruples the risk of developing preeclampsia.
- Extremes of age (under 18 or over 40 years)
- Certain autoimmune conditions, including antiphospholipid antibody syndrome are associated with an increased risk for preeclampsia.
- African-American or Hispanic ethnicity.
- *A change of male partner:* Having a male partner whose previous partner had preeclampsia may increase the woman's risk of developing preeclampsia during her future pregnancies.
- Nulliparity.
- Multifetal gestation.
- *History of smoking:* Although smoking is associated with an increased risk of various adverse pregnancy-related outcomes, ironically it is associated with a reduced risk of hypertension during pregnancy.
- A time duration of more than or equal to 10 years since the last pregnancy.
- Raised BP at the time of booking.

*Past Medical History*

- Ask for the past history of chronic hypertension, diabetes, renal disease, etc.

*Family History*

- History of hypertensive disorders of pregnancy in the patient's mother or sister.

*Past Obstetric History*

- History of preeclampsia-eclampsia in previous pregnancies, especially the first one, particularly if its onset was before the third trimester.

for 3 years, resident of ABC, primigravida patient with 39 completed weeks gestation, with a single live fetus in cephalic presentation, flexed attitude, with vertex as the presenting part, which is free floating along with history and clinical examination suggestive of hypertensive disorders of pregnancy. The possible differential diagnoses in this case could be gestational hypertension, preeclampsia, chronic hypertension or gestational hypertension superimposed on chronic hypertension. This can be confirmed by estimation of proteinuria and performing other investigations (described later in the text).

**Q. What is the correct method of measuring the blood pressure?**

**Ans.** According to the current consensus, BP during pregnancy must be measured after 5 minutes of rest. The right upper arm must be used and the arm must be taken out of the sleeve. The BP cuff should be of the appropriate size (12 cm wide and 35 cm in length) and should be placed at the level of the heart. If the arm is very fat, a wider cuff must be used to obtain a correct reading. An ideal cuff should have a bladder length of 80% and width of at least 40% of the arm circumference (i.e. a length to width ratio of 2:1). The cuff

**Table 5.5:** Various findings elicited at the time of clinical examination in case of hypertensive disorders of pregnancy

*General Physical Examination*

*Increased blood pressure:* BP may rise insidiously, but sometimes even abruptly. Presence of increased BP (> 140/90 mm Hg) for the first time during pregnancy, after 20 weeks of gestation can be considered as one of the diagnostic features of preeclampsia. BP should be taken in both supine and left lateral positions. In case of increased BP, another reading must be taken after giving the patient at least 6 hours of rest.

*Presence of proteinuria:* The usual screening test for proteinuria is visual assessment of dipstick or a regent strip. Dipstick is a device in which a strip of paper impregnated with a reagent (used for testing proteins) is dipped into urine in order to measure the quantity of proteins present in the urine.

*Other features on GPE suggestive of preeclampsia:* The other features on GPEs which are suggestive of severe preeclampsia are described below:
- *Edema:* The clinician must specifically look for vulvar edema, facial edema, pedal edema and edema over the fingers. Clinical grading of edema is as follows:
  - 1+ Pitting lasts for 0–15 seconds
  - 2+ Pitting lasts for 16–30 seconds
  - 3+ Pitting lasts for 31–60 seconds
  - 4+ Pitting lasts more than 60 seconds
- *Weight gain:* The weight of a patient with suspected or diagnosed preeclampsia must be taken at each antenatal visit because preeclampsia is associated with a significant weight gain. Weight gain of more than 2 pounds per week or 6 pounds in a month or a sudden weight gain over 1–2 days can be considered as significant.
- *Petechiae:* Presence of petechiae may reflect a bleeding tendency, which may serve as an indicator of HELLP syndrome. Platelet count may fall below $100 \times 10^6$/L.
- *Ankle clonus:* Presence of ankle clonus is indicative of excessive neuromuscular irritability, which can progress to seizures (eclampsia).
- *Knee jerks:* Evaluation of knee jerks is especially important in patients receiving magnesium sulfate as reduced or absent knee jerks in a patient on magnesium sulfate therapy is usually indicative of magnesium toxicity.
- *Papilledema:* This can be described as the swelling of optic disk diagnosed on ophthalmoscopy or slit-lamp examination in very severe cases of hypertension. Papilledema occurs due to increased intracranial pressure, usually in association with malignant hypertension.

*Specific Systemic Examination*

*Abdominal examination*
- On abdominal examination, there may be evidence of placental insufficiency in the form of oligohydramnios or/and IUGR. Findings on abdominal examination suggestive of oligohydramnios are as follows:
  - The fundal height is less than that estimated on the basis of last menstrual period (LMP).
  - Uterus may appear full of fetus and/or evidence of IUGR may be present.
  - Findings suggestive of IUGR on abdominal examination are described later in text.

must be applied firmly around the arm, not allowing more than one finger between the cuff and the patient's arm. The woman should not have used tobacco or caffeine within 30 minutes of the measurement. RCOG recommends that mercury sphygmomanometers should be used at least to establish baseline BP as a reference, since this reading is supposed to be most accurate.

Korotkoff phase 5 (disappearance of heart sounds and not simply muffling of sounds) is considered as the appropriate measurement of diastolic BP. In cases where K5 is absent, 4th Korotkoff sound should be accepted. On the other hand, the systolic BP is taken at Korotkoff phase 1 (the first sound heard after the cuff pressure is released). It is also recommended that elevation of gestational BP must be defined on the basis of at least two readings of high BP obtained at least 6 hours apart within a span of 1 week.

### Q. How can proteinuria be assessed through dipstick method?

**Ans.** Visual dipstick assessment is most commonly used method for estimation of proteinuria, despite of being associated with high false positive and false negative test results. The approximate equivalence of the dipstick result and amount of proteins in the urine is as follows, with the results of trace = 10 mg/day; 1+ = 0.3 g/L; 2+ = 1 g/L; 3+ = 3 g/L; and 4+ = 10g/L. Proteinuria is defined as significant if the excretion of proteins exceeds 300 mg/24 hours or there is persistent presence of the protein (30 mg/dL or 1+ dipstick) in random urine sample in absence of any evidence of urinary tract infection.

In view of the high false-positive rates with visual dipstick assessment, a 24-hour urine collection for protein estimation or a timed collection corrected for creatinine excretion is sometimes recommended by the clinician to confirm significant proteinuria.

### Q. How should the clinician take the history of edema?

**Ans.** The best way to ask the patient about development of edema is to enquire if she has been experiencing tightening of rings on the fingers of her hands or facial puffiness and swelling of feet on getting up from the bed. Some swelling of the feet and ankles is considered normal with pregnancy.

Nondependent edema such as facial or hand swelling (the patient's ring may no longer fit her finger) is more specific than dependent edema. Vulvar edema, sacral edema or the presence of edema over ankles in the morning on getting up from the bed is also pathological.

### Q. What are hypertensive disorders during pregnancy?

**Ans.** According to the classification system proposed by the International Society for the Study of Hypertension in Pregnancy (ISSHP, 2001) and National High Blood Pressure Education Program (NHBPEP, 2000) working group hypertensive disorders in pregnancy can be classified as gestational hypertension, preeclampsia-eclampsia, chronic hypertension in pregnancy, and preeclampsia superimposed on chronic hypertension (Flow chart 5.1).

- *Preeclampsia:* Preeclampsia is defined as a pregnancy-specific, multifactorial disease, which presents as a syndrome of specific signs and symptoms. Preeclampsia can be considered as a potentially serious disorder, which is characterized by high BP (>140/90 mm Hg) and proteinuria. It usually develops after the 20th week of pregnancy and goes away after the delivery. Proteinuria is defined by excretion of protein more than or equal to 300 mg/24 hours, a urine protein/creatinine ratio of greater than or equal to 0.3, or a reading of more than or equal to 1 "+" on dipstick. Preeclampsia may also be accompanied by rapid weight gain and/or edema and appearance of abnormalities of coagulation or liver function tests. This condition is characterized by placental dysfunction and a maternal response highlighting systemic inflammation with activation of the endothelium and coagulation. Clinical classification of preeclampsia is based on its time of onset (early onset, prior to 34 weeks or late onset, after 34 weeks).

Occurrence of hypertension and proteinuria before 20 weeks of gestation (e.g. in gestational trophoblastic disease), can be designated as atypical preeclampsia.

- *Gestational hypertension:* This form of high BP develops after the 20th week of pregnancy and goes away after the delivery. Affected women do not have proteinuria.
- *Chronic hypertension:* This can be defined as high BP that is diagnosed before pregnancy or before the 20th week of pregnancy in absence of gestational trophoblastic disease. The condition does not return to normal following delivery.
- *Preeclampsia superimposed upon chronic hypertension:* There is ample evidence that preeclampsia may occur in women already suffering from chronic hypertension prior to pregnancy. This condition holds importance because the prognosis for mother and fetus is much worse than with either condition alone.

### Q. What is preeclampsia-eclampsia?

**Ans.** Preeclampsia-eclampsia can be considered as a serious multisystemic disorder having a broad clinical spectrum with preeclampsia at one end and the most severe manifestation of preeclampsia, i.e. eclampsia at the other. Clinical course of preeclampsia can vary from one patient to the other. Preeclampsia always presents potential danger to the mother and baby. Sometimes, mild preeclampsia (especially if remains untreated) can progress into severe preeclampsia. Severe preeclampsia may ultimately result in development of eclampsia, which can be defined as the occurrence of seizures, which cannot be attributed to other causes, in a woman with preeclampsia.

Flow chart 5.1: Classification of hypertensive disorders in pregnancy

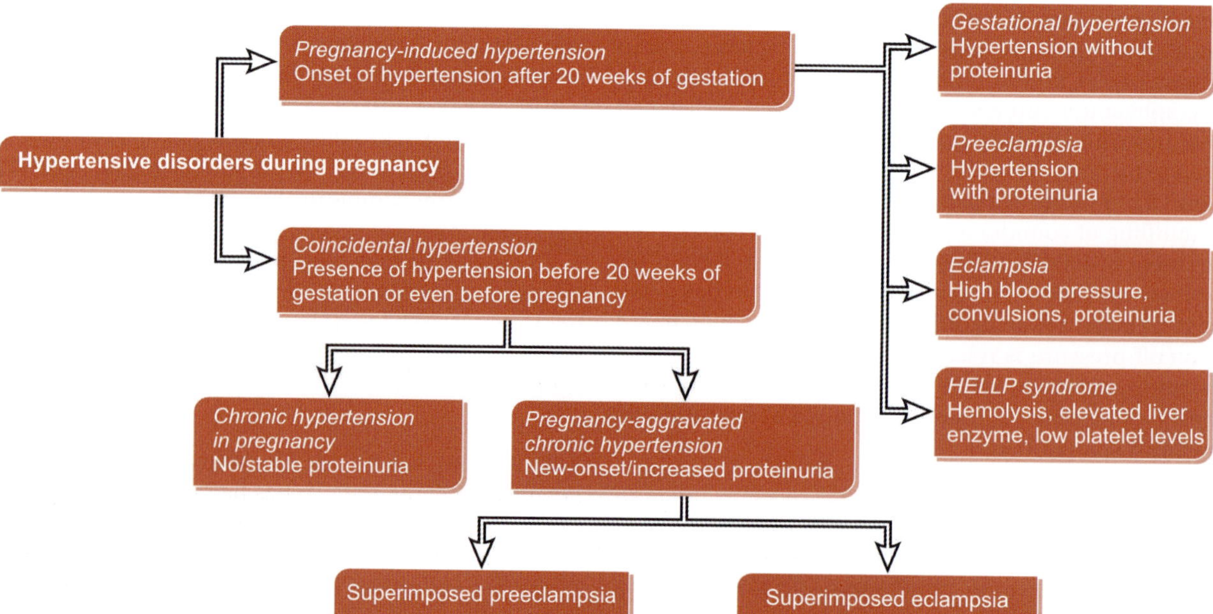

**Q. What are the cardiovascular and volume changes occurring during normal pregnancy? How are they different in a patient with preeclampsia?**

**Ans.** There is a fall in the systemic vascular resistance during normal pregnancy. Also, due to an increase in the plasma volume, accompanied by marked increases in intravascular and extracellular volume there is an increase in cardiac output during normal pregnancy. Despite of an increase in the cardiac output, there is a fall in BP due to a reduction in systemic vascular resistance. As a result, there is an overall fall in the diastolic pressure and mean arterial pressure during pregnancy, with the decrease starting in early gestation and reaching a nadir near mid-pregnancy.

On the other hand, patient with preeclampsia is characterized by reduced plasma volume and hemoconcentration. Also, there is associated intravascular volume depletion with high peripheral vascular resistance.

**Q. What are the investigations, which must be done in the cases of preeclampsia?**

**Ans.** Laboratory tests, which must be performed in these patients, include the following:

- *Complete blood count (CBC) and hematocrit:* The decrease in blood volume in preeclampsia can lead to an increase in maternal hemoglobin concentration resulting in increased hematocrit.
- *Platelet count:* In preeclampsia, the platelet count can fall below $200 \times 10^9/L$ and is associated with progressive disease.
- *Liver function tests:* Liver function tests including the measurement of ALT and AST, and lactate dehydrogenase (LDH) activities must be performed. An AST level of above 75 IU/L is seen as significant and a level above 150 IU/L is associated with increased morbidity to the mother.
- *Measurement of serum electrolytes, blood urea nitrogen (BUN).*
- *Kidney function tests:* These include the following:
  - Serum creatinine levels: In normal pregnancy, there is an increase in creatinine clearance with a concomitant decrease in serum creatinine and urea concentrations. In severe preeclampsia, serum creatinine can be seen to rise and is associated with a worsening outcome.
  - Serum uric acid levels: Serum concentrations of uric acid fall in normal pregnancy because renal excretion increases. In preeclampsia, there can be a rise in uric acid concentrations. Increased serum uric acid levels are usually related to poorer outcomes both for the mother and baby.
- *Urinalysis.*
- *Ophthalmoscopic examination.*

**Q. What is the management in cases of preeclampsia?**

**Ans.** Immediate hospitalization is recommended even in cases where there is suspicion of preeclampsia because of the disease's potential to accelerate rapidly. There is no role for domiciliary management in cases of preeclampsia. Immediate delivery is indicated irrespective of the period of gestation if severe hypertension remains uncontrolled for 24–48 hours or whenever there is appearance of certain "ominous" signs such as coagulation abnormalities, signs of worsening renal/hepatic function, signs of impending eclampsia (headache, epigastric pain and hyperreflexia), or the presence of severe growth restriction or nonreassuring fetal testing. Immediate delivery of the baby remains the only known "cure". Preeclampsia remote from term is a special situation in which the patients should be hospitalized and closely monitored in tertiary obstetric care centers. Pregnancy may be allowed to continue as long as BP remains controlled, no ominous signs of life-threatening maternal complications occur, and there are no signs of imminent danger to the fetus (e.g. nonreassuring fetal heart rate). Medical treatment must be initiated when diastolic BP is above or equal to 105 mm Hg.

## Case Study 2

Mrs XYZ, 26-year-old married for 5 years, resident of ABC, G2P1L1 woman presented at 36 weeks of gestation in the ANC clinic with the complaints of pedal edema since last 7 days. Her BP was 144/94 mm Hg. All the BP recordings during her previous ANC visits were WNL. She had never been diagnosed to be suffering from hypertension previous to the present pregnancy. Dipstick examination revealed 1+ proteinuria.

**Q. What is the likely diagnosis in the above-mentioned case study?**

**Ans.** Based on the findings of the previous and present ANC visits, she was diagnosed as a case of mild preeclampsia. The most likely diagnosis in this case is Mrs XYZ, a 26-year-old woman, married for 5 years, resident of ABC, G2P1L1 with 36 completed weeks of gestation having a single live fetus in cephalic presentation along with mild preeclampsia (as suggested by history, clinical examination and results of proteinuria estimation).

**Q. How would you define mild and severe preeclampsia?**

**Ans.** Classification of hypertension based on the degree of severity is described in Table 5.6. Difference between mild and severe preeclampsia has been described in Table 5.7.

**Q. What is the management in cases of mild preeclampsia?**

**Ans.** Management of mild preeclampsia comprises of the following steps:

*Maternal Management*

When the mother is diagnosed with mild type of preeclampsia in the antenatal period, she should be admitted in the hospital in order to assess the severity of condition and decide further management. Domiciliary treatment has no role in an established case of preeclampsia and the patient must be hospitalized. In an under-resourced setting, where it might not be possible to admit every patient with mild preeclampsia,

**Table 5.6:** Classification of hypertension based on the degree of severity

| Degree of hypertension | Systolic blood pressure | Diastolic blood pressure |
| --- | --- | --- |
| Mild | 140–149 mm Hg | 90–99 mm Hg |
| Moderate | 150–159 mm Hg | 100–109 mm Hg |
| Severe | ≥ 160 mm Hg | ≥ 110 mm Hg |

**Table 5.7:** Difference between mild and severe preeclampsia

| Characteristics | Mild preeclampsia | Severe preeclampsia |
| --- | --- | --- |
| Time of presentation | Presents at gestational age ≥ 34 weeks | Presents at gestational age < 34 weeks |
| Diastolic BP | < 100 mm Hg | > 110 mm Hg |
| Symptoms showing neurological involvement such as headache, visual disturbances, hyperreflexia, etc. and abdominal pain | Absent | May be present |
| Presence of ominous features such as convulsions (eclampsia), congestive heart failure or pulmonary edema | Absent | May be present |
| Oliguria | Absent | Present |
| Elevated liver enzymes (LDH, AST) | Absent | Present |
| Thrombocytopenia (platelet count < 1,00,000 per µL) | Absent | May be present |
| Serum creatinine levels | Normal | Elevated |
| Proteinuria | Mild to moderate | Severe (in nephrotic range) > 3 g/24 hours (especially in association with ominous features) |
| Nonreassuring fetal heart rate with or without fetal growth restriction | Absent | Present |

the patient must be at least referred to an antenatal day unit for further investigations. The following assessments need to be carried out in the patients who are admitted:

- Daily detailed examination for the symptoms indicative of severe preeclampsia, including history of headache, visual disturbances, epigastric pain, edema, etc.
- Regular weight measurement at weekly intervals to assess if the woman is gaining weight at a rapid rate.
- Daily examination of urine for the presence of proteins by dipstick. If proteinuria of 2+ or more on dipstick is present, 24-hour urine protein estimation may be required.
- Blood pressure measurement to be done every 4 hourly (at least four times a day).
- The investigations, which need to be done on weekly basis, include hematocrit with platelet count, KFT (blood urea; serum uric acid; and serum creatinine); LFT (AST, ALT and LDH) and ophthalmoscopic examination.
- Rest in left lateral position to avoid vena caval compression is advised. Absolute bed rest, as recommended in the past is not required. No salt or fluid restriction is required.
- Prescription of the sedatives or tranquilizers is not required.
- Well-balanced diet, rich in proteins and calories is prescribed. A diet containing at least 100 g of proteins and 1,600 calories/day is usually advised.

- Low-dose aspirin in the dose of 60–150 mg daily can be prescribed.
- Calcium supplementation: Though no definite role of calcium supplementation in prevention of preeclampsia has been shown during pregnancy, supplementation with 300–600 mg of exogenous calcium preparations from 20th week of gestation has been significantly shown to increase the density of fetal bones.

Most cases of the gestational hypertension and mild preeclampsia respond to conservative management. However, fetal surveillance is required until the baby has attained maturity because the underlying pathophysiology behind preeclampsia would be corrected only following delivery of the baby. The pregnancy should not be allowed to continue beyond expected date of delivery (EDD).

### Fetal Management

Until the fetal maturity is attained, fetal surveillance comprises of the following tests:

- Daily fetal movement count (DFMC).
- Weekly measurement of fundal height and abdominal girth in order to detect IUGR.
- Nonstress test (NST) weekly.

- Ultrasound examination for evaluating the period of gestation in early pregnancy and in the third trimester at every 2 weekly intervals.
- BPP after every 2 weeks.
- Doppler ultrasound at every 3–4 weekly intervals

### Q. What should be the mode of delivery in the above-mentioned case study?

**Ans.** The clinician can continue until term if the patient is stabilized on the above-mentioned conservative management. However, the pregnancy must not be allowed to exceed the EDD. There is no advantage of performing a cesarean over normal delivery in cases of preeclampsia unless there is an additional obstetric indication for cesarean delivery. There is no need to hasten the delivery in cases of mild preeclampsia.

### Q. What precautions must be taken in the postpartum period for the women with preeclampsia?

**Ans.** The clinician must remain vigilant regarding the high chances for the occurrence of PPH following delivery of the baby in the postnatal period.

This is all the more important since the routine use of methergine at the time of delivery of the baby's anterior shoulder is contraindicated in hypertensive women. Following delivery, the ACE inhibitors can be restarted. Use of methyldopa is to be stopped due to risk of development of psychological changes, like depression in the mother.

## Case Study 3

Mrs XYZ, a 24-year-old married for 4 years, resident of ABC, G2P1L1 patient with 20 weeks of gestation visited the ANC clinic with the complaints of headache, blurred vision and epigastric pain since past 4–5 days. She gives history of being hypertensive during her first pregnancy. However, her BP normalized soon after delivery. In the present pregnancy, her BP is 160/104 mm Hg; pulse is 100 beats per minute and there is mild pedal edema on both sides.

### Q. What are the indicators of severe preeclampsia during pregnancy?

**Ans.** Some indicators of severe preeclampsia during pregnancy are as follows:

- Diastolic BP above or equal to 110 mm Hg and/or systolic BP above or equal to 160 mm Hg.
- Proteinuria 2+ or more on the dipstick.
- Presence of symptoms like headache, visual disturbances, oliguria (urine volume ≤ 500 mL/24 hours), convulsions, etc.
- Investigations show presence of thrombocytopenia (platelet count < 1,00,000 cells/mm$^3$), elevated serum creatinine levels (> 1.2 mg/dL), serum uric acid of more than 4.5 mg percent, elevated liver enzymes (ALT or AST), evidence of microangiopathic hemolytic anemia, fetal IUGR, etc.

### Q. What is the goal of antihypertensive therapy?

**Ans.** The goal of antihypertensive therapy is to maintain BP at a level so as to prevent cardiovascular and central nervous system consequences related to severe hypertension in the mother without compromising uteroplacental blood flow and fetal perfusion. Eventually, this protects the mother and fetus from the dangers of severe hypertension and related morbidity, thereby allowing the pregnancy to continue and the fetus to grow and mature. However, antihypertensive medicines do not prevent preeclampsia nor do they reverse the primary pathogenic process of placental underperfusion and severe preeclampsia.

### Q. What is the management in cases of severe preeclampsia?

**Ans.** The aim of treatment in cases of severe preeclampsia is to protect both the mother and the fetus from the adverse effects of high BP and to prolong the pregnancy as far as possible in order to prevent the risk of fetal prematurity. Management of severe preeclampsia must be preferably done in tertiary unit, following a multidisciplinary team approach involving the clinician, physician, pediatrician and the anesthetist. Management of cases with severe preeclampsia is all the more important because there is danger of progression to eclampsia (a stage in which the patient experiences fits), if the BP remains uncontrollably high. The management of severe preeclampsia is to be based on careful fetal assessment, maternal stabilization, continued monitoring and delivery at an optimal time for the mother and her baby. The only cure for preeclampsia is the delivery of the baby. Therefore, while deciding the time for delivery, a fine balance between fetal maturity and maternal well-being needs to be maintained.

### *Maternal Stabilization*

The following steps also need to be taken for stabilizing the mother in cases of severe preeclampsia:

- Patients with severe preeclampsia must be hospitalized to a tertiary unit.
- Senior obstetric and anesthetic staff and experienced midwives should be involved in the care of such patients.
- *Continuous maternal BP monitoring:* The BP should be checked at every 15 minutes in the beginning, until the woman has stabilized and then after every 30 minutes in the initial phase of assessment. Once the patient has become stable and asymptomatic, the BP may be checked at 4-hourly intervals, especially if a conservative management plan is in place.
- Urine should be carefully monitored for proteinuria twice daily. In presence of significant proteinuria, a 24-hour estimation of urine proteins may be done.
- Maternal weight must be measured every day.
- Tests like platelet count, KFT (serum uric acid concentration, blood urea and serum creatinine concentration) and tests of liver function must be done at the time of admission and then twice weekly.

- Antihypertensive drugs must be used to keep the diastolic BP below 110 mm Hg. Prescription of antihypertensive medicines helps to prevent the development of the complications related to high BP (e.g. intracranial hemorrhage).
- Prophylactic use of magnesium sulfate helps in prevention of eclampsia and help buy time until the fetus has gained sufficient maturity so that it can be delivered.

### Fetal Management in Case of Severe Preeclampsia

If conservative management is planned, until fetal maturity is attained, the following investigations need to be done:

- *Daily fetal movement count:* The fetus responds to chronic hypoxia by conserving energy and the subsequent reduction of fetal movements.
- Weekly measurement of fundal height and abdominal girth in order to detect IUGR.
- Ultrasound measurement of fetal growth after every 2 weeks.
- *Umbilical artery Doppler analysis:* Serial assessment of umbilical blood flow velocity by Doppler ultrasonographic assessment must be done after every 2 weeks. Umbilical artery Doppler analysis showing absent or reversed end diastolic flow is consistent with placental dysfunction as a cause of fetal growth restriction (FGR). This is usually associated with poor neonatal outcomes and mandates immediate delivery. Abnormalities on uterine artery Doppler velocimetry may also be useful in hypertensive pregnant women in supporting a placental origin for the hypertension.
- *Electronic fetal heart rate monitoring (EFHRM):* At present, most authorities recommend a weekly NST for women with hypertensive diseases of pregnancy and twice weekly for women with severe disease or evidence of fetal compromise (growth restriction or oligohydramnios).
- *Amniotic fluid index (AFI) and biophysical profile (BPP):* The fetal BPP is usually performed at weekly or twice weekly intervals depending on the clinical situation. Reduced liquor volume is also associated with placental insufficiency and FGR. Serial estimations of liquor volume can help to detect fetal compromise.

The frequency of various tests for fetal and maternal surveillance is not fixed. It can vary from patient to patient based on the clinical situation.

### Q. What steps must be taken in case the preterm delivery is planned for a woman suffering from severe preeclampsia?

**Ans.** In case the delivery of a preterm fetus is planned, the following steps need to be undertaken:

- Administration of corticosteroids.
- Measurement of L:S ratio in the amniotic fluid; L:S ratio greater than 2 is indicative of fetal maturity.

- Fetus should be closely monitored at the time of labor, preferably with continuous electronic fetal monitoring.
- Delivery must be conducted in an obstetric unit, which can offer a reasonable chance of survival to the neonate in terms of outcomes of prematurity.

### Q. What is the rationale for fetal assessment in cases of severe preeclampsia?

**Ans.** In cases of severe preeclampsia, the fetuses are at risk particularly due to prematurity as premature delivery may be required to save mother's life. On the other hand, if the pregnancy is allowed to continue, placental insufficiency resulting from preeclampsia may cause IUGR and poor fetal reserves. IUGR occurs in approximately 30% of pregnancies with preeclampsia. Therefore, fetal monitoring forms an important aspect of management of patients with preeclampsia. There are high chances of abnormal fetal heart rate pattern, meconium stained amniotic fluid and overall poor fetal outcomes in labor, which may be at times related to severe complications such as placental abruption and fetal death.

The rationale behind fetal assessment is that if there is even a slight evidence of poor perinatal outcome; obstetric intervention must be undertaken immediately before irreversible damage occurs. The obstetric intervention in such situations is usually delivery. An earlier period of gestation may be associated with prematurity-related complications such as respiratory distress, intraventricular hemorrhage, necrotizing enterocolitis, metabolic disturbances, sepsis, etc. A balance has to be maintained between intervention and conservation following fetal assessment. In cases of hypertensive disorders in pregnancy, it is also important to identify fetuses, which may be at a risk of growth restriction. Surveillance and monitoring in these fetuses should be then undertaken by umbilical artery Doppler.

### Q. What should be the timing of delivery in cases of severe preeclampsia?

**Ans.** The only way to cure preeclampsia is to deliver the baby. Therefore, termination of pregnancy is the treatment of choice in all patients with severe preeclampsia where the fetus has attained maturity. The timing of delivery based on the period of gestation in cases with severe preeclampsia is described below:

- *More than 32 weeks of gestation:* In cases of severe preeclampsia, when the pregnancy is more than 32 weeks of gestation, delivery is the treatment of choice. In case the period of gestation is less than 32 weeks, prophylactic steroids should be given to induce fetal lung maturity. A policy of administering corticosteroids, 12 mg betamethasone IM every 24 hours for two doses or 6 mg dexamethasone IM every 12 hours for four doses to women who are likely to have a preterm delivery can be expected to achieve substantial reduction in neonatal morbidity and mortality.

- *Before 26 weeks of gestation:* In women with severe preeclampsia before 26 weeks of gestation, prolonging the pregnancy at this gestational age may result in grave complications for the mother. Therefore, labor must be induced for pregnancies less than 26 weeks, although it is quite unlikely that the fetus would survive at this time.
- *Between 26 weeks and 32 weeks of gestation:* Pregnancies between 26 weeks and 32 weeks represent a "gray zone". The clinician needs to balance the risk of prolonging the pregnancy, thereby increasing the maternal risk of developing complications related to severe preeclampsia against the risk of delivering a premature fetus which may not even survive.

  The timing of delivery is guided by the nursery facilities and the gestational age at which the baby can be saved. If the clinician decides to continue pregnancy, close maternal and fetal monitoring requires to be done, because simply lowering the BP under conservative management will not slow down the disease process.

### Q. How should the fetus be delivered in case of preeclampsia?

**Ans.** Severe preeclampsia per se is not an indication for cesarean section (CS). If the cervix is ripe, labor can be induced by using intravenous oxytocin and ARM. Labor may be immediately induced in presence of any of the following conditions:

- Signs of impending eclampsia including abdominal pain, blurring of vision, severe persistent headache, etc.
- Abnormal BPP; nonreassuring results on electronic fetal monitoring.
- Diastolic BP over 110 mm Hg.
- Abnormal liver function tests (LDH > 1,000 IU/L).
- Eclampsia.
- IUGR
- HELLP syndrome
- Rising serum creatinine levels
- Fetal death
- Placental abruption
- Urine output < 500 mL/24 hours

In presence of unfavorable cervix or other complications (e.g. breech presentation, fetal distress, etc.), a cesarean section needs to be done.

### Q. How should the mother be managed during labor?

**Ans.** The parameters, which need to be taken care of at the time of labor in a patient with severe preeclampsia, are as follows:

- *Maternal vitals monitoring:* This involves monitoring of vitals especially maternal pulse and BP at hourly intervals. Urine protein levels using a dipstick must be monitored at every 6-hourly intervals.
- *Choice of anesthesia:* An epidural analgesia, by allowing adequate pain relief, can reduce the rise in BP commonly associated with labor. It also allows a planned delivery and easy transition to CS, if necessary.

- *Use of intravenous fluid in women with severe preeclampsia or eclampsia:* While in normal pregnancy, there is an increase in plasma volume, in preeclampsia there is contracted plasma volume and hemoconcentration. These patients usually have intravascular volume depletion, with high peripheral vascular resistance. Therefore, administration of intravenous fluids in women with severe preeclampsia and eclampsia must be monitored carefully. Infusion of excessive fluid may result in the development of pulmonary edema and adult respiratory distress syndrome.
- *Use of antihypertensive medication:* Antihypertensive agents are used to control persistent increase in BP, especially when diastolic BP is above 110 mm Hg. Antihypertensive therapy should be continued throughout labor. Presently, there is little evidence regarding the antihypertensive drug of choice to be used for lowering BP in case of women with severe preeclampsia. The aim of treatment must be to maintain diastolic BP between 95 mm Hg and 105 mm Hg. When the BP remains uncontrollable despite the use of antihypertensive medications, delivery is the only option.

  The most commonly used drugs include hydralazine, alpha-methyldopa, labetalol and nifedipine. Nevertheless, methyldopa and labetalol remain the most widely used drugs, followed by nifedipine as the second-line agent for the treatment of hypertension in pregnancy. While these medications to lower BP are safe during pregnancy, others, including drugs like ACE inhibitors, β-blockers (atenolol), ARBs and diuretics can harm the fetus. Other rapidly acting agents, like nitroglycerine, diazoxide and sodium nitroprusside are usually preserved for use in an ICU setting or in the OT. Drugs used for control of chronic hypertension in pregnancy are listed in Table 5.8.
- *Use of magnesium sulfate in severe preeclampsia:* Magnesium sulfate should be considered for women with preeclampsia, especially those with severe preeclampsia in whom there is concern about the risk of eclampsia. Magnesium sulfate is now also considered as an anticonvulsant of choice for treating eclampsia. A total dose of 14 g is administered in the form of loading and maintenance dose. The following regimens can be given:
- *Pritchard's regimen:* A loading dose of 4 g magnesium sulfate is administered slowly intravenously over 10 minutes. The intravenous dose must be immediately followed by 5 g (i.e. 10 mL 50% magnesium sulfate) by deep IM injection into each buttock.
  - *Maintenance dose:* The maintenance dose comprises of 5 g intramuscularly in each buttock at every 4-hourly intervals.
- *Zuspan's regimen:* A loading dose of 4 g should be given by infusion pump over 5–10 minutes, followed by a further

| **Table 5.8:** Different types of antihypertensive drugs used for controlling hypertension | | |
|---|---|---|
| *Drug* | *Dose* | *Comments* |
| Methyldopa | 0.5–3.0 g/day in 2 divided doses | Drug of choice according to NHBPEP working group. The safety of this drug after the first trimester has been well documented. |
| Labetalol | Labetalol is given as a 20 mg IV bolus dose, followed by 40 mg after 10 minutes. If the first dose is not effective, then 80 mg is administered every 10 minutes. Maximum total dose of 220 mg can be administered. It can also be administered in the form of a continuous infusion—250 mg of labetalol in 250 mL of normal saline, administered at the rate of 20 mg/hour (20 mL/minute). Orally, labetalol is administered in the dose of 100 mg 8-hourly, which may be increased to 800 mg/day. | Labetalol, a nonselective β-blocker that also has vascular α1 receptor blocking capabilities, has gained wide acceptance in pregnancy. It helps in lowering BP smoothly but rapidly, without causing tachycardia. The use of this drug during pregnancy is gaining popularity because no real adverse effects have been demonstrated. The onset of action of intravenous dosage is within 5–10 minutes. |
| Nifedipine | Nifedipine should be given in the dose of 5–10 mg orally, which can be repeated after 30 minutes, if necessary, followed by 10–20 mg every 3–6 hours. The slow release preparation is given in the dosage of 30–120 mg/day. Nifedipine can also be administered via intragastric route using a Ryle's tube. The dose should not exceed 10 mg at a time and should not be repeated more frequently than every 30 minutes. | Nifedipine is a calcium-channel blocker, which should be given orally and not sublingually for control of high BP. There has been little experience with other calcium-channel blockers. |
| Hydralazine | It is used for urgent control of severe hypertension or as a third-line agent for multidrug control of refractory hypertension in the dosage of 50–300 mg/day in 2–4 divided doses. For controlling hypertensive crisis during pregnancy, hydralazine is given in the dose of 5–10 mg intravenously, repeated every 20 minutes until the desired response is achieved. It can also be administered in the form of continuous infusion, given at the rate of 0.5–10 mg/hour. | Hydralazine is a directly acting arterial vasodilator, which is the preferred antihypertensive for the treatment of hypertensive crisis during pregnancy. |
| β-receptor blockers | Dosage varies with different agents. Propranolol is initiated at a dosage of 40–60 mg daily. The maximum dosage is 480–640 mg/day. Dosage of labetalol has been previously mentioned. | Use of atenolol must be avoided during pregnancy. Presently labetalol is being considered safer than other β-blockers during pregnancy, and it is rapidly becoming the first-line therapy for treatment of chronic hypertension during pregnancy. Propranolol can also be considered as an effective drug for treatment of chronic hypertension during pregnancy. |
| ACE inhibitors and AT1-receptor antagonists | To be avoided in all trimesters of pregnancy | |

*Abbreviations:* NHBPEP, National High Blood Pressure Education Program; ACE, angiotensin-converting enzyme; AT 1, angiotensin 1
*Source:* Alpern RJ, Hebert SC. The Kidney: Physiology and Pathophysiology, 4th edition. San Diego, California: Academic Press, Elsevier; 2008. p. 2386

infusion of 1 g/hour maintained for 24 hours after the last seizure.

- *Sibai's regimen:* A loading dose of 6 g should be given by infusion pump over 5–10 minutes, followed by a further infusion of 1 g/hour maintained for 24 hours after the last seizure.

When magnesium sulfate is administered, the maternal parameters such as urine output, deep-tendon reflexes, respiratory rate and oxygen saturation must be regularly assessed. If available, serum levels of magnesium should also be regularly monitored. The therapeutic levels of magnesium range from 4 mEq/L to 7 mEq/L. If the IM regime is used, it is important to ensure the following parameters before the administration of a repeat dose: urine output is more than 30 mL/hour; patellar reflexes are intact and respiratory rate is above 16/minute. An overdose of magnesium sulfate causes respiratory and cardiac depression.

Toxicity to magnesium sulfate is a life-threatening emergency and intubation with bag and mask ventilation must be done immediately. External cardiac massage may also be required. Ten milliliters of 10% calcium gluconate must be slowly administered intravenously. This serves as an antidote for magnesium sulfate poisoning.

In case of nonavailability of $MgSO_4$ drugs like diazepam (valium) or phenytoin (dilantin) must be used.

### Q. When are diuretics prescribed during pregnancy?

**Ans.** Most commonly used diuretic during pregnancy is furosemide (Lasix), which is prescribed orally in the dosage of 40 mg after breakfast for 5 days in the week. Diuretics are prescribed only under the following circumstances:

- Cardiac failure.
- Pulmonary edema.
- Along with some antihypertensive agents (e.g. diazoxide group) where BP reduction is associated with fluid retention.
- Massive edema, which is not relieved by taking rest and is producing major discomfort to the patient.

### Q. How is the hypertension controlled in the postpartum period?

**Ans.** Postpartum hypertension commonly occurs 3–6 days after delivery, with the maximum increase in BP occurring towards the end of the first postpartum week. Therefore, continued close monitoring must be done following delivery.

- Antihypertensive drugs should be given if the BP exceeds 150 mm Hg systolic or 100 mm Hg diastolic in the first 4 days of the puerperium. The medication may then be discontinued when BP normalizes.

### Q. What are the various maternal and fetal complications, which can occur as a result of preeclampsia?

**Ans.** Some of the maternal and fetal complications related to preeclampsia are as follows:

#### Fetal Complications

- *Prematurity*: Premature babies born before 37 completed weeks of pregnancy.
- *Intrauterine growth restriction:* Uteroplacental insufficiency in patients with preeclampsia restricts the placental blood flow limiting the supply of essential nutrients and oxygen to the fetus. Blood flow in the baby may get restricted to the limbs, kidney and abdomen in an effort to preserve the blood supply to the vital areas like the brain and heart, resulting in the development of growth-restricted fetuses. Intrauterine growth restriction (IUGR) in the long run can result in the development of fetal acidosis and hypoxia.
- Oligohydramnios
- Intrauterine death (IUD)/infant death.
- Prematurity.
- Intrauterine asphyxia and acidosis.

#### Maternal Complications

- *Abruption placenta:* Preeclampsia is an important cause for development of abruption placenta, which refers to the premature separation of a normally implanted placenta.
- *Cerebral hemorrhage*: Untreated high BP serves as an important cause for the development of cerebral hemorrhage and stroke.
- *HELLP syndrome:* About 20% of women with severe preeclampsia may develop a complication called HELLP syndrome (an abbreviation which stands for hemolysis, elevated liver enzymes and a low platelet count).

- Eclampsia.
- Risk of recurrence of preeclampsia in subsequent pregnancies.
- Impaired renal/liver function.
- Pulmonary edema, maternal death.
- Preterm labor.
- Acute respiratory distress syndrome.
- *Postpartum hemorrhage:* This may be due to coagulation failure.
- *Remote complications:* These may include complications such as residual hypertension, which may persist for even 6 months following delivery in about 50% of cases and recurrent preeclampsia, where there are nearly 25% chances of recurrence in subsequent pregnancies.
- Chronic renal disease.

## Case Study 4

Mrs XYZ, a 29-year-old married for 4 years, resident of ABC, G3P2L2 patient with 38 weeks of gestation presented to the emergency department with the history of throwing a fit at home, 2 hours back. On examination, the per abdominal examination revealed a single live fetus in cephalic presentation. Her BP was 180/100 mm Hg. The patient at the time of examination was conscious and well-oriented in time, place and person. No other abnormality was observed on general physical examination.

### Q. What is eclampsia?

**Ans.** Eclampsia is one of the most serious complications of preeclampsia. This can be defined as the onset of tonic and clonic convulsions in a pregnant patient with preeclampsia, usually occurring in the third trimester of pregnancy, intrapartum period or more than 48 hours postpartum.

Eclampsia is thought to be related to cerebral vasospasm, which can cause ischemia, disruption of the blood brain barrier and cerebral edema. Once the seizures and severe hypertension has been controlled, delivery is required for the treatment of eclampsia.

### Q. How is eclampsia prevented?

**Ans.** In order to prevent the occurrence of eclampsia, the clinician needs to remain vigilant regarding the appearance of signs of imminent eclampsia in patients with severe preeclampsia. The decision for delivery must be made as soon as possible in patients with severe preeclampsia.

Women with severe preeclampsia (BP > 160/100 mm Hg along with proteinuria) should be given magnesium sulfate as a prophylactic measure. Magnesium sulfate should be continued for 24 hours after delivery or 24 hours after the last convulsion, whichever is later.

### Q. How should eclampsia be managed?

**Ans.** Every maternity unit must be equipped to deal with this obstetric emergency and must institute emergency management effectively. There should preferably be a separate eclampsia room in each obstetric ward. This room should be especially reserved for patients with severe preeclampsia or eclampsia and should be free from noise. It should have a railed bed and equipment like suction machine, equipment for resuscitation, syringes, tongue blade and drug tray with drugs such as magnesium sulfate, nifedipine, diazepam, etc. Early involvement of consultant clinician, anesthetic staff and other specialists including a hematologist, ophthalmologist, neonatologist, etc. may be required. Care of patients with eclampsia requires the following steps:

- Immediate care involves maintenance of airway, oxygenation and prevention of trauma or injury to the patient. Injury to the patient can be prevented by placing her on a railed bed. A tongue blade can be used to prevent her from biting her tongue.
- The patient should be placed in the left lateral position and the airway must be secured. Oxygen should be administered through a face mask.
- Monitoring of vitals including pulse, BP, respiratory rate and oxygen saturation needs to be done every 15 minutes. Knee jerks and urine output need to be monitored every half hourly.
- An IV line must be secured and the patient must be given IV ringer lactate or 0.9% normal saline solution. Fluids should be restricted to 80 mL/hour or 1 mg/kg body weight.
- Close monitoring of fluid intake and urine output at every half hourly interval is mandatory.
- Treatment of choice to treat convulsions is the administration of magnesium sulfate.
- Once the patient has stabilized, an obstetric examination must be performed and fetal status must be evaluated. An obstetric evaluation and plan to deliver the patient is required.
- Continued fetal monitoring, preferably through continuous electronic monitoring is required until the baby is delivered.

Though definitive treatment of eclampsia is delivery, the maternal wellbeing gets priority over fetal condition. Once the mother has stabilized, delivery should be undertaken as soon as possible. However, it is inappropriate to deliver an unstable mother even if there is fetal distress. Once seizures and severe hypertension has been treated and hypoxia has been corrected, delivery can be expedited. The mode of delivery, either by vaginal or abdominal route depends on obstetric evaluation of the individual patient. If the cervix appears unfavorable, vaginal prostaglandins can be used for induction of labor. Strict BP monitoring must be continued throughout labor. If the maternal condition stabilizes, convulsions are absent and the fetus is preterm, the delivery can be delayed. During this time, corticosteroids should be administered to attain fetal maturity and continuous fetal surveillance needs to be done. The patient can be shifted to a tertiary care center having adequate neonatal resuscitation facilities.

### Q. What should be the mode of delivery in patients with eclampsia?

**Ans.** Eclampsia per se is not an indication for cesarean delivery. In case the cervix is not favorable, labor can be induced using vaginal prostaglandins and oxytocin infusion. Indications for CS in cases of eclampsia are as follows:

- Any obstetric indication [cephalopelvic disproportion (CPD), placenta previa, etc.].
- Fetal distress.
- Vaginal delivery is unlikely to occur within a reasonable time frame after the first eclamptic fit.

### Q. How is the management of women with eclampsia done in the postpartum period?

**Ans.** Since most postnatal convulsions occur within the first 24 hours after delivery, following precautions must be observed in the postpartum period:

- Anticonvulsant therapy is generally continued for at least 24 hours after delivery.
- Clinicians must remember that nearly half the cases of eclampsia occur postpartum, especially at term, so women with signs or symptoms compatible with preeclampsia should be carefully observed postnatally at least for 4 days or more following delivery.
- Antihypertensive medication should be continued after delivery depending on the BP recordings. During this time, BP should not be allowed to exceed 160/110 mm Hg. Currently, there is insufficient evidence to recommend any particular antihypertensive. The most commonly used drugs in the postpartum period include β-blockers (e.g. atenolol 50–100 mg OD), with addition of a calcium antagonist (e.g. slow-release nifedipine 10–20 mg OD) and/or an ACE inhibitor (e.g. enalapril 5–10 mg BD).
- A regular assessment of BP and proteinuria by the general practitioner at the 6th and 12th weeks following delivery is recommended.

# Breech Presentation

### Case Study 1

Mrs XYZ, a 30-year-old married for 7 years, resident of ABC, primi patient with 39 completed weeks of gestation having breech presentation as diagnosed by ultrasound examination had presented for regular antenatal check-up. No other abnormality was detected on the ultrasound.

### Q. What is the most likely diagnosis in the above-mentioned case study?

**Ans.** The most likely diagnosis in the above-mentioned case study is Mrs XYZ, a 30-year-old woman, married for 7 years, resident of ABC, primi patient with 39 weeks of amenorrhea, corresponding to 39 weeks of gestation having a single live fetus in longitudinal lie, flexed attitude, breech presentation and buttocks as the presenting part. The questions to be asked at the time of taking history and the parameters to be assessed at the time of examination in such a case are described in Tables 5.9 and 5.10 respectively.

**Q. What is breech presentation and what are different types of breech presentations?**
**Ans.** In breech presentation, the fetus lies longitudinally with the buttocks and/or the feet presenting in the lower pole of the uterus. Different types of breech presentations are described next:
- *Frank breech:* This is the most common type of breech presentation (50–70% cases). Buttocks present first with hips flexed and legs extended on the abdomen. This position is also known as the pike position.
- *Complete breech:* Also known as the cannonball position, this type of presentation is present in 5–10% cases. In this, the buttocks present first with flexed hips and flexed knees. Feet are not below the buttocks.
- *Footling breech:* One or both feet present as both hips and knees are in extended position. As a result, feet are palpated at a level lower than the buttocks. This type of presentation is seen in 10–30% cases.

**Q. What are the findings observed on ultrasound examination in case of breech presentation?**
**Ans.** Ultrasound examination helps in confirming the type of breech presentation. The other things which can be observed on the ultrasound include the following:
- Presence of uterine and/or fetal anomalies.
- Extension of fetal head: "Star gazing sign" on ultrasound examination can be observed if the degree of extension of fetal head is greater than 90°.
- Fetal maturity.
- Placental location and grading.

**Table 5.9:** Symptoms to be elicited at the time of taking history in a case of breech presentation

*History of Presenting Complains*
- There are no specific symptoms suggestive of breech presentation.

*Medical History*
- Past history of gynecological disorders, e.g. uterine anomalies (bicornuate or septate uterus) or presence of space occupying lesions (e.g. fibroids in the lower uterine segment), pelvic tumor, etc. could act as a risk factor for breech presentation.

*Obstetric History*
- Presence of cephalopelvic disproportion or contracted maternal pelvis in the previous pregnancy and presence of liquor abnormalities (polyhydramnios, oligohydramnios) in the present pregnancy or placental abnormalities (placenta previa, cornuofundal attachment of placenta); multiparity (especially grand multiparas); could act as the likely risk factors for breech presentation.
- Previous history of breech delivery.

**Table 5.10:** Various findings elicited at the time of clinical examination in a case of breech presentation

*Specific Systemic Examination*

*Abdominal Examination*
*Inspection of the abdomen:* A transverse groove corresponding to the fetal neck may be seen above the umbilicus. In a patient with thin built, the fetal head may be seen as a localized bulge in one hypochondrium.

*Abdominal Palpation*
- Fetal lie is longitudinal with fetal head on one side and breech on the other side.
- *First Leopold maneuver/fundal grip:* Smooth, hard, ballotable structure, often tender, is suggestive of fetal head.
- *Second Leopold maneuver/lateral grip:* Firm, smooth board-like fetal back is identified on one side and knob-like structures suggestive of fetal limbs on other side. A depression corresponding to the fetal neck may also be identified.
- *Leopold's third maneuver:* If the engagement has yet not occurred, the breech is movable above the pelvic brim. The breech is felt as a smooth soft mass continuous with the back.
- *Leopold's fourth maneuver:* Head is not felt in pelvis; instead an irregular, soft, nonballotable structure suggestive of fetal buttocks and/or feet may be felt.
- *Fetal heart auscultation:* In case the engagement has not occurred, fetal heart sound (FHS) is just heard above the umbilicus; if the engagement has occurred, the FHS is heard just below the umbilicus.

*Vaginal Examination*
Following features may be observed on vaginal examination:
- Palpation of three bony landmarks of the breech, namely, ischial tuberosities and sacral tip.
- Feet may be felt besides the buttocks in cases of complete breech.
- Fresh meconium may be found on the examining fingers; presence of thick, dark meconium is a normal finding in cases of breech presentation.
- Palpation of the male genitalia.

- Adequacy of liquor.
- Estimation of gestational age and fetal weight.
- Ruling out multiple gestation (diagnosis of unsuspected twins).
- Exclusion of congenital abnormalities

### Case Study 2

Mrs XYZ, a 30-year-old married for 8 years, resident of ABC, G4P3A1L2 patient with 35 completed weeks of gestation was seen in the clinic for a routine ANC visit. Her general physical examination was WNL and vitals were stable. Per abdominal examination showed a uterus of 36 weeks size with a single live fetus in breech presentation. She had been diagnosed as having breech presentation by ultrasound examination, when she had presented for last antenatal check-up. No other abnormality was detected on the ultrasound. She has been planned for an external cephalic version (ECV) at 37 weeks of gestation.

**Q. How can the above-mentioned case study be managed during pregnancy?**

**Ans.** The management options for breech presentation include ECV during pregnancy to convert breech presentation into cephalic presentation or delivery by CS or a breech vaginal delivery at term. In the above-mentioned case study, the option of ECV had been planned as the woman was not willing for cesarean delivery. All the factors which are likely to result in a successful version were present in this patient. The external version score was 8 in this case. Moreover, there were no contraindications for ECV.

**Q. What is external cephalic version?**

**Ans.** External cephalic version is a procedure in which the clinician externally rotates the fetus from a breech presentation into a cephalic presentation. The use of ECV helps in producing considerable cost savings in the management of the breech fetus at term by reducing the rate of CS.

**Q. What is the external version score in this patient?**

**Ans.** The external version score (Table 5.11) helps in predicting the success rate of ECV. Five factors (parity, placental location, dilatation, station and estimated fetal weight) are used for calculating this score. A higher version score ($\geq 4$) is associated with an increased likelihood of successful breech version. In the above-mentioned case study, the parity was more than 2; the cervical os permitted one finger; station was more than –3; estimated fetal weight was between 2.5 kg and 3 kg; and the placenta was fundal in location. The total score was 8 in the above-mentioned case study.

**Q. What are the indicators for a successful external cephalic version?**

**Ans.** Some of the indicators for successful ECV include the following:

- *Multiparity:* ECV is more likely to be successful in multiparous women.
- *Nonfrank breech:* ECV is more likely to be successful in nonfrank breech (complete breech) pregnancies in comparison to frank breech pregnancies. This is so as the splinting action of the spine in a frank breech gestation is likely to prevent easy movement of the fetus.
- *Unengaged breech:* Fetus in breech presentation which has engaged is less likely to undergo version in comparison to the unengaged fetus in breech presentation.
- *Adequate liquor:* Presence of reduced (oligohydramnios) or excessive liquor (polyhydramnios) is also likely to interfere with successful version.

**Q. When should the external cephalic version be performed?**

**Ans.** It is preferable to wait until term (37 completed weeks of gestation) before external version is attempted because of an increased success rate and avoidance of preterm delivery if complications arise. Ideally the ECV should be performed as close to 37 weeks as possible, but after 36 weeks. If external version is performed in preterm gestations, the success rate is believed to be 80%. However, small-sized fetuses with preterm gestation may undergo spontaneous reversion back to breech presentation in about 16% cases. A small preterm fetus has more room to be turned and therefore, can revert on its own. When ECV is performed at term, though the success rate falls to 63%, the reversion rate improves to 6–7%. This is so because the larger fetus has less freedom of movement and therefore is less likely to revert back to breech presentation. The most important reason to wait until the fetus is at term is to avoid iatrogenic prematurity in case emergency delivery is required. This can happen if an attempt at external version results in complications like active labor, ruptured membranes, fetal compromise, etc.

**Q. Describe the procedure of ECV.**
**Ans.** Kindly refer to Chapter 6.

**Q. What are the contraindications of ECV?**
**Ans.** Kindly refer to Chapter 6.

**Q. What are the complications of ECV?**
**Ans.** Kindly refer to Chapter 6.

**Table 5.11:** The external version score

|  | 0 | 1 | 2 |
|---|---|---|---|
| Parity for ECV | 0 | 1 | $\geq 2$ |
| Dilatation | $\geq 3$ cm | 1–2 cm | 0 cm |
| Estimated fetal weight | < 2,500 g | 2,500–3,500 g | > 3,500 g |
| Placenta | Anterior | Posterior | Fundal |
| Station | $\geq$ –1 | –2 | $\geq$ –3 |

*Abbreviation:* ECV, external cephalic version

## Case Study 3

Mrs XYZ, a 32-year-old married for 10 years, resident of ABC, G4P2A2L2 woman with 38 weeks of gestation with diagnosis of breech presentation at the time of her previous visit presented to the ANC with the complaints of labor pain. Her general physical examination was WNL and vitals were stable. Per abdominal examination showed a uterine size corresponding to 38 weeks of gestation. Per vaginal examination revealed soft patulous cervix which was two fingers dilated. Soft presenting part suggestive of breech presentation was felt at 0 station.

### Q. If the breech presentation persists till term, what is the mode of delivery?

**Ans.** There are two choices regarding mode of delivery for patients with breech presentation: breech vaginal delivery (also known as trial of breech) or an elective CS. There has been much controversy for choosing the best option for delivery. Parents must be informed about potential risks and benefits to the mother and neonate for both vaginal breech delivery and cesarean delivery. Presently, the trend for term breech presentation is elective CS. However, in the above-mentioned case study, since the patient was a multigravida and already in labor, the option of breech vaginal delivery was considered. Though she was also given an option for cesarean delivery she did not give her consent for it.

### Q. What is the Zatuchni and Andros breech scoring system?

**Ans.** The breech scoring system by Zatuchni and Andros (Table 5.12) can be also used for deciding whether to perform a vaginal or an abdominal delivery. If the woman has a score of 3 or less in this scoring system, it means that she should probably be delivered by a CS, which would be associated with a lower degree of fetal morbidity and mortality in comparison to vaginal delivery. Higher scores, although not guarantying a safe vaginal delivery, suggest that a trial of labor (TOL) with close monitoring can be considered.

### Q. What are the various indications for breech vaginal delivery?

**Ans.** Various indications for breech vaginal delivery are as follows:
- Frank or complete breech (not footling).
- Estimated fetal weight between 1.5 kg and 3.5 kg.
- Gestational age (36–42 weeks).
- Well-flexed fetal head (no evidence of hyperextension of the fetal head).
- Adequate pelvis (no fetopelvic disproportion).
- Normal progress of labor on partogram.
- Uncomplicated pregnancy (No other obstetric contraindications for vaginal birth, e.g. placenta previa, severe IUGR, etc.).
- Multiparous women.
- No obstetric indication for CS, (e.g. fetopelvic disproportion, placenta previa, etc.).
- An experienced clinician.
- Presence of severe fetal anomaly or fetal death.
- Mother's preference for vaginal birth.
- Delivery is imminent.

### Q. What are different types of breech vaginal deliveries?

**Ans.** Three types of vaginal breech deliveries have been described:
- *Spontaneous breech delivery:* No traction or manipulation of the infant by the clinician is done. The fetus delivers spontaneously on its own. This occurs predominantly in very preterm deliveries.
- *Assisted breech delivery:* This is the most common mode of vaginal breech delivery. In this method, a "no-touch technique" is adopted in which the infant is allowed to deliver spontaneously up to the umbilicus, and then certain maneuvers are initiated by the clinician to aid in the delivery of the remainder of the body, arms, and head. Various such maneuvers have been described in Chapter 4.
- *Total breech extraction:* In this method, the fetal feet are grasped, and the entire fetus is extracted by the clinician. Total breech extraction should be used only for a noncephalic second twin. It should not be used for singleton fetuses because the cervix may not be adequately dilated to allow passage of the fetal head.

### Q. What type of vaginal delivery was adopted in the above-mentioned case study?

**Ans.** Assisted breech delivery was planned in this patient. Various maneuvers adopted at the time of assisted breech delivery are described in Chapter 4.

| **Table 5.12:** Zatuchni and Andros scoring system | | | |
|---|---|---|---|
| *Parameter* | *0 point* | *1 point* | *2 points* |
| Parity | Primigravida | Multigravida | |
| Gestational age | 39 weeks or more | 38 weeks | 37 weeks |
| Estimated fetal weight | > 8 pounds (3,690 g) | 7–8 pounds (3,176–3,690 g) | < 7 pounds (< 3,176 g) |
| Previous breech > 2,500 g | None | One | Two or more |
| Cervical dilatation on admission by vaginal examination | 2 cm or less | 3 cm | 4 cm or more |
| Station at the time of admission | –3 or higher | –2 | –1 or lower |

**Q. List the steps of intrapartum care for patients undergoing breech vaginal delivery.**

**Ans.** Intrapartum care for patients undergoing breech vaginal delivery is as follows:

- Informed consent must be taken from the patient after explaining that the trial of breech can fail in 20% of cases, thereby requiring a CS.
- Plan for vaginal breech delivery must be clearly documented in the mother's notes.
- Care should be provided by an experienced clinician and midwife. Anesthetist and pediatrician must also be present. Women should be given the choice of analgesia. Ranitidine 150 mg orally must be administered every 6 hours in case cesarean delivery is required in future.
- At the time of labor, the risk factors for presence of breech presentation should be reviewed again (presence of placenta previa, twins, etc.) and a complete abdominal and vaginal examination needs to be carried out.
- Close monitoring of maternal vital conditions, uterine contractions and FHR needs to be done.
- Maternal intravenous line must be set up as the mother may require emergency induction of anesthesia at any time.
- Women should be advised to remain in bed to avoid PROM and the risk of cord prolapse. The fetal membranes must be left intact as long as possible; they must not be ruptured artificially, but allowed to rupture on their own in order to prevent the hazard of overt cord prolapse. In case the bag of membranes ruptures spontaneously, a per vaginal examination must be performed immediately to rule out cord prolapse. It is also advisable to do continuous FHR recording for 5–10 minutes following rupture of membranes (ROM) to rule out occult cord prolapse.
- Active management of labor preferably using a partogram needs to be done.
- Breech presentation should be confirmed by an ultrasound examination in the labor ward.
- Use of oxytocin induction and augmentation for breech presentation is controversial.
- Labor must be preferably monitored using cardiotocographic examination.
- Mother should be in dorsal lithotomy position for breech vaginal delivery.
- Lumbar epidural analgesia must be used to provide pain relief and to prevent voluntary bearing down efforts prior to complete dilatation of cervix.
- Routine episiotomy for every breech vaginal delivery is not required. However, if the clinician feels that the birth passage is too small, he/she must use his/her own discretion in giving an episiotomy.
- Delivery should be preferably conducted in the operation theater so that a CS should be considered if there is delay in the descent of the breech in the first or second stage of labor.

**Q. What are the various maternal and fetal complications associated with breech vaginal delivery?**

**Ans.** Various maternal and fetal complications associated with breech vaginal delivery are as follows:

*Fetal Complications*

- *Low APGAR Scores:* Low APGAR scores, especially at 1 minute are more common with vaginal breech deliveries and could be related to birth asphyxia. Increased risk of birth asphyxia in cases of breech vaginal delivery could be due to the following causes:
  - Cord compression/cord prolapse.
  - Premature attempts by the baby to breathe while the head is still inside the uterine cavity.
  - Delay in the delivery of the head may be due to head entrapment.
- *Fetal head entrapment:* Fetal head entrapment may result from an incompletely dilated cervix and head that lacks time to mold to the maternal pelvis. In most of the cases, fetal head entrapment is also associated with umbilical cord compression. Therefore, this condition must be dealt with urgently.
- *Preterm birth:* Preterm birth (delivery of baby at < 28 weeks) commonly occurs in breech presentation. Preterm birth can often result in complications related to prematurity.
- *Neonatal trauma/injuries:* Neonatal trauma including brachial plexus injuries, hematomas, fractures, visceral injuries, etc. can occur in about 25% of cases. There can be fractures of humerus, clavicle and/or femur. Hematomas of sternocleidomastoid muscle can also commonly occur. However, they disappear spontaneously. Testicular injury resulting in anorchia may also sometimes follow breech vaginal delivery. Successive compression and decompression of unmolded after-coming head of the breech and increased risk of head entrapment can result in intracranial hemorrhage and tentorial tears.
- *Cord prolapse:* Cord prolapse is a condition associated with abnormal descent of the umbilical cord before the descent of the fetal presenting part. The cord could be lying by the side of the fetal presenting part or it could have slipped down below the presenting part. In extreme cases, the cord could be lying totally outside the vagina. Cord prolapse occurs in 7.5% of all breeches. This incidence varies with the type of breech: 0–2% with frank breech, 5% with complete breech and 10–15% with footling breech. Cord prolapse occurs twice as often in multiparas (6%) than in primigravidas (3%). This condition can be diagnosed on Doppler ultrasound.

*Maternal Complications*

- Increased rate of maternal morbidity and mortality due to increased incidence of operative/difficult delivery.
- Traumatic injuries to the genital tract.

**Q. What is the management plan in cases of cord prolapse?**
**Ans.** Cord prolapse is an obstetric condition which must be urgently dealt with in order to prevent fetal mortality. If the cord has already prolapsed at the time of examination, no attempt must be made to replace the cord back. Urgent delivery of the baby (by any route) is required in these circumstances. If urgent vaginal delivery is not possible or is contraindicated, immediate preparations for an emergency cesarean delivery must be made. While preparations for cesarean delivery are being made, attempts must be made to minimize cord compression. For more information related to this, kindly refer to Chapter 4.

## Case Study 4

Mrs XYZ, a 28-year-old married for 2 years, resident of ABC, primi patient with 39 weeks of gestation who had been diagnosed with breech presentation and placenta previa on the ultrasound examination, presented with complaints of vaginal spotting since past 1 hour. Her general physical examination was WNL and vitals were stable. The abdominal examination revealed a uterus 38 weeks in size with a single live fetus in breech presentation and normal fetal heart rate.

**Q. What is the management in above-mentioned case study?**
**Ans.** Presently, the management of term breech fetus has largely shifted from routine vaginal breech delivery to elective cesarean delivery for all. However, in this case there was also an associated placenta previa. Therefore, cesarean delivery was the most suitable option.

**Q. When is cesarean delivery considered in cases of breech presentation?**
**Ans.** Presently, the management of term breech fetus has largely shifted from routine vaginal breech delivery to elective cesarean delivery for all. Some of the absolute indications for CS in cases of breech presentation are as follows:
- Cephalopelvic disproportion (any degree).
- Placenta previa.
- Estimated fetal weight more than 4 kg.
- Hyperextension of fetal head (as detected on ultrasound examination).
- Susceptibility to cord prolapse.
- Footling breech (danger of entrapment of head in an incompletely dilated cervix).
- Severe IUGR.
- Clinician not competent with the technique of breech vaginal delivery.
- Presence of an additional obstetric indication for cesarean delivery.

Most clinicians also consider a cesarean delivery in cases of primigravidas because in these cases, the maternal passages have not been tested for delivery before. Cesarean delivery is also considered in pregnancies complicated with diabetes, hypertension, placenta previa, prelabor PROM ($\geq$ 12 hours), post-term pregnancy, IUGR, placental insufficiency, etc.

# Previous Cesarean Delivery

## Case Study 1

Mrs XYZ, a 24-year-old married for 4 years, resident of ABC, G3P2L1 woman attended the booking antenatal clinic with a previous history of a CS at term due to fetal distress. Prior to this delivery, she also gives history of normal vaginal delivery. She is sure of her last menstrual period (LMP) and her period of gestation is 14 weeks both by dates and on abdominal examination.

**Q. What is the most likely diagnosis in the above-mentioned case study?**
**Ans.** The diagnosis in above-mentioned case study is Mrs XYZ, a 24-year-old woman, married for 4 years, resident of ABC, G3P2L1 with 40 weeks amenorrhea, corresponding to term pregnancy having a single live fetus in longitudinal lie, flexed attitude, cephalic presentation with previous history of one cesarean delivery performed for a nonrecurrent indication. The questions to be asked at the time of taking history and the parameters to be assessed at the time of examination in such a case are described in Tables 5.13 and 5.14 respectively.

**Q. What is a cesarean section and what are the different indications for cesarean delivery?**
**Ans.** Cesarean section is removal of a fetus from the uterus by abdominal and uterine incisions, after 28 weeks of pregnancy. If the removal of fetus is done before 28 weeks of pregnancy, the procedure is known as hysterotomy. Presently, there has been a considerable rise in the rate of cesarean delivery. Some of the common indications for cesarean delivery are as follows:
- A term singleton breech pregnancy (if ECV is contraindicated or has failed).
- Dystocia (secondary arrest of cervical dilatation, arrest of descent, CPD, etc.).
- A twin pregnancy with first twin in noncephalic presentation.
- HIV positive women (who are not receiving any antiretroviral therapy or those who are receiving any antiretroviral therapy and have a viral load of 400 copies/mL or more—in these women cesarean delivery helps in reducing the risk of mother-to-child transmission).
- Grade 3 and 4 placenta previa.
- Women suspected to have morbidly adherent placenta on color Doppler and/or magnetic resonance imaging examination.
- Fetal distress.
- Co-infection with both HIV and hepatitis C (to reduce the risk of mother-to-child transmission).
- Primary genital herpes in the third trimester.
- Maternal request for cesarean delivery (vaginal birth is unacceptable to the mother even after provision of adequate counseling and mental support).

**Table 5.13:** Symptoms to be elicited at the time of taking history in a case with previous history of cesarean delivery

*History of Presenting Complains*

The following questions regarding the previous cesarean section (CS) need to be asked:

- What was the indication for the surgery?
  - Was it for a repetitive or a nonrepetitive cause. For example, if the indication for cesarean delivery is breech presentation, it is a nonrepetitive cause. However cephalopelvic disproportion (CPD) can be a repetitive cause requiring a repeat CS during future pregnancies.
  - Was the CS elective one or an emergency surgery?
  - Place where the previous surgery was performed.
  - The period of gestation at which the CS was performed and the skill of the clinician who had performed the surgery.
  - What was the type of the scar given (classical or the lower segment)?
  - Were there any technical difficulties encountered during the procedure? Was there any lateral extension of the uterine scar or uncontrolled bleeding during the surgery?
  - Suturing method: If the operative notes of previous surgery are available, the following information can be gathered: two verus three layers method of suturing; suture material used, vicryl versus catgut; any extension of the uterine incision; inverted T-scar, etc.
  - Postoperative convalescence: What was the duration of stay in the hospital following surgery?
  - After how many days were the sutures removed?
  - History of wound healing: Was there any history of wound breakdown, history of re-suturing, history of postoperative fever, infection, etc.
  - History of any normal vaginal delivery before or after the previous CS. If yes, was it full term or preterm?
  - Previous history of any other uterine surgery, especially myomectomy for myoma uterus needs to be enquired. This is especially important as vaginal delivery following myomectomy may be complicated by uterine rupture.

**Table 5.14:** Various findings to be elicited at the time of clinical examination in a case with previous history of cesarean delivery

- The routine obstetric abdominal examination.
- Examination of the abdominal scar.
  - *Position of the scar:* Vertical or transverse; corresponding to the lower or upper uterine segment.
  - *Appearance of the scar:* Presence of hypertrophy or keloid formation over the scarred region. Presence of incisional hernia.
  - *Scar tenderness:* The scar tenderness is palpated using the ulnar border of right hand in the region above the public symphysis for a few centimeters.

### Q. What are the various management plans available for pregnant women with a previous section?

**Ans.** There are two options for delivery in the pregnant patients with the history of previous cesarean delivery: Vaginal birth after cesarean delivery (VBAC) or elective repeat cesarean section (ERCS). More than 80% of women are likely to have a vaginal birth following cesarean delivery. The risks and benefits of both CS and vaginal delivery need to be explained to the patient.

### Q. What is TOLAC?

TOLAC refers to trial of labor in a woman who had previous cesarean delivery, irrespective of the outcome, i.e. whether vaginal birth would be successful or not.

## Case Study 2

Mrs XYZ, a 30-year-old married for 8 years, resident of ABC, G3P2L2 patient with the history of previous cesarean delivery for placenta previa was admitted at 38 weeks gestation with history of labor pains since past 6–8 hours. Ultrasound examination during the previous ANC visit had revealed a fundal placenta. Abdominal examination showed a term fetus in cephalic presentation. The fetal head was free floating with fetal heart rate of 140 beats per minute. On pervaginal examination, the cervix was 80% effaced; 4 cm dilated, with fetal head at –3 station. No CPD was present.

### Q. What is the management plan in the above-mentioned case study?

**Ans.** In the past, management of the patient with a history of cesarean scar was considered as "once a cesarean, always a cesarean". This dictum has now been changed to "once a cesarean always hospitalization". In the above-mentioned case study, the woman gave a history of previous lower segment cesarean delivery. There was no recurrent cause for cesarean delivery and the patient was willing for VBAC. There was availability of adequate resources and no other obstetric indications for a cesarean delivery were present. CPD had been ruled out. As a result of these above-mentioned factors, a decision for VBAC was taken in this case study.

### Q. What are the various criteria before considering vaginal birth after cesarean section?

**Ans.** The decision for VBAC is usually taken after considering the parameters described next:

- *Indication for the previous cesarean (recurrent or a nonrecurrent cause):* If the indication of previous CS was a nonrecurrent cause (e.g. fetal distress or nonprogress of labor), which may or may not recur in future pregnancies, the option of VBAC can be considered. However, if the indication for previous cesarean is a recurrent cause like CPD, the option of ERCS would be more suitable.

- *Any associated obstetrical complications in the present pregnancy:* If the present pregnancy is associated with some other obstetrical indication for CS (e.g. grade III, IV placenta previa; breech presentation; etc.), the patient must be considered for ERCS.
- *Ultrasound estimated weight of the baby:* If the ultrasound estimated fetal weight is more than or equal to 4.0 kg, the option of ERCS should be considered due to the increased risk of shoulder dystocia and fetal injuries with vaginal delivery.
- *Number of the previous sections:* According to recommendations by RCOG (2007), women with the history of previous two uncomplicated low transverse CS can be considered for a planned VBAC. Women with a prior history of two uncomplicated low transverse cesarean sections, in an otherwise uncomplicated pregnancy at term, with no contraindication for vaginal birth, need to be adequately counseled by a consultant clinician before being considered for VBAC.
- *Strength of the scar as elicited from history and the clinical examination:* If the scar appears to be healthy and strong as elicited from the history and clinical examination, the option of VBAC can be considered.
- *Informed consent of the patients:* VBAC should be undertaken only if the patient is herself satisfied with the decision and is willing to give an informed consent for the same.
- *Previous vaginal birth:* Previous history of vaginal birth, particularly previous VBAC can be considered as the single best predictor for successful VBAC and is associated with a planned VBAC success rate of approximately 90%.
- *Presence of adequate resources:* VBAC should be undertaken in settings where facilities for emergency CS are present and facilities for continuous fetal monitoring during labor are available.

### Q. What are the various advantages of VBAC?

**Ans.** The vaginal birth after CS is associated with the following advantages:

- Prevention of surgery related complications such as blood loss, infection, injury to various organs including bowel, urinary bladder, thromboembolism, etc.
- Breastfeeding is generally easier after a vaginal birth.
- Vaginal birth is usually associated with reduced health care costs in comparison to cesarean births.
- VBAC is also associated with lower fetal mortality and morbidity in comparison to elective repeat cesareans.

### Q. What are the contraindications for vaginal birth after cesarean section?

**Ans.** Vaginal birth after CS is contraindicated in the presence of the following conditions:

- Previous history of uterine rupture (risk of recurrent rupture is unknown).

- Previous history of J-shaped or an inverted T-shaped uterine incision (variants of the lower segment transverse incision).
- Previous history of high vertical classical CS, with the uterine incision involving almost the whole length of the uterine corpus (associated with approximately 200–900/10,000 risk of uterine rupture).
- History of previous three or more lower segment uterine scars in the past.
- Presence of an obstetric indication for cesarean including CPD, placenta previa, malpresentation, etc.
- Limited resource setting, where it might not be possible to continuously monitor the patient.
- Patient refuses to give consent for VBAC.

### Q. What are the possible risks of VBAC?

**Ans.** The possible risks of VBAC are as follows:

- If VBAC turns out to be unsuccessful, an emergency CS may be required.
- There is a risk of the scar dehiscence and rupture, which may be associated with an increased rates of maternal and perinatal mortality.
- Failure of vaginal trial may end up in requirement for an emergency CS. It may also cause uterine rupture or pelvic floor dysfunction.

### Q. How should the women be counseled for vaginal birth after cesarean section?

**Ans.** All the women with a previous history of uncomplicated lower segment cesarean delivery, in an otherwise uncomplicated pregnancy at term, with no contraindication for vaginal birth, need to be counseled regarding both the delivery options (VBAC and ERCS). Women considering the option for vaginal birth after a single previous cesarean should be informed that the chance of successful planned VBAC is approximately 70%. Women who want VBAC should be encouraged and supported and should be counseled regarding the advantages and disadvantages of both the procedures. They should also be informed about the slightly increased chances of uterine rupture during VBAC in comparison with ERCS (about 1 per 10,000 risk of uterine rupture in cases with ERCS vs. 50 per 10,000 with VBAC). Though occurrence of intrapartum fetal death is rare, it is slightly more in cases with VBAC compared with those with ERCS.

### Q. What are the steps to be taken in the intrapartum period of patients undergoing VBAC?

**Ans.** The following steps must be observed during the intrapartum period:

- Blood should be sent for grouping, crossmatching and CBC (including hemoglobin and hematocrit levels). One unit of blood should be arranged.
- Intravenous access to be established and Ringer's lactate can be started.

- Clinical monitoring of the mother for the signs of scar dehiscence needs to be done. This includes monitoring of vitals, especially the pulse rate and scar tenderness, which must be done every 15 minutes.
- Careful monitoring of fetal heart rate (FHR), preferably using continuous external cardiotocograph (CTG). There is no role of intermittent auscultation in these cases.
- Facilities for emergency CS should be available.
- Although induction or augmentation of labor is not contraindicated in these cases, it should be preceded by careful obstetric assessment and appropriate maternal counseling.
- Epidural analgesia can be safely given at the time of labor.
- Intrapartum monitoring regarding the progress of labor must be done using a partogram.
- Second stage of labor can be cut short by using prophylactic forceps or ventouse.
- Routine uterine exploration following VBAC is not recommended. If the patient shows signs of uterine rupture including tachycardia, hypotension, vaginal bleeding, etc. uterine exploration may be done. Laparotomy may be required if a uterine rent is found on the uterine exploration.

## Case Study 3

Mrs XYZ, a 40-year-old married for 15 years, resident of ABC, G2P2L1 patient with the previous history of CS for oblique lie presented to the A & E at 36 weeks of gestation with the complaints of severe abdominal pain since a few hours. On general physical examination, the pulse was 120 beats/minute and BP was 116/84 mm Hg. On per abdominal examination, there was a 36-week-sized fetus in cephalic presentation. Fetal heart sound could not be heard. There was scar tenderness. On per vaginal examination, cervix was 2 cm dilated and 10% effaced; the presenting part could not be felt, it was high up.

### Q. What is the likely diagnosis in the above-mentioned case study and how can it occur?

**Ans.** The clinical presentation in the above-mentioned case study is suggestive of uterine rupture in a case with previous CS, posted for VBAC. However, this diagnosis can only be confirmed by exploratory laparotomy. Nevertheless before undertaking laparotomy, steps must be taken to resuscitate the patient.

In a patient with a previous CS, TOLAC (trial of labor after cesarean delivery) may cause the previous uterine scar to separate. Disintegration of the scar, also known as scar rupture is one of the most disastrous complications associated with VBAC. Risk of scar rupture after vaginal delivery following one previous lower transverse segment CS on an average is estimated to be about 0.8–1%. However, the exact risk of scar rupture depends upon the type of uterine incision given at the time of previous CS. The weakest type of scar that may give way at the time of VBAC is the previous classical incision in the upper segment of the uterus, which is associated with almost 10% risk of development of scar rupture. Uterine rupture can result in complete extrusion of the fetus into the maternal abdominal cavity. In other cases, rupture is associated with fetal distress or severe hemorrhage from the rupture site.

### Q. What are the symptoms of impending scar rupture?

**Ans.** The most important complication associated in a patient with previous history of CS is the possibility of scar rupture during future pregnancies, especially if given trial is for vaginal delivery. Thus, it is the prime duty of the clinician to remain vigilant and at the earliest detect the signs related to impending scar rupture. Symptoms of impending scar rupture during the labor include the following:

- Dull suprapubic pain or severe abdominal pain, especially if persisting in between the uterine contractions.
- Slight vaginal bleeding or hematuria.
- Bladder tenesmus or frequent desire to pass urine.
- Unexplained maternal tachycardia.
- Maternal hypotension or shock.
- Abnormal FHR pattern.
- Scar tenderness.
- Interruption of previously efficient uterine activity.
- Chest pain or shoulder tip pain, or sudden onset of shortness of breath.
- On vaginal examination, there may be a failure of normal descent of the presenting part and the presenting part may remain high up. There also may be a sudden loss of station of the presenting part.

None of the above-mentioned signs and symptoms are a definite proof of the impending scar rupture. However, presence of any of these symptoms must raise caution in the clinician's mind and he/she must become more vigilant. The diagnosis of scar rupture is ultimately confirmed at the time of emergency cesarean delivery or exploratory laparotomy.

### Q. What is uterine rupture and what are the various types of scar rupture?

**Ans.** Uterine rupture is defined as a disruption of the uterine muscle. It may or may not extend uptill the uterine serosa. The uterine rupture can be of two types: complete rupture and incomplete rupture.

- *Complete rupture:* Complete rupture describes a full-thickness defect of the uterine wall and serosa resulting in direct communication between the uterine cavity and the peritoneal cavity.
- *Incomplete rupture:* Incomplete rupture describes a defect of the uterine wall that is contained by the visceral peritoneum or broad ligament. Incomplete rupture is also known as uterine dehiscence and can be described as

partial disruption of the uterine muscle with the uterine serosa remaining intact.

- The identification or suspicion of uterine rupture is a medical emergency and must be followed by an immediate and urgent response from the clinician. An emergency laparotomy is usually required to save the patient's life.

### Q. How would you manage a case of ruptured uterus?

**Ans.** When uterine rupture is diagnosed or strongly suspected, surgery (laparotomy) is necessary. While in the previous days, most cases of uterine rupture were managed with hysterectomy, nowadays most cases are managed by controlling the bleeding surgically and repairing the defect.

A decision must be made regarding whether to perform hysterectomy or to repair the rupture site. If future fertility is desirable and the rent in the uterus appears to be repairable (straight-cut scar, rupture in the body of uterus; pelvic blood vessels are intact), repair of the rupture site must be performed. If future fertility is not desirable or the uterine rent appears to be unrepairable (multiple rents, with ragged margins; injury to the iliac vessels, etc.), hysterectomy should be performed.

### Case Study 4

Mrs XYZ, a 28-year-old married for 7 years, resident of ABC, G3P2L1 woman with previous history of cesarean delivery for CPD presented to the ANC clinic with 38 weeks of gestation with history of labor pains since past few hours. Per abdominal examination showed a single live fetus in cephalic presentation. On per vaginal examination, cervix was 30% effaced; 4 cm dilated and head was at –2 station. Moderate degree CPD was present.

### Q. What was the likely management in the above-mentioned case study?

**Ans.** Though the woman had been initially posted for ERCS at 39 weeks in lieu of the recurrent cause for previous cesarean delivery, she was now immediately admitted because she was in active labor. She was posted for an emergency cesarean delivery as vaginal delivery appeared impossible in this case.

### Q. What are the advantages of elective repeat cesarean section over VBAC?

**Ans.** For the physician, ERCS may offer a few advantages including convenience, saving of time, increased monetary compensation and reduced fear of legal litigation in case of complications with VBAC. Though CS is safe, it is a major surgical intervention and would be therefore associated with some complications in comparison to normal vaginal delivery. Nevertheless it is associated with the following advantages:

- Reduced incidence of perineal pain.
- Reduced incidence of urinary incontinence.
- Reduced incidence of uterovaginal prolapse.

### Q. What are the disadvantages of ERCS?

**Ans.** Cesarean delivery is associated with an increased risk of complications, which are as follows:

- Abdominal pain.
- Injury to bladder, ureters, etc.
- Neonatal respiratory morbidity.
- Requirement of hysterectomy.
- Thromboembolic disease.
- Increased duration of hospital stay.
- Antepartum or intrapartum IUDs in future pregnancies.
- Patients with a previous history of cesarean delivery are more prone to develop complications like placenta previa and adherent placenta during future pregnancies.

### Q. When should a woman with previous cesarean section delivered by repeat cesarean section?

**Ans.** In case of previous history of classical scar, the woman must preferably be hospitalized at 36 weeks and posted for an elective CS at 38 weeks. In patients with previous history of lower segment uterine scar as in the above-mentioned case study, the planned surgery should be preferably done after 39 weeks. This is so as the risk of respiratory morbidity considerably increases in babies born by CS before 39 weeks of gestation.

## Multifetal Gestation

### Case Study 1

Mrs XYZ, a 24-year-old woman, married for 5 years, resident of ABC, G3P2L2 with 36 completed weeks of gestation and previous history of normal vaginal delivery at term presented for an ANC check-up. There is no history of taking any fertility treatment. On per abdominal examination, multiple fetal parts could be palpated. She gives history of being diagnosed with twin gestation on an ultrasound examination done at 8 weeks.

### Q. What is the most likely diagnosis in the above-mentioned case study?

**Ans.** The diagnosis in above-mentioned case study is Mrs XYZ, a 24-year-old married for 5 years, resident of ABC, G3P2L2 with 36 weeks' amenorrhea, corresponding to 36 weeks of gestation, with multiple fetal parts palpated on per abdominal examination suggestive of multifetal gestation. The exact number of fetuses and their presentation needs to be confirmed by an ultrasound examination. The questions to be asked at the time of taking history or the parameters to be assessed at the time of examination in such a case are described in Tables 5.15 and 5.16 respectively.

### Q. What is multifetal gestation?

**Ans.** Development of two or more embryos simultaneously in a pregnant uterus is termed as multifetal gestation. Development of two fetuses simultaneously is known as twin gestation; development of three fetuses simultaneously as triplets; four fetuses as quadruplets; five fetuses as quintuplets and so on.

| **Table 5.15:** Symptoms to be elicited at the time of taking history in a case of multifetal gestation |
|---|
| *History of Presenting Complains* |
| • Exaggeration of symptoms of early pregnancy, including symptoms like nausea, piles, varicosities, heartburn, shortness of breath, backache, ankle swelling, piles, varicose veins, etc. due to higher levels of circulating hormones. The woman may also be experiencing excessive abdominal enlargement.<br>• Pregnancy complications like preterm labor, preeclampsia, placenta previa, polyhydramnios, anemia, etc. are also more common in twin pregnancies.<br>• With increasing period of gestation, the woman may experience increased frequency of heartburn; indigestion and urinary frequency as the enlarging uterus presses on other organs.<br>• Back pain is common because of the extra load of the enlarging uterus in combination with the relaxation of muscles and ligaments produced by the pregnancy hormones.<br>• The women with multifetal gestation may experience early onset of preeclampsia.<br>• History of painless bleeding pervaginum must be elicited because multifetal fetal gestation is likely to be associated with a large placenta, which may encroach til the cervical os.<br>• History of excessive fetal movements: This could be related to the presence of multiple fetuses. |
| *History of the Likely Risk Factors* |
| • Increased maternal age and parity.<br>• Previous history of twin gestation.<br>• Family history of twin gestation (especially on maternal side).<br>• Conception following a long period of infertility.<br>• Pregnancy attained through use of ART (IVF or use of clomiphene citrate).<br>• Racial origin (twin gestation is more common amongst the women of West African ancestry, less common in those of Japanese ancestry). |

*Abbreviations:* ART, assisted reproductive technology; IVF, in vitro fertilization

| **Table 5.16:** Various findings elicited at the time of clinical examination in a case of multifetal gestation |
|---|
| *General Physical Examination* |
| • Exaggeration of the signs of anemia in a woman with multifetal gestation. She may exhibit pallor of extreme degrees.<br>• There may be early onset of preeclampsia in these women. As a result, they may show high blood pressure and proteinuria before 20 weeks of gestation.<br>• Excessive weight gain.<br>• Edema of feet.<br>• Varicosities over the vulva and vagina. |
| *Specific Systemic Examination* |
| *Abdominal Examination*<br>Inspection<br>• Abdominal overdistension (barrel-shaped abdomen) may be present.<br>• Skin over the abdomen may be tense and shiny with broad stria gravidarum.<br>• Umbilicus is everted.<br><br>Palpation<br>• The uterus may be palpable abdominally earlier than 12 weeks of gestation.<br>• In the second half of pregnancy, the women may present with a uterine size more than the period of gestation and/or higher than expected weight gain in comparison to singleton pregnancies. Height of the uterus is greater than period of amenorrhea (fundal height is typically 5 cm greater than the period of amenorrhea in the second trimester).<br>• Abdominal girth at the level of umbilicus is greater than the normal abdominal girth at term.<br>• Palpation of multiple fetal parts (e.g. palpation of two fetal heads or three fetal poles).<br>• Presence of hydramnios. This may be suggested by the presence of fluid thrill in all directions over the uterus, fetal parts may not be easily felt and the fetal heart sounds may appear muffled.<br><br>Auscultation<br>• Two FHS can be auscultated, located at two separate spots separated by a silent area in between.<br>• Arnaux's sign: At times, the superimposition of two FHS produces a galloping rhythm. |
| *Vaginal Examination* |
| • Vaginal examination may help in identifying the presenting parts of one or more fetuses.<br>• Cervix may be pulled up or partly taken up.<br>• Tense bulging membranes may be felt on per vaginal examination if the cervical os is even slightly open. |

*Abbreviation:* FHS, fetal heart sound

**Q. What is Hellen's rule?**

**Ans.** According to the Hellen's rule, the frequency of twins is 1 in 80; frequency of triplets 1 in 80$^2$; frequency of quadruplets 1 in 80$^3$ and so on.

**Q. What are different types of twin gestation?**

Multifetal twin gestation can be of two types: monozygotic twins and dizygotic twins. The differences between these two are described in Table 5.17:

- *Dizygotic twins:* When two or more ova are fertilized by sperms, the result is development of dizygotic twins or nonidentical twins or fraternal twins. As a result of being fertilized by two separate sperms, the two embryos can be of different sexes. Furthermore, in dizygotic twins the two embryos have separate placentae and there is no communication between the fetal vessels of the two embryos.
- *Monozygotic twins:* Monozygotic twins are formed due to the division of a single fertilized egg. In monozygotic multiple pregnancies, different types can result depending on the timing of the division of the ovum.

**Q. What are different types of monozygotic twins?**

**Ans.** Different types of monozygotic twins are as follows:

- *Diamniotic dichorionic monozygotic twin pregnancy:* The embryo splits at or before 3 days of gestation. This results in development of two chorions and two amnions. There is development of two distinct placentae or a single fused placenta. This type of monozygotic twin accounts for nearly 8% of all twin gestations.
- *Diamniotic monochorionic monozygotic twin pregnancy:* The cleavage division is delayed until the formation of inner cell mass and the embryo splits between 4 and 7 days of gestation. This results in development of a single chorion and two amnions. Nearly 20% of all twins are of this type.
- *Monoamniotic monochorionic monozygotic twin pregnancy:* The embryo splits between 8 and 12 days of gestation. This results in development of one chorion and one amnion. Such types of monozygotic twins are rare, accounting for less than 1% of all twin gestations.
- *Conjoined or Siamese monozygotic twin pregnancy:* The embryo splits at or after 13 days of gestation, resulting in development of conjoined twins, which share a particular body part with each other. Development of such type of monozygotic twins is extremely rare. Joining of the twins can begin at either pole and may be dorsal, ventral and lateral.

**Q. What are the various causes where the fundal height is more than the period of amenorrhea?**

**Ans.** Other than multifetal gestation, various other causes for fundal height being more than period of amenorrhea are as follows:

- Hydramnios
- Wrong dates

**Table 5.17:** Difference between monozygotic and dizygotic twins

| Parameter | Monozygotic twins (identical twins) | Dizygotic twins (nonidentical or fraternal twins) |
|---|---|---|
| Etiology | Division of a fertilized ovum into two | Fertilization of two or more ova by sperms |
| Sex | Same | Can be different |
| Placenta | Single | Each fetus has a separate placenta |
| Communication between fetal vessels | Present | Absent |
| Genetic features (DNA fingerprinting) | Same | Different |
| Blood group | Same | Different |
| Skin grafting | Acceptance by the other twin | Rejection by the twin |
| Intervening membrane between the two fetuses | Composed of three layers: a fused chorion in the middle surrounded by amnion on two sides | Composed of four layers: two chorions in the middle surrounded by amnion on two sides |
| Fetal growth and congenital malformations | More common | Less common |
| Incidence | Comprises of one-third of total cases of twins | Comprises of two-thirds of total cases of twins |
| Frequency | The frequency of monozygotic twin births is relatively constant worldwide and is approximately one set per 250 live births | Variable |
| Influence of various factors | Though the occurrence of monozygotic twins is largely independent of factors such as race, heredity, age, and parity, there is now increasing evidence that assisted reproductive technology increases the incidence of zygotic splitting | The incidence of dizygotic twinning is greatly influenced by factors such as race, heredity, maternal age, parity, nutrition and, fertility treatment |

- Hydatidiform mole
- Uterine fibroids
- Adnexal masses
- Fetal macrosomia
- Elevation of the uterus by a distended bladder.
  Ultrasound examination can help in ruling out various conditions which cause the fundal height to be more than the period of gestation and also help in confirming the diagnosis of multifetal gestation.

### Q. What are the various findings which can be observed on ultrasound examination in case of multifetal gestation?

**Ans.** Various findings suggestive of multifetal gestation on ultrasound examination are as follows:

- *Multiple fetuses:* There may be presence of two or more fetuses or gestational sacs.
- *Multiple placentas:* There may be two placentas lying close to one another or presence of a single large placenta with a thick dividing membrane. This dividing layer could be composed of maximum up to four membranes (two layers of chorion fused in the middle, surrounded by amnion). In case of dichorionic pregnancies, the dividing membrane is usually 2 mm or more in thickness. On the other hand, in case of monochorionic pregnancies, the dividing membrane is composed of only two layers of amnion and may be so thin (less than 2 mm) that it may not be visualized until the second trimester.
- *Other features:* Other features that can be observed on ultrasound examination include fetal maturity, placental localization and grading, adequacy of liquor and presence of any fetal or uterine congenital anomalies.

### Q. How are the cases of multifetal gestation managed during the antenatal period?

**Ans.** Management of multifetal gestation during the antenatal period comprises of the following steps:

- Prevention of preterm labor.
- *Increased daily requirement for dietary calories, proteins and mineral supplements:* There is an increase in requirement for total dietary calories and proteins. There is an additional calorie requirement to the extent of 300 kcal/day above that required for a normal singleton gestation or 600 kcal more in comparison with the nonpregnant state. There is a requirement for increased iron and folic acid supplements in order to meet the demands of twin pregnancy. Iron requirement must be increased to the extent of 60–100 mg/day and folic acid to 1 mg/day. Calcium also needs to be prescribed above the requirements for a normal singleton gestation.
- *Increased frequency of antenatal visits:* The patient should be advised to visit the ANC clinic every 2 weeks, especially if some problem is anticipated. Attention should be focused on evaluation of BP, proteinuria, uterine fundus height and fetal movements. The patient should be advised to maintain a DFMC chart. The fetal growth should be monitored using an ultrasound examination every 3–4 weeks. Vaginal and bladder infections should be recognized and treated promptly to prevent the risk of preterm labor. The patient should be advised to stop doing extraneous activities and rest in the lateral decubitus position for a minimum of 2 hours each morning and afternoon.

- *Increased fetal surveillance:* Since presence of multifetal gestation can produce numerous complications for the fetuses, which can result in significant neonatal morbidity and mortality, stringent fetal surveillance becomes mandatory. Failure of one or both fetuses to thrive must be identified. Fetal monitoring can be done with the help of following tests: assessment of amniotic fluid volume or index (AFI), NST or BPP, and Doppler evaluation of vascular resistance.

### Q. What steps must be taken for the prevention of preterm labor?

**Ans.** Since preterm labor is the common complication associated with multifetal gestation, steps should be taken to avoid the risk of preterm labor. Some of these are as follows:

- *Bed rest*: Studies have shown that routine hospitalization or bed rest during the antenatal period does not help in prolonging pregnancy or improving fetal growth in cases of multifetal gestation.
- Administration of tocolytic agents (β-mimetic agents, calcium-channel blockers, etc.).
- Regular monitoring of uterine activity, if possible using external cardiotocography in which uterine contractions along with the fetal heart rate are continuously monitored.
- *Prophylactic cervical cerclage*: The success of this procedure has not yet been proven.
- *Weekly injections of 17-α hydroxyprogesterone caproate:* Progesterone therapy has also not been found to be helpful in preventing preterm births among women with multifetal gestation.
- The woman should be advised to contact her midwife or clinician as soon as she experiences a contraction.
- *Corticosteroids for lung maturation:* According to ACOG, (2004) the guidelines for the use of corticosteroids for attaining pulmonary maturity in cases of multifetal gestation are same as that used for singleton gestation.

### Q. How should the woman with multifetal gestation managed during the intrapartum period?

**Ans.** The following precautions need to be observed in the intrapartum period:

- Blood to be arranged and kept crossmatched.
- Pediatrician/anesthesiologist needs to be informed.
- A clinician skilled in intrauterine identification of fetal parts and in intrauterine manipulation of a fetus should be present.

- Patient should be advised to stay in bed as far as possible in order to prevent PROM.
- Labor should be monitored with help of a partogram and the heart rate of both the fetuses must be monitored preferably using a cardiotocogram. If the membranes have ruptured, the first twin can be monitored with help of internal cardiotocography, whereas the second twin can be monitored with help of external cardiotocography.
- Prophylactic administration of corticosteroids for attaining pulmonary maturity in cases of anticipated preterm deliveries.
- Intravenous access in the mother must be established. In the absence of hemorrhage or metabolic disturbances during labor, lactated Ringer or an aqueous dextrose solution may be infused at a rate of 60–120 mL/hour.
- Fetal trauma at the time of labor and delivery should be avoided.
- Expert neonatal care must be available.
- Epidural analgesia for relief from pain is preferred as it can be rapidly extended in caudal direction in case a procedure like internal podalic version or CS is required.
- Vaginal examination must be performed soon after the ROM to exclude cord prolapse and to confirm the presentation of first twin.
- The labor ward where the deliveries of the babies have to take place should be equipped with fetal monitoring equipment. An ultrasonography machine should be readily available to help evaluate the position and status of the remaining fetus(es) after delivery of the first one.
- An experienced anesthesiologist should be immediately available in case some intrauterine manipulation or cesarean delivery is required.
- Two health care professionals (one clinician and one pediatrician) should be available for each anticipated fetus. At least one of these persons should be well-versed in neonatal resuscitation.

### Q. What is the mode of delivery of the fetuses in twin gestation?

**Ans.** The optimal mode of delivery in case of multifetal gestation is enumerated in Table 5.18. If both the twins are in cephalic presentation, delivery can usually be accomplished through vaginal route, either spontaneously or with help of forceps. In cases where the first twin is noncephalic and the second twin is cephalic or in cases where both the twins are in noncephalic presentation, CS appears to be the most appropriate method of delivery, except in cases where the fetuses are dead or may not be salvageable. The optimal route for delivery in cases where the first twin is in cephalic presentation and the second twin is in noncephalic presentation, currently remains controversial. When the estimated fetal weight (EFW) is greater than 1,500 g, vaginal delivery of a nonvertex second twin is reasonable. If the EFW is less than 1,500 g, the vaginal delivery can still be tried based on clinical circumstances.

**Table 5.18:** Mode of delivery in case of twin gestation

| Type of twins | Mode of delivery |
| --- | --- |
| Both cephalic | Vaginal delivery |
| First twin cephalic, second twin noncephalic | The clinician needs to decide between vaginal delivery and cesarean delivery |
| First twin noncephalic, second twin cephalic | Cesarean section |
| Both twins noncephalic | Cesarean section |

### Q. What precautions must be observed following the vaginal delivery of the first baby?

**Ans.** Following precautions must be observed following the vaginal delivery of the first baby:
- Delivery of the first baby in cephalic presentation should be conducted according to guidelines for normal pregnancy.
- Ergometrine is not to be given at the birth of first baby.
- Cord of the first baby should be clamped and cut to prevent exsanguination of the second twin in case communicating blood vessels between the two twins exist.

### Q. What precautions must be observed at the time of vaginal delivery of the second baby?

**Ans.** After the delivery of the first baby, the following steps must be taken:
- An abdominal and vaginal examination should be performed to confirm the lie, presentation and FHS of the second baby. External version can be attempted at the time of abdominal examination, in case the lie is transverse. Internal podalic version at the time of vaginal examination can be attempted in the cases of transverse lie.
- Vaginal examination also helps in diagnosing cord prolapse, if present.
- If following the delivery of first twin, contractions do not resume within approximately 10 minutes, dilute oxytocin may be used to stimulate contractions.
- Monitoring of fetal heart rate of second twin and observation of mother for presence of vaginal bleeding must be performed. Vigilant monitoring in case of nonreassuring fetal heart rate or active vaginal bleeding is required. Hemorrhage may be indicative of placental abruption.

### Q. How should the delivery of second twin be timed?

**Ans.** According to the ACOG (1998), the interval between the deliveries of twins is not critical in determining the outcome of twins delivered. The clinician must still try to expedite the delivery of second twin as far as possible. However, an urgent delivery of the fetus is not required unless any of the following conditions are present:
- Severe bleeding per vaginum.
- Cord prolapse of second baby.

- Fetal distress of second baby.
- Inadvertent use of intravenous ergometrine with the delivery of anterior shoulder of the first baby.
- Delivery of the first baby under general anesthesia.

### Q. How should be the mode of vaginal delivery in case of second twin?

**Ans.** Depending on the presentation of second twin, various options can be adopted as described next:

#### Lie is Longitudinal

- *Cephalic:* Low ROM is done after fixing the presenting part on the pelvic brim. If the patient is not having good contractions, labor can be induced with the help of syntocinon. If the head has reached pelvic brim, i.e. the head has engaged and is not progressing beyond this point, outlet forceps or vacuum can be applied.
- *Breech:* In case of breech presentation, delivery is completed by breech extraction.

#### Lie is Transverse

If the lie is transverse, external version must be attempted in order to correct the fetal lie. If the external version fails, internal version under general anesthesia can be attempted. *The only indication for internal podalic version in modern obstetrics is the transverse lie of second twin.*

### Q. What are the indications for cesarean section in twin pregnancy?

**Ans.** Cesarean section is not required in routine clinical practice for every case of twin gestation. However, in case of presence of an obstetric or fetal indication, a cesarean delivery may be required. There is no need for a routine CS in all cases of second twin with noncephalic presentation. Cesarean section is usually required in cases where the first twin or both the twins are in noncephalic presentation. Some of the fetal indications for CS are same as that for singleton pregnancy and include the following: first fetus with noncephalic presentation, (i.e. the first fetus shows either breech or transverse presentation), fetal distress, IUGR, etc.

There are some indications specific to twin gestation for CS, which are as follows: monochorionic twins with twin-to-twin transfusion syndrome (TTTS); conjoined twins; locking of twins, etc.

### Q. What is the locking of twins?

**Ans.** The locking of twins usually takes place when the first fetus presents as breech, whereas the second twin presents as cephalic presentation. The after-coming head of the fetus in breech presentation locks between the neck and chin of the second fetus. Cesarean section is usually recommended in case the potential for locking is identified.

### Q. How should the third stage of labor be managed?

**Ans.** There is an eminent risk for PPH due to uterine atony in cases of multifetal gestation. Some of steps, which can be taken to prevent PPH, include the following:

- Intravenous methergine (0.2 mg) must not be administered with the delivery of anterior shoulder of first twin as this can result in the trapping of second twin inside the uterine cavity.
- However, intravenous methergine must be definitely administered with the delivery of anterior shoulder of the second twin. Oxytocin drip can be continued for about 1 hour following delivery.
- Delivery of placenta must be by controlled cord traction.
- In case of excessive blood loss, blood transfusion may be required.

### Q. What are the various complications associated with multifetal gestation?

**Ans.** Various complications associated with multifetal gestation are as follows:

## Maternal Complications

*During antenatal period:* Multifetal gestation is associated with an increased frequency of pregnancy-related complications in the antenatal period such as:

- Spontaneous abortion
- Anemia: Due to increased iron requirement by two fetuses, early appearance of anemia is a common complication. This problem can be avoided by increasing the dose of daily iron supplementation.
- Fatty liver of pregnancy: It is rare complication that occurs more often in multifetal than in singleton pregnancies.
- Hyperemesis gravidarum.
- Polyhydramnios.
- Preeclampsia.
- Antepartum hemorrhage.
- Preterm labor.
- Varicosities, dependent edema.

*During labor:* Multifetal gestation is also associated with a higher rate of complications during labor, such as:

- Fetal malpresentation.
- Vasa previa.
- Cord prolapse.
- Premature separation of placenta, resulting in abruption placenta.
- Cord entanglement.
- Postpartum hemorrhage.
- Dysfunctional uterine contractions.
- Increased operative interference.

*Puerperium:* Multifetal gestation can also result in a high rate of complications during the puerperium including complications like:

- Subinvolution
- Infection
- Failure of lactation.

## Fetal Complications due to Twin Gestation

- Miscarriage
- *Prematurity:* Premature labor (onset before 37 completed weeks of gestation) is the main risk of twin pregnancy, probably resulting from overstretching of the uterine cavity. The most frequent neonatal complications of preterm birth are hypothermia, respiratory difficulties, persistent ductus arteriosus, intracranial bleeding, hypoglycemia, necrotizing enterocolitis, infections and retinopathy of prematurity, low birthweight babies, etc.
- *Congenital anomalies:* A 2–4 folds increase in the risk of congenital abnormalities has been found to be associated with multiple pregnancies, especially the monozygotic twin pregnancies.
- Intrauterine death
- Intrauterine growth restriction often resulting in low birthweight babies
- Low birthweight babies due to IUGR and preterm delivery.

## Fetal Complications Specific to Twin Gestation

### Discordant Growth

Discordancy refers to the difference in growth rates between the two twins.

### Abnormalities Specific to Monozygotic Twins

Spectrum of abnormalities associated with monozygotic, specifically monoamniotic twin include the following:

- *Twin-to-twin transfusion syndrome (TTTS):* This is a rare complication that can occur in monozygotic monochorionic diamniotic twins, which causes the blood to pass from one twin to the other. This usually occurs due to the presence of abnormal placental vascular communications. As a result of the vascular communication, one of the twins, which donates blood (donor twin) becomes thin and undernourished, while the other twin who receives blood (recipient twin) grows at the expense of donor twin. The donor twin in TTTS usually shows poor growth, oliguria, anemia and hyperproteinemia, low or absent liquor, resulting in development of oligohydramnios, etc. On the other hand, recipient twin shows polyuria, polyhydramnios, polycythemia, biventricular cardiac hypertrophy and diastolic dysfunction with tricuspid regurgitation. Death of this twin eventually occurs due to congestive heart failure.
- *Neurological damage:* Abnormal vascular communication between twins could be responsible for causing neurological complications such as cerebral palsy, microcephaly, porencephaly, multicystic encephalomalacia, etc. This is usually caused by ischemia.
- *Acardiac twin or twin reversed arterial perfusion syndrome:* This is an unusual form of TTTS, occurring in about 1 in 15,000 pregnancies. In these monochorionic twins, one twin develops normally while the other twin fails to develop a heart as well as other body structures. This abnormal twin, called an acardiac fetus, shows characteristic features, in which the cardiac structures are absent or nonfunctioning and the head, upper body and upper extremities are poorly developed. The lower body and lower extremities are, however, more or less normal. The acardiac twin acts as a recipient and depends on the normal donor (pump) twin for obtaining its blood supply via transplacental anastomoses and retrograde perfusion of the acardiac umbilical cord. The perfusion pressure of the donor twin overpowers that of the recipient twin, who thus receives reverse blood flow from its twin sibling. Deoxygenated umbilical arterial blood from the donor, thus, flows into the umbilical artery of the recipient, with its direction reversed. This blood flow is reversed from the normal direction leading to the name for this condition—twin reversed arterial perfusion syndrome.
- *Conjoined twins:* Conjoined twins are the least common form of monozygotic twinning, which is always, associated with monochorionic monoamniotic twins.
- *Death of one fetus:* In case of death of one of the fetuses, prognosis for the surviving twin depends on the gestational age at the time of the demise, the chorionicity, and the length of time between the demise and delivery of the surviving twin. Death of one of multiple fetuses later in gestation could theoretically trigger coagulation defects in the mother resulting in the development of twin embolization syndrome, (explained next in text).
- *Twin embolization syndrome:* Twin embolization syndrome is a rare complication of monozygotic twins where in utero death of one of the twins has occurred. This may be associated with the passage of thromboplastic material from the dead twin into the circulatory system of surviving twin. This is likely to result in the ischemic structural defects of central nervous system, gastrointestinal and genitourinary tract of the surviving twin.
- *Cord entanglement:* Cord entanglement is a rare complication of monochorionic monoamniotic monozygotic twin pregnancy. Due to the absence of any intervening membrane between the two twins, the umbilical cords of these twins are likely to get entangled with each other. The clinician must remain vigilant against the probability of the development of this complication. In case of development of cord entanglement, the clinician may have to resort to immediate cesarean delivery, to save the twins.

- *External parasitic twin:* In this abnormality, the defective fetus or merely a part of it is attached externally to a relatively normal twin.
- *Long-term complications:* Complications related to multiple gestations do not end with the birth of the babies. Long-term complications like language and speech delay, cognitive delay or motor problems, behavioral problems and difficulty in parent-child interactions all appear to be more commonly associated with babies born as a result of multifetal gestation.

# Abnormalities of Liquor

## OLIGOHYDRAMNIOS

### Case Study 1

Mrs XYZ, a 26-year-old, primigravida woman, married for 2 years, resident of ABC, at 36 weeks gestation presented to the ANC clinic with the history of experiencing reduced fetal movements since past 1 day. On per abdominal examination, the fundal height corresponded to 34 weeks gestation. On palpation, the uterus appeared full of fetus. A single live fetus in cephalic presentation was palpated. Per abdominal examination done at the time of previous ANC visit, 1 month back was WNL. In the present visit, fetal heart rate was found to be 140 beats/minute having a regular rate, using a hand-held-Doppler. An ultrasound examination was performed which showed AFI of 3 cm. The ultrasound showed a single live fetus having maturity corresponding to 36 weeks. No congenital anomaly could be found.

### Q. What is the likely diagnosis in the above-mentioned case study?

**Ans.** The most likely diagnosis in this case is Mrs XYZ, a 26-year-old, primigravida patient, married for 2 years, resident of ABC, with 36 weeks amenorrhea corresponding to 36 weeks period of gestation, with findings of history, clinical examination and ultrasound examination suggestive of oligohydramnios in pregnancy. No probable cause for oligohydramnios could be identified. Normally, diagnosis of oligohydramnios can only be confirmed only after performing an ultrasound examination. The questions to be asked at the time of taking history or the parameters to be assessed at the time of abdominal examination in such a case are described in Tables 5.19 and 5.20 respectively.

### Q. What is oligohydramnios?

**Ans.** Oligohydramnios can be defined as having less than 200 mL of amniotic fluid at term or an AFI of less than 5 cm or presence of the largest pocket of fluid, which does not measure more than 1 cm at its largest diameter. In comparison to oligohydramnios, normal amount of amniotic fluid varies from 700 mL to 1L, whereas the normal AFI ranges between 5 cm and 25 cm. Early onset of oligohydramnios, in comparison to that with a late onset, often results in poor outcomes.

| **Table 5.19:** Symptoms to be elicited at the time of taking history in a case of oligohydramnios |
|---|
| • The patient may give a history of experiencing reduced fetal movements.<br>• Fundal height is less than that estimated on the basis of LMP.<br>• Evidence of intrauterine growth restriction (IUGR) may be present. |

| **Table 5.20:** Various findings elicited at the time of clinical examination in a case of oligohydramnios |
|---|
| • Fundal height is less than that estimated on the basis of LMP.<br>• Uterus appears full of fetus due to scanty liquor.<br>• Evidence of intrauterine growth restriction (IUGR) may be present.<br>• Malpresentation (e.g. breech) may be present |

### Q. What is the normal volume of amniotic fluid diagnosed on ultrasound examination?

**Ans.** Volume of amniotic fluid inside the amniotic cavity (based on ultrasound findings) is described in Table 5.21.

### Q. What are the causes of oligohydramnios?

**Ans.** Known causes of oligohydramnios include the following:
- Premature rupture of the membranes.
- *Birth defects:* Birth defects, especially those involving the kidneys and urinary tract, e.g. renal agenesis, or obstruction of the urinary tract (posterior urethral valves) etc.
- Post-term pregnancy (> 40 weeks).
- *Placental dysfunction:* Presence of amnion nodosum (squamous metaplasia of amnion) on the placenta.
- *Maternal health conditions:* GDM, preeclampsia, chronic hypertension, uteroplacental insufficiency, etc.
- *Certain medications:* Medications including ACE inhibitors, prostaglandin inhibitors (aspirin, etc.) can cause oligohydramnios.
- Fetal chromosomal abnormalities.
- Intrauterine infections.
- IUGR associated with placental insufficiency.

### Q. How can oligohydramnios be diagnosed?

**Ans.** Oligohydramnios is diagnosed on ultrasound examination.

### Q. What should be the likely management in the above-described case study?

**Ans.** The likely steps of management in the above-described case study are as follows:
- Women with otherwise normal pregnancies who develop oligohydramnios near term probably require no treatment because in most of these cases, oligohydramnios would resolve itself without treatment.
- In case of presence of congenital malformations, the woman must be delivered irrespective of the period of gestation.

**Table 5.21:** Volume of amniotic fluid inside the amniotic cavity (based on ultrasound findings)

| Amount of amniotic fluid | Total amount of amniotic fluid | Maximum vertical pool of liquor | Amniotic fluid index (AFI) |
|---|---|---|---|
| Normal | 700 mL to 1L at full term | Adequate fluid, seen everywhere | AFI of 5–25 cm |
| Oligohydramnios | Less than 200 mL of amniotic fluid | Maximum vertical pool of liquor less than 2 cm | AFI < 5 cm |
| Polyhydramnios | Amniotic fluid volume of 2,000 mL or greater at term | Presence of maximum vertical fluid pocket seen is greater than 8 cm in diameter | AFI > 25 cm |

- Induction of labor may not always be the best option in all cases of oligohydramnios due to increased chances of fetal distress.
- Hospitalization may also be sometimes required in severe cases.
- *Reduced physical activity:* Many providers advise women to observe bed rest.
- *Maternal hydration:* Simple maternal hydration has been suggested as a way of increasing amniotic fluid volume.
- *Amnioinfusion:* This method involves infusion of sterile water through the cervix into the uterine cavity. This treatment may help to reduce complications during labor and delivery and reduce the requirement for CS.
- *Fetal surveillance:* Close fetal surveillance of these patients in the form of weekly (or more frequent) ultrasound examinations to measure the level of amniotic fluid, tests of fetal wellbeing, such as the NST, BPP, etc. may also be required. If one of these tests shows abnormality, early delivery by the fastest route may be required even if the fetus is preterm.

### Q. What are the likely complications related to oligohydramnios?

**Ans.** Complications related to oligohydramnios are as follows:
*Complications during early pregnancy include:*

- Restriction of the amount of free space inside the uterine cavity.
- Amniotic adhesions causing deformities or constriction of the umbilical cord.
- Pressure deformities such as clubfeet, amputation of limbs, abnormal shape of skull, wry neck, etc.

*Complications during the late pregnancy:* These include the following:

- Fetal distress, IUGR.
- Fetal pulmonary hypoplasia.
- Cord compression, resulting in fetal hypoxia and asphyxia.
- Prolonged ROM.
- Fetal malformations (renal agenesis, polycystic kidneys, urethral obstruction, etc.).
- Postmaturity syndrome.
- Birth defects (compression of fetal organs, resulting in lung and limb defects).
- Miscarriage, premature birth, stillbirth.
- Prolonged labor due to uterine inertia.
- Increased risk of meconium aspiration syndrome.
- Increased requirement for operative delivery.

# Polyhydramnios

## Case Study 1

Mrs XYZ, a 38-year-old married for 12 years, resident of ABC, G3P2L2 woman at 32 weeks of gestation presented to the ANC clinic with massive abdominal distension and no perception of any fetal movements. On general physical examination, the abdomen was tense and shiny and the uterus was enlarged up to the level of xiphisternum. Fetus, probably in cephalic presentation was palpated. However, the fetal parts could not be easily palpated. Fetal heart sound also appeared muffled.

### Q. What is the likely diagnosis in the above-mentioned case study?

**Ans.** The likely diagnosis in this case is Mrs XYZ, a 38-year-old, G3P2L2 woman, married for 12 years, resident of ABC, with 8 months period of amenorrhea corresponding to 32 weeks period of gestation, with history and clinical examination showing an abdomen disproportionately enlarged in accordance with the period of gestation as calculated on the basis of LMP. The various differential diagnoses possible in these cases include, multifetal gestation, polyhydramnios, wrong dates, presence of a pelvic tumor, macrosomic baby, hydatidiform mole, concealed abruption placenta, etc. Exact diagnosis can only be confirmed after performing an ultrasound examination. In this case, an ultrasound examination was performed which showed a single live fetus in cephalic presentation having a maturity of 32 weeks. amniotic fluid index was 30 cm. The fetal heart rate was 142 beats/minute and no congenital anomaly was detected. Diagnosis of polyhydramnios was therefore, established. No likely cause of oligohydramnios could be identified. The questions to be asked at the time of taking history and the parameters to be assessed at the time of abdominal examination in such a case are described in Tables 5.22 and 5.23 respectively.

### Q. What is polyhydramnios and how can it be defined?

**Ans.** Polyhydramnios is defined as presence of amniotic fluid volume of 2,000 mL or greater at term. The excessive amount of liquor may cause discomfort to the patient and may also require ultrasound examination for confirmation of fetal lie and presentation. Amniotic fluid index in cases of polyhydramnios is greater than 24 cm and the largest vertical pocket is greater than 8 cm. The varying degrees of polyhydramnios are based on the measurement of the largest vertical pocket of liquor (Table 5.24).

**Table 5.22:** Symptoms to be elicited at the time of taking history in a case of polyhydramnios

*Clinical Presentation*
- Women with minor polyhydramnios experience few symptoms. Those who are more severely affected may experience the following symptoms:
  - Difficulty in breathing (patient may be able to breathe easily in sitting position).
  - Palpitations.
  - Presence of large varicosities in the legs and/or vulva.
  - Presence of new hemorrhoids or the worsening of those present previously.

**Table 5.23:** Various findings elicited at the time of clinical examination in a case of polyhydramnios

*General Physical Examination*
- Patient may get dyspneic on lying down.
- Evidence of preeclampsia (pedal edema, facial puffiness, vulval edema, weight gain, etc.).
- Varicosities in leg or vulva.
- Presence of hemorrhoids.

*Specific Systemic Examination*
*Abdominal Examination*
Inspection
- Abdomen is markedly enlarged and globular in appearance, along with fullness of flanks
- The skin of the abdominal wall appears to be tense, shiny and may show appearance of large striae.

Palpation
- Clinically, the patients have a fundal height greater than the period of amenorrhea.
- Abdominal girth at the umbilicus is more than normal.
- Fetal heart sounds may appear muffled as if coming from a distance.
- A fluid thrill and/or shifting dullness may be commonly present.
- It may be difficult to palpate the uterus or the fetal presenting parts due to presence of excessive fluid.

Auscultation
- The fetal heart sound may appear inaudible when tried to be heard using a stethoscope of a fetoscope. However, it may be possible to hear them on Doppler.

*Vaginal Examination*
- Cervix may be pulled up and partially taken up
- Cervix os may be slightly dilated
- Tense bulging membranes can be felt through the cervical os

**Table 5.24:** Degrees of polyhydramnios

| Grading | Criteria |
| --- | --- |
| Mild | Largest vertical pocket of liquor measures 8–11 cm |
| Moderate | Largest vertical pocket of liquor measures 12–15 cm |
| Severe | Largest vertical pocket of liquor measures > 16 cm |

**Q. What are the likely causes of polyhydramnios?**

**Ans.** In about two-thirds of cases, the cause of polyhydramnios is unknown. It most likely occurs due to defective absorption as well as excessive production of liquor amnii.

Polyhydramnios is more likely to occur due to the following causes:

*Fetal causes*: These include the following:
- *Congenital abnormalities:* The most common birth defects that cause polyhydramnios are those that hinder fetal swallowing, such as birth defects involving the gastrointestinal tract and central nervous system (e.g. esophageal atresia, anencephaly, etc.)
- Twin-to-twin transfusion syndrome.
- Parvovirus B19 infection.

*Maternal causes:* These include multiple gestations, maternal diabetes, and Rh blood incompatibilities between mother and fetus.

**Q. What are the various congenital anomalies, which could be associated with polyhydramnios?**

**Ans.** Various congenital anomalies which could be associated with polyhydramnios include neural tube defects (anencephaly, spina bifida, etc.), polydactyly, gastric defects like gastroschisis, anterior abdominal wall defects, esophageal atresia, duodenal atresia, sacrococcygeal tumors, facial clefts, hydrops fetalis (due to Rhesus isoimmunization), chorioangioma of placenta, multifetal gestation (especially the monozygotic twins), Down's syndrome, Edward's syndrome, etc.

**Q. What are the findings of polyhydramnios on ultrasound examination?**

**Ans.** The various grades of polyhydramnios based on the ultrasound findings have been previously described in Table 5.24.

Ultrasound examination also shows presence of fetal anomalies, placental location, any other anomaly like placental tumor, etc., amount of liquor, AFI, number of fetuses and estimated fetal weight.

**Q. What are the various steps of management in a case of polyhydramnios?**

**Ans.** Mild degree of hydramnios usually resolves on its own without any treatment. No active management may be required in patients with asymptomatic hydramnios. The treatment in symptomatic cases aims at obtaining symptomatic relief, to find out the causative factor, and to avoid and deal with complications. For patients showing symptomatic/severe degrees of hydramnios, the following treatment options are available:
- *Treatment of the underlying cause:* Three most important causes of polyhydramnios include gestational diabetes, fetal anomalies and multifetal gestation.
- *Decompression by amniocentesis:* Amniocentesis is a procedure involving the removal of a sample of amniotic

fluid in order to provide relief against symptoms, such as respiratory embarrassment, excessive uterine activity or premature opening of cervical os, etc.

- *Supportive therapy:* This involves bed rest, treatment of associated conditions such as preeclampsia or diabetes.
- *Diuretics:* Use of diuretics is of little value in these cases.
- *Indomethacin:* Indomethacin is administered orally in the dosage of 25 mg every 6 hourly to reduce the amount of amniotic fluid as it helps in reducing the urine output.
- Further management depends upon response to treatment, period of gestation, presence of fetal malformations and associated complicating factors.
- In uncomplicated cases where there is no fetal malformation and there is a positive response to treatment, pregnancy may be continued awaiting spontaneous delivery at term.
- In symptomatic cases, if the period of gestation is less than 37 weeks, serial amnioreductions (removal of some amount of amniotic fluid using amniocentesis) are performed until the fetal maturity is attained.
- In case there is presence of fetal malformations, pregnancy is terminated irrespective of the period of gestation.
- In case the patient is unresponsive or there is presence of complications (e.g. severe maternal distress), delivery of the baby is based on the period of gestation.
- If period of gestation is greater than 37 weeks or the fetal pulmonary maturity has been attained, the labor is induced. The following steps are taken prior to the induction of labor:
  - Amniocentesis is done to drain the amount of liquor so that the clinician can accurately assess the fetal lie and presentation.
  - Stabilizing infusion of oxytocin is started following which an ARM is done in a controlled manner.

**Q. What steps must be taken for management of such patients during labor?**

**Ans.** The following steps must be taken at the time of labor in such patients:

- Management of such patients is similar to those with multifetal gestation.
- Vaginal examination must be performed immediately following ROM to exclude cord prolapse.
- Oxytocin infusion can be utilized in case of weak uterine contractions.
- Steps must be taken to prevent PPH (administration of IV methergine at the time of delivery of anterior shoulder).
- The delivered baby must be carefully examined for the presence of any congenital anomalies.

**Q. What are the various investigations, which must be done in these cases?**

**Ans.** The various investigations, which must be done in these cases, are as follows:

- *Blood (ABO and Rh typing):* Rh isoimmunization may be associated with hydrops fetalis and fetal ascites.
- *Blood sugar levels:* Post prandial blood glucose levels and glucose tolerance test need to be done.
- *Amniotic fluid alpha fetoproteins estimation:* Levels of alpha fetoproteins are elevated in presence of a fetus with open neural tube defects.
- *Ultrasound examination:* It is for detection of fetal congenital anomalies.

**Q. What are the various steps for management of respiratory distress in these patients?**

**Ans.** The following steps should be taken for management of respiratory distress in these patients:

- Propped up position.
- Oxygen by face mask.
- Intravenous line.
- Ultrasound examination for diagnosis of hydramnios.
- Amniocentesis with drainage of excessive fluid if required.
- Indomethacin can be tried at 31 weeks of gestation. Indomethacin should not be given after 32 weeks of gestation due to the risk of premature closure of ductus arteriosus.

**Q. What are the various complications related to polyhydramnios?**

**Ans.** Various complications related to polyhydramnios are as follows:

### Maternal Complications

*During pregnancy:* The following complications can occur:
- Respiratory compromise.
- Antepartum/accidental hemorrhage.
- Abnormal fetal presentations.
- Gestational diabetes, preeclampsia.
- Increased incidence of operative intervention.

*During labor:* The following complications can occur:
- Increased risk of premature delivery and PROM.
- Increased risk of placental abruption, cord prolapse and stillbirth.
- Increased risk of uterine dysfunction and uterine inertia.
- Increased risk of retained placenta, PPH and shock.

*During puerperium:* The following complications can occur:
- Subinvolution.
- Increased puerperal morbidity.

### Fetal Complications

- Increased perinatal morbidity and mortality. Deaths are mainly due to prematurity and congenital anomalies.

# Transverse Lie

## Case Study 1

Mrs XYZ, a 28-year-old married for 6 years, resident of ABC, primi patient with 36 completed weeks of gestation having fetus with shoulder presentation (diagnosed by ultrasound examination at previous antenatal visit) presented for a routine antenatal check-up.

### Q. What is the most likely diagnosis in the above-mentioned case study?

**Ans.** The most likely diagnosis in the above-mentioned case study is Mrs XYZ, a 28-year-old married for 6 years, resident of ABC, primi patient with 36 completed weeks of amenorrhea, corresponding to 36 weeks of gestation having a single live fetus in shoulder presentation. The questions to be asked at the time of taking history and the parameters to be assessed at the time of examination in such a case are described in Tables 5.25 and 5.26 respectively.

### Q. How can you define transverse lie?

**Ans.** Transverse lie is an abnormal fetal presentation in which the fetus lies transversely with the shoulders presenting in the lower pole of the uterus. Most fetuses in transverse lie early in pregnancy, convert to a cephalic (or breech) presentation by term. In shoulder presentation, long axis of the fetus is perpendicular to the maternal spine. As a result, the presenting part becomes the fetal shoulder. The denominator is the fetal back. Depending on whether the position of the fetal back is anterior, posterior, superior or inferior, the following positions are possible:

- *Dorsoanterior:* The most common position where the fetal back is anterior.
- *Dorsoposterior:* Fetal back is posterior.
- *Dorsosuperior or "back-up":* Fetal back is directed superiorly. In this case the small fetal parts present at the cervix.
- *Dorsoinferior or "back-down":* Fetal back is directed inferiorly. In this case the fetal shoulder presents at the cervix.

Depending on the position of the fetal head, the fetal position can be described as right or left.

### Q. What is the role of ultrasound examination in cases of transverse lie?

**Ans.** Ultrasound examination is used for confirming the diagnosis of transverse lie and determining the precise fetal position. Besides confirming the transverse lie, other things which can be observed on the ultrasound include the following:

- Presence of uterine and/or fetal anomalies
- Fetal maturity
- Placental localization and grading
- Adequacy of liquor
- Ruling out multiple gestations.

### Q. How should the cases of transverse lie be managed?

**Ans.** There is no mechanism of labor for a fetus in transverse lie, which remains uncorrected until term. The management options for transverse lie during pregnancy include ECV in the antenatal period, which involves the conversion of transverse presentation to cephalic presentation. For the procedure of performing ECV, kindly refer to Chapter 6. If ECV is unsuccessful or is contraindicated, delivery by CS (elective or an emergency) remains the only option.

### Q. What are the various complications associated with transverse lie?

**Ans.** Though in modern obstetrics much of the morbidity and mortality associated with this condition has been considerably reduced, nevertheless, these pregnancies are at an increased risk of maternal and perinatal morbidity in comparison to pregnancies in which the fetus is a cephalic or breech presentation. In developed countries, the most important causes of morbidity in cases of transverse lie are related to conditions such as placenta previa, prolapse of the umbilical cord, fetal trauma, prematurity, etc. In developing countries, increased morbidity and mortality is related to complications of neglected transverse lie such as arm prolapse, obstructed labor, ruptured uterus, etc. Some of these are described next:

*Maternal Complications*

*Arm prolapse:* Due to the ill-fitting fetal part, sudden ROM can result in the escape of large amount of liquor and the prolapse of fetal arm. Prolapse of fetal arm is often accompanied by a loop of cord. A neglected arm prolapse often results in obstructed labor. This in primigravida causes the uterus to become inert. In these cases, though the uterus does not rupture,

---

**Table 5.25:** Symptoms to be elicited at the time of taking history in a case of transverse lie

*History of Presenting Complains*
- There are no specific symptoms suggestive of shoulder presentation.

*Medical History*
- Past history of gynecological disorders, e.g. uterine anomalies (bicornuate or septate uterus) or presence of space occupying lesions (e.g. fibroids in the lower uterine segment), pelvic tumor, etc. could act as a risk factor for shoulder presentation.

*Obstetric History*
- Presence of cephalopelvic disproportion or contracted maternal pelvis in the previous pregnancy and presence of liquor abnormalities (polyhydraminos, oligohydramnios) in the present pregnancy or placental abnormalities (placenta previa, cornuofundal attachment of placenta); multiparity (especially grand multiparas); could act as the likely risk factors for shoulder presentation.
- History of prematurity, multifetal gestation, hydramnios, intrauterine fetal death, fetal anomalies, etc. in the present pregnancy.

| **Table 5.26:** Various findings elicited at the time of clinical examination in a case of transverse lie |
| --- |

*General Physical Examination*

No specific finding is observed on general physical examination.

*Specific Systemic Examination*

*Abdominal Examination*
Abdominal Palpation
On abdominal palpation, the following findings can be elicited:
• Fetal lie is in the horizontal plane with fetal head on one side of the midline and podalic pole on the other.
• The abdomen often appears barrel-shaped and is asymmetrical.
• Fundal height is less than the period of amenorrhea.
The diagnosis of transverse lie can be made by abdominal palpation utilizing Leopold's maneuvers:
– *First Leopold maneuver/fundal grip:* No fetal pole (either breech or cephalic) is palpable on the fundal grip. In case of dorsoinferior (back-down) position, nodulations due to presence of baby's feet may be palpated on fundal grip. In case of dorsosuperior position, a wide convexity of fetal back may be palpated on fundal grip.
– *Second Leopold's maneuver/lateral grip:* Soft, broad, smooth irregular part suggestive of fetal breech is present on one side of the midline, while a smooth hard globular part suggestive of the fetal head is present on the other side of the midline. The fetal head is usually placed at a level lower than the rest of the body and is usually confined to one iliac fossa. In case of dorsoanterior position, back may be felt anteriorly in the midline on the lateral grip. In case of dorsoposterior position, small irregular knob-like structures, suggestive of the fetal limbs, are felt anteriorly in the midline while performing lateral grip.
– *Leopold's third maneuver:* Pelvic grip appears to be empty during the antenatal period. It may be occupied by the shoulder at the time of labor.
– *Leopold's fourth maneuver:* No appreciable mass to indicate fetal descent may be identified on Leopold fourth maneuver.

Fetal Heart Auscultation
Fetal heart rate is easily heard much below the umbilicus in dorsoanterior position. On the other hand in dorsoposterior position, the fetal heart may be located at a much higher level and is often above the umbilicus.

*Vaginal Examination*

If transverse lie is suspected by abdominal palpation, a vaginal examination should be postponed until placenta previa has been excluded.

*Vaginal examination during the antenatal period*
• Pelvis appears to be empty.
• Even if something is felt on vaginal examination, no definite fetal part may be identified.

*Vaginal examination during labor*
• Fetal shoulder including scapula, clavicle, humerus and grid iron feel of fetal ribs can be palpated.
• Due to ill-fitting fetal part, an elongated bag of membranes may be felt on vaginal examination. If the membranes have ruptured, the fetal shoulder can be identified by feeling the acromion process, the scapula, clavicle, axilla, ribs and intercostal spaces. Ribs and intercostal spaces upon palpation give feeling of grid iron.
• If the arm prolapse has occurred, the fetal arm might be observed to be lying outside the vagina. If still inside the vagina, a prolapsed arm must be distinguished from a leg. The elbow is sharper than the knee. Moreover, there is no heel and abduction of the thumb will help in distinguishing hand from the foot.

complications such as maternal exhaustion, ketoacidosis, sepsis, etc. can occur. These result in an increased maternal morbidity. On the other hand, in multigravidae, the uterus responds vigorously in face of obstruction. In order to push out the fetus, the upper uterine segment thickens, whereas the lower uterine segment distends. A retraction ring forms at the junction of upper and lower uterine segments. If the uterine obstruction is not immediately relieved, the intensity of uterine contractions increases. As the frequency of uterine contraction increases, there is a progressive reduction in the relaxation phase. This results in setting up of a phase of tonic contractions. Retraction of upper uterine segment continues. This causes the lower uterine segment to elongate, become progressively thinner in order to accommodate the fetus which is being pushed down from the upper segment resulting in formation of a circular groove between the upper and lower uterine segment. This is known as the pathological retraction ring or Bandl's ring. As the degree of obstruction increases, the retraction ring becomes more prominent. Eventually, there is rupture of uterus as the lower segment gives way due to marked thinning of the uterine wall. This results in an increased incidence of dehydration, ketoacidosis, septicemia, rupture uterus, PPH, shock, peritonitis, injury to the genital tract, etc. All these factors result in an increased rate of both maternal and fetal morbidity and mortality.

*Long-term complications:* Long-term maternal complications include development of genitourinary fistulas, secondary amenorrhea (related to Sheehan's syndrome associated with PPH), hysterectomy, etc.

*Fetal Complications*

*Fetal asphyxia:* Tonic uterine contractions can interfere with uteroplacental circulation resulting in fetal distress. Other fetal complications may include preterm birth, PROM, intrauterine fetal death and increased fetal mortality.

# Intrauterine Growth Restriction

## Case Study 1

Mrs XYZ, a 28-year-old married for 8 years, resident of ABC, G4P3L3 patient, who is 34 weeks pregnant, presented for a regular antenatal check-up. She has no particular problems and has been experiencing normal fetal movements. The symphysis-fundus (S-F) height had not shown any increase over the past three antenatal visits. The estimated fetal weight (EFW) taken at the time of last antenatal visit had fallen below the 10th centile of the average for that particular gestational age. The patient is a farm laborer and she smokes.

### Q. What is the most likely diagnosis in the above-mentioned case study?

**Ans.** The most likely diagnosis in the above-mentioned case study is Mrs XYZ, a 28-year-old married for 8 years, resident of ABC, G4P3L3 patient, with 34 weeks amenorrhea, corresponding to 34 weeks of gestation. Abdominal examination showed symphysis-fundal height corresponding to 32 weeks with a single live fetus in cephalic presentation. The likely diagnosis at the time of taking history and doing a clinical examination points towards IUGR because the patient is sure of her LMP. The diagnosis of IUGR needs to be confirmed upon ultrasound examination. The questions to be asked at the time of taking history and the parameters to be assessed at the time of examination in such a case are described in Tables 5.27 and 5.28 respectively.

### Q. How can you ascertain the accuracy for the prediction of gestational age?

**Ans.** It is important for the clinician to estimate the patient's accurate gestational age at the time of taking history, especially in the cases suspected to be having IUGR. If the patient is unsure about the date of her LMP, the clinician can rely on some ultrasound report, which had been performed on the patient early in gestation (in case such a report is available). If several previous sonograms are available, the age must be calculated from the earliest sonogram available.

The best time to determine gestational period based on a single ultrasound parameter is between 18 to 24 weeks of gestation. Crown-rump-length of 15–60 mm (corresponding to gestational period varying from 8–12.5 weeks) is found to have the greatest accuracy in determining the period of

| **Table 5.27:** Symptoms to be elicited at the time of taking history in a case of IUGR |
|---|
| *Accurate Estimation of Gestational Age* |
| Accurate estimation of the gestational age is the first prerequisite before making a diagnosis of IUGR. Therefore, accurate estimation of LMP needs to be done at the time of taking history. History must aim at identifying the probable risk factor for IUGR. The following points need to be asked in the history:<br>• History of maternal malnutrition, chronic illness, drug abuse, bleeding, etc.<br>• Low maternal weight gain during the antenatal visits.<br>• History of reduced fetal movements. |
| *Personal History* |
| • *Tobacco smoking:* Poor placental function is uncommon in a healthy woman who smokes.<br>• Excessive alcohol intake.<br>• Intake of any drugs of abuse.<br>• *Occupation:* It is important to ask about the patient's occupation because strenuous physical work may be associated with IUGR. |
| *Socioeconomic History* |
| • Poor socioeconomic conditions. |
| *Medical History* |
| • Previous history of any medical disorder (e.g. essential hypertension, chronic renal disease, etc.).<br>• Preeclampsia and chronic hypertension: preeclampsia resulting in poor placental function (placental insufficiency or inadequacy) could act as an important risk factor for preeclampsia.<br>• Maternal anemia, especially sickle cell anemia. |
| *Nutritional History* |
| • Detailed nutritional history from the mother needs to be elicited because malnutrition is an important cause of IUGR. |
| *Obstetric History* |
| • Past history of giving birth to IUGR fetuses.<br>• History of multifetal gestation, presence of any chromosomal abnormalities, (e.g. trisomy 21), severe congenital malformations, chronic intrauterine infection, e.g. congenital syphilis, TORCH infections [especially rubella and cytomegalovirus (CMV)], viral, bacterial, protozoal and spirochetal infection in the present pregnancy needs to be asked because these could act as the risk factors for the development of IUGR. |

*Abbreviations:* IUGR, intrauterine growth restriction; TORCH, Toxoplasmosis, Other infections, Rubella, Cytomegalovirus, Herpes simplex virus

**Table 5.28:** Various findings elicited at the time of clinical examination in a case of IUGR

*General Physical Examination*

- There may be no specific findings on general physical examination.
- Constitutionally small mothers: Constitutionally small-sized mothers may give birth to small-sized babies.
- Low maternal weight, especially a low body mass index resulting from undernutrition may be associated with IUGR. Poor maternal weight gain, however, is of very little value in diagnosing IUGR.
- She may be showing signs of poor nutritional status such as anemia, chronic malnutrition, etc. However, use of repeated maternal weight check-ups has not been proved to be a good predictor of IUGR.

*Specific Systemic Examination*

*Abdominal Examination*
The approximate size of the fetus can be estimated on abdominal examination. Palpation of fetal head gives an estimation of fetal size and maturity. The diagnostic accuracy of abdominal palpation in predicting IUGR is limited. Thus, abdominal palpation itself should not be used for diagnosing IUGR. Instead, it should be used in combination with ultrasound parameters for diagnosing IUGR.
- *Estimation of symphysis-fundus height:* Symphysis-fundus height is measured in centimeters from the upper edge of the symphysis pubis to the top of the fundus of the uterus. If the uterus is deviated towards one side, it should be stabilized in the middle using one hand, before taking measurement. While taking the measurement, the readings of the measurement tape should be facing the patient's abdomen and not the examiner in order to prevent the measurement bias. After 24 weeks of gestation, S-F height corresponds to the period of gestation. A lag of 4 cm or more is suggestive of FGR.
- There may be reduced amount of liquor amnii and the fetus may clinically appear to be of small size.

*Abbreviations:* IUGR, intrauterine growth restriction; FGR, fetal growth restriction

gestation in the first trimester, but then biparietal diameter (BPD) (at least 21 mm) is found to be more precise after this period of gestation, i.e. in the second trimester. In the early third trimester, no significant difference in accuracy is seen amongst various ultrasound parameters. All predictors have been found to be imprecise late in the third trimester, so gestational age assigned on the basis of a sonographic measurement made during this stage of pregnancy is not reliable.

### Q. What is fetal growth restriction?

**Ans.** Fetal growth restriction refers to low birthweight infants whose birthweight is below the 10th percentile of the average for the particular gestational age. Previously, the term fetal growth retardation was used. However, this term has now been discarded because it implies abnormal mental functioning. The fetal weight is estimated using ultrasound parameters like BPD, head circumference (HC), abdominal circumference (AC), femur length (FL), etc.

### Q. What is a small-for-gestational-age fetus? How is it different from an IUGR fetus?

**Ans.** Small-for-gestational-age (SGA) fetus is defined as one, which has failed to achieve a specific weight or biometric size in accordance with the gestational age (constitutionally small babies). Even if the infant's birthweight is less than 10th percentile, he/she may not be pathologically growth restricted. Not all fetuses, which are SGA, have pathological growth restriction and not all fetuses, which have growth restriction, are SGA. The small size of the infant could be related to normal biological factors.

The pathologically growth restricted fetus is unable to reach its genetically determined potential size, which is detrimental to its health and may be associated with significant neonatal mortality and morbidity. The difference between the SGA infants and infants with pathological growth restriction is described in Table 5.29.

### Q. What are the causes of pathological growth restriction?

**Ans.** Intrauterine growth restriction is usually due to some pathological process (either intrinsic or extrinsic). Intrinsic FGR usually occurs due to some fetal problem like fetal infections or chromosomal abnormalities. On the other hand, extrinsic FGR is due to placental conditions or maternal disease, such as hypertension, anemia, etc.

### Q. What is symmetric and asymmetric growth restriction?

**Ans.** Pathologically, growth restricted infants can be of two types, i.e. symmetric intrauterine growth retarded and asymmetric intrauterine growth retarded, depending on the stage of fetal growth at which the pathological insult occurred. If the pathological insult occurs at stage 1 of fetal growth, the process of cellular hyperplasia is mainly affected. This results in symmetrically growth-restricted infants. If the pathological insult occurs at stage 3 of fetal growth, cellular hypertrophy is mainly affected. This results in asymmetrically affected growth-restricted infants. The other differences between symmetric IUGR and asymmetric IUGR infants are enumerated in Table 5.30.

### Q. What are the investigations, which need to be done in cases of growth restricted babies?

**Ans.** Two types of tests—the biometric tests (which help in measuring fetal size and gestational age) and biophysical tests (which help in assessing fetal wellbeing) are usually done in growth-restricted babies.

**Table 5.29:** Difference between the small-for-gestational-age infants and infants with pathological growth restriction

| Characteristics | Small-for-gestational-age infants (normal) | Infants with pathological growth restriction |
|---|---|---|
| Birthweight | Less than 10% of the average weight. Birthweight is usually less than 2.5 kg. | Less than 10% of the average weight, but may also be less than 25%. Birthweight is usually less than 2.5 kg, but may be larger. |
| Etiology | Constitutionally small baby due to normal biological factors | Due to some pathological process (intrinsic or extrinsic) |
| Ponderal index | Normal | Low |
| Amount of subcutaneous fat | Normal | Reduced |
| Neonatal course | Usually uneventful | May develop complications like hypoglycemia, hypocalcemia, hyperviscosity, hyperbilirubinemia, necrotizing enterocolitis, etc. |
| RBC count | Normal RBC count | Elevated number of nucleated RBCs |
| Platelet count | Normal | Thrombocytopenia is usually present |
| Investigations | Fetal biometric tests which help in measuring fetal size are usually abnormal. Results of Doppler waveform analysis are within normal limits. | Fetal biophysical tests, which help in assessing fetal well-being are usually abnormal. Doppler waveform analysis of umbilical and uterine arteries may be associated with reduced diastolic flow; absent or sometimes even reversed flow. |
| Intervention | No intervention is required | Identification of the underlying cause and its appropriate management is required |

**Table 5.30:** Differences between symmetric and asymmetric intrauterine growth restriction

| Symmetric IUGR | Asymmetric IUGR |
|---|---|
| Growth is affected before 16 weeks of gestation | Fetal growth is affected later in gestation |
| Fetus is proportionately small | Fetus is disproportionately small |
| Cell hyperplasia is affected | Cellular hypertrophy is mainly affected |
| Causes of symmetric IUGR mainly include congenital abnormalities, chromosomal aberrations, intrauterine infections, etc. | Causes of asymmetric IUGR include hypertension, anemia, heart disease, accidental hemorrhage, etc. |
| Pathological process is intrinsic to the fetus | Pathological process is extrinsic to the fetus |
| Such neonates are small in all parameters | Head circumference is not as much affected as is abdominal circumference |
| Catch-up growth occurs poorly after birth | Catch-up growth occurs reasonably well after birth |
| Neonatal prognosis is usually poor | Neonatal prognosis is usually good |
| Ponderal index is normal | Ponderal index is low |
| HC/AC and FL/AC ratios are normal. | These ratios are elevated. HC and FL remains unaffected, whereas AC is reduced. As a result HC/AC and FL/AC are elevated |
| This type of IUGR is also termed as type II | Also termed as type I |
| Less common: Usually responsible for 20% cases of IUGR | More common: Usually responsible for 80% cases of IUGR |

*Abbreviations:* HC, head circumference; AC, abdominal circumference; FL, femur length; IUGR, intrauterine growth restriction

### Biometric Tests

According to the RCOG, 2002, of the various available biometric tests, fetal AC and expected fetal weight are most accurate parameters for predicting IUGR. Various biometric tests are as follows:

- *Head circumference/abdominal circumference ratio:* The use of HC/AC ratio in diagnosis of IUGR is based on the idea that the HC is usually preserved in asymmetric IUGR babies, whereas the AC is reduced. Pathological growth restriction is diagnosed when HC/AC ratio is above the 95th percentile for the gestational age.
- *Femoral length/abdominal circumference ratio:* The normal value of FL/AC ratio remains 22 ± 2, irrespective of the period of gestation. IUGR can be suspected if the ratio is more than 24.

- *Fetal ponderal index:* Fetal ponderal index (FPI) is another ultrasound measured fetal index, which is used for diagnosing IUGR. FPI is calculated with help of the formula as described below:

FPI = Estimated fetal weight/(Femur length)$^3$

## Measures of Fetal Surveillance/Biophysical Tests

Fetal surveillance measures include the biophysical tests, which aim at identifying the fetus with IUGR before it becomes acidotic. The schedule for conducting various antepartum surveillance tests in patients with IUGR is shown in Table 5.31.

Fetal surveillance is of utmost importance in cases of IUGR. The patient must be instructed to maintain a daily count of number of fetal movements she experiences. NST should be done biweekly. If NST is abnormal, BPP must be performed on weekly basis. Ultrasound for measuring fetal growth velocity must be carried out on bimonthly basis. Frequency of Doppler monitoring in IUGR fetuses need not be more than once every fortnightly.

### Q. What are the changes occurring in various Doppler velocity waveforms in IUGR fetuses?

**Ans.** The evaluation of fetal wellbeing by Doppler velocimetry in cases of IUGR is of great importance as it is very useful in detecting those IUGR fetuses that are at high risk because of hypoxemia. Several Doppler studies, which were initially performed on fetal arteries (umbilical arteries, uterine arteries, middle cerebral arteries, etc.) and recently on the fetal venous system (ductus venosus) provide valuable information for the clinicians concerning the optimal time of delivery.

The major Doppler detectable modifications in the fetal circulation associated with IUGR and fetal hypoxemia include increased resistance in the umbilical artery, fetal peripheral vessels and maternal uterine vessels, in association with decreased resistance in the fetal cerebral vessels. The various types of Doppler indices calculated are tabulated in Table 5.32.

### Q. What is the sequence of various changes occurring in various Doppler velocity waveforms in IUGR fetuses?

**Ans.** Doppler velocimetry is one of the best methods of fetal surveillance during IUGR and helps in diagnosing the associated fetal acidosis and hypoxia. The sequences of changes occurring in fetal vessels occur in parallel to the extent of the fetal compromise. Initially there is appearance of changes on fetal artery Doppler analysis, followed by changes on fetal venous Doppler analysis. This is followed by changes on BPP and CTG. The usual order of the findings on CTG trace indicating fetal hypoxia include the initial loss of acceleration, followed by decreasing variability and presence of late decelerations.

**Table 5.31:** Schedule for conducting various antepartum surveillance tests in patients with IUGR

| Test | Timing |
| --- | --- |
| Fetal movement count | Daily |
| Amniotic fluid volume | Weekly |
| Nonstress test (NST) | Twice weekly |
| Biophysical profile (BPP) | Weekly if NST is abnormal |
| Oxytocin challenge test | Every fortnightly, if BPP is less than 8 |
| Umbilical artery Doppler | Every 2–3 weeks |

**Table 5.32:** Types of Doppler indices

| Doppler index | Calculation of Doppler index |
| --- | --- |
| S/D ratio (Stuart, 1980) | Peak systolic blood flow/end diastolic velocity |
| PI (Pourcelot, 1974) | (Peak systolic velocity – end diastolic velocity)/mean systolic velocity |
| RI (Gosling and King, 1977) | (Peak systolic velocity – end diastolic velocity)/peak systolic velocity |

### Q. How is the amniotic fluid volume affected in the IUGR fetuses?

**Ans.** Measurement of amniotic fluid volume is an important method of fetal surveillance. Estimation of amniotic fluid can be done in two ways: maximal vertical pocket depth of amniotic fluid and AFI. Determination of maximal vertical pool of liquor involves the measurement of maximum vertical diameter of the deepest pocket of amniotic fluid identified upon ultrasound examination. AFI is obtained by measuring the vertical depth of the largest fluid pockets in each of the four uterine quadrants. These four measurements are added in order to obtain a total AFI. Use of amniotic fluid volume evaluation has become important in the assessment of pregnancy at risk for an adverse pregnancy outcome as it forms basis of two important tests of fetal wellbeing used commonly, namely the BPP and the modified BPP both of which include ultrasound estimation of amniotic fluid volume.

### Q. What is the nonstress test?

**Ans.** The fetal NST is a simple, noninvasive test performed in pregnancies over 28 weeks of gestation. The test is named "nonstress" because no stress is placed on the fetus during the test. The test involves attaching one belt to the mother's abdomen to measure fetal heart rate and another belt to measure uterine contractions. Fetal movement, heart rate and "reactivity" of fetal heart (acceleration of fetal heart rate) are measured for 20–30 minutes.

The mother is handed a probe, which she is asked to press whenever she feels a fetal movement. NST is defined as reactive if there is a presence of two or more accelerations that peak 15 beats/minute above the baseline each lasting for 15 seconds or more and all occurring in association with fetal movements within a 20-minute period from beginning of the test. The test is defined as nonreactive if there is no fetal heart rate acceleration over a 40-minute period.

### Q. What is the biophysical profile?

**Ans.** The BPP was first described by Manning in 1980. It utilizes multiple ultrasound parameters of fetal wellbeing and the NST. It is more accurate than a single test as it correlates five measurements to give a score. The ultrasound parameters of the test are fetal tone, fetal movement, fetal breathing and amniotic fluid volume. An NST, which is not an ultrasonic measurement, is also performed. Two points are given if the observation is present and zero points are given if it is absent. The various components of BPP are as follows:

- *Fetal breathing movements:* Normal fetal breathing movements are defined as presence of one or more episodes of rhythmic fetal breathing movements of 30 seconds or more within a period of 30 minutes.
- *Fetal movement:* Normal fetal movement is defined as three or more discrete body or limb movements within a period of 30 minutes.
- *Fetal tone:* Normal fetal tone is defined as one or more episodes of extension of a fetal extremity with return to flexion, or opening or closing of a hand.
- *Determination of the amniotic fluid volume:* A single vertical pocket of amniotic fluid exceeding 2 cm is considered as an indicator of adequate amniotic fluid volume.

    A total score of 8 or 10 is considered as normal, a score of 6 is considered equivocal and a score of 4 or less is abnormal. If the BPP falls below 4, the patient should be urgently prepared for delivery.

### Q. What is modified biophysical profile?

**Ans.** In the late second or third trimester fetus, amniotic fluid volume reflects fetal urine production. Placental dysfunction may result in diminished fetal renal perfusion, leading to oligohydramnios. Amniotic fluid volume assessment can therefore be used to evaluate long-term uteroplacental function. This observation encouraged the development of "modified BPP" as a primary method for antepartum fetal surveillance. The modified BPP combines NST with the AFI. An AFI greater than 5 cm generally is considered to represent an adequate volume of amniotic fluid. Thus, the modified BPP is considered normal if the NST is reactive and the AFI is more than 5 and abnormal if either the NST is nonreactive or the AFI is 5 or less. If the results of a modified BPP indicate a possible abnormality, then the full BPP is performed.

### Q. How should the growth-restricted babies be managed during the antenatal period?

**Ans.** If FGR is diagnosed, one of the most important tasks of the clinician is to identify and treat the underlying cause and observation of adequate fetal surveillance. Some of the steps, which can be taken to identify the underlying cause for IUGR, are described below:

- Screening for congenital infections may be important in cases of symmetrical IUGR.
- Preeclampsia needs to be excluded as the cause for IUGR. This requires regular maternal BP monitoring and urine analysis (for ruling out proteinuria).
- Fetal karyotyping for chromosomal defects.
- Maternal assessment for the presence of nutritional deficiency.
- Since smoking and alcohol abuse or other substances of abuse is commonly associated with IUGR, it is important to rule out these causes of IUGR. Many women may not be open about their smoking or drinking habits. The clinician may need to maintain a lot of tact to elicit this history.

### Q. What instructions must be given to the woman with suspected growth-restricted babies in the antenatal period?

**Ans.** The woman must be advised to take the following precautions in the antenatal period:

- To take rest in the left lateral position for a period of at least 10 hours every day (8 hours in the night and 2 hours in the afternoon).

    Presently there is no evidence regarding the effect of various modalities such as bed rest, maternal nutritional supplementation, plasma volume expansion, maternal medications (low-dose aspirin), oxygen supplementation, etc. in improving perinatal outcome in cases with IUGR.

- If the gestational age is 28 weeks or more, the patient must be instructed to count her fetal movements daily and maintain it in the form of a chart. If she is able to perceive at least ten or more movements within 2 hours, the test can be considered as normal. She should continue with DFMC. In case she perceives less than six fetal movements within 2 hours, she should be advised to immediately consult her doctor.
- The patient should be advised to quit smoking, drinking alcohol or taking drugs of abuse.
- Smoking cessation programs, particularly those using behavioral strategies can be effective for preventing IUGR in women who smoke.
- Women must be counseled to abstain from alcohol and other drugs of abuse. The women may be enrolled in de-addiction programs if they are unable to quit their habit of drug addiction.
- If undernutrition is suspected as a cause of IUGR, the patient should be given nutritional supplements.

- Antepartum/fetal surveillance by ultrasound (BPP) and fetal heart monitoring (NST) must be done to decide on timing and mode of delivery.
- Despite the lack of good quality evidence, low-dose aspirin therapy (colsprin) in the dose of 1–2 mg/kg body weight is commonly prescribed to the women in whom IUGR is suspected.

### Q. What precautions must be observed during the intrapartum period in case of growth-restricted babies?

**Ans.** Since the growth-restricted fetus is especially prone to develop asphyxia, continuous fetal monitoring using external or internal cardiotocographic examination needs to be done in the intrapartum period. If at any time, the fetal heart rate appears to be nonreassuring, emergency cesarean may be required. However, elective CS is not justified for delivery of all IUGR fetuses. Precautions which need to be taken at the time of labor during the intrapartum period include the following:

- Delivery must be carried out in the unit with optimal neonatal expertise and facilities.
- The patient should be lying on bed as far as possible in order to prevent PROM.
- Continuous electronic fetal monitoring either external (if membranes are intact) or internal (if membranes have ruptured) needs to be done.
- Administration of strong analgesic or sedatives to the mother must be avoided due to the risk of transmission of the drugs to the fetus.
- Amnioinfusion may be required in cases with low AFI and meconium stained liquor.
- A skilled pediatrician, who is trained in neonatal resuscitation techniques, must be present at the time of delivery.
- Administration of IM corticosteroids is required in case the delivery takes place between 24 weeks and 36 weeks of gestation. The dosage regimen of corticosteroids is as follows:
  - Two doses of 12 mg each of betamethasone IM at intervals of 24 hours.
  - Four doses of 6 mg each of dexamethasone IM at intervals of 12 hours.

### Q. When should elective cesarean delivery be considered in case of IUGR fetuses?

**Ans.** Elective CS is not justified for delivery of all IUGR fetuses. Various indications for emergency CS in growth-restricted babies are as follows:

- Intrauterine growth restriction along with reduced fetal movements.
- Presence of an obstetric complication (placenta previa, abruption placenta, etc.).
- Nonreassuring fetal heart sound.
- Meconium stained liquor.
- IUGR fetus with breech presentation.

- Absent or reversed umbilical artery blood flow on Doppler examination.

### Q. What is the appropriate timing for delivery in these cases?

**Ans.** There is wide variation in practice in the timing of delivery of growth-restricted fetuses. The most important goal of management is to deliver the most mature fetus in the least compromised position and at the same time causing minimum harm to the mother.

Presently, the RCOG (2002) recommends that the clinician needs to individualize each patient and decide the time for delivery by weighing the risk of fetal demise due to delayed intervention against the risk of long-term disabilities resulting from preterm delivery due to early intervention. The two main parameters for deciding the optimal time of delivery include results on various fetal surveillance techniques and gestational age. Also, the patient needs to be counseled regarding the potential risks associated with the two strategies.

Preterm delivery could be associated with future disabilities, intraventricular hemorrhage, sepsis and retinopathy of prematurity, etc. Delayed delivery on the other hand may be associated with ischemic brain injury, periventricular leukomalacia, intraventricular hemorrhage and IUD.

### Q. What are the various complications associated with growth-restricted pregnancies?

**Ans.** Various complications associated with growth-restricted pregnancies are as follows:

#### Fetal Complications

*Antepartum complications:* These may include the following:
- Fetal hypoxia and acidosis.
- Meconium aspiration/infection.
- Stillbirth.
- Oligohydramnios.
- Iatrogenic prematurity.

*Intrapartum complications:* Neonatal asphyxia and acidosis is especially common in these fetuses. Some of the neonatal complications associated with this include the following:

- *Respiratory distress syndrome:* The pulmonary system of the growth-restricted babies is often immature at birth resulting in the development of respiratory distress syndrome.
- *Meconium aspiration syndrome:* Aspiration of meconium is a significant cause of mortality and morbidity in a FGR baby.
- *Persistent fetal circulation:* This condition is characterized by severe pulmonary vasoconstriction and persistent blood flow through the ductus venosus even after birth. This is responsible for producing hypoxia, hypercarbia and signs of right-to-left shunting.

- *Intraventricular bleeding:* This condition is produced as a result of bleeding inside or around the cerebral ventricles in a growth-restricted baby.
- *Neonatal encephalopathy:* This condition can occur as a consequence of severe birth asphyxia and can produce a constellation of neurological signs and symptoms (seizures, twitching, irritability, apnea, etc.).

### Neonatal Complications

The newborn child typically shows an old man like appearance. There are signs of soft tissue wasting including reduced amount of subcutaneous fat and loosened, thin skin. The muscle mass of arms, buttocks and thighs is greatly reduced. The abdomen is scaphoid and the ribs are protuberant. The HC may appear to be obviously larger than the AC. Some of the metabolic complications which can be frequently encountered in these babies include the following:

- *Hypoglycemia:* Neonatal hypoglycemia can be defined as blood glucose levels of less than 30 mg/dL. It can be associated with symptoms like jitteriness, twitching, apnea, etc. It can occur due to reduced glycogen stores/glycogenolysis/gluconeogenesis, increased metabolic rate and deficient release of catecholamines in an IUGR baby. Early feeding of the newborn baby can help prevent hypoglycemia.
- Hypoinsulinemia.
- Hypertriglyceridemia.
- *Hypocalcemia:* Hypocalcemia is often associated with perinatal stress, asphyxia and prematurity in the newborn baby.
- Polycythemia.
- Meconium aspiration.
- Hyperphosphatemia.
- Birth asphyxia.
- *Hypothermia:* The growth-restricted fetus has a poor temperature control due to which there is an increased tendency to develop hypothermia. Other factors responsible for producing hypothermia include reduced amount of subcutaneous fat, increased surface-volume ratio, decreased heat production, etc.
- Hyperbilirubinemia.
- Sepsis.
- Thrombocytopenia.
- Respiratory distress.
- Necrotizing enterocolitis.
- *Hyperviscosity syndrome:* It is mainly associated with polycythemia and increased hematocrit levels above 65%.

### Long-Term Sequel of IUGR

- *Postnatal growth:* In some cases catch-up growth may occur in first 6 months of life.
- Cerebral palsy.

- *Adult disease:* These children are supposed to be at an increased risk of developing disorders such as obesity, diabetes mellitus, hypertension, cardiovascular disease, ischemic heart disease, etc. later in life.

# Antepartum Hemorrhage

## Case Study 1

Mrs XYZ, a 32-year-old married for 10 years, resident of ABC, G3P2L2 woman presented to the emergency department at 32 weeks of gestation with a sudden onset of bleeding since past few hours. Bleeding occurred suddenly, was painless, profuse, bright red in color and not initiated by any preceding trauma. She had soaked several clothes and beddings. On examination, her pulse was 100 beats per minute, BP was 120/80 mm Hg, and respiratory rate was 20 beats per minute. She appeared very pale and had a clear chest. Per abdominal examination revealed a single, live fetus in transverse lie corresponding to 30 weeks of gestation.

**Q. What is the most likely diagnosis in the above-mentioned case study?**

**Ans.** The most likely diagnosis in the above-mentioned case study is Mrs XYZ, a 32-year-old married for 10 years, resident of ABC, G3P2L2 woman, with 32 weeks amenorrhea, corresponding to 32 weeks of gestation with the diagnosis of antepartum hemorrhage (APH). The definite cause of APH can only be diagnosed following an ultrasound examination. The questions to be asked at the time of taking history and the parameters to be assessed at the time of examination in such a case are described in Tables 5.33 and 5.34 respectively.

**Q. What is antepartum hemorrhage?**

**Ans.** APH can be defined as hemorrhage from the genital tract occurring after the 28th week of pregnancy, but before the delivery of baby. It does not include the bleeding which occurs after the delivery of the baby; this bleeding which occurs in the postpartum period after the birth of the baby is known as PPH. The 28 weeks interval is arbitrarily taken as a limit while defining APH because the fetus is supposed to have attained viability by that time.

**Q. What are the causes of antepartum hemorrhage?**

**Ans.** The antepartum bleeding could be due to placental or extraplacental causes. Besides this, some cases of APH could be due to unexplained causes and are also termed as indeterminate APH. The placental causes of bleeding are termed as true APH and can be due to placenta previa or placental abruption. Extraplacental cause of bleeding is also termed as false APH and includes bleeding related to the presence of cervical polyps, carcinoma cervix, cervical varicosities, cervical trauma, etc. Placental causes of bleeding are the most common cause of APH, accounting for nearly 70–75% cases; whereas the extraplacental causes account for 5% cases and unexplained causes for the remaining 20–25%.

| **Table 5.33:** Symptoms to be elicited at the time of taking history in a case of antepartum hemorrhage |
| --- |

### History of Presenting Complains

*Bleeding per vaginum:* The bleeding in cases of antepartum hemorrhage (APH) usually occurs after 28 weeks of gestation. It is important to elicit the characteristics of bleeding in order to arrive at a diagnosis. As previously described, true APH occurs due to two main causes—placenta previa and placental abruption. History is one of the most important parameter for differentiating between these two most important causes for bleeding, late in pregnancy. Difference in the clinical presentation between these two conditions has been tabulated in Table 5.35. The following characteristics need to be taken into consideration at the time of taking history:

- *Type of bleeding:* Placenta previa is typically associated with sudden, painless, apparently causeless, recurrent and profuse bleeding, which is bright red in color. Abruptio placenta, on the other hand is associated with bleeding, which is dark red in color.
- *Amount of bleeding:* The amount of bleeding in cases of placenta previa may range from light to heavy. It may stop, but it nearly always recurs days or weeks later. The patient may also give a history of experiencing small "warning hemorrhages" before the actual episode of bleeding. The occurrence of these warning hemorrhages must be viewed with greatest suspicion and caution and appropriate steps must be taken to exclude placenta previa. Bleeding in placental abruption may not be proportional to the amount of placental separation as in many cases the bleeding may be concealed.
- *Timing of bleeding:* In cases of placenta previa, bleeding usually occurs late in the third trimester. The earlier in pregnancy, the bleeding occurs, more likely it is due to severe degree of placenta previa.
- *Abdominal pain:* While the bleeding in cases of placenta previa is virtually painless, bleeding in cases of abruption placenta is typically accompanied by abdominal and/or back pain. Some women may experience slightly different symptoms including, faintness and collapse, nausea, thirst, reduced fetal movements, etc.
- *Backache:* In cases of placenta previa, if the placenta is present posteriorly, the women may experience severe backache. Otherwise, in other cases of placenta previa, there is hardly any back pain. On the other hand, most important symptom in case of placental abruption is vaginal bleeding in combination with abdominal and back pain.
- *Presence of any factor which triggers bleeding:* While the bleeding related with placenta previa is causeless, bleeding due to abruption placenta is preceded by some triggering factor such as abdominal trauma, road traffic accident or hypertension.

### Obstetric History

Some risk factors, which are associated with an increased incidence of placenta previa or abruptio placenta, need to be elicited at the time of taking the history:

- *Previous history of cesarean delivery:* Previous history of cesarean delivery is associated with an increased risk of placenta previa in future pregnancies. Also this risk further increases with the number of previous pregnancies involved. It is important to elicit the history of previous uterine surgery, because presence of a uterine scar along with placenta previa may be often associated with placenta accreta, increta or percreta.
- *Advanced maternal age:* The risk of placenta previa also increases with advancing maternal age. Increased maternal age and parity is also associated with an increased risk of abruption placenta.
- History of placenta previa in the previous pregnancy is also associated with an increased risk of placenta previa in the present pregnancy.
- *Previous history of placental abruption:* If the woman has a history of experiencing placental abruption in past, she is at a high risk of experiencing the same condition during her present pregnancy as well. As the number of previously affected pregnancies increase, the risk further increases, with the risk of recurrence increasing to 25% with previous two affected pregnancies.
- *Smoking and/or substance abuse especially cocaine abuse:* Placental abruption is more common in women who smoke, drink alcohol, or abuse drugs like cocaine or methamphetamine during pregnancy.
- History of multiple gestations, fetal malpresentation and fetal congenital anomaly in the present pregnancy is associated with an increased risk of placenta previa as well as abruption placenta.
- *Trauma or injury to the abdomen:* Injury resulting due to a motor vehicle accident or fall is a common cause for placental abruption. Rarely, placental abruption may be caused by an unusually short umbilical cord or sudden uterine decompression (as in cases of polyhydramnios), which may cause sudden placental detachment. Sudden preterm rupture of membranes is also likely to cause placental separation, resulting in placental abruption.

### Medical History

- *High blood pressure associated with preeclampsia and chronic hypertension:* High BP increases the risk of placental abruption.
- *Blood clotting disorders:* Blood clotting disorders, e.g. thrombophilias (both inherited and acquired) may also act as risk factors for placental abruption.

### Gynecological History

*Presence of uterine leiomyomas:* Presence of uterine leiomyomas especially at the site of placental implantation is supposed to be associated with an increased incidence of placental abruption.

### Q. How can you clinically assess the amount of blood loss?

**Ans.** It is also important to take the history regarding the amount of blood loss. Most of the times, it is difficult to rely upon the patient's own estimation regarding the amount of bleeding. An important parameter to help decide the severity of hemorrhage is to ask the patient regarding the number of pads she had to use during the episode of bleeding. A history of passage of clots is also indicative of severe hemorrhage.

**Table 5.34:** Various findings elicited at the time of clinical examination in a case of APH

*General Physical Examination*

- The difference between placenta previa and placental abruption is described in Table 5.35.
- The patient's physical condition is proportional to the amount of blood loss in cases of placenta previa. However, it may not be proportional to the amount of blood loss in cases of concealed abruption placenta.
- *Signs of hemodynamic compromise:* Hemodynamic compromise may be present in cases of severe placental abruption and severe cases of placenta previa. Anemia and oliguria may also be sometimes present in cases of abruption placenta.
- *Anemia or shock:* Repeated bleeding can result in anemia, whereas heavy bleeding may cause shock. Profuse hemorrhage can result in hypotension and/or tachycardia.
- There may be signs and symptoms suggestive of preeclampsia (increased BP, proteinuria, etc.) in cases of abruption placenta.

*Specific Systemic Examination*

*Abdominal Examination*
*Uterine Palpation*

- Uterus is soft, relaxed and nontender in cases of placenta previa. Size of the uterus is proportional to the period of gestation. The fetal presenting part may be high and cannot be pressed into the pelvic inlet due to the presence of placenta. There may be an abnormal fetal presentation (e.g. breech presentation, transverse lie, etc.)
- Uterine hypertonicity and frequent uterine contractions are commonly present in cases of abruptio placenta. It may be difficult to feel the fetal parts due to presence of uterine hypertonicity. Uterine rigidity may become apparent on abdominal palpation. The uterus may either be tense and tender upon palpation or it may feel doughy or woody hard due to persistent hypertonus.

*Auscultation*

- Fetal heart rate is usually within normal limits in cases of placenta previa. Fetal heart tones may be rarely absent in cases of APH due to placenta previa as a result of maternal shock. Slowing of fetal heart rate can sometimes result in cases of dangerous placenta previa (marginal degree of placenta previa, located posteriorly).
- *Stallworthy's sign:* In cases of placenta previa, when the head is pushed into the pelvis, there is slowing of fetal heart rate due to compression of placenta and cord, in cases of dangerous placenta previa.
- *Absent or slow fetal heart sound:* Severe degree of placental abruption may be associated with fetal bradycardia and other fetal heart rate abnormalities. In extreme cases, fetal demise may even be detected at the time of examination.

*Vaginal Examination*

- Vaginal examination must never be performed in cases of antepartum hemorrhage with the suspected diagnosis of placenta previa. Though presence of placental abruption is not a contraindication for vaginal examination, vaginal examination should ideally not be performed in patients with history of APH due to the risk of placenta previa.

*Rectal Examination*

A rectal examination is more dangerous than a vaginal examination and must never be performed in cases of suspected placenta previa.

**Table 5.35:** Difference between placenta previa and abruption placenta on history and clinical examination

| Characteristics | Placenta previa | Placental abruption |
|---|---|---|
| **Clinical Features** | | |
| Patient's general condition | Proportional to the amount of blood loss. Blood loss is always revealed in these cases | Out of proportion to the amount of visible blood loss (especially in cases of concealed hemorrhage). Blood loss in these cases could be revealed, concealed or mixed |
| Nature of vaginal bleeding | Bleeding is painless, apparently causeless and recurrent. Bleeding is usually bright red in color | Bleeding is painful, often attributed to some underlying cause (e.g. trauma, preeclampsia, etc.) and continuous. Blood loss is usually dark-colored |
| Features of preeclampsia | Not relevant | May be present in up to one-third cases |
| Amount of blood loss | Profuse, may be preceded by small amounts of warning hemorrhages | Blood loss may vary from slight in amount to large |
| **Abdominal Examination** | | |
| Fundal height | Proportionate to the period of gestation | Uterus may be disproportionately enlarged in cases of concealed hemorrhage |
| Feel of uterus | Soft and relaxed | Tense, tender and rigid |
| Malpresentation | Commonly encountered | May or may not be present |
| Engagement of head | Head is usually unengaged and free floating | Head may be engaged |
| Fetal heart sound | Present | May be absent in cases of fetal jeopardy |

Presence of blood at the sides of patient's legs, at the time of examination often extending up to the heels is also indicative of severe hemorrhage. Severe hemorrhage may be associated with signs of shock (tachycardia, reduced BP, etc.).

### Q. Should vaginal or a rectal examination be performed in cases of antepartum hemorrhage?

**Ans.** *Vaginal and/rectal examination must never be performed in suspected cases of placenta previa.* Instead, an initial inspection must only be performed. On inspection, the following points must be noted:

- To see if bleeding is occurring or not.
- In case the bleeding is occurring, to note the amount and color of the bleeding.
- A per speculum inspection using a Cusco's speculum can be performed once the patient has become stable. Performance of per speculum examination helps in ruling out the local causes (e.g. cervical erosions, polyps, etc.) of bleeding per vaginum.
- Nowadays, the diagnosis of placenta previa can be confirmed on ultrasound examination. In case, facilities for ultrasound examination are not available and a vaginal examination is required, it must be performed in the operating room under double set-up conditions (i.e. arrangements for an emergency cesarean delivery are in place).

## Case Study 2

Mrs XYZ, a 32-year-old married for 8 years, resident of ABC, G2P1L1 woman with 33 weeks of gestation, presented with painless bleeding per vaginum since last 2 hours. This was the first time during the pregnancy that she has experienced this bleeding. According to her, the bleeding was severe and she gave a history of soaking nearly 5–6 pads in last 2 hours. Her pulse rate was 90 beats/minute and her BP was 110/70 mm Hg.

### Q. What is the likely diagnosis in the above-mentioned case study? Why does this patient need to be assessed urgently?

**Ans.** Since the bleeding in this patient has occurred after 28 weeks of gestation, the most probable diagnosis of APH can be made. Most common causes for APH include placenta previa and placental abruption. In this case, the history of painless, causeless bleeding, points in the direction of placenta previa. However, the diagnosis needs to be confirmed by ultrasound examination. This patient needs to be urgently managed because APH due to any cause must always be regarded as an emergency, until the exact cause for the bleeding has been found. After the ultrasound examination, correct management can be given.

### Q. What is the first step in the management of a patient with APH?

**Ans.** The first step in the management of such a patient is to stabilize the patient. The clinical condition of the patient must be assessed. The priority should be towards the resuscitation of the patient with the emphasis on maintenance of ABC (airway, breathing and circulation).

Since the patient is likely to be hypovolemic, two wide bore cannulae must be inserted and IV fluids be started. The patient's blood must be sent for blood grouping and typing, hematocrit and coagulation profile. At least four units of blood needs to be arranged as urgent transfusion may be required at any time.

### Q. What is the next step in the management of a patient with APH?

**Ans.** After the maternal condition has stabilized, the fetal condition must be assessed. Arrangements for an urgent ultrasound must be made in order to confirm the fetal well-being and presentation, and placental localization. Placental localization helps in differentiating between the two most common causes of APH: placenta previa and abruptio placenta. Further management needs to be decided based on the exact diagnosis.

### Q. Can engagement of the head occur if placenta previa is present?

**Ans.** No. Presence of a major degree placenta previa is usually associated with a free floating head in case of cephalic presentation. If two-fifths or less of the fetal head can be palpated above the pelvic brim, the possibility of a major degree placenta previa can be nearly excluded.

### Q. What do you understand by a "warning bleed"?

**Ans.** This bleeding refers to small episodes of hemorrhage which occur prior to the episode of the major hemorrhage in cases with placenta previa. The bleeding occurs at about 34 weeks of gestation or earlier when the lower uterine segment begins to form.

### Q. How do you go about doing a double setup vaginal examination in an OT?

**Ans.** Double setup examination is rarely done nowadays for the danger of provoking torrential hemorrhage. It may be sometimes done in cases where there are no facilities for ultrasound examination. The double setup examination is done while all the preparations for an emergency CS are in place, in case it is required. The double setup vaginal examination involves the following steps:

- The clinician must scrub up and put on double pair of gloves. If on vaginal examination placenta is felt, the first pair of gloves would be discarded so that the clinician can immediately proceed for an emergency CS.
- The OT nurse must be scrubbed up with her trolley ready.
- The patient must be preferably under GA or epidural anesthesia. In case an emergency CS is required, the anesthetist must be ready to extend the anesthesia.
- A careful digital examination involving the following steps is done by the clinician:
  - Firstly, the index finger must be gently introduced inside the vagina. The vaginal fornices must be

palpated for presence of any bogginess between the fetal presenting part and the finger.

- If the fetal presenting part can be palpated through the fornix, the finger can be introduced with some confidence into the cervical canal and a careful examination is done through the cervix.
- If the placental edge is felt at any point, the examination must be stopped and the finger must be withdrawn. In these cases, an emergency CS needs to be performed. If no placental edge is palpable, the entire lower segment can be gradually explored. In such cases with term gestation, the membranes can be ruptured with the aim of allowing a vaginal delivery.

### Q. Why do patients with a placenta previa have an increased risk of PPH?

**Ans.** In cases of placenta previa, the placenta is implanted in the lower segment which, normally does not have the same ability as the upper segment to contract and retract after delivery. Due to this, the chances of bleeding following the delivery of the baby are increased. Therefore, measures must be taken in advance to prevent the occurrence of PPH.

### Q. What is placenta previa?

**Ans.** Placenta previa is one of the important placental causes of APH and can be defined as abnormal implantation of the placenta in the lower uterine segment. Depending on the location of placenta in the relation of cervical os, there can be four degrees of placenta previa, which are as follows:

- *Type 4 placenta previa:* This is also known as total or central placenta previa. In total placenta previa, the placenta completely covers the cervix as observed on transvaginal sonography.
- *Type 3 placenta previa:* This is also known as partial placenta previa. In partial placenta previa, the placenta partly covers the cervical os.
- *Type 2 placenta previa:* This is also known as marginal placenta previa. In marginal placenta previa, the placenta does not in any way cover the cervical os, but it approaches the edge of the cervix.
- *Type 1 placenta previa:* This is also known as low-lying placenta. Low-lying placenta is a term used to describe a placenta which is implanted in the lower uterine segment, but is not as close enough to the cervix to qualify as marginal placenta previa. Though the placenta does lie in close proximity to the internal os, the placental margin does not approach the cervical edge in any way. Though a low-lying placenta usually does not cause intrapartum bleeding, it does increase the risk of PPH because of lower uterine segment atony.

### Q. Why does placenta previa cause bleeding?

**Ans.** The cause of bleeding in cases of placenta previa is related to mechanical separation of the placenta from the site of implantation. This usually occurs at the time of formation of the lower uterine segment, during third trimester, or during effacement and dilatation of the cervix at the time of labor. As the lower uterine segment progressively enlarges in the later months of pregnancy, the placenta gets sheared off from the walls of the uterine segment. This causes opening up of uteroplacental sinuses which can initiate an episode of bleeding. Since the growth of the lower uterine segment is a physiological process, the episode of bleeding becomes inevitable in cases of placenta previa. The episode of bleeding is also triggered off, if placenta is separated from the lower uterine segment due to traumatic acts like vaginal examination, sexual intercourse, etc.

### Q. What is dangerous placenta previa?

**Ans.** Marginal placenta previa when implanted over the posterior uterine wall is termed as dangerous placenta previa. This is so, as the placental thickness (about 2.5 cm) overlying the sacral promontory greatly diminishes the anterior posterior diameter of the pelvic inlet, thereby preventing the engagement of fetal presenting part. Since the engagement of the presenting part does not take place, effective compression of the separated placenta cannot take place and the vaginal bleeding continues to occur. In fact if the vaginal bleeding is allowed to occur, fetal distress may develop soon.

### Q. What are the various investigations which need to be done in these cases of placenta previa?

The various investigations which need to be done in these cases are as follows:

- *ABO/Rhesus compatibility:* At least four units of blood need to be crossmatched and arranged. At any time, if severe hemorrhage occurs, the patient may require a blood transfusion.
- *Imaging studies:* The main way of confirming the diagnosis of placenta previa is by imaging studies, especially transvaginal sonography. Sonography also helps in determining the placental position, fetal maturity, fetal wellbeing, fetal presentation and presence of congenital anomalies. Transvaginal examination need not be performed in all the women. A reasonable antenatal imaging policy would be to perform a transvaginal ultrasound scan on all women in whom a low-lying placenta is suspected from their transabdominal anomaly scan (at approximately 20–24 weeks).
- *Magnetic resonance imaging:* Magnetic resonance imaging (MRI) has been reported as a safe technique in the diagnosis of placenta previa when the images obtained by ultrasound (both TAS and TVS) have been unsatisfactory.
- *Doppler ultrasound:* Antenatal imaging by color flow Doppler ultrasonography is especially useful in women with placenta previa who are at an increased risk of placenta accreta. Women with placenta previa having a

previous history of uterine scar are at an increased risk of having a morbidly adherent placenta, especially when there has been a short cesarean to conception interval. Doppler ultrasound examination should be preferably done in such individuals.

**Q. What factors should be taken into consideration before deciding the final treatment plan for patients with placenta previa?**

**Ans.** The factors to be taken into consideration before deciding the final treatment plan for patients with placenta previa include the following:

- Amount of vaginal bleeding
- Whether bleeding has stopped or is continuing
- Gestational age
- Fetal condition
- Maternal health
- Position of the placenta and baby.

**Q. What should be the management of patients with severe bleeding?**

**Ans.** Patients with severe bleeding need to be carefully monitored in the hospital. These women must be transferred to tertiary care units as soon as possible. In cases of severe bleeding, the most important step in management is to stabilize the patient; arrange and cross-match at least four units of blood and start blood transfusion if required. All efforts must be made to shift her to the operating theater as soon as possible for an emergency cesarean delivery. The following steps need to be taken:

1. One or two large bore IV cannula need to be inserted and IV fluids like ringer lactate must be started.
2. Monitoring of pulse, BP and amount of vaginal bleeding to be done at every half hour intervals.
3. Input-output charting at hourly intervals.
4. If the bleeding is severe, a blood transfusion may be required in order to replace the lost blood.
5. Once the patient has stabilized, electronic fetal monitoring needs to be initiated.
6. Sedative analgesics like pethidine can be administered.
7. Rhesus (Rh) immunoglobulins must be administered, when appropriate, to Rh-negative, nonimmunized women.
8. The definitive cause of the bleeding needs to be addressed after the maternal and fetal conditions have stabilized. If the definitive diagnosis of placenta previa is made and the period of gestation is greater than or equal to 36 weeks, delivery is appropriate. In case the bleeding is excessive or continuous or the fetal heart tracing is nonreassuring, the patient needs to be delivered irrespective of the period of gestation.
9. Severe bleeding is usually due to a major degree of placenta previa. The definitive treatment in these cases would be delivery by CS.

**Q. What should be the management of patients with moderate bleeding?**

**Ans.** The initial five steps as mentioned in patients with severe bleeding must be applied in the patient with moderate bleeding at the same time using clinical discretion.

- The timing for delivery in these patients must be based upon the period of gestation as follows:
- *Period of gestation 36 weeks or more:* If the period of gestation is 36 weeks or more, the women must be delivered by performing a CS.
- *Period of gestation is less than 36 weeks:* If the period of gestation is between 32 and 36 weeks, assessment of fetal lung maturity needs to be done using the lecithin-sphingomyelin (L:S) ratio. The L:S ratio of greater than or equal to 2 indicates fetal lung maturity, implying that the fetus can be delivered in these cases. If L:S ratio is less than 2, the fetal lungs have yet not attained maturity. Intramuscular corticosteroid injection must be given to the mother. Until the complete dose of corticosteroids has been administered, the delivery should be preferably delayed.
- During this waiting period, the patient must be kept under intensive monitoring. Though the role of tocolysis remains controversial, tocolytic agents such as β-mimetics and magnesium sulfate can be used to prevent uterine activity. If the patient remains stable for next 24–48 hours, she becomes a candidate for expectant management. If the patient does not remain stable for the next 24–48 hours, she must be delivered by a CS.

**Q. What is the management of patients with mild bleeding?**

**Ans.** Similar to the patients with moderate bleeding, in the patients with mild bleeding the management is based on period of gestation and fetal pulmonary maturity. If the period of gestation is less than 36 weeks or the fetal lungs are immature (i.e. L:S ratio is < 2), the woman who has stabilized after an initial episode of bleeding becomes a candidate for expectant management. If the fetus has attained maturity, the women can be delivered. The mode of delivery depends upon the grade of placenta previa.

**Q. What steps does the expectant management comprise of?**

**Ans.** The expectant management was introduced by McAfee and Johnson and is often also known as McAfee and Johnson's regime. The aim of expectant management is to delay pregnancy until the time fetal maturity is reached.

*Prerequisites for expectant management:* The prerequisites for expectant management are as follows:

- Stable maternal health (Hb > 10%).
- Period of gestation is less than 37 completed weeks.
- Fetal wellbeing is assured on ultrasound examination.
- No active bleeding is present.
- Facilities for emergency CS are there, in case it is required.

*Steps to be taken:* The expectant management includes the following steps:

- If there is little or minimal bleeding, the woman is advised to limit her physical activity and take bed rest. Bed rest helps in reducing pressure on the cervix, which may help in stopping preterm contractions or vaginal bleeding. Bed rest also helps in increasing blood flow to the placenta, thereby stimulating fetal growth.
- The woman must be asked to avoid sexual intercourse, which can trigger vaginal bleeding by initiating contractions or causing direct trauma.
- The woman is also advised not to engage in any type of physical exercise as far as possible.
- The woman should be prescribed iron tablets throughout pregnancy in order to keep the blood hemoglobin levels within the normal range.
- In case preterm delivery is anticipated, the mother must be administered corticosteroids intramuscularly.
- Placenta previa is likely to result in fetomaternal hemorrhage. Therefore, all Rh-negative women with placenta previa who bleed must be offered anti-D immunoglobulin injections in order to prevent the risk of Rh isoimmunization.
- Thromboprophylaxis may be offered to women who are advised prolonged bed rest in order to reduce the risk of thromboembolism.

### Q. Should the patient with placenta previa be hospitalized or managed in outpatient setting?

**Ans.** Once the patient presents to the hospital with an episode of bleeding, she should be observed in the hospital until she is free of bleeding for at least 48 hours. Following the initial period of observation, the expectant management plan can be carried out at home or in the hospital. The indications for hospitalization are as follows:

- Hospitalization at 32–34 weeks is required for asymptomatic women with major degrees of placenta previa, who had been previously stable, because she might suddenly start bleeding heavily at any time, requiring urgent delivery.
- Severe bleeding irrespective of the period of gestation.
- Patient perceives reduced fetal movements.

### Q. What is the mode of delivery in cases of placenta previa?

**Ans.** Cesarean delivery is necessary for most cases of placenta previa, especially the major degree placenta previa including type II (posterior); type III and type IV. Severe blood loss may require a blood transfusion. Indications for immediate delivery by CS in cases of placenta previa irrespective of the period of gestation or degree of placenta previa are as follows:

- Bleeding is heavy.
- Bleeding is uncontrolled.
- Fetal distress.
- Obstetric factors like CPD, fetal malpresentation, etc.

Prior to delivery, the clinician needs to have detailed antenatal discussions with the woman and her partner, regarding the need for cesarean delivery, possibility of hemorrhage, possible blood transfusion and requirement for major surgical interventions, such as hysterectomy.

### Q. What steps must be taken to control bleeding at the time of cesarean section?

**Ans.** Steps which must be taken to control bleeding at the time of cesarean delivery are as follows:

- Use of uterotonic agents to reduce the blood loss.
- Application of CHO sutures or B-lynch sutures.
- Bilateral uterine artery or internal iliac artery ligation.
- Intrauterine packing.
- Hydrostatic balloon catheterization.
- Aortic compression.
- Pelvic artery embolization.

    If all above described conservative measures fail and the patient continues to bleed, the clinician may have no other alternative left, but to resort to cesarean hysterectomy in order to save the mother's life.

### Q. What kind of maternal and fetal complications can occur in cases of placenta previa?

**Ans.** Various maternal and fetal complications, which can occur in cases of placenta previa are as follows:

#### *Maternal Complications*

*Bleeding:* One of the biggest concerns with placenta previa is the risk of severe vaginal bleeding (hemorrhage) during labor, delivery or the first few hours after delivery. The bleeding can be heavy enough to cause maternal shock or even death.

*Placenta accreta, increta, percreta:* Pathological adherence of the placenta is termed as invasive placenta. In this condition, the trophoblastic invasion occurs beyond the normal boundary established by the Nitabuch's fibrinoid layer. While the term "accreta" refers to abnormal attachment of the placenta to the uterine surface, the terms "increta" and "percreta" refer to much deeper invasion of the placental villi into the uterine musculature. In placenta increta, the invasion by the placental villi is limited to approximately half the myometrial thickness. On the other hand, in cases of placenta percreta there is through and through invasion of the uterine wall. Abnormally adherent placenta can result in severe bleeding and, may often require cesarean hysterectomy.

*Anemia and infection:* Excessive blood loss can result in anemia and increased susceptibility to infections.

#### *Fetal Complications*

Placenta previa can be commonly associated with neonatal complications such as fetal growth impairment, neurodevelopmental delay, sudden infant death syndrome (SIDS) and iatrogenic prematurity.

*Premature birth:* Severe bleeding may force the clinician to proceed with an emergency preterm cesarean delivery.

*Fetal death or fetal distress:* Though chances of fetal distress and fetal death are much less in cases with placenta previa in comparison to that in cases with placental abruption, severe maternal bleeding in cases with placenta previa is sometimes also responsible for producing fetal distress.

## Case Study 3

Mrs XYZ, a 32-year-old woman, married for 12 years, resident of ABC, G4P3L2 patient, who is 36 weeks pregnant, presented with a history of severe vaginal bleeding and abdominal pain. The blood contained dark colored clots. Since the hemorrhage, the patient has also been complaining of reduced fetal movements. The patient's BP is 80/60 mm Hg and the pulse rate is 120 beats/minute.

### Q. What is placental abruption?

**Ans.** Placental abruption can be defined as abnormal, pathological separation of the normally situated placenta from its uterine attachment. As a result, bleeding occurs from the opened sinuses present in the uterine myometrium. "Abruptio placentae" is a Latin word meaning, "rending asunder of placenta", which denotes a sudden accident. Thus, placental abruption is also known as accidental hemorrhage. Separation of the normally situated placenta results in hemorrhage into the decidua basalis. A retroplacental clot develops between the placenta and the decidua basalis, which interferes with the supply of oxygen to the fetus. As a result, fetal distress can also develop in the cases of abruptio placenta.

### Q. What should be the initial steps for management in the above-mentioned patient?

**Ans.** The initial step in the management of this case is the emergency active resuscitation of the mother. The other steps which need to be taken include the following:

- Two IV infusion lines are usually needed, one of which can be a central venous pressure line.
- Blood needs to be sent for investigations, such as CBC, ABO and Rh typing and crossmatching, and blood coagulation profile.
- Two units of FFP and at least four units of whole blood need to be urgently arranged and cross-matched. This is usually required for effective resuscitation.
- The pulse rate and BP must be checked every 15 minutes until the patient's condition stabilizes and every half hourly thereafter.
- A Foley's catheter must be inserted into the bladder and half hourly input-output charting needs to be done.
- An urgent ultrasound examination needs to be performed to confirm placental position, fetal viability and presentation.
- Pain relief in the form of IM injection of pethidine must be administered.

### Q. In this case, on ultrasound examination, a retroplacental clot was observed and placenta was located posteriorly in the upper uterine segment. Ultrasound showed a single live fetus, 36 weeks of gestation in cephalic presentation. Cardiotocography trace showed nonreassuring fetal heart trace. What would be the next step of management in this case?

**Ans.** In this case, a diagnosis of placental abruption in association with fetal distress was made. The baby needs to be delivered as soon as possible. Since the diagnosis of placenta previa has been excluded, a vaginal examination can be safely performed. Further management needs to be decided based on the findings of the vaginal examination. If the cervix is 9 cm or more dilated and the fetal head is on the pelvic floor, ARM can be done and oxytocin infusion can be started so that the fetus can be delivered vaginally as quickly as possible.

If the cervical dilatation is found to be less than 9 cm, an emergency CS must be performed as soon as the patient has been resuscitated. Immediately before starting the CS, the FHS must be auscultated.

In this case since the patient is stable and is not experiencing severe bleeding, the membranes should be ruptured and the fetus delivered vaginally, if possible.

### Q. What is the most likely cause of APH with fetal distress?

**Ans.** The most likely cause of APH in association with fetal distress is placental abruption. Intrauterine death also can commonly occur in cases of placental abruption, whereas it is relatively less common in cases of placenta previa.

### Q. How would you manage this patient if a fetal heart beat is not heard?

**Ans.** If placental separation is so severe that the fetus is dead, vaginal delivery is preferred unless hemorrhage is so severe that it cannot be managed even by vigorous blood replacement or there is the presence of some other obstetrical factor.

### Q. What are the likely causes for renal failure in patients with placental abruption?

**Ans.** In cases with placental abruption, the renal failure could result from numerous causes including the following:

- Acute tubular necrosis.
- Massive hemorrhage resulting in impaired renal perfusion.
- Frequent coexistence of preeclampsia which is an important cause of renal vasospasm.

### Q. What are the causes of PPH in a case of placental abruption?

**Ans.** If the woman has suffered a placental abruption, there might be presence of intramuscular hemorrhages within the uterine musculature, which may prevent effective uterine contractions thereby resulting in development of PPH.

Due to onset of disseminated intravascular coagulation (DIC) in cases with severe placental abruption, there might be failure of coagulation due to which the blood may fail to clot. This may be another cause for PPH.

**Q. What steps should be taken to prevent the occurrence of PPH?**

**Ans.** Active management of the third stage of labor is the most important step for the prevention of PPH. This incorporates the following steps:

- 0.5 mg of ergometrine must be administered at the delivery of anterior shoulder. This can be supplemented with five units of oxytocin, if required. If necessary, these drugs may be repeated several times.
- An IV line must be running and typed and cross-matched blood should be available. Any time, severe hemorrhage occurs, or the mother appears to be in shock, blood must be transfused immediately.
- Bimanual compression of the uterus may be tried after ruling out the traumatic causes of bleeding.

**Q. Describe the clinical classification of placental abruption.**

**Ans.** Depending on the severity of clinical features, the placental abruption could be of the following types (Table 5.36):

- *Grade 0:* No obvious clinical features are present. Diagnosis is made after the inspection of placenta following the delivery of the baby. Sometimes placental abruption is not diagnosed until after delivery, when an area of clotted blood may be found behind the placenta.
- *Grade 1 (Mild):* There may be slight external bleeding. Uterus may be irritable; uterine tenderness and abdominal pain may or may not be present. FHS is good and shock is absent (no signs of low BP in the mother). The perinatal outcome is usually favorable and volume of retroplacental clot is usually less than 200 mL.
- *Grade 2 (Moderate):* In this type of placental abruption, the external bleeding is mild to moderate in amount. The uterus is tender and the abdominal pain is often present. Maternal shock is absent; the patient may have tachycardia but does not have signs of hypovolemia. FHS may be present or absent and often there are signs of fetal distress. The perinatal outcome may or may not be favorable and fetal death often occurs. The volume of retroplacental clot may vary from 150–500 mL.
- *Grade 3 (Severe):* This type of placental abruption is associated with moderate to severe amount of revealed bleeding or concealed (hidden) bleeding. In this condition, more than half of the placenta separates and the volume of retroplacental clot is often more than 500 mL. Retroplacental clot volume more than 2.5 L is usually sufficient to cause fetal death. Tonic uterine contractions (called tetany), abdominal pain and marked uterine tenderness may be present. The abdominal pain is very severe. On examination, the uterus is tender and rigid; it may be impossible to feel the fetus. Maternal shock is pronounced and the BP may become extremely low. Fetal death commonly occurs. Complications related to severe disease like coagulation failure or anuria may be present.

**Q. What are the different types of placental abruption?**

**Ans.** Based on the type of clinical presentation, there can be three types of placental abruption:

- *Concealed type:* In this type of placental abruption, no actual bleeding is visible. The blood collects between the fetal membranes and decidua in the form of the retroplacental clot. Though this type of placental abruption is usually rarer than the revealed type, it carries a higher risk of maternal and fetal hazards because of the possibility of consumptive coagulopathy, which can result in the development of DIC.
- *Revealed type:* In this type of placental abruption, following the placental separation, the blood does not

**Table 5.36:** Clinical classification of placental abruption

| Parameter | Grade 0 | Grade 1 | Grade 2 | Grade 3 |
|---|---|---|---|---|
| External bleeding | Absent | Slight | Mild to moderate | Moderate to severe |
| Uterine tenderness | Absent | Uterus irritable, uterine tenderness may or may not be present | Uterine tenderness is usually present | Tonic uterine contractions and marked uterine tenderness |
| Abdominal pain | Absent | Abdominal pain may or may not be present | Abdominal pain is usually present | Severe degree of abdominal pain may be present |
| FHS | Present, good | Present, good | Fetal distress | Fetal death |
| Maternal shock | Absent | Absent | Generally absent | Present |
| Perinatal outcome | Good | Good | May be poor | Extremely poor |
| Complications | Absent | Rare | May be present | Complications like DIC and oliguria are commonly present |
| Volume of retroplacental clot | – | Less than 200 mL | 150–500 mL | More than 500 mL |

*Abbreviations:* FHS, fetal heart sound; DIC, disseminated intravascular coagulation

collect between the fetal membranes and decidua but moves out of the cervical canal and is visible externally. This type of placental abruption is more common than the concealed variety.

- *Mixed type:* This is the most common type of placental abruption and is associated with both revealed and concealed hemorrhage.

### Q. What is the role of ultrasound examination in cases of placenta previa?

**Ans.** The diagnosis of placental abruption is usually made on the basis of history and clinical examination. Ultrasound examination must be performed in order to confirm the diagnosis. Ultrasonography examination helps in showing the details described next:

- Ultrasound examination may help in showing the location of the placenta and thus would help in establishing or ruling out the diagnosis of placenta previa.
- Ultrasound examination also helps in visualization of retroplacental clot, which may appear as a sonolucent area, thereby confirming the diagnosis of placental abruption. Blood or collection of blood and clots may be identified on ultrasound examination. There may be presence of "Jello sign". This implies that there may be jiggling of the intrauterine clots when bounced by the transducer.
- Ultrasound also helps in checking the fetal viability and presentation.
  - Ultrasound examination is especially important in cases of placental abruption as it may become extremely difficult to palpate the fetal parts due to uterine hypertonicity. Also, it is important to record the fetal heart rate as the fetus is quite likely to be at jeopardy in the severe cases of placental abruption.
- Negative findings with ultrasound examination do not exclude placental abruption. There may be no retroplacental collection in revealed type of placental abruption.

### Q. What steps can be taken for preventing the development of placental abruption?

**Ans.** Once placental detachment has occurred, there is no treatment to replace the placenta back to its original position. However, some of the following steps can be taken to help reduce its occurrence:

- Early detection and treatment of preeclampsia
- Avoidance of smoking, drinking alcohol or using illicit drugs during pregnancy
- Avoidance of trauma
- Avoidance of sudden uterine decompression.

### Q. What should be the treatment plan in a patient with abruptio placenta?

**Ans.** The management plan in cases with abruptio placenta depends on grade of placental abruption (extent and severity of the disease process) and fetal maturity. Other factors which need to be considered before deciding the specific treatment for placental abruption include maternal condition, amount of maternal bleeding and fetal condition.

*Mild placental abruption:* In cases with mild abruption, where fetal maturity has yet not been attained, expectant management can be undertaken until the fetus attains maturity. If at any time severe bleeding occurs; fetal distress appears or maternal condition worsens, an emergency cesarean delivery may be required.

*Moderate placental abruption:* A moderate case of placental abruption requires hospitalization and constant fetal monitoring. The expectant management can be continued if the mother and fetus remain stable.

In case the maternal condition deteriorates or fetal distress develops, an emergency cesarean delivery may be required. If the uterus remains soft, the pregnancy must be terminated by induction of labor by ARM and oxytocin infusion. If during labor, the FHR becomes nonreassuring or if the uterus becomes hypertonic, an emergency CS is usually required.

*Severe placental abruption:* If the woman presents with severe placental abruption, the following steps need to be urgently undertaken:

- The patient requires an urgent admission to the hospital.
- Insertion of a central venous pressure line, IV line and a urinary catheter.
- Blood needs to be sent for ABO and Rh typing, cross-matching and CBC. At least four units of blood need to be arranged.
- Blood transfusion must be started if signs of shock are present. Once the patient has stabilized the following investigations need to be sent—clotting time, fibrinogen levels, prothrombin time, activated partial thromboplastin time (APTT) and platelet count.
- Analgesia can be administered.
- Intravenous fluids and blood should be administered in such a way as to maintain hematocrit at 30% and a urine output of at least 30 mL/hour.
- Inspection of vaginal pads and monitoring of vitals (pulse, BP, etc.) at every 15–30 minutes intervals depending upon the severity of bleeding.
- Blood coagulation profile (fibrinogen, FDP, APTT, prothrombin time, platelet count, etc.) needs to be done at every 2 hours intervals.
- The placental position must be localized using an ultrasound scan. After the patient has stabilized, the cervix must also be inspected with the help of a speculum in order to rule out the local causes of bleeding.
- The FHS must be monitored continuously with external cardiotocography.
- Intramuscular corticosteroids need to be administered to the mother in case of fetal prematurity.

- As the chances of the baby being distressed at birth are high, pediatrician and neonatologist need to be informed for resuscitation of the baby, immediately after the delivery.
- Definitive treatment in these cases is the delivery of the baby. In case of severe abruption, delivery should be performed by the fastest possible route. Cesarean delivery needs to be performed for most cases with severe placental abruption. If the baby is alive, a CS is often the best mode of delivery especially when the cervical os is closed. In conditions where the baby has already died in the womb, urgent delivery is still warranted keeping in view the development of possible maternal complications particularly DIC. In cases of IUD, delivery by vaginal route appears to be the best option. In patients with fetal death and unripe cervix, misoprostol 400 µg intravaginally or high-dose oxytocin (50–100 mIU/minute) may be required in order to accelerate vaginal delivery.

### Q. What are the indications for emergency cesarean delivery in cases of placental abruption?

**Ans.** Indications for emergency CS in cases of placental abruption are as follows:
- Appearance of fetal distress
- Bleeding continues to occur despite of ARM and oxytocin infusion
- Labor does not seem to progress well, despite ARM and oxytocin infusion
- Deterioration of maternal or fetal condition
- Presence of fetal malpresentation
- Associated obstetric factors
- Appearance of a complication (DIC, oliguria, etc.).

### Q. What are the various complications of placental abruption?

**Ans.** Various maternal and fetal complications of placental abruption are as follows:

#### Maternal Complications

*Maternal shock due to severe bleeding:* Placental abruption is a serious complication of pregnancy that requires immediate medical attention. Placental abruption can cause life-threatening hemorrhage for both mother and baby.

*Maternal death:* Severe bleeding, shock and DIC associated with placental abruption can sometimes result in maternal death.

*Renal failure:* Severe shock resulting from grade 3 placental abruption and/or DIC can be responsible for development of renal failure.

*Couvelaire uterus or uteroplacental apoplexy:* This condition has been found to be associated with severe forms of concealed placental abruption and is characterized by massive intravasation of blood into the uterine musculature up to the level of serosa. The blood gets infiltrated between the bundles of muscle fibers. As a result, the uterus becomes port wine in color. This is likely to interfere with uterine contractions and may predispose to the development of severe PPH. However, couvelaire uterus per se is not an indication for cesarean hysterectomy.

*Risk of recurrence of abruption in future pregnancies:* Recurrence risk of placental abruption varies from 8% to 15%.

*Postpartum uterine atony and postpartum hemorrhage*

*Disseminated intravascular coagulation:* Disseminated intravascular coagulation is a syndrome associated with both thrombosis and hemorrhage. Most common sign of DIC is bleeding. It can be manifested in the form of ecchymosis, petechiae and purpura. There can be oozing or frank bleeding from multiple sites. Extremities may become cool and mottled. Pleural and pericardial involvement may be responsible for producing dyspnea and chest pain respectively. Hematuria is commonly produced. Bleeding and renal failure are the most important manifestations in cases with DIC.

#### Fetal Complications

*Fetal distress:* Placental abruption can deprive the baby of oxygen and nutrients and cause heavy bleeding in the mother. If left untreated, placental abruption puts both mother and baby in jeopardy. Decreased oxygen to the fetal brain leads to later development of neurological or behavioral problems. In severe cases, stillbirth is possible.

*Premature delivery:* Peak incidence of abruption occurs between 24 and 26 weeks of gestation and is associated with nearly 10% cases of preterm birth. The preterm babies have been found to be at an increased risk of perinatal asphyxia, intraventricular hemorrhage, periventricular leukomalacia, and cerebral palsy.

*Stillbirth and fetal death:* Placental abruption is an important cause of fetal distress, asphyxia and ultimately IUD. Premature delivery in cases with placental abruption is an important cause of fetal morbidity.

# Intrauterine Death

## Case Study 1

Mrs XYZ, a 35-year-old married for 10 years, resident of ABC, G3P2A0L2 patient presented to the accident and emergency department (A&E) with the history of massive fall over her abdomen a few hours back. She has been experiencing pain in the abdomen and has not felt any fetal movements since that time. There is a history of slight vaginal bleeding.

Period of gestation according to her LMP was calculated to be 33 weeks. Her antenatal period had been otherwise normal and the clinical findings during her previous antenatal visits were within the normal limits.

### Q. What is the most likely diagnosis in the above-mentioned case study?

**Ans.** Mrs XYZ, a 35-year-old G3P2A0L2 patient with 33 weeks amenorrhea, corresponding to 33 weeks of gestation, married for 10 years, resident of ABC, with a single fetus in cephalic presentation, with absent fetal heart sounds. A probable diagnosis of abruptio placentae and IUD due to abdominal trauma was made because the fetal heart sound could not be heard even with the hand-held Doppler. The definitive diagnosis, however, needs to be confirmed by an ultrasound examination to locate the absent fetal heart movements and establish the diagnoses of placental abruption. The questions to be asked at the time of taking history and the parameters to be assessed at the time of examination in such a case are described in Tables 5.37 and 5.38 respectively.

### Q. How would you define IUD and what are the likely causes for IUD?

**Ans.** Intrauterine fetal death can be defined as "death prior to the complete expulsion or extraction of the products of human conception from the mother, regardless of the duration of pregnancy". This definition also does not include an induced termination of pregnancy. Fetal deaths may be divided into two: (1) antepartum IUD (fetal deaths occurring in the antenatal period) and (2) intrapartum IUD (fetal deaths occurring during labor).

For statistical purposes, intrauterine fetal demise can be defined as the diagnosis of the stillborn infant (with the period of gestation being > 20 weeks and fetal weight > 350 g).

A death that occurs prior to 20 weeks of gestation is classified as a spontaneous abortion. The likely causes of IUD are listed in Table 5.39.

### Q. What steps can be taken for prevention of intrauterine deaths?

**Ans.** Intrauterine death can be prevented by observing the following precautions:
- Regular antenatal care
- Screening out the high-risk patients to carefully monitor the fetal wellbeing and to terminate the pregnancy at the earliest evidences of fetal compromise. Regular antepartum surveillance is required in these cases in order to prevent fetal death.

### Q. What are the various investigations required to confirm the diagnosis of intrauterine death?

**Ans.** Some of the commonly performed tests for confirming the diagnosis of IUDs are as follows:
- *Absent fetal heart:* Inability to detect a fetal heartbeat via Doppler.
- *Sonography:* Definitive diagnosis of IUD is made by observing the lack of fetal cardiac motion during a 10-minute period of careful examination with real-time ultrasound. Late signs of IUD are oligohydramnios and collapse of cranial bones.
- *X-ray abdomen:* Abdominal X-ray may show presence of Spalding sign (irregular overlapping of the cranial bones), which usually occurs approximately within 7 days after death; hyperflexion of the spine; and crowding of ribs and appearance of gas shadows in the heart and great vessels (Robert's sign), which usually appears by 12 hours after birth. Spalding sign can be also observed on ultrasound examination.

---

**Table 5.37:** Symptoms to be elicited at the time of taking history in a case of intrauterine death

*History of Presenting Complains*
- Absence of interpretation of the fetal movements by the mother for more than a few hours
- Retrogression of the positive pregnancy changes (disappearance of breast changes, fundal height becomes smaller than the period of amenorrhea, reduction of uterine tone and the uterus becomes flaccid).
- No perception of fetal movements by the patient.

*Obstetric History*
- History of hypertensive disorders, fetal chromosomal anomalies, antepartum hemorrhage (placenta previa, abruptio placentae, etc.), Rh incompatibility, severe anemia, hyperpyrexia, maternal/fetal infection, antiphospholipid syndrome, etc. in the present pregnancy need to be elicited because these are likely to act as the possible risk factors for IUD.
- History of any iatrogenic uterine manipulation, e.g. external version.

*Medical History*
- *Pre-existing medical diseases:* The clinician must take the history of pre-existing medical diseases such as chronic hypertension, chronic nephritis, diabetes, severe anemia, hyperpyrexia, syphilis, hepatitis, toxoplasmosis, etc. in the mother because these pre-existing medical diseases can act as the underlying risk factors for IUD.
- *History of fever with rash:* Fever in association with a rash can be encountered in TORCH group of infections, viral fever, malaria, drug reaction, and allergy to any food or medications. The characteristics of the rash, whether maculopapular or vesicular; transient or permanent and painful or not needs to be enquired. Rash associated with rubella is maculopapular in appearance whereas rash associated with herpes is small vesicular with an erythematous base and painful.

*Abbreviations:* IUD, intrauterine death; TORCH, Toxoplasmosis, Other infections, Rubella, Cytomegalovirus, Herpes simplex virus

**Q. What tests must be performed in cases of IUD for diagnosing the underlying etiology?**

**Ans.** Various tests which need to be performed in cases of IUD for identifying the underlying etiology are as follows:

- Fetal autopsy
- Placental evaluation
- Fetal karyotype
- Indirect Coombs' test
- Serologic test for syphilis
- Testing for fetal-maternal hemorrhage (Kleihauer-Betke test)
- Parvovirus serology

| **Table 5.38:** Various findings elicited at the time of clinical examination in a case of intrauterine death |
|---|
| *General Physical Examination* |
| No specific finding is observed on GPE except that there may be retrogression of the positive breast changes (normally seen during pregnancy). |
| *Specific Systemic Examination* |
| *Abdominal Examination*<br>• Gradual retrogression of the height of the uterus<br>• Uterine tone is diminished<br>• Fetal movements are not felt during palpation<br>• Fetal heart sounds are not audible<br>• Fetal head shows egg-shell cracking feeling upon palpation (late sign). |

*Abbreviation:* GPE, general physical examination

- Lupus anticoagulant, anticardiolipin anticoagulant, for antiphospholipid testing
- Anti-$\beta_2$-glycoprotein 1 IgG or IgM antibodies
- Diabetes testing using hemoglobin A1c and a fasting blood glucose
- Syphilis screening using the VDRL or rapid plasma reagin test
- Thyroid function testing (i.e. TSH, FT4)
- Urine toxicology screening
- Factor V Leiden
- Prothrombin mutation
- TORCH titers
- Protein C, protein S, and antithrombin III deficiency (useful in some circumstances)
- Coagulation profile: Clotting profile, including tests, such as blood fibrinogen levels and partial thromboplastin time, may especially be required, if the fetus has been retained for more than 2 weeks.

**Q. If the patient gives history of fever with rashes, what extra investigations need to be performed in this case?**

**Ans.** The extra tests which must be performed in these cases include assessment for TORCH and HIV infections, and CBC with peripheral smear.

**Q. What are the steps of management in cases of intrauterine death?**

**Ans.** Management in these cases comprises of the following steps:

- Reassurance to be provided to the bereaving parents.

| **Table 5.39:** Causes of intrauterine death | |
|---|---|
| *Maternal causes* | *Fetal causes* |
| • Older mother, multiparity<br>• Hypertensive disorders<br>• Chromosomal anomalies<br>• Antepartum hemorrhage: Placenta previa, abruptio placentae, etc.<br>• Pre-existing medical disease such as chronic hypertension, chronic nephritis, diabetes, severe anemia, hyperpyrexia, syphilis, hepatitis, toxoplasmosis, hyperthyroidism, etc.<br>• Thrombophilias: Factor V Leiden mutation, protein C, protein S deficiency, hyperhomocysteinemia<br>• Rh incompatibility<br>• Severe anemia<br>• Hyperpyrexia<br>• Abnormal labor (prolonged or obstructed labor, ruptured uterus)<br>• Post-term pregnancy<br>• External version<br>• Maternal infection [TORCH infections, viral infections, malaria, ascending genital infections ( especially, bacterial and viral)]<br>• Antiphospholipid syndrome<br>• Systemic lupus erythematosus | • Chromosomal anomalies<br>• Fetal infections<br>• Rh incompatibility |
| *Iatrogenic causes* | *Placental causes* |
| • External cephalic version, drugs (e.g. quinine in toxic doses) | • Placental causes: Placental insufficiency, antepartum hemorrhage, cord accidents, twin-to-twin transfusion syndrome, etc. |

*Abbreviation:* TORCH, Toxoplasmosis, Other infections, Rubella, Cytomegalovirus, Herpes simplex virus

- Diagnosis and treatment of abnormality, if possible. In most of the cases, spontaneous expulsion occurs within 2 weeks of birth. In cases where spontaneous expulsion does not occur, induction by oxytocin infusion or prostaglandins (PGE2 gel or 25–50 µg of misoprostol) may be required.
- Fibrinogen levels to be estimated on a weekly basis. Falling fibrinogen levels to be arrested by controlled infusion of heparin.
- *Postmortem examination:* Examination of the dead baby and placenta (placental cultures for suspected infection) needs to be done in order to detect the cause of death. Autopsy and chromosomal analysis for detection of fetal anomalies and dysmorphic features needs to be done.

### Q. What should be the mode of delivery of the dead fetus?

**Ans.** Once the fetal death has been diagnosed, the options of expectant or active management must be discussed with the patient. These are as follows:

### Expectant Management

The following need to be done in case expectant management is planned:

- The clinician must await spontaneous onset of labor during the coming 4 weeks.
- The woman must be assured that in 90% of cases the fetus would be expelled spontaneously during the waiting period with no complications.
- If platelet levels are found to be decreasing on serial examinations or 4 weeks have passed without onset of spontaneous labor or fibrinogen levels are found to be low or the woman requests active management, the clinician must consider induction of labor.

### Induction of Labor

- In case induction of labor is planned, cervix must be firstly assessed.
- If the cervix is favorable, labor can be induced with oxytocin. If cervix is unfavorable, it must be ripened using vaginal prostaglandin E2 or synthetic prostaglandin E1 analog (misoprostol).
- In women with fetal death before 28 weeks of gestation, cervical ripening may be attained using prostaglandin E2 vaginal suppositories (10–20 mg q4–6h), or misoprostol vaginally or orally (400 µg q4–6h). In women with fetal death after 28 weeks of gestation, lower doses should be used. Infusion of oxytocin may be required if the woman is not experiencing uterine contractions of sufficient intensity. Misoprostol must preferably not be used in a woman with previous uterine scar due to the risk of uterine rupture.
- The membranes must be preferably not ruptured.

### Q. What are the various complications associated with IUD?

**Ans.** Various complications associated with IUD are as follows:

- Psychological upset.
- Infection (typically with anaerobic infections such as *Clostridium welchii*) resulting in septic shock.
- Blood coagulation disorder (disseminated intravascular coagulation).
- Renal shutdown.
- Amniotic fluid embolism.
- *During labor*: Uterine inertia, retained placenta and PPH.

### Q. What is the next step of immediate management in the previously-described case study?

**Ans.** The patient was immediately admitted in the emergency ward. On GPE, her vitals were stable. An IV line was secured and blood samples were collected for blood grouping and crossmatching, and a coagulation profile.

On per abdominal examination, fundal height corresponded to 34 weeks of gestation and there was extreme abdominal tenderness. Fetal heart sounds were not heard on fetal Doppler examination. On vaginal examination, slight vaginal bleeding was present, the cervical os was dilated by 2–3 cm and was about 50% effaced and fetal membranes were present. An ultrasound examination was performed immediately. Fetal heart rate was found to be absent. The placenta was fundal, but a retroplacental clot was detected.

### Q. What mode of delivery should be chosen in this patient?

**Ans.** Since the cervix was favorable, vaginal mode of delivery was chosen. An ARM was performed. In the absence of good uterine contractions, an oxytocin infusion was started.

### Q. What are the warning signs of fetal demise?

**Ans.** Some warning signs of fetal demise are as follows:

- Fetal tachycardia or fetal bradycardia.
- Fetal hypoactivity and hyperactivity.
- Poor or nonreactive NST.
- Biophysical score below 4.
- Reduced liquor.

## Preterm Labor, PROM

### Case Study 1

Mrs XYZ, a 28-year-old married for 6 years, resident of ABC, G2P1A0L1 unbooked patient presented at 32 weeks of gestation with complaints of experiencing abdominal cramps at every 5 minute intervals since the morning (last 2–3 hours). Initially, the pain was coming at the intervals of 15–20 minutes. However, it progressively increased in intensity and frequency since morning. There is no history of leakage of any fluid or passage of any kind of vaginal discharge or bleeding. Previous baby was born at 34 weeks of gestation. He is presently healthy and 3 years old.

**Q. What is the most likely diagnosis in the above-mentioned case study?**

**Ans.** Mrs XYZ, a 28-year-old married for 6 years, resident of ABC, G2P1A0L1 unbooked patient with 32 weeks of amenorrhea corresponding to 32 weeks of gestation with a single live fetus in cephalic presentation with the most likely diagnosis of preterm labor as suggested by history and clinical examination. The questions to be asked at the time of taking history and the parameters to be assessed at the time of examination in such a case are described in Tables 5.40 and 5.41 respectively.

**Table 5.40:** Symptoms to be elicited at the time of taking history in a case of preterm labor

*History of Presenting Complains*
- The patient may give history of experiencing symptoms such as menstrual cramps, pelvic pressure, backache and/or vaginal discharge or bleeding.
- Increase in the amount of vaginal discharge: There may be copious amount of vaginal discharge, which may be watery, bloody or mucoid in nature.
- There may be pelvic or lower abdominal pressure.
- There may be constant low backache or mild abdominal cramps with or without diarrhea.
- Uterine tightening or contractions (often painless)
- Patient may give a history of breaking her membranes, followed by a sudden gush of watery fluid (in cases of PROM)
- Rupture of membranes may be associated with the history suggestive of chorioamnionitis. These may include fever (temperature greater than 100.4°F or 37.8°C); tachycardia [greater than 120 beats per minute (bpm)], foul smelling vaginal discharge, uterine tenderness and maternal leukocytosis (total leukocyte blood count > 15,000–18,000 cells/mL.
- *Extremes of maternal age:* Maternal age less than 18 years or greater than 35 years can be considered as a risk factor for preterm labor.
- *Race and ethnicity:* Black women are twice at risk in comparison to the white women.

*Obstetric History*
- *Previous history of preterm births:* Previous history of preterm births or second trimester pregnancy loss may be associated with 17–20% risk of recurrence. Previous history of three or more miscarriages may be associated with presence of cervical incompetence. Of the various risk factors for preterm birth, past obstetric history of preterm birth may act as one of the strongest predictors for recurrent preterm birth.
- *Previous history of multiple births:* An increased incidence of multiple births is associated with an increasing risk of preterm labor.
- *Preterm premature rupture of membranes:* Nearly 30% of preterm births could be due to PPROM. It usually results from intra-amniotic infections.
- *Preeclampsia:* History of preeclampsia in the previous pregnancy serves as an important risk factor.
- Antepartum hemorrhage (especially that associated with abruption placenta resulting in hemorrhage at decidual-chorionic interface) also serves as a risk factor.
- Second trimester bleeding not associated with placental causes is also another risk factor.
- *Iatrogenic causes for inducing preterm labor:* Iatrogenic causes where labor is induced or infant is delivered by a prelabor cesarean section can include preeclampsia, fetal distress, intrauterine growth restriction, abruption, intrauterine death, etc.
- Previous history of fetal complications such as congenital malformations and intrauterine death.
- Previous history of placental complications such as infarction, thrombosis, placenta previa or abruption.
- *Recurrent midtrimester loss:* Midtrimester pregnancy losses may be associated with many causes such as infection (e.g. syphilis), antiphospholipid syndrome, diabetes, substance abuse, genetic disorders, congenital Müllerian abnormalities, cervical trauma, and cervical incompetence.

*Past Medical History*
- Past history of medical and surgical illnesses such as chronic hypertension, acute pyelonephritis, diabetes, renal diseases, acute appendicitis, etc.
- *Stressful life event:* Stressful life events such as anxiety, depression and negative life events could be responsible for triggering preterm labor. Maternal or fetal stress can precipitate preterm labor by increasing the secretion of corticotropin-releasing hormone.
- Drug abuse, smoking, alcohol consumption.

*Gynecological History*
- *Vaginal infection:* History of any vaginal discharge or symptoms suggestive of vaginal infection, e.g. asymptomatic bacterial vaginosis (BV), *Trichomonas vaginalis*, infection by *Chlamydia trachomatis, Ureaplasma urealyticum, Mycoplasma hominis,* etc. Infections such as asymptomatic bacteriuria, pyelonephritis, pneumonia, acute appendicitis, etc. may also be responsible for producing intra-amniotic inflammatory response, which may trigger uterine contractions.
- *Cervical trauma:* Cervical trauma and injury resulting in cervical incompetence may act as another risk factor for preterm labor. The most common causes for cervical injury may include procedures for elective abortion, surgeries to treat cervical dysplasia, and cervical injury occurring at the time of normal delivery. Patients with a history of multiple first-trimester elective terminations or one or more second-trimester elective abortions may be at an increased risk for preterm delivery. Cervical dilatation with laminaria tents or cervical ripening agents, such as misoprostol, appears to be less traumatizing to the cervix than mechanical dilation. Surgeries for treating cervical dysplasia, e.g. cold knife cone, cryoconization, laser cone, loop electrical excision procedure (LEEP), etc. may increase the risk of subsequent preterm deliveries. Since obstetric trauma is an important risk factor for mid-trimester loss or preterm birth, the cervix must be visually inspected to assess the degree of injury and risk.
- Pregnancy with an intrauterine contraceptive device in situ.

*Abbreviations:* PROM, premature rupture of membranes; PPROM, preterm premature rupture of membranes

| **Table 5.41:** Various findings elicited at the time of clinical examination in a case of preterm labor |
| --- |
| *General Physical Examination* |
| • *Body mass index:* Women with low body mass index and poor maternal weight gain during pregnancy are at an increased risk. |
| *Specific Systemic Examination* |
| *Abdominal Examination* <br> • Uterine contractions of greater than or equal to 4 per 20 minutes or greater than or equal to 8 per hour, lasting for more than 40 seconds |
| *Per Speculum Examination* <br> • Collection of vaginal swabs <br> • Collection of escaping liquor for confirmation of PROM |
| *Vaginal Examination* <br> • Cervical dilatation of greater than or equal to 1 cm and effacement of 80% or more <br> • Cervical length on TVS less than or equal to 2.5 cm and funneling of internal os <br> • Bishop's score may be 4 or greater. <br> • Lower uterine segment may be thinned out and the presenting part may be deep in the pelvis. |

*Abbreviations:* PROM, premature rupture of membranes; TVS, transvaginal sonography

## Q. What is the next step of management in the above-mentioned case study?

**Ans.** The patient's history in this case was suggestive of preterm labor. Firstly a general physical and abdominal examination was performed. This was followed by per speculum and vaginal examination. Before performing the cervical examination, vaginal fluid sample was collected to be sent for fetal fibronectin (fFN) estimation, if required. On cervical examination, the cervix was 3–4 cm dilated and 80% effaced. Since the cervical examination findings confirmed the diagnosis of preterm labor, the vaginal fluid sample previously collected for fFN estimation was discarded.

## Q. What is preterm labor?

**Ans.** Preterm labor can be defined as onset of labor prior to the completion of 37 weeks of gestation, once the period of viability (20 weeks) has been attained. The mortality rates amongst these infants are high and the surviving infants may have a high rate of complications such as bronchopulmonary dysplasia, necrotizing enterocolitis, intraventricular hemorrhage (IVH), and sepsis. Diagnosis of preterm labor is established in case of presence of uterine contractions of at least 4 in 20 minutes or 8 in 60 minutes along with cervical changes showing effacement of 80% or more and cervical dilatation of more than 1 cm. Babies born before 37 weeks of pregnancy are called premature babies. Premature delivery may be preceded either by contractions or PROM. Based on the findings of clinical examination, preterm labor can be of two types:

*Early preterm labor:* In cases of early preterm labor, cervical effacement is greater than or equal to 80% and cervical dilatation is greater than or equal to 1 cm, but less than 3 cm.

*Advanced preterm labor:* In cases of advanced preterm labor, cervical dilatation is greater than or equal to 3 cm.

## Q. What investigations must be done in these cases?

**Ans.** The following investigations must be done in cases of preterm labor:

- *Clinical examination:* Diagnosis of preterm labor is usually made at the time of clinical examination. Uterine contractions of sufficient frequency and intensity causing progressive effacement and dilation of the cervix prior to 37 weeks of gestation are indicative of active preterm labor. Following the suspicion of preterm labor on clinical examination, the diagnosis of preterm labor can be predicted with the help of following tests:
  - Fetal fibronectin (fFN) levels
  - Ultrasound measurement of cervical length.

Investigations which must be done to identify the probable cause of preterm labor are as follows:

- *Assessment of lower genital tract infection:* Presence of the lower genital infection could serve as the probable underlying cause for preterm labor. Patients with preterm labor may be assessed for the presence or absence of lower genital tract infection. The presence of asymptomatic bacteriuria, sexually transmitted disease, and symptomatic bacterial vaginosis (BV) may be investigated with the help of tests such as endocervical sampling for gonorrhea and chlamydia, vaginal fluid pH, wet smear for BV and trichomonal infection, *Group B Streptococcus* (GBS) culture, urinalysis and culture, etc. Positive results are treated with appropriate antibiotics.
- *Investigations for midtrimester loss:* Laboratory tests, which may be required in cases of midtrimester loss, include the following:
  - Rapid plasma reagent test
  - Gonorrheal and chlamydial screening
  - Vaginal pH/wet smear/whiff test
  - Anticardiolipin antibody, lupus anticoagulant antibody
  - Activated partial thromboplastin time
  - One-hour glucose challenge test
  - Screening for TORCH infections
  - *Tests for cervical incompetence:* A preconceptual hysterosalpingogram may be of benefit in patients with a history of two or more midtrimester losses. One can also attempt to pass a No. 8 Hegar's dilator into the nonpregnant cervix; easy passage may be a sign of cervical incompetence. Baseline transvaginal ultrasonography scan must be performed to assess cervical length, especially at 13–17 weeks' gestation; abnormal findings include a length less than 2.5 cm, funneling greater than 5 mm, or dynamic changes.

**Q. How is the measurement of cervical length done with the help of ultrasound examination?**

**Ans.** Transvaginal screening of cervical length with an empty bladder during mid-gestation (19–24 weeks) is the gold standard test for predicting preterm labor, which must be offered to all pregnant women. Cervical length of less than 2.5 cm and/or cervical score [cervical length (cm) – cervical dilation (cm) at the internal os] of less than 0 in the second trimester is associated with high chances of having preterm birth at less than 35 weeks of gestation.

**Q. What is the significance of measuring fetal fibronectin levels?**

**Ans.** Fibronectin is a glycoprotein, secreted by the chorionic tissue at the maternal-fetal interface, which acts as biological glue, and helps in binding blastocyst to endometrium. It is normally present in the cervicovaginal secretions up to 20–22 weeks of gestation. From around 22 weeks, the chorion fuses completely with the underlying decidua. Therefore, this prevents the leakage of fibronectin into the vaginal secretions until at the time of labor when the membranes rupture or the cervix dilates. Therefore, presence of fibronectin in the vaginal secretions between 27 weeks and 34 weeks serves as an important marker of preterm labor. A cut-off value of 50 ng/mL is considered positive. Presence of fibronectin is associated with sensitivity of 89% and specificity of 86%. On the other hand, absence of fibronectin from the cervicovaginal secretions is associated with a low risk for preterm delivery.

**Q. How should the patient be managed, once the diagnosis of preterm labor is confirmed?**

**Ans.** The patient must be immediately admitted to the hospital and administered analgesic drugs. Corticosteroids must be administered in the dosage of 12 mg betamethasone, to be given 24 hours apart through intramuscular route. Nifedipine can also be started in the dosage of 20 mg orally. A repeat dose of nifedipine must be administered by intramuscular route after 1.5–2 hours. Thereafter, nifedipine can be administered in the dosage of 20 mg TDS orally for 3 days. High vaginal swab must be taken to rule out *Group B streptococcal* infection and continuous fetal cardiotographic monitoring is to be performed.

After a week of above-mentioned expectant management, the uterine contractions had stopped in this case. The fetus also appeared fine. NST was found to be reactive. Since the patient stayed very close to the hospital and was very compliant, she was discharged home after giving strict instructions of coming for biweekly check-ups in the OPD or to come to the hospital immediately in case she experiences any of the symptoms suggestive of preterm labor.

**Q. If the above case study had been accompanied by rupture of membranes, in what way would the management change?**

**Ans.** In case of accompanying PROM, the following course of management must be followed:

Fetal pulmonary maturity must be assessed. If the lungs have matured, the patient can be delivered.

If the fetal lungs have yet not attained maturity, the patient must be hospitalized (bed rest with bathroom privileges). IV antibiotics must be administered for 48–72 hours. During this time, the fetal heart rate and maternal condition (to rule out chorioamnionitis) must be monitored. Single course of corticosteroids must be at least administered prior to the birth of baby.

**Q. How would you decide the time for delivery in cases of preterm labor?**

**Ans.** For a majority of patients, prolonging pregnancy does not offer any benefit because in a majority of cases, preterm labor serves as a protective mechanism for fetuses threatened by problems such as infection or placental insufficiency. Preterm labor is often associated with PROM. The following considerations should be given regarding delivery in women with preterm labor:

*Period of Gestation less than 34 Weeks*

For pregnancies less than 34 weeks of gestation in women with no maternal or fetal indication for delivery, expectant management comprising of the following may be used:

- Close monitoring of uterine contractions.
- Fetal surveillance.
- Corticosteroids may be used for enhancing pulmonary maturity.
- *Magnesium sulfate:* Use of magnesium sulfate infusion for 12–24 hours, helps in providing neuroprotection.
- *Antibiotic therapy:* Prophylactic therapy for *Group B streptococcal* infection should be administered, especially in the cases where the membranes have also ruptured.
- *Progesterone therapy:* This can be used to reduce the occurrence of preterm birth.
- *Tocolytic therapy:* This may be required to delay delivery for up to 48 hours, thereby buying time to allow the maximum benefit of corticosteroids in order to reduce the incidence of respiratory distress syndrome.
- *Corticosteroid therapy:* The administration of glucocorticoids is recommended in patients with preterm labor, whenever the gestational age is between 24 weeks and 34 weeks.

*Period of Gestation 34 Weeks or More*

For pregnancies at 34 weeks or more, women with preterm labor must be monitored for labor progression and fetal wellbeing.

**Q. What should be the steps for intrapartum management in these cases?**

**Ans.** Intrapartum management in these cases comprises of the following steps:

- Delivery should preferably be undertaken in a tertiary care setting.

- *Fetal surveillance and monitoring:* Since the preterm babies are susceptible to the development of fetal hypoxia and acidosis, these fetuses must be carefully monitored for signs of hypoxia during labor, preferably by continuous electronic fetal monitoring.
- *Antibiotic prophylaxis:* This may be particularly useful in cases of *Group B streptococcal* infection.
- *Tocolysis:* Most commonly used tocolytic agents are indomethacin and nifedipine.
- Magnesium sulfate is administered for neuroprotection of the premature neonate in some countries.
- *Delivery:* This must be conducted in presence of an expert neonatologist capable of dealing with the complications of prematurity. Ventouse application is contraindicated in preterm deliveries. Cesarean delivery is indicated only in case of obstetrical indications.
- At the time of delivery, an episiotomy may be given to facilitate the delivery of fetal head. However, there is no need for routine administration of an episiotomy.

### Q. What is the role of tocolysis in such patients?

**Ans.** The goals of tocolytic therapy are as follows:

- Primary purpose of tocolytic therapy today is to delay delivery for 48 hours to allow the maximum benefit of glucocorticoids to decrease the incidence of respiratory distress syndrome.
- Delay in delivery to optimize the place, time, and type of delivery.
- Antibiotic administration in labor to reduce neonatal infection, specifically *Group B Streptococcus* infection.
- Administration of magnesium sulfate before the anticipated delivery for fetal neuroprotection.

### Q. What is the role of corticosteroid therapy in cases of preterm labor?

**Ans.** Corticosteroid therapy helps in reducing the incidence of complications such as respiratory distress syndrome, IVH and neonatal mortality. This therapy is recommended in the absence of clinical infection whenever the gestational age is between 24 and 34 weeks. An attempt should be made to delay delivery for a minimum of 12 hours to obtain the maximum benefits of antenatal steroids. The recommended dosage of corticosteroids includes the following:

- Two 12-mg doses of betamethasone 24 hours apart (to be administered intramuscularly).
- Four doses of 6 mg of dexamethasone should be administered at 6-hour intervals (to be administered intramuscularly).

### Q. What complications can occur in cases of preterm labor?

**Ans.** Maternal and fetal complications related to preterm labor are as follows:

*Maternal Complications*

- Premature rupture of membranes and/or preterm delivery
- Chorioamnionitis
- Placental abruption
- Retained placenta
- Postpartum hemorrhage
- Endometritis.

*Neonatal Complications*

- Prematurity
- Pneumonia and early neonatal sepsis
- Pulmonary hypoplasia
- Fetal death.

### Q. How can you define premature rupture of membranes (PROM)?

**Ans.** Premature rupture of membranes can be defined as spontaneous rupture of membranes, beyond 28 weeks of pregnancy, but before the onset of labor. ROM occurring beyond 37 weeks of gestation, but before the onset of labor is known as term PROM. On the other hand, ROM occurring before 37 completed weeks of gestation but before the onset of labor is called preterm premature rupture of membranes (PPROM). If the ROM is present for more than 24 hours before delivery, it is known as prolonged ROM. PROM is not actually a complication; rather a cause for preterm labor because this condition may be followed by a preterm delivery.

### Q. How should the cases with PROM be managed?

**Ans.** Management of PROM basically depends on gestational age and fetal status. Main aim of management in case of PROM is to avoid delivery prior to 34 weeks of gestation.

Expectant management may be considered if the period of gestation is less than 34 weeks or the pulmonary maturity has not been attained. It comprises of the following steps:

- Patient must be hospitalized for strict bed rest with bathroom privileges.
- She should be given a sterile vulval pad.
- Women should be observed for signs of clinical chorioamnionitis (fever, tachycardia, foul smelling vaginal discharge, etc.) at least every 12 hourly.
- A weekly high vaginal swab and at least a weekly maternal full blood count should be considered.
- Fetal monitoring using cardiotocography should be considered where regular fetal surveillance is required.
- Women with PPROM and uterine activity who require antenatal corticosteroids should be considered for tocolysis. The tocolytic agent of choice for women with PPROM is nifedipine. It is given in the initial dosage of 20–30 mg followed by 10–20 mg at every 6 hours interval.
- Digital cervical examination should be avoided in patients with PROM unless they are in active labor or unless imminent delivery is anticipated.

- Cesarean section is not routinely required, but may be required in the presence of an obstetric indication.
- A single course of antenatal corticosteroids should be given to women with PROM at 24–31 weeks of gestation to reduce the risk of perinatal mortality, respiratory distress syndrome, and other morbidities.

**Q. When is immediate delivery required in the cases of PROM?**

**Ans.** Women who need to be delivered irrespective of the period of gestation include the following:
- Those with acute chorioamnionitis/subclinical infection/inflammation or those at a high risk of infection.
- Patients with placental abruption, or evidence of fetal compromise.
- Those with mature lungs or with period of gestation greater than 36 weeks.
- Nonreassuring fetal heart sounds.
- Fetuses with lethal congenital anomalies.
- Women in advanced labor, with cervical effacement of 80% or more and cervical dilatation of 5 cm or more.

**Q. What are the various complications associated with PROM premature birth?**

*Maternal Complications*

These are as follows:
- *Infection:* Infection could be related to acute or chronic chorioamnionitis. There are high chances of ascending infection if ROM is present for greater than 24 hours.
- *Preterm labor:* PROM is an important cause for preterm labor. In about 80–90% of the cases, labor starts within 24 hours.
- *Cord prolapse:* Sudden gush of amniotic fluid may be associated with an increased incidence of cord prolapse and/or premature placental separation (placental abruption) and/or oligohydramnios.

*Fetal/Neonatal Complications*

These are as follows:
- *Respiratory distress syndrome/hyaline membrane disease:* The newborn infant may suffer from severe respiratory distress, thereby requiring ventilator support after birth. There also may be bronchopulmonary dysplasia.
- *Nonreassuring fetal heart rate pattern:* Most common abnormality is variable decelerations associated with umbilical cord compression as a result of oligohydramnios. Moderate or severe variable/late decelerations may be present as a result of placental insufficiency and are indicative of intrapartum fetal distress.
- *Pulmonary hypoplasia:* This condition may be characterized by the presence of multiple pneumothoraces and interstitial emphysema.

- *Cerebral palsy:* This may be the result of intraventricular bleeding, intrapartum fetal acidosis and hypoxia.
- *Fetal deformities:* These may especially include facial and skeletal deformities.
- *Fetal trauma:* This could be related to fetal macrosomia, which may be responsible for producing injury to the brachial plexus, fracture of humerus or clavicle, cephalic hematomas, skull fracture, etc.
- *Gastrointestinal complications:* Hyperbilirubinemia, necrotizing enterocolitis, failure to thrive, etc.
- *Central nervous system complications:* Intraventricular hemorrhage (IVH), hydrocephalus, cerebral palsy, neurodevelopmental delay and hearing loss.
- *Ophthalmological complications:* Retinopathy of prematurity, retinal detachment, etc.
- *Cardiovascular complications:* Hypotension, patent ductus arteriosus, pulmonary hypertension, etc.
- *Renal complications:* Water and electrolyte imbalance, acid-base disturbances, etc.
- *Hematological complications:* Iatrogenic anemia, requirement for frequent blood transfusions, anemia of prematurity, etc.
- *Endocrinological complications:* Hypoglycemia, transiently low thyroxine levels, cortisol deficiency and increased insulin resistance in adulthood.

**Q. What is chorioamnionitis and how is it diagnosed?**

**Ans.** Chorioamnionitis can be defined as inflammatory reaction of the fetal membranes, amnion and chorion due to ascending vaginal infection (bacterial and/or viral). Diagnosis of chorioamnionitis is made in case of temperature above 38.0°C (100.0°F) and presence of two out of the five following signs:
- White blood cell (WBC) count greater than 15,000 cells/mm$^3$
- Maternal tachycardia greater than 100 BPM.
- Fetal tachycardia greater than 160 BPM.
- Tender uterus.
- Foul smelling vaginal discharge.

**Q. Describe the physical appearance of a preterm baby.**

**Ans.** The preterm baby is usually deficient in subcutaneous fat. As a result, the baby's skin appears pink in color, feels very thin and can easily wrinkle. The preterm baby's head circumference may exceed the waist circumference. Birthweight of a normal term infant varies from 2,500 g to 3,999 g. Most preterm babies are of low weight. Low birthweight can be defined as weight less than 2,500 g. Length of a preterm baby may be less than 47 cm.

# Post-Term Pregnancy

## Case Study 1

Mrs XYZ, a 28-year-old married for 5 years, resident of ABC, primiparous patient presented to the obstetrics and gynecology clinic with the pregnancy, which was postdated by 2 weeks both according to dates and according to an ultrasound examination done during the first trimester. She has yet not started feeling any labor pain. She is, however, experiencing normal fetal movements.

### Q. What is the most likely diagnosis in the above-mentioned case study?

**Ans.** The most likely diagnosis in this case is Mrs XYZ, a 28-year-old married for 5 years, resident of ABC, primiparous woman with 42 weeks of amenorrhea corresponding to 42 weeks of gestation. The pregnancy was postdated by 2 weeks both according to dates and according to an ultrasound examination done during the first trimester. Though the fetus does not appear to be compromised on the basis of history, the fetal wellbeing needs to be confirmed by various tests. The questions to be asked at the time of taking history and the parameters to be assessed at the time of examination in such a case are described in Tables 5.42 and 5.43 respectively.

### Q. What is post-term pregnancy and what are the likely causes?

**Ans.** Post-term or postmature pregnancy can be defined as any pregnancy continuing beyond 2 weeks of the EDD (> 294 days). Postdated pregnancy, on the other hand, can be defined as pregnancy with period of gestation greater than 40 completed weeks (> 280 days).

Although the exact causes of post-term pregnancy remain unknown, some likely causative factors are as follows:

- *Wrong dates:* This can be considered as the most common cause of postmaturity. In these cases, use of ultrasonography helps in determining the accurate estimation of gestational age.
- *Maternal factors:* These include factors such as primiparity, previous history of prolonged pregnancy, sedentary habits and elderly multipara.
- *Fetal congenital anomalies:* Fetal congenital anomalies such as anencephaly and adrenal hypoplasia may be implicated in the causation of postmaturity.
- *Placental factors:* Placental factors such as sulfatase deficiency may be involved.

### Q. What investigations must be done in these cases?

**Ans.** The investigations which require to be done in these cases include those which aim at confirming fetal maturity and those which aim at confirming fetal wellbeing. The following investigations need to be done:

- *Confirming fetal maturity:* The most important test which helps to confirm fetal maturity is ultrasonography. Ultrasound parameters, such as crown-rump length (CRL), biparietal diameter (BPD) and femur length (FL), help in the assessment of gestational age. Ultrasound scans performed early in gestation are more helpful in the accurate assessment of gestational age. Amniotic fluid pocket of less than 2 cm and AFI less than or equal to 5 cm on ultrasound examination is an indication for induction of labor or delivery. Absent end-diastolic flow on umbilical artery Doppler is another indicator of fetal jeopardy.
- *Tests for fetal wellbeing:* These include tests, such as NST, BPP or modified BPP (NST plus amniotic fluid volume estimation), contraction stress testing (CST) and a combination of these modalities. However, none of these methods have been shown to be superior to the other. While presently there is no recommendation regarding the frequency of antenatal fetal surveillance,

---

**Table 5.42:** Symptoms to be elicited at the time of taking history in a case of post-term pregnancy

*History of Presenting Complains*

*Calculation of accurate gestational age:* The most important parameter which needs to be evaluated in a case of suspected postdated pregnancy is the calculation of gestational age. LMP tends to be reliable in calculation of period of gestation if the patient definitely remembers her LMP, she had been experiencing normal, regular menstrual cycles, there is no history of intake of oral contraceptives during the past 3 months and the pregnancy was planned.

In case of any discrepancy between the period of gestation calculated by applying Naegele's rule and that estimated using clinical examination in the first trimester, the following pointers can be used:

- *Time at which the mother can perceive quickening:* Maternal perception of fetal movements normally occurs at about 16–20 weeks.
- *Ultrasound examination:* Fetal heart sound can be heard by 11 weeks of gestation.

*Obstetric History*

- Previous history of prolonged pregnancy.
- Diagnosis of congenital anomalies (e.g. anencephaly, adrenal hypoplasia, etc.) in the present pregnancy.

*Abbreviation:* LMP, last menstrual period

---

**Table 5.43:** Various findings elicited at the time of clinical examination in a case of post-term pregnancy

*General Physical Examination*

*Maternal weight record:* Stationary or falling maternal weight

*Systemic Examination*

*Abdominal Examination*

- *Abdominal girth:* Gradually diminishing abdominal girth due to the gradually reducing liquor volume.
- *False labor pains:* Appearance of labor pain which quickly subside.
- *Abdominal palpation:* The uterus may feel "full of fetus" due to the diminishing volume of the liquor. Also, the fetus may be large in size.

*Vaginal Examination*

- *Internal vaginal examination:* Ripe cervix could be suggestive of fetal maturity. Hard skull bones may be felt through the cervix or vaginal fornix, thereby suggesting fetal maturity. Per vaginal examination also helps in assessing cervical inducibility by calculation of the Bishop's score.

most practitioners follow twice-weekly testing regime. According to ACOG (1997), antenatal surveillance should be initiated by 42 weeks of gestation.

### Q. What are the steps of management in these cases?

**Ans.** The obstetric management is based on two principles, the first being determination of accurate gestational age and second being increased fetal surveillance. Delivery is recommended when the risks to the fetus as a result of continuing the pregnancy are greater than those faced by the neonate after birth. High-risk pregnancies must be particularly not allowed to become post-term. In these cases delivery is preferred around 38–39 weeks of gestation. Management of low-risk patients is more controversial and is usually based on the results of antepartum fetal assessment and cervical favorability:

- If the patient is sure of dates and the cervix is favorable, and no benefit is likely to occur to either fetus or the mother from waiting, labor can be induced with intravenous oxytocin and ARM.
- If the patient is sure of dates, but cervix is unfavorable, and fetal jeopardy or fetal macrosomia is suspected, labor must be induced with intravaginal instillation of PGE2. Cesarean delivery may be required in cases of failed induction.
- If there is no fetal jeopardy or macrosomia, expectant management with fetal surveillance in the form of weekly NSTs and AFI must be done, while awaiting spontaneous onset of labor.
- Expectant management is appropriate between 40 weeks and 41 weeks of gestation. Delivery becomes mandatory when the period of gestation reaches 42 weeks, because the risk of antepartum stillbirths and maternal complications is significant enough.

### Q. What precautions must be observed at the time of labor and delivery in these patients?

**Ans.** The following precautions must be observed at the time of labor and delivery in these patients:

- Patient must be made to lie in the left lateral position.
- Continuous electronic fetal monitoring must be done in anticipation of intrapartum asphyxia.
- Initiating ARM in the early active phase helps in hastening progress and also helps in an early detection of meconium.
- *Amnioinfusion:* This is a procedure, involving the infusion of 500–1,000 mL of isotonic fluid through intrauterine catheter to dilute the meconium present in the uterine cavity in case of presence of meconium stained liquor. The infusion of fluid is thought to dilute meconium and reduce the risk of meconium aspiration.
- Pediatrician must be present at the time of delivery in view of macrosomia and meconium-stained liquor.
- When fetal macrosomia is suspected, ultrasound should be performed to estimate fetal weight. In case of vaginal delivery, clinician should always be prepared to deal with a potential shoulder dystocia. Most clinicians favor cesarean delivery for infants in whom expected fetal weight is more than 4.5 kg.

### Q. What are precautions, which must be taken at the time of delivery in case of meconium-stained liquor?

**Ans.** The precautions, which must be taken at the time of delivery in case of meconium-stained liquor, are as follows:

- Prior to delivery of the fetal head, amnioinfusions can be performed.
- Following the delivery of fetal head, meconium can be suctioned out from the nose and pharynx to prevent aspiration.
- After delivery of entire fetus, but before the first neonatal breath, neonatal tracheal meconium can be aspirated out using a laryngoscope.

### Q. What are the likely complications in cases of post-term pregnancy?

**Ans.** The following complications are likely to occur:

- *Fetal distress:* Diminished placental function and oligohydramnios due to PROM may result in fetal hypoxia and distress.
- *Macrosomia:* Macrosomia can be defined as a newborn with an excessive birth weight. This is associated with an increased incidence of shoulder dystocia and operative delivery.
- *Birth trauma:* There is an increased incidence of traumatic birth deliveries due to large size of the baby and nonmolding of fetal head due to hardening of skull bones.
- *Respiratory distress:* Respiratory distress can occur due to chemical pneumonitis, atelectasis and pulmonary hypertension. This may occur following meconium aspiration and eventually result in hypoxia and respiratory failure.
- *Neonatal problems:* After birth, many neonatal complications can arise, such as hypothermia, poor subcutaneous fat, hypoglycemia, hypocalcemia, and increased incidence of injuries such as brachial plexus injuries.
- *Increased perinatal mortality and morbidity:* These complications result in an overall increased rate of perinatal morbidity and mortality.

# Bad Obstetric History/Recurrent Pregnancy Loss

### Case Study 1

Mrs XYZ, a 32-year-old woman, married for 9 years, resident of ABC, G4P0A3L0 with previous history of three miscarriages (all in the first trimester) presented with 14 completed weeks of gestation for regular ANC check-up.

**Q. What is the most likely diagnosis in the above-mentioned case study?**

**Ans.** The most likely diagnosis in the above-mentioned case study is Mrs XYZ, a 32-year-old woman, married for 9 years, resident of ABC, G4P0A3L0 with previous history of three miscarriages (all in the first trimester) presenting with 14 weeks of amenorrhea corresponding to 14 weeks of gestation with the diagnosis of recurrent pregnancy loss likely to be due to an unidentified cause on the basis of history and clinical examination. The questions to be asked at the time of taking history and the parameters to be assessed at the time of examination in such a case are described in Tables 5.44 and 5.45 respectively.

**Q. What is recurrent pregnancy loss and bad obstetric history? What are the likely risk factors for it?**

**Ans.** RCOG, 2011 has defined recurrent miscarriage as the clinically recognized loss of three or more pregnancies with the same partner before 24 weeks of gestation. Bad obstetric history (BOH), on the other hand, can be defined as an obstetric condition where the woman's present obstetric history is likely to be adversely affected by the nature of previous obstetric disasters. Bad obstetric history could be related to recurrent miscarriage or a history of previous unfavorable fetal outcome in terms of two or more consecutive spontaneous abortions, early neonatal deaths, stillbirths, IUDs, congenital anomalies, etc.

Some important causes of BOH are as follows:

- Genetic causes (Robertsonian translocations).
- Abnormal maternal immune response.
- Hormonal causes (luteal phase defect, polycystic ovary syndrome, hypothyroidism, diabetes mellitus, hyperprolactinemia, etc.).
- Maternal infection (infections by TORCH complex, syphilis, bacterial vaginosis, etc.).
- Environmental factors (radiation exposure, occupational hazards, addictions, etc.).
- Autoimmune causes (antiphospholipid syndrome).
- Inherited thrombophilias (factor V Leiden mutation, deficiency of protein C and S, hyperhomocysteinemia).
- Structural anomalies of cervix (septate uterus, cervical incompetence).
- Anatomical causes (uterine malformations, Asherman's syndrome, uterine fibroids).

**Q. What investigations must be performed in these cases?**

**Ans.** The following investigations need to be done:

- *Parental karyotype:* All couples with a history of recurrent miscarriages should have peripheral blood karyotyping and cytogenetic analysis of the products of conception.
- *Thyroid function test:* Tests for thyroid function include tests for thyroid hormones (T3, T4 and TSH) and detection of antibodies (antithyroid antibodies). Measurement of TSH levels in the second trimester is a sensitive indicator of thyroid function.

- *Serum prolactin levels:* Normal serum prolactin levels in nonpregnant women vary from 2 ng/mL to 29 ng/mL. During pregnancy, the prolactin levels normally increase and may lie in the range of 10–209 ng/mL.
- *Blood glucose levels:* Blood sugar levels (both fasting and postprandial) need to be carried out. For ruling out diabetes mellitus and gestational diabetes, tests like oral glucose tolerance test (OGTT) and glucose challenge test (GCT) also need to be carried out respectively.
- *Blood grouping:* ABO and Rh typing of both the parents must be done as Rh isoimmunization is an important cause for repeated pregnancy losses.
- *Tests for syphilis:* The most common tests for detection of syphilis using nonspecific antibodies are rapid plasma reagin (RPR) and Venereal Disease Research Laboratory (VDRL) tests.
- *TORCH test:* Confirmation of maternal infection by TORCH screening is recommended.
- *High vaginal swab:* High vaginal swab helps in detection of infections like Chlamydia, bacterial vaginosis, etc.
- *Testing for lupus anticoagulant or anticardiolipin antibodies:* Presence of moderate to high levels of anticardiolipin antibodies (IgG or IgM) in serum or plasma (i.e. > 40 IgG phospholipid units (GPL)/mL or IgM phospholipid units (MPL)/mL or > 99th percentile) on two or more occasions at least 12 weeks apart is considered to be positive for APAS.
- *Diagnosis of uterine anomalies:* All women with recurrent miscarriage should undergo an ultrasound examination for assessment of uterine anatomy and morphology. Ultrasound, especially a vaginal scan helps in detection of abnormalities inside the uterus (uterine septa, intrauterine adhesions, submucosal adhesions, leiomyomas), testing the ovarian reserve and making diagnosis of polycystic ovaries.
  - Sonohysterography is a new technique which helps in imaging of the uterine cavity in order to better diagnose the uterine anomalies. In this technique, sterile saline solution is infused inside the uterine cavity with help of a plastic catheter in conjunction with transvaginal ultrasound.
  - Hysterosalpingography is a procedure, which involves taking X-ray of the pelvis following the instillation of radiopaque contrast agent. This technique helps in delineating the shape of the uterine cavity and in confirming the patency of the fallopian tubes. HSG also helps in diagnosing causes of recurrent miscarriage including uterine malformations, cervical incompetence, Asherman's syndrome etc.
  - If ultrasound examination does not prove useful, hysteroscopic examination also helps in visualization of the interior of the uterine cavity (presence of structural uterine anomalies, e.g. adhesions, uterine septa, etc.), the endometrial lining and shape of

| **Table 5.44:** Symptoms to be elicited at the time of taking history in a case of recurrent pregnancy loss |
| --- |

*History of Presenting Complains*
- History of excessive vaginal discharge suggestive of incompetent os.
- Pain/discomfort in the abdomen.
- Bleeding/spotting per vaginum.
- *Maternal age:* Maternal age is an important risk factor for a further miscarriage

*Obstetric History*

History of previous obstetric losses has to be taken in great details and must be presented in the chronological order in relation to the obstetric events. The following need to be asked:
- Number of years that have passed since her marriage.
- Time after marriage when she first conceived.
- Whether she had any problems in conceiving (infertility could be associated with PCOS).
- The period of gestation at which she suffered a loss, early pregnancy loss (pregnancy loss at ≤ 12 weeks) or a late pregnancy loss (pregnancy loss between 12 to 20 weeks).
- Had the fetus attained the stage of viability when the fetal loss first occurred?
- Weight and sex of the baby.
- Presence of any malformations in the fetus.
- Was the fetus dead or alive at the time of miscarriage?
- If alive at the time of birth, how long did it survive after birth?
- Was the baby jaundiced (suggestive of Rh isoimmunization)?
- If stillbirth, was it fresh or macerated?
- Was there a history of fetal malpresentations (breech or transverse lie) in recurrent pregnancies because this could be suggestive of some underlying uterine malformation?
- Was check curettage done following the fetal loss?
- Was there any hispopathological evaluation of the curetted tissue? If yes, are the results available?
- Whether the loss was accompanied by pain or not?
- Was there any accompanying fever, with or without chills, suggestive of malaria?

*Menstrual History*
- Menorrhagia could be due to presence of fibroids/uterine malformations.
- Irregular shortened cycles could be due to luteal phase defects.
- Polycystic ovary syndrome could be associated with a variety of menstrual abnormalities such as amenorrhea, oligomenorrhea, dysfunctional uterine bleeding (DUB), etc.

*Past Medical History*
- History of chronic hypertension, diabetes mellitus, tuberculosis, hyperthyroidism and hypothyroidism (Tables 5.46 and 5.47).
- History of any sexually transmitted disease.
- History suggestive of previous episodes of thrombosis: Symptoms suggestive of DVT include sudden unilateral swelling of an extremity; presence of pain or aching of an extremity, etc. This would help in ruling out thrombophilia as the cause for recurrent miscarriage.
- History suggestive of antiphospholipid antibody syndrome (APAS): Signs and symptoms suggestive of APAS have been enumerated in Table 5.48.

*Surgical History*

History of any gynecological surgery in the past, e.g. D&C (which may cause injury to the internal os), metroplasty (for correction of congenital uterine malformations) or myomectomy.

*Family History*
- Ask for any family history suggestive of chronic hypertension, diabetes mellitus and tuberculosis.
- Family history related to the presence of genetic disorders: Stepwise genetic evaluation of couples with recurrent miscarriage comprises of the following:
  - Detailed medical, antenatal, and family history especially about history of mental retardation, learning disabilities, progressive muscle weakness, early cataracts, infertility, stillbirth, recurrent miscarriage, and coagulation disorders needs to be taken in order to ascertain the genetic etiology.
  - A three generation pedigree chart must be made.
  - Enquiry must be made regarding the history of consanguinity.

*Personal History*
- Ask for any history suggestive of smoking, tobacco chewing, caffeine consumption, alcohol consumption or drug abuse (e.g. cocaine).
- Exposure to various drugs and toxins such as antiprogestogens, antineoplastic agents, anesthetic gases, petroleum products, ionizing radiation, exposure to organic solvents, environmental toxins (heavy metals), exposure (of the mother) to diethylstilbestrol, etc.

*Abbreviations: DVT, deep vein thrombosis; PCOS, polycystic ovary syndrome*

**Table 5.45:** Various findings elicited at the time of clinical examination in a case of recurrent pregnancy loss

*General Physical Examination*
- *Body mass index:* While a low BMI could be suggestive of poor nutritional status, high BMI could be associated with PCOS
- *Pallor*
- *Blood pressure:* There may be accompanying hypertension.
- *Milk secretion from the breasts:* Look for any evidence of galactorrhea.
- Hirsutism, and other signs of hyperandrogenism.
- Stigma of endocrinological disorders.
- *Thyroid enlargement:* Hypothyroidism is an important cause of fetal death after 16 weeks of gestation.

*Respiratory System*
- Look for the presence of any chronic pulmonary disease.

*Cardiovascular System*
- Look for the presence of any underlying cardiac disease

*Systemic Examination*

*Abdominal Examination*
- Irregular contour of the abdomen or nodular uterus (this could be suggestive of fibroids with pregnancy or bicornuate uterus).
- Look for malpresentations like breech or transverse lie.

*Per Speculum Examination*
- *Examination of external genitalia:* This would help in detecting the presence of blisters, sores, chancres, ulcers, etc., which could be associated with genital tract infection.
- *External appearance of the cervix:* Whether the cervix is healthy, amputated or conized.
    - Presence of cervical abnormalities, vaginal septum, etc.
- *External os:* Whether opened or closed
- If external os is open
    - Can fetal membranes be seen bulging out?
    - Presence of cervicovaginal infection: Infections of the genital tract could be associated with the presence of abnormal vaginal discharge.

*Per Vaginal Examination*
Tests for cervical incompetence
- *Shirodkar's digital palpation test:* If the cervical os is open, insert a finger inside and while withdrawing it, check for the tone of internal os
- *Passage of No. 6-8 Hegar's dilator:* If the clinician is able to pass No 6–8 Hegar's dilator through the internal os without any pain or resistance especially in the premenstrual period, this test is indicative of cervical incompetence. Also, there is absence of a snapping sound as the Hegar's dilator is suddenly withdrawn out of cervical canal in cases of cervical incompetence.

*Abbreviations:* BMI, body mass index; PCOS, polycystic ovary syndrome

**Table 5.46:** Symptoms suggestive of hyperthyroidism

- Palpitations, nervousness, breathlessness
- Heat intolerance
- Insomnia
- Increased bowel movements
- Light or absent menstrual periods
- Tachycardia
- Tremors in hands
- Weight loss
- Muscle weakness
- Warm moist skin
- Hair loss

**Table 5.47:** Symptoms suggestive of hypothyroidism

- Weight gain or increased difficulty in losing weight
- Fatigue, weakness
- Hair loss; coarse, dry hair; dry, rough, pale skin
- Reduced thermogenesis resulting in cold intolerance
- Muscle cramps and frequent muscle aches
- Constipation
- Memory loss
- Husky, low-pitched and coarse voice
- Abnormal menstrual cycles, decreased libido
- Depression, irritability
- Pitting edema in the lower extremities

**Table 5.48:** Clinical features of APAS depending on the organ system affected

| Organ system affected | Symptom |
|---|---|
| Peripheral venous system | Deep venous thrombosis |
| Central nervous system | Cerebrovascular accident, stroke, etc. |
| Hematologic system | Thrombocytopenia, hemolytic anemia |
| Effect on pregnancy | Recurrent pregnancy losses, IUGR, preeclampsia, etc. |
| Pulmonary system | Pulmonary embolism, pulmonary hypertension |
| Dermatologic effect | Livedo reticularis, purpura, infarcts, ulceration |
| Cardiovascular system | Libman-Sacks valvulopathy, myocardial infarction |
| Ocular effects | Amaurosis, retinal thrombosis |
| Adrenal system | Infarction, hemorrhage, etc. |
| Musculoskeletal | Avascular necrosis of bone |

the uterus. Laparoscopic examination helps in the visualization of external surface of the uterus (e.g. presence of bicornuate uterus, unicornuate uterus, etc.).

- *Thrombophilia screening:* This includes screening for factor 5 Leiden mutation, prothrombin G20210A mutation and thrombophilia screening.

- *Tests for cervical incompetence:* Ultrasound examination and other tests for diagnosing the cases of cervical incompetence have been described previously in the text.
- However, all the above-mentioned investigations are not required to be performed in all the patients. A planned and systemic approach should be adopted and evaluation of every case must be individualized.

**Q. What are the principles of management in cases of bad obstetric history?**

**Ans.** The principles of management in the case of BOH are as follows:

- To find out the causative factor.
- To rectify the underlying abnormality as soon as possible. If the causative agent is identified, appropriate therapy must be instituted.
- To remain vigilant throughout the antenatal period until the delivery of the baby. Any complicating factor in present pregnancy is likely to recur in future pregnancies. If an adverse obstetric event has occurred in previous two pregnancies, there is a high probability that it might recur again in the third pregnancy.

**Q. When should the clinician start investigating the women presenting with a history of recurrent abortions?**

**Ans.** The clinician should start investigating the woman presenting with a history of recurrent abortions in the following cases:

- More than or equal to three abortions
- Unexpected fetal death after 16 weeks
- Severe IUGR
- Severe preeclampsia/eclampsia before 34 weeks.

**Q. What are the steps of management in the previous-mentioned case study?**

**Ans.** Since there was no history suggestive of any cause pertaining to recurrent miscarriage in the previous-mentioned case study, some of the investigations, which need to be done include the following: ABO/Rh, blood glucose levels (fasting/postprandial), GCT, TFT, VDRL, TORCH, LA and aCL antibodies, and a transvaginal ultrasound scan. Abnormalities on ultrasound examination should be followed by hysteroscopy, laparoscopy, sonohysterography and/or HSG depending on the type of abnormalities detected.

**Q. In this case, all investigations were found to be within normal limits and a diagnosis of unexplained recurrent miscarriage was made. What should be the next line of management in women with unexplained recurrent miscarriage?**

**Ans.** In significant proportion of cases of recurrent miscarriage, the causative factor remains unexplained, despite detailed investigations. These women can be reassured that the prognosis for a successful future pregnancy with supportive care alone is approximately 75%. Women with unexplained recurrent miscarriage have an excellent prognosis for future pregnancy outcome without pharmacological intervention, if offered supportive care (tender loving care) alone. The prognosis in cases with recurrent pregnancy losses worsens with increasing maternal age and the number of previous miscarriages.

**Q. How should the patient with recurrent miscarriage be treated if a causative factor is identified?**

**Ans.** The treatment comprises of the following steps depending upon the results of various investigations:

- *Psychological support:* It is important to alleviate patient's anxiety and to provide psychological support. About 40–50% of the total cases of recurrent abortion remain unexplained. For these cases, tender loving care especially by the family and the partner, reassurance and supportive care are all that are usually required. All clinicians should be aware of the psychological sequel associated with miscarriage and should provide adequate psychological support and follow-up, as well as access to formal counseling when required.
- *Genetic counseling:* Genetic abnormalities require referral to a clinical geneticist. In case of detection of a chromosomal anomaly, genetic counseling, familial chromosomal studies, and appropriate prenatal diagnosis in future pregnancies gives the couple a good prognosis for future pregnancies. These couples should also be offered the options of preimplantation genetic diagnosis, IVF, donor gametes, adoption, etc. Preimplantation genetic diagnosis or prenatal diagnosis (amniocentesis and chorionic villus sampling) helps in identifying embryos having or not having chromosomal abnormalities.
- *Control of diabetes and thyroid dysfunction:* Prepregnancy glycemic control is particularly important for women with overt diabetes mellitus. Replacement with thyroid hormone analogs may be required in hypothyroid women.
- *Operative hysteroscopy:* Operative hysteroscopy can help in treatment of the following anomalies: removal of submucous leiomyomas, resection of intrauterine adhesions, resection of intrauterine septa, etc.
- *Treatment of luteal phase defects (LPD):* Treatment of LPD is done using micronized progesterone in the dosage of 100 mg/day. Progesterone supplementation must continue until 10–12 weeks following gestation.
- *Antiphospholipid antibody syndrome:* Treatment of cases of APAS comprises of the following:
  - *Prevention of thrombosis:* Patients with recurrent pregnancy loss must be administered a prophylactic dose of subcutaneous heparin [preferably low molecular weight heparin (LMWH) because it is associated with fewer side-effects] and low dose aspirin.
  - *Termination of pregnancy:* Termination of pregnancy must be considered at 37 completed weeks of gestation.
- *Cervical incompetence:* Various surgical procedures for cervical incompetence are described as follows:
  - *McDonald procedure:* In McDonald procedure, a 5-mm band of permanent purse string suture using

4–5 bites is placed high on the cervix. It is usually removed at 37 weeks, unless there is a reason (e.g. infection, preterm labor, preterm rupture of membrane, etc.) for an earlier removal. Kindly refer to Chapter 6 for details.

- *Shirodkar technique:* In Shirodkar procedure, a permanent purse string suture, which would remain intact for life, is applied. Therefore, the patient is delivered by a CS.

- *Inherited thrombophilias:* Antithrombotic therapy with heparin has been found to be effective. Antithrombotic therapy is usually administered up to 34 weeks of gestation.

- *Polycystic ovary syndrome:* Treatment of PCOS involves weight reduction, use of insulin sensitizing agents (metformin) and ovulation induction with clomiphene citrate.

- *Infections:* For cases in which an infectious organism has been identified, appropriate antibiotics should be administered, e.g. penicillin (syphilis); ganciclovir (cytomegalovirus); acyclovir (genital herpes); pyrimethamine and sulfadiazine (toxoplasmosis). Post treatment cultures must be done in order to verify eradication of the infectious agent before the patient is advised to attempt conception.

# Rh Isoimmunization

## Case Study 1
## Rh-negative (Nonimmunized) Pregnancy

Mrs XYZ, a 34-year-old patient (Rh negative, G3P2A0L1) with 28 weeks period of gestation, married for 8 years, resident of ABC, presents for antenatal check-up. She gives history of receiving some kind of injection related to Rh-negative blood (probably Rh immunoglobulins) in the previous pregnancy.

**Q. What is the likely diagnosis in the above-mentioned case study?**

**Ans.** The most likely diagnosis in the above-mentioned case study is Mrs XYZ, a 34-year-old patient (Rh negative, G3P2A0L1), married for 8 years, resident of ABC, with 28 weeks period of amenorrhea, corresponding to 28 weeks period of gestation with the clinical history most likely suggestive of Rh isoimmunization. The questions to be asked at the time of taking history and the parameters to be assessed at the time of examination in such a case are described in Tables 5.49 and 5.50, respectively.

**Q. Describe the Rh blood group system.**

**Ans.** Rh blood group system (rhesus blood group classification system) is the most important blood group system after the ABO blood group system. Although the Rh system contains five main antigens (C, c, D, E and e), antigen D is considered to be the most immunogenic. According to the rhesus classification, the blood groups can be classified as Rh positive (those having D antigen) and Rh negative (those not having D antigen).

**Q. What is Rh isoimmunization/alloimmunization and how can it occur during pregnancy?**

**Ans.** Isoimmunization can be defined as the production of immune antibodies in an individual in response to the foreign red cell antigens derived from another individual of the same species. It can occur in two stages: (1) sensitization and (2) isoimmunization.

Rh incompatibility may develop when a woman with Rh-negative blood marries a man with Rh-positive blood and conceives a fetus with Rh-positive blood group (who has inherited the Rh factor gene from the father). Rh-positive

| **Table 5.49:** Symptoms to be elicited at the time of taking history in a case of Rh-negative pregnancy |
| --- |
| *History of Presenting Complains* |
| The following risk factors must be elicited on history:<br>• Rh-negative (dd) blood type<br>• Younger (< 16 years) or older (> 35 years) maternal age<br>• Rh-negative woman partnered with Rh-positive father<br>• History of previous blood transfusions<br>• Reduction in fetal movements in the present pregnancy |
| *Obstetric History* |
| It is important to elicit detailed past obstetric history from the patient. Previous history of neonatal deaths or stillbirths and history of previous successive fetuses affected by jaundice, anemia, etc. is quite suggestive of Rh isoimmunization. Women may typically give a history of having received injections of anti-Rh immunoglobulins in previous pregnancies or following miscarriage, and invasive procedures like amniocentesis, CVS, etc. The following need to be enquired from the woman:<br>• History of jaundice, congenital malformations, stillbirths or intrauterine deaths in previous pregnancies<br>• Previous history of hydrops fetalis<br>• Previous history of fetomaternal transfusion<br>• History of receiving anti-Rh immunoglobulins in previous pregnancies<br>• History of unrecognized miscarriage with transplacental hemorrhage<br>• History of jaundice, hyperbilirubinemia and kernicterus in previous pregnancies |

| **Table 5.50:** Various findings elicited at the time of clinical examination in a case of Rh-negative pregnancy |
| --- |
| *General Physical Examination* <br> • No specific finding is observed on general physical examination |
| *Specific Systemic Examination* <br> • *Abdominal Examination* <br>    – Normal abdominal and vaginal examination should be carried out as described in Chapter 1 |

fetal RBCs from the fetus leak across the placenta and enter the woman's circulation. Throughout the pregnancy, small amounts of fetal blood can enter the maternal circulation (fetomaternal hemorrhage), with the greatest transfer occurring at the time of delivery or during the third trimester. This transfer stimulates maternal antibody production against the Rh factor, which is called isoimmunization. The process of sensitization has no adverse health effects for the mother. During the time of first Rh-positive pregnancy, the production of maternal anti-Rh antibodies is relatively slow and usually does not affect that pregnancy. Therefore, Rh incompatibility is not a factor in a first pregnancy, because few fetal blood cells reach the mother's bloodstream until delivery. The antibodies that form after delivery cannot affect the first child. However, if the mother is exposed to the Rh D antigens during subsequent pregnancies, the immune response is quicker and much greater. The anti-D antibodies produced by the mother can cross the placenta and bind to Rh D antigen on the surface of fetal RBCs, causing lysis of the fetal RBCs, resulting in development of hemolytic anemia. Severe anemia can lead to fetal heart failure, fluid retention, and hydrops and IUD. Depending on the degree of erythrocyte destruction, various types of fetal hemolytic diseases can result. An umbrella term for these hemolytic disorders is known as "erythroblastosis fetalis". Clinical manifestations of erythroblastosis fetalis include hydrops fetalis, icterus gravis neonatorum and congenital anemia of the newborn.

### Q. What are the two types of antibodies which can be formed as a result of Rh isoimmunization?

**Ans.** The two types of antibodies that can be formed as a result of Rh isoimmunization are as follows:

- *IgM antibodies:* These are the first type of antibodies to appear in the maternal circulation and agglutinate the red cells (containing D antigen) when suspended in saline. IgM antibodies are larger than the IgG antibodies and they cannot cross the placenta.
- *IgG antibodies:* They are the incomplete or blocking antibodies and they appear in the maternal circulation later than the IgM antibodies. They agglutinate the RBCs containing D antigen only when they are suspended in 20% albumin. Since they are smaller than IgM antibodies in size, they can cross the placental barrier, resulting in fetal damage.

### Q. What is the management protocol in a pregnant patient with Rh-negative blood group married to an Rh-positive blood group husband?

**Ans.** Firstly, the Rh blood group of the husband needs to be determined. If the father is also Rh negative, no problem is likely to occur with Rh factor. However, if the husband is found to be Rh positive, further investigations need to be carried out because in this case, the woman may bear an Rh-positive child. The investigations mainly involve at finding out if the woman has been already immunized to Rh antigen. In all cases of Rh-negative women, the anti-Rh antibody can be detected with the help of indirect Coombs' test. In case the woman has already been immunized to Rh antigen, the clinician needs to forecast the likely affection on the baby. Following this, the management plan for baby's treatment needs to be formulated.

### Q. What investigations must be carried out in an Rh-negative woman married to an Rh-positive man?

**Ans.** The following investigations must be done:

- Blood grouping (both ABO and Rh)
- *Coombs' test:* This can be of two types: (1) direct Coombs' test and (2) indirect Coombs' test.
  - *Direct Coombs' test:* This test aims at detecting the maternal antibodies that may be bound to the surface of fetal RBCs and is performed after baby's birth. In the direct Coombs' test, washed infant's RBCs are incubated with the Coombs' serum (antiglobulin antibodies). If agglutination is produced, the direct Coombs' test is positive. This is indicative of the presence of antibodies on the surface of RBCs.
  - *Indirect Coombs' test:* This test is used for measuring the presence of antibodies, which are present unbound in the maternal serum. In this test, the maternal serum is incubated with Rh-positive erythrocytes and Coombs' serum (antiglobulin antibodies). The red cells will agglutinate, if anti-Rh antibodies are present in the maternal plasma.
- *Kleihauer-Betke test:* This is a blood test for measuring the amount of fetal hemoglobin transferred from a fetus to mother's bloodstream as a result of fetomaternal hemorrhage.

  Kleihauer-Betke test involves acid elution to detect the fetal RBCs. This test is based on the principle that fetal hemoglobin is resistant to acid. Exposure of a standard blood smear prepared from the mother's blood to an acid bath helps in removing adult hemoglobin, but not fetal hemoglobin, from the RBCs. Subsequent staining, using Shepard's method, causes the fetal cells (containing fetal hemoglobin) to become rose-pink in color, whereas adult RBCs are only seen as "ghosts". Fetal RBCs are counted per 50 low power fields. Presence of 80 fetal erythrocytes in 50 low power fields in maternal peripheral blood films represents a transplacental hemorrhage to the extent of 4 mL of fetal blood.

- *Newer/advanced tests:* Newer, advanced and more accurate tests for measuring fetomaternal hemorrhage include immunofluorescence and flow cytometry.

### Q. What should be the plan of management in an Rh-negative nonimmunized woman?

**Ans.** In an Rh-negative nonimmunized woman, the indirect Coombs' test is performed at 20, 24 and 28 weeks of gestation in order to detect the presence of any new antibodies, which may develop during the antenatal period. In case, the antibody screen is negative, the patient should be administered 300 µg (1,500 IU) of immunoglobulins at 28 weeks of gestation. After delivery of the baby, the Rh status of the newborn is to be checked. If the baby is Rh positive, 300 µg of anti-D immunoglobulins must be administered within 72 hours of delivery.

In case the antibody screen turns out to be positive, the woman must be further managed as Rh-sensitized pregnancy. In these cases, routine anti-D prophylaxis is not required.

### Q. Can Rh-positive ABO compatible blood be transfused to an Rh-negative individual?

**Ans.** Rh-positive ABO compatible blood can be transfused to Rh-negative males in case of emergency as a life-saving procedure. However, such transfusions must be avoided in Rh-negative females from birth until menopause due to the risk of acceleration of the process of Rh isoimmunization in case the Rh-negative woman marries an Rh-positive man and conceives an Rh-positive child.

### Q. After what kind of sensitizing event is anti-D Ig prophylaxis required and in what dosage?

**Ans.** In the presence of a sensitizing event, minimum recommended doses of anti-D Ig at less than 12 weeks of gestation to an Rh-negative unsensitized woman is 50 µg and at more than 12 weeks of gestation is 300 µg. Various sensitizing events occurring in the first trimester include induced or spontaneous abortion, ectopic or molar pregnancy, chorionic villus sampling in the first trimester, etc. Other sensitizing events which can occur throughout after the first trimester include invasive prenatal diagnosis (amniocentesis, CVS, cordocentesis, intrauterine transfusion, etc.), other intrauterine procedures (e.g. insertion of shunts, embryo reduction, laser, etc.), antepartum hemorrhage, ECV of the fetus, any kind of abdominal trauma (direct/indirect, sharp/blunt, open/closed), fetal death, etc.

Three hundred micrograms of immunoglobulins protect a woman from fetal hemorrhage of up to 30 mL of whole fetal blood. For successful immunoprophylaxis, anti-D Ig should be administered as soon as possible after the potentially sensitizing event but always within 72 hours.

## Case Study 2
## Rh-negative (Immunized Pregnancy)

Mrs XYZ, a 28-year-old patient (Rh negative, G3P2A0L1) with 28 weeks period of gestation, married for 8 years, resident of ABC, history of previous pregnancy being affected by anemia presents for antenatal check-up. In her last pregnancy (2 years back), she had delivered a child having severe anemia and jaundice. The baby survived for only 10 days after birth in the neonatal ICU. She gives history of receiving some kind of injection related to Rh-negative blood (probably Rh immunoglobulins) during her first pregnancy. She does not remember receiving any injections during her past pregnancy.

### Q. What steps can be taken for minimizing fetomaternal bleed?

**Ans.** Various steps which can be taken for minimizing fetomaternal bleed are as follows:

- *Precautions to be taken at the time of cesarean delivery:* Spilling of blood in the peritoneal cavity must be avoided; manual removal of placenta must not be done as a routine
- Prophylactic ergometrine with the delivery of anterior shoulder must be withheld as it may cause more fetomaternal bleed
- Amniocentesis (if required) must be performed after the sonographic localization of placenta to prevent its injury
- Forcible attempts to perform external version under anesthesia must be avoided
- Manual removal of the placenta must be gently performed
- Abdominal palpation should be avoided as far as possible in case of abruption placenta
- Transfusion of Rh-positive blood to an Rh-negative mother must be preferably avoided from birth till menopause.

### Q. What would be the next step of management in the above-mentioned case study?

**Ans.** This woman should be managed as a case of Rh-negative sensitized pregnancy with a history of previously affected pregnancy. Amniocentesis for the estimation of fetal bilirubin levels was performed. Spectrophotometric analysis of amniotic fluid was performed and ΔOD 450 values were plotted on Liley's chart (Fig. 5.1). The values were in zone I and remained in zone I even when a repeat amniocentesis was performed after 4 weeks. This implies that the infant needs to be delivered at term in anticipation of the delivery of a healthy fetus.

### Q. What should be the plan of management in Rh-negative immunized women?

**Ans.** In Rh-negative immunized women, the main objective of the management is to diagnose and treat fetal anemia as soon as possible. In case of Rh-negative immunized women, the next step of management depends on whether or not there is a previous history of affected fetus.

### Q. What should be the plan of management in Rh-negative immunized women with no previous history of affected babies?

**Ans.** In women where there is no previous history of affected babies, serial determination of maternal anti-Rh

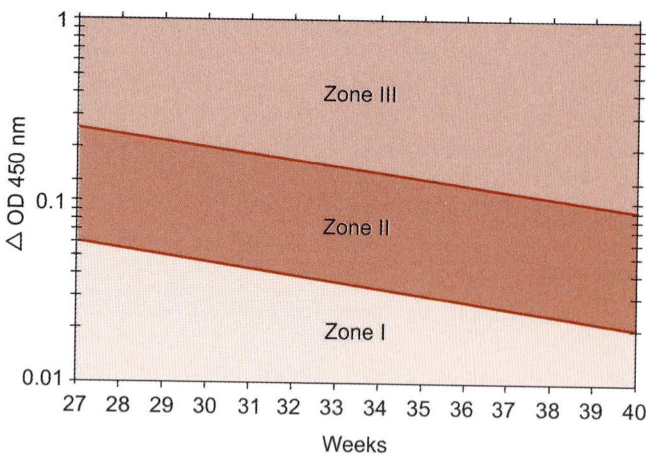

**Fig. 5.1:** Liley's chart

antibody titers is done at 3 to 4 weekly intervals, starting at 30–32 weeks of gestation. Pregnancy can be continued till term if the antibody titer remains under the critical level. If there is a sudden increase in the antibody titer and pregnancy has attained 34 weeks gestation, mother is induced and delivered. However, in case the period of gestation is less than 34 weeks, amniocentesis is to be done at weekly intervals. If serum bilirubin levels are less than 0.05 and lungs are immature, amniocentesis is continued at weekly intervals. If the serum bilirubin is greater than 0.05 or lungs are mature, the fetus is delivered.

**Q. What should be the plan of management in Rh-negative immunized women with previous history of affected babies?**
**Ans.** Woman who previously had an affected pregnancy is likely to experience a recurrence in her present pregnancy, if not treated. Therefore, monitoring for fetal anemia in these cases must commence at least 10 weeks earlier than the time of her previously affected pregnancy. Fetal anemia can be diagnosed through one of the following ways: measurement of the peak systolic velocity (PSV) of the fetal middle cerebral artery; Doppler ultrasound; amniocentesis and amniotic fluid analysis; ultrasound examination of the fetus and percutaneous umbilical cord blood sampling (cordocentesis).

**Q. What is amniotic fluid analysis?**
**Ans.** Amniotic fluid analysis involves determination of bilirubin concentration in the amniotic fluid and spectropho-tometric analysis. The optical density (OD) of the liquor (containing bilirubin pigment) is observed at the wavelength between 250 nm and 700 nm. Optical density readings of normal amniotic fluid when analyzed by spectrometry form an almost straight line between 350 nm and 650 nm. If bilirubin is present in the amniotic fluid, a "deviation bulge" peaking at the wavelength of 450 nm is observed. The bigger the deviation bulge, more severe would be fetal affection. Instead of doing continuous spectrophotometry, OD readings

are selectively measured at 375 nm, 450 nm and 525 nm. The results are then plotted on a semilogarithmic paper and a straight line is drawn between the readings at 375 nm and 525 nm. The $\Delta$OD 450 values are calculated next, which are equal to the difference between the expected value (point at which the line crosses the 450 nm mark) and the actual reading at this wavelength. The $\Delta$OD 450 values can, therefore, be simply defined as the deviation bulge. The $\Delta$OD 450 values are then plotted on Liley's chart. For any given period of gestation, the height of spectrophotometric "deviation bulge" at $\Delta$OD 450 falls within one of the three zones, when plotted on the Liley's chart.

**Q. What is the significance of three zones on the Liley's chart?**
**Ans.** Zone III on the Liley's curve corresponds to severely affected infants, zone II to moderately affected infants and zone I to unaffected or mildly affected infants. If bilirubin levels in amniotic fluid lie in zone I, pregnancy can be allowed to continue to term and the clinician can await spontaneous labor. If bilirubin levels lie in zone II or zone III, management is based upon the period of gestation. If period of gestation is greater than 34 weeks, the fetus can be delivered. If the period of gestation is less than 34 weeks, fetal hematocrit must be determined.

If at any time, the $\Delta$OD 450 value lies in the zone III or shows a rising trend, the fetus is in imminent danger of the IUD. In these cases, cordocentesis must be done and fetal hemoglobin values must be determined. If fetal hematocrit values are less than 30%, intrauterine transfusion is indicated. Treatment of fetal anemia can be in the form of in-utero transfusion (intraperitoneal or intravascular), if fetal anemia is severe or exchange transfusion after birth.

**Q. How is the timing of delivery decided in these cases?**
**Ans.** In case no detectable antibody can be found, an expectant attitude is followed until term. Tendency of the pregnancy to overrun the EDD should not be allowed.

In case there is an evidence of the hemolytic process in the fetus in utero, patient should be shifted to an equipped tertiary center having a neonatal ICU with facilities for exchange transfusion and an expert neonatologist. Intrauterine fetal transfusion could be of two types: (1) intraperitoneal and (2) intravascular. Sometimes, exchange transfusion can be used as a life-saving procedure in severely affected newborn babies with hemolytic disease of the newborn.

**Q. How does management change based on the fetal hematocrit values?**
**Ans.** If fetal hematocrit is greater than 30%, the baby must be followed up with fetal blood sampling and ultrasound examination at weekly intervals. Decision for delivery is based on fetal condition and maturity.

In case fetal hematocrit is less than 30%, intrauterine blood transfusion at 10 days to 2 weekly intervals is indicated. Fetus must be delivered at 34–36 weeks of gestation.

**Q. What should be the timing of amniocentesis in Rh-negative immunized women?**

**Ans.** Timing for amniocentesis is based on the previous history of affected baby.

In case there is no history of previously affected baby, amniocentesis is done at 30–32 weeks of gestation. In case there is a history of previously affected baby, amniocentesis is done at least 10 weeks prior to the date of previous stillbirth.

**Q. What are the various manifestations of the hemolytic disease?**

**Ans.** Depending upon the degree of agglutination and destruction of fetal RBCs, various types of fetal hemolytic diseases may appear. These include hydrops fetalis, icterus gravis neonatorum and congenital anemia of the newborn.

*Hydrops fetalis:* This is the most serious form of hemolytic disease associated with excessive red cell destruction, which may result in severe anemia, tissue anoxemia and metabolic acidosis. As a result, there occurs hyperplasia of the placental tissues in an effort to increase the transfer of oxygen. Anoxemia also results in damage to liver causing hypoproteinemia. This is characterized by an accumulation of fluids within the baby's body, resulting in development of ascites, pleural effusion, pericardial effusion, skin edema, etc. Fetal death commonly occurs due to cardiac failure.

*Icterus gravis neonatorum:* The baby is born without any clinical evidence of jaundice, but it soon develops within 24 hours of birth. If the bilirubin levels rise to more than 20 mg/100 mL, it may cross the blood–brain barrier resulting in kernicterus.

*Congenital anemia of the newborn:* This is the mildest form of the disease where the hemolysis occurs slowly. Anemia occurs slowly within a few weeks of life, but jaundice does not usually occur. The destruction of red cells continues up to 6 weeks. The sites of extramedullary erythropoiesis (i.e. liver and spleen) are enlarged.

**Q. What is cordocentesis?**

**Ans.** Cordocentesis is a diagnostic test which aims at detection of fetal anomalies (e.g. chromosomal anomalies like Down's syndrome; blood disorders like hemolytic anemia, etc.) through direct examination of fetal blood.

**Q. What steps should be taken in the intrapartum period in such patients?**

**Ans.** The steps, which must be taken in the intrapartum period in patients with Rh-negative pregnancy, are as follows:

*Precautions to be taken at the time of delivery:* Following steps must be taken to minimize the chances of fetomaternal bleeding during the time of delivery:
- Prophylactic ergometrine with the delivery of the anterior shoulder must be withheld.
- If the manual removal of the placenta is required, it should be performed gently.

- Invasive procedures, like amniocentesis, chorionic villus sampling, etc., should be followed by administration of 300 µg of anti-Rh immunoglobulins, except for the cases of first-trimester abortion where the dose required is 50 µg.
- Careful fetal monitoring needs to be performed during the time of labor in order to detect fetal distress at the earliest.
- Delivery should be as nontraumatic as possible.
- The clinician should remain vigilant regarding the possibility for the occurrence of PPH.
- Umbilical cord should be clamped as soon as possible to minimize the chances of fetomaternal hemorrhage.
- While cutting the cord, care should be taken that it remains long (15–20 cm) so that it would be possible to carry out exchange transfusion in the baby, if required in future.
- About 5 mL of blood sample (2 mL oxalated and 3mL clotted) must be collected from the placental end of the cord for the purpose of the following tests:
  - ABO/Rh, direct Coombs' test and serum bilirubin levels in clotted blood
  - Hemoglobin estimation and blood smear examination for the presence of immature RBCs in oxalated blood.
- At the time of CS, all precautions should be taken to prevent any spillage of blood into the peritoneal cavity.
- Rh-positive blood transfusion must be preferably avoided in Rh-negative women right from birth until menopause: Rh-positive ABO compatible blood can be transfused to Rh-negative males in case of emergency as a lifesaving procedure. However, such transfusions must be avoided in Rh-negative females from birth until menopause due to the risk of acceleration of the process of Rh isoimmunization process in case the Rh-negative woman marries an Rh-positive man and conceives an Rh-positive child.

**Q. What are the various complications, which can occur, in an Rh-negative woman during her pregnancy?**

**Ans.** The various complications which can occur in an Rh-negative woman during her pregnancy are as follows:

*Maternal Complications*

- Recurrent miscarriages and IUDs
- Increased incidence of complications such as preeclampsia, polyhydramnios, large-sized babies, PPH (due to a large placenta), hypofibrinogenemia (due to prolonged retention of a dead fetus), etc.
- Maternal syndrome is characterized by generalized edema, proteinuria and pruritus due to cholestasis
- Complications, such as abortion and preterm labor, are related to procedures, such as fetal cord blood sampling.

*Fetal Complications*

- *Erythroblastosis fetalis:* Clinical manifestations of erythroblastosis fetalis include hydrops fetalis, icterus gravis neonatorum and congenital anemia of the newborn. Each of these conditions has been described in details previously in the text.

- Excessive destruction of fetal RBCs results in hyperbilirubinemia, jaundice and/or kernicterus, which can lead to deafness, speech problems, cerebral palsy or mental retardation.

# Cardiac Disease in Pregnancy

## Case Study 1

Mrs XYZ, a 34-year-old married for 6 years, resident of ABC, primigravida patient gives a history of having valve prosthesis 1 year back and presently is on warfarin. She presents for the first time in the antenatal clinic at 38 weeks of gestation. Presently, she is asymptomatic.

### Q. What is the most likely diagnosis in the above-mentioned case study?

**Ans.** The most likely diagnosis in above-mentioned case study is Mrs XYZ, a 34-year-old married for 6 years, resident of ABC, primigravida patient with 38 weeks amenorrhea, corresponding to 38 weeks of gestation having a history of getting valve prosthesis 1 year back for mitral stenosis, with a single live fetus in cephalic presentation, presently asymptomatic in normal sinus rhythm and no congestive cardiac failure. The questions to be asked at the time of taking history and the parameters to be assessed at the time of examination in such a case are described in Tables 5.51 and 5.52 respectively.

### Q. How can dyspnea be graded?

**Ans.** According to the Medical Research Council classification, dyspnea can be graded into five categories:

- *Grade 1:* No dyspnea at rest; dyspnea is present only while doing strenuous exercise (e.g. walking up the hill).
- *Grade 2:* Shortness of breath when walking with the people of same age group on ground level
- *Grade 3:* Limitation of walking pace (slower than others) as a result of dyspnea. The individual has to stop in between to catch breath.
- *Grade 4:* The individual needs to stops to catch for breath after walking nearly every 100 meters on level ground.
- *Grade 5:* Severe degree of dyspnea, which severely limits the individual's activities of daily living and prevents her from leaving her house.

### Q. What are the hemodynamic changes during normal pregnancy?

**Ans.** The following hemodynamic changes occur during normal pregnancy:

- There is a 30–50% increase in cardiac output. Normally the cardiac output starts increasing by around 5th week and increases rapidly until the 34th week of gestation, following which it plateaus or continues to increase slightly. The increase in cardiac output is achieved by three factors:
  1. An increase in preload because of greater blood volume. Blood volume increases by 40–50% during normal pregnancy. The increase in plasma volume is greater than the increase in red blood cell mass, contributing to the fall in hemoglobin concentration (i.e. the "physiological anemia in pregnancy").
  2. Reduced afterload due to reduction in systemic vascular resistance; and
  3. A rise in the maternal heart rate by 10–15 beats/minute.
- Stroke volume increases during the first and second trimesters, but declines in the third trimester due to the compression of inferior vena cava by the uterus.
- Both plasma and interstitial colloid oncotic pressure decrease throughout pregnancy. There is an accompanying increase in the capillary hydrostatic pressure. Increase in capillary hydrostatic pressure or decrease in colloid oncotic pressure is likely to cause edema.
- A decline in systemic arterial pressure begins to occur during first trimester, reaches a nadir in mid-pregnancy and returns towards pregestational level before term. Blood pressure typically falls by about 10 mm Hg below baseline by the end of the second trimester because of reduction in systemic vascular resistance and the addition of new blood vessels in the uterus and placenta.

  During labor, there is further increase in cardiac output, heart rate, blood pressure and systemic vascular resistance due to the stress and anxiety of labor and delivery and uterine contractions. Moreover, there is a sudden increase in the cardiac output in the immediate postpartum period due to autotransfusion of approximately 600–800 mL of uteroplacental blood into the peripheral circulation. Cardiac output also increases during labor due to squeezing out of blood from uterus at the time of uterine contractions. Therefore, while preparing a woman with cardiac disease for labor and delivery, it is important to anticipate that there will be important changes in maternal hemodynamic parameters.

### Q. What are the most common types of heart diseases encountered during pregnancy?

**Ans.** The most common cardiac lesions encountered during pregnancy are rheumatic ones followed by the congenital ones. Rheumatic valvular lesion encountered in nearly 80% of cases is mitral stenosis. Chronic mitral regurgitation, another common lesion encountered as a result of rheumatic heart disease is usually well-tolerated during pregnancy. The common congenital lesions include, patent ductus arteriosus, atrial or ventricular septal defects, pulmonary stenosis, coarctation of aorta and Fallot's tetralogy.

| **Table 5.51:** Symptoms to be elicited at the time of taking history in a case of cardiovascular disease in pregnancy |
| --- |
| *History of Presenting Complains* |
| Women with preexisting cardiac dysfunction usually experience cardiac deterioration during the end of the second trimester. Typical signs and symptoms include fatigue, dizziness, dyspnea on exertion, orthopnea, nonspecific chest pain, light-headedness or fainting, peripheral edema and abdominal discomfort and distension. It is important to elicit the history of the following symptoms:<br>• *Dyspnea:* Though some amount of exertional dyspnea or breathlessness can commonly occur during normal pregnancy, severe dyspnea, especially that occurring at rest or while sleeping or that resulting in inability to perform normal activities may be suggestive of heart disease. Dyspnea can commonly result from left ventricular failure (LVF), pulmonary embolism, etc. While taking the history of dyspnea it is important to enquire the circumstances under which the patient experiences breathlessness. The dyspnea can be graded into four categories depending on whether dyspnea occurs during exertion, while doing daily activities, or at rest. The history of orthopnea or shortness of breath while sleeping at night can be elicited by asking about the number of pillows the patient uses at night in order to prevent breathlessness. Paroxysmal nocturnal dyspnea can be diagnosed if the patient gives history of waking up at night, gasping for breath.<br>• *Peripheral edema:* Presence of cardiac disease can further aggravate the physiological edema in pregnancy.<br>• *Palpitation:* Palpitations may be due to ectopic beats, atrial fibrillations, supraventricular tachycardia and ventricular tachycardia, thyrotoxicosis, anxiety, etc. The clinician must take the history about previous episodes of palpitations; precipitating/relieving factors; duration of symptoms and presence of associated symptoms like chest pain, dyspnea or dizziness.<br>• *Chest pain:* Acute history of chest pain radiating to shoulders/neck may be suggestive of myocardial infarction. Chest pain in association with headache, dysarthria, limb weakness, etc. may be indicative of central nervous system (CNS) causes.<br>• *Light-headedness or fainting:* Owing to the normal pregnancy-related cardiovascular changes, many healthy pregnant women may show symptoms mimicking those of cardiac disease, including fatigue, dyspnea, light-headedness, fainting, etc. |
| *Medical History* |
| • History of fleeting joint pains and/or fever in the past (suggestive of rheumatic heart disease), congenital heart disease since childhood.<br>• Previous history of congestive cardiac failure, infective endocarditis, etc. also needs to be asked. |
| *Surgical History* |
| • History of any cardiac surgery in the past and if yes, details related to it (e.g. type of cardiac surgery, if valvular replacement was done, types of valves replaced; how long ago was the surgery done? |
| *Dietary History* |
| • Has the woman been ever prescribed a special diet (e.g. restriction of salt, saturated fat, etc.) in the diet. |
| *Drug History* |
| • History of receiving IM injections of benzathine penicillin G (Penidure 12LA) could be suggestive of prophylaxis for rheumatic heart disease.<br>• History of intake of any other medicines for cardiac diseases (e.g. digoxin, anticoagulants, etc.) also needs to be taken. |

## Q. What are the effects of cardiac lesions on pregnancy?

**Ans.** Cardiac lesions are associated with an increased tendency of preterm delivery and prematurity. IUGR may be commonly observed in cases of cyanotic congenital heart diseases.

## Q. What is New York Heart Association functional classification of heart diseases?

**Ans.** The New York Heart Association (NYHA) functional classification of heart disease is as follows:

1. *Class I:* Patients with cardiac disease, but without resulting limitations of physical activity. Ordinary physical activity does not cause fatigue, palpitations, dyspnea or anginal pain.
2. *Class II:* Patients with cardiac disease resulting in slight limitation of physical activity. They are comfortable at rest. Ordinary physical activity results in fatigue, palpitations, dyspnea or anginal pain.
3. *Class III:* Patients with cardiac disease resulting in marked limitation of physical activity. They are comfortable at rest. Less than ordinary physical activity results in fatigue, palpitations, dyspnea or anginal pain.
4. *Class IV:* Patients with cardiac disease resulting in an inability to carry on any physical activity without discomfort. Symptoms of cardiac insufficiency may be even present at rest. If any physical activity is undertaken, discomfort is increased.

## Q. How should such patients be managed during the antenatal period?

**Ans.** The following steps must be taken during the antenatal period:

- *Supervision in a tertiary healthcare setting:* Such patients should be preferably supervised in a tertiary healthcare setting.
- *Management of mitral stenosis:* Drugs, like digoxin and β-blockers, can be used to reduce heart rate, and diuretics can be used to reduce the blood volume and left atrial pressure. With development of atrial fibrillations and hemodynamic deterioration, electrocardioversion can be performed safely. Anticoagulation must be initiated with the onset of atrial fibrillations in order to reduce the risk of stroke.
  - Heart surgery may be necessary when medical treatment fails to control heart failure or symptoms remain intolerable to the patients despite medical therapy. While open heart surgery may be associated with risks to the fetus, closed mitral valvuloplasty

**Table 5.52:** Various findings elicited at the time of clinical examination in a case of cardiac disease in pregnancy

*General Physical Examination*

- *Pulse:* The rate, volume and rhythm must be assessed. The pulse must be recorded in both the upper limbs. Abnormalities in pulse pattern may be suggestive of underlying cardiac disease. Presence of radiofemoral delay could be suggestive of coarctation of aorta.
- *Blood pressure:* There may be accompanying hypertension.
- *Respiratory rate:* Look for any signs, which suggest that the patient has difficulty in breathing (dyspnea).
- *Finger clubbing:* Clubbing of fingers may be associated with the diseases of heart or lungs.
- *Cyanosis:* Cyanosis is bluish discoloration of the skin and mucous membranes due to presence of at least 5 g % of deoxygenated hemoglobin in the blood. The place to look for peripheral cyanosis is the fingertips including underneath the nail beds. The places to look for central cyanosis are the lips and tongue.
- *Features indicative of infective endocarditis:* These include the following:
  - Splinter hemorrhages (areas of hemorrhage under the fingernails or toenails).
  - Janeway lesions (small, nontender, erythematous or hemorrhagic macular or nodular lesions, occurring most commonly on the palms and soles including the thenar and hypothenar eminences).
  - Osler's nodes (tender, transient nodules commonly present in the pulp of fingers; at times also may be present in the sole of the feet), etc.
- *Hepatomegaly:* Presence of hepatomegaly or ascites on abdominal examination could be due to congestive heart failure.
- *Peripheral edema:* Presence of edema in the feet or sacral edema could occur due to congestive cardiac failure.
- *Pallor*
- *Jugular venous pressure (JVP):* Raised JVP could be suggestive of cardiac disease.

*Specific Systemic Examination*

*Examination of the Cardiovascular System*

Inspection
- Precordium must be inspected for any of the following:
  - Visible pulsations
  - Apex beat
  - Masses/scars/lesions
  - Signs of trauma/ previous surgery
  - Precordial bulge (left parasternal lift due to right ventricular dilation).

*Palpation*
The cardiac apex may be shifted downwards and outwards in cases of LV enlargement.

*Auscultation*
Upon auscultation of the precordial area, normal heart sounds (S1 and S2) can be heard. Upon auscultation, it is important to note whether or not an additional sound (e.g. murmur, opening snap, click, third or fourth heard sounds, etc.) are present. The cardiac areas, which are most commonly auscultated, include the following:
- *Mitral area (at the point of cardiac apex):* Corresponds to the left fifth intercostal space and is 1 cm medial to the midclavicular line.
- *Tricuspid area:* The lower left parasternal border is the tricuspid area.
- *Pulmonary area:* The left second intercostal space.
- *The aortic area:* The right second intercostal space.
- *The second aortic area or the Erb's area:* The left third intercostal space.
  Functional murmurs are frequently heard during pregnancy due to the increased cardiac output and do not require further investigation or management. The functional murmur needs to be distinguished from a pathological one. Characteristics of some common pathological murmurs are described in Table 5.53.
A detailed examination of the cardiovascular system is beyond the scope of this book. The reader needs to refer to a standard medical text book for that.

*Abdominal and Vaginal Examination:* Normal abdominal and vaginal examination must be carried out as described in Chapter 1.

(CMV), a relatively safe procedure, may be performed in case of severe pulmonary congestion unresponsive to drugs, profuse hemoptysis and any episode of pulmonary edema before pregnancy.
- *Mode of delivery:* Most patients with mitral stenosis can undergo vaginal delivery.
- *Prevention of the recurrence of rheumatic heart disease:* For preventing the recurrence of rheumatic heart disease, injection penidure LA12 (benzathine penicillin) is given at the intervals of 4 weeks throughout pregnancy.
- *Fetal surveillance:* Careful fetal monitoring, mainly in the form of clinical and ultrasound examinations may be required when signs of hemodynamic compromise are present.
- *Increased frequency of antenatal visits:* In general, prenatal visits should be scheduled every month in women with mild disease and every 2 weeks in women with moderate

**Table 5.53:** Characteristics of some common pathological murmurs

| Type of lesion | Location | Character | Shape | Duration | Radiation |
|---|---|---|---|---|---|
| Mitral stenosis | Mitral area | Low pitched, rough and rumbling | Plateaus with presystolic accentuation | Mid diastolic and presystolic | |
| Tricuspid stenosis | Tricuspid area | Low pitched, rumbling | Plateaus | Mid diastolic | – |
| Mitral regurgitation | Apex | High pitched | Plateaus | Holosystolic | Radiates to axilla |
| Tricuspid regurgitation | Tricuspid area | High pitched | Plateaus | Holosystolic | – |
| Ventricular septal defect | Lower left sternal border | High pitched | Plateaus | Holosystolic | Heard across the sternum |
| Aortic stenosis | First aortic area | High pitched, harsh or musical | Crescendo-decrescendo | Mid systolic | Radiates to carotids |
| Pulmonary stenosis | Pulmonary area | High pitched, harsh or musical | Crescendo-decrescendo | Mid systolic | – |
| Aortic regurgitation | Second aortic area | High pitched, blowing | Decrescendo | Early diastolic | Towards apex |
| Pulmonary regurgitation | Pulmonary area and one interspace below | High pitched, blowing | Decrescendo | Early diastolic | – |

or severe disease, until 28–30 weeks and weekly thereafter until delivery.

- *Use of antiarrhythmic medicines during pregnancy:* Pharmacologic treatment is usually reserved for patients with severe symptoms.
- *Use of anticoagulants during pregnancy:* Anticoagulants may be required in case of patients with congenital heart disease who have pulmonary hypertension, mechanical prosthetic valves or atrial fibrillation. Despite their own set of advantages and disadvantages, both heparin and warfarin are used for anticoagulation during pregnancy.
- Management must be by a multidisciplinary team.
- *Bed rest:* At least 10 hours each night and half an hour after each meal must be advised. Light house work and walking is permitted, but no heavy work must be done.
- Weight gain during pregnancy must not exceed 12 kg.
- She should be advised to avoid contact with persons who have respiratory tract infections including common colds and flu. Pneumococcal and influenza vaccines are usually recommended.
- Cigarette smoking is prohibited.
- Anemia should be treated actively during pregnancy, hemoglobin levels should be preferably kept at or above 12 g/dL throughout pregnancy.
- Risk factors which might precipitate cardiac failure need to be treated. Some of these risk factors include infections (dental infections, infections of the urinary tract, respiratory tract, etc.), anemia, hypertension, arrhythmias, hyperthyroidism, etc.

**Q. In the above-mentioned case study what should be the next line of management?**

**Ans.** This is a very tricky and controversial situation. Presence of prosthetic valves is associated with a significant risk of maternal thrombosis or thromboembolism. As previously mentioned, the two most commonly used anticoagulant drugs during pregnancy include warfarin and heparin (either unfractionated or low molecular weight). Assuming that the woman and her partner wish to proceed with the pregnancy, they should first be educated about the hazards of warfarin or heparin anticoagulation, alone or in sequence, throughout pregnancy and in the peripartum period. Whatever strategy is chosen, they should be told that neither of the strategies are perfect and may be associated with some amount of maternal or fetal risk. The parents should be counseled that while warfarin crosses the placenta and can be teratogenic, heparin is not. However, warfarin has greater efficacy than heparin in preventing an episode of thromboembolism.

One approach for obtaining effective anticoagulation is to consider using low molecular weight heparin, on a dose-adjusted basis, throughout the pregnancy. The second option would be to use heparin (either unfractionated or low molecular weight) during the first trimester instead of warfarin. This strategy appears to be useful because the risk of warfarin related embryopathy seems to be the highest with exposure between week 6 and week 12. Warfarin should again be started in the second trimester and continued until approximately 36 weeks of pregnancy. After that time, it would be appropriate to substitute heparin for warfarin leading up to labor and delivery, with resumption of warfarin after delivery.

**Q. When should the patients with heart disease preferably be admitted?**

**Ans.** The patients with class I heart disease must preferably be admitted in the hospital (tertiary health care unit) at least 2 weeks prior to the EDD. Patients with class II heart disease must be admitted at 28 weeks of gestation, particularly in cases of unfavorable social surroundings. Patients with class

III and IV heart disease must be admitted as soon as the pregnancy is diagnosed. Such patients should be monitored in the hospital settings throughout their pregnancy. Emergency admission may be required in the following cases: deterioration of the functional grading; appearance of dyspnea or cough or sudden crepitation; appearance of any pregnancy complications such as anemia, preeclampsia, etc.

### Q. What are the goals of management during labor and delivery in such patients?

**Ans.** Intrapartum care in these cases comprises of the following goals:

- The main objective of management should be to minimize any additional load on the cardiovascular system from delivery and puerperium by aiming for spontaneous onset of labor and providing effective pain relief with low-dose regional analgesia.
- Vaginal delivery over CS is the preferred mode of delivery for most women with heart disease—whether congenital or acquired.
- Cesarean section is considered only in the presence of specific obstetric or cardiac considerations.
- Positioning the patient on the left lateral side helps in reducing associated hemodynamic fluctuations.

### Q. What steps must be taken for managing the patients with class I and II heart disease during labor?

**Ans.** Steps to be taken for managing class I and II patients during labor are as follows:

- Patient must be placed in a semi-recumbent position with lateral tilt.
- Vital signs must be monitored every 15–20 minutes during the first stage and every 10 minutes during the second stage.
- Pulse rate greater than 100 beats/minute and respiratory rate greater than 24/minute may be indicative of impending heart failure. In these cases rapid digitalization is done using intravenous digoxin 0.5 mg.
- Epidural analgesia appears to be the best form of analgesia.
- Oxygen (5–6 L/minute) may be administered by face mask.
- Pulse oximetry and cardiac monitoring may be done for early detection of arrhythmias and hypoxemia.
- Intravenous fluids must be restricted to about 75 mL per hour.
- *Intrapartum antibiotic prophylaxis:* AHA guidelines (2007) do not recommend the routine use of endocarditis prophylaxis for CS delivery or for uncomplicated cases of vaginal delivery without infection. However, in developing countries prophylactic antibiotics are usually given in all cases of operative delivery and to women at increased risk, e.g. patients with rheumatic heart disease, valvular prosthesis, previous endocarditis, cardiac surgery and cyanotic heart disease. The most commonly used regimen includes intravenous ampicillin 2 g and gentamycin 1.5

mg/kg body weight (not to exceed 80 mg) at the onset of induction of labor followed by a repeat dosage at 8-hourly interval.

Such women must also be prescribed antibiotic prophylaxis (especially for *Streptococcus viridians*) before undergoing oral, dental or an upper respiratory tract procedure. In high-risk patient who can take oral medicines, 2 g of oral amoxicillin can be prescribed.

- Thromboprophylaxis may be required in patients with mitral stenosis, heart failure, valvular prosthesis and other general risk factors.
- Straining during the second stage of labor must be avoided as far as possible.
  - Outlet forceps or ventouse delivery can be used to shorten the second stage of labor. Ventouse is preferable to forceps because it can be applied without placing the patient in lithotomy position. This is especially important in these cases because raising the patient's legs is likely to increase cardiac overload.
- No bolus oxytocin must be administered because it can result in sudden hypotension. Ergot alkaloids (methergine) must also be avoided to prevent sudden overloading of the heart due to additional blood which may be squeezed out of the uterus as a result of uterine contractions due to this drug.

### Q. How should the third stage of labor be managed in these patients?

**Ans.** During the third stage of labor in women with heart disease, bolus doses of oxytocin can cause severe hypotension and should therefore be avoided. Low-dose oxytocin infusions are safer and may be equally effective. Ergometrine is best avoided in most cases as it can cause acute hypertension. Misoprostol may be safer but it can cause problems such as hyperthermia. Furosemide can be administered in cases where there is a risk of cardiac overload.

### Q. What are the indications for therapeutic termination during pregnancy?

**Ans.** Termination of pregnancy is rarely done and if required, it is usually performed within 12 weeks of gestation, preferably using suction/vacuum aspiration.

Indications for therapeutic termination of pregnancy are listed next:

*Absolute Indications*
- Primary pulmonary hypertension
- Eisenmenger's syndrome
- Pulmonary veno-occlusive disease.
- Marfan's syndrome with an abnormal aorta.
- Severe uncorrected valvular stenosis.

*Relative Indications*
- Parous women with grade III and IV cardiac lesion.
- Women having grade I or grade II cardiac lesion with previous history of cardiac failure in early pregnancy.
- History of peripartum cardiomyopathy.

**Q. What are the indications for cesarean delivery?**
**Ans.** Indications for cesarean delivery in these patients are as follows:

- Marfan's syndrome with dilated aortic root (> 4 cm)
- Aortic aneurysm/dissection
- Women with a mechanical Bjork-Shiley mitral valve who have opted for warfarin anticoagulation should also be considered for elective section to reduce the time off warfarin
- Taking warfarin within 2 weeks of labor.

**Q. What advice regarding the contraceptive method must be given to these patients?**
**Ans.** Barrier methods are safe for all cardiac patients and clearly have the added benefit of providing protection against sexually transmitted diseases. Subdermal progestogen implants and progestogen-loaded intrauterine devices are efficacious and are safe method for most women with significant heart disease. Combined oral contraceptive pills (COCPs) are relatively contraindicated in women with heart disease because the estrogen component of the combined oral contraceptive confers an increased risk of thrombosis. These women must also be educated regarding the importance of emergency contraception in case she does have an unprotected sexual intercourse. Sterilization by tubal ligation may be appropriate for women in whom pregnancy would be at high risk.

**Q. What are the various complications related to the heart disease during pregnancy?**
**Ans.** Various complications related to heart disease during pregnancy are as follows:

- *Maternal complications:* These include the following:
  - Pulmonary edema and arrhythmias.
  - Increased maternal morbidity.
  - An increased risk for cardiac complications, such as heart failure, arrhythmias and stroke.
- *Fetal complications:* These include the following:
  - IUGR (mild in cases of patients with rheumatic heart valve disease and severe in cases of lesions associated with cyanosis in the mothers).
  - Neonatal asphyxia.
  - Respiratory distress and fetal or neonatal death.

# Diabetes in Pregnancy

## Case Study 1

Mrs XYZ, a 30-year-old married for 5 years, resident of ABC, G2P1L1 with previous history of giving birth to a baby with birthweight of 4.8 kg presented for routine ANC checkup at 20 weeks. The first baby was born by normal vaginal delivery. The diagnosis of gestational diabetes was confirmed in the previous pregnancy. However, the oral glucose tolerance test (OGTT) performed at 6 weeks postpartum at the time of previous pregnancy was found to be WNL. The questions to be asked at the time of taking history and the parameters to be assessed at the time of examination in such a case are described in Tables 5.54 and 5.55 respectively.

**Q. What is the most likely diagnosis in the above-mentioned case study?**
**Ans.** Mrs XYZ, a 30-year-old married for 5 years, resident of ABC, G2P1L1 woman with amenorrhea of 20 weeks, corresponding to 20 weeks of gestation with the history of gestational diabetes in her previous pregnancy. Though the risk of gestational diabetes in this pregnancy is quite high, this needs to be confirmed by doing various investigations.

**Q. What is gestational diabetes mellitus?**
**Ans.** Gestational diabetes is defined by the WHO as "carbohydrate intolerance resulting in hyperglycemia of variable severity with onset or first recognition during pregnancy". Gestational diabetes now includes both gestational impaired glucose tolerance and gestational diabetes mellitus (GDM).

Impaired glucose tolerance or isolated abnormal plasma glucose in pregnancy can be defined as a prediabetic state of dysglycemia, characterized by insulin resistance and an increased risk of cardiovascular pathology. It is also associated with an increased incidence of lower segment cesarean section (LSCS), preeclampsia and macrosomia.

**Q. What are the likely risk factors for the development of gestational diabetes?**
**Ans.** The risk factors, which predispose a woman to develop gestational diabetes, are as follows:

- Body mass index above 30 kg/m$^2$.
- Previous history of macrosomic baby weighing 4.5 kg or above.
- Previous history of gestational diabetes.
- Family history of diabetes.
- Ethnic origin with a high prevalence of diabetes (e.g. South Asian, Middle Eastern, etc.).
- Previous history of unexplained perinatal loss.
- Presence of polyhydramnios or recurrent vaginal candidiasis in the present pregnancy
- Persistent glycosuria
- Age over 30 years
- History of previous stillbirth with pancreatic islet hyperplasia on autopsy

**Q. What is the screening test for gestational diabetes mellitus? How is it performed?**
**Ans.** Glucose challenge test (GCT) is a screening test for gestational diabetes, in which plasma blood glucose levels are measured 1 hour after giving a 50 g glucose load to the woman, irrespective of the time of the day or last meals. It is not necessary for the woman to follow a special diet

**Table 5.54:** Symptoms to be elicited at the time of taking history in a case of gestational diabetes

*History of Presenting Complains*
- History of polyuria (increased frequency of micturition), polydipsia (increased amount of thirst) and polyphagia (increased appetite).
- Age over 30 years is associated with high risk for gestational diabetes
- Ethnic origin with a high prevalence of diabetes (e.g. South Asian, Middle Eastern, etc.) is also another risk factor for diabetes.

*Medical History*
- Is she a known diabetic?
- If yes, since how long?
- What kind of therapy has she been taking for controlling her blood sugar levels?
- Had she been monitoring her blood glucose levels?
- What was her last blood glucose level?
- Have her blood glucose levels been fluctuating?
- Have there been any complications related to diabetes [cardiomyopathy (history suggestive of complaints related to the cardiovascular system), retinopathy (history suggestive of any complaints pertaining to the eyes), nephropathy (history suggestive of renal complaints), etc.
- Attacks of fainting (hypoglycemia).
- History of excessive vaginal discharge (with or without pruritis), history suggestive of recurrent infection of the urinary tract.
- Past history of chronic hypertension.

*Obstetric History*
- History suggestive of hyperemesis gravidarum, excessive abdominal distension (suggestive of polyhydramnios) in the present pregnancy.
- Previous history of macrosomic baby weighing 4.5 kg or above.
- Previous history of gestational diabetes.
- Previous unexplained perinatal loss.
- History of previous stillbirth with pancreatic islet hyperplasia on autopsy
- Presence of polyhydramnios or recurrent vaginal candidiasis in the present pregnancy.
- Persistent glycosuria in the present pregnancy.

*Family History*
- Family history of diabetes.

*Dietary History*
Dietary history is to be taken in great details especially if she is a known diabetic and is taking insulin's or oral hypoglycemic drugs.

**Table 5.55:** Various findings elicited at the time of clinical examination in a case of gestational diabetes

*General Physical Examination*
There are no specific findings related to gestational diabetes on general physical examination.
- *BMI:* Body mass index above 30 kg/m$^2$ acts as a risk factor for the development of gestational diabetes.
- Presence of pedal edema (could be related to preeclampsia or be a normal physiological change related to pregnancy).
- Lymphadenopathy.
- Signs suggestive of preeclampsia must be looked for as the women with GDM are especially prone to develop preeclampsia. There also may be the presence of underlying hypertension.

*Specific Systemic Examination*
*Abdominal Examination*
Women with GDM are especially prone to develop polyhydramnios. Some signs suggestive of polyhydramnios on abdominal examination are as follows:
- Abdomen is markedly enlarged along with fullness of flanks. The skin of the abdominal wall appears to be tense, shiny and may show appearance of large stria.
- The patients have a fundal height greater than the period of amenorrhea and fetal parts may not be easily palpable.
- Fetal heart sounds may appear muffled as if coming from a distance.
- A fluid thrill may be commonly present.
- It may be difficult to palpate the uterus or the fetal presenting parts due to presence of excessive fluid.
  - Since women with GDM are prone to develop macrosomic or intrauterine growth restriction (IUGR) fetuses, signs for both these features must be observed on clinical abdominal examination. Macrosomic fetus is suggested in case expected fetal weight on Leopold's maneuver appears to be more than 4.0 kg. (However, estimation of fetal weight on Leopold's maneuver has been observed to be grossly inaccurate).

*Per Speculum Examination*
- Evidence of discharge indicative of candiadiasis.
- Look for any premature opening of the cervical os.

*Abbreviation:* GDM, gestational diabetes mellitus

before test or to be in the fasting stage. The timing for this test depends on the woman's likely risk of developing gestational diabetes during her pregnancy. This test need not be routinely performed in women at low risk for diabetes, must be performed at 24–28 weeks in women with average risk of diabetes and as soon as possible in women at high risk for diabetes (Table 5.56). A value of 140 mg/dL or higher indicates high risk for development of gestational diabetes. An abnormal result on GCT must be followed by a 100-g OGTT.

### Q. What is oral glucose tolerance test?

**Ans.** An abnormal result on GCT should be followed by an OGTT. This test involves measurement of blood glucose levels at fixed time intervals following the intake of prefixed quantities of glucose. While a 100-g, 3-hour OGTT is a standard in the United States, in the United Kingdom a 75-g, 2-hour OGTT is preferred. If the 100-g 3-hour OGTT is used, the diagnosis can be made either using the Carpenter and Coustan criteria (Table 5.57) or criteria defined by the National Diabetes Data Group (Table 5.58). On the other hand, if the 2-hour 75-g OGTT is used, the diagnosis can be made using the criteria defined by the WHO (Table 5.59) or the criteria by the ADA (Table 5.60). A 75-g OGTT is performed in the morning after the patient has had at least 3 days of unrestricted diet comprising of greater than 150 g of carbohydrates. Firstly, a fasting blood sample, i.e. the patient had no caloric intake for at least 8–14 hours, is taken. Following this, the patient is advised to drink 75-g of anhydrous glucose in 150–300 mL of water over the course of 5 minutes. The second blood sample is taken 2 hours following the glucose load. Measurement of venous glucose levels is usually recommended. If one or more of these values on the WHO OGTT are abnormal, the patient has gestational diabetes.

**Q. What should be the steps for management of diabetic patients during the antenatal period?**
**Ans.** The following steps must be taken for the management of diabetic patients during the antenatal period:

- *Diabetes education and information:* Education and information regarding diabetes, hypoglycemia, self-monitoring of blood glucose levels, etc. needs to be provided to the patient.
- *Diet:* In woman with BMI within the normal range, the recommended calorie intake is about 2,000–2,500 Kcal/day. Total calorie intake must be restricted to 1,200–1,800 Kcal/day for overweight women.
- *Exercise program:* A daily exercise program in the form of brisk walking, aerobic exercises, etc. are safe in pregnancy and may help in avoiding the requirement for insulin therapy during pregnancy.
- *Maintenance of blood glucose levels:* This can be done with the help of monthly measurement of the glycosylated hemoglobin levels and self-monitoring of blood glucose levels using a glucose meter.

**Table 5.56:** Timing for glucose challenge test based on the woman's likely risk of developing gestational diabetes during pregnancy

| Low risk | Average risk | High risk |
|---|---|---|
| • Member of an ethnic group with a low prevalence of gestational diabetes mellitus (GDM) <br> • No known history of diabetes in first degree relatives <br> • Age < 25 years <br> • Normal weight before pregnancy <br> • No history of abnormal glucose metabolism <br> • No previous history of poor obstetrical outcome | • Member of an ethnic group with a high prevalence of GDM <br> • Overweight before pregnancy <br> • Diabetes in first degree relatives <br> • Age > 25 years | • Marked obesity <br> • Strong family history of type 2 diabetes mellitus <br> • Previous history of GDM, impaired glucose metabolism or glucosuria <br> • Previous history of giving birth to an infant with macrosomia |
| *Blood glucose screening not routinely required* | *Blood glucose testing at 24–28 weeks (one- or two-step procedure)* | *Perform glucose testing as soon as possible* |

*Source:* Metzger BE, Coustan DR. Summary and recommendations of the fourth internal workshop-conference on gestational diabetes mellitus. Diabetes Care. 1998;21(2):B161-7.

**Table 5.57:** 100 g glucose load by O'Sullivan and Mahan: criteria modified by Carpenter and Coustan

| Status | Plasma/serum glucose (mmol/liter) | Plasma/serum glucose levels (mg/dL) |
|---|---|---|
| Fasting | ≥ 5.8 | 95 |
| 1 hour | ≥ 10.0 | 180 |
| 2 hour | ≥ 9.1 | 155 |
| 3 hour | ≥ 8.0 | 140 |

*Source*: Carpenter MW and Coustan DR. Criteria for screening tests for gestational diabetes. Am J Obstet Gynecol. 1982;144:768-73.

**Table 5.58:** National Diabetes Data Group criteria for 100 gm OGTT

| Status | Plasma/serum glucose levels (mmol/liter) | Plasma/serum glucose levels (mg/dL) |
|---|---|---|
| Fasting | ≥ 5.3 | 105 |
| 1 hour | ≥ 10.0 | 190 |
| 2 hour | ≥ 8.6 | 165 |
| 3 hour | ≥ 7.8 | 145 |

*Source*: National Diabetes Data Group. Classification and diagnosis of diabetes mellitus and other categories of glucose intolerance. Diabetes. 1979;28:1039-57.

**Table 5.59:** World Health Organization criteria for 75-g oral glucose tolerance test

| Status | Whole blood venous | Whole blood capillary | Plasma venous | Plasma capillary |
|---|---|---|---|---|
| Fasting | ≥ 6.1 mmol/L | ≥ 6.1 mmol/L | ≥ 7.0 mmol/L (126 mg/dL) | ≥ 7.0 mmol/L |
| 2-hour | ≥ 6.7 mmol/L | ≥ 6.7 mmol/L | ≥ 7.8 mmol/L (140 mg/dL) | ≥ 8.9 mmol/L |

*Source:* WHO consultation: Definition, diagnosis and classification of diabetes mellitus and its complications: Report of a WHO consultation. Part I: Diagnosis and classification of diabetes mellitus. World Health Organization, Geneva; 1999.

**Table 5.60:** American Diabetes Association criteria for 75-g oral glucose tolerance test

| Status | Plasma venous/ serum glucose levels (mg/dL) | Plasma venous/ serum glucose levels (mmol/L) |
|---|---|---|
| Fasting | ≥ 95 mg/dL | 5.25 mmol/L |
| 1-hour | ≥180 mg/dL | 10.00 mmol/L |
| 2-hour | ≥153 mg/dL | 8.50 mmol/L |

*Source:* American Diabetes Association. Standards of medical care in diabetes—2013. Diabetes Care. 2013;36(Suppl 1):S11-S66.

- *Requirement for hypoglycemic therapy:* In case of previously diabetic women, oral diabetes medication needs to be changed to insulin. In case of women with gestational diabetes, initial control of blood glucose levels must be through exercise and nutritional advice. If these options do not work, insulin may be advised. The objective of the antidiabetic treatment is to maintain the fasting capillary glucose values under 95 mg/dL and 1 or 2 hour postprandial values under 140 mg/dL and 120 mg/dL respectively. The aim should be to maintain her HbA1c levels below 7.0% and glucose levels within 4–7 mmol/liter.
- *Maintenance of adequate body weight:* Women with diabetes who are planning to become pregnant and who have a BMI above 27 kg/m$^2$ should be offered advice on how to lose weight.
- *Regular intake of folic acid:* Women with diabetes who are planning to become pregnant should be advised to take folic acid in the dose of 5 mg/day, starting right from the periconceptional period and extending throughout the period of gestation.
- *Insulin therapy:* Insulin therapy may include regular insulin, or rapid-acting insulin analogs (aspart and lispro). During pregnancy, women are usually prescribed 4-daily insulin injections (3 injections of regular insulin to be taken before each meal and one injection of isophane insulin to be taken at night time).
- *Fetal monitoring:* These include tests, such as DFMC, NST, fetal BPP and monthly ultrasound scans for estimation of fetal weight starting at 32–36 weeks of gestation.
- *Screening for congenital malformations:* First trimester ultrasound scan at 11–13 weeks must be done to measure the nuchal translucency as there is an increased risk of neural tube defects. Maternal serum screening for α-fetal proteins at 16–18 weeks must be done to rule out the risk for neural tube defects. Second trimester ultrasound scan for detailed scanning of fetal congenital anomalies must be performed at 18–20 weeks.

### Q. When should such patients be delivered?

**Ans.** Low-risk women may be allowed to develop spontaneous labor and to deliver by 38–40 weeks of gestation. High-risk gestational diabetic patients should have their labor induced when they reach 38 weeks. Diabetes should not in itself be considered a contraindication for attempting VBAC. The ACOG recommends an elective CS in women with sonographically estimated fetal weight of 4.5 kg.

### Q. How should such patients be managed during the intrapartum period?

**Ans.** The two main goals of intrapartum management include avoidance of shoulder dystocia and maintenance of blood glucose levels. Management during the intrapartum period comprises of the following steps:

- During the time of labor and birth, capillary blood glucose should be monitored on an hourly basis in women with diabetes and maintained at levels between 4 mmol/liter and 7 mmol/liter by using intravenous dextrose and insulin infusion.
- Babies born with gestational diabetes are particularly at risk of developing neonatal hypoglycemia. Early feeding of the neonate is recommended for reducing the risk of neonatal hypoglycemia.
- A pediatrician must be present at the time of baby's delivery. The clinician must be well-versed with the management of shoulder dystocia.
- Beta mimetic drugs should not be used for tocolysis in women with diabetes due to the tendency of betamimetics to cause hyperglycemia and ketoacidosis. Tocolytic agents of choice in these cases are nifedipine and magnesium sulfate.
- Delivery should be by the vaginal route unless there are obstetric contraindications.
- Since fetal distress is more common in diabetic women, continuous external or internal cardiotocographic monitoring is required at the time of labor. Fetal scalp blood may also be analyzed in case of nonreassuring fetal heart trace.
- Capillary blood glucose levels must be checked frequently using finger stick at every 1–2 hourly intervals and regular insulin must be administered accordingly to maintain the glucose concentration in the target range of 4.0–8.0 mmol/L.

### Q. What steps can be taken for management of neonatal hypoglycemia?

**Ans.** Development of hypoglycemia (i.e. blood glucose less than 2.6 mmol/L or less than 40 mg/dL) in the babies of diabetic mothers is a major concern. In a woman with gestational diabetes, placental transfer of glucose to the baby may occur. This is likely to result in the development of fetal hyperinsulinemia, which through various mechanisms may eventually result in the development of fetal hypoglycemia. The following steps need to be taken for its management:

- Blood glucose testing should be carried out routinely at birth in babies of women with diabetes. This should be repeated at every 2–4 hours intervals.

- Early breastfeeding must be encouraged.
- These babies should be fed as soon as possible after birth (within 30 minutes) and then at frequent intervals (every 2–3 hours) in order to maintain blood glucose concentration of at least 2.0 mmol/L.

### Q. What are the indications for cesarean delivery in these cases?

**Ans.** Some of the indications for cesarean delivery in these cases are enumerated as follows:

- Expected fetal weight greater than 4.5 kg.
- Previous history of shoulder dystocia/stillbirths.
- Presence of other obstetric indications for cesarean delivery.

### Q. What are the various complications related to diabetes during pregnancy?

**Ans.** Diabetes in pregnancy is associated with numerous risks to the mother and the developing fetus, which are as follows:

*Maternal Complications*

- Miscarriage.
- Preeclampsia.
- Preterm labor
- Prolonged labor.
- Polyhydramnios (could be associated with fetal polyuria).
- About 35–50% risk of developing type 2 diabetes later in the life.
- Increased risk of traumatic damage during labor.
- Increased risk of shoulder dystocia.
- Diabetic retinopathy and nephropathy can worsen rapidly during pregnancy.

*Fetal Complications*

- Fetal distress and birth asphyxia.
- Brachial plexus injuries.
- Macrosomia (birthweight more than 4 kg).
- Increased risk for perinatal death, birth trauma and rates of CS.
- Cephalohematoma, resulting in more pronounced neonatal jaundice.
- Stillbirth, congenital malformations, macrosomia, birth injury, perinatal mortality.
- Hypoxia and sudden intrauterine death after 36 weeks of gestation.
- Congenital malformations (caudal regression sequence; congenital heart diseases; GI abnormalities; renal defects; neural tube defects; cystic fibrosis, etc.).
- Fetal/neonatal hypoglycemia, polycythemia, hyperbilirubinemia and renal vein thrombosis.
- An increased long-term risk of obesity and diabetes in the child.

## FURTHER READINGS


1. Bonow RO, Carabello BA, Chatterjee K, et al. 2008 Focused update incorporated into the ACC/AHA 2006 guidelines for the management of patients with valvular heart disease: a report of the American College of Cardiology/American Heart Association Task Force on Practice Guidelines (Writing Committee to Revise the 1998 Guidelines for the Management of Patients With Valvular Heart Disease): endorsed by the Society of Cardiovascular Anesthesiologists, Society for Cardiovascular Angiography and Interventions, and Society of Thoracic Surgeons. Circulation. 2008;118(15):e523-661
2. Society for Maternal Fetal Medicine Publications Committee. ACOG Committee Opinion number 419 October 2008 (replaces no. 291, November 2003). Use of progesterone to reduce preterm birth. Obstet Gynecol. 2008;112(4):963-5.
3. ACOG Practice Bulletin No. 102: management of stillbirth. Obstet Gynecol. 2009;113(3):748-61.
4. ACOG Committee on Practice Bulletins-Obstetrics. ACOG Practice Bulletin. Clinical management guidelines for obstetricians-gynecologists. Number 55, September 2004 (replaces practice pattern number 6, October 1997). Management of Postterm Pregnancy. Obstet Gynecol. 2004; 104(3):639-46.
5. ACOG Technical Bulletin. Diagnosis and management of fetal death. Int J Obstet Gynecol. 1998;42:291-9.
6. ACOG Committee on Obstetric Practice. ACOG practice bulletin. Diagnosis and management of preeclampsia and eclampsia. Number 33, January 2002. American College of Obstetricians and Gynecologists. Int J Gynaecol Obstet. 2002;77(1):67-75.
7. American College of Obstetricians and Gynecologists. ACOG Practice bulletin no. 115: Vaginal birth after previous cesarean delivery. Obstet Gynecol. 2010;116(2 Pt 1):450-63.
8. American College of Obstetricians and Gynecologists Committee on Practice Bulletins--Obstetrics. ACOG Practice Bulletin. Clinical management guidelines for obstetrician-gynecologists. Number 30, September 2001 (replaces Technical Bulletin Number 200, December 1994). Gestational diabetes. Obstet Gynecol. 2001;98(3):525-38.
9. Committee on Obstetric Practice. ACOG Committee Opinion No. 435: postpartum screening for abnormal glucose tolerance in women who had gestational diabetes mellitus. Obstet Gynecol. 2009;113(6):1419-21.
10. American College of Obstetricians and Gynecologists. ACOG practice bulletin. Management of recurrent pregnancy loss. Number 24, February 2001. (Replaces Technical Bulletin Number 212, September 1995). American College of Obstetricians and Gynecologists. Int J Gynaecol Obstet. 2002;78(2):179-90.
11. American College of Obstetricians and Gynecologists. ACOG Guidelines on Premature Rupture of Membranes. Am Fam Physician. 2008;77(2):245-6.
12. American College of Obstetricians and Gynecologists. ACOG Practice Bulletin. Assessment of risk factors for preterm birth. Clinical management guidelines for obstetrician-gynecologists. Number 31, October 2001. (Replaces Technical Bulletin number 206, June 1995; Committee Opinion number 172, May 1996; Committee Opinion number 187, September 1997; Committee Opinion number 198, February 1998; and Committee Opinion number 251, January 2001). Obstet Gynecol. 2001;98(4):709-16.
13. American College of Obstetricians and Gynecologists. Postpartum hemorrhage. ACOG Educational Bulletin 1998; Number 243. In 2001 Compendium of selected publications.
14. ACOG practice bulletin. Prevention of Rh D alloimmunization. Number 4, May 1999 (replaces educational bulletin Number 147, October 1990). Clinical management guidelines for

obstetrician-gynecologists. American College of Obstetrics and Gynecology. Int J Gynaecol Obstet. 1999;66(1):63-70.

15. American Diabetes Association: Clinical practice recommendations 1999. Diabetes Care. 1999;22 (Suppl 1): S1-114.

16. American Diabetes Association: Gestational diabetes mellitus. Diabetes Care. 2003;26 (Suppl 1):S103-5.

17. American Diabetes Association: Gestational diabetes mellitus. Diabetes Care. 2004;27 (suppl 1):S88-90.

18. American Diabetes Association: Report of the expert committee on the diagnosis and classification of diabetes mellitus. Diabetes Care. 2004;27:5.

19. American Diabetes Association. Standards of medical care in diabetes 2013. Diabetes Care. 2013;36 (Suppl 1):S11-66.

20. Carpenter MW, Coustan DR. Criteria for screening tests for gestational diabetes. Am J Obstet Gynecol. 1982;144(7):768-73.

21. Centers for Disease Control and Prevention. Recommendations to prevent and control iron deficiency in the United States. MMWR. 1998;47(No. RR-3):51 [online] Available from www. cdc. gov/ [Accessed November, 2014].

22. Centre for Maternal and Child Enquiries (CMACE). Saving Mothers' Lives: reviewing maternal deaths to make motherhood safer: 2006–08. The Eighth Report on Confidential Enquiries into Maternal Deaths in the United Kingdom. BJOG. 2011;118 (Suppl 1):1-203.

23. Committee on Obstetric Practice. Committee Opinion no. 514: emergent therapy for acute-onset, severe hypertension with preeclampsia or eclampsia. Obstet Gynecol. 2011;118(6):1465-8.

24. Department of Health. National Service Framework for Diabetes: Standards. London: Department of Health; 2002.

25. Department of Health. Why Mothers Die: Report on Confidential Enquiries into Maternal Deaths in the United Kingdom 2000–2002 Triennial Report. London: RCOG Press; 2004. pp. 94-103.

26. Duley L, Henderson-Smart D. Magnesium sulfate versus diazepam for eclampsia. Cochrane Database Syst Rev. 2000;(2):CD000127.

27. Duley L, Henderson-Smart D. Magnesium sulfate versus diazepam for eclampsia (Cochrane Review). Cochrane Database Syst Rev. 2003;(4):CD000127.

28. Duley L, Henderson-Smart D. Magnesium sulfate versus phenytoin for eclampsia (Cochrane Review). Cochrane Database Syst Rev. 2003;(4):CD000128.

29. Duley L, Henderson-Smart DJ, Meher S. Drugs for treatment of very high blood pressure during pregnancy. Cochrane Database Syst Rev. 2006;3:CD001449.

30. Eclampsia Trial Collaborative Group. Which anticonvulsant for women with eclampsia? Evidence from the collaborative eclampsia trial. Lancet. 1995;345(8963):1455-63.

31. Federation International of Obstetrics and Gynecology (2012). FIGO Misoprostol for post-partum haemorrhage in low resource settings initiative. [online] Available from www. figo. org/projects/misoprostol [Accessed November, 2014].

32. Hannah ME, Hannah WJ, Hewson SA, et al. Planned caesarean section versus planned vaginal birth for breech presentation at term: a randomised multicentre trial. Term Breech Trial Collaborative Group. Lancet. 2000;356(9239):1375-83.

33. International Confederation of Midwives, International Federation of Gynecology and Obstetrics; Society of Obstetricians and Gynaecologists of Canada. Management of the third stage of labour to prevent postpartum hemorrhage. J Obstet Gynaecol Can. 2003;25(11):952-3.

34. Liabsuetrakul T, Choobun T, Peeyananjarassri K, et al. Prophylactic use of ergot alkaloids in the third stage of labour. Cochrane Database Syst Rev. 2007;18(2):CD:005456.

35. Lowe SA, Brown MA, Dekker GA, et al. Society of Obstetric Medicine of Australia and New Zealand. Guidelines for the management of hypertensive disorders of pregnancy 2008. Aust N Z J Obstet Gynaecol. 2009;49(3):242-6.

36. Magee L, Sadeghi S. Prevention and treatment of postpartum hypertension. Cochrane Database Syst Rev. 2005;1:CD004351.

37. National High Blood Pressure Education Program. The seventh report of the Joint National Committee on prevention, detection, evaluation, and treatment of high blood pressure. Bethesda (MD): Dept. of Health and Human Services, National Institutes of Health, National Heart, Lung, and Blood Institute; 2004. NIH Publication No. 04-5230.

38. Ministry of Health and Family Welfare (Government of India, 2013). Guidelines for control of iron deficiency anemia. [Online] Available from www.unicef.org/india/10._National_Iron_Plus_Initiative_Guidelines_for_Control_of_IDA.pdf [Accessed November, 2014].

39. National Collaborating Centre for Women's and Children's Health guidelines. London: RCOG Press; 2004.

40. Classification and diagnosis of diabetes mellitus and other categories of glucose intolerance. National Diabetes Data Group. Diabetes. 1979;28(12):1039-57.

41. National high blood pressure education programme: Working group report on high blood pressure in pregnancy. Am J Obstet Gynecol. 2000;183(1):S1-22.

42. National Institute for Health and Clinical Excellence. Diabetes in pregnancy: Management of diabetes and its complications from preconception to the postnatal period. London: RCOG Press; 2008.

43. National Institute of Health and Care Excellence. Hypertension in Pregnancy: The Management of Hypertensive Disorders During Pregnancy (NICE clinical guideline 107). London: RCOG press; 2011.

44. Neilson JP, Hickey M, Vazquez J. Medical treatment for early fetal death (less than 24 weeks). Cochrane Database Syst Rev. 2006;(3):CD002253.

45. Pedersen J, Pedersen LM. Prognosis of the outcome of pregnancy in diabetes. A new classification. Acta Endocrinol. 1965;50(1):70-8.

46. Practice Committee for the American Society for Reproductive Medicine. Definitions of infertility and recurrent pregnancy loss. Fertil Steril. 2008;89(6):1603.

47. RCOG. Green Top Guideline No. 17. The Investigation and Treatment of Couples with Recurrent Miscarriage. Revised April 2011. [online] Available from www.rcog.org.uk/ resources/ Public/pdf/Recurrent_Miscarriage_ No17.pdf [Accessed November, 2014].

48. Ressel G, American College of Obstetricians and Gynecologists. ACOG issues recommendations on assessment of risk factors for preterm birth. Am Fam Physician. 2002;65(3):509-10.

49. Royal College of Clinicians and Gynaecologists (RCOG). External cephalic version and reducing the incidence of breech presentation. London (UK): Royal College of Clinicians and Gynaecologists; 2006. p. 8 (Green-top guideline; no. 20a).

50. Royal College of Obstetricians and Gynaecologists (RCOG). Birth after previous caesarean birth. London (UK): Royal College of Obstetricians and Gynaecologists (RCOG); 2007. p. 17. (Green-top guideline; no. 45).

51. Royal College of Obstetricians and Gynaecologists. (2002). The investigation and management of the small-for-gestational-age fetus. Guideline No. 31. [online] Available from www.gestation. net/RCOG%20Small_Gest_Age_Fetus_No31. pdf. [Accessed November, 2014].

52. Royal College of Obstetricians and Gynaecologists. RCOG Green-top Guideline No. 1b. Tocolysis for women in preterm labor. London: RCOG Press; 2002.

53. Royal College of Obstetricians and Gynaecologists. Placenta previa and placenta previa accreta: Diagnosis and management. Guideline No. 27. Revised October 2005.

54. Royal College of Obstetricians and Gynaecologists. Prevention of postpartum haemorrhage. Clinical Guideline no 52. London: RCOG Press; 2009.

55. Royal College of Obstetricians and Gynaecologists. The Investigation and Treatment of Couples with Recurrent Miscarriage. Guideline No. 17. London: RCOG Press; 2003.

56. Royal College of Obstetricians and Gynaecologists. The Management of Early Pregnancy Loss. Guideline No. 25. London: RCOG Press; 2006.

57. Royal College of Obstetricians and Gynaecologists. The management of severe preeclampsia and eclampsia. Green Top Guidleine No.10A. London: RCOG Press; 2006.

58. Royal College of Obstetricians and Gynecologists. (Nov, 2006). Preterm Prelabour Rupture of Membranes Guideline No 44. [online] Available from www.neonatalformulary.com/pdfs/uk_ guidelines/AMPICILLIN-RCOG_guideline_ on_PPROM.pdf [Accessed October, 2013].

59. Royal college of Obstetricians and Gynecologists. The Use of Anti-D Immunoglobulin for Rhesus D Prophylaxis. Green-top Guideline No. 22. 2011.

60. Scottish Executive Committee of the RCOG (2000). Scottish Obstetric Guidelines and Audit Project. The Management of Postpartum Hemorrhage. [online] Available from www. nhshealthquality.org/nhsqis/ files/MATERNITYSERVICES_ Postpartum Haemorrage_SPCERH6_JUN98.pdf. [Accessed November, 2014]

61. Shakur H, Elbourne D, Gülmezoglu M, et al. The WOMAN Trial (World Maternal Antifibrinolytic Trial): tranexamic acid for the treatment of postpartum haemorrhage: an international randomised, double blind placebo controlled trial. Trials. 2010;11:40.

62. ACOG Committee on Practice Bulletins—Obstetrics. ACOG practice bulletin. Management of preterm labor. Number 43, May 2003. Int J Gynaecol Obstet. 2003;82(1):127-35.

63. Society of Obstetricians and Gynecologists of Canada. (2007). SOGC clinical practice guideline: Prenatal screening for fetal aneuploidy. [online] Available from http://www.sogc.org/ guidelines/public/187E-CPG-February2007[1].pdf. [Accessed November, 2014].

64. Clinical Practice Obstetrics Committee, Maternal Fetal Medicine Committee, Delaney M, et al. Guidelines for the Management of Pregnancy at 41+0 to 42+0 Weeks. J Obstet Gynaecol Can. 2008;30(9):800-23.

65. SOGC clinical practice guideline. Diagnosis and Management of Placenta Previa. No. 189. 2007.

66. The Reproductive Health Access Project. First trimester bleeding algorithm. [online] Available from www.reproductiveaccess. org/m_m/downloads/First_trimester_bleeding_algorithm.pdf. [Accessed November, 2014].

67. US Department of Health and Human Services, Centers for Disease Control and Prevention, National Center for Health Statistics. Procedures for coding cause of fetal death under ICD-10. 2005.

68. Women's Hospitals Australasia. Management of Early Pregnancy Loss Clinical practice guidelines. March 2008. [online] Available from www.clinicalguidelines.gov.au/browse. php?treePath=&p ageType=2&fldglrID=1281& [Accessed November, 2013].

69. World Health Organization (2006). International statistical classification of diseases and related health problems, Tenth revision (ICD-10). Geneva, Switzerland.

70. American College of Cardiology, American Heart Association Task Force on Practice Guidelines. ACC/AHA 2006 guidelines for the management of patients with valvular heart disease: a report of the American College of Cardiology/American Heart Association Task Force on Practice Guidelines (writing Committee to Revise the 1998 guidelines for the management of patients with valvular heart disease) developed in collaboration with the Society of Cardiovascular Anesthesiologists endorsed by the Society for Cardiovascular Angiography and Interventions and the Society of Thoracic Surgeons. J Am Coll Cardiol. 2006;48(3):e1-148.

71. De Swiet M. Cardiac disease. In: Lewis G, Drife J, (Eds). Why mothers ie 1997–1999. The Confidential enquiries into maternal deaths in the United Kingdom. London: RCOG. 2001. pp. 153-64.

72. Cantwell R, Clutton-Brock T, Cooper G, et al. Saving Mothers' Lives: Reviewing maternal deaths to make motherhood safer: 2006-2008. The Eighth Report of the Confidential Enquiries into Maternal Deaths in the United Kingdom. BJOG. 2011;118 (suppl 1):1-203.

# CHAPTER

# Routine Labor Room Procedures



## Obstetric Forceps

Vaginal instrumental delivery involves the use of either forceps or vacuum to facilitate the delivery of fetal head. Both the types of assisted vaginal deliveries aid the delivery of fetal head through application of manual traction (forceps) or suction force (vacuum cup). Although, the most important function of forceps is application of traction, they also prove useful for rotating the fetal head, particularly those lying in the occiput transverse or occiput posterior positions. The force produced by the forceps on fetal skull is a complex function of the strength of pull and compression exerted by the forceps and friction produced by maternal tissues. It is impossible to determine the exact amount of force exerted by the forceps for an individual patient.

### Indications for Application of Forceps

Indications for application of forceps are as follows:

#### Maternal Indications

- *Cutting short the second stage of labor:* This may be required in case of conditions which are threatening to the mother (severe preeclampsia, severe bleeding, cardiac or pulmonary disease, history of spontaneous pneumothorax, chorioamnionitis, acute pulmonary edema, etc.).
- *Prolonged second stage:* If the second stage of labor is too prolonged, it requires to be terminated. Prolonged second stage of labor has been described by Friedman, as nulliparous woman, who fail to deliver after 3 hours with and 2 hours without regional anesthesia. It also includes multiparous woman, who fails to deliver even after 2 hours with or 1 hour without regional anesthesia. Prolonged second stage of labor may be related to inadequate uterine contractions, ineffective maternal efforts, etc.
- Malrotation of fetal head (e.g. occiput posterior position), perineal rigidity, epidural analgesia, etc.
- *When maternal efforts fail to effect delivery:* For example, maternal exhaustion.

#### Fetal Indications

- *Fetal distress:* Suspicion of immediate or potential fetal compromise in the second stage of labor, in the form of nonreassuring fetal heart sounds on continuous cardiotocographic trace (particularly fetal heart decelerations with reduced or absent variability) could be indicative of fetal distress. This may be related to conditions, such as fetal umbilical cord prolapse, premature separation of placenta, etc. While forceps are usually used for speeding up the delivery, occasionally they can also be used for slowing down delivery, for example while delivering the after-coming head of the breech.
- *Fetal malposition:* In the hands of an experienced surgeon, fetal malpositions, such as the after-coming head in breech vaginal delivery and occipitoposterior positions can be indications for forceps delivery.

Presently there is no evidence regarding the beneficial use of prophylactic forceps application in otherwise normal term labor and delivery.

## SURGICAL EQUIPMENT USED

### Forceps

Forceps are instruments, which help in the delivery of the fetus, by applying traction to the fetal head. The credit for the invention of the precursor of the modern forceps, which is presently used for the delivery of live infants, goes to Peter Chamberlen of England (1600 c). Modifications in the forceps design have led to the development of more than 700 different types and shapes of forceps. Presently, the use of forceps has reduced considerably in the clinical practice due to an improvement in the fetal monitoring and surveillance techniques. Many different types of forceps are being used at different centers (Fig. 6.1A). Wrigley's forceps are most commonly used for outlet forceps delivery (Fig. 6.1B), whereas Keilland's forceps are commonly used for the rotation of fetal head (Fig. 6.1C). Another type of forceps commonly used is the Piper forceps (Fig. 6.1D), which is used for the delivery of the after-coming head in cases of breech vaginal deliveries. Use of Piper's forceps helps in reducing traction on the fetal neck during breech vaginal delivery.

### Different Types of Forceps

Different types of forceps commonly used in the clinical setup are described below:

*Wrigley's forceps:* Wrigley's forceps is designed for use when the head is on the perineum and local anesthesia is being used. It is a short light instrument, having a slight pelvic and marked cephalic curves and an English lock. The size of this forceps is small due to reduced length of the shanks and the handle.

*Kielland's forceps:* The Kielland's forceps were introduced in 1915 by Dr Christian Kielland. This forceps was originally designed to facilitate rotation and extraction of the fetal head, arrested in the deep transverse or occipitoposterior position. In order to achieve this objective, this instrument has been designed with several significant modifications, which help in differentiating it from the classic forceps. Some of these are:
- The blades of Kielland's forceps have only a slight pelvic curve. The minimal pelvic curve of the blades enables the operator to safely rotate the forceps blade inside the vaginal canal. The anterior (superior) blade is applied first.
- The shanks of the forceps blades are overlapping and joined by a sliding lock in comparison to the English lock, which is present in most classical forceps.
- The knobs on the finger grips of the forceps handle help in identifying the anterior surface of the instrument.

*Piper's forceps:* Piper's forceps was introduced by Dr Edmund B Piper in 1924. This forceps was designed to facilitate delivery of the after-coming fetal head in breech deliveries. Piper's forceps (Fig. 6.1D) have long shanks with a backwards curve.

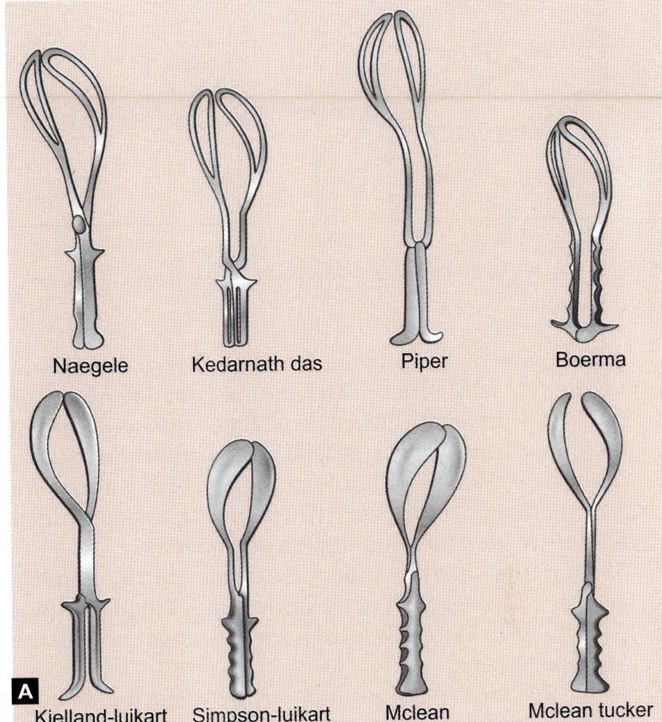


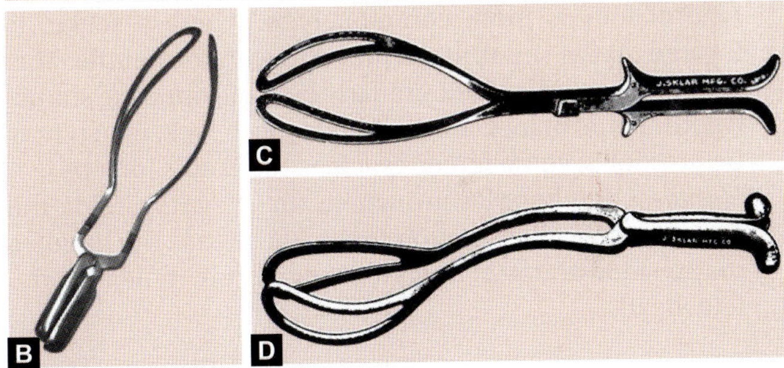


**Figs 6.1A to D:** (A) Different types of forceps used in clinical practice; (B) Wrigley's forceps: most commonly used outlet forceps; (C) Keilland's forceps: used for rotation of fetal head; (D) Piper's forceps: used for the delivery of the after-coming head of the breech

This causes the handles to fall below the level of the blades, which help the surgeon to directly apply the forceps blades to the baby's after-coming head, without the necessity of elevating the baby's body above the horizontal.

### Parts of Forceps

Forceps are composed of two branches, each of which has four major components: blades, shank, lock and handle (Fig 6.2). Each of these are described as follows:
- *Blades:* The blades help in grasping the fetus and have two curves, the pelvic curve and the cephalic curve. While the pelvic curve corresponds to the axis of birth canal, the cephalic curve conforms to the shape of fetal head.

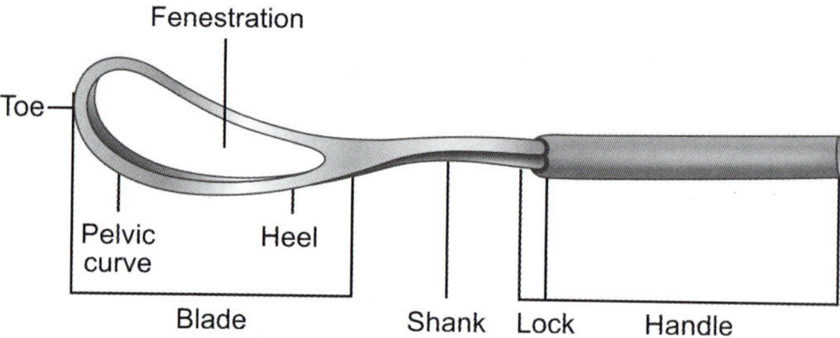



**Fig. 6.2:** Different components of a forceps

The forceps blades may be fenestrated (e.g. Simpson's, Wrigley's); solid (Tucker McLane) or pseudofenestrated (Luikart's forceps). Presence of fenestrations helps in providing firmer grip of the fetal head. Fenestrated blades are best used for providing traction; solid blades are useful for rotational purposes, whereas pseudofenestrated blades are used for both rotation and traction.

- *Shanks:* The shanks connect the blades to the handles and provide the length of the device. They could be either parallel (as in Wrigley's forceps) or crossing (as in Tucker McLane forceps).
- *Lock:* The lock is the articulation between the shanks. Many different types have been designed. The English type of lock is more common type, where a socket is located on the shank at the junction with the handle. This fits into a socket located similarly over the opposite shank. Another type of lock is the sliding type of lock, which may be present in some forceps such as Kielland's forceps.
- *Handles:* The handles are where the operator holds the device and applies traction to the fetal head. The handles may be fenestrated at times to allow a firmer hold over the fetal head.

## Curves of Forceps Blades

The forceps blades have two curves, i.e. the cephalic curve and the pelvic curve (Figs 6.3A and B). The cephalic curve is adapted to provide a good application to the fetal head. In cephalic application, the forceps blades are applied along the sides of the head, grasping the biparietal diameter in between the widest part of the blades. The long axis of the blades corresponds more or less to the occipitomental plane of the fetal head. Since this method of application results in negligible compression effect on the cranium, this method of application is favored over pelvic method of application. On the other hand, the pelvic curve conforms to the axis of birth canal and allows the blades to fit in with the curve of the birth canal. Pelvic application consists of application of forceps blades along the sides of lateral pelvic wall, ignoring the position of fetal head. Therefore, this type of application can result in serious compression on the cranium, especially in case of unrotated head.

## Identification of the Forceps Blades

In order to identify the blade of the forceps, whether left or right, the blades must be articulated and then placed in front of the pelvis with the tip of the blades pointing upwards and the concave side of the pelvic curve forwards.

In this position, the forceps blade which corresponds to the left side of the maternal pelvis is the left blade and the one which corresponds to the right side of the maternal pelvis is the right blade.

In order to identify the isolated forceps blade, the tip of the blade must point upwards; the cephalic curve must be directed inwards and the pelvic curve must be directed forwards.

## ACOG Criteria for Types of Forceps Deliveries

The ACOG (2007) criteria for classification of instrumental delivery (both forceps and vacuum) according to the station and rotation of fetal head are described in Table 6.1. The revised classification uses the level of the leading bony point of the fetal head in centimeters, measured from the level of the maternal ischial spines to define station (±5 cm). High forceps deliveries, used in previous classification systems, defined them as procedures performed when the head was not engaged. High forceps application is not included in the present classification system. According to ACOG

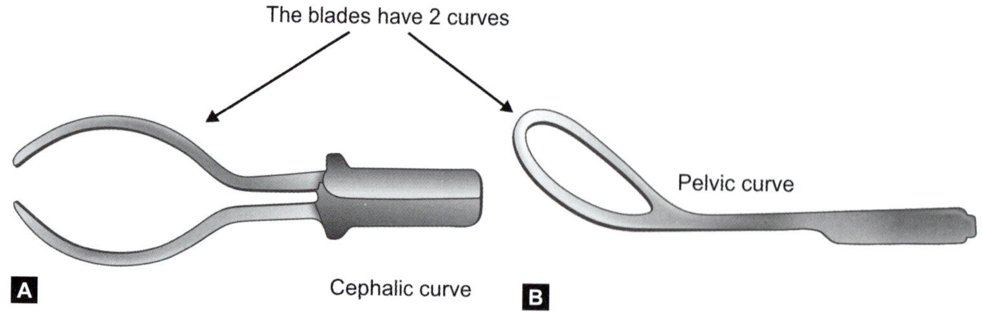



**Figs 6.3A and B:** Different curves of the forceps. (A) Cephalic curve; (B) Pelvic curve

**Table 6.1:** ACOG criteria for classification of instrumental delivery

| Procedure | Criteria |
|---|---|
| Outlet forceps | • The fetal scalp is visible at the introitus without separating the labia<br>• The fetal skull has reached the pelvic floor<br>• The sagittal suture is in anteroposterior diameter or right or left occiput anterior or posterior positions<br>• The fetal head is at or on the perineum<br>• The rotation does not exceed 45° |
| Low forceps | • Leading point of fetal skull is at station +2 and not on the pelvic floor<br>• The degree of rotation does not matter. It could be either:<br>  – Rotation is 45° or less (left or right occiput anterior to occiput anterior or left or right occiput posterior to occiput posterior)<br>  – Rotation is 45° or more |
| Midpelvic | Station is above +2 cm, but the head is engaged |
| High-pelvic application | Not included in the classification system |

*Source:* American Academy of Pediatrics and American College of Obstetricians and Gynecologists. Guidelines for Perinatal care, 6th edition. Washington DC; AAP and ACOG: 2007. p.158.

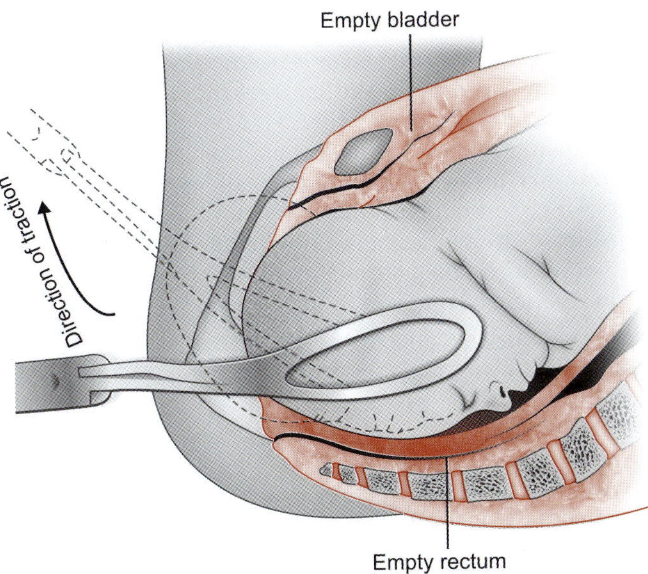


**Fig. 6.4:** Application of outlet forceps

(1994) and SOGC (2005), "high forceps deliveries are not recommended in modern obstetric practice." Outlet forceps application where the forceps are applied when the head is on the perineum is the most common application of forceps (Fig. 6.4). Another commonly used forceps application is the low forceps application. This type of application is done when the head is near the pelvic floor or may be visible at the introitus. In modern day obstetrics, outlet forceps are mainly used.

Use of midforceps is presently associated with much controversy regarding its safety. High midforceps deliveries are also best avoided. In cases of low midforceps application, manual rotation of the fetal head may be required prior to the application of forceps. Application of rotational forceps (Keilland's forceps) is best done by the experts. Otherwise, it is best to wait for the head to descend and rotate completely prior to the application of forceps.

Application of the forceps when the head is not "engaged" is known as "high forceps". In our setup only low forceps and outlet forceps are used and midforceps are usually replaced by cesarean section. Indications for operative vaginal deliveries are identical for forceps and vacuum extractors. No indication for operative vaginal delivery is absolute and largely depends upon the skill and preference of the operator. Many a times, the surgeon may prefer a cesarean section rather than a difficult forceps delivery.

## Prerequisites for Forceps Delivery

Before the application of forceps, it is important for the operator to review the indications for operative vaginal delivery and confirm the presence of all the prerequisites for forceps application.

Prerequisites for forceps delivery include the following:
- *Maternal verbal consent:* Maternal verbal consent should be obtained prior to the application of forceps. However, in some circumstances, it may not be possible to take the maternal consent, especially if the procedure needs to be performed as an emergency or if the mother is sedated. In these cases, consent may be taken from the patient's partner or relatives. If a forceps delivery has been planned in advance (i.e. for maternal medical indications), it is possible to counsel the patient and take her consent prior to the onset of active labor.
- *Assessment of the maternal pelvis:* The maternal pelvis must be adequately assessed before proceeding with a forceps delivery. The type of pelvis (i.e. gynecoid, android, anthropoid or platypoid) and adequacy of the pelvis for delivery of the baby must be clinically assessed prior to undertaking delivery. It should be emphasized that adequate pelvic size depends not just on the pelvic assessment, but also on the size and presentation of the fetus.
- *Engagement of fetal head:* The fetal head must be engaged before application of forceps. Engagement of the fetal head implies that the largest diameter of the fetal presenting part (biparietal diameter in case of cephalic presentation) has passed through the pelvic inlet. Engagement of the fetal presenting part is of great importance, as it helps in ruling out fetopelvic disproportion.

- *The presentation, position and station of the presenting part:* The presentation, position and station of the fetal presenting part must be reconfirmed just before the procedure. The fetus must present as vertex or face with the chin anterior. The station of the fetal head must be at or below the zero station. If the leading part of the fetal head is at zero station or below, the fetal head is said to be engaged. This implies that the biparietal plane of the fetal head has passed through the pelvic inlet.

  However in the presence of excessive molding or caput formation, engagement may not have taken place, even if the head appears to be at zero station. In these cases, the clinician can improve their clinical estimate of engagement by using the abdominal palpation to estimate how much of the fetal head is above the upper level of the pubic symphysis. A recently engaged fetal head may be two-fifths palpable per abdominally.

  The presence of the sagittal sutures in the antero-posterior diameter of the pelvic outlet must be also confirmed before application of forceps. Determination of fetal position by examination of sagittal sutures and fontanels is possible when the head is low in the pelvis. However, when the head is at a higher station, an absolute determination of the position of fetal head may not be possible. In these cases, fetal position can be determined by locating the fetal ear. Forceps are applied across the ears to the mandibular region.

- *Cervical dilatation and effacement:* The cervix must be fully dilated and effaced. If the forceps are applied before complete cervical dilatation and effacement has been attained, the procedure may produce severe maternal lacerations and hemorrhage.

- *Status of the membranes:* The fetal membranes must have ruptured prior to the application of forceps.

- *Bladder to be emptied:* The bladder should be emptied in preparation for forceps operative deliveries, regardless of the type of anesthesia used. Except for the cases, where the fetal head is on the perineum, the bladder should be emptied with help of a catheter.

- *The woman's position:* The laboring woman, in whom forceps have to be applied, should be preferably placed in the "lithotomy position". However, some practitioners prefer to use the left lateral position instead. After placement in the proper position, the woman must be adequately cleaned and draped, while observing aseptic precautions in order to minimize the chances of maternal infection.

- *Adequate analgesia:* The patient must be administered adequate analgesia prior to the application of forceps. The decision regarding the type of anesthesia to be used should be made before initiating the delivery. An adequate level of anesthesia is an important prerequisite before forceps application. Attempts to undertake the instrumental delivery without adequate anesthesia may be extremely painful for the mother and may end up in failure. While some surgeons use only local infiltration of anesthesia to the perineal body prior to forceps application, others may prefer to use pudendal block anesthesia augmented with intravenous sedation. In some cases adequate anesthesia may also be obtained using regional or general anesthesia. Regional anesthesia using epidural or spinal block is more commonly used, while general anesthesia is usually reserved for very complicated situations.

- *Operator's competence and facilities for operative delivery:* Adequate facilities for cesarean section should be available in case the delivery by forceps fails. Operator's skill, training and competence in the use of forceps, play an important role in the eventual success of the procedure. The operator should not only be competent in the use of the forceps but he/she should be promptly able to recognize and manage potential complications. It is very important for the operator to know when he/she must abandon the attempts at forceps delivery and resort to cesarean section.

## Contraindications for Forceps Application

The following are contraindications for the forceps-assisted vaginal deliveries:

- Any contraindication for normal vaginal delivery (a total placenta previa, cephalopelvic disproportion, etc.).
- Refusal of the patient to give verbal consent for the procedure.
- Cervix is not fully dilated or effaced.
- Inability to determine the fetal presentation or position of fetal head.
- Inadequate pelvic size or cephalopelvic disproportion.
- Previous unsuccessful attempts of vacuum extraction (relative contraindication).
- Absence of adequate anesthesia/analgesia.
- Setup with inadequate facilities and support staff.
- Inexperienced operator.

In general, evaluation of the patient for forceps delivery is purely clinical and no laboratory or imaging evaluations are required.

## APPLICATION OF THE FORCEPS

The success of instrumental vaginal delivery, using forceps largely depends upon the technique of forceps application. Knowledge regarding the exact position of the fetal head is of utmost importance before the application of forceps. The term "pelvic application" is used when the left blade is applied on the left side of the pelvis and the right blade is applied on the right side of the pelvis, regardless of the fetal position. The "cephalic application", on the other hand, involves application of blades of forceps on the two sides of fetal head. Since pelvic application is more dangerous due to the risk of significant maternal injury involved, this type of forceps application is not commonly used in clinical practice. The cephalic application of forceps is largely preferred over the pelvic application. Figures 6.5A to H represent a pictorial demonstration of a simple outlet-forceps delivery for an occipitoanterior position and is described below in details:

- *Checking the prerequisites for forceps application:* After ensuring proper anesthesia, an empty bladder and other prerequisites for forceps application (as described previously), the fetal position and fetal heart rate (FHR) is checked again.
- *Application of the left blade of forceps:* Before the application of forceps blades, the clinician places his or her back towards the maternal right thigh and holds the left handle of the left branch of forceps between the fingers of left hand, as if holding a pencil. The shank is held perpendicular to the floor and under the guidance of the fingers of the right hand, the left blade is inserted into the posterior half of the left side of the pelvis along the left vaginal wall. The force necessary to insert the blade is exerted by the pressure of the thumb, which is placed over the heel of the forceps blade. The left hand guides the handle in a wide arc until the blade is in place. As the blade is introduced into the vagina, it is brought to a horizontal position. This blade may be either left in place to stand freely on its own or is held in place without pressure by an assistant.

  The blades of the forceps are usually applied when the uterus is relaxed and not when the woman is experiencing uterine contraction. However, once properly applied, the blades may be left in place, if a contraction occurs at the time of placement.
- *Application of the right blade of forceps:* The right blade of the forceps is held in the right hand and introduced into the right side of the pelvis in the similar manner, with the operator's back towards the patient's left thigh.
- *Checking the proper application of forceps:* The forceps blades must be applied directly to the sides of fetal head along the occipitomental diameter. In case of occiput anterior position, appropriately applied blades are equidistant from the sagittal sutures. The shanks of the blades must be perpendicular to the sagittal suture and there must be only a fingertip or less space between the heel of the blade and sagittal suture.

  On the other hand, in case of occiput posterior position, the blades would be equidistant from the midline of the face and brow.

  The biparietal diameter of the fetal head corresponds to the greatest distance between the appropriately applied blades. Consequently, in a proper cephalic application, the long axis of the blades corresponds to the occipitomental diameter, with the ends of the blades lying over the posterior cheeks. When the forceps have been correctly applied, the blades lie over the parietal eminence, the shank should be in contact with the perineum and the superior surface of the handle should

be directed upwards. In this position, the forceps should lock easily without any force and stand parallel to the plane of the floor.

- *Locking the blades of the forceps:* In case there is trouble locking the blades of forceps, it implies that they have not been properly applied. Even if the blades do get locked up, they might just slip off when the traction is applied. Therefore, before locking the forceps blades and application of traction, it is important to check, if the blades have been properly applied or not.
- *Application of traction:* When the operator is sure that the blades have been placed appropriately and locked, traction can be applied. At all times, the surgeon should be careful towards avoiding the use of undue force.

The traction is usually applied in the direction of pelvic axis (Figs 6.5F and G) and at all times must be gentle and intermittent. The operator should be seated in front of the patient with elbows kept pressed against the sides of the body. To avoid excessive force during traction, the force should be exerted only through the wrist and forearms. Initially, the traction is applied in downwards and backwards direction and then in a horizontal direction until the perineum begins to bulge. With the application of traction, as the vulva starts getting distended by the fetal occiput, an episiotomy may be performed, if the operator feels that it would facilitate the delivery process. As the fetal occiput emerges out, the handles of forceps are gradually elevated, eventually pointing almost directly upwards as the parietal bones emerge. As the handles are raised, the head delivers by extension. While applying traction in the upwards direction, the surgeon's four fingers should grasp the upper surface of the shanks and handles, while the thumbs must exert the necessary force on their lower surface. Traction should be applied intermittently, synchronous with the uterine contractions and the fetal head should be allowed to recede inside during the periods of uterine relaxation. This helps in simulating normal delivery, as much as possible and helps in preventing undue compression over the fetal head. In an emergency, applying continuous traction may be necessary until the fetal head delivers. The safe limit for the amount of traction to be applied, in order to accomplish safe fetal head descent has been considered to be about 45 pounds in primiparas and 30 pounds in multiparas.

Though, there is no fixed limit for the number of traction attempts to be applied before abandoning the procedure, in case there is no descent of the fetal head, abdominal delivery should be considered following three unsuccessful attempts at the forceps. Once the vulva has been distended by the fetal head, we prefer to remove the forceps blades and complete the delivery of fetal head by modified Ritgen's maneuver. Some clinicians prefer to keep the forceps blades in place, while the fetal head is emerging out. We do not use this practice because we believe that this practice increases the total fetal dimension, thereby increasing the likelihood of causing injury to the vulval outlet.

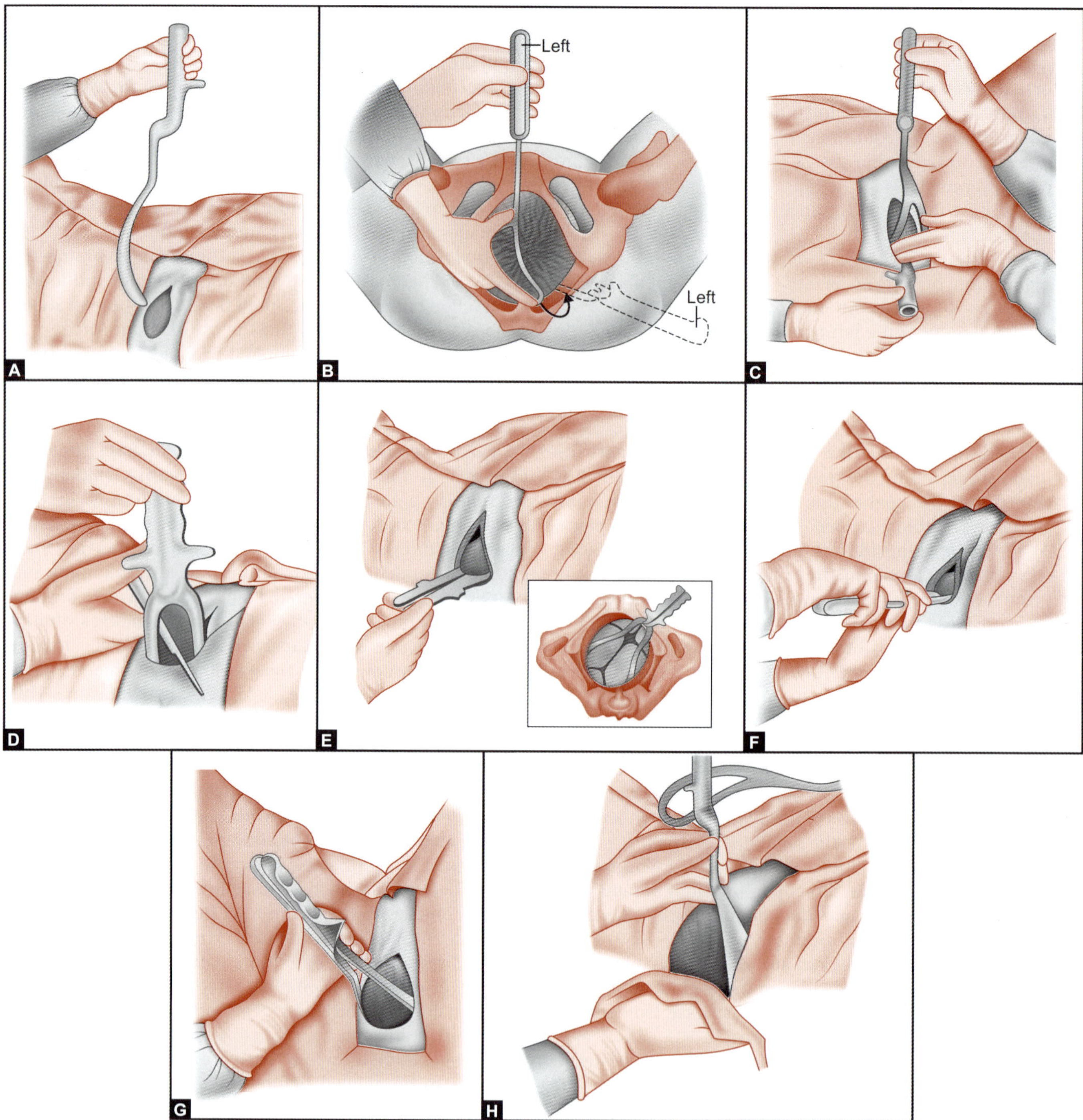

**Figs 6.5 A to H:** (A) The left handle is held in the left hand; (B) The left blade is introduced into the left side of the pelvis; (C) The left blade is in place and the right blade is introduced by the right hand; (D) A median or mediolateral episiotomy may be performed at this point. A left mediolateral episiotomy is shown here; (E) The forceps have been locked. The inset shows a left occipitoanterior fetal position, where appropriately applied blades are equidistant from the sagittal sutures; (F) Application of horizontal traction with the operator seated; (G) As the fetal occiput bulges out, the traction is applied in the upwards direction; (H) Following the distension of vulval outlet by the fetal head, the branches of forceps are disarticulated and delivery of rest of the head is completed by modified Ritgen's maneuver

- *Episiotomy:* With the application of traction, as the vulva is distended by the fetal occiput, an episiotomy may be performed, if the operator feels that it would facilitate the delivery of fetal head. In our setup, an episiotomy is usually performed in all cases of forceps deliveries. With the application of metallic blades of forceps, less opportunity exists for the maternal tissues to stretch. Therefore, we believe that performance of an episiotomy would help in allowing a more rapid delivery, even though it may result in increased blood loss at times. However, the utility of episiotomy in preventing short- and long-term maternal injury is controversial.

## Examination Post-Forceps Application

Following forceps delivery, thorough examination of both the mother and the newborn is advisable.

### Maternal Examination

The mother's external genitalia must be carefully examined, in order to rule out presence of any cervical, vaginal, perineal and paraurethral lacerations or tears. In case of presence of significant maternal vulvar edema, measures such as perineal ice application and pain killers may prove to be useful. A postoperative hemogram should be obtained in patients who experience excessive bleeding. Before discharging patients, who had undergone forceps delivery, a pelvic and rectal examinations must be performed in order to exclude any bleeding and presence of entities, such as pelvic hematoma, rectal tears, misplaced sutures, unrecognized lacerations, etc.

### Neonatal Examination

The newborn must be examined for lacerations, bruising and other injuries over the scalp and face.

## Follow-Up

In case no forceps-related complications are found at the time of discharge, the mother should be asked to come for a follow-up postpartum examination within 4–6 weeks, where the usual protocol for postpartum care, including a thorough pelvic examination must be performed.

## FUNCTIONS OF THE FORCEPS

The forceps help to perform the following functions:
- *Application of traction:* The use of forceps helps in avoiding abdominal cesarean delivery. It may be especially useful in cases of prolonged second stage of labor or in cases, where the clinician wants to cut short the second stage of labor due to maternal condition.
- *Rotation:* Forceps can be used for rotation of fetal head, which may be in occipitotransverse or occipitoposterior

positions. Scanzoni's maneuver can be used for rotation of fetal head using forceps. The original Scanzoni's method was a double application method where the forceps are first applied conforming to the pelvic curve, resulting in the reverse cephalic position in case of occipitoposterior positions. Following the completion of rotation, the blades are removed and reapplied conforming to both the cephalic curve and the pelvic curves. New forceps are used for the second application. The forceps most appropriate for this maneuver are the tucker McLane or Elliot type forceps with solid shanks.

*Modified Scanzoni's method:* Following the application of forceps blades along the pelvic curve, the blades are rotated to make the occiput transverse. Following this, the blades are removed and reapplied in the reverse direction and rotated till the pelvic curve corresponds to the pelvic axis and then the fetal extraction is completed.

- *Protection of the fetal head:* The forceps help to protect the soft fetal head by forming a protective cage around it.
- *Dilator action:* It helps to dilate the vulva through advancement of the fetal head.
- *Stimulator action:* The forceps help to perform stimulator action through the following:
  - Stimulation of uterine contractions
  - Lever action
  - Single branch of the forceps can be used as a vectis to help deliver fetal head in cases of lower segment cesarean section (LSCS).

## Other Applications of Forceps

- Delivery of the head in the occiput posterior position.
- If the head is deep transverse arrest, in experienced hands, rotation by Kielland's forceps is a better option in comparison to manual rotation or delivery by cesarean section.
- In cases of breech presentation, the safest method of delivering the after-coming head, once it has entered the pelvis, is by application of the forceps.
- In a face presentation (mentoanterior) the forceps may be applied directly. Mentoposterior face positions must be rotated prior to application of forceps.

## Piper Forceps

As discussed previously, the Piper forceps are used to facilitate delivery of the after-coming fetal head in cases of breech presentation (Figs 6.6A and B).

### Procedure

In cases of breech vaginal delivery, if the Mauriceau-Smellie-Veit or Burns Marshall maneuvers fail to deliver the head

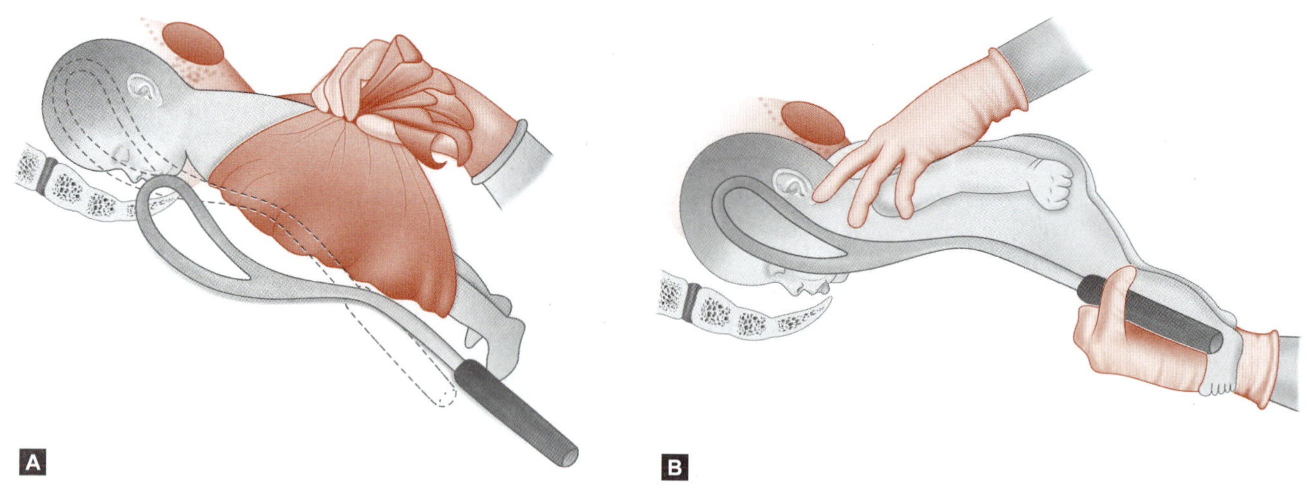

**Figs 6.6A and B:** (A) Application of piper forceps on the after-coming head of the breech; (B) Application of the downwards traction to deliver the fetal head

easily, Piper forceps should be promptly applied. The steps for forceps application are described next:

1. Prior to the application of forceps, the infant should be supported by an assistant, and the operator should sit on a low stool for the forceps insertion.
2. After checking the prerequisites for forceps application, the left blade is applied directly to the right side of the baby's face (Fig. 6.6A). The opposite blade is then applied and the forceps locked.
3. A deep episiotomy should be performed to prevent damage to the vagina and perineum.
4. After rechecking for the prerequisites for forceps application, the head is delivered by downwards traction (Fig. 6.6B). Once the face appears at the introitus, the forceps handles are elevated to flex and deliver the rest of the head by flexion.

The use of forceps has been found to be associated with long-term maternal and fetal morbidity. Midforceps application is associated with higher rate of maternal and neonatal morbidity in comparison to outlet forceps or low-forceps application.

### Kielland's Forceps

The use of Kielland's forceps carries additional risks compared with other types of forceps and requires specific expertise and training. The methods for application of Kielland's forceps are classic application and the wandering method.

The classical method of forceps application is condemned because rotation in the birth canal is likely to cause potential damage to the birth canal. The wandering method is more commonly used where the anterior blade is first inserted laterally and then wondered over the face to make it lie anteriorly. This is followed by insertion of the posterior blade, which is inserted directly under guidance of the fingers of

right hand placed between the fetal head and hollow of the sacrum. The handle tips are depressed down and the handle tips are brought into alignment to help correct asynclitism. Following this the blades of the forceps are locked. Once the blades of the forceps are locked, they are rotated through 90°–180° until the fetal head lies in the occipitoanterior position. The traction is then applied.

## COMPLICATIONS

### Maternal Complications

- *Injury to the maternal tissues:* Even with use by an experienced surgeon, forceps deliveries may be associated with an increased risk of perineal tears and lacerations (both vaginal and cervical). This could be related to the more rapid and extensive stretching of the maternal tissues with delivery of the fetal head. Perineal tears are likely to especially occur in the cases where the episiotomy is not given at the right time.
- *Hemorrhage:* Severe maternal tissue injury and lacerations due to forceps application can sometimes result in extensive bleeding and maternal hemorrhage.
- *Febrile morbidity:* This could be the manifestation of postpartum uterine infection and pelvic cellulitis, resulting from the infection caused by trauma to the tissues.
- *Urinary retention and bladder dysfunction:* Damage to the urethral sphincters may result in urinary retention and bladder dysfunction.
- *Late maternal complications:* Late maternal complications could be related to damage caused to the pelvic support tissues. This damage could manifest in the form of genitorurinary fistulae or pelvic organ prolapse. Injury caused by forceps may in the long-term result in the development of fecal incontinence due to damage to the

rectal sphincter function or urinary incontinence due to damage to the urethral sphincters.

### Fetal Complications

*Fetal injury:* Various fetal injuries, which can be caused by the application of forceps, include cephalohematoma, facial nerve injury, depressed skull fractures, intracranial bleeding, shoulder dystocia, etc. Additionally, cerebral palsy and subtly lower IQ (2.5 points) levels have been described in infants delivered by forceps.

Over the past two decades, the uses of vacuum extraction and forceps delivery have been declining both in low and high income countries. At the same time, there has been an increase in the rate of cesarean delivery. The objection to the use of forceps mainly includes, the presence of a high rate of complications associated with its use. Forceps delivery is likely to cause potential harm both to the mother and the infant. In fact, some medical schools no longer train their junior doctors in the skills to perform instrumental delivery. At most places, the art of performing instrumental delivery is largely restricted to specialists and consultants. The art of instrumental delivery, especially vacuum extraction needs to be taught to practitioners, such as midwives, nurse practitioners, resident doctors and general physicians, so that it can be useful to provide emergency obstetric care at the periphery. This allows women to give birth closer to home in midlevel facilities, when hospitals may not be easily accessible or in cases of emergency, when facilities for cesarean delivery are not available. Use of forceps delivery helps in potentially reducing the risks associated with cesarean delivery and overall costs of obstetric care.

### Failed Forceps

The term implies that an attempt to deliver with forceps had been unsuccessful. If the surgeon is not sure regarding, whether the attempt at forceps delivery would be successful or not, the attempt is considered to be a trial of forceps delivery. The patient undergoing trial of forceps must be delivered in a setup, well equipped with facilities for an emergency cesarean delivery, in case the need arises. In case the satisfactory application of the forceps cannot be achieved or there is no descent of fetal head even after three attempts of traction application through forceps, the procedure must be abandoned and delivery accomplished with the help of vacuum extraction or cesarean section. Some of the causes of failed forceps are as follows:

- Unsuspected cephalopelvic disproportion.
- Misdiagnosis of the position of the head.
- Incomplete dilation of the cervix.
- Outlet contraction (very rare in an otherwise normal pelvis).

Over the years, the use of forceps to facilitate delivery has been advocated in order to avoid abdominal (cesarean) delivery. Even though the rate of cesarean delivery has increased, while that of instrumental vaginal delivery has fallen over the past decade, the ACOG (2001) recommends forceps delivery as an acceptable and safe option for delivery. However, presently there has been a decline in the rate of forceps delivery. This has resulted in a decline in the level of experience and training of the young doctors in the skill of operative vaginal delivery. The complete obstetrician must be well trained and capable of using all of the modalities of vaginal deliveries, both instrumental (forceps and vacuum) and spontaneous vaginal, in order to ensure a safe maternal and fetal outcome.

## Obstetric Vacuum Application

Vacuum application is emerging as an important procedure for assisted vaginal delivery. Vacuum delivery has been rapidly replacing forceps as the more predominant method of instrumental vaginal delivery. The term ventouse is derived from a French word meaning a soft cup. This devise is known as vacuum extractor in the US, while it is referred to as ventouse in Europe.

The increasing interest in the use of vacuum extractor can be largely considered due to the fact that it is relatively safer for both the mother and infant in comparison to forceps delivery. Suction force by the vacuum creates an artificial caput or chignon within the cup. This helps in the firm hold of vacuum cup and allows adequate traction. The original vacuum extractor was designed by Sir John Young at Edinburgh in 1849. Soon after, Malmström developed the prototype of the modern vacuum extractor in Sweden. The Malmström extractor consisted of a metal cup with a flat plate inside it and a chain attached to the plate. The chain was placed inside a rubber tube, which was necessary to develop the vacuum, and was attached to a traction bar. Traction is applied to the vacuum cup by the chain and plate. The metal cup comes in four sizes and it is recommended that the largest cup possible should be used for delivery.

It was not until 1973, when Kobayashi developed the soft silastic cup in the USA. The silastic cup has many advantages over the metal cup. Compared with metal-cup vacuum extractors, soft-cup devices are easier to use and cause fewer neonatal scalp injuries. The chance of injury to the fetal scalp is relatively less because the vacuum can be developed quickly and, therefore, can be released between contractions. However, the major disadvantage associated with the use of vacuum extractors is that they are likely to detach more frequently in comparison to the metallic cups, which detach less frequently.

Today, more and more clinicians are showing preference towards the use of silastic vacuum extractor as an alternative to delivery, when the fetal head is stuck up in the midpelvis rather than proceeding directly with cesarean section. While forceps is an instrument, which helps in the delivery of fetal head through transmission of the mechanical force to the base of skull, ventouse is an instrument, which assists in delivery by creating a vacuum between it and the fetal scalp. The pulling force in case of vacuum extraction helps in dragging the cranium.

## SURGICAL EQUIPMENT USED

### Types of Vacuum Devices

Originally, vacuum devices as invented by Malmström had a rigid metal cup with a separate suction catheter attached laterally and connected to a foot- or hand-operated pedal. The instrument as devised by Malmström comprised of three parts: (1) suction cup, (2) vacuum generator and (3) traction tubing devise (Fig. 6.7).

The devices available nowadays have soft or semi-rigid cups in different shapes and sizes. Newer devices are based on the use of soft or semi-rigid cups. Most of these devices use hand-pump suction, which requires an assistant or can be used by the clinician (herself or himself) (Fig. 6.8). In the United States, the handheld devices are intended for single use and are disposable.

Examples of different types of cups include soft or rigid anterior cups and rigid posterior cups. Posterior cups are flatter, which allow for better placement at the flexure point on the fetal head, which is usually much further back in the sacral hollow during occipitoposterior presentation.

### Indications for Application

The classification, indications and contraindications for vacuum delivery are almost same as that utilized for forceps delivery. However, unlike the forceps, vacuum extractors

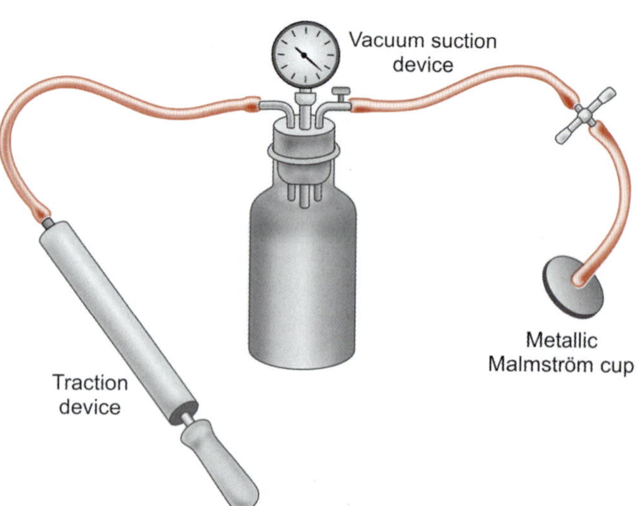


**Fig. 6.7:** An illustration showing various parts of the Malmström vacuum extractor

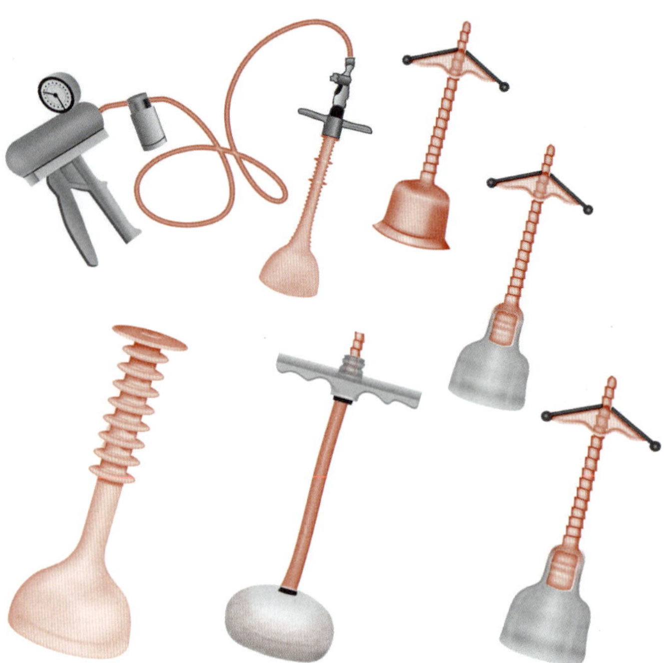

**Fig. 6.8:** Different types of vacuum cups

cannot be used in cases of face presentation or after-coming head of breech. The vacuum must never be applied to an unengaged head, i.e. above zero station.

Indications for vacuum application are more or less similar to that of forceps and include the following:

- As an alternative to forceps operation (e.g. occipitotransverse or occipitoposterior position).
- Shortening of the second stage of labor for maternal benefit (e.g. maternal exhaustion).
- Delay in descent of the head in the second stage of labor (e.g. case of the second baby of twins).
- Prolonged second stage of labor.
- Nonreassuring fetal heart tones or other suspicion of immediate or potential fetal compromise.

### Prerequisites for Vacuum Delivery

Before application of vacuum, the obstetrician must ensure that the prerequisites required before application of forceps are fulfilled. These have been previously described with forceps delivery.

### Contraindications for the Use of Vacuum for Operative Vaginal Delivery

- *Absolute contraindications:* Some absolute contraindications for the use of vacuum for operative vaginal delivery are as follows:
  - Cephalopelvic disproportion.
  - Nonengagement of fetal head or presence of the head at a high station.

- Any presentation other than the vertex (face, brow, breech, etc.).
- Patient has not given consent.
- Operator inexperience.
- *Relative contraindications:* Some relative contraindications to vacuum delivery are as follows:
  - Fetal prematurity: Gestational age less than 34 weeks has been considered as a relative contraindication to vacuum delivery due to an increased risk for intracranial hemorrhage and injury to the fetal scalp.
  - Known fetal conditions that affect bone or disorders of fetal bone mineralization.
  - Fetal coagulation defects or active bleeding disorders.
  - Fetal macrosomia.

### Steps for Vacuum Extraction

The actual steps of vacuum extraction in case of occiput anterior position are shown in Figures 6.9A to D and are described as follows:

- *Strict asepsis:* Under all aseptic precautions, the patient's perineum and external genitalia are cleaned and draped.

The patient's labia are separated, following which the vacuum (soft) cup, which has been compressed and folded, prior to insertion, is applied. The cup is inserted gently by pressing it in inwards and downwards direction, so that the inferior edge of the cup lies close to the posterior fourchette.

- *Positioning of the vacuum cup:* The vacuum cup should be so positioned as to prevent the deflexion and asyncylitism of fetal head. The correct or ideal cup application is the flexing median application (Fig. 6.10). In this type of application, the vacuum cup should be placed in such a way that the center of the cup lies directly over the sagittal suture, 3 cm in front of the posterior fontanel. This point is known as the flexion or the pivot point (Fig. 6.11). The distance between the leading anterior edge of the cup and the anterior fontanel should be about 3 cm (two-finger breadth); this is known as the application distance. As a general rule, the cup must be placed as far posteriorly as possible. This implies that the edge of the cup would be approximately over the posterior fontanel as most of the cups have a diameter of 5–7 cm. This positioning helps in maintaining flexion of the fetal head and avoids

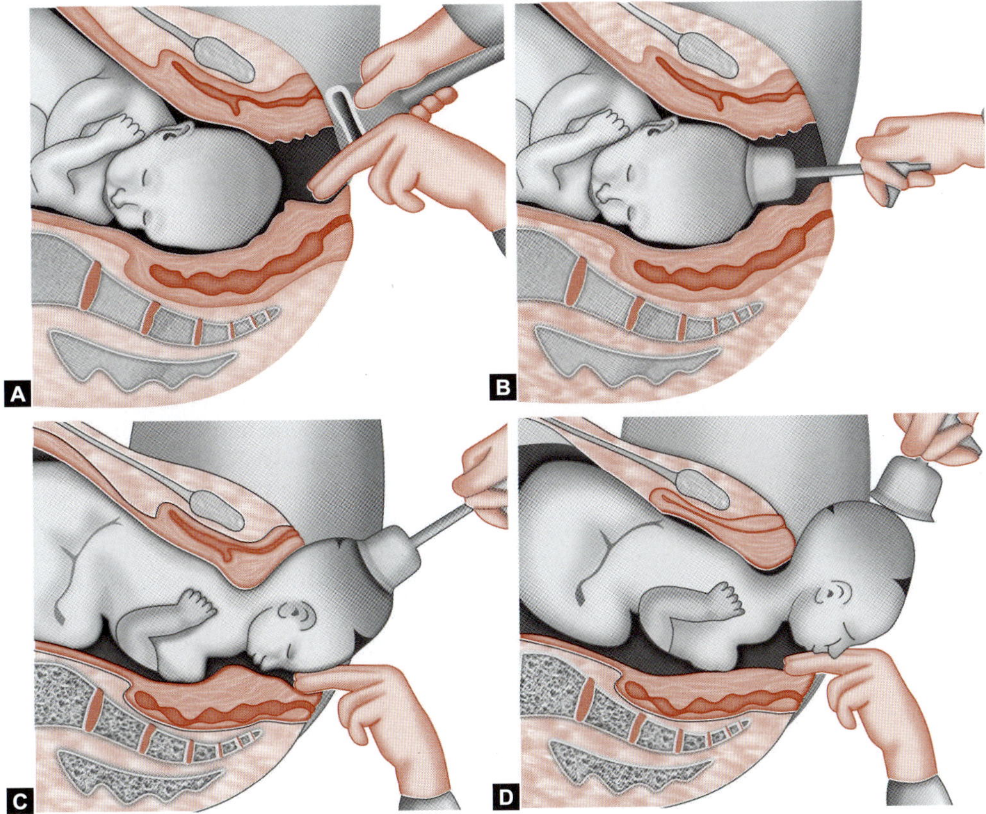

**Figs 6.9A to D:** (A) Insertion of the vacuum cup into the vagina; (B) Application of the vacuum cup over the fetal head; (C) Creation of vacuum suction; (D) Application of traction to facilitate the delivery of fetal head

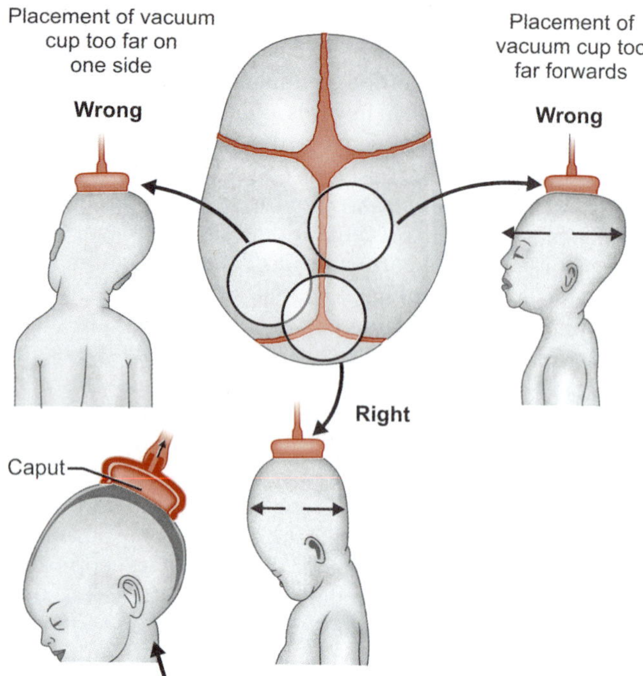



**Fig. 6.10:** Correct placement of vacuum cup over the fetal head

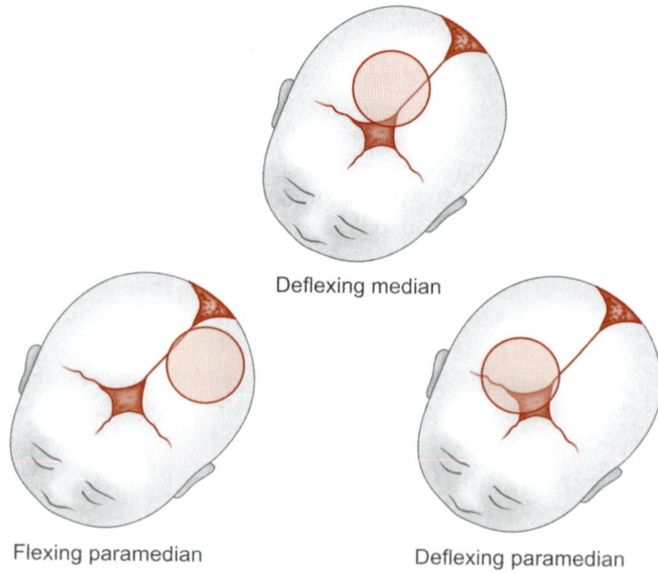



**Fig. 6.12:** Incorrect placements of the vacuum cup

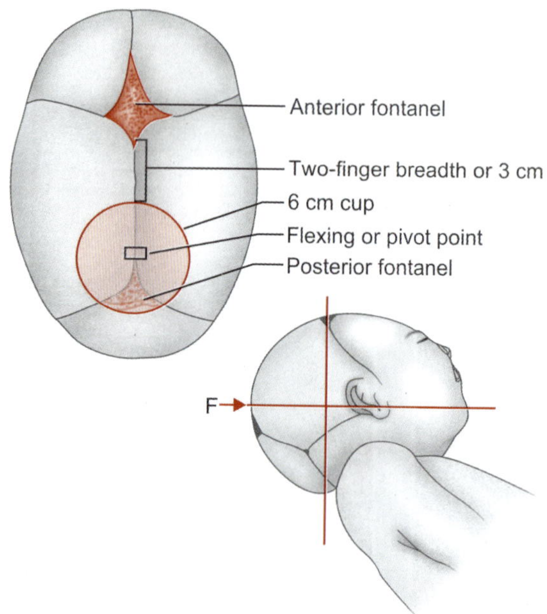



**Fig. 6.11:** Flexing median application showing the flexion point (F)

traction over the anterior fontanel. If the cup is placed anteriorly on the fetal cranium near the anterior fontanel rather than over the occiput, this may result in undue extension of the cervical spine. Similarly, if the cup is asymmetrically placed in relation to the sagittal suture, it is likely to worsen asynclitism.

Other types of cup applications, which are incorrect or not ideal and must not be used include the following (Fig. 6.12):

*Flexing paramedian:* When the center of the cup is situated more than 1 cm to the either side of the sagittal suture, but the application distance is 3 cm.

*Deflexing median:* When the center of the cup is over the sagittal suture, but the application distance is less than 3 cm.

*Deflexing paramedian:* When the center of the cup is more than 1 cm to the either side of sagittal suture, but application distance is less than 3 cm.

While positioning the cup, the clinician must be careful that no maternal soft tissues get trapped between the vacuum cup and fetal head. Moreover, the cup should not be twisted because this is likely to result in lacerations or injury to the fetal head. In order to prevent the entrapment of maternal tissues within the vacuum cup, the full circumference of the vacuum cup must be palpated, both before and after the vacuum has been created, as well as prior to the application of traction.

- *Creation of vacuum suction:* Once the cup has been properly placed, vacuum must be created. The clinician must place the fingers of one hand against the suction cup and grasp the handle of the instrument with the other hand, following which the vacuum is applied. In order to achieve effective traction, a pressure of at least 0.6–0.8 kg/cm$^2$ must be created. The pressure must be gradually created, by increasing suction by 0.2 kg/cm$^2$ every 2 minutes. The pressure is gradually raised at the rate of 0.1 kg/cm$^2$/minute until the effective vacuum of 0.8 kg/cm$^2$ has been created in about 10 minutes. With the use of soft cups, it is possible to create negative pressure of 0.8 kg/cm$^2$ over as little as 1 minute. Prior to the application of traction, an episiotomy may be performed. With the vacuum extractor a midline or mediolateral episiotomy is adequate and a pudendal nerve block serves as an optimal form of anesthesia. As a result of creation of vacuum, the scalp is sucked inside and an artificial caput succedaneum (chignon) is produced. Chignon usually disappears within a few hours after birth.

- *Force of traction:* As soon as the vacuum has been built up and the operator has checked that no vaginal tissue is trapped inside the silastic cup, traction should be applied with each uterine contraction in line of pelvic axis. The direction of traction should be at right angle to the plane of the cup. The patient is encouraged to push at the same time, so that a minimum amount of traction is required to complete the delivery. In case the cup gets dislodged, it should be reapplied only after careful inspection of fetal scalp for any injury. Traction should be repeated with each contraction, until crowning of the fetal head occurs. As the head clears the pubic symphysis, the delivery of head is completed by modified Ritgen's maneuver. Once the fetal head has delivered, suction is released and the cup is removed. Delivery can then proceed as usual. Vacuum extraction should not be attempted for more than 20 minutes. It usually becomes obvious within six to eight pulls, whether delivery would be successful or not. The procedure should be abandoned, if delivery is not achieved or the labor does not progress. Under ordinary circumstances, the procedure must be abandoned after three successive cup detachments. In these cases forceps delivery or abdominal delivery must be considered. The procedure should also be stopped, if there appears any evidence of maternal or fetal trauma.
- *Using the "ABCDEFGHIJ" mnemonic:* The steps performed in vacuum extraction can be described using the mnemonic "ABCDEFGHIJ". This acronym has been reviewed in Table 6.2.

A: Prior to delivery, the obstetrician should address the patient and discuss the risks and benefits of operative vaginal delivery. At the time of delivery, extra assistance is required. This includes nursing care professionals, midwives, anesthetists, pediatricians and neonatal resuscitation team. Adequate analgesics should be administered before carrying out vacuum delivery. Though pudendal anesthesia suffices in most of the cases, regional anesthesia may be sometimes required for vacuum delivery.

B: The bladder should be emptied prior to the application of vacuum in order to avoid risk of injury.

C: Prior to the application of vacuum, the cervix should be completely dilated.

**Table 6.2:** Using the mnemonic "ABCDEFGHIJ" for vacuum extraction

| Letter of acronym | Interpretation |
|---|---|
| A | **A**ddressing the patient to discuss the risks and benefits of vacuum application<br>**A**sk for help: assistants must be present (nursing care professionals, midwives, anesthetists, pediatricians, etc.)<br>**A**nalgesic requirements to be taken care of (pudendal anesthesia is usually sufficient) |
| B | **B**ladder to be empty |
| C | **C**omplete cervical dilatation |
| D | **D**etermination of fetal position prior to vacuum application |
| E | **E**quipment to be checked and kept ready prior to the application |
| F | **F**lexion point: vacuum cup to be placed at the flexion point |
| G | **G**entle traction |
| H | **H**alting the procedure |
| I | **I**ncision for episiotomy (needs to be individualized) |
| J | **R**emove the vacuum cup when the **j**aw is reachable |

D: The position of the fetal head should be determined prior to vacuum application.

E: The vacuum equipment should be checked by the obstetrician to ensure adequate suction.

F: The center of the cup should be placed at the flexion point, which can be defined as a point over the sagittal suture, approximately 3 cm in front of the posterior fontanel and approximately 6 cm from the anterior fontanel. The placement of cup over the flexion point is important, as it helps in maximizing traction and minimizing detachment of the cup.

G: The clinician must apply gentle traction and increase the force of vacuum suction with the manometer at the recommended range. While some clinicians prefer to lower the force of suction between contractions to decrease rate of scalp injury, others prefer to maintain continuous suction, especially in cases, where rapid fetal delivery is required, e.g. in cases of nonreassuring fetal heart tones.

H: It is important for the clinician to know when to halt the procedure for instrumental delivery. Use of vacuum should be halted, when there are three disengagements of the vacuum (or "pop-offs") or more than 20 minutes have elapsed or three consecutive pulls result in no progress or delivery.

I: The clinician must evaluate each individual patient, regarding whether or not to give an incision for a possible episiotomy, when the perineum gets distended by the fetal head.

J: The vacuum cup must be removed as soon as the fetal jaw is reachable.

### Postoperative Steps

The postoperative steps for vacuum delivery are same as that of forceps delivery. It must involve the inspection of maternal tissues (cervix, vagina, vulva and paraurethral tissues) for the presence of any tears, lacerations, injury, etc. The newly delivered infant must be also carefully examined for the presence of any injuries.

### COMPLICATIONS

Some of the complications for vacuum application are as follows:

### Neonatal Injury

Use of vacuum can result in development of injuries, such as scalp lacerations, bruising, subgaleal hematomas, cephalo-hematomas, intracranial hemorrhage (Figs 6.13 and 6.14A and B), neonatal jaundice, subconjunctival hemorrhage, clavicular fracture, shoulder dystocia, injury of sixth and seventh cranial nerves, Erb's palsy, retinal hemorrhage and fetal death. Signs and symptoms of serious intracranial injury in a neonate include apnea, bradycardia, bulging fontanels, convulsions, irritability, lethargy and poor feeding. Various neonatal injuries, which can occur as a result of vacuum application, would be now described in detail:

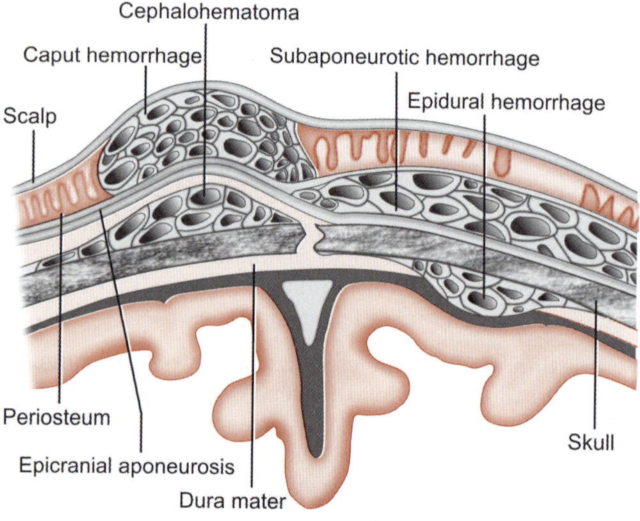


**Fig. 6.13:** Various types of fetal injuries which can occur as a result of vacuum application

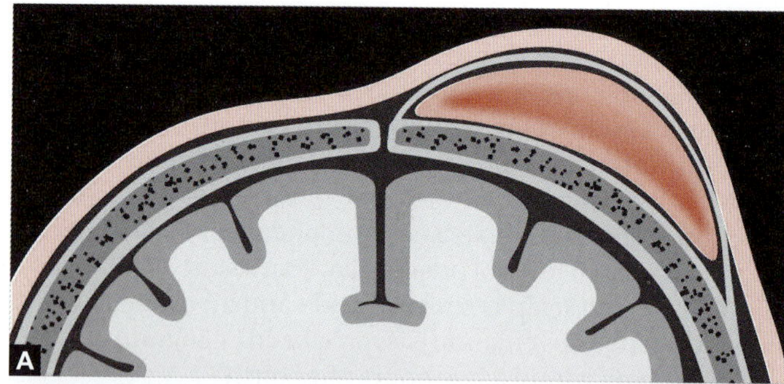


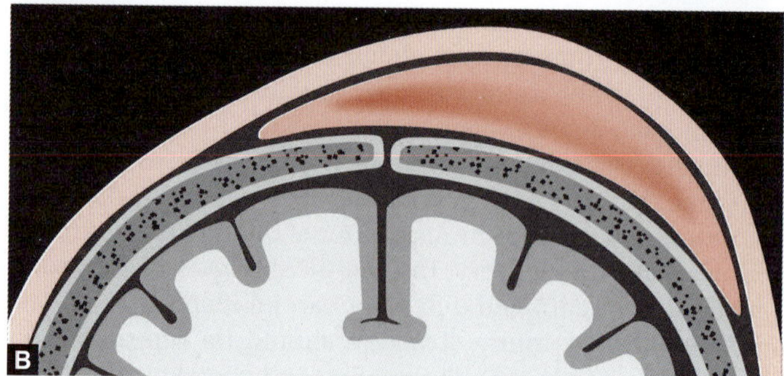


**Figs 6.14A and B:**  (A) Cephalohematoma; (B) Subgleal hematoma

*Cephalohematomas:* Vacuum deliveries are associated with higher chances of development of neonatal cephalo-hematoma in comparison with forceps delivery. The resolution of cephalohematomas can result in the development of hyperbilirubinemia over long-term. In case of cephalohematoma, bleeding occurs beneath the periosteum, between the skull and the periosteum. As a result, the boggy swelling associated with cephalohematoma is limited by the suture lines in contrast to the subgaleal hematomas, which are not limited by the suture lines.

*Subgaleal or subaponeurotic hematomas (Fig. 6.14B):* Sub-galeal hematoma occurs as a result of bleeding in the potential space between the skull periosteum and epicranial aponeurosis. Since the collection occurs above the periosteum, it can cross the sutures lines. Subgaleal hematoma must be suspected in case of boggy scalp swelling, swelling crossing the suture lines and an expanding head circumference. The diffuse head swelling shifts with repositioning and indents on palpation. Swelling is not limited by suture lines (unlike in the cases of cephalohematoma). The infants may also have signs of hypovolemia (hypotension, pallor, tachycardia, tachypnea and a falling hematocrit).

*Intracranial hemorrhage:* These can be of various types, depending upon the location of the blood collection. Epidural hematoma occurs in the potential space between the dura mater and the skull. Subdural hematoma occurs in the potential space between the dura mater and arachnoid mater. Subarachnoid hemorrhage occurs in the subarachnoid space between the arachnoid mater and pia mater.

*Shoulder dystocia:* Operative vaginal delivery is a risk factor for shoulder dystocia and it occurs more commonly with vacuum delivery, in comparison to the forceps delivery. The incidence of shoulder dystocia increases in cases of fetal macrosomia.

*Retinal hemorrhage:* These usually resolve within several weeks and are unlikely to be associated with long-term morbidity.

*Transient neonatal lateral rectus palsy:* Since this usually resolves spontaneously, it is unlikely to have much clinical importance.

## Forceps versus Vacuum Delivery

Similar to forceps delivery, the use of vacuum helps in avoiding the need of abdominal delivery (cesarean section). The "ventouse" delivery is considered to be more physiological and similar to normal vaginal delivery in comparison to the forceps delivery. The comparison between vacuum and forceps delivery has been tabulated in Table 6.3 and illustrated in Figure 6.15. Theoretically, the use of vacuum extractor has several advantages over obstetric forceps. The use of vacuum helps in avoiding the insertion of space-occupying steel blades within the vagina. On the other hand, with a forceps delivery, the fetal biparietal diameter is increased by the thickness of each forceps blade. Unlike forceps, the vacuum cup takes up no space in a mother's birth canal and therefore, it is less likely to result in accidental maternal injuries.

Additionally, with the use of vacuum extractor, there is no requirement for precise rotation of fetal head prior to the application of the vacuum cup. Thus the vacuum can be used, even if the obstetrician is unsure about the exact fetal position. Since the vacuum extractor helps in the application of traction only, therefore, even if the occiput is not directly anterior or the head is an unrotated position, it is most likely to rotate, when it reaches the perineum, similar to the case of spontaneous vaginal delivery. Moreover, even if the fetal head is deflexed, vacuum extraction often helps in flexing it. Vacuum application is associated with a much reduced maternal trauma. The amount of traction applied to the fetal head remains uncontrollable with forceps delivery, but it can be controlled with the use of a vacuum extractor. As a result, a high incidence of third and fourth degree maternal lacerations is associated with the use of forceps. However, use of vacuum is likely to result in serious fetal complications, including significant cranial injuries. An increased incidence of cephalohematomas and retinal hemorrhages has also been noted after vacuum deliveries. The incidence of fetal injuries is likely to be higher with the use of Malmström vacuum cup, in comparison to the use of soft silastic cups.

**Table 6.3:** Comparison between forceps and vacuum delivery

| *Parameters* | *Delivery by forceps* | *Delivery by vacuum extraction* |
|---|---|---|
| Effect on BPD of fetal head | Space-occupying steel blades within the vagina cause an increase in the fetal BPD | Vacuum cup is not a space occupying device, therefore no change in fetal BPD |
| Amount of traction required | More traction force is required. Traction force in a primigravida is about 20 kg and in a multigravida is about 13 kg | Lesser traction force is needed |
| Maternal injuries | More chances of perineal injuries and lacerations | Lower chances of perineal injuries and lacerations |
| Fetal injuries | Lesser chances of injury to the fetal scalp and brain | More chances of injury to the fetal scalp and brain |
| Technical skill required | More technical skill is required on the part of the operator | Less technical skill is required on part of the operator |
| Use in case of unrotated fetal head or occipitoposterior position | Must not be used in cases of unrotated fetal head or occipitoposterior position | Can be used in cases of unrotated fetal head or occipitoposterior position. Vacuum helps in autorotation |
| Cervical dilation | Must be applied only in cases of fully dilated cervix | Can be applied even through incompletely dilated cervix |
| Use in other fetal presentations | Can be used in cases of mentoanterior position and after-coming head of the breech | Cannot be used in cases of mentoanterior position and after-coming head of the breech |
| Safety in case of delivery of a premature baby | Delivery with forceps is safer because head remains in a protective cage | More chances of injury to the fetal scalp in case of a premature head |
| Failure rate | Lower. If the blades of the forceps have been properly applied, they do no detach that easily (unlike the vacuum cup) | Higher. Cup detachments or pop offs occur when the vacuum is not maintained |

*Abbreviation:* BPD, biparietal diameter

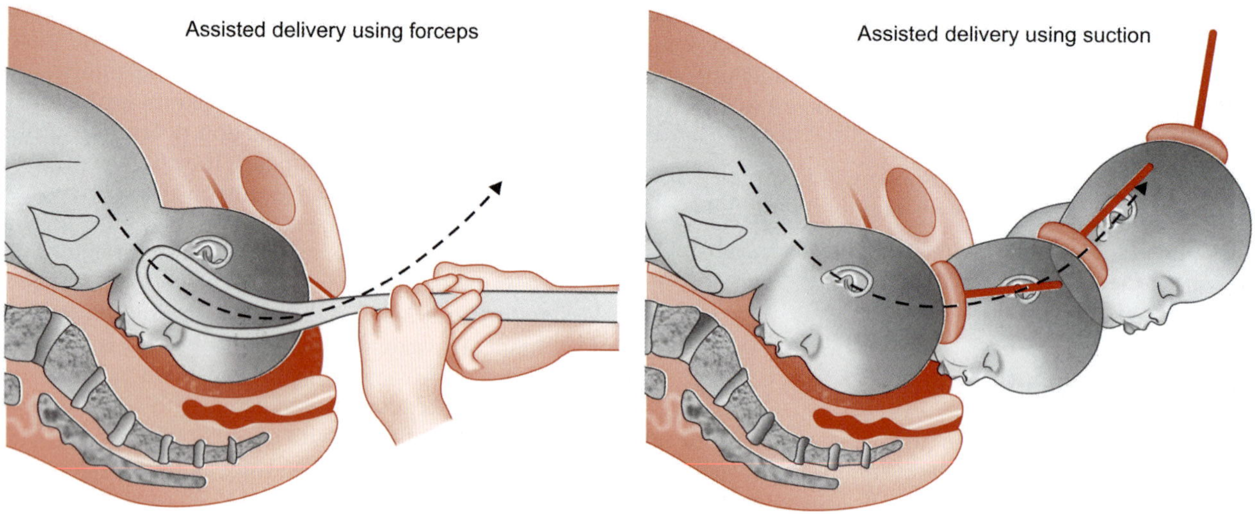



**Fig. 6.15:** Comparison between forceps and vacuum delivery

The modern, soft, silastic vacuum cup, which can be used nowadays can be safely applied to the fetal scalp without much chances of causing injury or fetal scalp trauma. Also, the vacuum can be built up and released in between contractions, thereby further reducing the chances of fetal head injury. Vacuum extractors have replaced forceps for many situations, in which instrumental vaginal delivery is required, in order to avoid abdominal cesarean delivery. These devices are usually employed in cases of nonprogress of fetal head in the second stage of labor or for a nonreassuring fetal heart tracing. Vacuum extraction is associated with a higher rate of neonatal injury in comparison to the forceps delivery. In comparison with metal-cup vacuum extractors, soft-cup devices are easier to use and are associated with fewer neonatal scalp injuries. However, the soft cups are likely to detach more frequently.

### Conclusion

From the above discussion, it has become apparent that the use of silastic vacuum extractor is gaining popularity in various parts of the world. However, the procedure must be performed by an experienced clinician and it must be immediately abandoned, if it does not proceed smoothly or the cup dislodges more than three times. The clinician must consider vacuum extraction as a trial. There should be a progressive descent of fetal head with each traction attempt. If there is no clear evidence regarding the descent of fetal head, an alternative delivery approach must be considered. Delivery by vacuum extractor is considered less traumatic for the mother, in comparison to the forceps delivery. Moreover, complications to the fetus may be minimized, if the physician recognizes contraindications to the use of vacuum extraction and follows the procedure correctly.

# Management of Shoulder Dystocia

Shoulder dystocia can be defined as the inability to deliver the fetal shoulders after the delivery of the fetal head without the aid of specific maneuvers (other than the gentle downwards traction on the head). Shoulder dystocia occurs as a result of disproportion between the bisacromial diameter of the fetus and the anteroposterior diameter of the pelvic inlet, which causes the impaction of the anterior shoulder behind the symphysis pubis.

Shoulder dystocia can occur both during a normal vaginal delivery or an assisted instrumental (ventouse or forceps) delivery. Shoulder dystocia occurs in about 0.5% births and can be of two types: (1) high shoulder dystocia and (2) the low shoulder dystocia. Low shoulder dystocia results due to the failure of engagement of the anterior shoulder and impaction of anterior shoulder over the maternal symphysis pubis. This type of the shoulder dystocia is also known as unilateral shoulder dystocia. This is the more common type and is easily dealt with using standard techniques. There can be a high perinatal mortality and morbidity associated with this complication and therefore it needs to be managed appropriately. Since it is difficult to predict shoulder dystocia or prevent its occurrence, all the clinicians must be well-versed with its management.

### Risk Factors

Shoulder dystocia is a largely unpredictable and unpreventable event as a large majority of cases occur in the children or women with no risk factors. Nevertheless, the clinicians must be aware of the probable risk factors and remain alert regarding the possibility of shoulder dystocia with any delivery.

| **Table 6.4:** Risk factors for shoulder dystocia | |
| --- | --- |
| *Prelabor factors* | *Intrapartum factors* |
| • Previous history of shoulder dystocia<br>• Macrosomia (fetal weight of over 4.5 kg)<br>• Diabetes mellitus<br>• Maternal body mass index > 30 kg/m$^2$<br>• Multiparity | • Prolonged first stage of labor<br>• Secondary arrest<br>• Oxytocin augmentation<br>• Prolonged second stage of labor<br>• Failure of descent of the head |

| **Table 6.5:** Mnemonic for describing initial management in the cases of shoulder dystocia | |
| --- | --- |
| **H** | Call for **h**elp |
| **E** | Evaluate for **e**pisiotomy |
| **L** | **L**egs (the McRoberts maneuver) |
| **P** | Suprapubic **P**ressure |
| **E** | **E**nter the pelvis maneuvers (internal rotation): such as Rubin II maneuver, Wood's screw maneuver and reverse Wood's screw maneuver |
| **R** | **R**emove the posterior arm |
| **R** | **R**oll the patient |

Some important risk factors associated with occurrence of shoulder dystocia are listed in Table 6.4.

## Diagnosis

There are two main signs that indicate the presence of shoulder dystocia:

1. The baby's body does not emerge out even after the application of routine traction and maternal pushing following the delivery of baby's head. Routine traction is defined as "that traction required for delivery of the shoulders in a normal vaginal delivery where there is no difficulty with the shoulders". There is also difficulty with the delivery of fetal face and chin in these cases.
2. The "Turtle sign": The fetal head suddenly retracts back against the mother's perineum after it emerges from the vaginal introitus. The baby's anterior shoulder is caught on the back of the maternal pubic bone, causing retraction of the fetal head and preventing delivery of the remainder of the baby. The baby's cheeks bulge out, resembling a turtle pulling its head back into its shell. There is failure of restitution of the fetal head and the descent of shoulders.

## MANAGEMENT OF SHOULDER DYSTOCIA

Shoulder dystocia drill should form an important part of training for the junior doctor and the nurses. Drill is a practice run-through of the labor and delivery team for a simulated case of shoulder dystocia. The initial management in the cases of shoulder dystocia has also been summarized by the mnemonic HELPERR, which is described in Table 6.5. Management of shoulder dystocia has been summarized in Flow chart 6.1.

The immediate steps which need to be taken in case of an anticipated or a recognized case of shoulder dystocia include the following:

- After recognition of shoulder dystocia, extra help should be summoned immediately. This should include further midwifery assistance, an experienced obstetrician, a pediatric resuscitation team and an anesthetist. One person should be assigned the task of recording the time since the time of onset of dystocia and saying it loud after every 30 seconds.
- As soon as the shoulder dystocia has been identified, maternal pushing and fetal pulling and pivoting should be discouraged, as this may lead to further impaction of the shoulders.
- The woman should be maneuvered to bring her buttocks to the edge of the bed.
- Fundal pressure should not be employed. It is associated with a high rate of neonatal complications and may sometimes even result in uterine rupture.
- Enlarging the episiotomy may facilitate the delivery of shoulders in some cases. However, the routine use of episiotomy is not necessary in all cases. The clinicians should apply their own discretion regarding whether an episiotomy needs to be given or not; or if already given, does it need to be enlarged or not.
- Management of shoulder dystocia needs to be done within 5–7 minutes of the delivery of the fetal head in order to prevent irreversible fetal injury.
- After delivery of baby, the clinicians should be alert regarding the possibility of maternal complications such as PPH and third- and fourth-degree perineal tears. If the above-mentioned steps do not prove to be useful, the following maneuvers can be undertaken:

## McRoberts Maneuver

McRoberts maneuver is the single most effective intervention, which is associated with success rate as high as 90% and should be the first maneuver to be used. It causes the pubic symphysis to rotate in cephalad direction and straightening of the lumbosacral angle. Prophylactic McRoberts position may also be recommended in cases where shoulder dystocia is anticipated. The McRoberts maneuver (Figs 6.16A and B) involves sharp flexion and abduction of the maternal hips and positioning the maternal thighs on her abdomen. This maneuver helps in cephalad rotation of the symphysis pubis

**Flow chart 6.1:** Management of shoulder dystocia

Shoulder dystocia
- Avoid 3P's: Pushing, pulling and pivoting
- Documentation of events, their timing and management
- Call for help (an experienced obstetrician, midwife, neonatologist)
- Consider episiotomy, if required
- Move buttocks to the edge of bed

↓

McRoberts maneuver

↓

Suprapubic pressure and routine traction

→ Throughout, all these maneuvers, the shoulders must be rotated using pressure on the scapula or clavicle. The fetal head per se must never be rotated

↓

Try second-line maneuvers depending on clinical circumstances

← Deliver posterior arm

→ Internal rotational maneuver (Wood's Screw)

↓

Inform consultant obstetrician and anesthesist

→ The obsterician must be prepared for the maternal and neonatal complications such as postpartum hemorrhage and fetal asphyxia

↓

Consider all four position if all other maneuvers fail

Third-line maneuvers

↓

Consider cleidotomy, Zavanelli maneuver or symphysiotomy if nothing works

and the straightening of lumbosacral angle. This maneuver, by straightening the sacrum tends to free the impacted anterior shoulder. In a large number of cases, this maneuver by itself helps to free the impacted anterior shoulder.

## Suprapubic Pressure

Suprapubic pressure (also known as Rubin I maneuver) in conjunction with McRoberts maneuver is often all that is required to resolve 50–60% cases of shoulder dystocias. By application of suprapubic pressure, the clinician makes an attempt to manually dislodge the anterior shoulder from behind the symphysis pubis. In this maneuver the attendant makes a fist and places it just above the maternal pubic bone and pushes in a downward and lateral direction to push the posterior aspect of the anterior shoulder towards the fetal chest for a period of at least 30 seconds (Fig. 6.17). Since shoulder dystocias are caused by an infant's shoulders entering the pelvis in a direct anteroposterior orientation instead of the more physiologic oblique diameter, pushing the baby's anterior shoulder to one side or the other from above often helps in changing its position to the oblique, which would facilitate its delivery.

If these simple measures (the McRoberts maneuver and suprapubic pressure) fail, then a choice needs to be made between the all-four position and internal manipulation.

Some of the maneuvers for internal manipulation include Wood's screw maneuver, Rubin II maneuver, and reverse Wood's screw maneuver. These maneuvers are more commonly used in comparison to the all-four position.

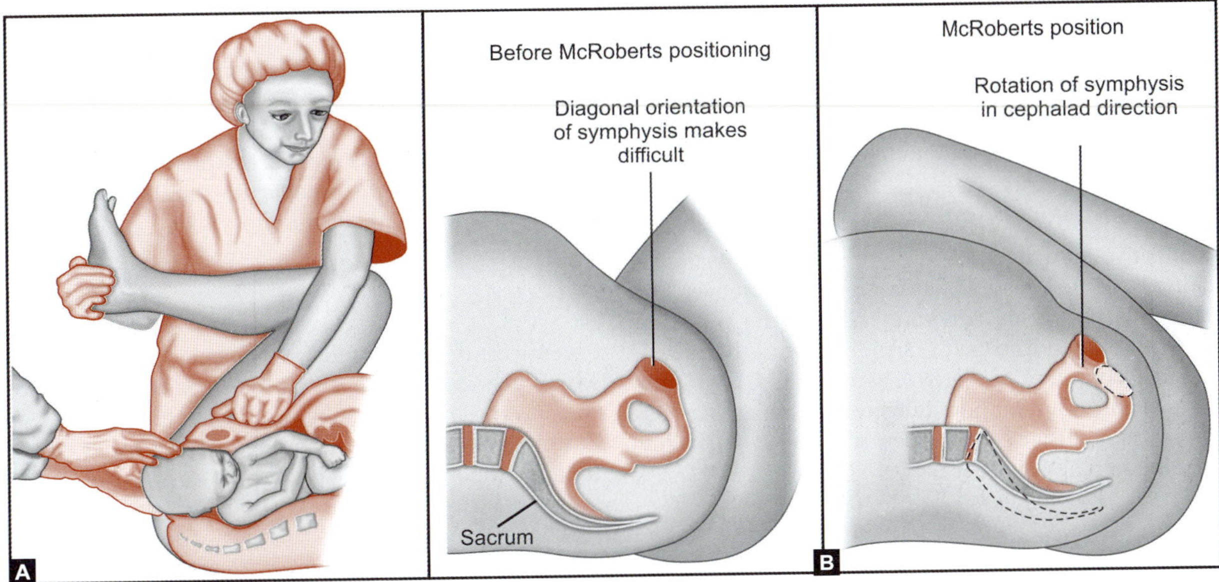



**Figs 6.16A and B:** (A) McRoberts maneuver (exaggerated hyperflexion of the thighs upon the maternal abdomen) and application of suprapubic pressure; (B) McRoberts maneuver causes the pubic symphysis to rotate in the cephalad direction and the straightening of lumbosacral angle

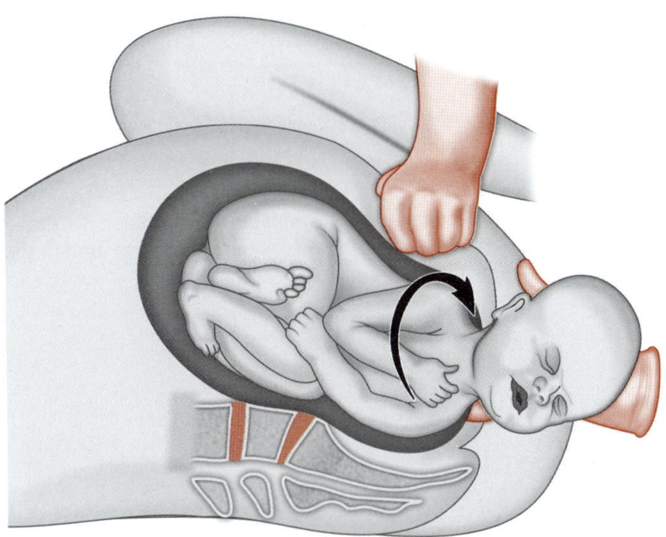

**Fig. 6.17:** Application of suprapubic pressure in the direction of fetal face

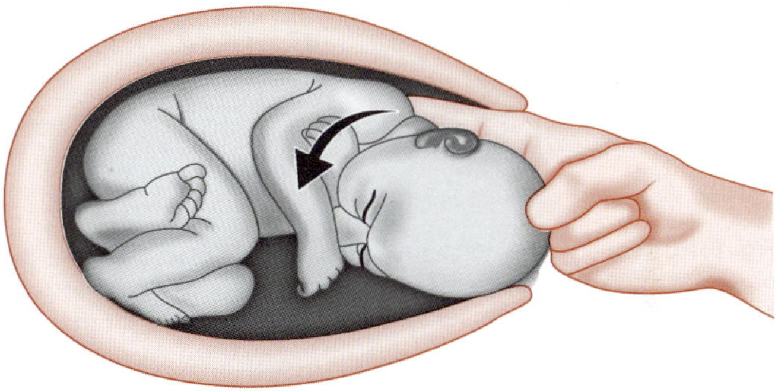

**Fig. 6.18:** Rubin II maneuver

into the more favorable oblique diameter. The delivery is likely to be successful, if attempted, after the application of this maneuver.

## Wood's Screw Maneuver

In this maneuver, the clinician's hand is placed behind the posterior shoulder of the fetus (Fig. 6.19). The shoulder is rotated progressively by 180° in a corkscrew manner so that the impacted anterior shoulder is released.

A variation of this is the Rubin's II maneuver, which involves pushing on the posterior surface of the posterior shoulder. In addition to the corkscrew effect, pressure on the posterior shoulder has the advantage of flexing the fetal shoulders across the chest. This decreases the distance between the shoulders, thereby reducing the dimension that must come out through the pelvis.

## Enter the Pelvis Maneuvers

### Rubin II Maneuver

In this maneuver, the clinician inserts the fingers of his/her right hand into the vagina and applies digital pressure on to the posterior aspect of the anterior shoulder, making an attempt to push it towards the fetal chest (Fig. 6.18). This rotates the shoulders (or the shoulder which is more accessible) forwards

### Reverse Wood's Screw Maneuver

In this maneuver the obstetrician applies pressure to the posterior aspect of the posterior shoulder and attempts to rotate it through 180° in the direction opposite to that described in the Wood's screw maneuver (Fig. 6.20).

### Delivery of the Posterior Arm

Another effective maneuver for resolving shoulder dystocias is the delivery of the posterior arm. In this maneuver, the obstetrician places his or her hand behind the posterior shoulder of the fetus and locates the arm. This arm is then swept across the fetal chest and delivered (Figs 6.21A to C). With the posterior arm and shoulder now delivered, it is relatively easy to rotate the baby, dislodge the anterior shoulder and allow delivery of the remainder of the baby.

### All-Four Maneuver

In this maneuver the patient is instructed to roll over from her existing position and to take a knee chest position on all her four limbs. This allows rotational movement of the sacroiliac joints, resulting in a 1–2 cm increase in the sagittal diameter of the pelvic outlet. It disimpacts the shoulders, allowing them to slide over the sacral promontory.

## Third-Line Maneuvers

Several third-line methods have been described for cases, which are resistant to all simple measures. Some of these maneuvers include cleidotomy, symphysiotomy and the Zavanelli maneuver. These maneuvers are rarely employed in today's modern obstetric practice.

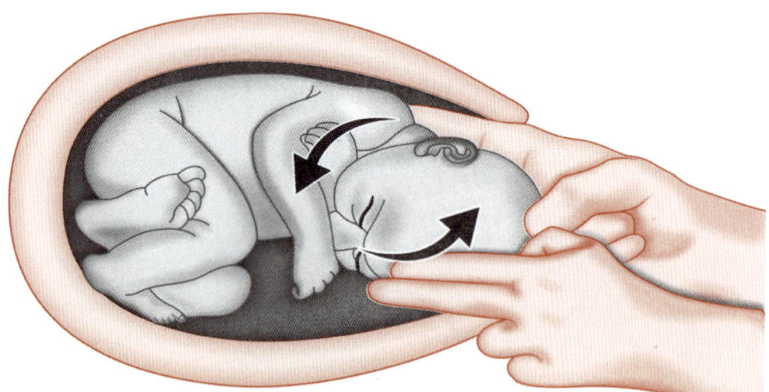

**Fig. 6.19:** Wood's screw maneuver: the hand is placed behind the posterior shoulder of the fetus. The shoulder is rotated progressively by 180° in a corkscrew manner so that the impacted anterior shoulder is released

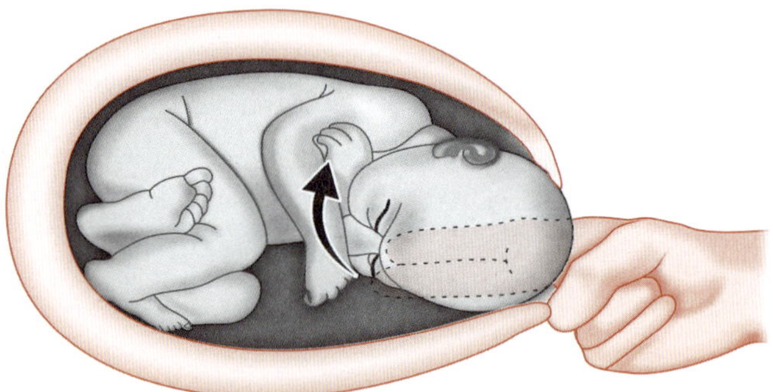

**Fig. 6.20:** Reverse Wood's screw maneuver: the shoulder is rotated progressively by 180° in a direction opposite to that described in the Wood' screw maneuver

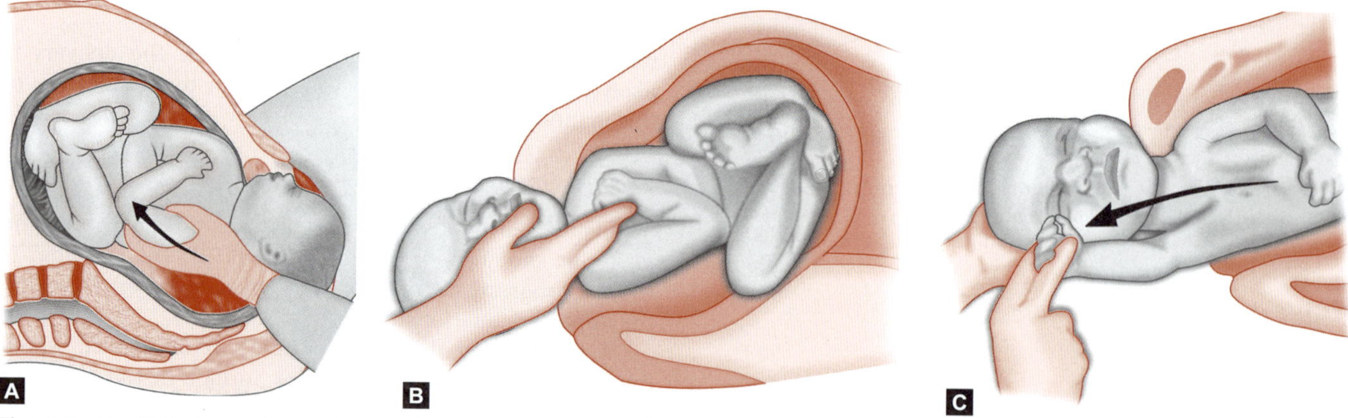

**Figs 6.21 A to C:** Delivery of posterior arm: (A) The clinician's hand is introduced into the vagina along the posterior shoulder. Keeping the arm flexed at the elbow, it is swept across the fetal chest; (B) The fetal hand is grasped and the arm is extended out along the side of the face; (C) The posterior arm and shoulder are delivered from the vagina

## COMPLICATIONS

### Fetal and Neonatal Complications

Following shoulder dystocia deliveries, 20% of babies may suffer some sort of injury, either temporary or permanent. The most common of these injuries are damage to the brachial plexus nerves, fracture of clavicles, fracture of humerus, contusions and lacerations and birth asphyxia.

### Maternal Complications

Besides the fetal complications, shoulder dystocia can also produce some complications in the mother. The most common maternal complications include PPH, second- and third-degree perineal tears, cervical lacerations and vaginal and vulvar lacerations.

### Conclusion

Presently, there is no way for the obstetricians to determine with any degree of accuracy, which babies are likely to be macrosomic or to experience shoulder dystocia at the time of delivery. Since both the prediction and prevention of shoulder dystocia is difficult, it is important for the obstetricians to be well-versed with this technique for immediately managing this condition in case it occurs.

Following the delivery of fetal head, as the baby's anterior shoulder passes under the mother's pubic bone, an effort must be made to deflect the baby's head in the downwards direction and traction must be applied to release the anterior shoulder. An important thing for the obstetricians is not to apply undue traction over the fetal head at the time of delivery as it is likely to result in fetal injuries such as injury to the brachial plexus. Another important thing for the obstetrician to remember is not to panic when faced with such a situation. Most cases of shoulder dystocia can be resolved by practicing the above described maneuvers with a cool mind.

# Episiotomy

An episiotomy is a surgical incision given through the perineum in order to enlarge the vagina for assisting the process of childbirth. Episiotomy is one of the most commonly performed surgical procedures in the United States. However, the prevalence of episiotomy has reduced gradually over the past few years. This is primarily due to the controversy related to the efficacy and safety of the procedure. Although episiotomy is commonly performed in our setup, there is no strong medical evidence supporting its use. Episiotomy can be considered as one of the most controversial operations in obstetric practice.

Giving an episiotomy is one of the ways of preventing the pelvic floor muscles against the harm caused by the genital tract trauma during the process of childbirth. The

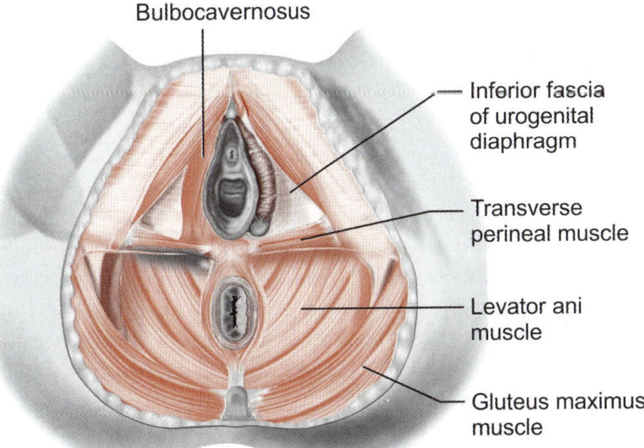


**Fig. 6.22:** Normal anatomy of the pelvic floor muscles

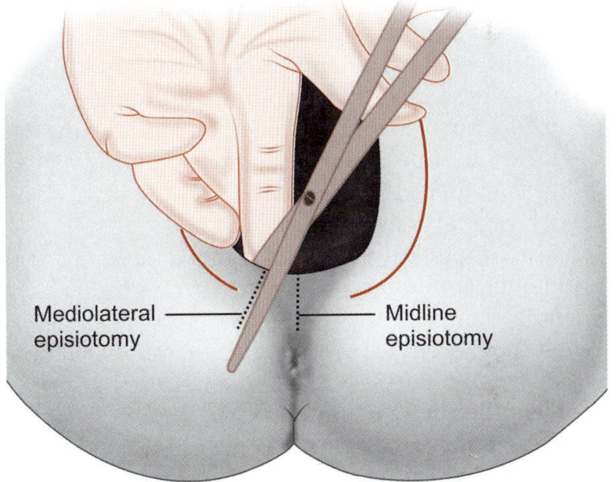


**Fig. 6.23:** Direction of giving different types of episiotomies

muscles of the pelvic floor form the major support on which the uterus and vagina rest, related anteriorly to bladder and urethra and posteriorly to rectum and anal canal (Fig. 6.22). Episiotomy is a surgical incision, which is believed to guard the muscles of the pelvic floor by protecting them against stretching related to childbirth and delivery. Episiotomy is believed to confer protection to the woman by substituting a ragged laceration with a straight surgical incision, thereby protecting the pelvic floor against trauma and injury related to childbirth. There are two different types of episiotomies depending upon the direction of the surgical incision (Fig. 6.23): midline episiotomy and the mediolateral episiotomy. The midline episiotomy extends medially in the midline, directly from the lower most edge of the vaginal opening towards the anus. The mediolateral episiotomy, on the other hand, begins in the midline and is directed laterally, either towards the right or the left.

## Aims of the Episiotomy

Previously it was believed that an episiotomy must routinely be performed at the time of vaginal delivery, especially in the primigravidas. However, according to the current recommendations by ACOG, an episiotomy must be only performed in the situations it is indicated. Some of the conditions in which an episiotomy is indicated are as follows:

- As a prophylactic method to spare the strain on the pelvic floor muscles when it becomes apparent that natural vaginal delivery may cause straining of the pelvic floor muscles resulting in second or third degree perineal tears.
- Rigidity of perineal muscles, which is responsible for causing an arrest in the natural progress of labor. An episiotomy must be performed if, at the time of normal vaginal delivery, the tissues around the vaginal opening begin to tear or do not seem to be stretching enough to allow the baby to be delivered.
- The baby is very large.
- To prevent complete perineal tears in cases where the perineum is short.
- In cases where instrumental vaginal delivery is indicated.
- Shoulder dystocia: Although the performance of episiotomy does not resolve the problem of shoulder dystocia, it does allow the operator more room to perform maneuvers to free shoulder from the pelvis.
- Breech vaginal delivery.
- In cases where a woman has undergone female genital mutilation, a midline or a mediolateral episiotomy may be indicated.
- When the patient is actively pushing, but rapid delivery is still required due to fetal distress (prolonged late decelerations or fetal bradycardia).
- Episiotomy may also be at times given in cases of extremely premature babies in order to prevent compression of fetal head.
- Episiotomy may be given in cases of high-risk pregnancy to shorten the duration of the second stage of labor. This

may help prevent undue bearing down efforts on the part of the mother in cases where she is suffering from medical disorders such as preeclampsia, heart disease, etc.

## Performance of Episiotomy

An episiotomy is a surgical incision, usually made with sterile scissors in the perineum as the baby's head is being delivered (Figs 6.24A to C). The following steps are observed while performing an episiotomy:

- Under all aseptic precautions after cleaning and draping the perineum, the proposed site of incision is infiltrated with 10 mL of 1% lignocaine solution (Figs 6.24A).
- Before performing the incision, two fingers of the clinician's left hand are placed between the fetal presenting part and the posterior vaginal wall.
- The incision is made using a curved scissors at the point when the woman is experiencing uterine contractions; the perineum is being stretched by the maternal presenting part and is at its thinnest.
- The cut should be made starting from the center of fourchette extending laterally either to the right or left. This type of episiotomy is known as the mediolateral type of episiotomy, which is most commonly performed in our setup. In many centers, a median episiotomy is performed extending from the center of fourchette towards the anus.
- The structures which are cut while performing the episiotomy include: posterior vaginal wall, superficial and deep transverse perineal muscles, bulbospongiosus and part of levator ani muscle, fascia covering these muscles, transverse perineal branches of pudental nerves and vessels, and subcutaneous tissues and skin.

## Repair of an Episiotomy Incision

- Following the delivery of the baby after the placenta has been expelled, the episiotomy incision is repaired. In case

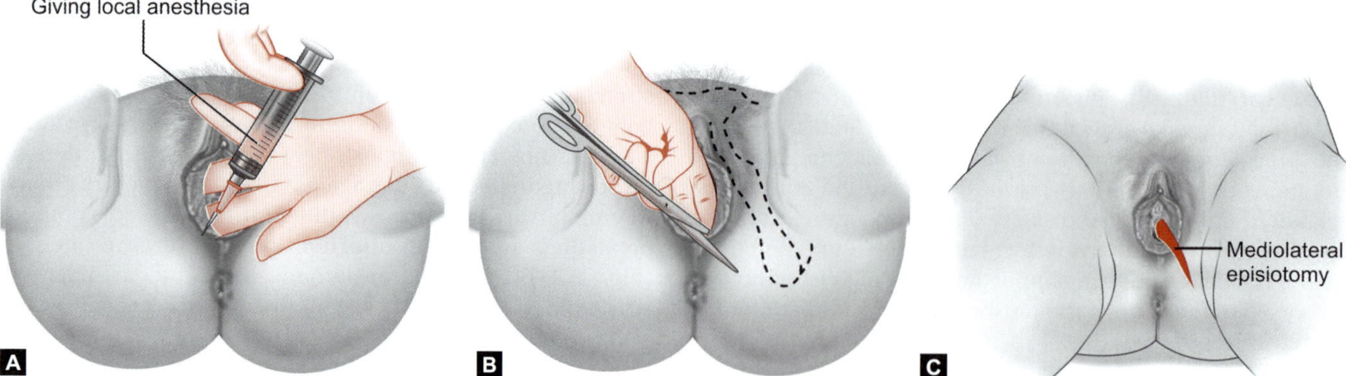



**Figs 6.24 A to C:** Procedure of giving a mediolateral episiotomy. (A) Infiltration of the perineum with local anesthesia before giving a mediolateral episiotomy; (B) The procedure of giving a mediolateral episiotomy incision; (C) Cut in the skin and muscles after giving a mediolateral episiotomy

of presence of vaginal tears or lacerations, their repair is also performed essentially in the same manner as that of the episiotomy.

- Prior to the repair of an episiotomy incision, the patient is placed in a lithotomy position with a good source of light, illuminating the area of incision. The area to be repaired must be cleaned with an antiseptic solution. The surgeon must examine the cervix, the vaginal walls, the vulval outlet and paraurethral areas for any suspected injuries or tears, which also need to be repaired.
- Under all aseptic precautions after cleaning and draping the perineum, the proposed site of repair is infiltrated with 10 mL of 1% lignocaine solution. If proper visualization of lower genital tract does not appear to be possible, it may be necessary to take the woman to theater for examination under anesthesia.
- The obstetrician must ensure that adequate assistance and instruments are also available in order to provide adequate exposure of the genital tract.
- The entire genital tract including the vulva, vagina, cervix and perineum must be inspected for trauma. Per speculum examination helps in the visualization of cervix and lower genital tract to exclude lacerations.
- Any injury, if found, must adequately be sutured and repaired.
- Before performing the repair, the perineum along with the site of incision must be well swabbed with an antiseptic solution.
- The repair of an episiotomy or vaginal lacerations (tears) is performed in three layers (Figs 6.25A to C): first layer comprising of the vaginal mucosa and submucosal tissues, second layer comprising of the perineal muscles, and the third layer comprising of the skin and subcutaneous tissues. The vaginal mucosa is repaired using continuous sutures with chromic 2-0 and 3-0 chromic catgut sutures. The first vaginal suture is placed just above or at the apex of the incision. After closing the vaginal incision and reapproximating the cut margins of the hymenal ring, the sutures are tied and cut. Next the fascia and the muscles of incised perineum are reapproximated with interrupted sutures of 2-0 or 3-0 chromic catgut. Lastly the skin is closed using interrupted matrix stitches with silk or subcuticular stitches.
- Small, nonbleeding lacerations of the cervix can be left unsutured. Lesions larger than 2 cm in size or those with a bleeding vessel need to be sutured.
- After stitching the laceration, the obstetrician must look for any continuing bleeding. Pressure or packing over the area of repair may help in achieving hemostasis.

## Postoperative Care of an Episiotomy

While repairing the episiotomy incision, the following steps must be observed:
- If infection is suspected, combinations of broad spectrum antibiotics can be administered.
- Application of an ice-pack over the stitches may help in reducing inflammation in the area, thereby reducing pain and swelling.
- Regular use of warm Seitz bath is also helpful in reducing pain and inflammation over the site of incision.
- The patient must be advised to ambulate around as much as possible and regularly perform the pelvic floor exercises in order to stimulate circulation and speed-up the process of healing.
- Use of pain killers, such as paracetamol may help in providing pain relief.

## Complications

Episiotomy can be associated with extensions or tears into the muscle of the rectum or even the rectum itself. Some of the complications which are likely to occur as a result of an episiotomy are as follows:
- Bleeding
- Infection
- Pain: While a slight amount of pain which gets relieved on taking pain killers is a common occurrence with an episiotomy, persistent severe pain at the episiotomy site could be an indicator of presence of a large vulvar, paravaginal or ischiorectal hematoma, thereby necessitating a thorough exploration in these cases.
- Extension of the episiotomy into third and fourth degree vaginal lacerations.
- Longer healing times.
- Increased discomfort when intercourse is resumed.
- Swelling.

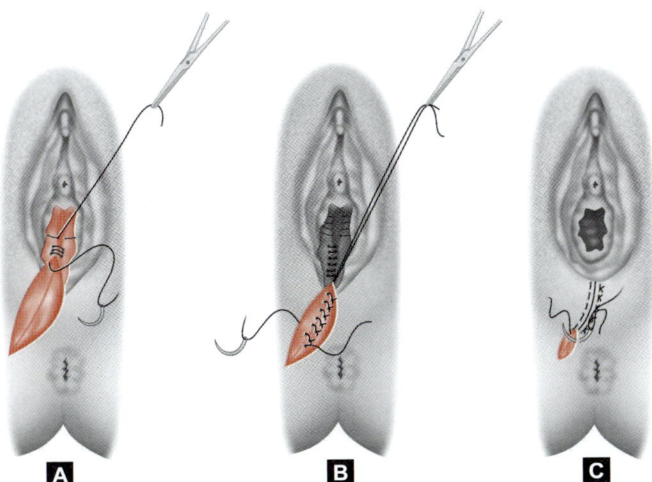

**Figs 6.25A to C:** Repair of an episiotomy incision: (A) Vaginal mucosa being repaired using continuous stitches; (B) Muscle layer being repaired using interrupted stitches; (C) Skin being repaired using interrupted matrix sutures

## Mediolateral versus Midline Episiotomy

Presently there also remains a controversy regarding the type of episiotomy to be performed: midline or mediolateral. Surgical repair and postoperative healing of a midline episiotomy is better in comparison to a mediolateral one. A midline episiotomy is also associated with better anatomical results, minimal postoperative pain, reduced blood loss and dyspareunia. Despite of these advantages, a midline episiotomy is associated with greater risk of extension into the third and fourth degree tears. This may be associated with the development of rectovaginal fistula in the long run, resulting in considerable morbidity.

As a result, midline episiotomy is considered to be superior to the mediolateral episiotomy except for the issue that it is more commonly associated with third and fourth degree extensions.

## Timing of an Episiotomy

If performed too early, an episiotomy may result in considerable amount of bleeding. If performed too late, it may not be able to prevent the lacerations. The episiotomy must be performed when the fetal head distends the vaginal introitus by 3–4 cm. When used with forceps application, episiotomy must be preferably performed following the application of the blades.

## Conclusion

Although the procedure of episiotomy was originally invented to reduce the risk of the genital tract injuries and lacerations, the exact benefit of the procedure still remains controversial.

According to recommendations of ACOG, an episiotomy should not be considered routine and only be performed if deemed necessary. The use of an episiotomy should be only restricted to the situations where there is likely to be a high risk of severe lacerations or there is a requirement for rapid delivery of the fetus. The women must be advised to exercise their pelvic muscles through Kegel exercises, which can help to prevent the requirement for an episiotomy.

# Perineal Tear Repair

## Perineal Injury

The perineal injury can be defined as the injury, which occurs to the perineum during the process of childbirth and can be classified into the following degrees (Figs 6.26A to D):

- *First degree:* Injury to the vaginal mucosa not involving the perineal muscles.
- *Second degree:* Injury to the perineum involving the perineal muscles, but not the anal sphincters.
- *Third degree:* Injury to the perineum involving the anal sphincter complex (external and internal anal sphincter):
    - 3a: Less than 50% of external anal sphincter is torn
    - 3b: More than 50% of external anal sphincter is torn
    - 3c: Internal anal sphincter also gets involved
- *Fourth degree:* Injury to the perineum involving the anal sphincter complex (external and internal anal sphincters) and rectal mucosa.

## Repair of Perineal Tears

Perineal tears and/or lacerations must be immediately repaired following the delivery of placenta in order to

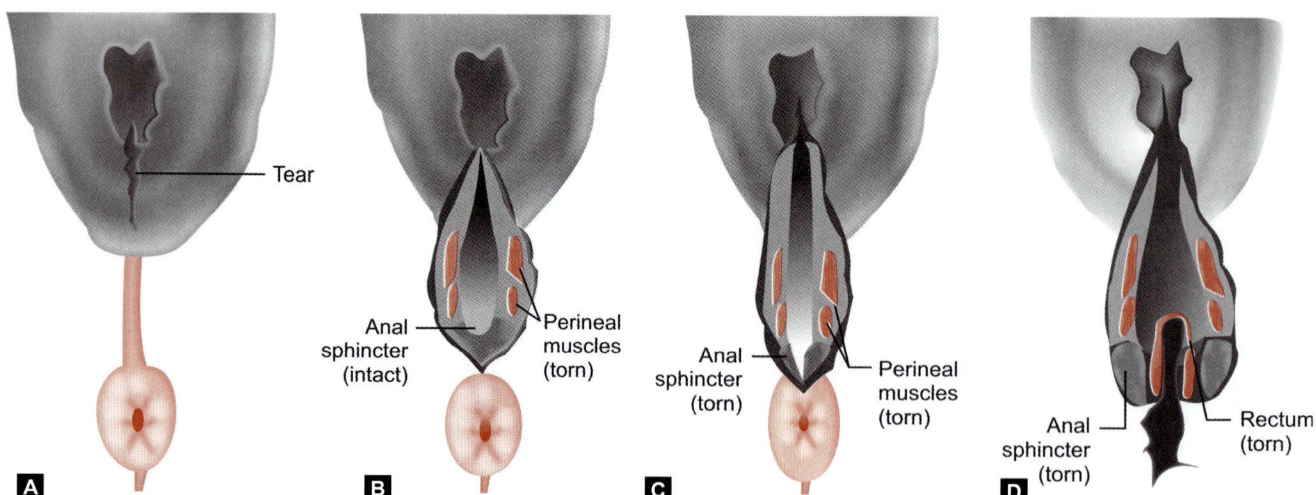


**Figs 6.26A to D:** (A) First degree perineal tear involving only the vaginal mucosa and not the perineal muscles; (B) Second degree perineal tear involving the perineal muscles as well; (C) Third degree perineal tear involving the anal sphincter complex; (D) Fourth degree perineal tear involving the rectal mucosa as well

minimize the blood loss and reduce the chances of infection. The repair of perineal tears is withheld if there is a delay of more than 24 hours. In these cases antibiotics must be instituted.

In case of lacerations, the steps of repair are essentially the same as that of an episiotomy except in the cases of third degree and fourth degree lacerations where there might be an extension up to the anal sphincters and rectal mucosa respectively. The preoperative preparation is same as that described for episiotomy before. The steps of surgery are as follows:

- In case of fourth degree laceration, it is important to approximate the torn edges of the anorectal mucosa with the fine absorbable sutures.
- Approximation of the anorectal mucosa and submucosa is done using 3-0 or 4-0 chromic catgut or vicryl sutures in a running or an interrupted manner (Fig. 6.27A).
- The superior extent of the anterior anal laceration is identified and sutures are placed through the submucosa of the anorectum starting above the apex of the tear and extending down until the anal verge.
- A second layer of sutures is placed through rectal muscularis using 3-0 vicryl or catgut sutures in a running or interrupted fashion (Fig. 6.27B). This layer of sutures acts as a reinforcing layer and incorporates the anal sphincter at the distal end.
- Finally, the torn edges of the anal sphincter are isolated, approximated and sutured together with 3 or 4 interrupted

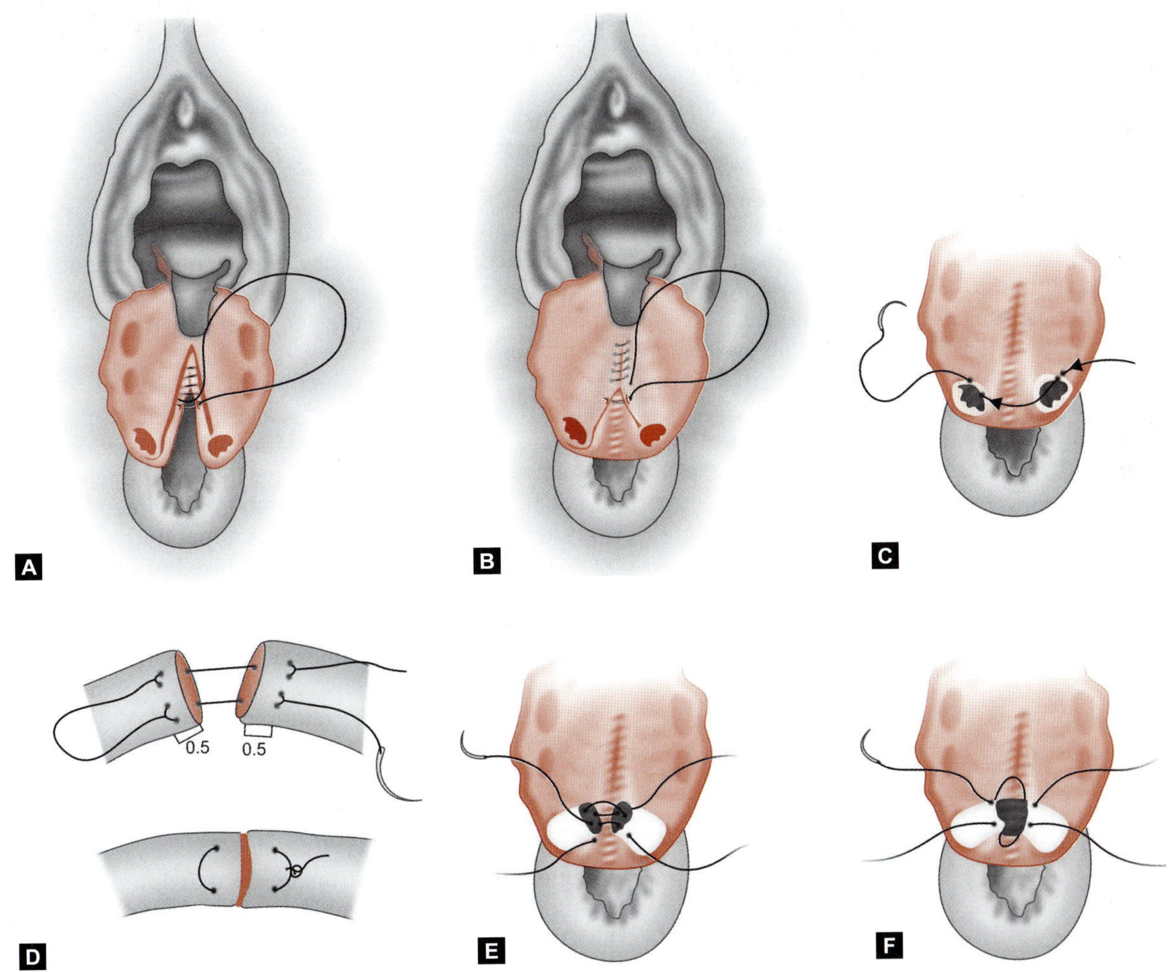

**Figs 6.27A to F:** (A) Approximation of anorectal mucosa and submucosa using continuous sutures; (B) Second layer of sutures placed through the rectal muscularis; (C) End-to-end approximation of the external anal sphincter. Sutures being placed through the posterior wall of external anal sphincters (these would be tied in the end); (D) Close-up view of the external anal sphincters showing end-to-end approximation; (E) End-to-end sutures taken through the interior of external anal sphincter (shown in whitish blue); (F) Approximation of the anterior wall of external anal sphincter

stitches. The anal sphincters need to be repaired in case of fourth degree tears as well as some third degree tears. The internal anal sphincter is identified as the thickening of the circular smooth muscle layer at the distal 2–3 cm of the anal canal. It appears as the glistening white fibrous structure lying between the anal canal submucosa and the fibers of external anal sphincter. In case the internal anal sphincters have retracted laterally, they need to be sought and brought together.

- Following the repair of internal anal sphincters, the torn edges of external anal sphincters are identified and grasped with allies clamp. The repair of these sphincters can be performed either using end-to-end repair (Figs 6.27C to F) or the overlap method (Fig. 6.28). For end-to-end approximation of the external anal sphincters, 4–6 simple interrupted sutures using 2-0 or 3-0 vicryl are placed through the edges of external anal sphincter and its connective tissue capsule at 3, 6, 9 and 12 O'clock positions. The sutures are first placed through the inferior and posterior portions of the sphincter; these stitches are tied last in order to facilitate the repair. The overlap method involves taking two sets of sutures: The first row of sutures is taken 1.5 cm from the edge on one side and 0.5 cm on the other side in such a way that when the sutures are tied, the free ends overlap one another. The free end is then sutured to the rest of the sphincter. The overlap method was considered to be superior to the end-to-end method as it was thought to be associated with fewer postoperative complications such as fecal urgency and anal incontinence.
- The remainder of repair is same as that described for a midline episiotomy previously.

### Postoperative Care of a Fourth Degree Laceration

The postoperative steps are essentially the same as described for an episiotomy. Due to the involvement of anal sphincters and rectal mucosa, additional steps may be required, which are described below:

- In case of fourth degree tears where the injury has extended until the rectal mucosa, the patient should be prescribed stool softeners for about a week or two. In these cases the use of enemas must be avoided.
- Immediately following the surgery, the patient must be advised to take liquid diet for a day and then gradually convert to low-residue diet over a few days.
- Lactulose in the dosage of 8 mL twice daily is administered from the second day onwards. This dosage is increased to 15 mL as the solid diet is started.
- Vaginal/rectal examination and sexual intercourse must be avoided for at least two weeks following the repair.
- Prophylactic intravenous antibiotics in the dose of cefuroxime (1.5 mg) and metronidazole (500 mg) must be administered either during the intraoperative or postoperative period.

# Cervical Tear Repair

### Introduction

Minor degree of tears can invariably occur in the cervix at the time of delivery and usually require no treatment. However, neglected cervical tears are the most common causes for traumatic PPH, with the left lateral tears being the most common.

The cervix must be explored in cases of unexplained hemorrhage after the third stage of labor, especially if the uterus is firmly contracted. In many cases, the deep cervical tears may be the likely cause for PPH. Although most of the cervical tears are less than 0.5 cm in size, deep cervical tears may at times even extend into the upper third of vagina. If the cervix is partially or completely avulsed from the vagina, the condition is known as colporrhexis. Rarely such tears may also extend up to the lower uterine segment and uterine artery or its branches and sometimes even through the peritoneum. This may result in extensive external hemorrhage. In such cases laparotomy may be required.

### Repair of Cervical Tears

*Preoperative Preparation*

Preoperative preparation is same as that described previously for repair of episiotomy and vaginal tears and laceration.

- Anesthesia is usually not required prior to the repair of cervical tears.
- An assistant should be asked to massage the uterus and provide fundal pressure.
- In order to detect the cervical tears, proper visualization of the cervix under good source of light is essential.

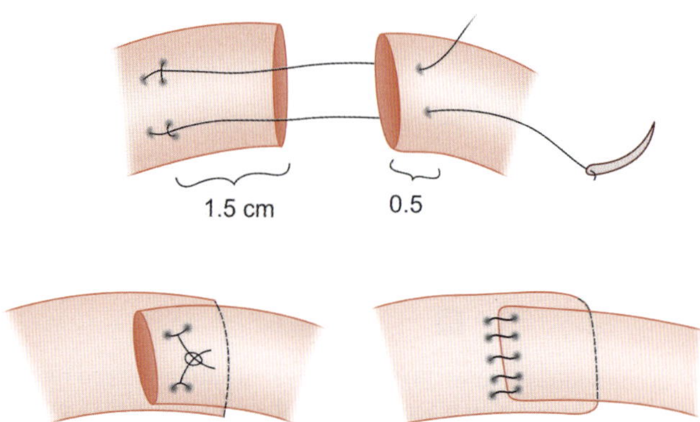


**Fig. 6.28:** Overlap method of suturing the anal sphincters

*Steps of Surgery*

An assistant must be asked to apply firm pressure in the downwards direction over the uterus, while the surgeon must exert downwards traction on the lip of cervix with the help of sponge-holding forceps. The procedure of repair comprises of the following steps (Fig. 6.29):

- Direct visualization and inspection of the cervix is done using three sponge-holding forceps. The anterior lip of cervix is grasped with one forceps at 12 O'clock position, the second forceps is placed at 2 O'clock position and the third one is placed at 4 O'clock position. The position of these three forceps is progressively changed, i.e. the first forceps is placed at 2 O'clock position, second one is placed at 4 O'clock position and third one at 6 O'clock position.
- The changes in the position of forceps are done until the entire cervical circumference has been inspected.
- Small, nonbleeding lacerations of the cervix can be left unsutured. Lesions larger than 2 cm in size or those with a bleeding vessel need to be sutured.
- The lacerations can be stitched with the help of continuous interlocking No. 0 chromic catgut sutures or polyglycolic sutures.
- The stitch must begin 1cm above the apex of the tear. If the apex cannot be visualized, gentle traction must be applied to bring the apex into the view. The stitch must be placed as high as possible.
- After stitching the laceration, the clinician must look for any continuing bleeding. Pressure or packing over the area of repair may help in achieving hemostasis.

## Complications

The complications, which can occur as a result of cervical tears, are tabulated in Table 6.6.

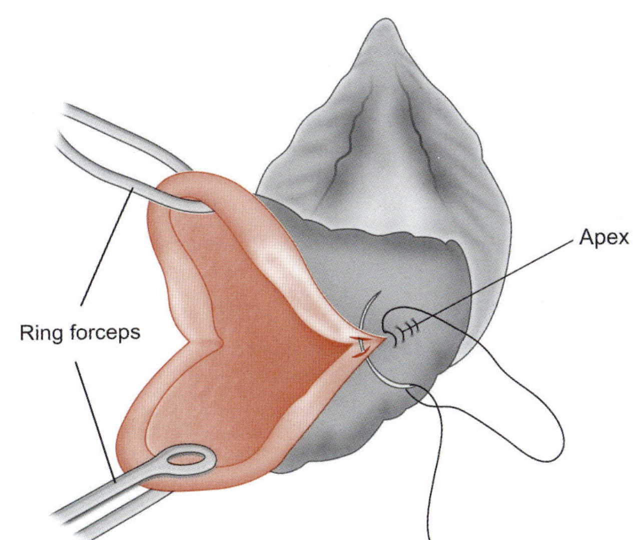


**Fig. 6.29:** Repair of a cervical tear

| **Table 6.6:** Complications occurring due to cervical tears | |
|---|---|
| *Early* | *Late* |
| • Severe PPH | • Ectropion |
| • Broad ligament hematoma | • Cervical incompetence |
| • Pelvic cellulitis | |
| • Thrombophlebitis | |

*Abbreviation:* PPH, postpartum hemorrhage

# Induction of Labor

Induction of labor can be defined as commencement of uterine contractions before the spontaneous onset of labor with or without ruptured membranes. It is indicated when the benefits of delivery to the mother or fetus outweigh the benefits of continuing the pregnancy. Induction of labor comprises of cervical ripening (in case of an unfavorable cervix) and labor augmentation. While cervical ripening aims at making the cervix soft and pliable, augmentation refers to stimulation of spontaneous contractions, which may be considered inadequate due to failed cervical dilation or fetal descent. Dilatation and effacement of cervix associated with cervical ripening and labor augmentation ultimately results in delivery of the baby.

Cervical ripening is complex process, primarily occurring under the influence of prostaglandins whereby prostaglandins cause the breakdown of the cervical proteoglycan ground substance, scattering of the collagen fibers, an increase in the content of substances such as elastase, glycosaminoglycan, dermatan sulfate and hyaluronic acid levels in the cervix. Induction of labor must be considered only when vaginal delivery appears to be an appropriate route of delivery and no contraindications for the vaginal route are present.

## Indications

Induction of labor is indicated only in those situations where it becomes apparent that both the mother and the fetus would be associated with a higher likelihood of better outcome if the fetal birth is expedited. Before taking the decision for induction of labor the clinician must weigh the benefits of labor induction against the potential maternal and fetal risks. Though there are no absolute indications for induction of labor, some common indications for the induction of labor are as follows:

### Maternal Indications

*Indications specific to pregnancy:* These include the following:
- Oligohydramnios
- Polyhydramnios

- Ruptured membranes with preeclampsia or eclampsia or nonreassuring fetal heart status
- Abruptio placenta
- Chorioamnionitis
- Rh isoimmunization.

*Maternal diseases:* These include the following:
- Diabetes mellitus
- Renal disease
- Chronic pulmonary disease
- Chronic hypertension.

### Fetal Indications

- Postmaturity
- Intrauterine growth restriction
- PROM
- Fetus with congenital anomalies
- Intrauterine fetal death.

## Prerequisites

Prior to the induction of labor, following steps must be performed:
- *Patient counseling:* Before induction of labor is undertaken, the patient must be carefully counseled. She should be explained about the reason for induction, end points of the process, requirement for LSCS in case the induction fails, options of mode of delivery, neonatal outcomes and complications, etc. All relevant information should be made available to the women and she should be helped to be able to make an informed choice regarding her care or treatment plan.
- *Evaluation of state of cervix:* This is done by calculation of the Bishop's score (Table 6.7). A maximum score of 13 is possible with this scoring system. Labor is most likely to commence spontaneously with a score of 9 or more, whereas lower scores (especially those < 5) may require cervical ripening and/or augmentation with oxytocin.
- *Ultrasound assessment of gestational age:* This would help to prevent induction in premature babies.
- *Assessment of fetal lung maturity:* This may not be required in case where induction is medically indicated and the

risk of continuing the pregnancy is greater than the risk of delivering a baby before lung maturity has been attained.

## Methods for Induction of Labor

Methods for induction of labor comprise of both methods for cervical ripening and as well as augmentation of labor. Methods of cervical ripening include pharmacological methods, nonpharmacological methods and use of mechanical cervical dilators.

### Pharmacological Methods

Medical methods for labor induction commonly comprise of prostaglandins [Dinoprostone (PGE2), or misoprostol (PGE1)] and/or oxytocin.

*Dinoprostone:* Dinoprostone helps in cervical ripening and is available in the form of gel (prepidil or cerviprime) or a vaginal insert (cervidil). Prepidil comprises of 0.5 mg of dinoprostone in a 2.5 mL syringe. The gel is injected intracervically every 6 hours for up to three doses in a 24-hour period. Cervidil, on the other hand is a vaginal insert containing 10 mg of dinoprostone. The main advantage of cervidil is that it can be immediately removed in case it causes hyperstimulation.

*Misoprostol:* Misoprostol (Cytotec) is a synthetic PGE1 analog. This drug has not been currently approved by the US FDA for cervical ripening or induction of labor. Misoprostol, however, has been approved for the prevention of peptic ulcers. Use of misoprostol for cervical ripening is an off-label use, which is still considered controversial by some clinicians. However, its use is recommended by the ACOG. A dose of 25 mg is placed transvaginally at every 3 hourly intervals for a maximum of 4 doses or it may be prescribed in the oral dosage of 50 mg orally at every 4 hourly intervals. Also, presently, the available evidence supports the intravaginal or oral use of 25–50 µg of PGE1 for cervical ripening/induction of labor. The same dosage can be repeated after 4–6 hours, if required.

*Oxytocin:* Oxytocin is a uterotonic agent, which stimulates uterine contractions and is used for both induction and

| | **Table 6.7:** Bishop's score (modified) | | | | |
|---|---|---|---|---|---|
| *Score* | *Dilation (cm)* | *Effacement (%)* | *Station of the* | *Cervical consistency* | *Position of cervix presenting part* |
| 0 | Closed | 0–30 | –3 | Firm | Posterior |
| 1 | 1–2 | 40–50 | –2 | Medium | Mid-position |
| 2 | 3–4 | 60–70 | –1,0 | Soft | Anterior |
| 3 | > 5 | > 80 | +1,+2 | — | — |

augmentation of labor. It can be started in low dosage regimens of 0.5–1.5 MIU/minute or the high dosage regimen of 4.5–6.0 MIU/minute with incremental increases of 1.0–2.0 MIU/minute at every 15–40 minutes. If an intrauterine pressure catheter is in place, measurement of intrauterine pressure ranging between 180–200 Montevideo units/period is an indicator of adequate oxytocin dosing. For further details related to oxytocin, kindly refer to Chapter 15.

*Other pharmacological methods for induction of labor:* Mifepristone (Mifeprex) is an antiprogesterone agent, which is able to stimulate the uterine contractions. Isosorbide mononitrate is another agent, which can be used for cervical ripening without stimulating uterine activity.

Breast massage with nipple stimulation is a nonpharmacologic method, which is thought to stimulate uterine contractions by facilitating the release of oxytocin from the posterior pituitary gland.

The most commonly used technique involves gentle massage of the breasts or application of warm compresses to the breasts for 1 hour, three times a day.

### Surgical Management

Various nonpharmacological methods for labor induction comprise of the following:
- Low rupture of membranes.
- Stripping of membranes.

*Low rupture of membranes:* Artificial rupture of membranes is used as a method of induction only in the patients where the cervix is favorable. ARM induces labor by causing the release of prostaglandins. Procedure for rupture of membranes has been described later in the text.

*Stripping of membranes:* As the name implies, the process involves stripping of membranes by inserting the examining finger through the internal cervical os and moving it in a circular direction to detach the inferior pole of the membranes from the lower uterine segment. The process is thought to augment labor by causing the release of prostaglandins (PG F2$\alpha$) and phsospholipase A2.

### Mechanical Methods

This may include natural osmotic dilators (e.g. laminaria tents) and synthetic osmotic dilators. The natural dilators are hygroscopic in nature and are capable of absorbing endocervical and local tissue fluids, which cause the device to enlarge within the endocervical canal, thereby exerting controlled mechanical pressure. Balloon devices such as 24/26-French Foley's balloon can also be used to provide mechanical pressure directly in the cervix as the balloon is inflated.

## Contraindications

Contraindications for induction of labor are the similar to that for spontaneous labor and vaginal delivery. Some of the absolute contraindications for induction of labor include:
- Transverse lie.
- Vasa previa, placenta previa.
- Previous history of uterine surgery (especially with the involvement of uterine cavity).
- Previous history of classical cesarean section.

Certain relative contraindications for induction of labor are as follows:
- Previous LSCS.
- Breech presentation.
- Multiple pregnancy.
- Maternal heart disease.

## Complications

Induction of labor in general can be associated with the following complications:
- Uterine hyperstimulation (with oxytocin and misoprostol), may result in uteroplacental hypoperfusion and fetal heart rate deceleration.
- Prostaglandins may produce tachysystole, which may be controlled with terbutaline.
- Maternal systemic effects, such as fever, vomiting and diarrhea, may be infrequently observed.
- Failure of induction.
- Uterine atony and PPH.
- Increased rate of cesarean delivery.
- Chorioamnionitis.
- Oxytocin may be sometimes responsible for producing water intoxication.

Complications associated with ARM are as follows:
- Reduction in amniotic fluid may result in cord compression and/or head compression
- The intensity of pains may increase to undesirable levels, adversely affecting the fetus
- There may be a danger of cord prolapse and limb prolapse
- Predisposition to a premature separation of the placenta
- The risk of ascending infection, which further increases with the passage of time
- The clinician is compelled to accomplish delivery within a reasonable period of time.

Complications associated with sweeping and stretching of membranes include risk of infection, bleeding, accidental rupture of the membranes and discomfort to the patient.

## Summary

Induction of labor helps in expediting the process of vaginal delivery. Induction and augmentation of labor appear to be the two parts of the same continuum merging imperceptibly into one another. Induced labors are associated with higher rate of operative interference and an increased demand for pain relief. It can be done both using medical and surgical methods. However, any induced labor must be carefully monitored. It is especially important for the clinician not to leave any patient with induced labor unattended. All induced labors must be monitored with help of a partogram. Continuous electronic fetal monitoring is not essential. In case of suspicious/pathological findings on cardiotocography, oxytocin infusion must be decreased or discontinued. In suspected or confirmed cases of acute fetal compromise, the delivery should be accomplished as soon as possible (preferably within 30 minutes).

# Version

Version is a manipulative procedure aimed at changing the lie of fetus or bringing the comparatively favorable fetal pole towards the lower pole of the uterus mainly to facilitate vaginal delivery. Version could be external or internal. In external version, the manipulative procedure is performed externally. On the other hand, in the procedure of internal version, the maneuver is performed by introducing one hand inside the uterine cavity and keeping the other hand over the abdomen. The version is known as cephalic when the cephalic pole of the fetus is brought down towards the lower pole of the uterus. The version is known as podalic when the podalic pole of the fetus is brought down towards the lower pole of the uterus. The most common type of version employed in modern obstetric practice is the external cephalic version (ECV). Internal podalic version is also rarely employed in modern obstetric practice.

## EXTERNAL CEPHALIC VERSION

### Definition

External cephalic version is a procedure in which the clinician externally rotates the fetus from a breech/transverse presentation into a cephalic presentation. The use of ECV helps in producing considerable cost savings in the management of the fetus in breech or shoulder presentation

at term by reducing the rate of cesarean section. The most common indications for cesarean section in obstetric practice include history of previous cesarean section and labor dystocia, followed by malpresentations (breech presentation and transverse lie). Routine use of external version has been observed to reduce the rate of cesarean delivery by about two-thirds. Therefore, this procedure must become a routine part of obstetric practice.

Efficacy of ECV varies between 48% and 77%, with an average of 62%. Use of ECV is associated with minimal risks, including rare complications like umbilical cord entanglement, abruption placenta, preterm labor, premature rupture of the membranes (PROM), transient fetal heart changes and severe maternal discomfort.

## Indications for ECV

The indications for ECV are as follows:
- Breech presentation
- Transverse lie (if version fails in cases of transverse lie, the only option for delivery is via cesarean section.

## Timing for ECV

It is preferable to wait until term (37 completed weeks of gestation) before external version is attempted because of an increased success rate and avoidance of preterm delivery if complications arise. Ideally the ECV should be performed as close to 37 weeks as possible, but after 36 weeks.

## Contraindications

ECV should not be performed in the women having contra-indications mentioned in Table 6.8.

## Prerequisites for ECV

Before the performance of ECV, the following prerequisites should be fulfilled:
- The place where ECV is being performed should have all facilities available for cesarean section or emergency breech vaginal delivery, in case it is required. There is

**Table 6.8:** Contraindications for external cephalic version

| *Absolute contraindications* | *Relative contraindications* |
|---|---|
| • Multiple gestation with a fetus presenting as a transverse lie/ breech presentation<br>• Herpes simplex virus infection<br>• Placenta previa<br>• Nonreassuring fetal heart rate tracing<br>• Premature rupture of membranes<br>• Significant third-trimester bleeding (placenta previa, etc.) | • Uterine malformations<br>• Evidence of uteroplacental insufficiency (IUGR, preeclampsia, etc.)<br>• Fetal anomaly<br>• Maternal cardiac disease |

*Abbreviation:* IUGR, intrauterine growth restriction

always a possibility for emergency cesarean section during the procedure in case there is a decline in FHR.

- Blood grouping and crossmatching should be done in case an emergency cesarean section is required.
- In case the mother is Rh-negative, administration of 50 µg of anti-D immunoglobulin is required after the procedure in order to prevent the risk of isoimmunization. Anesthetists must be informed well in advance.
- Maternal intravenous access must be established.
- The woman is not required to be nil by mouth for the procedure.
- An ultrasound examination must be performed to confirm the fetal presentation, check the rate of fetal growth, amniotic fluid volume and to rule out anomalies associated with breech or shoulder presentation.
- A nonstress test or a biophysical profile must be performed prior to ECV to confirm fetal well-being.
- Though ECV can be performed by a clinician single handedly, an assistant is also required.
- Before performing an ECV, a written informed consent must be obtained from the mother.
- A tocolytic agent such as terbutaline in a dosage of 0.25 mg may be administered subcutaneously. By producing uterine relaxation, administration of this drug is supposed to help increase the success rate of the procedure. The use of general anesthesia should be avoided due to an increased risk of complications. However, ECV can be performed under epidural or spinal analgesia.
- Whether the process has been successful or has failed, a nonstress test and an ultrasound examination must be performed after each attempt of ECV and after the end of the procedure in order to rule out fetal bradycardia and to confirm successful version.

If ECV is unsuccessful, then the clinician can discuss further options with the woman. These include repeat ECV attempt, vaginal breech delivery or an elective cesarean section.

## Procedure

- The patient is placed in a supine or slight Trendelenburg position to facilitate disengagement/mobility of the presenting part.
- Ultrasonic gel/talcum powder, almond or vegetable oil is applied liberally over the abdomen in order to decrease friction and to reduce the chances of an over-vigorous manipulation. External version can be performed by a clinician experienced in the procedure along with his/her assistant.
- Initially, the degree of engagement of the presenting part should be determined and gentle disengagement of the presenting part is performed, if possible.

### Manipulation in Breech Presentation

While performing ECV in cases of breech presentation, the clinician helps in gently manipulating the fetal head towards the pelvis while the breech is brought up cephalad towards the fundus. Two types of manipulation of fetal head can be performed: a forward roll or a backward roll. The clinician must attempt a forward roll first and then a backward roll, if the initial attempt is unsuccessful. Though it does not matter in which direction the fetus is flipped, most physicians tend to start with a forward roll.

The forward roll (Figs 6.30A to D) is usually helpful if the spine and head are on opposite sides of the maternal midline.

If the spine and head of the fetus are on the same side of the maternal midline, then the back flip may be attempted (Figs 6.31A to C). If the forward roll is unsuccessful, a second attempt is usually made in the opposite direction.

### Manipulation in Cases of Transverse Lie

- Version in transverse lie is much easier than in cases of breech presentation. While performing the ECV in case of transverse lie, the clinician helps in gently manipulating the fetal head towards the pelvis while the podalic pole

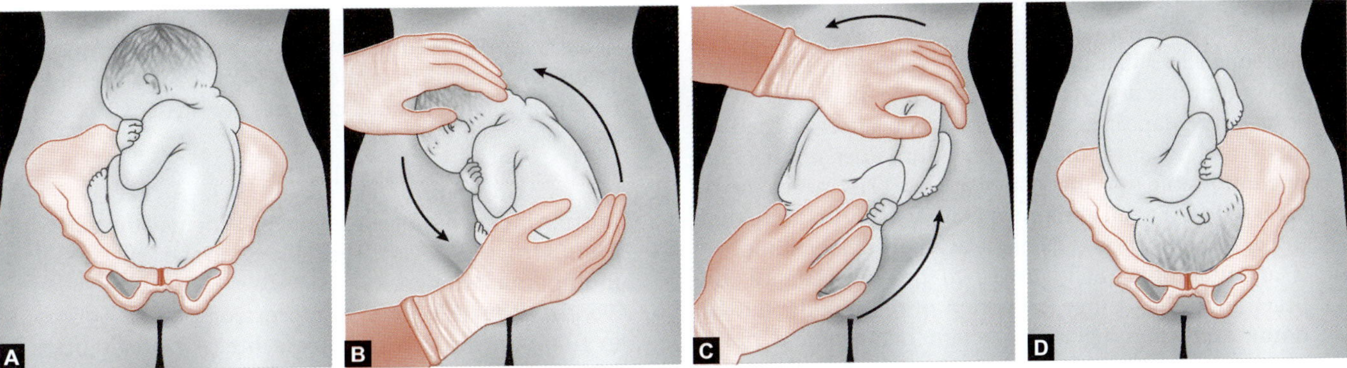

**Figs 6.30A to D:** External cephalic version through forward roll. (A) Baby in breech presentation; (B) Forward roll: The breech is disengaged and simultaneously pushed upwards; (C) The vertex is gently pushed towards the pelvis; (D) Forward roll is completed

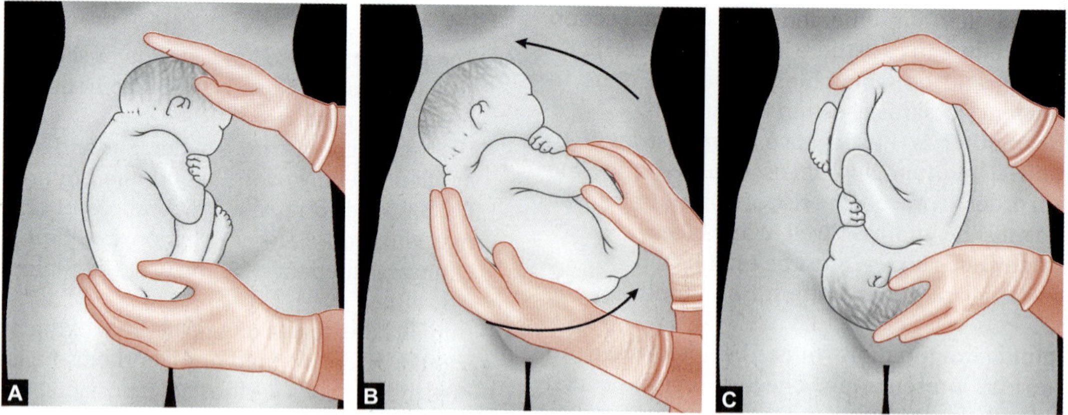

**Figs 6.31A to C:** External cephalic version through back flip. (A) Disengaging the breech; (B) Pushing the breech upwards and gently guiding the vertex towards the pelvis; (C) Completing the back flip

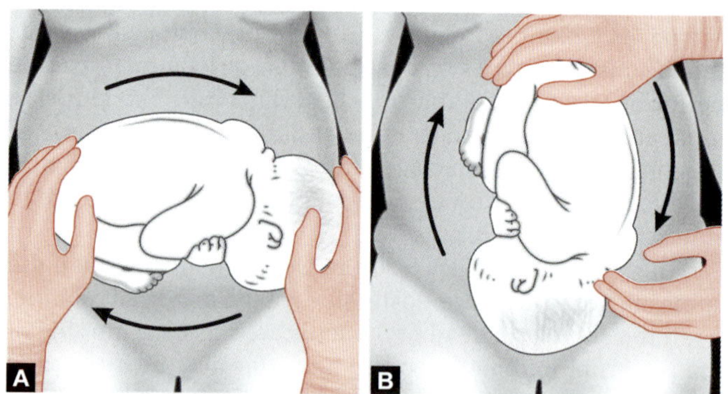

**Figs 6.32A and B:** Procedure for external cephalic version in case of transverse lie

is brought up cephalad towards the fundus (Figs 6.32A and B).

- While doing the ECV, the fetus should be moved gently rather than using forceful movements.
- If unsuccessful, the version can be reattempted at a later time. The procedure should only be performed in a facility equipped for emergency cesarean section.
- No consensus has been reached regarding how many ECV attempts are appropriate at one particular time. At a particular time setting, multiple attempts can be made making sure that the procedure does not become uncomfortable for the patient. Also FHR needs to be assessed after each attempt at ECV. Usually no more than three attempts should be made at a particular sitting.
- If an attempt at ECV proves to be unsuccessful, the practitioner has either the option of sending the patient home and adopting an expectant management policy or proceeding with a cesarean delivery. Expectant management also involves repeat attempts of ECV at weekly intervals. With expectant management there is also

a possibility that the fetus would undergo spontaneous reversion into cephalic position.

## Complications of ECV

Though ECV is largely a safe procedure, it can rarely have some complications, including the following:

- Premature onset of labor.
- Premature rupture of the membranes.
- A small amount of fetomaternal hemorrhage. This is especially dangerous in cases of Rh-negative pregnancies as it can result in the development of Rh isoimmunization. Therefore, in cases of Rh-negative pregnancy, anti-D immunoglobulins must be administered to the mother following the procedure of ECV.
- Fetal distress leading to an emergency cesarean delivery.
- Failure of version: The baby might turn back to the breech position after the ECV is done. ECV is associated with high rate of spontaneous reversion into breech presentation, if performed before 36 weeks of gestation.
- Risk of cord entanglement: If fetal bradycardia is detected after a successful version, it is recommended that the infant be returned to its previous breech presentation with the hope of reducing the risk of a tangled cord.
- Transient reduction of the FHR is probably due to vagal response related to head compression with ECV.

## Indicators of Successful ECV

Some of the indicators for successful ECV include the following:

- *Multiparity:* ECV is more likely to be successful in multiparous women.
- *Nonfrank breech:* ECV is more likely to be successful in nonfrank breech (complete breech) pregnancies in comparison to frank breech pregnancies. This is so as the splinting action of the spine in a frank breech gestation is likely to prevent fetal movement.

- *Unengaged breech:* Fetus in breech presentation which has engaged is less likely to undergo version in comparison to the unengaged fetus in breech presentation.
- *Adequate liquor:* Presence of reduced (oligohydramnios) or excessive liquor (polyhydramnios) is likely to interfere with successful version.

## INTERNAL PODALIC VERSION

### Introduction

Internal podalic version involves manipulating the fetus with the help of operator's one hand introduced inside the uterus to help bring down the podalic pole of the fetus into the lower pole of the uterus. This is completed with the breech extraction of the baby.

### Indication

In modern obstetrics the only indication for internal version is fetus in transverse lie in case of second baby in twin gestation. Besides this indication, this technique is rarely employed in obstetric practice. Also, this technique must never be employed in case of obstructed labor.

### Technique for Internal Podalic Version

*Prerequisites for Internal Podalic Version*

Before undertaking the procedure of internal podalic version, the obstetrician must make sure that the following conditions are fulfilled:
- Cervix must be completely dilated.
- Liquor amnii must be adequate for intrauterine manipulation.
- Fetal lie, presentation and FHR must be assessed by an experienced obstetrician before undertaking the procedure.

*Actual Procedure*

- The technique of internal version is shown in Figure 6.33. The procedure must be ideally performed under general anesthesia with the uterus sufficiently relaxed.
- Under all aseptic precautions, the clinician introduces one of his/her hands into the uterine cavity in a cone-shaped manner.
- The hand is passed along the breech to ultimately grasp the fetal foot, which is identified by palpation of its heel. While the foot is gradually brought down, clinician's other hand present externally over the abdomen helps in gradually pushing the cephalic pole upwards.
- Rest of the delivery is completed by breech extraction.

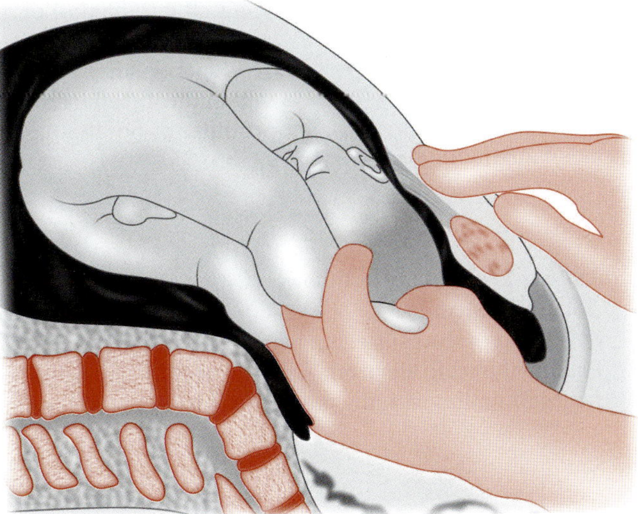

**Fig. 6.33:** Technique for internal podalic version

**Table 6.9:** Complications due to internal podalic version

| *Maternal* | *Fetal* |
|---|---|
| • Placental abruption | • Asphyxia |
| • Rupture uterus | • Cord prolapse |
| • Increased maternal mortality and morbidity | • Intracranial hemorrhage |

*Postdelivery*

Following the delivery of the baby, routine exploration of the cervicovaginal canal must be done to exclude out any injuries.

### Complications

Various complications, which can occur as a result of internal podalic version, are described in Table 6.9.

## Artificial Rupture of Membranes

### Definition

As the name implies, "artificial rupture of membranes" or amniotomy involves breaking the fetal membranes below the fetal presenting part overlying the internal os in order to drain out some amniotic fluid. The procedure acts as a method for surgical induction of labor. In this process, the labor can be induced through the following mechanisms:
- Stretching of the cervical os.
- Stretching of fetal membranes resulting in the release of prostaglandins.

- Escape of amniotic fluid resulting in the reduction of the volume of liquor

Effectiveness of the procedure depends upon several factors, i.e. state of cervix (cervical dilatation and effacement); station of the presenting part and whether or not the patient has been augmented with oxytocin.

## Indications

Indications for ARM are as follows:
- Abruptio placenta.
- Severe preeclampsia/eclampsia.
- Placing the scalp electrode for electronic fetal monitoring.
- In combination with the medical methods of induction.

## Contraindications

Contraindications of ARM are as follows:
- High presenting part (care must be taken while performing ARM to reduce the risk of cord prolapse).
- Preterm labor.
- Maternal AIDS.
- Caution must be observed in cases of polyhydramnios or any malposition or malpresentation.
- Placenta previa.
- Vasa previa.
- Active genital herpes infection.

## Procedure

### Preoperative Preparation

Following precautions should be taken while performing an ARM:
- Before performing an ARM, the patient must be asked to empty her bladder.
- The procedure is usually conducted in the labor ward, but should be conducted in the operation theater if the risk of cord prolapse is high.
- An abdominal examination must be performed prior to the procedure to confirm the fetal lie, presentation, position and degree of engagement.
- The patient is made to lie in a lithotomy position prior to the procedure.
- Before doing an ARM, the fetal head must be stabilized using the abdominal hand in order to minimize the chances of cord prolapse.
- Complete surgical asepsis must be observed prior to the procedure.

### Actual Procedure

- The index finger and the middle fingers of the clinician's gloved right hand (smeared with antiseptic) are introduced inside the vagina. The index finger is passed through the cervical canal beyond the internal os. As far as can be reached by the fingers, the fetal membranes are swept free from the lower uterine segment.
- After sweeping and stretching of membranes the fingers are still kept inside, keeping their palmer surface upwards. Along with the guidance of these fingers, a long Kocher's forceps or an amnion hook is introduced inside up till the membranes are reached (Figs 6.34 and 6.35).
- The forceps blades are opened to grasp the membranes, which are torn with help of twisting movements.
- If an amnion hook is used, the nonexamining hand is used for carefully sliding the amnion hook with its hook pointing downwards between the examining hand and

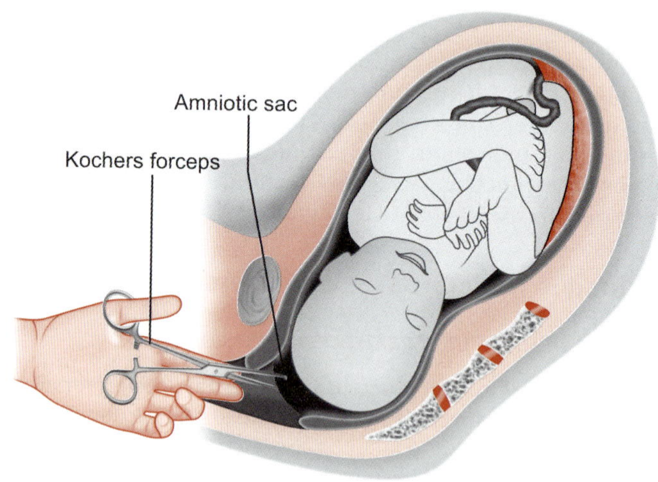



**Fig. 6.34:** Artificial rupture of membranes using Kocher's forceps

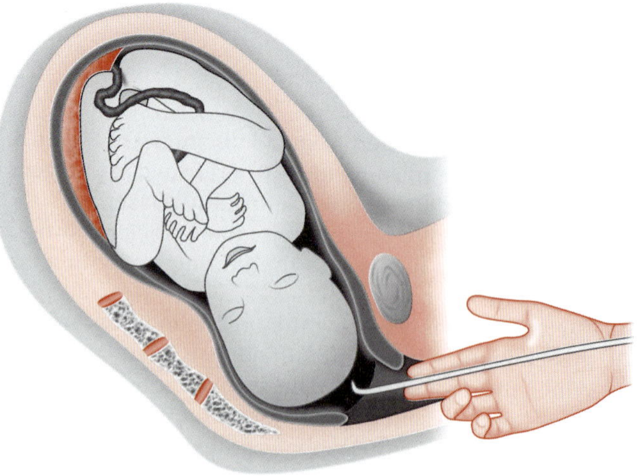

**Fig. 6.35:** Artificial rupture of membranes using amnion hook

the vaginal wall. The amnion hook is then guided into place against the fetal membranes. The amnion hook is twisted against the bulging fore-waters at the height of a contraction, thereby rupturing the membranes. Rupture of membranes is evidenced by a visible escape of amniotic fluid.

- If the head is not engaged, an assistant must be asked to push the fetal head into the pelvic cavity using external manipulations. This is likely to prevent the occurrence of cord prolapse.

### *Postoperative Steps*

- Fetal heart rate should be heard following ARM. Decline in FHR could be indicative of fetal distress resulting from cord prolapse.
- A vaginal examination must be performed following ARM, in order to exclude the possibility of cord presentation. Membranes are normally not ruptured in HIV positive patients unless there is poor progress of labor. Other things which must be assessed at the time of vaginal examination include status of the cervix, station of the head and color of amniotic fluid. For example, meconium-stained liquor could be indicative of fetal distress.
- A sterile vulval pad is applied.
- Prophylactic antibiotics are prescribed.

## Complications

Various complications associated with ARM include the following:

- Cord prolapse: Risk of cord prolapse is usually low if the head is engaged or if the fetal membranes are ruptured with the head fixed at the brim.
- Sudden escape of amniotic fluid can result in placental abruption.
- Injury to the cervix and/or the presenting part/placenta, etc.
- Amnionitis: Observation of strict asepsis during the procedure helps in reducing the risk of infection. Careful selection of cases with favorable preinduction score helps shorten the induction-delivery interval, thereby further reducing the risk for development of infection.
- Rupture of vasa previa resulting in fetal blood loss.
- Rarely amniotic fluid embolism.

# Amnioinfusion

## Introduction

Amnioinfusion is a technique, which involves infusion of crystalloids inside the amniotic cavity with the aim of diluting the meconium if present, thereby reducing the risk of meconium aspiration. This technique is commonly being used in under-resourced settings in pregnancies complicated by meconium-stained liquor and/or oligohydramnios or fetal distress or nonreassuring fetal heart trace. Therapeutic amnioinfusion is a simple and effective intervention that reduces the rate of cesarean section for intrapartum non-reassuring fetal heart tracing and fetal distress.

## Principle of Amnioinfusion

The process of amnioinfusion functions by exerting the following beneficial actions:

- Increasing the volume of amniotic fluid: Amnioinfusion in the cases of oligohydramnios may help in diluting the meconium, correcting oligohydramnios, and relieving umbilical cord compression.
- Dilution of meconium.
- Prevention of cord compression.
- Prevention of development of subsequent hypoxia.

## Procedure of Performing Amnioinfusion

The technique of amnioinfusion (Figs 6.36 and 6.37A, B) as described by Weismiller is outlined below:

- Attach the drip administration set to a vac of normal saline or Ringer's lactate at one end and to the sterile catheter at the other end.
- While maintaining strict aseptic precautions, tip of the catheter must be passed through the cervix into the uterine cavity, preferably beyond the presenting part.
- The saline must be approximately at body temperature.
- The saline must be allowed to run through the system.

Five hundred milliliters of saline is infused over half-an-hour, followed by 180 mL hourly.

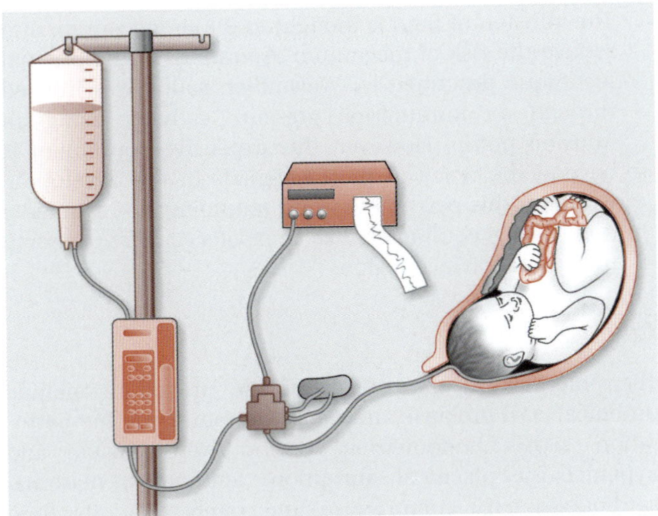

**Fig. 6.36:** Technique of amnioinfusion

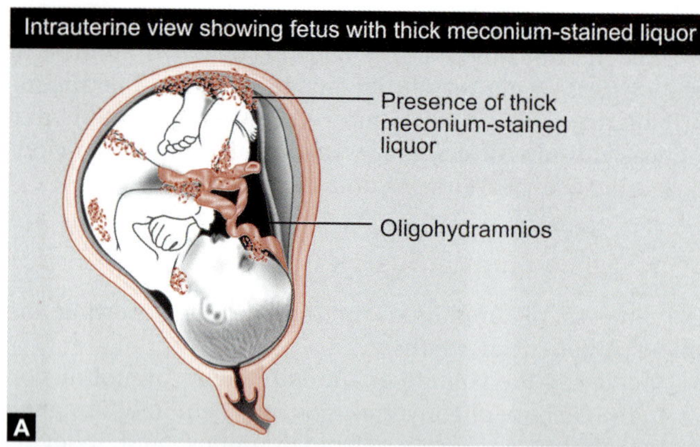



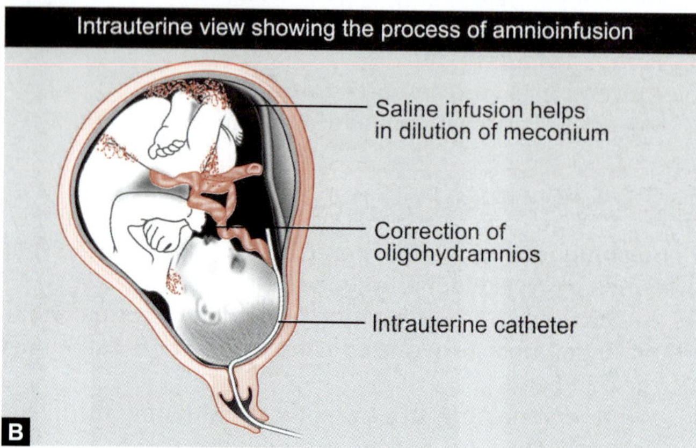



**Figs 6.37A and B:** The procedure of amnioinfusion and its outcome

- Evaluation of fetal well-being must continue while the fluid is being infused.
- Uterine pressure and FHR (via scalp electrode) must be monitored constantly.
- The infusion of fluid is thought to dilute meconium and reduce the risk of meconium aspiration. In the original technique described by Weismiller, saline was infused through an intrauterine pressure catheter using an infusion pump. However, this expensive equipment is beyond the reach of most hospitals in the developing world. In this part of the world amnioinfusion is mainly done using equipment like inexpensive infant feeding tubes and gravity infusion.

## Adverse Effects

The potential adverse effects of the procedure include umbilical cord prolapse, uterine scar rupture, uterine perforation, sepsis, endometritis, uterine overdistension and hyperactivity, placental abruption, amnionitis, maternal cardiopulmonary compromise and rarely amniotic fluid embolism.

## Contraindications

Contraindications for amnioinfusion are as follows:
- Active maternal genital herpes infection
- Diminished FHR variability or reactivity
- Fetal scalp pH below 7.20
- Late decelerations in the FHR
- Presence of fetal anomalies
- Placenta previa
- Multiple gestations
- Prior uterine rupture.

## Conclusion

Use of amnioinfusion in the antenatal period appears to be a lucrative alternative for reducing the risk of meconium aspiration syndrome. It has also been found to be useful for reducing the rate of cesarean section and neonatal morbidity associated with meconium-stained liquor. Amnioinfusion is able to cause a significant reduction in the incidence of the diagnosis of meconium aspiration syndrome. Thus, the present evidence indicates that amnioinfusion should become a standard practice in the management of meconium-stained liquor in labor, especially in low resource settings.

# Cervical Cerlage for Cervical Incompetence

## Cervical Incompetence

Cervical incompetence is a common cause of recurrent second trimester miscarriages and has been defined as a condition in which the pregnant woman's cervix starts dilating and effacing before her pregnancy has reached term, usually between 16 and 28 weeks of gestation and is, therefore, unable to retain the products of conception during pregnancy. The cervical length is usually less than 25 mm. In cases of cervical incompetence, the woman gives history of recurrent second trimester pregnancy losses, occurring earlier in gestation in successive pregnancies and usually presents with a significant cervical dilatation of 2 cm or more in the early pregnancy. In the second trimester, cervix may dilate up to 4 cm in association with active uterine contractions. This may be associated with rupture of the membranes resulting in the spontaneous expulsion of the fetus. Cervical incompetence could be due to congenital or acquired causes. The most common acquired cause of cervical incompetence is a history of cervical trauma or the previous history of cervical lacerations. Therefore, history of any cervical procedure, which could be the potential cause of injury to the cervix, including cervical conizations, loop electrosurgical excision procedure (LEEP), instrumental vaginal delivery or forceful cervical dilatation during previous miscarriage needs to be elicited.

Other risk factors for development of cervical incompetence, which need to be elicited at the time of taking history are as follows:

- Diagnosis of cervical incompetence in a previous pregnancy.
- History of any cervical cerclage performed at the time of previous pregnancy also needs to be elicited.
- Previous history of preterm premature rupture of membranes.
- History of diethylstilbestrol exposure, which can cause anatomical defects in uterus and cervix.

## Diagnosis

### Clinical Examination

The patient may give a history of complaints such as pelvic pressure and/or vaginal discharge. On clinical examination, the cervical canal may be dilated and effaced. Fetal membranes may be visible through the cervical os. Sonographic serial evaluation (every two weeks) of the cervix for funneling and shortening in response to transfundal pressure has been found to be useful in the evaluation of incompetent cervix. Recently, ultrasound examination has become a gold standard in the diagnosis of cervical incompetence. Findings observed on ultrasound examination include the following:

- Cervical length less than 25 mm.
- Protrusion of the fetal membranes.
- Presence of the fetal parts in the cervix or vagina.
- Cervical dilation and effacement with the changes in the form of T, Y, V, U (can be remembered using the mnemonic "Trust Your Vaginal Ultrasound") (Figs 6.38A and B).

T-shaped cervix on ultrasound examination points towards a normal cervix. As the internal cervical os opens and the membrane starts herniating into the upper part of endocervical canal, the cervical shape on ultrasound changes into a Y. With the further progression of above-mentioned cervical changes, Y shape changes into V and ultimately into U.

- Another important finding on TVS examination suggestive of cervical incompetence is funneling. Funneling implies herniation of fetal membranes into the upper part of endocervical canal.

### Other Tests

Some of the tests for diagnosing cervical incompetence, which were previously used and are still used at some places, include the following:

- Passage of a No. 8 (8 mm) Hegar dilator without any pain or resistance and absence of any snapping on its withdrawal is indicative of cervical incompetence.
- Foley's catheter (No 16) is placed inside the uterine cavity. The balloon of the catheter is inflated with 5 cc saline following which traction is applied. In case of cervical incompetence, the inflated catheter comes out easily.

## Cervical Cerclage

The treatment of cervical incompetence involves placement of a surgical suture to reinforce the cervical muscles. At present, the surgical approaches form the treatment of choice for cervical incompetence. Surgery involves placement of a cervical cerclage suture, either transabdominally or transvaginally. Different types of surgical procedures that can be performed include the following:

- McDonald's procedure
- Shirodkar's operation

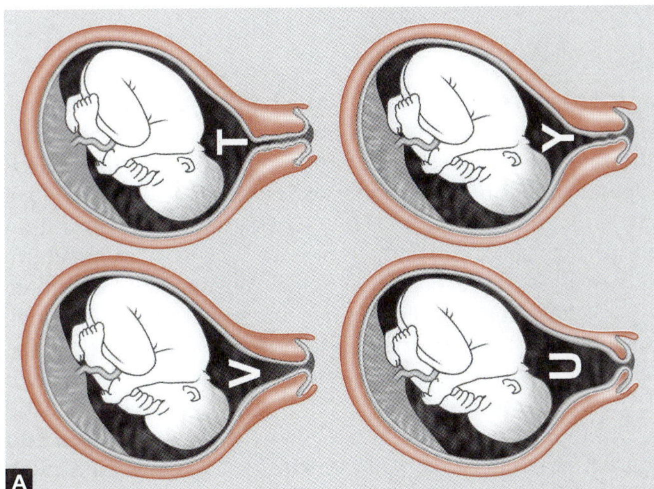
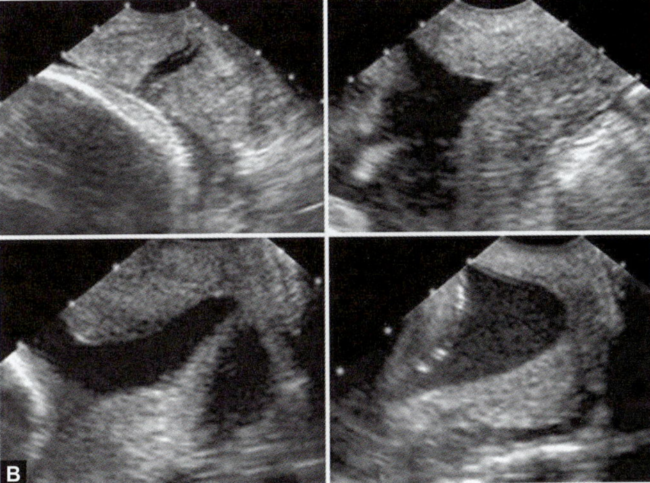

**Figs 6.38A and B:** (A) Anatomical changes in the endocervical canal associated with cervical incompetence; (B) Ultrasound changes in endocervical canal with cervical incompetence

- Wurm's procedure (Hefner cerclage)
- Transabdominal cerclage
- Lash procedure.

Out of the above-mentioned surgical procedures, McDonald's procedure and Shirodkar's procedures are most commonly performed. Cerclage could be performed either as an emergency or prophylactic procedure.

Prophylactic cerclage is placed at 12–16 weeks of gestation. These patients should be followed up with periodic vaginal sonography to assess stitch location and funneling. No additional restrictions are recommended as long as the stitches remain within the middle or upper third of the cervix without the development of a funnel and the length of the cervix is greater than 25 mm.

Emergency or rescue cerclage is used in cases of patients with acute presentation of incompetent cervix. Placement of emergency cerclage is both difficult as well as controversial. This surgery must be undertaken when there is still 10–15 mm or more of cervical canal left.

### Indications

Indications for cerclage are as follows:
- History compatible with incompetent cervix.
- Sonogram demonstrating funneling.
- Clinical evidence of extensive obstetric trauma to the cervix or the history of cervical cone biopsy, which involved removal of large portions of cervix that may weaken it considerably.

### Contraindications for Cerclage

Contraindications for cerclage are as follows:
- Uterine contractions/active labor
- Unexplained vaginal bleeding
- Chorioamnionitis
- Premature rupture of membranes
- Cervical dilatation of more than 4 cm
- Polyhydramnios
- Fetal anomaly incompatible with life
- Intrauterine fetal death
- Gestational age more than 28 weeks
- Placenta previa with mucopurulent discharge and fetal membranes protruding out through the cervical os.

### SURGERY

Two types of vaginal surgeries are most commonly performed during pregnancy. These include McDonald's surgery and Shirodkar's surgery. McDonald's surgery is the simpler one, while Shirodkar's surgery is relatively more complicated. In both these surgeries, after the confirmation of the diagnosis of cervical incompetence, a surgical reinforcement procedure, which involves placement of a purse-string suture as close to internal cervical os as possible, is performed. With these surgeries, success rate as high as 85–90% has been reported. Most clinicians prefer to use McDonald's surgery in cases of cervical incompetence and perform the more complicated Shirodkar's procedure only in cases where there has been previous failure of McDonald's procedure.

### Preoperative Preparation

The following preoperative steps must be observed prior to undertaking any of the previously mentioned cerclage procedures:
- Any contraindications for performance of cerclage procedure (as described before) must be ruled out before performing the procedure.
- Sonography must be performed to confirm a living fetus and to exclude any major congenital anomalies.
- Presence of cervical infection must be ruled out. For this, cervical specimen must be tested for presence of infections such as gonorrhea and chlamydia.
- Sexual intercourse must be prohibited for at least 1 week prior to and after the surgery.
- The procedure is usually performed under regional anesthesia; although, at times the surgeon might prefer to perform the surgery under paracervical block.
- Under all aseptic precautions the vagina and cervix are swabbed with an antiseptic solution (usually savalon or betadine) and a sterile vaginal Sim's speculum is placed inside the vagina over the posterior vaginal wall. An anterior vaginal wall retractor is used for cervical visualization. The anterior lip of cervix is grasped at 12 O'clock and 9 O'clock positions with the help of sponge-holding forceps.

Various types of surgeries which can be performed are described below.

### McDonald's Procedure

In McDonald's procedure, a 5-mm band of permanent purse string using 4–5 bites is placed high on the cervix (Fig. 6.39). The first bite is taken at 12 O'clock position at the cervico-vaginal junction. The needle exits a little above 9 O'clock position, re-enters at 9 O'clock position, exits again a little above 6 O'clock position, re-enters at 6 O'clock position, exits again a little below 3 O'clock position and re-enters at 3 O'clock position. Finally, it comes out at the 12 O'clock position, the site of original insertion. Following this, the needle is removed and the suture drawn closed in the form of a purse string suture. A surgeon's knot is placed tightly and the ends are trimmed to 2–3 cm to allow easy identification and manipulation of the stitch at the time of removal. The stitch is usually removed at 37 weeks, unless there is a reason (e.g.

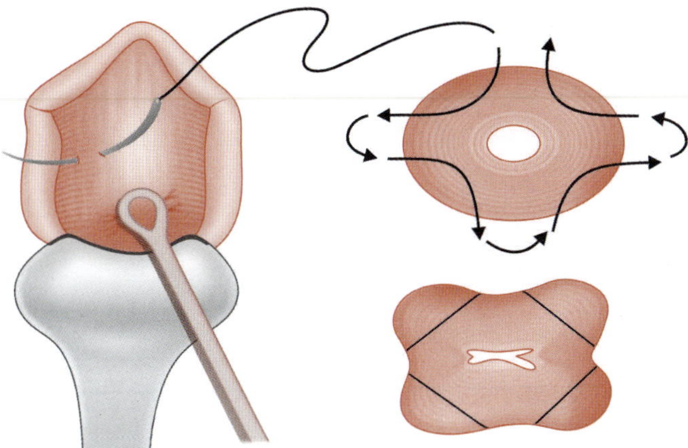

**Fig. 6.39:** McDonald's procedure

infection, preterm labor, preterm rupture of membrane, etc.) for an earlier removal. In McDonald's procedure no bladder dissection is required. It is associated with the success rate of approximately 80%. The advantages of McDonald's procedure over Shirodkar's procedure include the following:

- Simplicity of the procedure (does not involve bladder dissection or complete burial of the sutures).
- Reduced blood loss at the time of surgery.
- Ease of removal at the time of delivery. Therefore there is no requirement for a compulsory cesarean delivery during future pregnancies.
- The stitch can also be applied when the cervix is effaced or the fetal membranes are bulging.

The main disadvantage of the procedure is the occurrence of excessive vaginal discharge with the exposed suture material.

## Shirodkar Technique (Figs 6.40A to G)

The Shirodkar's procedure was first described in 1955. In this procedure, a permanent purse string suture, which would remain intact for life, is applied. As a result, the patient needs to be delivered by a cesarean section for all future deliveries. The suture is placed submucosally as close to the internal os as possible by giving incisions both over the mucosa on the anterior and posterior aspects of the cervix. This is followed by dissection and separation of the bladder and the rectum from both anterior and posterior surface of the cervix respectively. Although, the original Shirodkar's procedure involved the dissection of both bladder and rectal mucosa, the Shirodkar's procedure performed nowadays mainly involves opening of the anterior fornix and dissection of the adjacent bladder. The knot is tied anteriorly and buried by suturing the mucosal opening in the anterior fornix. Some

clinicians prefer tying a posterior knot in order to prevent erosion into the bladder.

The advantages of the procedure include that the stitch can be placed high on the cervix near the internal os. Since the sutures are buried under the mucosa, this considerably helps in reducing the chances of infection.

Initially, both Shirodkar and McDonald started suturing with the catgut but eventually Shirodkar turned to fascia lata and McDonald turned to silk. Presently, mersilene tape is used as an appropriate suture material. Both the procedures have been found to be equally effective. However, it is generally easier to perform McDonald suture as no bladder dissection is involved.

## Postoperative Steps

Following the procedure, the patient should be advised bed rest for at least 6–8 hours. If the procedure has been performed in the morning, she can be discharged by the evening provided that she is stable and there are no other complications. The following parameters need to be observed for the first 4–6 hours after surgery:

- Patient's vitals (pulse, blood pressure and temperature)
- Any bleeding through cervical os
- Presence of uterine contractions
- Fetal heart rate monitoring
- In case of uterine contractions, tocolysis with terbutaline can be administered.
- Although prescription of antibiotics is not essential, prophylactic antibiotics are usually prescribed.
- In our setup, broad spectrum antibiotics are usually started just before the procedure and continued 1–3 days orally postoperatively.
- *Removal of cerclage:* The cerclage (McDonald's stitch) is usually removed at 37 weeks of gestation when the fetus has attained sufficient maturity. In case of significant uterine activity, the sutures can be removed at 35 weeks of gestation.

## Complications

The performance of cerclage could be associated with the following risks:

- Premature rupture of the membranes (1–9%)
- Chorioamnionitis (1–7%)
- Puerperal fever
- Preterm labor
- Cervical laceration or amputation resulting in the formation of scar tissue over the cervix
- Bladder injury
- Maternal hemorrhage
- Cervical dystocia
- Uterine rupture, vesicovaginal fistula.

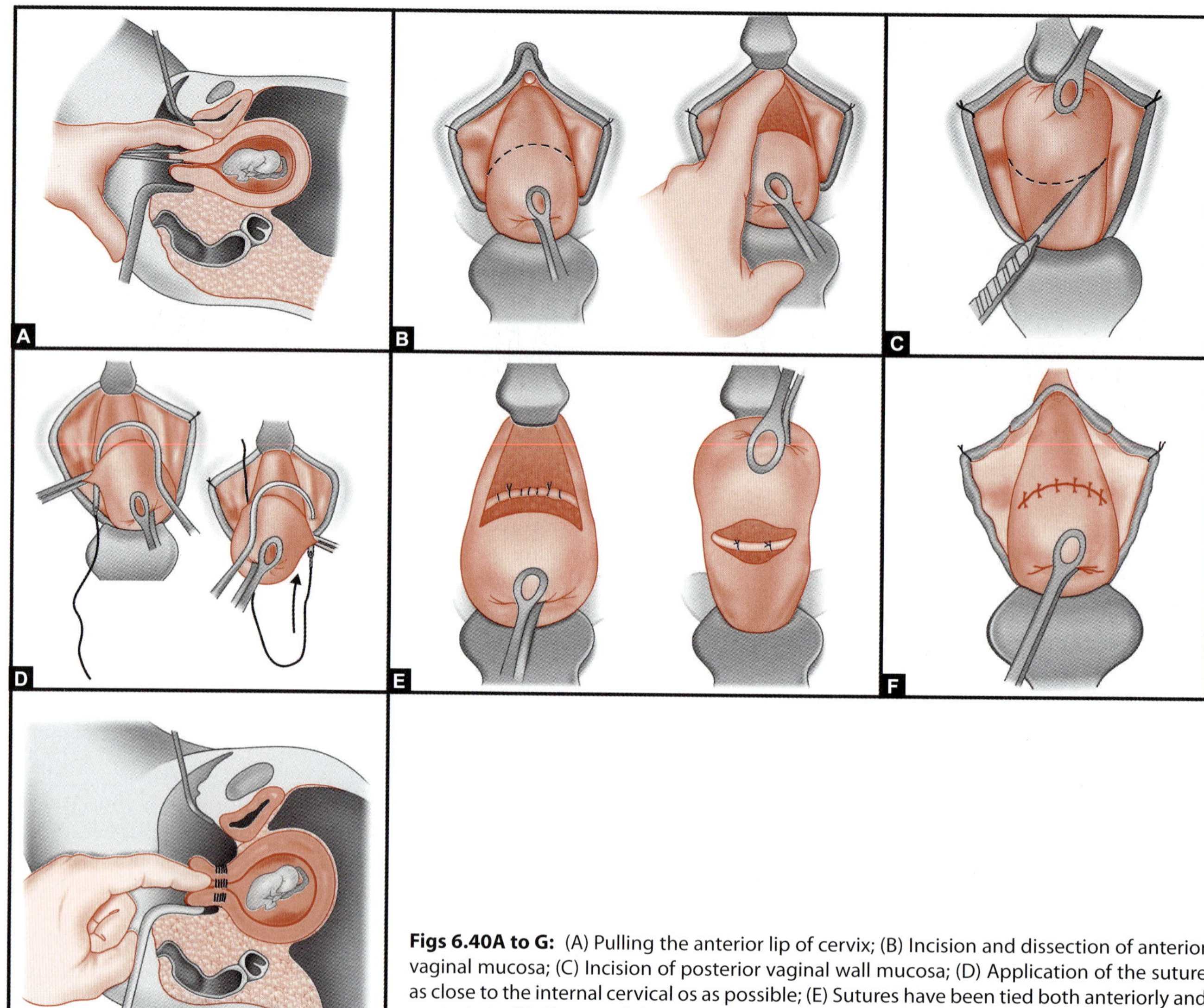

**Figs 6.40A to G:** (A) Pulling the anterior lip of cervix; (B) Incision and dissection of anterior vaginal mucosa; (C) Incision of posterior vaginal wall mucosa; (D) Application of the suture as close to the internal cervical os as possible; (E) Sutures have been tied both anteriorly and posteriorly; (F) Closure of the vaginal mucosa; (G) Appearance of cervix after application of Shirodkar's stitch

# Fetal Scalp Blood Sampling

## Introduction

Fetal scalp blood sampling is a widely used method for assessing fetal condition in the event of ominous FHR patterns on electronic fetal monitoring. Fetal blood sampling (FBS) has been considered as a gold-standard in order to identify fetal hypoxia. Concurrent use of fetal scalp sampling with electronic fetal monitoring (EFM) may not only help in improving the fetal outcome but also reducing the rate of operative delivery.

## Principle

Under normal conditions when the fetus receives sufficient supply of oxygenated blood from the mother via the placenta, aerobic metabolism occurs. Glucose is broken down through the aerobic pathway, which uses oxygen to produce energy in the form of adenosine triphosphate (ATP), along with carbon dioxide and water. Under normal circumstances, the $CO_2$ is removed from the fetus via the placenta. However, in cases of fetal hypoxia or in case of conditions like cord compression causing obstruction to blood flow, there is accumulation of $CO_2$ and deficiency of oxygen resulting in the development of respiratory acidosis.

In case of reduced oxygen supply to the fetus, it has to engage in anaerobic metabolism. The end product of anaerobic metabolism is lactic acid. Lactic acid is a strong monocarboxylic acid, which disassociates easily at the physiological pH into hydrogen ions ($H^+$) and lactate. The accumulation of these substances can result in the development of metabolic acidosis, and lactacidosis. Metabolic

**Table 6.10:** Interpretation of fetal scalp blood sampling

| Scalp blood pH | Pathology | Intervention |
| --- | --- | --- |
| $\leq 7.20$ | Fetal acidosis | Urgent intervention |
| 7.21–7.24 | Borderline (preacidemia) | Sampling to be repeated within 30 minutes |
| $\geq 7.25$ | Reassuring (normal) | Normal monitoring to be performed, repeat if CTG continues to deteriorate |

acidosis results in multiorgan dysfunction in the newborn resulting in long-term neonatal outcome.

Fetus blood sampling is a procedure in which the fetal scalp is pierced to collect blood sample for testing the pH of fetal blood. Fetal scalp pH of less than 7.20 indicates fetal acidemia and mandates urgent delivery. Scalp blood pH between 7.21 and 7.24 is borderline and needs to be repeated within 30 minutes. Scalp blood pH more than 7.25 is reassuring and the labor progress must be monitored. Interpretations of results of fetal blood sampling are described in Table 6.10.

### Prerequisites

- Fetal membranes must be absent
- Cervix must be at least 4–5 cm dilated.

### Procedure

- Under all aseptic precautions, the patient is cleaned and draped after placing her in lithotomy position. Ideally the sampling should be carried out with the women in left lateral position to avoid the weight of the uterus pressing on the inferior vena cava, which could result in the development of maternal hypotension syndrome and consequent fetal bradycardia.
- An amnioscope (a plastic cone like structure) is introduced first in the backwards direction and then both backwards and anteriorly inside the vagina (Fig. 6.41). This would help the amnioscope to be placed perpendicular to the fetal scalp. The narrow inner end of the amnioscope is firmly placed against the scalp of the fetus. The area of the fetal scalp from which the blood is to be withdrawn is firstly cleaned with help of gauze dipped in an antiseptic solution, introduced with help of a metal forceps through the amnioscope.
- Some silicone grease is then applied on the area to be pricked in order to facilitate the formation of a blood drop.
- Next, a small incision up to the depth of 0.2 mm is made on the fetal scalp with help of a special knife.
- The blood from the site of cut is collected in a preheparinized glass capillary tube. For the purpose of acid-base analysis, approximately 35–50 μL of fetal blood is usually enough. This capillary tube is either sent to

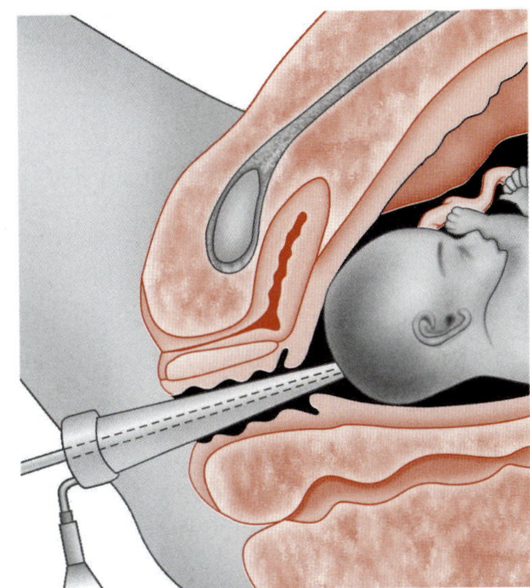

**Fig. 6.41:** Procedure of fetal scalp pH sampling

the hospital laboratory or analyzed by a machine in the labor and delivery department. In either case, results are available in just a few minutes.
- In order to prevent contamination from amniotic fluid, the edge of the amnioscope must be firmly pressed towards the fetal scalp. This would help in preventing contamination from amniotic fluid, which has high concentration of lactate.

### Complications

- The method of fetal scalp blood pH sampling has a high sampling/analysis failure rate, amounting to about 11–20%, with the failure rate being inversely proportional to the degree of cervical dilatation. Due to such high failure rate, fetal scalp blood pH sampling has been excluded from clinical practice in the US.
- This method does not discriminate between respiratory and metabolic acidosis.
- Contamination with maternal blood, secretions and amniotic fluid can lead to erroneous pH values.
- Application of ventouse after FBS: Rarely, if ventouse delivery is performed after FBS, the suction applied could cause severe fetal bleeding from the incision. Therefore, it

is recommended that transparent suction tubes be used in such cases so that fetal bleeding could be identified during the procedure.

- Continued bleeding can take place from the puncture site.
- Being an invasive procedure, it is associated with the risk of infection at the site of incision.
- Bruising and injury to the baby's scalp at the site of incision.

### Contraindications for Fetal Scalp Blood Sampling

- Face and brow presentation.
- Mother or fetus known or suspected to have bleeding disorders.
- HIV or hepatitis B positive mother—risk of transmission to fetus.

# Insertion of Dinoprostone (Cerviprime Gel)

Induction of labor can be defined as commencement of uterine contractions before the spontaneous onset of labor with or without ruptured membranes. It is indicated when the benefits of delivery to the mother or fetus outweigh the benefits of continuing the pregnancy. Induction of labor comprises of cervical ripening and labor augmentation. While cervical ripening aims at making the cervix soft and pliable, augmentation refers to stimulation of spontaneous contractions, which may be considered inadequate due to failed cervical dilation or fetal descent. Pharmacological methods for labor induction commonly comprise of using prostaglandins [Dinoprostone (PGE2), or misoprostol (PGE1)] and/or oxytocin. Of the various agents used for cervical ripening, intracervical application of dinoprostone (PGE2 0.5 mg) can be considered as the gold standard for cervical ripening.

### Various Preparations of Dinoprostone

Dinoprostone helps in cervical ripening and is available in the form of gel (prepidil or cerviprime (Fig. 6.42) or a vaginal insert (cervidil). Prepidil comprises of 0.5 mg of dinoprostone in a 2.5 mL syringe. Cervidil, on the other hand is a vaginal insert containing 10 mg of dinoprostone. The main advantage

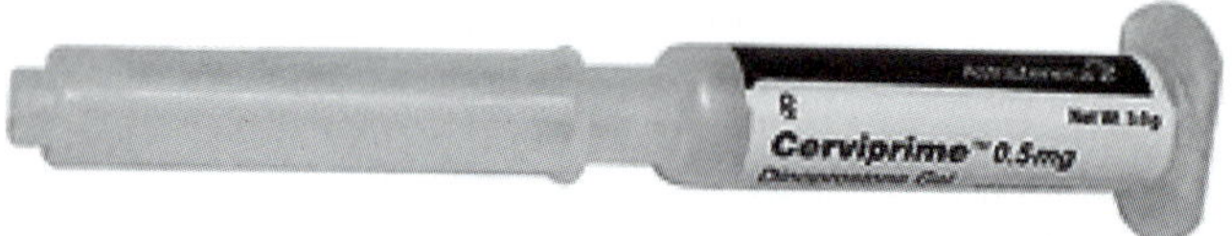

**Fig. 6.42:** Cerviprime gel

of cervidil is that it can be immediately removed in case it causes hyperstimulation. Dinoprostone is also available in form of oral preparations (Primiprost tablets). Refer to Chapter 15 for details related to Primiprost.

### Indications

Various indications for labor induction and cervical ripening with dinopstone are as follows:

*Maternal*

- Severe preeclampsia or eclampsia or nonreassuring fetal heart status.
- Postdated pregnancy.
- Diabetes mellitus.
- Renal disease.
- Abruptio placenta.
- Rh isoimmunization.
- Oligohydramnios.
- Polyhydramnios.

*Fetal*

- Postmaturity.
- Intrauterine growth restriction.
- PROM.
- Fetus with congenital anomalies.
- Intrauterine death.

### Contraindications

Various contraindications for use of cerviprime gel are as follows:
- Previous uterine surgery.
- Vaginal bleeding.
- Ruptured membranes.
- Cephalopelvic disproportion.
- Hypersensitivity to prostaglandins.
- History of allergy or asthma.

### Prerequisites

- Evaluation of maternal and fetal well-being prior to the insertion.
- To ensure that there are no contraindications (previously mentioned) for insertion of cerviprime gel.
- The cervipime gel is usually refrigerated and brought to the room temperature prior to its use.

### Actual Procedure

- Under all aseptic precautions, the pre-filled syringe containing cerviprime gel is introduced through the vagina into the cervix. The plunger is then pushed in order to instill the gel intracervically. Care must be taken that the gel does not go beyond the internal os into the lower uterine segment due to the risk of uterine hyperstimulation.

- The gel is injected intracervically every 6 hours for up to three doses in a 24-hour period.

### Postprocedural Steps

- The woman should be in bed for 30 minutes following its application.
- She should be monitored for uterine activity and FHR.
- Vaginal examination must be done 6 hours postinsertion and Bishop's score be calculated to assess the effectiveness of cerviprime insertion. Labor may be augmented with oxytocin if patient does not get adequate contractions despite of favorable cervix.

## Removal of Adherent Placenta

### Introduction

In normal cases, the mean time from delivery until placental expulsion is approximately 8–9 minutes. Longer intervals for placental delivery are associated with an increased risk of PPH, with rate doubling after 10 minutes. In a majority of patients, the placenta may have completely separated within a few minutes after the delivery of the baby. It may, however, not be able to deliver outside the uterine cavity. In these cases, manual removal of the placenta may be required. If the procedure of placental removal is delayed, it may result in intractable bleeding and hemorrhage. Even in the absence of any continuing bleeding, the surgeon must not wait for more than half an hour before attempting the manual removal of placenta. However, in the presence of continuing bleeding, the obstetrician must immediately proceed with the surgery. Adherent placenta, where the placenta fails to deliver outside the uterine cavity, could be of two types: simple adherent placenta and morbidly adherent placenta. In case of simple adhesion, although the placenta remains attached to the uterine wall, the placental attachments are not abnormal. In cases of simple adherent placenta, manual removal of the placenta is the most suitable option to facilitate the placental delivery.

In case of morbid adhesion, the placental attachment is definitely abnormal with chorionic villi being attached directly to the uterine muscle. This condition commonly occurs due to the deficiency of decidua basalis because of which the uterine musculature is exposed to the invasion by trophoblasts and chorionic villi. Three forms of morbidly adherent placenta have been identified: placenta accreta (placenta is adherent to the myometrium), placenta increta (placenta invades the myometrium) and placenta percreta (placenta penetrates the myometrium to or beyond the serosa). In these cases, as a result of inadequate development of the decidua there is an abnormal connection between the trophoblast and the myometrium. As a result, the condition can result in severe life-threatening hemorrhage. A timely diagnosis of morbidly adherent placenta is therefore of great importance for both mother and infant. In cases of suspicion, an exact diagnostic work-up especially sonography must be undertaken. It is then possible to plan therapy that in most cases comprises of hysterectomy. Hysterectomy helps in avoiding life-threatening complications such as PPH.

In case of a morbidly adherent placenta, manual removal of placenta may not prove to be successful because the placental tissue may have invaded the myometrium.

## MANUAL REMOVAL OF PLACENTA

### Preoperative Preparation

The preoperative care comprises of the following steps:

- *Anesthesia:* The procedure of manual placental removal must be performed under adequate anesthesia after taking complete aseptic precautions. Most clinicians prefer to use either general or regional anesthesia for the procedure.
- *Patient position:* At the time of induction of anesthesia, the woman must be placed in the dorsal position. However, the patient must be placed in lithotomy position for the manual removal procedure.
- The bladder must be catheterized before attempting the manual placental removal.
- Maternal vital signs must be assessed and, if unstable, immediate steps must be taken to bring them under control.
- Four units of blood must be arranged especially if woman is having PPH.
- Two wide-bore IV cannulae must be inserted and immediate resuscitation with crystalloids started.
- A broad spectrum antibiotic must be administered to the patient.
- An informed consent must be taken from the patient before starting the procedure.
- Under all aseptic precautions, vulva and vagina are swabbed with antiseptic solution and the patient is cleaned and draped with sterile towels. The operator should wear fresh sterile long cuffed gloves and a sterile gown, while observing all aseptic precautions.

### Actual Surgery

The steps of surgery are described in Figure 6.43 and are as follows:

- For the procedure, the patient is placed in a lithotomy position.
- One of the surgeon's hands must be placed over the patient's abdomen in order to steady the fundus and push the uterus downwards.
- At the same time, the surgeon's right hand, smeared with antibiotics, is introduced inside the vagina in a cone-shaped manner.

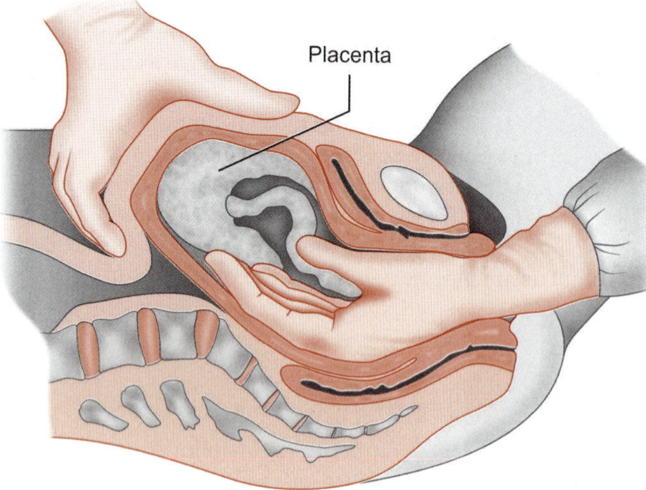



**Fig. 6.43:** Manual removal of the placenta

- It is then passed into the uterine cavity along the course of the umbilical cord. As soon as the lower placental margin is reached, the ulnar border of the hand is used to gradually separate the placenta from the uterine wall.
- The placental tissue is gradually separated by using the sideways slicing movements of the fingers. Once the placenta has separated, it can be grasped with the help of the entire hand and gradually taken out. The abdominal hand helps in stabilizing the uterine fundus and in guiding the movements of the fingers inside the uterine cavity until the placenta has completely separated out.
- Once the entire placenta has been separated, it should be withdrawn out with the help of gentle traction. Before withdrawing the hand, the surgeon must also look for any possible placental remnants or damage to the uterine wall. If the hand is removed and reintroduced once again inside the uterine cavity, the process is likely to add to the risk of infection.
- Before withdrawing the hand from vagina, bimanual compression of the uterus must also be done until the uterus becomes firm.

### Postoperative Care

The postoperative care in case of manual removal of placenta comprises of the following steps:
- In order to achieve sustained uterine contraction even after the surgery, the infusion of oxytocics must be continued.
- Intramuscular methergine/ergometrine 0.5 mg must be administered following the completion of the procedure.
- Blood transfusion may be required depending upon the patient's requirement.

- Broad-spectrum antibiotics must be administered to the patient.
- An informed consent must be taken from the patient before starting the procedure.
- Postoperatively, charting of the following parameters must be done: vital signs, input-output charting, evidence of fresh bleeding, etc.

### COMPLICATIONS

The following complications are likely to occur as a result of the procedure of manual removal:
- Perforation/uterine rupture.
- Incomplete placental removal.
- Hemorrhage.
- Infection: Inspite of strict aseptic precautions during the procedure, some uterine infection is inevitable; therefore a wide spectrum antibiotic cover must be provided for at least five days postoperatively.
- Secondary PPH.

## Pudendal Nerve Block

### Introduction

Pudendal nerve block is commonly used technique of attaining local anesthesia before performing vaginal deliveries (especially those involving the use of forceps) and for minor surgeries of the vagina and perineum. In this technique the pudendal nerve is infiltrated with a local anesthetic agent. Lidocaine 1% is most commonly used agent.

The pudendal nerve, which is derived from the 2nd, 3rd, and 4th sacral nerve is blocked with local anesthetic agent administered using a special needle introduced via a needle guide (Figs 6.44A and B). At the same time, perineal and vulval infiltration is also performed to block the perineal branch of posterior cutaneous nerve of the thigh and labial branches of the ilioinguinal and the genitofemoral nerves. Though the anesthesia may prove excellent for minor surgical procedures, the failure rate of the procedure is high, approaching almost 50%.

### Indications

- Analgesia for the second stage of labor.
- Repair of an episiotomy or perineal laceration.
- Breech vaginal delivery.
- Forceps delivery.
- Minor surgeries of the vagina and perineum.

### Contraindications

Various contraindications to the procedure are as follows:
- Patient refuses to give consent.
- Patient is noncompliant and is not willing to cooperate.

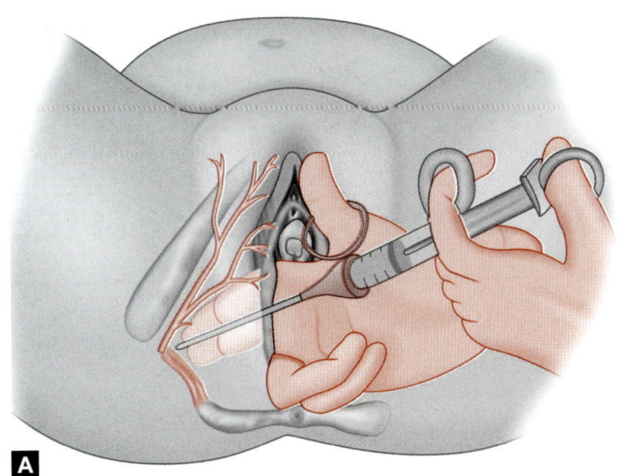
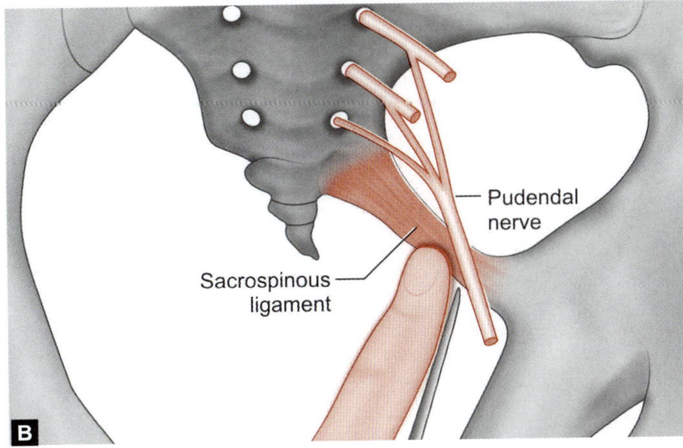


**Figs 6.44A and B:** Pudental nerve block. (A) Procedure of pudental nerve block; (B) Magnified view showing the site of nerve block

- Patient sensitivity to local anesthetic agents.
- Infection in the ischiorectal space, vagina or perineum.
- Presence of coagulation disorders.

## Procedure

### Preoperative Preparation

- Consent must be taken from the patient before performing this procedure.
- Vaginal preparation is usually not required prior to the procedure.
- Patient is placed in the lithotomy position.

### Actual Procedure

The procedure can be performed via transvaginal or transperineal route. Transvaginal route is the preferred route. In this, a 22-gauge needle, having a length of 15 cm is placed through the transducer, against the vaginal mucosa, with the tip of the needle aiming just medial and posterior to the ischial spine. This is the region where the pudendal nerve is most likely to be situated. Approximately 1 mL of 1% lidocaine solution is injected. The needle is next advanced through the sacrospinous ligament, which is then infiltrated with 3 mL of lidocaine solution. The needle is then advanced into the loose areolar tissues behind the ligament and another 3–5 mL of the solution is injected there. The needle is then withdrawn and moved to just above the ischial spine. Another 10 mL of the local anesthetic solution is deposited there. The block needs to be repeated on the opposite site.

## Complications

Some complications associated with the procedure are as follows:

- Hematoma formation.
- Infection (rarely).
- Intravascular injection (aspirate the syringe prior to the injection of local anesthetic agent to ensure that the injection is not given intravascularly).

## FURTHER READINGS


1. Sokol RJ, Blackwell SC, American College of Obstetricians and Gynecologists. Committee on Practice Bulletins-Gynecology. ACOG practice bulletin: Shoulder dystocia. Number 40, November 2002. (Replaces practice pattern number 7, October 1997). Int J Gynaecol Obstet. 2003;80(1):87-92.
2. American College of Obstetricians and Gynecologists. Practice Bulletin No. 13. External cephalic version. Washington, DC: ACOG. 2000.
3. Baskett TF. Shoulder dystocia. Best Pract Res Clin Obstet Gynecol. 2002;16:57-68.
4. Kettle C, Dowswell T, Ismail KM. Absorbable suture materials for primary repair of episiotomy and second degree tears. Cochrane Database Syst Rev. 2010;(6):CD000006.
5. Kettle C, Dowswell T, Ismail KM. Continuous and interrupted suturing techniques for repair of episiotomy or second degree tears. Cochrane Database Syst Rev. 2012;(11):CD000947.
6. Laufe LE, Berkus MD. Assisted vaginal delivery: obstetric forceps and vacuum application techniques. New York: McGraw-Hill; 1962.
7. O'Grady JP. Modern instrumental delivery. Baltimore: Williams and Wilkins, 1988: 150-152.
8. Royal College of Obstetricians and Gynecologists. Guidelines No. 42. Shoulder dystocia. London: RCOG Press; 2006.

# Operation Theater Procedures: Obstetrics



## Medical Termination of Pregnancy

Medical termination of pregnancy or induced abortion is often abbreviated as MTP. It is the medical procedure, which enables a couple to get free from the unwanted pregnancy.

Surgical techniques in the first trimester MTP practically comprise entirely of vacuum or suction techniques. The terms, "vacuum curettage", "uterine aspiration" or "vacuum aspiration" are often used interchangeably. They all refer to evacuation of the uterus by suction, regardless of the source of the suction.

### SURGICAL EQUIPMENT USED

The various surgical instruments used for the procedure of vacuum aspiration are shown in Figure 7.1. Prior to the surgical evacuation, the cervix is often dilated. Mechanical dilation using physical dilators is currently the most frequently used method of dilating the cervix. Other methods of dilatation include osmotic dilatation, using laminaria tents or use of pharmacological dilatation using medications such as misoprostol. Hegar dilators are the standard instruments for cervical dilation, which are commonly used in our setup. These are blunt-ended instruments having different sizes, of which different sizes vary by 1 mm.

Medical Termination of Pregnancy Act passed in 1971 in India has legalized abortion up to the duration of 20 weeks of gestation. This law holds true for all the Indian States except for the state of Jammu and Kashmir. Termination of pregnancy by registered medical practitioners can be done as follows:

- When the length of the pregnancy is less than 12 weeks, it can be terminated by a registered medical practitioner.
- If the length of the pregnancy is between 12 and 20 weeks, termination can be done if at least two registered medical

practitioners have given their approval for it in good faith. The termination of the pregnancy can be done on the basis of following grounds:

- *Medical grounds:* Continuation of the pregnancy is likely to put at risk, the life of the pregnant woman or cause grave injury to her physical or mental health.
- *Eugenic cause:* There is a substantial risk that if the child is born, it would suffer from such physical or mental abnormalities so as to be seriously handicapped.
- *Social cause:* These may include the following scenarios:
  - Pregnancy occurs as a result of a rape: When pregnancy is suspected to have been caused by rape, the distress caused by such pregnancy is

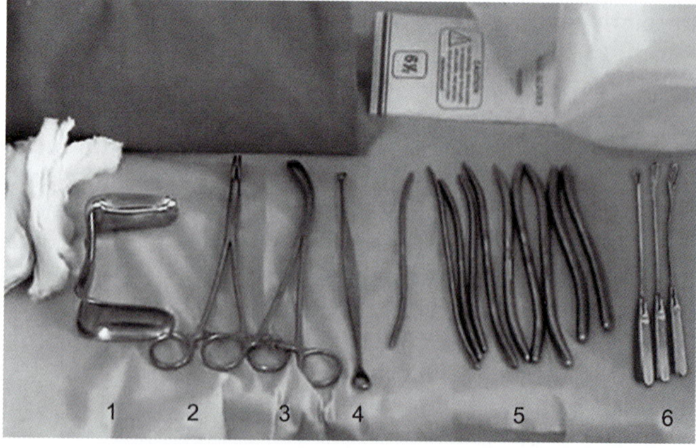

**Fig. 7.1:** Tray containing various equipment used for suction evacuation: (1) Sim's speculum; (2) Sponge holder; (3) Vulsellum; (4) Anterior vaginal wall retractor; (5) Hegar's dilators of increasing sizes; (6) Uterine curettes of varying sizes

presumed to be causing grave injury to the mental health of the pregnant woman.

- Pregnancy occurs as a result of failure of contraception: When the pregnancy occurs as a result of failure of any device or method used by the married woman or her husband for the purpose of contraception or limiting the number of children, the distress caused by such unwanted pregnancy may also be considered to constitute a grave injury to the mental health of the pregnant woman.

No pregnancy shall be terminated without taking consent of the pregnant woman, unless the woman has not attained the age of 18 years or who, having attained the age of 18 years, is a lunatic. In these cases the pregnancy must be terminated only after taking the consent in writing from her guardian.

## Place Where Pregnancy May Be Terminated

Medical termination of pregnancy should be only carried out in the hospital, which is established/maintained by the government. It can also be carried out at a place which has been approved for this purpose by the government or at a district level by a committee constituted by the government with the Chief medical officer acting as the chairperson.

## PROCEDURE

### Preoperative Preparation

- *Patient counseling:* Adequate counseling of the woman and her partner is essential in order to enable her to make a free and fully informed decision.
- *Estimation of the gestational age:* The clinician can estimate the gestational age by calculating the period of amenorrhea. The uterine size must be assessed by performing a bimanual examination. An ultrasound examination can also be performed to confirm the period of gestation.
- *Medical history:* A complete medical history must be taken in order to rule out the presence of the medical diseases, such as asthma, diabetes and the history of the drug allergy.
- Simple investigations, such as hemoglobin estimation, urine analysis and blood grouping (ABO, Rh), need to be done prior to the procedure.
- In case, where the procedure would be carried out under general anesthesia, investigations, such as blood sugar levels, kidney function tests, ECG and X-ray, may be required.
- Cervical priming using 400 µg of the vaginal or anal misoprostol can be done prior to the procedure.
- *Anesthesia:* The procedure is usually carried out under local anesthesia, using a paracervical block with 20 mL of 0.5% lignocaine. Short general anesthesia may be used in the patients, who are very apprehensive. In order to reduce the pain during and after the procedure, nonsteroidal anti-inflammatory drugs, such as naproxen 550 mg, may be commonly prescribed before the procedure.
- *Prophylactic antibiotics:* In cases where the possibility of intrauterine infection is suspected (e.g. history of prolonged bleeding per vaginum, patient at risk of bacterial endocarditis), antibiotics can be administered prior to the procedure.
- *Bladder catheterization:* Bladder must be emptied prior to the procedure.
- *Cleaning and draping:* Shaving the perineum is not required, but the perineal hair must be trimmed. After taking all aspectic precautions, the area of perineum, mons and lower part of the abdomen must be cleaned and draped, using povidone-iodine or chlorhexidine solution. The surgeon must use the "no-touch" technique, in which he/she must use sterile instruments and sterile gloves and take care never to touch that part of the instrument that would enter the uterus.

## Actual Procedure

The procedure of vacuum aspiration comprises of the following steps (Figs 7.2A to D):

- The cervix is exposed after retracting the posterior vaginal wall using Sims vaginal speculum.
- The anterior lip of the cervix is held, using a vulsellum or tenaculum. Once the cervix has been properly visualized, paracervical block is given.
- The cervix is then serially dilated, using a series of metallic or plastic dilators. Though a variety of dilators are available, Hegar's dilators are the most commonly used. While dilating the cervix, the dilators must be held in a pen-holding fashion and undue force must not be applied over the cervix. The dilatation is initially started using smaller dilators and then generally large dilators are used, one after the other. The dilators must be inserted slowly and gently. This practice is both safe and less painful. If resistance is experienced, the operator should return to the previous dilator, reinsert it and allow it to remain in place for a minute or so before attempting to insert the next large dilator. The rule normally followed is that "the size of the suction cannula to be used for the procedure must be equivalent to the size of the uterus". The dilation of the cervix must be approximately 0.5–1 mm more than the size of suction cannula to be used.
- Some clinicians prefer to use a uterine sound for determining the depth of the uterine cavity. We normally do not perform routine sounding of the uterine cavity in our setup.
- A plastic Karmans cannula is then inserted inside the uterine cavity. Once the cannula has been inserted, the

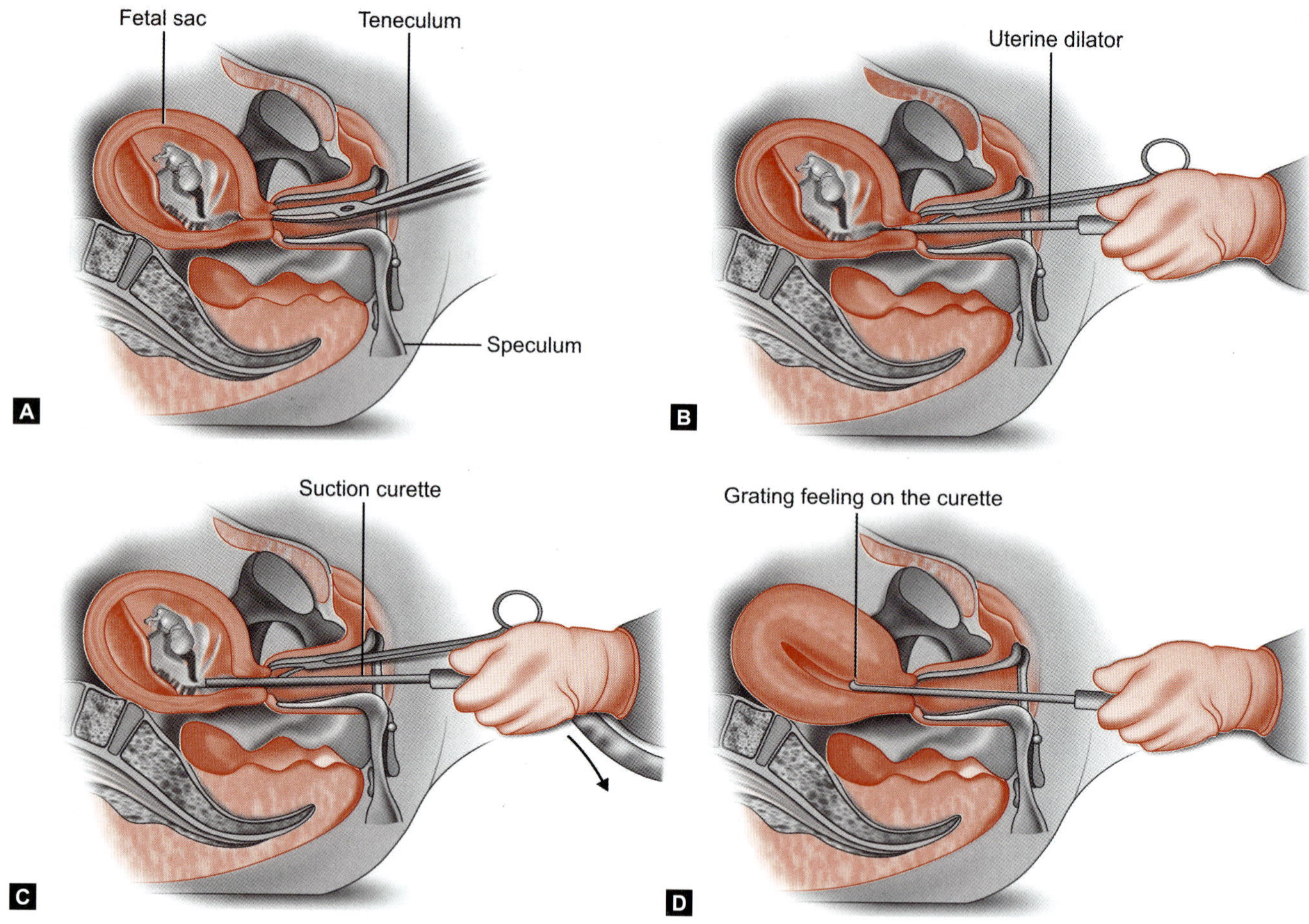



**Figs 7.2A to D:** Procedure of vacuum aspiration

clinician must connect the cannula to a suction machine, which generates pressure equivalent to 60–70 mm Hg. The cannula is rotated at an angle of 360° and moved back by 1–2 cm, back and forth, till the entire uterine cavity has been evacuated. The cannula can be gently rotated several times. Evacuation is said to be complete, when no more contents are seen coming out of the uterine cavity; instead of the uterine contents, air bubbles start appearing in the cannula and/or the uterine cavity appears to be firm and gritty. Once the surgeon is sure that the procedure is complete, the cannula is removed after disconnecting the suction.

- A sharp curettage is performed by some surgeons at the end of the procedure, just to confirm that the procedure has been completely performed. This step is considered as controversial and not everyone performs it, because the use of sharp curettage may slightly increase the blood loss.

## Postoperative Care

- Methergine 0.25 mg IM may be administered after the procedure.

- The aspirated tissue must be sent for histopathological examination to confirm for the presence of chorionic villi in the aspirated tissues.
- The patient must be observed in the recovery room for 2–3 hours before discharge.
- The patient's vital signs and blood loss must be regularly monitored.
- In case of pain, analgesic drugs may be prescribed.
- If the procedure is performed under general anesthesia, the patient can be discharged after a few hours, once she has stabilized.
- Women who are Rh-negative can be given Rh immune globulins immediately following the procedure.
- A woman who has undergone MTP must be counseled regarding the use of contraception in future, in order to prevent the reoccurrence of unwanted pregnancies. Immediate contraception in form of intra-uterine contraceptive device insertion or placement of a subdermal rod, intramuscular depot medroxy-progesterone acetate injections, etc. may be provided after the procedure depending on the patient's wishes.

- The patients are scheduled for a follow-up visit, 1–2 weeks after abortion to check for the presence of any potential MTP-related complications.

## COMPLICATIONS

Though small amount of cramping, pain and bleeding can commonly occur for 2–3 days after the procedure, severe degrees of persistent pain or amount of bleeding more than that associated with normal menstruation, especially in association with fever or fainting could be indicative of the underlying complications. Some of these are discussed hereunder.

### Uterine Perforation

The most dreaded complication of the procedure is uterine perforation because the procedure of suction evacuation is essentially a blind one. The risk of uterine perforation becomes greater with the increasing gestational age of the fetus. Most uterine perforations are thought to occur during the process of uterine sounding or cervical dilation because the most common site of perforation is the junction of the cervix and the lower uterine segment.

A uterine perforation must be suspected, when no tissue is obtained; when the instruments appear to be inserted deeper than the depth expected, on the basis of the gestational age; when hemorrhage occurs; or when obvious maternal tissues, such as omentum are obtained. Sometimes, if the procedure is being performed under ultrasound guidance, uterine instrument (such as a uterine sound) may be visualized outside the uterine cavity.

Treatment of perforation depends on the expected location, the woman's vital signs and condition and whether the abortion is complete or not. In case of a suspected perforation, the patient must be observed for a few hours for the signs of hypovolemia and shock. Intramuscular oxytocics (methergine) and antibiotics must be administered. If the patient's vitals are stable; the uterine perforation is midline; repeated pelvic examinations are negative; repeat hematocrit results are stable; the uterus is already empty and/or the amount of bleeding is minimal or none, then there is no need for patient hospitalization. The patient may be discharged home in the company of a responsible adult and instructed to visit the hospital immediately, in case she experiences excessive pain or bleeding or some other complication at any time. She must be scheduled for a repeat general physical and pelvic examination, the next day. In case the patient continues to experience bleeding, pain or her vitals continue to remain unstable; she should be admitted to a hospital for observation and a possible laparoscopic examination. Laparotomy may be required, in cases where intraperitoneal bleeding or bowel injury is suspected.

### Infection

This can be easily avoided by the administration of broad-spectrum antibiotics. In case the infection is as a result of incomplete evacuation, the clinician first needs to completely evacuate the uterine cavity. Following this, the antibiotics must be given. In the cases of serious infection, intravenous antibiotics can be given. Laparotomy may be required in cases of peritonitis.

### Incomplete Evacuation

The most common presentation in cases of incomplete evacuation is prolonged bleeding. In these cases the uterine contents have to be re-evacuated under the antibiotic coverage. Typical history suggestive of an incomplete evacuation is a woman returning several days after the procedure with the history of increased bleeding and cramping. On examination, she may have an enlarged uterus or tissue visible in the cervical os. Ultrasound examination is usually performed, but may not be always helpful.

Treatment of incomplete abortion may be pharmacologic. Uterotonic drugs, such as methylergonovine (methergine) may help contract the uterus and expel the residual tissue. This method is appropriate when the amount of retained tissue is small and there are no signs of infection. If this method is chosen, the woman should be called for a follow-up visit within a few days, to make sure that her symptoms have resolved. If the amount of retained tissue inside the uterine cavity is large or if the woman cannot return for follow-up, then repeat suction should be done. Repeat suction is usually easy because the cervix is dilated and a cannula smaller than that used for the original procedure is adequate.

### Bleeding during and Following the Abortion

Most women have minimal bleeding during first trimester abortion. Uterine atony is the most likely the cause of heavy and prolonged bleeding in these cases. Intravenous ergometrine (0.2 mg) or oxytocin (10–20 units) may be used to contract the uterus. Alternatively misoprostol, in the dosage of 400 µg may be prescribed either through oral or rectal route. Doses of misoprostol, as high as 1,000 µg, have been used per rectally in cases of atonic uterus. Prostaglandin F2α (carboprost) can be prescribed intramuscularly or into the uterus. In the absence of an obvious cervical or uterine injury, the surgeon should complete the abortion, evacuating the uterus rapidly, but gently. If the bleeding still continues to occur, the uterus is massaged between the two hands, e.g. bimanual compression. Surgical procedures for control of bleeding from an atonic uterus have been described later in the text.

## Failure of the Procedure

The procedure, if not performed properly, may result in the continuation of pregnancy. This may result in cases of very small sized uterus, where the suction cannula fails to suck out the product of conception.

## Hypotension

This could be related to excessive blood loss or due to a vasovagal response to pain. Management in these cases comprises of administration of IV fluids, oxygen, whole blood transfusion and corticosteroids.

## Minor Complications

Minor complications like postoperative nausea and vomiting can be managed with antiemetics such as metoclopramide or ondansetron.

## Ashermans Syndrome

This is a delayed complication, which can occur as a result of vigorous curettage. This complication is usually managed by hysteroscopic resection of interauterine adhesions, followed by insertion of an IUCD or a Foleys catheter, in order to keep the uterine wall apart.

## Cervical Lacerations/Cervical Incompetence

Rarely, vigorous dilatation may result in the development of cervical lacerations and/or cervical incompetence in the subsequent pregnancies. This complication can be avoided by taking a good history and correct estimation of gestational age during the bimanual examination. Overzealous cervical dilation must be avoided. Dilatation is carried out using the smallest sized dilator. Cervical priming using prostaglandins, prior to the procedure, facilitates the process of dilatation without the use of undue force.

# Drainage of Pelvic/Vulvar Hematoma

## Introduction

Pelvic hematoma can be defined as the collection of blood between the pelvic peritoneum and the perineal skin. Depending upon the location of hematoma above and below the levator ani muscle, hematoma can be classified as infralevator or supralevator. Infralevator hematoma is the most common cause of pelvic hematoma.

## Causes

Infralevator hematoma/vulvar hematoma can occur due to the following causes:

- Improper hemostasis during repair of vaginal or perineal tears or episiotomy wound: Blood from the rupture of deep vulvar and vaginal veins gets collected in a closed space. Since there is no opening for the blood to drain out, the swelling increases in size over the time and is extremely painful.
- Failure to include the apex of vaginal tear or episiotomy at the time of repair.
- Failure to obliterate the dead space at the time of repair.
- Rupture of paravaginal plexus spontaneously or following instrumental delivery (more commonly associated with forceps delivery in comparison with vacuum delivery).

Supralevator hematoma can occur due to the following causes:

- Extension of cervical lacerations.
- Vault rupture (primary colporrhexis).
- Lower uterine segment rupture.
- Spontaneous rupture of paravaginal venous plexus.

## Symptoms

Vulvar hematoma may be associated with the following symptoms:

- Severe pain in the perineal region. Vulvar hematoma is commonly associated with a swelling localized to one side of vulva, which may steadily increase in size over time.
- The woman complains of severe pain, which increases on sitting down. The pain may be unrelieved with mild painkillers.
- There may be difficulty in passing urine if the swelling presses on the urethra.
- Rectal tenesmus or bearing down efforts.
- Urinary retention.

## Clinical Signs

- Variable degrees of shock depending upon the amount of blood collection.
- In case of vulvar hematoma, there may be tense/tender swelling at the vulva which may be bluish-purple in color and highly tender to touch.
- In case of supralevator hematoma, on abdominal examination there may be a swelling above the inguinal ligament pushing the uterus to the contralateral side.
- *Vaginal examination:* On vaginal examination, the following may be observed:
    - Occlusion of the vaginal canal by a bulge.
    - Palpation of bogginess through the vaginal fornices.
    - Rectal examination confirms the presence of boggy swelling.

## Investigation

Ultrasound examination may reveal the exact location of the hematoma.

## Treatment

- Small hematomas (<5 cm) can be treated conservatively by application of cold compresses. This helps in controlling the pain and limiting the swelling. This also prevents further bleeding into the hematoma.
- Large hematomas must be surgically dealt with.

## SURGERY

### Preoperative Preparation

Immediate measures for the management of shock must be instituted.

- An IV line must be secured.
- Blood should be sent for ABO/Rh typing and crossmatching. At least four units blood must be arranged.
- Larger hematomas must be explored under general anesthesia.
- A Foley catheter is inserted and left in situ.

### Actual Surgery

#### Infralevator Hematoma

For drainage of vulvar hematoma, an incision is made at the most distended region of the hematoma. The incision is deepened following which, the blood clots are scooped out. The bleeding points, if visible, are secured and ligated.

#### Supralevator Hematoma

In case of supralevator hematoma, the anterior leaf of broad ligament is incised and the blood clots scooped out. Bleeding points are secured and ligated. However, random blind sutures must not be placed to prevent ureteric damage. Anterior division of anterior iliac artery may require ligation if the bleeding still continues. The dead space is obliterated by application of deep mattress sutures. Incision is then closed in layers.

### Postoperative Care

- A closed suction drain must be kept in place for 24 hours so that any blood which oozes out can flow out.
- Close monitoring of the patient's vital signs must be done for a time period depending on the patient's clinical condition.
- Antibiotics (third generation cephalosporins) must be prescribed.
- Appropriate analgesia in form of NSAIDs, oral narcotics or IV narcotics can be prescribed to the patient depending upon the severity of pain.
- Bladder must be catheterized with the help of Foley's catheter for 3–5 days.
- Blood transfusion may be given, if required.

| **Table 7.1:** Indications for cesarean section |
| --- |
| *Absolute Indications (situations where vaginal delivery is not possible)* |
| • Central placenta previa<br>• Absolute cephalopelvic disportion<br>• Abnormal presentation (transverse lie)<br>• Lower genital tract obstruction due to presence of a pelvic mass<br>• Advanced carcinoma cervix<br>• Vaginal obstruction (atresia, stenosis, etc.) |
| *Relative Indications* |
| • Dystocia<br>• Previous cesarean section<br>• Abnormal presentation (breech presentation)<br>• Fetal distress<br>• Preeclampsia<br>• Antepartum hemorrhage<br>• Failed surgical induction of labor<br>• Bad obstetric history with recurrent miscarriages |

- Patient is advised bed rest from a few days to a week following discharge.

# Cesarean Section

## OVERVIEW OF SURGERY

Cesarean section is a surgical procedure commonly used in the obstetric practice. In this procedure, the fetal delivery is attained through an incision made over the abdomen and uterus, after 28 weeks of pregnancy. If the removal of fetus is done before 28 weeks of pregnancy, the procedure is known as hysterotomy. Presently, there has been a considerable rise in the rate of cesarean delivery. The use of cesarean delivery helps in avoiding difficult cases of vaginal delivery, which may be associated with considerable maternal and fetal mortality and morbidity.

### Indications

Indications for cesarean section are listed in Table 7.1 and are described below in details.

#### Dystocia

In the US, dystocia is the most frequent cause of cesarean section. Dystocia could be related to secondary arrest of dilatation, arrest of descent, failure of progress of labor and cephalopelvic disproportion.

#### Previous Cesarean Section

Certain indications for a previous cesarean section, such as cephalopelvic disproportion, may make cesarean delivery

**Table 7.2:** Indications for cesarean section in case of a breech presentation

- Cephalopelvic disproportion
- Placenta previa
- Estimated fetal weight >4 kg
- Hyperextension of fetal head
- Footling breech (danger of entrapment of head in an incompletely dilated cervix)
- Severe IUGR
- Clinician not competent with the technique of breech vaginal delivery

*Abbreviation:* IUGR, intrauterine growth restriction

in future pregnancies inevitable. In the past, management of the patient with a history of cesarean scar was guided by the dictum "once a cesarean, always a cesarean".

As a result, there was a massive increase in the rate of cesarean deliveries. With the increasing rate of cesarean deliveries, interest in vaginal birth after cesarean (VBAC) was further revived. In 1988, ACOG recommended that most women with one previous low transverse cesarean delivery should be attempted for a trial of vaginal delivery in the subsequent pregnancies. The previous dictum has now been changed to "once a cesarean always hospitalization" due to a small, but definite risk of rupture associated with previous cesarean deliveries.

### Malpresentations

While cesarean delivery is the only likely available option in cases of transverse lie, vaginal delivery can be sometimes used in cases of breech presentation. Some of the absolute indications for cesarean section, in cases of breech presentation are enumerated in Table 7.2.

### Fetal Distress

Fetal distress as defined by the World Health Organization's International Classification of Diseases (ICD-10) includes fetal stress at the time of labor or delivery. It could be associated both with the presence of fetal heart-rate anomalies (fetal bradycardia, decelerations, etc.) and presence of meconium in amniotic fluid, resulting in complications at the time of labor and delivery. An emergency cesarean section may be required at any time, in cases of suspected or confirmed acute fetal compromise. In these cases, delivery should be accomplished as soon as possible, preferably within 30 minutes of the diagnosis of fetal distress (AAP, ACOG, 2007).

### Preeclampsia

Severe uncontrolled preeclampsia is another cause for cesarean delivery because the condition can be rectified only through the delivery of the baby.

## SURGERY

## Preoperative Preparation

The following steps should be taken for preoperative preparation:

*Empty stomach:* In order to prevent the risk of aspiration at the time of administration of anesthesia, the patient should be nil per mouth for at least 12 hours before undertaking a cesarean section. In case the patient is full stomach, she should be administered $H_2$ receptor blocker (ranitidine 150 mg) and an antiemetic (metoclopramide 10 mg) at least 2 hours prior to the surgery.

*Patient position:* The patient is placed with 15° lateral tilt on the operating table, in order to reduce the chances of hypotension.

*Anesthesia:* While cesarean section can be performed both under general or regional anesthesia, nowadays regional anesthesia is favored. Spinal and epidural anesthesia have become the most commonly used forms of regional anesthesia in the recent years.

*Clinical examination:* Before cleaning and draping the patient, it is a good practice to check the fetal lie, presentation, position and fetal heart sounds once again. Foley's or plain rubber catheter must be inserted, following which the cleaning and draping of the abdomen is done.

*Preparation of the skin:* The area around the proposed incision site must be washed with antiseptic soap solution (e.g. savlon and/or betadine solution). Antiseptic skin cleansing before surgery is thought to reduce the risk of postoperative wound infections. The antiseptic solution must be applied at least three times over the incision site, using a high-level disinfected sponge-holding forceps and cotton or gauze swab. The essential steps in a cesarean delivery are described next in details.

## Steps of Surgery

### Giving an Abdominal Skin Incision

A vertical or transverse incision can be given over the skin (Fig. 7.3). The vertical skin incision can be either given in the midline or paramedian location, extending just above the pubic symphysis to just below the umbilicus. Previously, vertical skin incision at the time of cesarean section was favored, as it was supposed to provide far more superior access to the surgical field in comparison to the transverse incision. Also, the vertical incision showed potential for extension at the time of surgery. However, it was associated with poor cosmetic results and an increased risk of wound dehiscence and hernia formation. Therefore, nowadays, transverse incision is mainly favored due to better cosmetic effect, reduced postoperative pain and improved patient recovery.

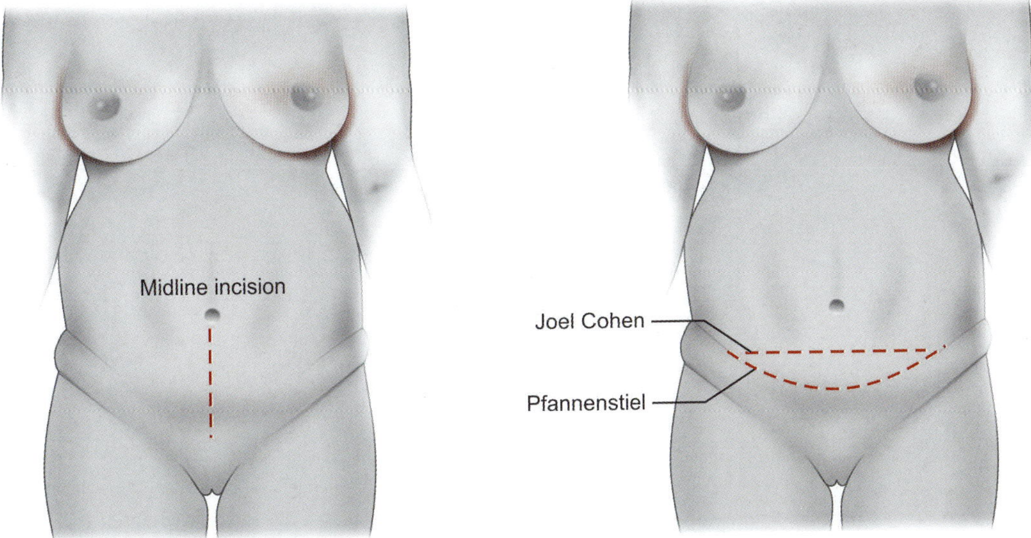


**Fig. 7.3:** Vertical or transverse skin incision

Two types of transverse incisions are mainly used, while performing cesarean section: (1) the sharp (Pfannenstiel) type and (2) the blunt (Joel Cohen) type.

*Sharp Pfannenstiel transverse incision:* While giving this type of incision, a slightly curved, transverse skin incision is made at the level of pubic hairline, about an inch above the pubic symphysis and is extended somewhat beyond the lateral borders of rectus abdominis muscle. The subsequent tissue layers, until the level of anterior rectus sheath are opened by using a sharp scalpel.

### Dissecting the Rectus Sheath

After dissecting through the skin, subcutaneous fat and fascia, as the anterior rectus sheath is reached, sharp dissection may be required. A scalpel can be used to incise the rectus sheath throughout the length of the incision. The cut edges of the incised rectus sheath are held with the help of allies forceps and then carefully separated out from the underlying rectus muscle and pyramidalis. These muscles are then separated with the help of blunt and sharp dissection to expose transversalis fascia and peritoneum.

### Opening the Peritoneum

The transversalis fascia and peritoneal fat are dissected carefully to reach the underlying parietal peritoneum. After placing two hemostats about 2 cm apart to hold the peritoneum, it is carefully opened. The layers of parietal peritoneum are carefully examined to be sure that omentum, bowel or bladder is not lying adjacent to it.

### Insertion of the Doyen's Retractor

Following the dissection of parietal peritoneum, the lower uterine segment is identified. Following the identification of lower uterine segment, some surgeons prefer to put a moistened laparotomy pack in each of the paracolic gutters. The loose fold of the uterovesical peritoneum over the lower uterine segment is then grasped with the help of forceps and incised transversely with the help of scissors. The lower flap of the peritoneum is held with artery forceps and the loose areolar tissue pushed down. The underlying bladder is then separated by blunt dissection. Finally, the lower flap of peritoneum and the areolar tissue is retracted by the Doyen's retractor to clear the lower uterine segment. The upper flap of the peritoneum is pushed up to leave about 2 cm wide strip on the uterine surface, which is not covered with visceral peritoneum.

*Giving a uterine incision:* An incision is made on the lower uterine segment about 1 cm below the upper margin of peritoneal reflection and about 2–3 cm above the bladder base. While making an incision in the uterus, a curvilinear mark of about 10 cm length is made by the scalpel, cutting partially through the myometrium. The uterine incision must be gently given, taking care to avoid any injury to the underlying fetus. Following this, a small cut (about 3 cm in size) is made, using the scalpel in the middle of this incision mark, reaching up to, but not through the membranes. The rest of the incision can be completed either by stretching the incision, using the tips of two index fingers along both the sides of the incision mark (Fig. 7.4A) or using bandage scissors, to extend the incision on two sides (Fig. 7.4B). The bandage scissor is introduced

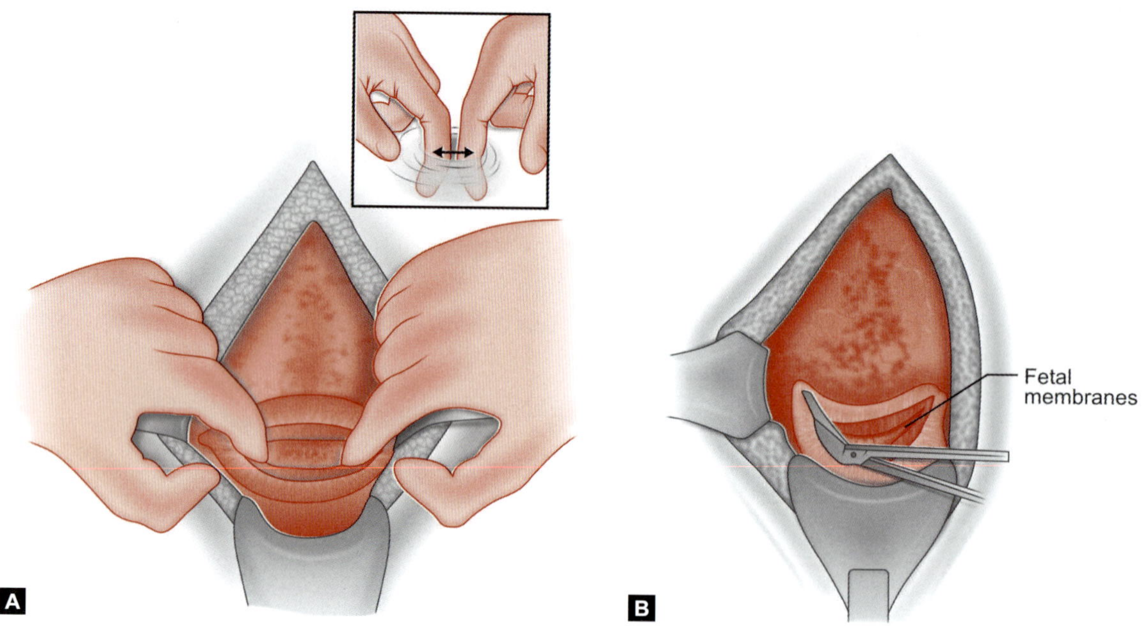



**Figs 7.4A and B:** (A) Extension of the uterine incision by manual stretching, using the index fingers;
(B) Extension of the uterine incision with the help of scissors

into the uterus over the two fingers, in order to protect the fetus. The use of bandage scissors may be especially required in cases, where the lower uterine segment is thickened and the uterine incision cannot be extended using the fingers. If the lower uterine segment is very thin, injury to the fetus can be avoided, by using the handle of the scalpel or a hemostat (an artery forceps) to open the uterus. The uterine incision must be large enough so as to allow the delivery of the head and trunk without the risk of extension of the incision laterally into the uterine vessels. As the fetal membranes bulge out through the uterine incision, they are ruptured. The amniotic fluid, which is released following the rupture of membranes, is sucked with the help of a suction machine.

*Location of the uterine incision:* The incision in the uterus is commonly given over the lower uterine segment. Sometimes a classical incision or an incision in the upper uterine segment can also be given. However, the classical incision has been found to be associated with high risk of scar rupture during future pregnancies. As a result, lower segment transverse scars are nowadays preferred. The lower segment uterine scar is considered to be stronger than the upper segment scar due to the reasons mentioned in Table 7.3.

### Delivery of the Infant

In case of cephalic presentation, once the fetal presenting part becomes visible through the uterine incision, the surgeon places his/her right hand below the fetal presenting part and grasps it. In case of cephalic presentation the fetal head is then elevated gently, using the palms and fingers of the hand. Delivery of the fetal head should be in the same way as during the normal vaginal delivery. The Doyen's retractor is removed, once the fetal presenting part has been grasped. In order to facilitate delivery, fundal pressure is applied by the assistant. Delivery is completed in the manner similar to normal vaginal delivery. Once the baby's shoulders have delivered, an IV infusion containing 20 IU of oxytocin per liter of crystalloids is infused at a rate of 10 mL/minute, until effective uterine contractions are obtained. Fundal massage, following the delivery of the baby, helps in reducing bleeding and hastens the delivery of placenta. Following the delivery of the baby, the cord is clamped and cut and the baby handed over to the clinician.

A single dose of prophylactic antibiotics in the dose of ampicillin 2 g or cefazolin 1 g administered intravenously after the cord is clamped and cut, helps in providing adequate prophylaxis. No additional benefit has been demonstrated with the use of multiple dose antibiotic regimens. If the woman shows signs of infection, e.g. fever, urinary tract infections, sepsis, etc., antibiotics must be continued until the woman becomes fever free for at least 48 hours.

### Placental Removal

At the time of cesarean, the placenta should be removed, using controlled cord traction (Fig. 7.5) and not manual removal as this reduces the risk of endometritis. Following the

**Table 7.3:** Reasons for greater strength of the lower segment uterine scar

| Criteria | Lower segment incision | Classical incision |
|---|---|---|
| Apposition of the margins of the incision. | The lower uterine segment is thinned out during labor. As a result, the thin margins of the lower segment can be easily apposed at the time of uterine repair without leaving behind any dead space pocket. | It may be difficult to appose the thick muscle layer of the upper segment. In these cases, blood filled pockets may be formed. This may be later replaced by fibrous tissues, resulting in further weakening of the scar. |
| Activity of the uterine segment in the postpartum period. | The lower segment usually remains inert in the postpartum period. | The upper segment undergoes rapid contractions and retractions, resulting in the loosening of the uterine sutures. This can result in imperfect healing and further weakening of the uterine scar. |
| Effect of the future pregnancy on the integrity of the scar. | When the uterus stretches in the future pregnancy, the stretch is along the line of the scar. | The uterus stretches in the direction perpendicular to the scar, thereby resulting in the scar weakness. |
| Chances of the placental implantation in the area of the scar at the time of the future pregnancy. | Highly unlikely. | Highly likely. Penetration and the invasion of the scar by the placental trophoblasts are likely to produce further weakening of the scar. |

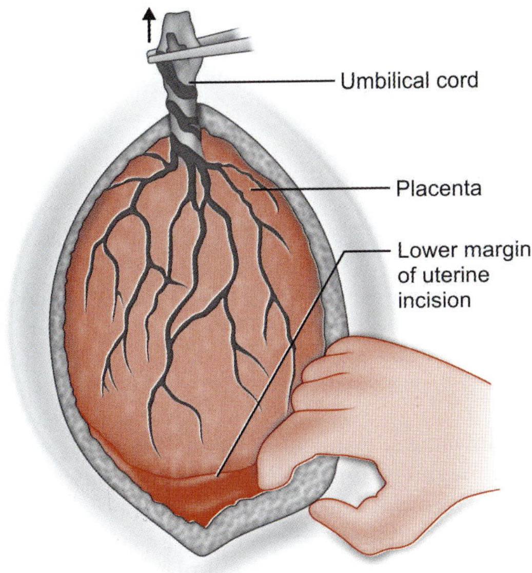


**Fig. 7.5:** Placental removal through controlled cord traction

delivery of the placenta, the remnant bits of membranes and decidua are removed using a sponge-holding forceps. The cut edges of the uterine incision are then identified and grasped with the help of Green Armytage clamps. The uterine angles are usually grasped with allies forceps.

### Closing the Uterine Incision

The main controversy related to the closure of the uterine incision is whether the closure should be in the form of a single-layered or a double-layered closure. Both single-layered and double-layered closure of uterine incision are being currently practiced. Though single-layered closure is associated with reduced operative time and reduced blood loss in the short term, the risk of the uterine rupture during subsequent pregnancies is increased. The current recommendation is to close the uterus in two layers, as the safety and efficacy of closing uterus in a single layer is presently uncertain. Individual bleeding sites can be approximated with the help of figure-of-eight sutures. If tubal sterilization has to be performed, it is done following the closure of uterine incision. Following the uterine closure, swab and instrument count is done. Once the count is found to be correct, the abdominal incision is closed in layers.

### Peritoneal Closure

The current recommendation by RCOG is that neither the visceral nor the parietal peritoneum should be sutured at the time of cesarean section, as this reduces the operative time and the requirement for the postoperative analgesia.

### Closure of the Rectus Sheath

Rectus sheath closure is performed after identifying the angles and holding them with allies forceps. The angles must be secured using 1-0 vicryl sutures. The rectus layer is closed with the help of continuous locked sutures placed no more than 1 cm apart. Hemostasis must be checked at all levels.

### Closure of Subcutaneous Space

There is no need for the routine closure of the subcutaneous tissue space, unless there is more than 2 cm of subcutaneous fat, because this practice has not been shown to reduce the incidence of the wound infection.

### Skin Closure

Clinicians should be aware that presently the differences between the use of different suture materials and methods of skin closure at the time of cesarean section are not certain. Skin closure can be either performed, using subcutaneous, continuous repair absorbable or nonabsorbable stitches or using interrupted stitches with nonabsorbable sutures or staples. In our setup the skin is closed with vertical mattress sutures of 3-0 or 4-0 silk. Following the skin closure, the vagina is swabbed dried and dressing applied to the wound.

## Postoperative Care

### Immediate Care

- After surgery is completed, the woman needs to be monitored in a recovery area.
- Monitoring of routine vital signs (blood pressure, temperature, breathing), urine output, vaginal bleeding and uterine tonicity (to check, if the uterus remains adequately contracted), needs to be done at hourly intervals for the first 4 hours. Thereafter, the monitoring needs to be done at every four hourly intervals for the first postoperative day at least. Adequate analgesia needs to be provided, initially through the IV line and later with oral medications.
- When the effects of anesthesia have worn off, about 4–8 hours after surgery, the woman may be transferred to the postpartum room.
- *Fluids and oral food after cesarean section:* As a general rule, about 3 liters of fluids must be replaced by IV infusion during the first postoperative day, provided that the woman's urine output remains greater than 30 mL/hour. If the urine output falls below 30 mL/hour, the woman needs to be reassessed to evaluate the cause of oliguria. In uncomplicated cases, the urinary catheter can be removed by 12 hours postoperatively. Intravenous fluids may need to be continued, until she starts taking liquids orally. The clinician needs to remember that prolonged infusion of IV fluids can alter electrolyte balance. If the woman receives IV fluids for more than 48 hours, her electrolyte levels need to be monitored every 48 hours. Balanced electrolyte solution (e.g. potassium chloride 1.5 g in 1 L IV fluids) may be administered.

  If the surgery was uncomplicated, the woman may be given a light liquid diet in the evening after the surgery. If there were signs of infection or if the cesarean section was for obstructed labor or uterine rupture, bowel sounds must be heard before prescribing oral liquids to the patient. In these cases, the woman can be given solid food, when she starts passing gas. Women who are recovering well and

who do not have complications after the surgery can be advised to eat and drink, whenever they feel hungry or thirsty. The clinician must ensure the woman is eating a regular diet before she is discharged from the hospital.

- *Ambulation after cesarean section:* The women must be encouraged to ambulate as soon as 6–8 hours following the surgery.
- *Dressing and wound care:* The dressing must be kept on the wound for the first 2–3 days after surgery, so as to provide a protective barrier against infection. Thereafter, dressing is usually not required. If blood or fluid is observed to be leaking through the initial dressing, the dressing must not be changed. The amount of blood/fluid lost must be monitored. If bleeding increases or the bloodstain covers half the dressing or more, the dressing must be removed and replaced with another sterile dressing. The dressing must be changed while using a sterile technique. The surgical wound also needs to be carefully inspected.

*Length of hospital stay:* Length of hospital stay is likely to be longer after a cesarean section (an average of 3–4 days) in comparison to that after a vaginal birth (average 1–2 days). However, women who are recovering well and have not developed complications following cesarean may be offered early discharge.

## Classical Cesarean Section

Classical cesarean section involves giving a vertical uterine incision. The classical uterine scar is worse than a transverse uterine scar for the reasons, which have already been discussed previously in this chapter.

### Indications

Though, nowadays, classical incisions are rarely performed, they might be rarely done in the following cases:

- *Cases where the lower segment is not easily accessible:* These may include cases such as bladder densely adherent to the lower segment, invasive carcinoma cervix, presence of an uterine myoma in the lower uterine segment, transverse lie of the fetus with the shoulder impacted in the birth canal, massive maternal obesity, cases of placenta previa in which the placenta penetrates through the lower uterine segment (placenta percreta).
- *Cases where lower uterine segment has not formed:* This is observed especially in association with a very small fetus having breech presentation or with multifetal gestation, etc.

### Procedure

In case of a classical cesarean section, the uterine incision is given vertically. The lower limit of the uterine incision is initiated as low as possible, usually above the level of bladder.

The uterine incision is extended in the cephalad direction using a bandage scissor, until the incision becomes large enough to facilitate delivery. The incision is deepened until the membranes are reached, which are then punctured. In case the placenta is encountered, fingers are slipped between the placenta and uterine wall until the membranes are reached. After rupturing the membranes, the baby is most commonly delivered as breech extraction. Following the delivery of the baby and the placenta, the uterine incision is closed in three layers. The deeper layers are approximated using a layer of continuous No. 0 or No. 1 chromic catgut or vicryl sutures. The outer layer is closed using figure-of-eight interrupted sutures using No. 1 chromic catgut or vicryl sutures. The edges of the uterine serosa are approximated using continuous 2-0 chromic catgut sutures.

## COMPLICATIONS

Various complications associated with cesarean delivery are tabulated in Table 7.4 and are described next in details.

## Uterine Rupture

Approximately 15% of all deliveries in the United State occur in women with previous cesarean sections. In a patient with a previous cesarean section, vaginal delivery may cause the previous uterine scar to separate. Disintegration of the scar, also known as scar rupture, is one of the most disastrous complications associated with VBAC. The reported incidence of scar rupture for all pregnancies is 0.05%. However, the exact risk of scar rupture depends upon the type of uterine incision, given at the time of previous cesarean (Table 7.5). The weakest type of scar that may give way at the time of VBAC is the previous classical incision in the upper segment of the uterus, which is associated with almost 10% risk of development of scar rupture.

The uterine rupture can be of two types: (1) complete rupture and (2) incomplete rupture. Details related to this and management of scar rupture has been described in Chapter 5.

**Table 7.4:** Complications associated with cesarean delivery

- Abdominal pain
- Injury to bladder, ureters, etc.
- Increased risk of rupture uterus and maternal death
- Neonatal respiratory morbidity
- Requirement for hysterectomy
- Thromboembolic disease
- Increased duration of hospital stay
- Antepartum or intrapartum intrauterine deaths in future pregnancies
- Patients with a previous history of cesarean delivery are more prone to develop complications, like placenta previa and adherent placenta during future pregnancies

**Table 7.5:** Risk of scar rupture based on the type of uterine scar, given at the time of previous cesarean delivery

| Types of previous cesarean scars | Estimated risk of rupture (%) |
| --- | --- |
| Classical cesarean | 4–9 |
| T-shaped incision | 4–9 |
| Low vertical | 1–7 |
| Low-transverse incision | 0.8–1 |

## Infection

Infection is a complication, which can commonly develop after cesarean section. Endometritis or infection of the endometrial cavity must be suspected, if there is excessive vaginal bleeding/discharge following the surgery. Infection of the urinary tract can result in symptoms like dysuria, increased urinary frequency, pyuria, etc.

## Trauma to the Urinary Tract

This complication can occur during the cesarean surgery and if not appropriately handled can result in development of urinary tract fistulas.

## Thromboembolism

Thromboembolism must be suspected, if the patient develops cough, swollen calf muscles or positive Homan's sign. A positive Homan's sign is associated with deep vein thrombosis and is said to be present when passive dorsiflexion of the ankle by the examiner elicits sharp pain in the patient's calf.

# Obstetric Hysterectomy

## Introduction

Obstetric hysterectomy refers to the removal of the uterus at the time of a planned or unplanned cesarean section. It involves either the removal of pregnant uterus with pregnancy in situ or a recently pregnant uterus due to some complications of delivery. Sometimes hysterectomy may be required following delivery, either vaginal or cesarean in order to save mother's life. Obstetric hysterectomy can be performed in the antepartum, peripartum or the postpartum periods. When hysterectomy is performed at the time of cesarean delivery, the procedure is termed as the cesarean hysterectomy. If performed within a short time after vaginal delivery, it is termed as postpartum hysterectomy.

The most common indication for hysterectomy at the time of cesarean section is ruptured uterus. In contrast, placenta accreta with or without an associated placenta previa is the most common indication for post-cesarean hysterectomy.

History of a previous cesarean section increases the likelihood of placenta previa, placenta accreta, scar dehiscence and overt uterine rupture. Each of these diagnoses increases the risk for emergency hysterectomy.

Obstetric hysterectomy could be performed as an emergency or an elective procedure depending upon the indications and circumstances under which it is performed. It could be of the subtotal/supracervical type (involving the removal of the uterus above the cervix); total (involving the removal of both uterus and cervix) or the radical type.

The procedure is usually performed as an emergency in order to control intractable primary PPH following childbirth and delivery. Before resorting to hysterectomy, a sequence of the conservative measures to control hemorrhage must be initiated.

## Indications

Some important causes for obstetric hysterectomy are enumerated in Table 7.6.

## SURGERY

### Preoperative Preparation

The preoperative investigations to be performed are as follows:

- *Hematocrit assessment:* Pregnant women should be offered a hemoglobin assessment before cesarean section to identify those who have anemia.
- *Blood transfusion:* Pregnant women having cesarean section for antepartum hemorrhage, abruption, uterine rupture and placenta previa are at an increased risk of blood loss greater than 1,000 mL and should have the cesarean section carried out at a maternity unit with on-site blood transfusion services.
- *Informed consent:* The indications for the procedure and its possible outcomes must be discussed with the patient and her partner and an informed consent should be obtained prior to labor and delivery.
- *Prophylactic antibiotics:* Antibiotics (single dose of first-generation cephalosporin or ampicillin) must be prescribed prior to the procedure.
- *Assessment of the risk for thromboembolic disease:* If the patient appears to be at a high risk of thromboembolic disorders, she can be offered graduated stockings, hydration, early mobilization and low molecular weight heparin.
- *Preanesthetic preparation:* In order to reduce the risk of aspiration pneumonitis, the patient must be kept nil per mouth at least 12 hours prior to the surgery. If performed as an emergency procedure, the patient must be given premedication with an antacid (sodium citrate 0.3%, 30 mL or magnesium trisilicate, 300 mg), $H_2$ antagonist

**Table 7.6:** Indications for obstetric hysterectomy

*Obstetric Emergencies*

- Postpartum hemorrhage
  - Intractable uterine atony
  - Inverted uterus
  - Coagulopathy
  - Laceration of a pelvic vessel
- Sepsis
  - Chorioamnionitis with sepsis
  - Myometrial abscesses

*Cesarean Delivery*

- Rupture uterus
  - Traumatic
  - Spontaneous
  - Extending pelvic hematoma
  - Lateral extension of the uterine incision with the involvement of uterine vessels
- Placental implantation in the lower segment (placenta accreta, increta or percreta)
- Presence of the large or symptomatic leiomyomas which may prevent effective uterine repair
- Presence of severe cervical dysplasia or carcinoma in situ
- Uncontrollable postpartum hemorrhage
- Unrepairable rupture uterus
- Operable cancer cervix: In stage one (I) cervical cancers with pregnancy, the treatment is by cesarean delivery followed by a radical hysterectomy
- Couvelaire uterus
- Severe uterine infection particularly that caused by *Clostridium welchii*

*Nonemergency Situations (Peripartum Hysterectomy)*

- Coexisting gynecological disorders
  - Leiomyomas
  - Stage I cervical carcinoma
  - Cervical intraepithelial neoplasia
  - Ovarian malignancy
- Previous gynecological disorders
  - Endometritis
  - PID
  - Heavy and irregular menstrual bleeding
  - Pelvic adhesions

(Cimetidine) IV and an antiemetic (perinorm), at least 1 hour prior to the procedure.

- *Catheterization:* In order to prevent injury to the urinary bladder at the time of surgery, it is important that the bladder be catheterized prior to undertaking the surgery.
- *Maternal position during cesarean section:* All obstetric patients undergoing cesarean section should be positioned with left lateral tilt to avoid aortocaval compression. This can be achieved by tilting the operating table to the left or by placing a pillow under the patient's right lower back.
- *Anesthesia:* The procedure can be performed either under general anesthesia or regional anesthesia (epidural

or spinal block). Regional anesthesia is regarded as considerably safer than general anesthesia and is most commonly used in our setup.

- *Preparation of the skin:* The area around the proposed incision site must be washed with soap and water. The woman's pubic hair must not be shaved as this increases the risk of wound infection. The hair may be trimmed, if necessary.
- *Cleaning and draping:* The skin at the operation site is routinely cleaned with antiseptic solutions before surgery because this practice is thought to reduce the risk of postoperative wound infections. An antiseptic solution (e.g. betadine) must be applied at least three times at the incision site using a high-level disinfected ring forceps and cotton or gauze swab.

## Actual Procedure

The surgery comprises of the following steps (Figs 7.6A to H):
- If a cesarean section has not been performed prior to the hysterectomy, a vertical midline incision must be given below the umbilicus until the pubic hairline, through the skin and to the level of the fascia.
- After giving a vertical fascial incision (about 2–3 cm in length), the edges of the fascia must be held with the forceps and the incision lengthened up and down using scissors.
- The rectus muscles must be separated using fingers or the scissors. Once the peritoneum has been identified, the fingers must be used for making an opening in the peritonium near the umbilicus. The incision must carefully be extended in the upwards and downwards direction, using scissors. In order to prevent bladder injury, the scissors must be used to carefully separate different layers of the peritoneum and to open the lower part of the peritonium.
- A bladder retractor must be placed over the pubic bone and self-retracting abdominal retractors must be placed to retract the abdominal skin.
- If a cesarean section has already been performed, there is no need for the above mentioned steps. In these women, following the delivery of the baby and the placenta, the uterine incision may be stitched in cases where appreciable amount of bleeding is occurring. Instead of stitching the uterine incision, sponge holding forceps or green armytage forceps can be applied at the margin of uterine incision for achieving hemostasis.
- The uterus is lifted out of the abdomen and gently pulled in order to maintain erection.
- The round ligaments are clamped, cut and double ligated with Kocher's clamps. In cases of emergency, the pedicle may be dropped initially, to be sutured later. In elective and nonemergent cases, the lateral pedicle must be secured with an absorbable suture.

- From the cut edge of the round ligament, the anterior leaf of the broad ligament is opened. The broad ligament is incised up to the point where the bladder peritoneum is reflected on to the lower uterine surface in the midline.
- The surgeon must use his/her two fingers in order to push the posterior leaf of the broad ligament forward, just under the tube and ovary, near the uterine edge. A hole of the size of a finger must be made in the broad ligament, using scissors.
- Through this hole, the right Fallopian tube and utero-ovarian ligaments are doubly clamped with a Kocher's clamp. The medial round ligament clamp is replaced to encompass the adnexal structures. The adnexal pedicle is then divided between the medial clamp and the two lateral clamps. The pedicle is dropped, and to be sutured later.
- The edge of the bladder flap must be grasped with forceps or a small clamp. The surgeon must dissect the bladder downwards off the lower uterine segment using finger or scissors. The pressure must be directed downwards, but inwards towards the cervix and the lower uterine segment.
- The uterine arteries and veins are then located on each side of the uterus. The uterine vessels are then doubly clamped at an angle of 90° on each side of the cervix and then ligated doubly with a No. 0 chromic catgut suture. Once the uterine vessels have been correctly ligated, the bleeding usually stops and the uterus starts looking pale. The surgeon must also feel for the joint between the uterus and cervix.
- In case of a subtotal hysterectomy the uterus must be amputated, above the level where the uterine arteries are ligated, using scissors.
- The cervical stump must be closed with interrupted 2-0 or 3-0 chromic catgut or polyglycolic sutures.
- In case of a total hysterectomy a few additional steps are required. These are as follows:
  - The posterior leaf of broad ligament is divided inferiorly towards the uterosacral ligament.
  - The bladder and the attached peritoneal flap are again deflected and dissected from the lower uterine segment and retracted out of the operative field. If the bladder flap is unusually adherent, a careful sharp dissection may be necessary.
  - The uterosacral and the cardinal ligaments are then clamped, cut and ligated.
  - As the upper 2 cm of the vagina gets free of the attachments, the vagina must be circumcised as close to the cervix as possible, clamping any bleeding points as they appear. Some surgeons prefer to close the vaginal cuff, while the others prefer to leave it open.
- Before closing the abdomen, the surgeon must carefully check various structures such as the cervical stump, leaves of broad ligament and other pelvic floor structures

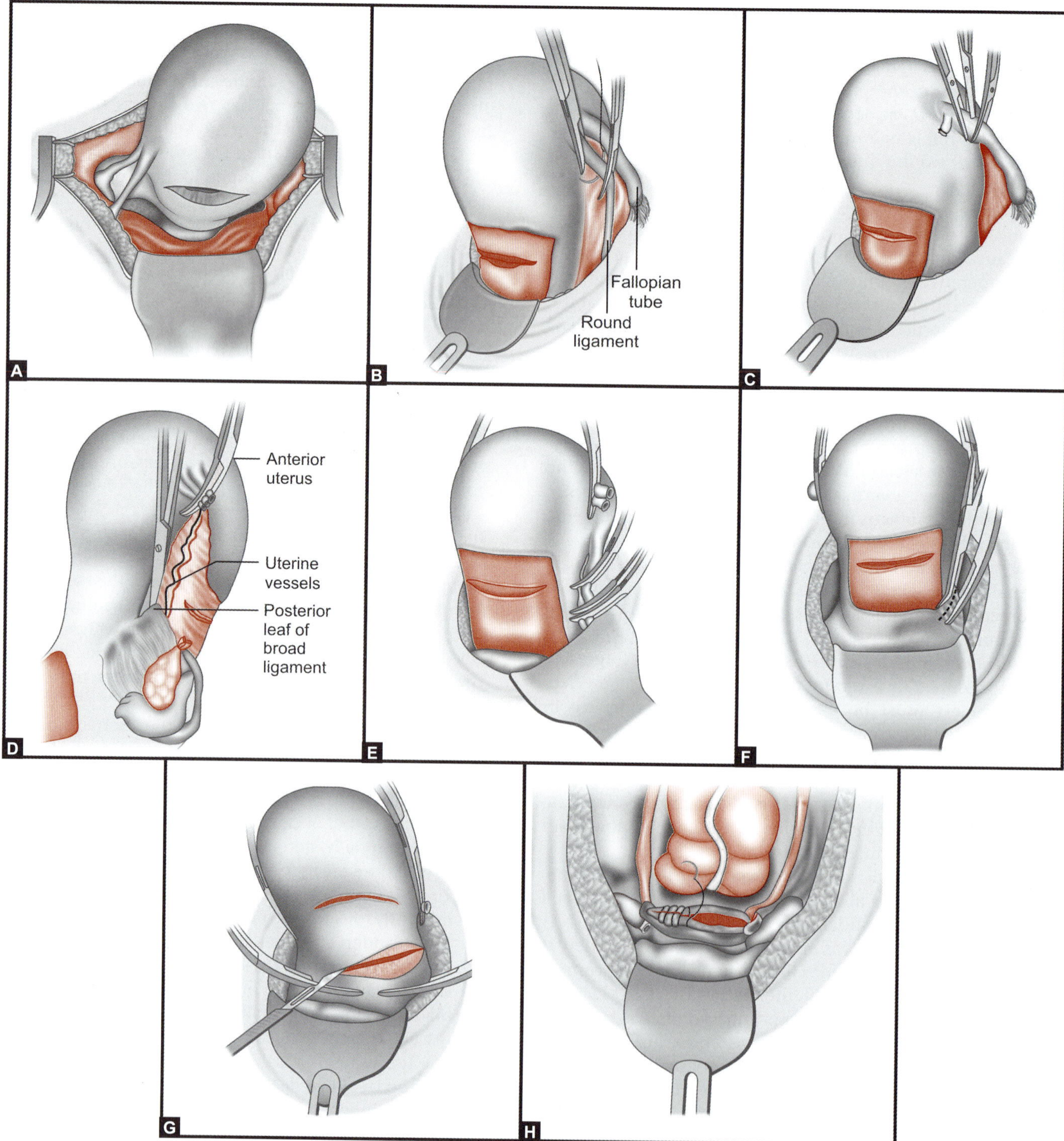



**Figs 7.6A to H:** (A) Incision in the uterus as a result of cesarean section; (B) Camping, cutting and ligating the round ligaments; (C) The utero-ovarian ligaments and Fallopian tubes are clamped and cut bilaterally; (D) Tracing the path of the uterine vessels; (E) Uterine vessels are clamped, cut and ligated bilaterally; (F) Cardinal and uterosacral ligaments are clamped, cut and ligated bilaterally; (G) Separating the uterus from the vaginal vault; (H) Closure of the vaginal vault

for any signs of bleeding. Bladder must also be checked for any signs of injury. Any injury, if identified, must be repaired before closing the abdomen.

- There is no need to close the bladder or abdominal peritoneum. Fascia must be closed using continuous No. 0 chromic catgut or polyglycolic sutures.
- If there are no signs of infection, the skin can be closed using vertical mattress sutures of 3-0 nylon or silk and a sterile dressing may be applied.

## Postoperative Care

- *Prophylactic antibiotics:* Immediately after the cord is clamped, a single dose of prophylactic antibiotics must be given intravenously. This could include ampicillin 2 g IV or cefazolin 1 g IV. No additional benefit has been demonstrated with the use of multiple-dose regimens. If signs of infection are present or the woman currently has fever, antibiotics must be continued until the woman is fever-free for at least 48 hours.
- *Monitoring the vitals:* After surgery is completed, the woman must be monitored in a recovery area for about 4–8 hours. The parameters which need to be monitored include the patient's vital signs such as pulse, blood pressure, temperature, respiratory rate, amount of bleeding per vaginum, bleeding from the incision site and whether the uterus remains well-contracted or not.
- *Analgesics:* Pain medication is also given, initially through the IV line, and later with oral medications. Adequate postoperative pain control is of prime importance.
- *Diet:* If the surgical procedure was uncomplicated, the woman can be started on a liquid diet from the next day onwards. If there are signs of infection, or if the surgery was performed for obstructed labor or uterine rupture, the surgeon must wait until bowel sounds are heard before giving liquids. When the woman begins to pass gas, she can be given solid food. If the woman is receiving IV fluids, they should be continued until she starts accepting liquids well. Prior to discharge, the surgeon must ensure that the woman is eating a regular diet. Women who are recovering well and who do not have complications after hysterectomy can eat and drink when they feel hungry or thirsty.
- *Early ambulation:* The woman must be encouraged to ambulate as soon as possible, usually within 24 hours in order to prevent the development of complications such as thromboembolism.
- *Dressing over the incision site:* The dressing over the incision site must be kept for the first few days after the surgery in order to protect the woman against infection, while re-epithelialization occurs. Thereafter, a dressing is not necessary.

The dressing must not be changed if there is blood or fluid leaking out through the initial dressing. In these cases, the dressing can be reinforced.

## Advantages of Cesarean Hysterectomy

The advantage of performing hysterectomy after cesarean section is the ease of development of the tissue planes in a pregnant uterus. Cesarean hysterectomy at times serves as the last resort for saving the pregnant woman's life.

This procedure may be unwelcome in women desirous of future conceptions.

## Complications

The complications associated with cesarean hysterectomy are typically high in cases where it is performed as an emergency procedure rather than an elective one. The procedure is associated with a high rate of mortality and morbidity. The high rate of mortality is usually not associated with the procedure per se, but with the underlying emergency condition for which the hysterectomy was performed in the first instant. The two most frequently encountered operative complications associated with the procedure include hemorrhage and injury to the urinary tract.

*Hemorrhage:* Obstetric hysterectomy in comparison to the normal elective hysterectomy is associated with an increased risk of the blood loss due to the presence of hypertrophied pelvic vessels in the pregnant women. This may be associated with an increased requirement for the blood transfusion. Control of blood loss during obstetric hysterectomy depends upon the surgical technique and careful management of all vascular pedicles. Unrecognized injuries before or during the surgery can develop into serious postoperative complications later on.

*Injury to the urinary tract:* Bladder injury may occur while dissecting the bladder from the scarred lower uterine segment. The bladder may also be injured due to the inclusion of bladder wall in a vaginal cuff clamp or a suture.

*Infections:* Infections can commonly occur following obstetric hysterectomy. These commonly include vaginal cuff cellulitis, abdominal incisional infections and urinary infections.

# Surgical Procedures for Controlling PPH

## INTRODUCTION

According to the WHO, PPH can be defined as excessive blood loss per vaginum (>500 mL in case of normal vaginal delivery or >1,000 mL following a cesarean section) from the time period within 24 hours of delivery of the baby lasting until the end of the puerperium. The PPH can be considered as a major obstetric emergency and a leading cause of maternal mortality and morbidity. Some amount of blood loss can occur normally during the process of childbirth. Approximate blood loss at the time of normal vaginal delivery is considered

| **Table 7.7:** Causes of postpartum hemorrhage |
| --- |
| • Tone: Atonic uterus<br>• Trauma: Cervical, vaginal and perineal lacerations, pelvic hematomas, uterine inversion, ruptured uterus<br>• Tissue: Retained tissue (placental fragments), invasive placenta<br>• Thrombin: Coagulopathies |

to be 500 mL; 1,000 mL at the time of cesarean section and 1,500 mL during postpartum hysterectomy.

The ACOG has defined PPH as a decrease in hematocrit by 10% or requirement of blood transfusion 24 hours after the delivery. The WHO has classified PPH into two: primary PPH and secondary PPH.

## Primary PPH

Primary PPH can be defined as blood loss, estimated to be greater than 500 mL, occurring from the genital tract, within 24 hours of delivery. Primary PPH can be considered as the most common cause for obstetric hemorrhage.

## Secondary PPH

Secondary PPH can be defined as abnormal bleeding from the genital tract, occurring 24 hours after delivery until 6 weeks of postpartum.

## Causes of PPH

The mnemonic "4 Ts" (tone, trauma, tissue and thrombin) help in describing the four important causes of PPH, which are enumerated in Table 7.7.

## MANAGEMENT OF PPH

Management of a patient with PPH is shown in Flow chart 7.1.

Once the maternal condition has stabilized, the cause of PPH must be identified and treated. The further management must be decided based on the fact whether the placenta has delivered on not. If the placenta has delivered, PPH could be due to uterine atonicity, uterine trauma, retained placental tissue, coagulation disorders, etc. In cases of atonic uterus, medical management usually suffices. Medical management of PPH includes use of uterotonic agents such as oxytocine (syntocinon) ergot alkaloids (methylergometrine), prostaglandin analogues (carboprost, misoprostol, etc.) (Table 7.8). Surgical options for controlling PPH vary depending on whether the placenta has delivered or not.

In earlier times, most cases of intractable PPH occurred due to uterine atony following normal vaginal delivery. However, nowadays, with increasing rate of cesarean deliveries, there has been an increase in the cases of PPH during cesarean section. Uterine rupture has also become an important cause of PPH, which makes sometimes require hysterectomy.

Surgical management in cases of PPH is usually required in severe cases experiencing life-threatening bleeding, which cannot be controlled by conservative or medical management. Surgical management becomes necessary if the uterus remains atonic and flabby despite of conservative management. The management of PPH at the time of cesarean delivery or uterine rupture is not greatly different from that following normal vaginal delivery. The most commonly used surgical approach in cases of PPH is the conservative type in which attempts are made to preserve the uterus and thereby future fertility. If the bleeding still remains uncontrollable, the surgeon may have to resort to more aggressive surgical approaches. If nothing seems to work, performing a hysterectomy may be the only option left to save life even in those women who require future fertility. Some of the indications for surgery in case of PPH are as follows:

- Atonic uterus not responding to uterotonic drugs.
- Severe uncontrollable bleeding following normal vaginal birth or cesarean delivery.

## Placenta Has Delivered

If the placenta has delivered, the main thing the clinician needs to see is whether the uterus has contracted or not.

### *Uterus Well Contracted*

If the uterus contracts, but the bleeding continues despite a well-contracted uterus, the clinician must look for other causes including traumatic causes and coagulation abnormalities.

### *Uterus Is Atonic*

If the placenta has delivered, but the uterus is not hard and contracted; instead appears to be atonic and flabby, the PPH is of atonic type. In this case, the following steps need to be carried out:

- The urinary bladder must be emptied.
- Exploration of the uterine cavity for any retained placental bits needs to be carried out.
- The vagina and cervix must still be inspected for presence of lacerations and tears (traumatic PPH is commonly present in association with atonic PPH).
- Administration of oxytocic drugs (Table 7.8).
- Uterine tamponade.
- Bimanual uterine massage.

*Bimanual uterine massage:* If the clinician finds the uterus to be soft upon bimanual examination, a bimanual uterine massage must be performed to contract the myometrial muscles. For more details related to bimanual uterine massage kindly refer to Chapter 3.

**Flow chart 7.1:** Management of a case of PPH

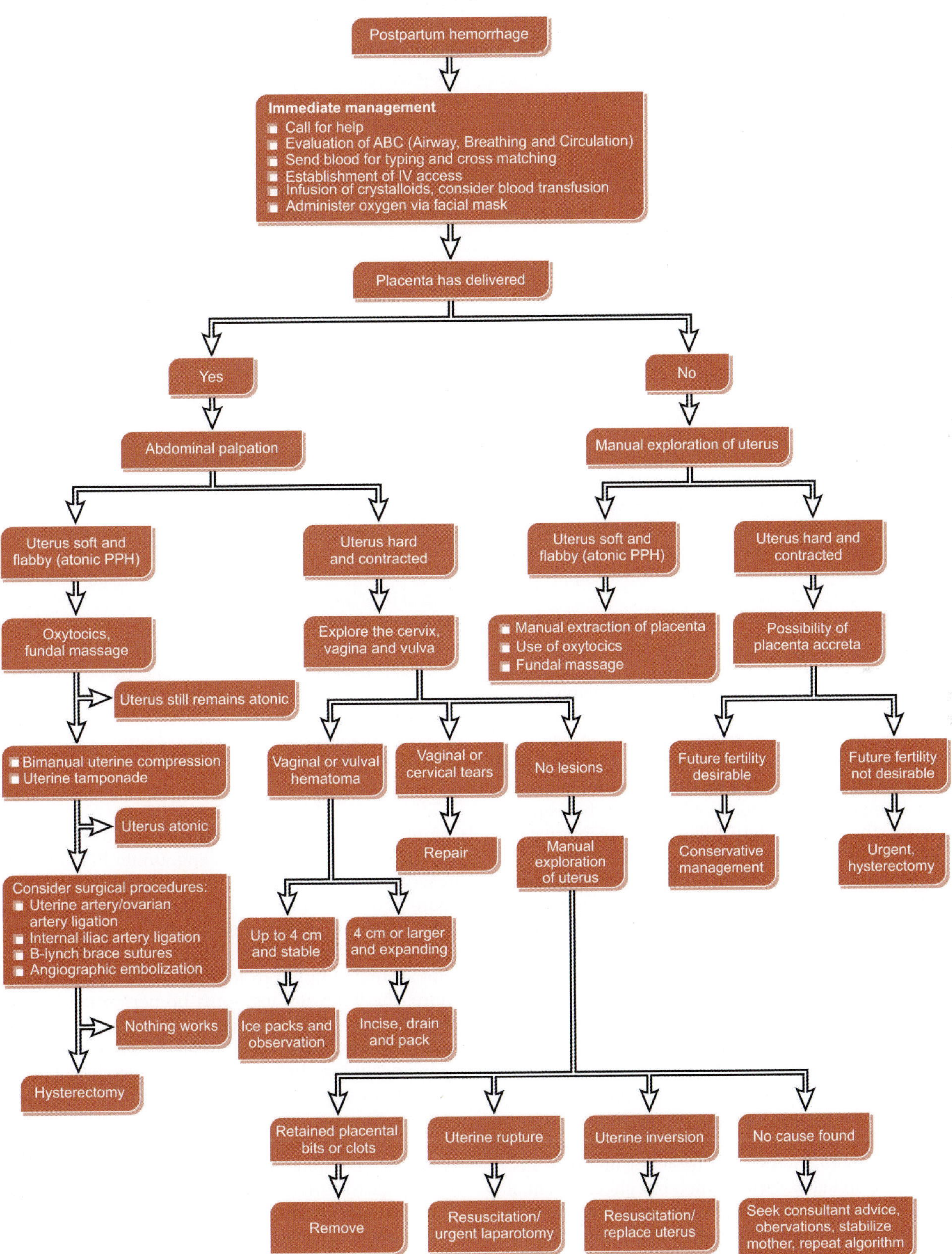

| Table 7.8: Various oxytocics used for controlling postpartum hemorrhage | | | |
|---|---|---|---|
| **Drug** | **Dosage** | **Side effects** | **Contraindications** |
| Oxytocin (used as a first-line drug in the active management of first stage of labor) | 20 IU in 1 L of saline may be infused intravenously at a rate of 125 mL/hour (over 4 hours) | Water intoxication (manifested by symptoms of hyponatremia such as confusion, coma, congestive heart failure, etc.) and nausea at high dosage | Nil |
| Methylergometrine (methergine) | 0.25 mg intramuscularly or intravenously (may be repeated as required at intervals of 2–4 hours) | Nausea, vomiting, hypertension, retained placenta, if given before placental separation, occurs | Hypertension, heart disease |
| Carboprost (15-methyl PGF2α) | 250 µg given as intramuscular injection every 15 minutes for a maximum of eight doses | Diarrhea, vomiting, flushing, pyrexia, hypertension, bronchoconstriction, etc. | Significant pulmonary, cardiac, hepatic or renal disease |
| Misoprostol | 600–1,000 µg perrectally or orally. Dose and frequency has yet not been standardized | Diarrhea, pyrexia (>40°C) | Significant pulmonary, cardiac, hepatic or renal disease |

If all the previously described conservative measures fail to control PPH, laparotomy may be required to save the mother's life. Application of aortal compression at the time of surgery must be considered. Most of the surgical methods for controlling PPH aim at controlling the blood supply to the uterus by ligation of some of the vessels, which supply blood to the uterus.

### Blood Supply to the Pelvic Structures

The blood supply to the pelvic structures is mainly by the common iliac vessels, which give rise to internal iliac artery (also known as the hypogastric artery) and external iliac artery (Fig. 7.7A). The blood supply to the uterus is mainly via the uterine and ovarian vessels (Fig. 7.7B). The ovarian arteries are direct branches of the aorta, which arise beneath the renal arteries. The uterine artery is the branch of internal iliac vessel. The uterine artery passes inferiorly from its origin into the pelvic fascia. It runs medially in the base of broad ligament to reach the uterus. It then reaches the junction of the body and cervix of the uterus (internal os) by passing superiorly. While taking such a course, the uterine artery passes above the ureter at right angles. It then ascends along the lateral margin of the uterus within the broad ligament. It continues to move along the lower border of the Fallopian tubes where it ends by anastomosing with the ovarian artery, which is a direct branch from the abdominal aorta. The uterine artery also gives off a small descending branch that supplies the cervix and the vagina. The uterine vein follows the uterine artery all along its course and ultimately drains into the internal iliac vein. Blood supply to anterior and posterior uterine walls is provided by the arcuate arteries, which run circumferentially around the uterus. The arcuate arteries give rise to the radial arteries, which enter the endometrium. The ultimate branches

of uterine artery which connect maternal circulation to the endometrium are the spiral and the basal arteries.

### TYPES OF SURGICAL OPTIONS

Various surgical options that can be used in a patient to control PPH are as follows:
- Brace sutures of uterus: B lynch sutures.
- Uterine artery or utero-ovarian artery ligation.
- Bilateral ligation of internal iliac (hypogastric arteries) vessels.
- Angiographic embolization.
- Hysterectomy (as a last option if nothing seems to work).

### B-Lynch Compression Sutures

Compression sutures can be considered as the best form of surgical approach for controlling atonic PPH as it helps in preserving the anatomical integrity of the uterus. The B-Lynch suture is the uterine bracing suture, which when tightened and tied helps in compressing the anterior and posterior uterine walls together. This technique is safe, effective and helps in retaining future fertility. Before using the B-Lynch suture, the following test must be performed to assess the effectiveness of these sutures:
- The uterus must be bimanually compressed followed by swabbing the vagina. If the bleeding is controlled temporarily in this fashion, the B-Lynch sutures are likely to be effective.

Presently, the uterine compression sutures have almost completely replaced uterine artery ligation, hypogastric artery ligation and postpartum hysterectomy for surgical treatment of atonic uterus. These brace like absorbable sutures help in controlling bleeding by

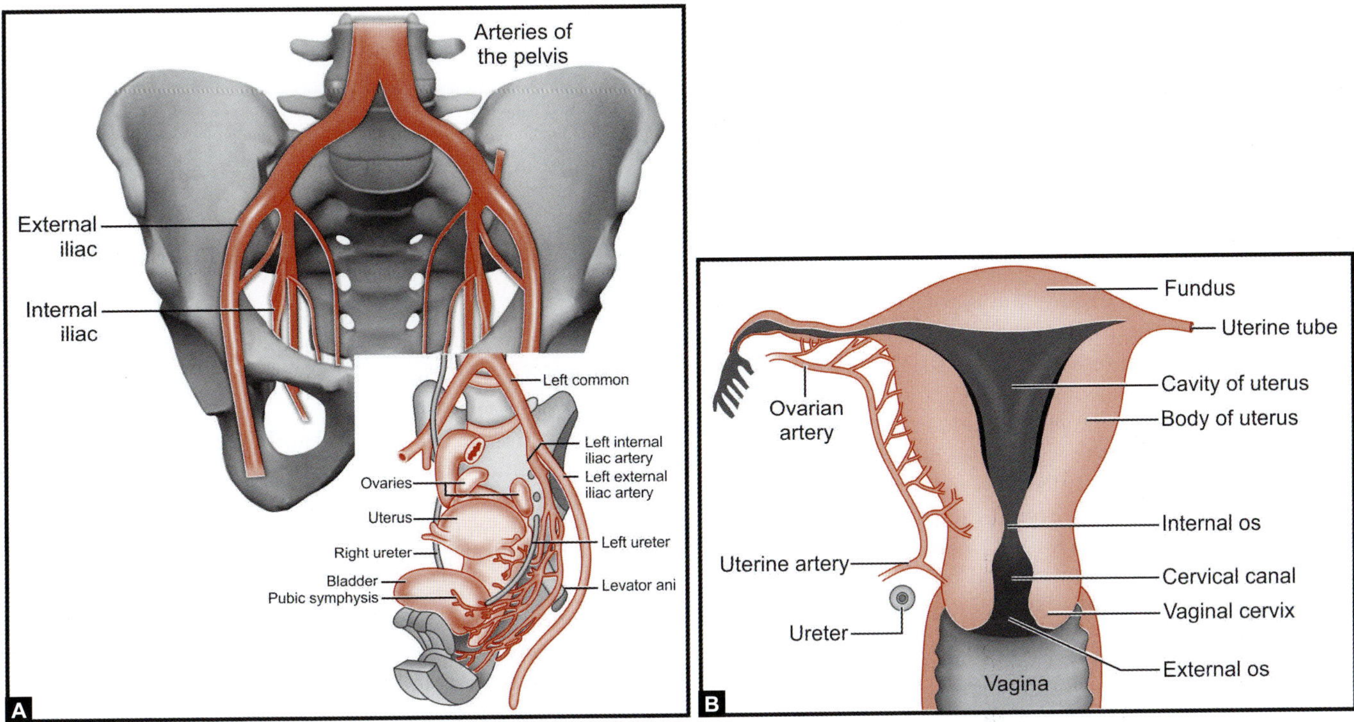



**Figs 7.7A and B:** (A) Blood supply to the pelvis (front view); (B) Blood supply to the uterus

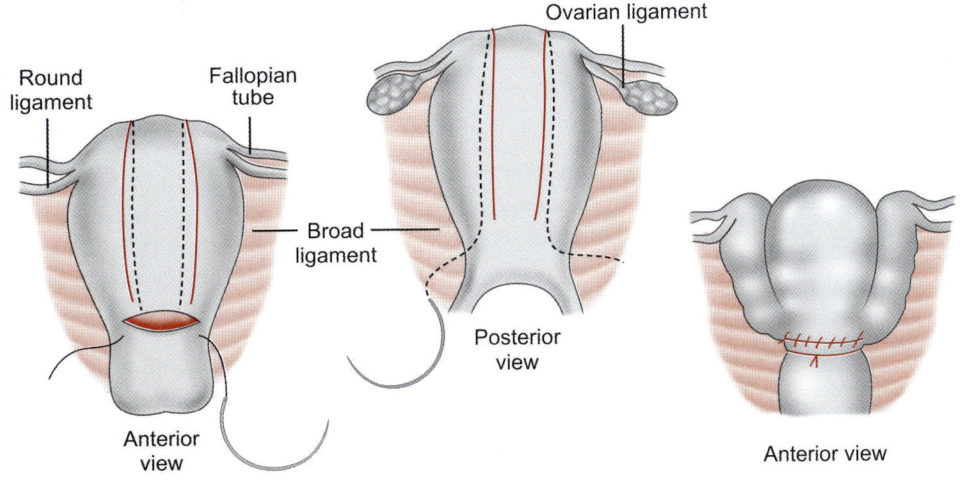



**Fig. 7.8:** B-Lynch suture
*Source*: B-Lynch C, Coker A, Lawal AH, et al. The B-Lynch surgical technique for the control of massive postpartum hemorrhage: an alternative to hysterectomy? Five cases reported. Br J Obstet Gynaecol. 1997;104(3):372-5.

causing hemostatic compression of the uterine fundus and lower uterine segment. The sutures are secured vertically around the anterior and posterior uterine walls giving appearance of suspenders. The sutures are first anchored in the anterior aspect of lower uterine segment, passed over the uterine fundus, anchored in the posterior aspect of the lower uterine segment, then again brought back anteriorly passing over the fundus of the uterus. These sutures are finally anchored near the entrance point on the anterior aspect of the lower uterine segment (Fig. 7.8). Simultaneously, the uterus is also massaged and manually compressed in order to reduce its size.

*Procedure*

- A No. 2 or No. 0 plain or chromic catgut absorbable sutures using a No. 2 sized needle are used for this procedure. The below-mentioned procedure describes the application of B lynch sutures when an incision has been given over the lower uterine segment.
- Using the above-mentioned sutures, a puncture is made in the uterus about 3 cm below the right hand corner of the lower uterine segment incision and brought out 3 cm above the incision. The suture is then passed 3–4 cm medial to the right cornu of the uterus. Here it may be fixed over the uterine fundus with the help of another suture to prevent it from slipping off.
- The suture is then placed posteriorly and brought down vertically to the same level where the suture had previously left the uterine cavity from the anterior side.
- The suture is passed through the posterior uterine wall into the cavity under the direct vision of the surgeon and back through the posterior wall for about 4–5 cm to the left of the previous site of entry.
- Then the suture is passed outside and posteriorly over the uterus 3–4 cm medial to the left cornual border and is brought out anteriorly and vertically down to the left of the left corner of the lower segment.
- The needle is then passed through the left corner in the same fashion as on the right hand side to emerge below the incision on the left side.
- When the sutures are in place, the assistant bimanually compresses the uterus while the chromic catgut sutures are pulled tightly by the surgeon.
    Another assistant/nurse is asked to look for any continuing vaginal bleeding.
- Some surgeons modify this technique by placing separate sutures over the main compression sutures in order to anchor it properly over the uterine fundus and prevent it from slipping.

This method has been found to be safe and effective and there have been reports of successful pregnancy following its use. A few complications, such as uterine ischemic necrosis with peritonitis, have been described with its use.

## Hypogastric Artery Ligation

Bilateral ligation of internal iliac vessels was first performed by Kelly in 1894. Appreciable reduction in the amount of bleeding can be achieved by the ligation of internal iliac vessels. The procedure, however, is technically difficult and may be successful only in 50% of cases in whom it is performed. This method causes nearly 85% reduction in pulse pressure in the arteries distal to the point of ligation. This is a highly effective method of controlling PPH, which is indicated in cases of PPH due to uterine atony, ruptured uterus and placenta accreta. This method also helps in preserving fertility of women desiring pregnancy in future.

*Procedure*

- The peritoneum between the Fallopian tube and the round ligament is incised to enter the retroperitoneal space.
- The common, internal and external iliac arteries must then clearly be identified.
- The external iliac artery on the pelvic side wall is identified and followed proximally until the bifurcation of common iliac artery. The ureter passes over the bifurcation of common iliac artery.
- The ureter must be identified and reflected medially along with the attached peritoneum.
- The peritoneum is opened over the common iliac vessels and dissection is continued for approximately 5 cm from the point of origin (i.e. the level of bifurcation of common iliac vessels). This site is ideal for ligation because the posterior division arises within 3 cm of the bifurcation and the ligature must be placed distal to the posterior division of the artery in order to reduce the risk of subsequent ischemic buttock pain.
- Following the dissection of the peritoneum over the internal iliac artery, a blunt-tipped, right angled clamp is gently placed around the hypogastric artery, 5.0 cm distal to the bifurcation of the common iliac artery (Figs 7.9A and B). The surgeon must pass the tip of the clamp from lateral to medial side under the artery in order to prevent injuries to the underlying hypogastric vein.
- The hypogastric artery is double-ligated with nonabsorbable sutures (1-0 silk or No. 2 chromic catgut) at two sites 1 cm apart. For this, a nonabsorbable suture is inserted into the open clamp, the jaws are locked and the suture is carried around the vessel. The vessel is then securely ligated. The vessel, however, must not be divided.
- The ligation is also performed on the contralateral side in the same manner.
- Following the ligation, the dorsalis pedis and femoral vessels must be palpated to ensure that external or common iliac arteries have not been inadvertently ligated.

## Uterine Artery Ligation

Since approximately 90% of the blood supply to the uterus is via the uterine artery, ligation of this vessel through the uterine wall at the level of uterine isthmus above the bladder flap is likely to control the amount of bleeding. If, despite of bilateral ligation of uterine vessels, bleeding remains uncontrollable, ligation of utero-ovarian anastamosis is done just below the ovarian ligament (Fig. 7.10).

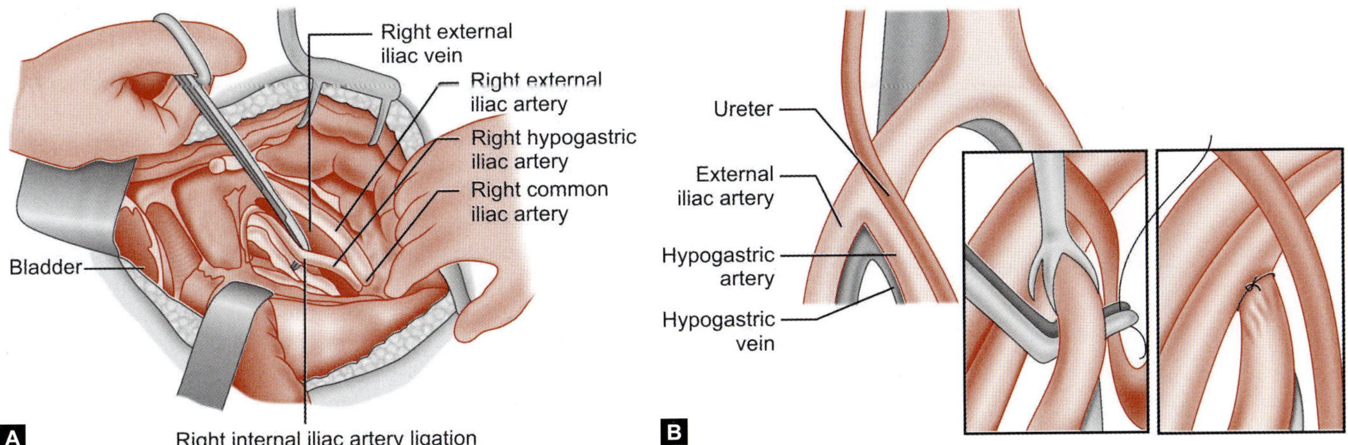



**Figs 7.9A and B:** Internal iliac artery ligation

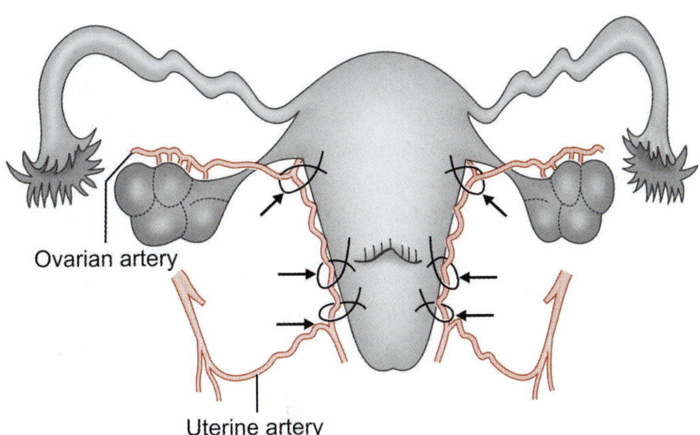



**Fig. 7.10:** Various sites of uterine artery ligation

## Uterine Artery Embolization

Nowadays, a commonly used alternative to uterine artery or internal iliac artery ligation is angiographic arterial embolization of the hypogastric vessel with small pledgets of gelfoam. Gelfoam acts as a selective occluding agent which dissolves within 2–3 weeks. This method has been found to be particularly useful in cases of retroperitoneal hematomas where surgery may be difficult. Success rate of up to 95% has been reported with this method.

## Uterine Packing

Packing of the uterine cavity can be considered in women with refractory PPH due to uterine atony who want to preserve their fertility. However, it can be associated with complications such as concealed bleeding and infection.

## Hysterectomy

If the above-mentioned surgical options are unable to control the hemorrhage, hysterectomy is the only choice left to save the woman's life.

## Repair of Genital Tract Tears and Lacerations

Presence of tears and lacerations in the genital tract is an important cause for continued bleeding following the birth of the baby.

# Surgical Management of Ectopic Pregnancy

## Introduction

In an ectopic (meaning "out of place") pregnancy, the fertilized ovum gets implanted outside the uterus as a result

*Procedure*

- The uterus is grasped and tilted in order to expose the blood vessels coursing through the broad ligament immediately adjacent to the uterus.
- The most common site of ligation is 2 cm below the level of transverse lower uterine incision site.
- While taking the stitch, maximum amount of myometrial thickness must be included in order to ensure complete occlusion of the artery and vein.
- The needle is then placed through an avascular portion of the broad ligament and tied anteriorly.
- There is no need for opening the broad ligament and the uterine artery ligation must be performed bilaterally.
- Following the ligation of uterine artery, ligation of the cervical branch must also be performed.
- For this, subsequent stitches are placed 2–3 cm below the initial stitches, following bladder mobilization.
- After the ligation of the cervical branch, the ligation of the ovarian branch may be also performed if the surgeon feels its requirement.

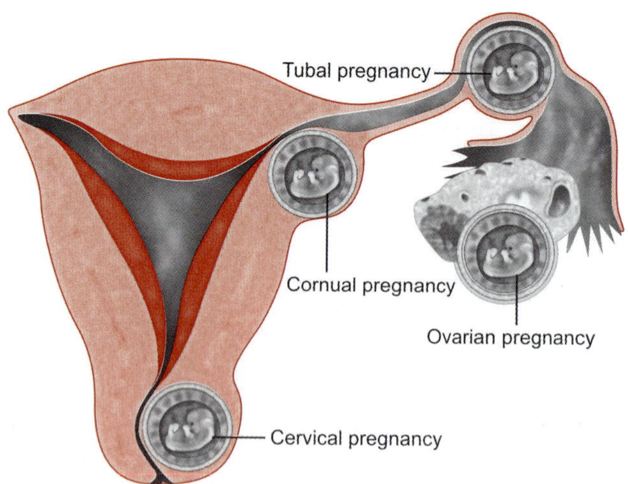


**Fig. 7.11:** Various sites of ectopic pregnancy

of which the pregnancy occurs outside the uterine cavity (Fig. 7.11). Ectopic pregnancy usually occurs as a result of delay or prevention in passage of the blastocyst to the uterine cavity resulting in its premature implantation in the extrauterine tissues. Most commonly, in nearly 95% of cases, the fertilized ovum gets implanted inside the Fallopian tube. Other less common extrauterine locations where an ectopic pregnancy can get implanted include the ovary, abdomen or the cervix.

The extrauterine locations do not have either sufficient space or nurturing tissues to support a growing pregnancy. A classical ectopic pregnancy normally does not develop into a live birth. Since none of these extra uterine areas have been equipped by nature to support a growing pregnancy, with the continuing growth of the fetus, the gestational sac and the organ containing it break open. This can result in severe bleeding, sometimes even endangering the woman's life. Although spontaneous resolution of ectopic pregnancy can occasionally occur, patients are at risk of tubal rupture and catastrophic hemorrhage. Ectopic pregnancy is estimated to occur in 2% of all pregnancies. It remains a major cause of maternal morbidity and mortality when misdiagnosed or left untreated.

## Management

Clinical symptoms of ectopic pregnancy are abdominal pain, amenorrhea and vaginal bleeding. Pregnancy test result is positive. Presence of a normal or slightly enlarged uterus and/or palpable adrenal mass on vaginal examination and symptoms such as vaginal bleeding and pelvic pain with clinical manipulation help increase the likelihood of an ectopic pregnancy. Imaging studies (both transabdominal and transvaginal ultrasound examination) help in establishing the diagnosis of ectopic pregnancy.

Various treatment options for ectopic pregnancy include expectant, medical and surgical management (Flow chart 7.2). In this chapter only the surgical management of ectopic pregnancy shall be discussed in details.

## Overview of Surgery

By the early 20th century, the standard treatment for ectopic pregnancy included laparotomy and ligation of the bleeding vessels with removal of the affected tube (salpingectomy). Since the 1980s and 1990s, medical therapy of ectopic pregnancy had been implemented and had replaced surgical treatment in many cases. However, now in the 21st century, the treatment modality has shifted towards minimal invasive surgery (operative laparoscopy) and salpingostomy, which have largely replaced laparotomy and salpingectomy.

## Aims of Surgery

Surgical therapy may be either in the form of open laparotomy or via the laparoscopic route. Surgical treatment in the form of open surgery (laparotomy) or minimal invasive surgery (laparoscopy) both are commonly used treatment options. The procedures which can be performed at the time of both laparotomy and laparoscopy include salpingectomy or salpingotomy. Numerous factors need to be considered before deciding the type of surgical approach to be used. Some of these factors include previous history of multiple prior surgeries, pelvic adhesions, skills of the surgeon and surgical staff, availability of the equipment, condition of the patient and size and location of ectopic pregnancy. A laparoscopic approach for the surgical management of tubal pregnancy must be used in the hemodynamically stable patients. On the other hand, management of tubal pregnancy in the presence of hemodynamic instability should be by laparotomy. Moreover, there is no role for medical management in the treatment of tubal pregnancy or suspected tubal pregnancy when a patient is showing signs of hypovolemic shock.

An early ectopic pregnancy can sometimes be treated with an injection of methotrexate, which stops the growth of the embryo. Medical therapy is commonly being employed nowadays in cases of ectopic pregnancy, especially if the patient is hemodynamically stable and does not have pelvic pain; patient desires future fertility; ectopic pregnancy is smaller than 4 cm in diameter and there is no fetal heart activity on TVS or the gestational sac is smaller than 3.5 cm with presence of cardiac activity and absence of any free fluid in the pouch of Douglas; there is no evidence of tubal rupture and the patient appears to be reliable and compliant who will return for post-treatment follow-up care; serum hCG or hCG is below 3,000 IU/L, with minimal symptoms; there is no coexisting intrauterine pregnancy; there is availability of facilities for follow-up care following the use of methotrexate; patient agrees to use reliable contraception for 3–4 months

**Flow chart 7.2:** Treatment plan for patients with ectopic pregnancy

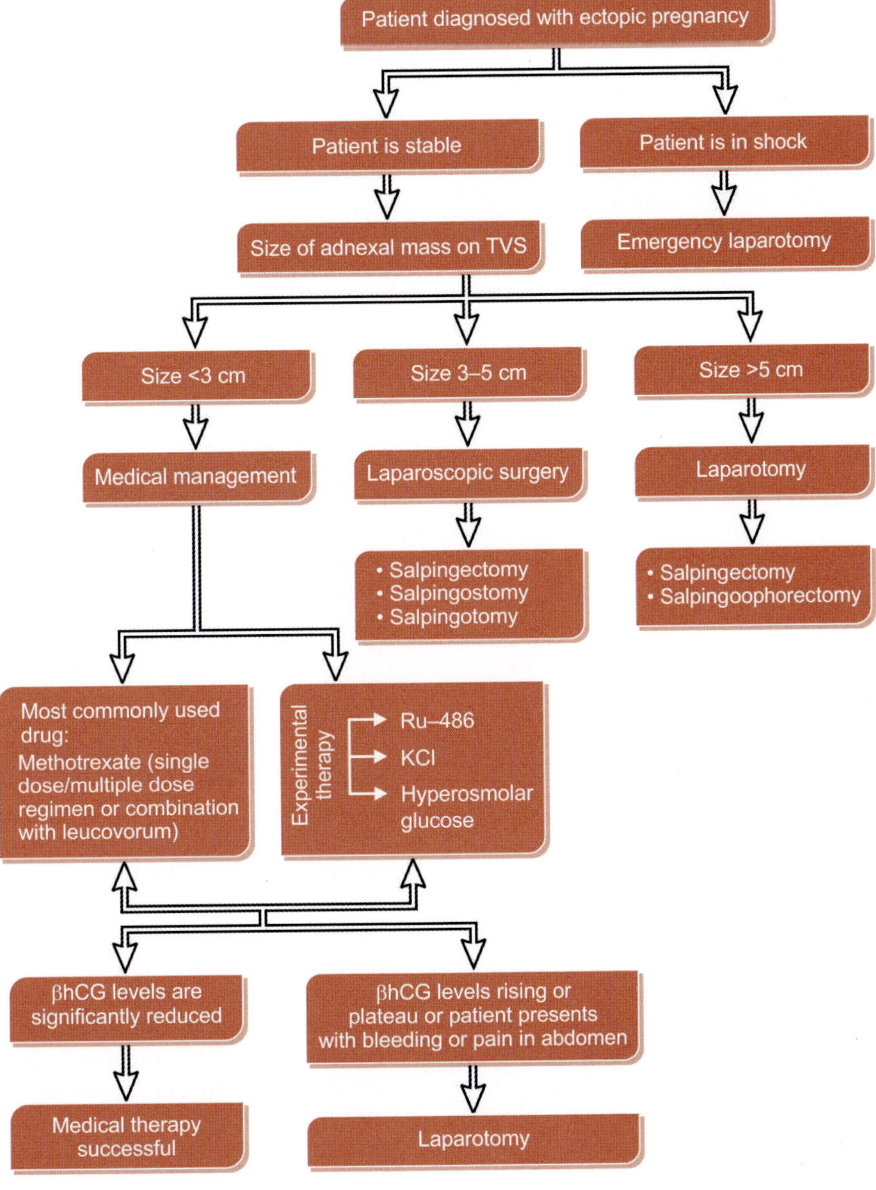


post-treatment; patient has no underlying severe medical condition or disorder and there is no underlying abnormality of liver function tests, kidney function test or full blood count suggestive of liver, renal or bone marrow impairment. In case any of the above-mentioned conditions are fulfilled, the patient may not be suitable for medical therapy. In these cases surgical treatment may be the only option left. Some of the indications for surgical therapy are described in Table 7.9. Surgery could be either in the form of laparoscopy or laparotomy.

## Laparotomy

The indications for laparotomy are summarized in Table 7.10. Laparotomy serves as the treatment of choice in patients who have completed their families or do not desire future fertility, have a history of previous ectopic pregnancy in the same tube or history of severely damaged tubes. The surgical procedure performed during laparotomy is usually sapingectomy, indications for which are described in Table 7.11. Sometimes instead of removal of tubes,

| **Table 7.9:** Indications for surgical therapy |
| --- |
| • Candidate not suitable for medical therapy<br>• Failed medical therapy<br>• Heterotopic pregnancy with a viable intrauterine pregnancy<br>• Patient is hemodynamically unstable and requires immediate treatment |

| **Table 7.10:** Indications for laparotomy |
| --- |
| • Patients are hemodynamically unstable<br>• Cervical, interstitial, cornual or abdominal ectopic pregnancy<br>• Patients having large hematoma due to large ruptured ectopic pregnancy<br>• Presence of more than 1,500 cc hemoperitoneum<br>• Patients with underlying cardiac diseases and chronic obstructive pulmonary diseases<br>• History of abdominal surgery in the past<br>• The surgeon is inexperienced in the laparoscopic techniques<br>• Laparoscopic approach may be difficult due to presence of dense adhesions and massive hemoperitoneum |

| **Table 7.11:** Indications for salpingectomy |
| --- |
| • The tube is severely damaged<br>• There is uncontrolled bleeding<br>• There is a recurrent ectopic pregnancy in the same tube<br>• There is a large tubal pregnancy of size >5 cm<br>• The ectopic pregnancy has ruptured<br>• The woman has completed her family and future fertility is not desired<br>• Ectopic pregnancy has resulted due to sterilization failure<br>• Ectopic pregnancy has occurred in a previously reconstructed tube<br>• Patient requests sterilization<br>• Hemorrhage continues to occur even after salpingotomy<br>• Cases of chronic tubal pregnancy |

| **Table 7.12:** Indications for laparoscopic management of ectopic pregnancy |
| --- |
| • Hemodynamically stable patients<br>• Unruptured ectopic pregnancy<br>• Absence of hemoperitoneum<br>• The ectopic pregnancy is not very small (<3 cm) or very large (>5 cm) in size |

a more conservative tube sparing approach in the form of salpingostomy may be performed.

## Laparoscopy

Laparoscopic management is the conservative surgical approach which is favored nowadays. Laparoscopic surgery is associated with reduced cost, reduced duration of hospital stay and a reduced convalescence period. Some of the indications for laparoscopic removal of ectopic pregnancy are described in Table 7.12.

## SURGERY

### Preoperative Preparation

Whenever the tubal ectopic pregnancy is diagnosed or suspected, the patient should be admitted immediately to the hospital. The further mode of management is based on numerous factors such as hemodynamic stability of the patient, patient's age, desire for future fertility, whether the diagnosed ectopic pregnancy is ruptured or unruptured, size of ectopic, state of contralateral tube (e.g. presence of tubal adhesions or blockage), and location of the pregnancy (i.e. interstitial, ampullary or isthmus). If the patient is in a state of shock, it needs to be treated first. The following steps need to be taken in women who are hemodynamically unstable:

- Immediate resuscitation.
- Immediate IV access must be secured by inserting large bore venous cannula.
- Blood should be sent for full blood count and cross matching and at least four units of blood must be arranged.
- The theater staff; anesthetist and on-call gynecology consultant must be immediately informed.
- Foley's catheter must be inserted prior to starting the procedure.
- Transfusion with blood, plasma or substitutes needs to be arranged as soon as possible.
- Immediate laparotomy and clamping of the bleeding vessels may be the only way of saving the life of a moribund patient.
- If in shock, resuscitation and surgery at the same time can be lifesaving. The urgency of the situation must be stressed to all concerned. The surgery must not be delayed and should be performed even before blood and fluid losses have been replaced. Irrespective of the type of surgery performed, whether salpingectomy or salpingotomy, via laparoscopy or laparotomy, the steps of preoperative preparation remain the same.
- Before deciding the treatment option in a woman with ectopic pregnancy, she and her partner must be fully involved in deciding the relevant management plan. They must be provided with the written information regarding the various treatment options and carefully explained about the advantages and disadvantages associated with each approach. The couple must be counseled about the likelihood of requirement for laparotomy or even hysterectomy with salpingectomy in case of uncontrollable bleeding or other unexpected surgical findings.

## Actual Procedure

### Salpingectomy

Salpingectomy involves removal of the ectopic pregnancy along with the Fallopian tube of the affected side. Salpingectomy may be done in cases of uncontrollable bleeding, tubal destruction, recurrent ectopic pregnancy, severe adhesions or presence of hydrosalpinx. The procedure of salpingectomy involves the following steps:

- The portion of tube between the uterus and the ectopic pregnancy is clamped and electrocoagulated. The pedicle is then cut and ligated.
- Progressive coagulation and cutting of the mesosalpinx can begin either at the proximal end or at the fimbrial end of the tube.
- The tubo-ovarian artery is also clamped, cut and ligated, while preserving the utero-ovarian artery and ligament.
- The mesosalpinx must be continued to be clamped, cut and ligated until the tube is free and can be removed.

### Partial Salpingectomy

Partial salpingectomy may be sometimes performed instead of complete salpingectomy if the pregnancy is in the midportion of the tube; none of the indications for salpingectomy are present, and the patient appears to be a candidate for tubal reanastomosis in future. In these cases, a clamp is placed through an avascular area in the mesosalpinx under the ectopic pregnancy.

This creates spaces through which two free ties are placed, which are tied around the tube on each side of the ectopic pregnancy. The isolated portion of the tube containing the ectopic pregnancy is then cut and removed.

### Salpingotomy

Tube-sparing salpingostomy or salpingotomy is a procedure in which the gestational sac is removed, without the removal of tube, through a 1 cm long incision on the tubal wall.

This surgery is preferred over salpingectomy because not only is salpingotomy less invasive, but is also associated with comparable rates of subsequent fertility and ectopic pregnancy. Laparoscopic salpingotomy should especially be considered as the primary modality of treatment if the woman has contralateral tube disease and desires future fertility. When salpingotomy is used for the management of tubal pregnancy, follow-up protocols (weekly serum hCG levels) are necessary for the identification and treatment of women with persistent trophoblastic disease. The steps of surgery are as follows:

- The mesosalpinx slightly inferior to the pregnancy and the antimesenteric surface of the tubal segment containing the pregnancy is infiltrated using a laparoscopic needle with 5–7 mL vasopressin (20 IU in 150 mL NS).

- A 1–2 cm incision is made on the antimesenteric side of the tube using laser scissors or a microelectrode. As the incision is given, the pregnancy begins to extrude out. This can be completed using hydrodissection or gentle traction with the forceps. A syringe filled with saline is inserted deep into the incision and the fluid is injected forcefully in such a way so as to dislodge the ectopic pregnancy and clots. The contents of ectopic pregnancy and clots are aspirated out.
- Following this, the bed of the ectopic pregnancy must be irrigated well. In case some trophoblastic tissue remains, the prior injection of vasopressin may lead to anoxia and death of the trophoblasts, preventing postoperative growth.
- Coagulation may occasionally be required for hemostasis. Oozing from the implantation site usually stops on its own.
- The incision on the Fallopian tube is left to heal by secondary intention. If the opening on the tube appears to be too large, it can be brought together using 4-0 absorbable sutures. In case the pregnancy is in the distal ampullary portion of the tube, it can be grasped with the help of forceps and the pregnancy can then be pulled out of the tubal fimbriae.

## Laparoscopic Surgery

*Laparoscopic salpingectomy:* Laparoscopic salpingectomy involves the use of bipolar cautery for desiccation of tube. The rest of the procedure is same as that performed during laparotomy. Products of conception can be removed from the abdomen using a 10 mm trocar port.

*Tube-sparing salpingotomy:* The procedure of laparoscopic salpingotomy (Figs 7.12A and B) is same as that described with laparotomy before.

## Postoperative Care

The postoperative care comprises of the following steps:
- *Weekly measurement of hCG levels:* Regular follow-up must be done following surgery in order to ensure that the patient's hCG levels have returned to zero. This may take several weeks. Although, the hCG levels come back to normal in 2–3 weeks' time, the period of observation must last for up to 6 weeks. Elevated hCG levels could mean that some ectopic trophoblastic tissue which was missed at the time of removal is still remaining inside.
- The patient must be instructed to visit the clinician after 1 week for removal of sutures.
- The patient must be counseled that she may experience mild bleeding or pain during the first postoperative week. In case of mild pain, she can use simple analgesic drugs available over the counter. In case of pain or bleeding of

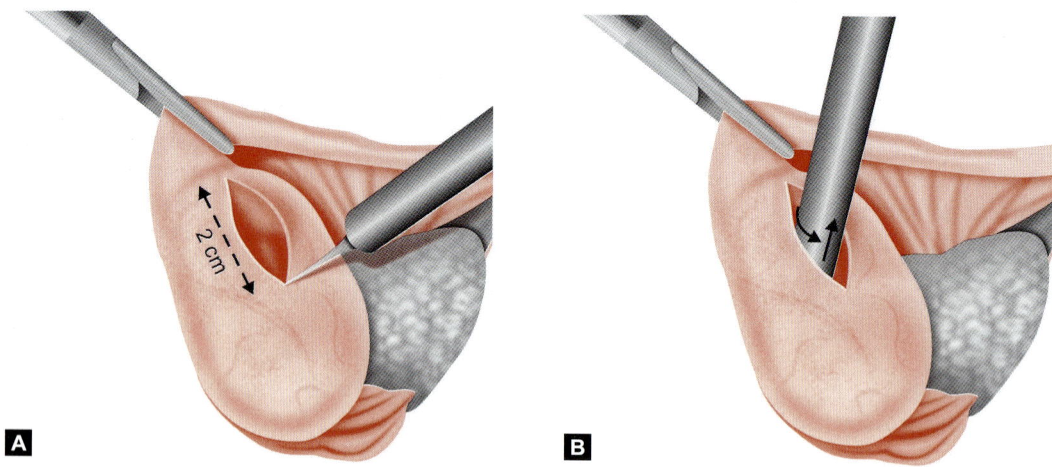

**Figs 7.12A and B:** Tube spacing salpingotomy: (A) A small incision given over the tubal ectopic; (B) Suction of the trophoblast tissue of the unruptured ectopic pregnancy

| **Table 7.13:** Advantages of laparoscopic surgery |
| --- |
| • Reduced amount of postoperative pain<br>• Faster recovery<br>• Shorter duration of hospital stay<br>• Lower rate of postoperative complications such as wound infection<br>• Cost-effectiveness<br>• Reduced postoperative analgesic requirement<br>• Reduced adhesion formation |

| **Table 7.14:** Complications due to laparoscopic surgery |
| --- |
| • Missed diagnosis<br>• Bleeding<br>• Incomplete removal of ectopic pregnancy<br>• Visceral injury<br>• Leakage of purulent exudates<br>• Intra-abdominal abscess<br>• Hernia |

severe intensity, she must be instructed to report to the clinician immediately.

## Benefits of Laparoscopic Management of Tubal Pregnancy

Laparoscopic management is a useful method for reducing hospital stay, complications and return to normal activity. The main advantages of laparoscopic surgery are enumerated in Table 7.13.

## Laparotomy

There are times when laparotomy is favored over the laparoscopic approach and the surgeon needs to perform laparotomy instead of laparoscopy.

## Complications

In the past few decades, ruptured ectopic pregnancy was amongst one of the leading causes of maternal mortality. With the improvement in imaging and minimal invasive procedures in cases of ectopic pregnancy, the mortality rate has considerably reduced. Nowadays, the trend is towards the use of minimal invasive surgery in cases of ectopic pregnancy.

Although, operative laparoscopy is associated with its own inherent complications, in experienced hands there are usually minimal complications related to the laparoscopic procedure. However, if the surgeon is not trained enough in laparoscopy then the chance of complications as described in Table 7.14 is there. In experienced hands, the chances of these complications are extremely rare. Altogether, laparoscopic procedure has a much lower complication rate in comparison to the conventional surgery.

# Destructive Procedures

## Introduction

In modern obstetrics, there is hardly any place for destructive obstetric procedures. Currently, these surgeries are almost never practiced in the developed countries. These may rarely be employed in settings with low resources, for example cases of obstructed/neglected labor in settings where there are no facilities for cesarean delivery. The aim of destructive operations is to reduce the fetal bulk, e.g. size of fetal head, shoulders or fetal body, thereby allowing its passage through the maternal pelvis. Some such destructive surgeries include:
• Craniotomy (perforation of the cranium).
• Cranioclasm (crushing of the brainstem).

- Cephalotripsy (crushing of the whole head including the base of skull).
- Decapitation (severing of the fetal head from trunk, following which the trunk is extracted first and then the head).
- Evisceration (incision of the abdomen and/or the thorax to evacuate its viscera to reduce its size, thereby allowing its vaginal delivery).
- Spondylotomy (division of the vertebral column).
- Cleidotomy (surgical division of one or both the clavicles with embryotomy scissors so as to reduce the bisacromial diameter).

## Indications

*Craniotomy:* Indications for craniotomy are as follows:
- Obstructed labor with vertex or face presentation and the fetus is dead.
- Hydrocephalus.
- Cephalopelvic disproportion with a dead fetus.
- Retained after-coming head of the breech (obstructed labor).
- Impacted head (malpresentations like mentoposterior, brow presentation or occipitoposterior positions).
- Interlocked head of the twin.
- Contracted pelvis.

*Decapitation:* Indications for decapitation are as follows:
- Selected cases of neglected impacted shoulder presentation: When the baby is dead and the obstetrician can reach the top of neck.
- Conjoined twins.
- Rare cases of locked twins.

*Evisceration and spondylotomy:* Indications for evisceration and spondylotomy are as follows:
- Transverse presentation of the fetus: If chest wall or the abdomen presents, evisceration may be required to reduce the fetal bulk. If the back presents, spondylotomy may be required.
- Dystocia due to the fetal malformations (e.g. fetal ascites, huge distended bladder, fetal tumors located in the fetal chest or abdomen, hydronephrosis, etc.).

*Cleidotomy:* Indications for cleidotomy are as follows:
- Large fetus with a shoulder dystocia.
- In conjunction with other embryotomy procedures (e.g. decapitation) to affect delivery of a dead baby which may be disproportionately large for maternal pelvis.

## SURGERY

## Preoperative Preparation

The following steps must be observed prior to the various destructive procedures:

- All the above-mentioned destructive procedures are performed under general anesthesia.
- Patient is placed in lithotomy position.
- Complete surgical asepsis must be maintained.
- Bladder must be catheterized prior to the procedure in order to empty it.
- Vaginal examination must be done prior to the procedure to ensure that the cervix is almost completely dilated (at least 7 cm).
- True conjugate must be more than 5 cm in case of craniotomy and cranioclasm.
- Patient should be experiencing uterine contractions.

## Steps of Surgery

### Craniotomy

The procedure of craniotomy is illustrated in Figures 7.13A to C and is described below:
- Simpson's/Oldham's perforator is used for the purpose of craniotomy. It is a long straight instrument with two triangular blades, long shanks, handles and two locks and has been described in details in Chapter 13.
- A careful per vaginal examination is performed to determine the site of perforation.
- Sites of perforation: Perforation can be performed at the following sites:
  - Vertex: Either parietal bone as close to the sagittal suture and anterior fontanel as possible (sutures are avoided to prevent collapse of the brain, thereby preventing the escape of brain tissue).
  - Face: Orbit.
  - Brow: Nasion or glabella.
  - After coming head of the breech: hard palate or posterolateral fontanel.
- Assistant steadies the fetal head per abdominally.
- Under the assistance of index finger and the middle finger of the left hand, the instrument is carefully inserted through the vagina up to the site of perforation and is applied perpendicular to it.
- Once the site of perforation has been identified, scratch marks are made on the skull so as to produce a groove where the blade can be fixed prior to the perforation to help prevent slipping and injury to the soft tissues.
- The skull is perforated by giving a thrust at right angle to the surface of skull.
- After piercing up to the shoulder gaurd of the blade, the blades are unlocked and separated by compressing them.
- The blades are again locked and their handle turned through 90°, following which they are again unlocked and separated in order to make a cruciate incision in the skull. Following this, the brain is churned.
- The closed instrument is then removed under the protection of fingers.

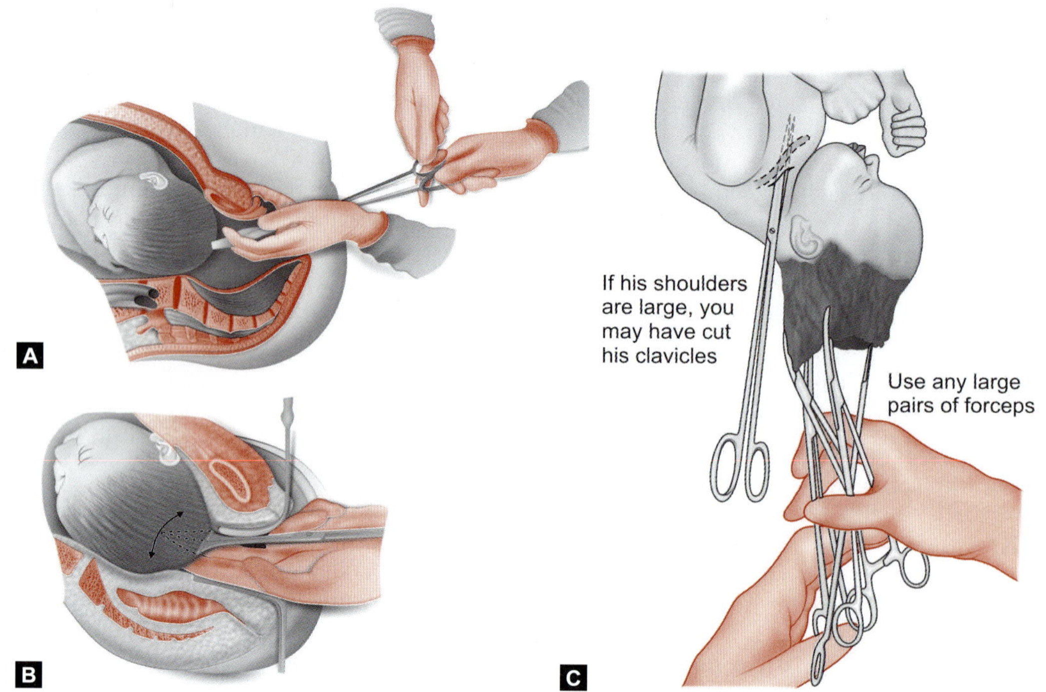



**Figs 7.13A to C:**  The process of craniotomy: (A) Introduction of the Oldham's perforator; (B) Perforation of the skull; (C) Removal of cranial contents and extraction of the collapsed skull

- Brain matter is then flushed out with the help of a blunt flushing curette.
- The projecting bone spicules are removed at the end of the procedure.
- Methods of extraction of head: The head can be then extracted through the various techniques, spontaneously, using the cranioclast or using together the cranioclast with cephalotribe, or use of the obstetric forceps.

## Cranioclasm

The instruments used for the procedure include a cranioclast or a cephalotribe or a combination of both cephalotribe and cranioclast. The cranioclast has one central perforating blade and one bone crushing blade. Cephalotribe on the other hand has only two crushing blades with no perforating blade. A combined cranioclast with a cephalotribe has three blades: one central perforating blade and two crushing blades on the either side. These instruments have been described in details in Chapter 13. The procedure involves following steps:

- The central perforating blade is introduced into the craniotomy hole with its serrated convex border towards the face.
- The first crushing blade, which goes towards the face, is introduced next. Firstly the face is crushed. This flexes the head which helps in crushing the base.

- The third blade is then introduced up to the occiput and the entire base then crushed.
- Before extraction, the instrument is rotated through 90° so that all the three blades lie in the anteroposterior diameter of the inlet.
- Extraction is performed as described previously.

## Decapitation

A decapitation hook (with knife or saw) or Blond Heidler's thimble and decapitating wire are used for the procedure (Figs 7.14A to D) which involves the following steps:

- If the hand is not prolapsed, it should be brought out for traction purposes.
- Under protection of the palm of left hand, the decapitation knife is introduced and brought in contact with the back of the fetal neck.
- Once the knob of the knife has gone beyond the neck, the handle is rotated in such a way that the blade comes to lie across the neck, front to back.
- A saw cutting motion of the knife helps in severing the neck.
- Once the head has been separated from the rest of the body, delivery of the baby is facilitated by applying traction on the prolapsed arm using a blunt hook.
- Alternatively, the operator hooks his fingers in the axilla to pull down the baby.

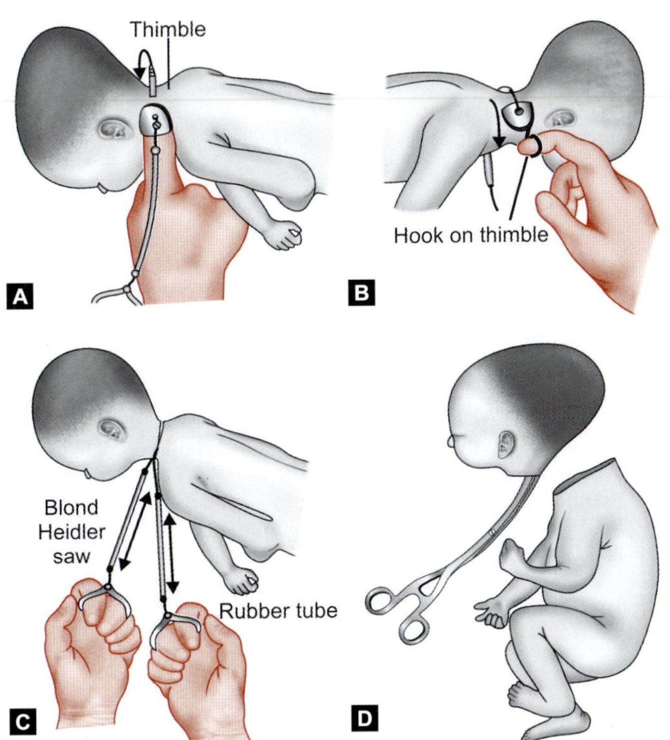



**Figs 7.14A to D:** Decapitation of the fetal head. (A) Pushing the thimble around the baby's neck; (B) Pulling the loop of the thimble down the other side of the neck; (C) Sawing motion to severe the baby's neck; (D) Removal of the cut head with forceps

- The severed head can be then delivered by traction (applied by putting two fingers in the mouth) or using a cranioclast with a cephalotribe. Traction can also be applied with the help of Willet's scalp forceps, etc.

## Spondylotomy

Spondylotomy is usually done with the help of an embryotomy scissors, which is a pair of long stout scissors.

- The closed blades of the evisceration scissors are introduced under the protection of two fingers of the other hand.
- The chest or the abdomen is opened by cutting the skin or the rib cage and the contents are then removed piecemeal.
- After this an attempt must be made to bring down the pelvis or the breech by hooking the fingers over lumbar vertebrae.
- After spondylotomy, spine can be pulled down by applying traction over the crochet. The fetus is usually delivered in two halves: one half is delivered by applying traction on the arm and on the other half, the traction is applied on the leg to deliver the other half.

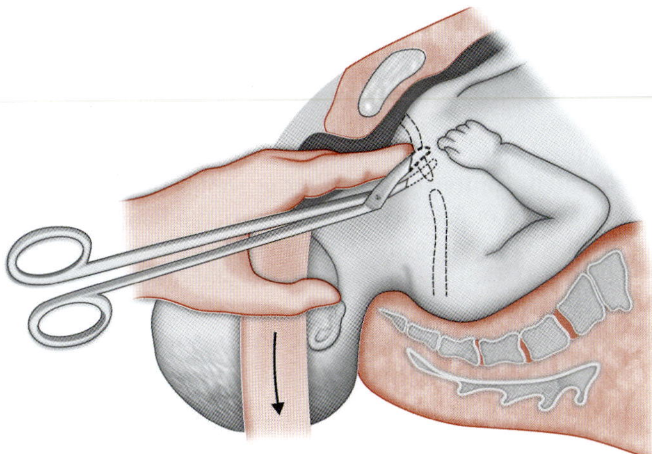

**Fig. 7.15:** Cleidotomy

## Cleidotomy

Cleidotomy (Fig. 7.15) involves the following steps:

- Division of the posterior clavicle is preferred first, because it is easier to reach the posterior shoulder as more room is afforded in the sacral hollow. Bilateral cleidotomy is rarely required.
- Embryotomy scissors are first introduced along the left wrist and hand (with extended index finger and middle finger) up to the posterior clavicle.
- Skin over the clavicle is cut first.
- Tip of the scissors is then introduced through the rent in the skin and the clavicle is cut.

## Postoperative Care

The following steps must be observed following surgery in these patients:

- Routine exploration of the uterovaginal canal must be done to exclude various injuries of the genital tract and adjacent viscera (e.g. rupture of the uterus, injuries to vagina/vulva/cervix, urethra/bladder and the adjacent tissues).
- Bladder is catheterized for a period of 3–5 days or until bladder tone is regained.
- Intravenous infusion of dextrose saline is continued until dehydration is corrected.
- Blood transfusion may be required in case the patient is in hemorrhagic shock.
- Antibiotics are to be prescribed (e.g. IV ceftriaxone infusion may be given twice daily).
- A proper per vaginal examination is done following the cranioclasm to look for any bony spicule. If present, they can be removed the help of a bone nibbler.

## Contraindications

- Severe infections
- Impending rupture of the uterus (laparotomy would be required in these cases).
- Scarred uterus.
- Severely contracted pelvis (true conjugate is less than 2.5 inches or 5.5 cm): In these cases the baby cannot be delivered because the bimastoid diameter of the skull (7.5 cm) cannot be compressed (for craniotomy and cranioclasm).
- Severely contracted pelvis with anteroposterior diameter of the inlet less than 5.5 cm.

## Complications

- Maternal traumatic injuries to the birth canal.
- Injury to the adjacent organs [e.g. uterus, cervix, vagina, bladder, rectum, resulting in the development of VVF (vesicovaginal fistula), RVF (rectovaginal fistula), UVF (urethrovaginal fistula), etc.].

- Rupture uterus.
- Postpartum hemorrhage.
- Shock (hemorrhagic, neurogenic).
- Puerperal sepsis.
- Maternal death.

## FURTHER READINGS


1. American College of Obstetricians and Gynecologists. ACOG Practice Bulletin No. 94: Medical management of ectopic pregnancy. Obstet Gynecol. 2008;111(6):1479-85.
2. Fernando RJ, Sultan AH, Kettle C, et al. Methods of repair for obstetric anal sphincter injury. Cochrane Database Syst Rev. 2006;3:CD002866.
3. Grimes DA. Management of abortion in TeLinde's Operative Gynecology, 9th edition. Philadelphia: Lippincot Williams & Wilkins; 1997. p. 8.
4. Practice Committee of the American Society for Reproductive Medicine. Medical treatment of ectopic pregnancy. Fertil Steril. 2006;86(Suppl 1):S96.
5. The Medical Termination of Pregnancy Act, 1971 (Act No 34 of 1971, 10th August 1971).

# SECTION 2

# Gynecology

# History Taking and Examination in Gynecology



## Introduction

The subject of gynecology pertains to the diseases of female genital organs. Some gynecological problems commonly encountered in clinical practice include abnormal menstrual bleeding, abdominal masses, gynecological cancers, pelvic pain, infertility, etc. For being able to diagnose the abnormal gynecological complaints, it is important for the clinician to be able to perform a normal gynecological examination. Since taking an adequate history and performing a complete pelvic examination is of utmost importance for detection of underlying pathology, this would be discussed in detail in this chapter.

## History and Clinical Presentation

The history must be taken in a nonjudgmental, sensitive and thorough manner. Importance must be given towards maintenance of patient-physician relationship. It is important for the clinician to maintain good communication with the patient in order to elicit proper history and to be accurately able to recognize her problems. The manner of speaking, the words used, the tone of speaking and the body language are important aspects of the patient-physician interaction. Kindness and courtesy must be maintained at all times. These aspects are especially important in case of male clinicians because the gynecological history entails asking some private and confidential questions from the female patients. Also, the woman may be reluctant while telling the history regarding her menstrual cycles to the male doctor. It is important for a male doctor to take history and perform vaginal examination in presence of a third party or a chaperone (a female nurse or the patient's female relative or friend). A chaperone must also be present while a female doctor is performing the clinical examination.

The clinician must begin taking the history, starting with open-ended questions to help alleviate the woman's anxiety. The woman should be encouraged to describe the problems in her own wordings. The doctor must attentively listen to the woman's history without making frequent interruptions.

The clinician must adopt both an empathetic and inquisitive attitude towards the patient. The patient's privacy must be respected at all costs. The clinician must refrain from asking personal questions until appropriate patient confidence has been established. The clinician needs to listen more and talk less while taking the patient's history. The clinician must avoid interrupting, commanding and lecturing while taking history. If any serious condition (e.g. malignancy) is suspected, the diagnosis must not be disclosed to the patient until it has been confirmed by performing investigations. Bad news must be preferably told to the patient when she is being accompanied by someone (relative, friend or spouse). The seriousness and urgency of the situation must be explained to the patient without causing undue alarm and fright to the patient. The clinician must never give false reassurance to the patient. Honest advice and opinion must always be provided.

Following the completion of examination, the patient must be informed about the likely gynecological diagnosis. Various available treatment options along with their associated advantages and disadvantages must be discussed with the patient to enable her make a right decision. The patient must be respected as an individual and the physician's opinion must not be forced upon her.

### History of Presenting Complaints

The patient must be asked to describe her complaints in her own wordings in the order of their chronological appearance. Asking the age of the patient is especially important. Risk factors related to a particular pathology in question (e.g.

postmenopausal bleeding) need to be asked. Some common gynecological problems with which the patient may present are described below.

### Abnormal Menstrual Bleeding

In cases of abnormal uterine bleeding (AUB), the clinician needs to ask questions to determine the pattern of bleeding: amount of bleeding; the time of bleeding (the days in the menstrual cycle during which the bleeding occurs); intermenstrual intervals (between the episodes of bleeding) and cycle regularity (whether the bleeding pattern is regular or irregular).

*Amount of bleeding:* Initially, the clinician needs to establish whether the woman is having heavy, light or moderate amount of blood loss.

Estimating the quantity of blood loss is a very subjective issue when considering vaginal bleeding. Accurate assessment of the menstrual blood loss may not be possible. Some questions which the clinician can ask in order to assess the amount of blood loss have been described in Chapter 9.

### Abdominal Pain

Pain in the abdomen is one of the most common clinical complaints in medical practice. Besides gastrointestinal pathology, underlying gynecological pathology is also a common cause of pain per abdomen. Gynecological problems like pelvic tuberculosis, pelvic inflammatory disease (PID) and endometriosis may be commonly associated with chronic pain. Acute lower abdominal pain may occur in association with gynecological abnormalities like ectopic pregnancy, torsion or rupture of an ovarian cyst and chocolate cyst. The following points need to be asked while taking history of pain:

*Exact site of pain:* Pain of ovarian or tubal origin is usually felt in the lower abdomen, above the inguinal ligament. Pain of uterine origin is diffusely present in the hypogastric region.

*Radiation of pain:* Pain of uterine origin is often referred to the inner aspect of the thighs, but does not usually extend beyond the knees. Pain due to appendicitis may initially start in the right iliac region and later radiate to the umbilicus.

*Nature of pain:* The nature of the pain, whether burning, gnawing, throbbing, aching or excruciating in nature, needs to be determined.

*Intensity of pain:* The degree of severity of pain, whether mild, moderate or severe needs to be determined. Pain of severe intensity may interfere with sleep and work.

*Aggravating and relieving factors for pain:* The history of various relieving and aggravating factors for pain must be taken.

*Relationship of other factors with pain:* Relationship of pain to other factors such as menstruation (dysmenorrhea), coital activity (dyspareunia), micturition (dysuria), defecation (dyschezia), posture and movement needs to be determined.

Dysmenorrhea or pain associated with menstruation can be of two types: spasmodic and congestive dysmenorrhea. Spasmodic dysmenorrhea usually has no cause and is seen on day 1 or 2 of menstruation. On the other hand, pain due to congestive dysmenorrhea is usually due to some underlying pathology (endometriosis, PID, etc.). This pain may be premenstrual, menstrual or postmenstrual in origin.

### Abdominal Lump

Questions which need to be asked at the time of eliciting the history in case of a lump in the abdomen are as follows:
- Time period since which the lump has been present.
- Has the lump been increasing in size or has it remained static?
- Is there any associated pain? Normally, the benign tumors cause no abdominal pain and are comfortably placed in the abdominal cavity which is distensible. Large intra-abdominal tumors, on the other hand, may cause abdominal discomfort and difficulty in walking. Acute abdominal pain may develop if the ovarian tumor undergoes torsion, rupture or hemorrhage.
- Is there presence of any pressure symptoms such as increased urinary urgency and frequency, constipation, etc.?

### Infertility/Amenorrhea

For taking detailed history regarding infertility and amenorrhea, kindly refer to Chapter 9.

### Hirsutism

Hirsutism refers to increased or excessive growth of hair in women. This is usually related to increased androgen production in the body.

### Urinary Problems and Sexual Dysfunction

Women may often present to the gynecology clinic with the main complaints of urinary problems, such as urinary incontinence (stress or urge incontinence), dysuria (related to urinary tract infection, etc.), voiding difficulties (due to pelvic prolapse, etc.), or sexual dysfunction (e.g. low sexual desire, reduced libido, sexual arousal disorders, orgasmic disorders, sexual pain disorders, vaginismus, etc.). Detailed history related to these complaints needs to be elicited.

*Vaginal Discharge*

History suggestive of pelvic, vaginal, or vulvar infections, e.g. vaginal discharge, vulvar or vaginal lesions, fever, pelvic pain, abnormal bleeding of the genital tract, previous history of having sexually transmitted infections or PID also needs to be asked.

*Pelvic Organ Prolapse*

For detailed information related to history and clinical presentation in cases of pelvic organ prolapse, kindly refer to Chapter 9.

## Past Medical History

Past history of medical illnesses, such as hypertension, hepatitis, diabetes mellitus, cancer, heart disease, pulmonary disease and thyroid disease needs to be taken. Patient's previous medical and surgical problems may have a bearing on her present complaints. For example, a history of longstanding diabetes could be responsible for development of genital candidiasis and associated pruritus. A patient with previous medical history of severe anemia or cardiovascular heart disease may require special anesthetic preparation (e.g. correction of anemia, or treatment of cardiovascular pathology) before undergoing a major gynecological surgery (e.g. hysterectomy).

Triad of diabetes, hypertension and obesity is associated with an increased risk of endometrial carcinoma. A history of sexually transmitted disease (especially infection with *Chlamydia*) may have a direct bearing on future infertility. Previous history of PID or puerperal sepsis could be responsible for producing gynecological complaints like menstrual disturbances, lower abdominal pain, congestive dysmenorrhea and infertility. Presence of endocrinological disorders (e.g. thyroid dysfunction) could be responsible for producing menstrual irregularities.

*History of Previous Surgery*

The patient should be asked about any surgery she has undergone in the past. The reason for undergoing surgery, particularly of abdominal or pelvic origin, type of incision (laparoscopy or laparotomy) and any history of postoperative complications needs to be enquired. History of undergoing previous abdominal surgery like cesarean section, removal of appendix, excision of ovarian cyst, myomectomy, etc. may be associated with the development of pelvic adhesions. These may not only make any subsequent surgery difficult, but also may be the cause of common gynecological problems like pelvic and abdominal pain, infertility, menstrual disturbances and dyspareunia.

*Past Medication History*

In the medication history, the patient should be asked about the various medicines she has been consuming. The details of various medicines including their dosage, route of administration, frequency and duration of use needs to be asked. The patient must be specifically asked about the various medicines she has been taking including prescription drugs, OTC drugs, herbal drugs and any therapy related to alternative medicine. History of allergy to any medication also needs to be asked.

## Family History

Certain gynecological cancers (e.g. cancer ovary, uterus and breast) have a genetic predisposition. A woman may be at a high risk of development of such cancers in the future if there is a positive family history of such cancers in her first degree relatives (especially mother and sister). Menstrual patterns, including age of menarche, frequency and regularity of cycle, associated dysmenorrhea and age of attaining menopause tend to be similar amongst the family members. The common gynecological problems like premature menopause, menorrhagia and premenstrual tension have been observed to run within families. Other medical disorders, like thyroid dysfunction, allergic diathesis and coagulation disorders, which may be responsible for development of gynecological complaints, are also often familial in nature.

## Marital and Sexual History

Details of the woman's marital life including her age at the time of marriage, how long she has been married and sexual history needs to be asked. Details of the woman's sexual history are particularly important. Some such details include her age at the time of first sexual intercourse; her current sexual activities (vaginal, oral, anal and manual); frequency of her sexual intercourses; is she currently seeking a pregnancy; is she presently using any method of contraception, if yes, the type of contraception used; is she or her partner experiencing any sexual dysfunction (frigidity in the woman or impotence or premature ejaculation in the male or problems with libido, arousal, lubrication or orgasm in both males and females); current frequency of her sexual activities, past sexual activities, number of sexual partners (currently and in the past), sexual preferences (heterosexual, homosexual or both), pain at the time of sexual intercourse (dyspareunia), etc. History regarding the use of any contraception (both in the past and present) needs to be asked. History related to sexual abuse also needs to be elicited.

## Obstetric History

Details of every pregnancy conceived irrespective of their ultimate outcome needs to be recorded. Number of previous live births, stillbirths, deaths, miscarriages (both spontaneous and induced), history of recurrent miscarriages, if any, medical termination of pregnancies and number of children living at present need to be noted. The ages of the youngest and eldest children also need to be enquired. The mode of delivery of each baby (normal vaginal delivery or cesarean section) and details of any obstetric complications encountered, e.g. puerperal or postabortal sepsis, postpartum hemorrhage, obstetrical interventions (use of forceps, vacuum, etc.) and other obstetric or gynecological complications (soft tissue injuries such as cervical tears, an incompetent cervical os, genital fistulae, complete perineal tear, genital prolapse, stress urinary incontinence) and chronic backache also needs to be enquired from the patient.

### Previous Gynecological History

History of other gynecologic problems in the past, such as previous history of ovarian cysts, uterine fibroids, infertility, endometriosis, polycystic ovarian syndrome, pelvic organ prolapse, urinary or anal incontinence, etc. needs to be asked. She also needs to be enquired if any treatment for these problems was instituted in the past. History of undergoing some gynecologic procedure (e.g. endometrial biopsy, laparoscopy, hysterectomy, etc.) in the past must be asked. Screening for intimate partner violence also needs to be done.

*Screening for Gynecological Malignancy*

History of screening tests done for screening gynecological malignancy, especially Pap test needs to be asked. History related to the date and results of the last test; diagnosis and follow-up of abnormal Pap smears must also be taken. For details related to screening for cervical pathology, kindly refer to Chapter 10.

### Menstrual History

The menstrual history needs to be taken in detail. The following details need to be recorded: age of menarche, date of last menstrual period, cycle length, whether regular or irregular, number of days the bleeding takes place, amount of bleeding (in terms of pads soaked), and presence of any associated symptoms, such as cramps, bloating or headache. Detailed menstrual history which needs to be asked in cases of AUB has been described in chapter 9.

# General Physical Examination

General physical examination involves the observation of the patient's general appearance, orientation in time, place and person, nutritional status and patient's demeanor (calm, anxious, or aggressive). The following features need to be observed at the time of general physical examination.

### Vital Signs

Patient's vital signs such as temperature, blood pressure, pulse, respiratory rate, height and weight need to be taken.

### Height and Weight

Height of the patient (in meters) and her weight (in pounds) can be used for calculation of BMI, which helps in categorizing woman as underweight, normal weight and obese. Calculation of BMI is especially important in women who appear underweight or overweight. Underweight women may commonly suffer from amenorrhea and other menstrual irregularities, whereas overweight women are at an increased risk for endometrial cancer.

### Anemia

Excessive blood loss may result in the development of anemia. Detailed clinical examination related to anemia has been described in Chapter 5.

### Signs Suggestive of Hyperandrogenemia

Signs suggestive of hyperandrogenemia such as hirsutism (presence of facial hair), deepening of voice, etc. may be related to the presence of androgen-secreting tumors or chronic anovulatory states (polycystic ovarian disease).

### Blood Pressure

Blood pressure that is persistently greater than or equal to 140 mm Hg (systolic) or greater than or equal to 90 mm Hg (diastolic) is considered as elevated. Patients with hypertension are at an increased risk for the development of endometrial cancer.

### Neck Examination

Local examination of the neck may reveal enlargement of thyroid gland or lymph nodes of the neck. Neck examination should also involve palpation of cervical and supraclavicular lymph nodes.

### Lymphadenopathy

Lymphadenopathy could be a sign of advanced metastatic disease associated with malignancy. The patient's neck, axilla and groins must also be palpated for the presence of enlarged lymph nodes.

### Thyroid Examination

It is important to examine the thyroid gland because menstrual abnormalities may be commonly associated with thyroid dysfunction. While hypothyroidism is commonly associated with oligomenorrhea, hyperthyroidism may be responsible for producing menorrhagia. Various signs and symptoms associated with hypothyroidism and hyperthyroidism are described in Chapter 5.

## Breast Examination

Examination of both the breasts should be carried out in three positions: with patient's hands on her hips (to accentuate the pectoral muscles), with her arms raised and then in supine position. Both the breasts must be inspected for symmetry, skin or nipple retraction, presence of any obvious growth or mass and skin changes such as dimpling, retraction, crusting or peau d'orange appearance. Both the breasts must be then palpated bilaterally for the presence of lumps, masses and tenderness. The nipples are assessed for presence of discharge. Axillary and supraclavicular regions are palpated for presence of any lymphadenopathy. The following points need to be particularly observed on examination of breasts:

- Breast examination may reveal changes indicative of early pregnancy. This is especially important in cases, where pregnancy is not suspected, e.g. in young unmarried girls.
- Staging of breast development: This could be important in women who have yet not attained sexual maturity. Tanner stages of breast development have been described in Chapter 9.
- In all women and especially those over the age of 30 years, breasts must be routinely palpated to exclude tumor formation.
- Bilateral milk discharge from the nipples may indicate galactorrhea due to hyperprolactinemia. Ruling out the presence of galactorrhea is especially important in cases that are infertile and suffer from oligomenorrhea or amenorrhea.
- Unilateral bloody nipple discharge could be associated with an intraductal papilloma.

## Examination of Back and Spine

Back must be assessed for symmetry, tenderness or masses. Flanks must be assessed for pain on percussion as it could be indicative of renal disease.

# Specific Systemic Examination

## ABDOMINAL EXAMINATION

### Inspection

The patient must be advised to breathe normally and relax. The examiner must stand on the right side of the patient. The following points need to be noted on inspection of the abdomen:

- *Abdominal shape:* The clinician must note for abdominal shape, whether symmetrical or asymmetrical.

- *Umbilical eversion or inversion:* In normal women, umbilicus is usually inverted (sunken) even if abdomen is distended due to obesity. Umbilical eversion can occur as a result of increased intra-abdominal pressure in conditions such as pregnancy, ascites, intra-abdominal tumors, etc.
- *Abdominal enlargement:* The specific region of abdominal distention (ascites, intra-abdominal lump) needs to be noted. The different abdominal quadrants are shown in Figure 8.1.
- *Organomegaly:* Very large spleen or liver arising from left or right hypochondriac regions respectively can be identified on abdominal inspection. Gross enlargement of the liver may produce a bulge in the right upper quadrant; whereas gross enlargement of the spleen may be seen as a bulge in the left upper quadrant.
- *Presence of dilated veins and varicosities:* Presence of prominent veins over the abdomen is abnormal and may be due to inferior cava obstruction or portal hypertension.
- *The mobility of abdominal wall with breathing:* If the abdominal mass moves up and down while breathing, it is likely to be intra-abdominal in origin. In case of a pelvic mass, the movements of the lower abdominal wall may be restricted.
- *Presence of striae or scar marks over the abdomen:* Abdominal striae (stripes over the abdomen) may be often present in parous women. Presence of striae could be indicative of previous pregnancies in the past or recent weight loss. Scars over the abdomen may indicate previous surgical operations and deserve further enquiry.
- *Signs of intraperitoneal and retroperitoneal hemorrhage:* The following signs are indicative of intraperitoneal and retroperitoneal hemorrhage:

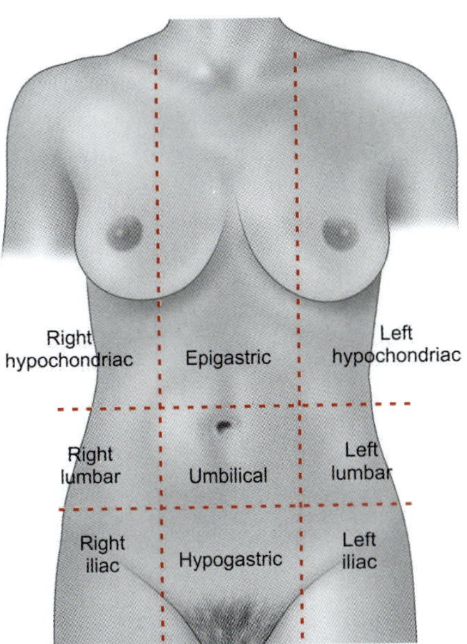


**Fig. 8.1:** Abdominal quadrants

– Grey-Turner's sign: This is the sign which is associated with discoloration (bruising) at the flanks.
– Cullen's sign: This is the sign which is associated with periumbilical bruising.

## Palpation

Normal abdomen should be soft and nontender, with no masses. It is important that the clinician warms his/her hands before palpating the patient's abdomen. The patient should be instructed to flex her hips and knees, which helps in relaxing the abdominal musculature, thereby making palpation easier.

If the patient does not relax sufficiently, the clinician may find it difficult to elicit relevant findings during the abdominal examination. Adequate relaxation can be achieved by making the patient comfortable and gaining her confidence. Asking the patient to take slow deep breaths can also help. The clinician must place his/her palm flat over the patient's abdomen.

Palpation must be done gently, while applying pressure by flexing the fingers in unison at the metacarpal-phalangeal joints. The following points must be noted while palpating the abdomen:

- *Tone of abdominal muscles:* Tone of the abdominal muscles can be assessed upon palpation. When muscle tone is increased, there may be resistance to depression of the abdominal wall by the palpating hand. This hypertonia is commonly accompanied with the presence of tenderness. Reduced tone of the abdominal muscles, on the other hand, could be associated with divarication of rectus muscles.
- *Abdominal tenderness:* There must be no tenderness or rebound tenderness present on abdominal palpation. Rebound tenderness refers to pain upon removal of pressure and may be indicative of localized peritonitis or appendicitis. Tenderness must be recorded on a scale of 0 to 3, where one corresponds to mild and three to most severe type of pain (Table 8.1).
- *Organomegaly:* In the absence of any pathology, most abdominal organs are not palpable in normal people. Palpation of all the abdominal quadrants for presence of any mass, firmness, irregularity or distention must be performed. The clinician should preferably adopt a systemic approach while palpating the abdomen. The clinician must start from the right upper quadrant and systemically palpate all the quadrants while moving down in a clockwise direction. Though a grossly enlarged organ (especially spleen and liver) can be visualized on inspection of the abdomen, organomegaly can be better appreciated on palpation. The normal edge of liver is sharp, smooth, soft and flexible. The liver can descend for up to 3 cm on deep inspiration. In some normal subjects, its edge can be palpable just below the right costal margin without being enlarged. The normal spleen in a healthy subject is not palpable.

*Abdominal mass:* If an abdominal mass is felt on abdominal palpation, the parameters which need to be determined are described next:

- *Location of the mass and its shape, size and texture:* Location of the mass in relation to the various abdominal quadrants needs to be determined. Shape of the mass (round, oval, irregular, etc.) and its size (in cm) also need to be determined. The surface texture of the mass whether smooth, nodular, regular and irregular, needs to be determined.
- *Margins of the mass:* The clinician must try to locate the margins of the mass. In case of the mass arising from the uterus, it may not be possible to localize the lower margin of the mass. Margins of a malignant tumor may be irregular and may not be well-defined.
- *Consistency of the mass:* Consistency of the mass whether hard, firm, rubbery, soft, fluctuant, indentable, or pulsating needs to be determined. Masses like leiomyomas usually have a firm consistency unless they have undergone degeneration. On the other hand, ovarian masses may have cystic consistency. In case of a malignant ovarian tumor, there may be variegated consistency. Furthermore, a malignant mass may be associated with indistinct margins, fixed or restricted mobility and presence of ascites. The pregnant uterus is soft in consistency and hardens with contractions. A full bladder may present as a tense and tender mass in the hypogastric region.
- *Mobility of the mass:* The mobility of the mass, whether free or fixed to adjacent tissues and its movement in relation to respiration needs to be determined. While a

| Table 8.1: Clinical grading of tenderness | | |
|---|---|---|
| *Grade* | *Degree* | *Description* |
| 0 | None | Palpation is not painful even when asked about it |
| 1 | Mild | Patient indicates that palpation is painful only when asked about it |
| 2 | Moderate | Patient indicates that palpation is painful by wincing during palpation |
| 3 | Severe | Patient withdraws his/her limbs at the time of examination or appears clearly distressed when the abdomen is palpated |

benign tumor is freely mobile, the malignant tumor may be fixed or has a restricted mobility.

- *Unilateral or bilateral mass:* Tumorous masses arising from both the ovaries are more likely to be malignant in comparison to the unilateral masses arising from a single ovary.
- *Tenderness on palpation:* Benign masses like fibroids and benign ovarian cysts are usually nontender on palpation. Tenderness upon palpation may be associated with conditions such as ectopic pregnancy, PID, twisted ovarian cysts and red degeneration of fibroids. In conditions like acute peritonitis, there may be guarding, rigidity and rebound tenderness of the lower abdomen.
- *Differentiating between the intra-abdominal masses from those arising from abdominal wall:* Masses arising from the abdominal wall can be distinguished from those inside the abdomen by asking the patient to tighten her abdominal wall muscles. The patient can tighten her abdominal wall muscles by lifting her head off the pillow and looking at her toes. When the patient tightens her abdominal wall muscles, the masses arising from the abdominal wall will remain palpable, while the intra-abdominal masses would no longer be palpable.

## Percussion

For percussion, the fingers of the clinician's left hand are spread slightly. He/she then places the palmar surface of the middle phalanx of the middle finger flat over the area, he/she wishes to percuss. The distal two phalanges of the middle finger of the clinician's right hand must be then flexed and its tip used to strike perpendicularly the middle phalanx of the middle finger of the left hand (already placed in an area wished to be percussed) (Fig. 8.2). The striking finger must be withdrawn as soon as the stroke is delivered. Delivery of the stroke is through flexion of the wrist and the finger at the metacarpophalangeal joint and not through any actions in the elbow or shoulder.

The percussion sound note is tympanitic when the site is over an area of air-filled bowel, whereas it is dull in presence of fluid. Shifting dullness on percussion can be used to determine whether the abdominal distention is due to the presence of fluid (ascites) or an intra-abdominal tumor.

Percussion of the abdomen is valuable in establishing the diagnosis of tumor and in distinguishing it from ascites and in deciding whether it is intraperitoneal or retroperitoneal. Most intraperitoneal tumors arising from the pelvic organs are dull to percussion, whereas a retroperitoneal tumor usually has one or more loops of bowel adherent to it in front, which may give a tympanitic note on percussion. Percussion also helps in differentiating between a large ovarian cyst and ascites. In case of an ovarian cyst, the tumor is dull on percussion, whereas both the flanks are tympanitic due to the presence of

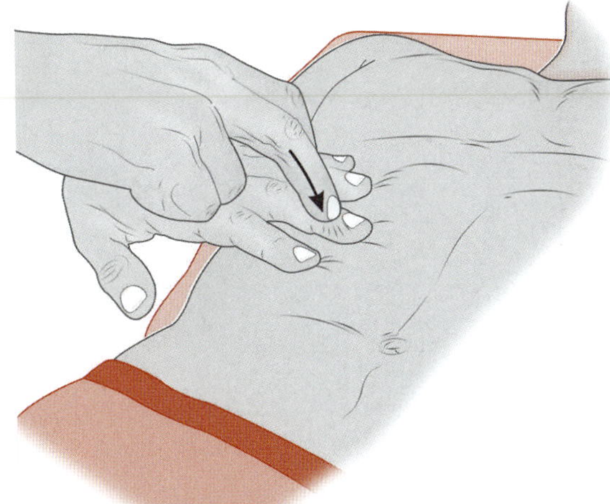

**Fig. 8.2:** Technique of percussion

intestines. In case of ascites, on the other hand, the abdomen is tympanitic in the midline due to the presence of intestines, whereas both the flanks are dull on percussion (Figs 8.3A and B). The technique of percussion also helps in the detection of the following:

*Liver dullness:* Measurement of liver dullness.

*Presence of ascites:* Ascites is commonly associated with malignant tumors. However, all malignant tumors may not be associated with ascites, because only epithelial ovarian malignancies produce ascites. Some benign conditions which may also be associated with ascites include tubercular peritonitis and pseudo-Meigs' syndrome. Presence of ascites is basically detected by two tests: fluid thrill and shifting dullness. Dullness in the flanks upon percussion and shifting dullness indicates the presence of free fluid in the peritoneal cavity.

### Shifting Dullness

Presence of dullness in both flanks when the patient is supine and dullness only in the dependent flank when the patient is on her side indicates the presence of ascites (Figs 8.4A and B). The ability to demonstrate shifting dullness increases with the volume of ascitic fluid. Shifting dullness may be absent if the volume of ascitic fluid is only small. This test comprises of the following steps:

- The patient is laid supine and the clinician starts percussing from the midline of the abdomen towards one of the flanks. The level at which the percussion note changes from tympanitic to dull is noted and then the patient is instructed to turn to the side opposite to the one where the percussion is being done. In normal individuals (without presence of any intra-abdominal

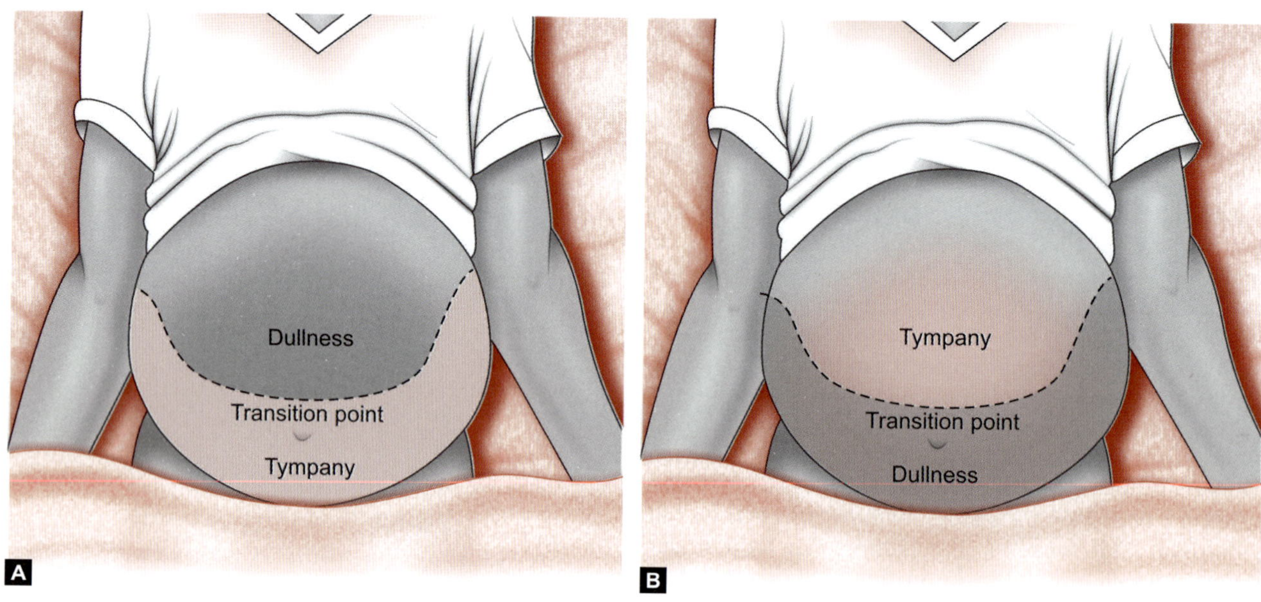



**Figs 8.3A and B:** Percussion of abdomen: (A) Shows presence of an ovarian or uterine tumor, whereas (B) shows ascites

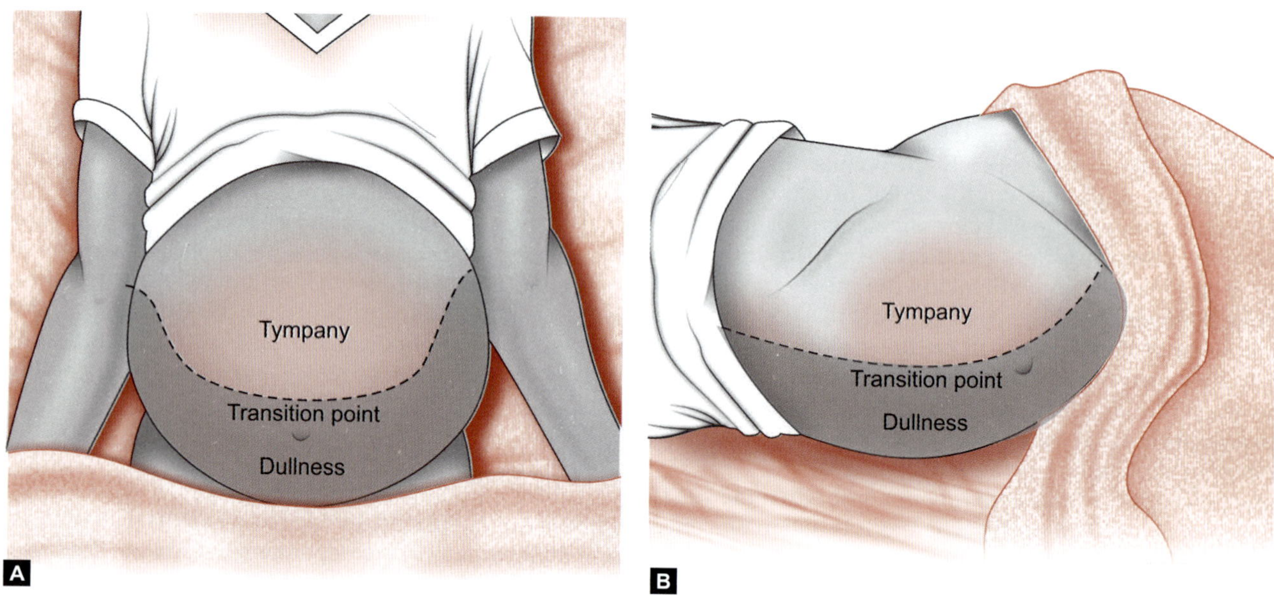



**Figs 8.4A and B:** Shifting dullness. (A) Dullness in both the flanks when the patient is supine; (B) Dullness only in the dependent flank when the patient is on her side

mass), gas-filled bowels float on top of the ascitic fluid when the patient is in supine position, whereas fluid gravitates in the flanks. This is responsible for producing tympanitic note in the midline of abdomen and a dull note in the flanks.

- The patient is then turned to her side and allowed time so that the fluid gravitates to the side of dependent flank.

Now the clinician performs the percussion once again.

The dependent flank where the fluid had gravitated would sound dull to percussion, while the nondependent flank would be tympanitic.

- The patient is then turned to the other side and the above mentioned step is again repeated.

*Fluid Thrill*

Another test for ascites is the demonstration of fluid thrill. The test comprises of the following steps (Fig. 8.5).

- The patient is laid supine and the clinician places one hand flat against her flank on one side.
- An assistant (e.g. a nurse) or the patient herself is asked to place the ulnar aspect of her hand firmly in the midline of the abdomen.
- Without crossing arms, the clinician taps the opposite flank of the abdomen with his/her other hand. In case the ascitic fluid is present, the impulse generated by the tap will be transmitted to the clinician's other hand on the flank. The hand on the abdomen helps in preventing the transmission of the impulse over the abdominal wall. Fluid thrill is demonstrable only if a large volume of ascitic fluid is present. Absence of shifting dullness or fluid thrill or both does not rule out the presence of a small volume ascites.

## Auscultation

Auscultation does not form an important part of abdominal examination. The purpose of auscultation of the abdomen is mainly to listen for bowel sounds produced by peristaltic activities and vascular sounds. Presence of bowel sounds in the abdomen of the patient who had undergone surgery is indicative of recovering bowel activity in the postoperative period.

## CARDIOVASCULAR SYSTEM EXAMINATION

Routine examination of the cardiovascular system involves palpation of cardiac impulse and auscultation of the heart at the apex for presence of any sounds, murmurs, clicks, etc.

Detailed examination of the cardiovascular system is required in cases of past history of cardiovascular disease or complaints suggestive of a possible cardiovascular pathology while taking history.

## EXAMINATION OF THE PULMONARY SYSTEM

Examination of the pulmonary system may be required to detect the presence of wheezes, rales, rhonchi and bronchial breath sounds.

# Pelvic Examination

Pelvic examination forms an important aspect of the gynecological check-up of a woman. The anatomy of female external and internal genitalia is shown in Figures 8.6 and 8.7 respectively. According to the current recommendations by ACOG (2011), annual pelvic examination must be performed for all women aged 21 years and older. In case the patient is asymptomatic, she needs to decide whether she should have a pelvic examination or not. Annual screening for chlamydial and gonorrheal infection is advised for women who are at high risk for infection (e.g. history of having a new sexual partner, multiple sexual partners, sexual partner having multiple sexual contacts, etc.).

Before starting a pelvic examination, the clinician must take verbal consent from the patient. Written consent is not required, except in cases of examination under anesthesia. In case of adolescents and children, parental consent is required for pelvic examinations unrelated to sexual contact. If pelvic examination is performed in the context of instituting treatment for sexually transmitted infections in case of an adolescent patient, parental consent is not required.

If the patient is virginal, the opening of the hymen may be wide enough to allow only one finger or narrow speculum (e.g. Pederson, Huffman, or pediatric) examination. As far as

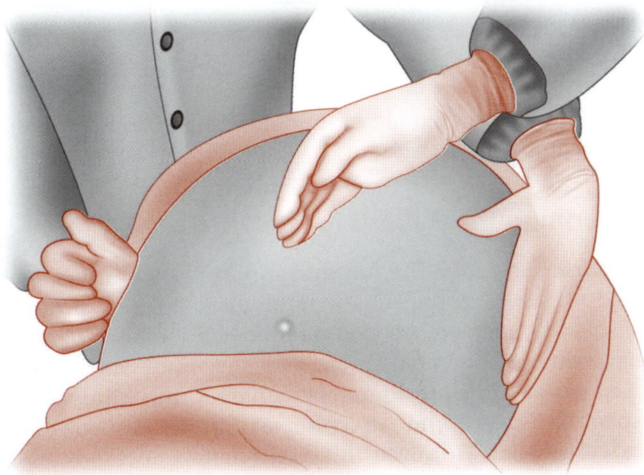

**Fig. 8.5:** Fluid thrill

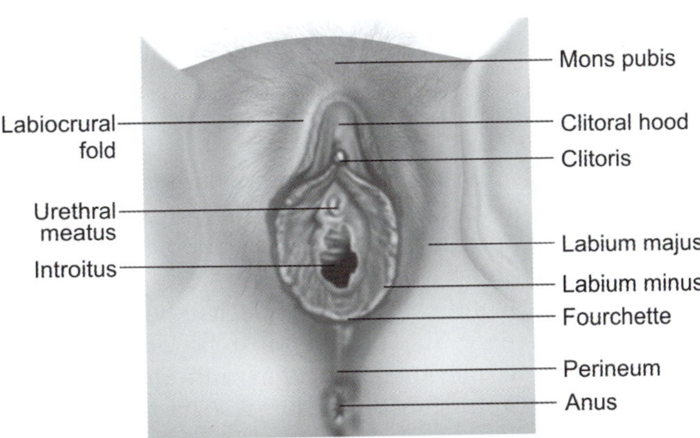


**Fig. 8.6:** Normal anatomy of female external genitalia

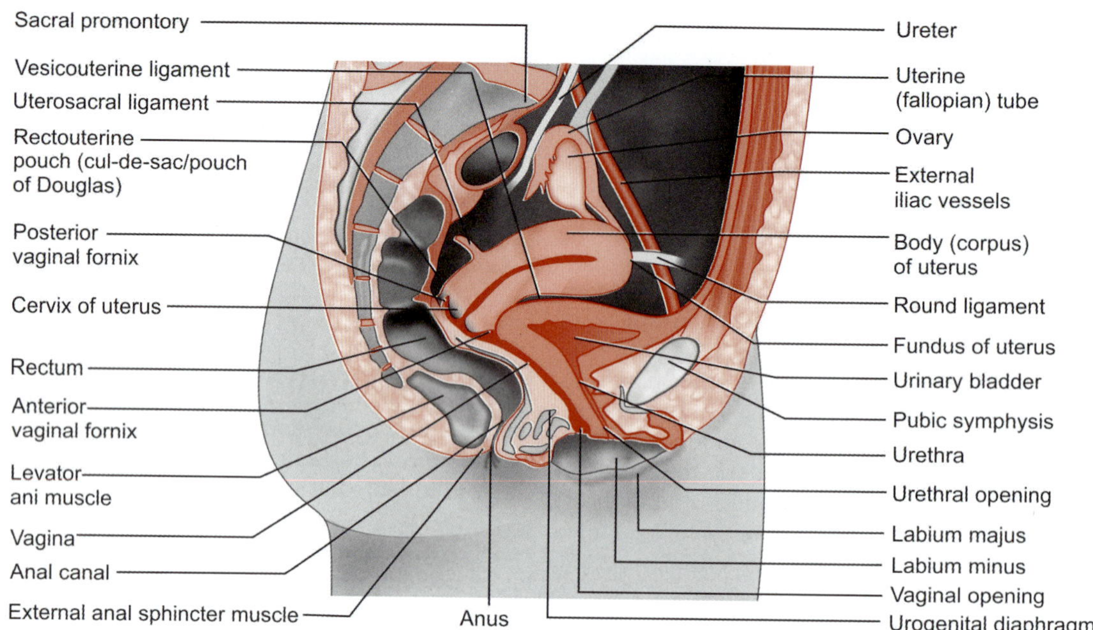



**Fig. 8.7:** Midsagittal view showing normal anatomy of female internal genitalia

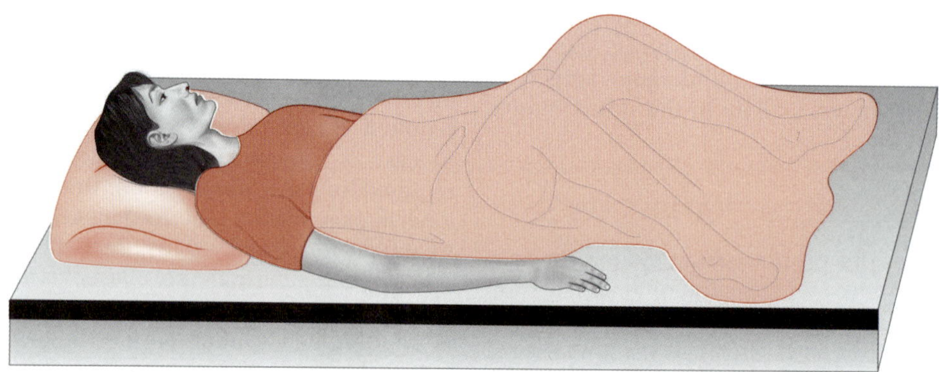

**Fig. 8.8:** Full dorsal position

possible, per vaginal examination must be avoided in virginal women.

The prerequisites before performing a pelvic examination are described below:

- The patient must be asked to empty her bladder before lying down on the table for the examination.
- Gloves and instruments, if not disposable, should be sterilized by autoclaving before reuse.
- Since this is an intimate examination, it requires patient's full cooperation. The patient must be described the procedure of pelvic examination and her informed consent be taken before proceeding with the examination.
- The clinician must wear nonsterile gloves on both hands before starting with the examination.
- Both male and female examiners should be chaperoned by a female assistant.

## Positioning the Patient for Pelvic Examination

*Full dorsal position:* The full dorsal position with the knees flexed (Fig. 8.8) is the most commonly employed position used for gynecological examination in clinical practice. This position allows adequate per speculum and vaginal examination. This position also enables the clinician to inspect the vagina and cervix for taking vaginal swabs and cervical smears. However, this examination does not allow adequate exposure of the lateral vaginal walls. The examiner stands to the right of the patient. The patient can be made to relax by partly covering her knees and thighs with a sheet. Elevating the head of the table 30–45° enables the woman to relax, thereby facilitating bimanual examination.

## Components of the Pelvic Examination

Pelvic examination comprises of the following components:
- Examination of the external genitalia
- Per speculum examination
- Bimanual vaginal examination
- Rectovaginal examination (if required)
- The abdomen and breasts are also commonly examined as a part of pelvic examination.

### *Inspection of the External Genitalia*

The clinician examines the external genitalia for the presence of any obvious lesions or signs of inflammation. Examination of external genitalia reveals areas of discoloration, ulceration and redness. Ulcerative areas could be indicative of herpetic infection, vulvar carcinoma, syphilis, etc. Examination of external genitalia involves inspection and palpation of the following:
- The hair distribution and skin over the vulva (presence of any lesions, ulcers, etc.)
- Labia minora and majora
- Perineal body
- Clitoris, urethral meatus, vestibule, and introitus
- Bartholin and paraurethral glands (the openings of Bartholin gland are located at the 4 O'clock and 8 O'clock positions just outside the hymenal ring. The glands are normally not palpable when healthy. The paraurethral glands lie adjacent to the distal urethra. If the glands appear enlarged or tender, an attempt should be made to express exudate, which could be suggestive of infection.

### *Per Speculum Examination*

Speculum examination of the vagina and cervix involves inspection of external genitalia, vagina and cervix (Fig. 8.9). Per speculum examination may reveal normal vaginal wall rugosities or smoothness of vaginal epithelium, which could be suggestive of atrophic vaginitis. Presence of masses, vesicles or any other lesions can also be assessed on per speculum examination. This examination should ideally precede the bimanual examination. This is primarily because the vaginal discharge can be seen and removed for examination before it gets contaminated with the lubricant used for vaginal examination; moreover, the cellular debris from the cervix and uterus remains undisturbed and can be obtained for cytological studies at the time of per speculum examination. Also, many superficial vaginal lesions may start bleeding following the vaginal examination and may not allow an optimal per speculum examination. A self-retaining,

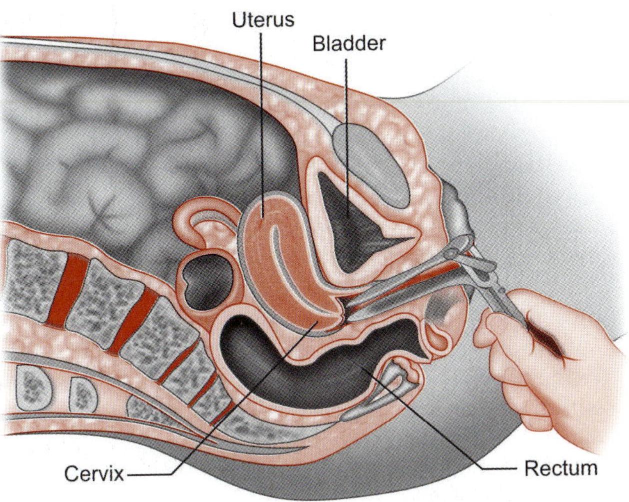


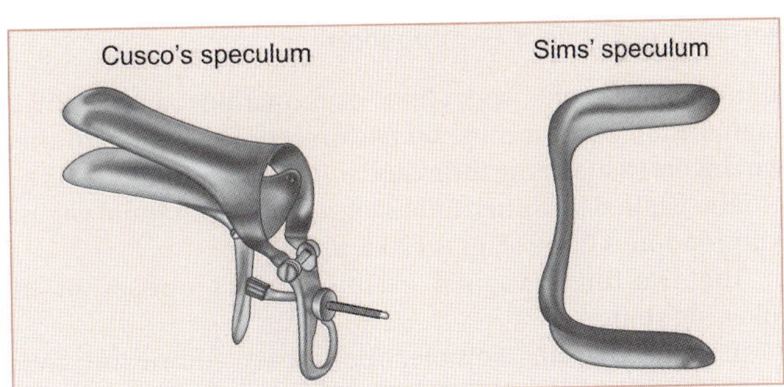


**Fig. 8.9:** Per speculum examination

bivalve speculum such as Cusco's speculum serves as an ideal equipment for vaginal examination. Cervical examination can also be performed using a Sims' vaginal speculum and an anterior vaginal wall retractor. This speculum allows the assessment of vaginal walls and evaluation of presence of uterine prolapse such as cystocele, or rectocele. However, cervical inspection using Sims' speculum is associated with two main disadvantages. The clinician needs to bring the patient to the edge of the table. Also, help of an assistant may be required while conducting a per speculum examination using a Sims' speculum. For detailed description of these equipment, kindly refer to Chapter 13.

### *Procedure of Insertion of Cusco's Speculum*

- The clinician must firstly warm and lubricate the speculum by holding it under running tap water.
- The vaginal introitus must be exposed by spreading the labia from below using the index and middle fingers of the left hand.
- The Cusco's bivalve speculum must then be inserted at an angle of 45°, pointing slightly downwards. Contact with any anterior structures must be avoided.

- Once past the introitus, the speculum must be rotated to a horizontal position and insertion continued until its handle is almost flush with the perineum.
- The blades of the speculum are opened up for a distance of approximately 2–3 cm using the thumb lever in such a way that the cervix "falls" in between the blades.
- The speculum can be secured in its position by using the thumb nut in case of a metal speculum. The speculum must not be moved while it is in a locked position.
- The cervical and vaginal walls must be observed for the presence of any lesions or discharge. Specimens for culture and cytology must also be obtained.
- While removing the speculum, the speculum must be withdrawn slightly to clear the cervix. As the cervix gets cleared off, the speculum must be loosened and its blades allowed to fall together. The speculum must then be rotated to an angle of 45° and continued to be withdrawn.

### Two-Finger Vaginal Examination

Following the per speculum examination, a two-finger vaginal examination must be performed. First one and then two fingers (usually the index and middle fingers) are inserted into the vaginal introitus, following which a bimanual vaginal examination is done (Figs 8.10A and B).

The two-finger vaginal examination comprises of the following steps:

- A water-based, soluble, nongreasy lubricant must preferably be used. A water soluble jelly is the best and if that is not available, cetrimide solution must be used.
- The labia are separated with the thumb and index finger of left hand.

- Following this, the two fingers of right hand, first one finger and then the second finger are gently inserted inside the vagina only when the patient relaxes the muscles around the vagina and when it is clear that a two-finger examination would be possible without causing any pain.
- Cervical shape, size, position, mobility, consistency and tenderness caused by pressure or movement needs to be assessed. The position and direction of the cervix are the guides to the position of the body of the uterus. If the cervix is pointing in the downward and backward direction, the anterior lip of the cervix would be encountered first on the vaginal examination. This indicates the anteverted position of the uterus. On the other hand, if the cervix is pointing in the upward and forward direction, the posterior lip of cervix would be encountered first on the vaginal examination. This indicates the retroverted position of the uterus.

A nonpregnant healthy cervix is usually firm in consistency. The cervix tends to soften during pregnancy. Under normal circumstances, the movement of cervix in any direction must not be painful. However, pain upon moving the cervix (also known as cervical motion tenderness) is a common symptom of PID (salpingo-oophoritis) and ectopic pregnancy.

### Bimanual Vaginal Examination

Since the vaginal examination provides only limited information, a bimanual vaginal examination must also be performed. In clinical scenario, the vaginal examination is immediately followed by a bimanual examination without removing fingers from the vaginal introitus. In bimanual

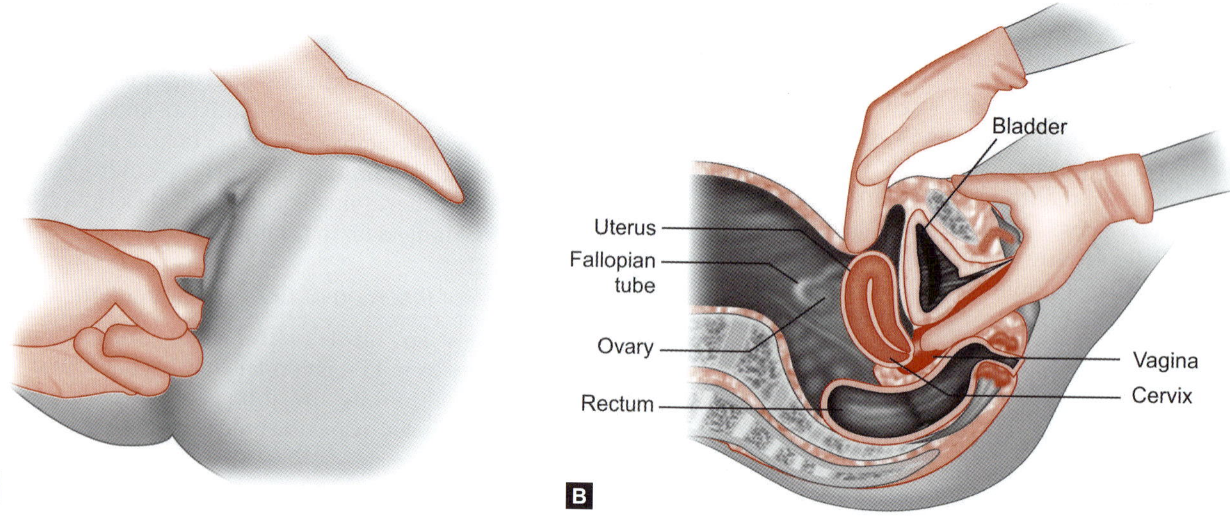


**Figs 8.10A and B:** (A) Two-finger vaginal examination, performed by inserting two fingers of right hand inside the vagina; (B) Bimanual vaginal examination performed with the palm of left hand over the abdomen and the fingers of right hand still inside the vagina

examination, the examiner also places palm of his/her left hand over the patient's abdomen, while the examiner's fingers are still inside the vaginal introitus. The success of bimanual examination primarily depends on the ability of the examiner to use the abdominal hand more often than the vaginal fingers. The procedure of bimanual vaginal examination comprises of the following steps:

- All the previously mentioned steps of a two-finger vaginal examination are firstly performed.
- To feel the uterus, the vaginal fingers should move the cervix as far backwards as possible to rotate the fundus downward and forward. The abdominal hand is then placed just below the umbilicus and gradually moved lower until the fundus is caught and pressed against the fingers in the anterior fornix.
- The following points are noted on bimanual examination: size of the uterus; its position, (anteverted or retroverted; anteflexed or retroflexed); mobility, (restricted mobility or fixed uterus). If a mass felt, its relation to the uterus is noted, like whether the mass is felt separate to the uterus or is continuous with it. When the mass is felt separate from the uterus, the origin of the mass is most likely from the adnexa or broad ligament. However, if the mass is continuous with the uterus, it probably arises from the uterus, like a fibroid.

*Size of the uterus:* Bulky uterus corresponds to 6-week pregnant size and is slightly larger than the normal. When the uterus appears to be filling all the fornices, it corresponds to 12 weeks size. The in-between size could be between 8 weeks and 10 weeks. Both the adnexa must then be palpated between the vaginal fingers in the lateral vaginal fornices and the abdominal hand to look for presence of any mass or abnormality.

### Rectovaginal Examination

Combined rectal and vaginal examination is done when required. Similar to the bimanual examination, the examiner inserts a lubricated, gloved finger into the rectum to feel for tenderness and masses, while the other finger remains inside the vagina. Per rectum examination will help reveal masses in the posterior pelvis. Rectovaginal examination allows optimal palpation of the posterior cul-de-sac and uterosacral ligaments, as well as the uterus and adnexa. Presence of nodularity in the pouch of Douglas and tenderness of uterosacral ligaments are signs of endometriosis. If a rectovaginal examination is performed, anorectal findings should also be documented (e.g. hemorrhoids, rectal mass) in the clinician's notes. At the time of rectovaginal examination, the same finger should not be used to examine both the vagina and rectum to avoid transmission of human papillomavirus or contamination with blood. Some practitioners include rectovaginal examination as part of the routine pelvic examination, while others do this procedure only in specific cases.

# Management

Following the completion of patient's history and physical examination, an appropriate management plan is formulated. Depending upon the suspected pathology, various investigations are ordered. Results of the various investigations help in formulating an appropriate management plan. The aims of management are the following:

- Making and confirming the patient's diagnosis
- Assessing the severity or stage of the disease
- Rendering treatment based on the stage of the disease
- Following up the patient's response to treatment.

### FURTHER READINGS

1. American College of Obstetricians and Gynecologists. ACOG Practice Bulletin. Clinical management guidelines for obstetrician-gynecologists: Number 41, December 2002. Obstet Gynecol. 2002;100(6):1389-402.
2. Committee on Ethics, American College of Obstetricians and Gynecologists. ACOG Committee Opinion No. 373: Sexual misconduct. Obstet Gynecol. 2007;110(2 Pt 1):441-4.
3. Committee on Gynecologic Practice. Committee opinion no. 534: well-woman visit. Obstet Gynecol. 2012;120(2 Pt 1):421-4.
4. Department for Education and Skills. Common core of skills and knowledge for the children's workforce, London: HM Government. Department of Health (2003) Confidentiality: NHS code of practice, London: DH; 2005.
5. Oakeshott P, Hay P. Best practice in primary care. BMJ. 2006; 333 (7560):173-4.
6. Padilla LA, Radosevich DM, Milad MP. Accuracy of the pelvic examination in detecting adnexal masses. Obstet Gynecol. 2000; 96(4):593-8.
7. Patient Care. In: Hillard, PJ, Berek, JS (Eds). Guidelines for Women's Health Care: A Resource Manual, 3rd edition. American College of Obstetricians and Gynecologists: Washington, DC; 2007. p.168.
8. Workowski KA, Berman S, Centers for Disease Control and Prevention (CDC). Sexually transmitted diseases treatment guidelines, 2010. MMWR Recomm Rep. 2010;59(RR-12):1-110.

# Cases in Gynecology

## CHAPTER OUTLINE

- Carcinoma Cervix
- Carcinoma Endometrium
- Fibroid Uterus
- Genital Prolapse
- Dysfunctional Uterine Bleeding
- Infertility
- Abnormal Vaginal Discharge
- Genitourinary Fistula
- Abdominal Lump
- Endometriosis
- Molar Gestation

## Carcinoma Cervix

### Case Study 1

Mrs XYZ, a 62-year-old woman, with an active married life of 23 years, resident of ABC, para 4 woman presented with the complaints of postcoital bleeding since past 2 months. She had been getting regular Pap smear examinations done in the past. The last smear done 1 year back had shown normal pathology. During this visit, a repeat Pap smear was performed, which was found to be within normal limits. After ruling out other likely causes of postcoital bleeding in this case, and detecting no significant finding on clinical examination, colposcopic examination was performed. Colposcopy revealed a lesion on the anterior surface of the ectocervix, showing irregular mosaic pattern, surface irregularity and an atypical blood vessel pattern after application of 5% acetic acid. A colposcopic-directed biopsy confirmed the diagnosis of squamous cell carcinoma. Based on clinical staging, the disease was assigned to be stage IA1 (FIGO staging system).

### Q. What is the likely diagnosis in the above-mentioned case study?

**Ans.** The above-mentioned case study corresponds to cervical cancer (FIGO stage IA1 as confirmed by clinical examination and investigations). The questions to be asked at the time of taking history and the parameters to be assessed at the time of examination are described in Tables 9.1 and 9.2 respectively. The most likely diagnosis in this case is Mrs XYZ, a 62-year-old woman, with an active married life of 23 years, resident of ABC, para 4 woman with chief complaints of postcoital bleeding since past 2 months. Diagnosis of invasive squamous cell cervical malignancy is confirmed on investigations, which had already been done in this case. If the results of various investigations had not been provided, the provisional diagnosis regarding the FIGO staging must be made on clinical examination.

### Q. What is cervix? What types of cancers are commonly found in the cervix?

**Ans.** The cervix is the lowermost, narrow portion of the uterus, which is joined with the upper portion of the vagina. It is anatomically composed of two parts: ectocervix and endocervix. The part of the cervix projecting into the vagina is known as the portio vaginalis or ectocervix, whereas the region of the cervix opening into the uterine cavity is known as the endocervix. The opening of ectocervix inside the vagina is known as the external cervical os, while the opening of the cervix inside the uterine cavity is known as the internal cervical os. The endocervical canal extends between the internal and the external cervical os.

The ectocervix is lined by squamous cells, while endocervical cells are mainly of the columnar type. The transformation zone (Fig. 9.1) lies at the junction of ectocervix and endocervix. Columnar cells are constantly changing into squamous cells in the transformation zone. Since cells in the transformation zone are constantly changing, this is the most common place for cervical malignancy to develop.

Of the various types of malignant tumors in the cervix, the most common types of cancer in the cervix is squamous cell carcinoma, which is responsible for nearly 80% cases of cancer. The next common type of cancer is adenocarcinoma, which develops from the glandular cells in the endocervical canal.

**Table 9.1:** Symptoms to be elicited at the time of taking history in a case of carcinoma cervix

*History of Presenting Complains*

- History of abnormal bleeding, spotting or watery discharge in between periods or after intercourse. A history of postcoital bleeding must specifically raise the suspicion of cervical cancer.
- Presence of a foul-smelling vaginal discharge and discomfort during intercourse.
- There may be history of postmenopausal bleeding.
- In advanced stages of cancer there may be symptoms like pelvic pain, loss of appetite, weight loss, fatigue, back pain, leg pain, leg swelling, bleeding from the vagina, leakage of urine or feces from the vagina and bone fractures.

*Age:* Cancer of the cervix is found most often in women older than 40 years, with the average age being 47 years. Though it can occur in younger women, it rarely occurs in women younger than 21 years.

*Obstetric History*

- Delivery of first baby at an early age (< 20 years)
- Multiparity with the history of giving births with poor spacing between pregnancies.

*Sexual History*

The factors which are associated with an increased risk of cervical cancer and need to be elicited at the time of taking sexual history include the following:
- Promiscuity or history of having multiple sexual partners.
- History of having a male sexual partner who has had sexual intercourse with more than one person (the more partners the person has, the greater is the risk).
- Young age (under 18 years) at the time of first sexual intercourse.
- Having a male sexual partner who has had a sexual partner with cervical cancer.
- History of having sexually transmitted diseases in the past including the diseases like HIV infection, herpes simplex 2 virus infection, HPV infection, etc. is associated with an increased risk of developing cancer of the cervix. Infection with HPV acts as an initiating event in cervical dysplasia and carcinogenesis. There are 100 different types of HPV, out of which, types 16 and 18 are most commonly found in cases of squamous cell carcinoma.

*Personal History*

- Smoking is associated with an increased risk for development of cancer of cervix.
- Women who do not come for regular health checkups and Pap tests are at an increased risk.

*Reduced immunity:* Women with reduced immunity are at an increased risk of developing cervical cancer. Some of the conditions associated with reduced immunity include the following:
- Human immunodeficiency virus infection
- Organ (especially kidney) transplant
- Hodgkin's disease

*Previous vaccination against cervical cancer:* Two HPV vaccines, quadrivalent Gardasil® and bivalent Cervarix™ have been approved by the US Food and Drug Administration for protection against the HPV subtypes 16 and 18. It is important to take history regarding such vaccination.

*Socioeconomic Status*

Individuals belonging to low socioeconomic classes or low income groups have been found to be at a high risk of developing cervical cancer.

*Treatment History*

It is important to elicit the history of intake of medicines like DES by the woman's mother, long-term use of OCPs, etc. because these could act as the risk factors.

*Dietary History*

Diets low in fruits and vegetables are linked to an increased risk of cervical and other cancers. Also, women who are overweight are at an increased risk of developing cervical cancer in the future.

*Family History*

Cervical cancer may run in some families. If the woman's mother or sister had cervical cancer, her chances of getting the disease in future are increased.

*Previous History of Cancerous Lesions in the Cervix*

The woman is at a high risk of developing cancer of cervix if she has a previous history of HSIL; history of cancer of the cervix, vagina, or vulva and has not been getting routine Pap tests done in the past.

*Abbreviations:* HIV, human immunodeficiency virus; HPV, human papillomavirus; HSIL, high-grade squamous intraepithelial lesions; OCPs, oral contraceptive pills; DES, diethylstilbestrol

**Table 9.2:** Various findings elicited at the time of clinical examination in a case of carcinoma cervix

*General Physical Examination*

- No specific finding may be detected on the general physical examination.
- *Signs of anemia:* Chronic bleeding may be associated with anemia.
- *Signs associated with advanced stages:* Advanced stages of cancer may be associated with cancer cachexia, lymphadenopathy or pedal edema.
- *Lymph node evaluation:* Evaluation of supraclavicular, axillary and inguinofemoral nodes is important to exclude the metastatic disease.

*Specific Systemic Examination*

At the time of systemic examination, efforts must be made to rule out the presence of any systemic anomaly (e.g. hypertension, diabetes, asthma, etc.), which could affect the patient's fitness for gynecological/surgical treatment of the diagnosed pathology.

*Per Speculum Examination*

- On per speculum examination, cervix must be carefully inspected for presence of any suspicious lesions. A per speculum examination also enables the clinician to simultaneously take the punch biopsy of the suspected lesion.
- Vaginal fornices must also be closely inspected.
- Squamous cell cancers of the ectocervix may appear as proliferative or cauliflower like, vascular, friable growth, which bleeds on touch; ulcerative lesions or as flat indurated areas. In case of an invasive cancer, the cervix may appear firm and expanded on per speculum examination.

*Vaginal Examination*

- On vaginal examination, both fungating and ulcerative cervical lesions may be identified.
- Uterus may appear bulky due to occurrence of pyometra in advanced stage when the cervix gets blocked by growth.

*Rectal Examination*

- The rectal examination may reveal thickening and induration of uterosacral ligaments and evaluation of parametrial extension of the disease (identified in form of parametrial nodularity).
- It is also useful for assessing cervical consistency and size, particularly in patients with endocervical disease.

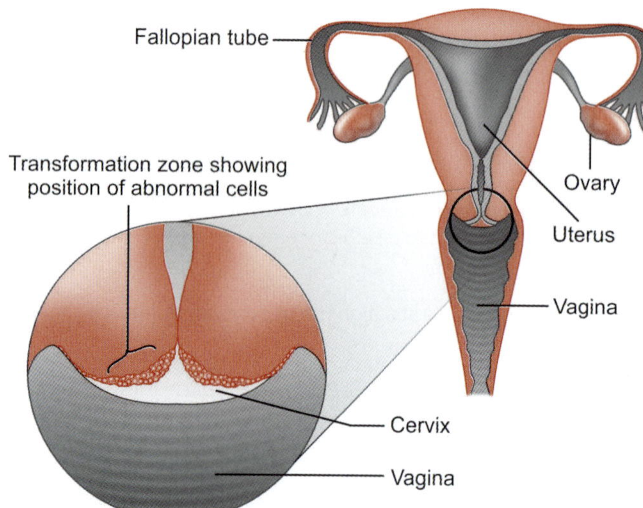


**Fig. 9.1:** Transformation zone

**Q. What investigations must be done in the above-mentioned case study to confirm the diagnosis?**

**Ans.** The investigations which need to be done in these cases to confirm the diagnosis are as follows:

- Pap smear (for details related to Pap smear, kindly refer to Chapter 10).
- Cervical biopsy.
- Test for acid fast bacillus.
- Enzyme linked immunosorbent assay (ELISA).
- Mantoux test.

**Q. Describe the staging systems for cervical cancer.**

**Ans.** Once the diagnosis of invasive cervical cancer has been established confidently by histological examination, the disease is clinically staged, which involves assessment of the degree of cancer dissemination. The most commonly used system for staging of cervical cancer is the staging system devised by FIGO, which is based on clinical examination, rather than surgical findings (Table 9.3). Once a clinical stage has been assigned and treatment is initiated, the cancer stage must not be changed because of consequent findings either by extended clinical or surgical staging.

Cancer grading is based on the results of the histopathological examination and gives an idea about the degree of malignancy. It can be classified as grade 1 (low grade malignancy), grade 2 (moderate grade malignancy) and grade 3 (higher grade malignancy). The more undifferentiated the malignancy, the higher would be its grading.

**Q. What investigations must be done to assess the spread of cervical cancer?**

**Ans.** Management of invasive cancer primarily depends on the stage of malignancy, which is essentially based on clinical

**Table 9.3:** International Federation of Gynecology and Obstetrics staging system for cervical cancer

| Stage | Characteristics |
|---|---|
| 0 | Carcinoma in situ, intraepithelial neoplasia |
| I | Carcinoma strictly confined to the cervix (extension to the corpus would be disregarded) |
| IA | Invasive cancer identified only microscopically. All gross lesions, even with superficial invasion, are stage IB cancers<br>Invasion is limited to measured invasion of stroma ≤ 5 mm in depth and ≤ 7 mm in width. Depth of invasion must not be greater than 5 mm taken from the base of the epithelium of vaginal tissue, squamous or glandular. The depth of invasion must always be reported in mm, even for those cases with "early minimal stromal invasion" (~ 1 mm). The involvement of lymphatic/vascular spaces should not change stage allotment |
| IA1 | Measured invasion of stroma ≤ 3 mm in depth and ≤ 7 mm in width |
| IA2 | Measured invasion of stroma > 3 mm and ≤ 5 mm in depth and ≤ 7 mm in width |
| IB | Clinical lesions confined to the cervix or preclinical lesions greater than IA |
| IB1 | Clinical lesions ≤ 4 cm in size |
| IB2 | Clinical lesions > 4 cm in size |
| II | Carcinoma extends beyond the cervix, but not to the pelvic wall; carcinoma involves the vagina but not as far as the lower one-third |
| IIA | No obvious parametrial involvement |
| IIA1 | Clinically visible lesion ≤ 4.0 cm in the greatest dimension |
| IIA2 | Clinically visible lesion > 4.0 cm in the greatest dimension |
| IIB | Obvious parametrial involvement |
| III | Carcinoma has extended to the pelvic wall; on rectal examination no cancer-free space is found between the tumor and the pelvic wall; the tumor involves lower one-third of the vagina; all cases with a hydronephrosis or nonfunctioning kidney should be included, unless they are known to be related to another cause |
| IIIA | No extension to the pelvic wall, but involvement of the lower one-third of the vagina |
| IIIB | Extension to the pelvic wall and/or hydronephrosis or nonfunctioning kidney, or both |
| IV | Carcinoma has extended beyond the true pelvis or has involved (biopsy proven) the mucosa of the bladder or rectum. A bullous edema as such does not permit the case to be allotted as stage IV |
| IVA | Spread to the adjacent organs |
| IVB | Spread to distant organs |

*Source:* Pecorelli S. Revised FIGO staging for carcinoma of the vulva, cervix and endometrium. Int Gynecol Obstet. 2009;105(2):103-4.

**Table 9.4:** Pretreatment investigations in a woman with histologic diagnosis of cervical cancer

- Physical examination
- Complete blood count, LFT, KFT
- Chest radiography
- Pelvic ultrasound
- Magnetic resonance imaging
- Computed tomography scans
- FDG-PET (positron emission tomography based on the use of radiolabeled compound fluorodeoxyglucose): Gold standard investigation for evaluation of metastasis to the lymph nodes
- Laparoscopy
- Intravenous pyelography or imaging of abdomen with intravenous contrast
- Barium enema, cystoscopy, rectosigmoidoscopy
- Cystoscopy: For visualization of the interior of the urethra and bladder
- Proctoscopy: For visualization of the interior of the rectum

*Abbreviations:* KFT, kidney function test; LFT, liver function test

findings and results of various imaging investigations as shown in Table 9.4. Management of cervical cancer changes based on lymph node involvement, the rate of which rises with increasing stage of the disease.

**Q. What are the various modes of treatments for invasive cervical cancer?**

**Ans.** The treatment of cervical cancer varies with the stage of the disease. While radiotherapy can be used for all stages of cervical cancer, for early invasive cancer (stage I and IIA disease), surgery is the treatment of choice. In more advanced cases, radiation combined with chemotherapy is the current standard of care. In patients with disseminated disease, chemotherapy or radiation provides symptom palliation. Palliative radiotherapy is often useful for controlling bleeding, pelvic pain and urinary or partial large bowel obstructions resulting from pelvic disease. Treatment of invasive cervical cancer is summarized in Table 9.5.

### Q. What are the various available surgical treatment options for cervical cancer?

**Ans.** Various types of surgical options which can be used in cases of cervical cancer are described in Table 9.6. Previously, surgery commonly included a radical hysterectomy (Wertheim's hysterectomy or Schauta vaginal hysterectomy, known as Mitra operation in India). Wertheim's hysterectomy involves removal of the entire uterus, both adnexa, medial one-third of parametrium, uterosacral ligaments, upper 2–3 cm cuff of the vagina, dissection of pelvic lymph nodes and selective removal of enlarged lymph nodes. This is in contrast to type II radical hysterectomy, which also includes pelvic lymphadenectomy. Para-aortic lymphadenectomy is performed if the pelvic nodes are found to be suspicious for metastatic disease at the time of pelvic lymphadenectomy.

### Q. What is the treatment in the above-mentioned case study (Stage IA tumors)?

**Ans.** As described before, stage IA tumors are mainly diagnosed by microscopic examination. The risk of nodal metastasis in the early invasive tumors (stage IA1) is quite low, only about 0.5%; therefore the prognosis in these cases is quite good. Five-year survival rate exceeds 95% with appropriate treatment. The recommended therapy for stage IA1 tumors without lymphovascular space invasion who are not desirous of future fertility is type I hysterectomy (extrafascial hysterectomy). If lymphovascular space invasion is found, a modified radical hysterectomy (type II hysterectomy) with pelvic lymphadenopathy is an appropriate and effective treatment option.

**Table 9.5:** Summary of treatment of invasive cervical carcinoma

| Cervical cancer stage | Therapeutic option |
| --- | --- |
| Stage 0 | LEEP, laser therapy, conization and cryotherapy |
| Stage IA1 | Conization or type I hysterectomy |
| Stage IA2 | Radical trachelectomy or radical type II hysterectomy with pelvic lymphadenectomy |
| Stage IB1 (invasion > 5 mm, < 2 cm) | Radical trachelectomy or radical type III hysterectomy with pelvic lymphadenectomy<br>Radical type III hysterectomy with pelvic lymphadenectomy |
| Stage IB2 | Radical type III hysterectomy with pelvic and para-aortic lymphadenectomy or primary chemoradiation |
| Stage IIA1 and IIA2 | Radical type III hysterectomy with pelvic and para-aortic lymphadenectomy or primary chemoradiation |
| Stage IIB, IIIA and IIIB | Primary chemoradiation |
| Stage IVA | Primary chemoradiation or primary exenteration |
| Stage IVB | Primary chemotherapy with or without radiotherapy |

*Abbreviation:* LEEP, loop electrosurgical excision procedure

**Table 9.6:** Classification of radical hysterectomy (as adopted by the Gynecological Cancer Group of the European Organization for Research and Treatment of Cancer)

| Classification | Description |
| --- | --- |
| Type I radical hysterectomy (Simple/extrafascial hysterectomy) | Removal of the uterus and cervix, but not the parametria or more than the upper vaginal margin |
| Modified radical or type II radical hysterectomy | Removal of the entire uterus, both adnexa, medial half of cardinal and uterosacral ligaments, upper 2–3 cm cuff of the vagina and pelvic lymphadenectomy |
| Type III radical hysterectomy (originally described by Meig in 1944) | Removal of the entire uterus, both adnexa, most of the cardinal and uterosacral ligaments, upper one-third of the vagina and pelvic lymphadenectomy |
| Type IV radical hysterectomy (Extended radical hysterectomy) | Periureteral tissues, superior vesical artery and as much as three-fourths of the vagina and paravaginal tissue are excised (in addition to structures removed in type III radical hysterectomy) |
| Type V radical hysterectomy (Partial exenteration) | In addition to the structures removed in type IV hysterectomy, portions of distal ureter and bladder are also removed |

Conization with clear margins may be considered adequate in young patients with stage IA disease who want to conserve their uterus. For effective treatment, there must not be any evidence of lymphovascular space invasion and both endocervical margins and curettage findings must be negative for cancer or dysplasia. The patients undergoing conization require close follow-up, including cytology, colposcopy and endocervical curettage.

**Q. What should be the next step of management in the above-mentioned case study?**

**Ans.** Since the woman had completed her family, did not want to conserve her uterus and there was no lymphovascular space invasion, a type I extrafascial hysterectomy was performed in this case.

**Q. What is the prognosis in the above-mentioned case study?**

**Ans.** Prognosis depends on the stage of the cancer, followed by the status of the lymph nodes. Outcomes are worse for women where there is involvement of pelvic or para-aortic nodes. If the earliest stage of invasive cervical cancer is treated, the 5-year relative survival rate is nearly 90–95% which was the scenario in this case study. With treatment, 80–90% of women with stage I cancer and 50–65% of those with stage II cancer remain alive for 5 years after diagnosis. Only 30–45% of women with stage III cancer and 15% or fewer of those with stage IV cancer remain alive after 5 years. With metastasis of cancer to other parts of the body, prognosis progressively worsens.

## Case Study 2

Mrs ABC, a 55-year-old woman, resident of XYZ, P5+0 presented to the gynecologic clinic with the complaints of postcoital bleeding and foul-smelling vaginal discharge since past 1 month. On per speculum examination, there was a large fungating growth on the left side of the cervix which bled on touching. On pelvic examination, the uterus was bulky, firm and mobile and the adnexa was not palpable.

**Q. What could be the likely differential diagnosis in the above-mentioned case study?**

**Ans.** The possible differential diagnoses in the above-mentioned case study are as follows:

- Cancer cervix
- Cervical ulcers (tubercular and syphilitic)
- Cervical pregnancy
- Cervicitis
- Ectropion
- Cervical erosion
- Cervical polyps (mucus, cervical, and fibroid polyps).

**Q. The diagnosis of cervical cancer was confirmed in this case. What would be the FIGO clinical staging?**

**Ans.** The most likely FIGO stage in the above-mentioned case study is IB.

**Q. What are the treatment options in the above-mentioned case study (Stage IB and IIA tumors)?**

**Ans.** The treatment option for early stage cervical cancer (stage IB1) is primarily surgical treatment. Treatment options for stage IB2 and stage IIA are surgical treatment or primary chemoradiation. Surgery in these cases comprises of radical type III hysterectomy with pelvic and para-aortic lymphadenectomy. Radiotherapy can be either in the form of external beam and intracavitary radiotherapy. Radiotherapy must be used as the primary treatment for only those women who are poor candidates for surgery due to presence of medical comorbidities or poor functional status.

## Case Study 3

Mrs ABC, a 60-year-old woman, resident of XYZ, P5+4 was admitted to the gynecology oncology ward with history of irregular vaginal bleeding and discharge since past few months. On per speculum examination study, a large irregular growth was observed on the anterior lip of cervix. The uterus was normal, retroverted and fixed. All the vaginal fornices appeared to be firm. However, the firmness was not observed to be extending up to the pelvic side wall. Cancer cervix was diagnosed following the biopsy of the fungating growth.

**Q. What is FIGO cancer staging in the above-mentioned case study?**

**Ans.** The cancer was likely to be in FIGO stage IIB.

## Case Study 4

Mrs ABC, a 51-year-old P4+4 woman, resident of XYZ, was admitted to the gynecology ward with the history of postcoital bleeding since last 3–4 weeks. On per speculum examination, a little bleeding, ulcerative growth was observed as 9 O' clock position. On pelvic examination, the uterus was retroverted and fixed. All the vaginal fornices felt firm and thickened up to the pelvic side wall. Per rectal examination was within normal limits. Diagnosis of cervical cancer was confirmed on biopsy.

**Q. What is the most likely FIGO cervical cancer stage in this case study?**

**Ans.** The most likely FIGO cancer stage is IIIB.

## Case Study 5

Mrs XYZ, a 60-year-old P6+3 woman, resident of ABC, presented to the emergency department with the history of bleeding per vaginum since last 2 days. On per speculum examination, a large fungating growth was observed on the posterior lip of cervix. On pelvic examination, the uterus was normal-sized, retroverted and fixed. All the vaginal fornices appeared to be thickened and firm up to the pelvic side walls. On rectovaginal examination, the rectal mucosa appeared to be immobile and fixed to the vaginal walls.

**Q. What is the most likely FIGO cervical cancer stage in this case study?**

**Ans.** The most likely FIGO cancer stage is IV, which needs to be confirmed by performing other investigations, such as CT, MRI, etc. Immobolity of rectal mucosa is indicative of involvement of the rectal mucosa in this case.

**Q. What should be the line of treatment in the above-mentioned case studies 3, 4 and 5 (stage IIB, III and IV)?**

**Ans.** In stage IIB, III and IV cancer as the tumor invades local organs, radiation therapy has become the mainstay of treatment. However, in some cases combination chemotherapy and radiotherapy is also employed. Patients with distant metastases (stage IVB) also require chemotherapy with or without radiotherapy to control systemic disease. Recently, the combination of cisplatin and topotecan is being preferred rather than use of single-agent cisplatin.

In advanced cases of cervical cancer, the most extreme surgery, called pelvic exenteration in which all of the organs of the pelvis including the bladder and rectum are removed, may be employed. This operation may also involve creating two stomas: a colostomy and a urostomy as well as reconstruction of a new vagina.

**Q. How is radiation therapy administered?**

**Ans.** Two types of radiation therapy can be administered in cases of carcinoma cervix: internal radiation therapy and external radiation therapy.

Internal radiation therapy also known as brachytherapy involves placing the selectron tubes inside the patient's vagina. This method helps in delivering radiation directly to the cervix and the surrounding areas.

External radiation therapy involves administration of radiation beams from a large machine onto the body where the cancer is located. External radiotherapy is normally administered on an outpatient basis. The treatments are usually given from Monday to Friday, with a rest at the weekend.

**Q. What complications can occur due to surgery?**

**Ans.** Complications which may occur due to radical hysterectomy are tabulated in Table 9.7.

**Q. What are the complications which can occur due to radiotherapy?**

**Ans.** During the acute phase of pelvic radiation, the surrounding normal tissues such as the intestines, the bladder and the perineum skin are often affected. As a result, radiotherapy to the pelvic area can cause side-effects such as tiredness, diarrhea and dysuria. These side-effects can vary in severity depending on the strength of the radiotherapy dose and the length of treatment. Some of the complications which can occur due to radiotherapy are described below:

- *Cystourethritis:* Inflammation of bladder and urethra can result in complications like dysuria, increased urinary frequency, and nocturia. Antispasmodic medicines are often helpful in providing symptomatic relief. Urine should be examined for possible infection. If urinary tract infection is diagnosed, therapy should be instituted without delay.
- *Gastrointestinal side effects:* Gastrointestinal side-effects due to radiotherapy include diarrhea, abdominal cramping, rectal discomfort, bleeding, etc. Diarrhea can be either controlled by loperamide (Imodium) or diphenoxylate (lomotil). Small, steroid-containing enemas are prescribed to alleviate symptoms resulting from proctitis.
- *Sore skin:* Radiotherapy can result in erythema and desquamation of skin.
- *Tiredness:* Radiotherapy can result in extreme tiredness. Therefore, the patient must be advised to take as much rest as possible.
- *Bowel complaints:* In a small number of cases, the bowel may be permanently affected by the radiotherapy resulting in continued diarrhea. The blood vessels in the bowel can become more fragile after radiotherapy treatment, resulting in hematochezia.
- *Vaginal stenosis:* Radiotherapy to the pelvis can cause narrowing and shortening of the vaginal orifice, thereby making sexual intercourse difficult or uncomfortable. This problem can be overcome by prescribing estrogen creams to the patient. Using vaginal dilators or having regular penetrative sex often helps in maintaining suppleness of the vaginal orifice.

| Table 9.7: Complications due to radical hysterectomy | |
|---|---|
| *Acute complications* | *Chronic complications* |
| • Hemorrhage, infection, shortened vagina, bowel obstruction | • Bladder dysfunction (particularly difficulty in voiding) |
| • Fistula formation (ureterovaginal/vesicovaginal, rectovaginal fistulas) | • Lymphocyst formation |
| • Pulmonary embolus | • Lymphedema |
| • Small bowel obstruction | • Premature menopause |
| • Febrile morbidity (due to pelvic infection, urinary tract infection, wound infection, pelvic abscess, phlebitis, etc. | • Stricture and fibrosis of the intestine or rectosigmoid colon and bladder |

- *Lymphedema:* Lymphedema resulting in the swelling of one or both the legs can commonly occur as a complication of radiotherapy or due to the cancer per se in advanced stages.

### Q. What is the significance of postcoital bleeding?

**Ans.** Postcoital bleeding usually indicates a structural lesion of the cervix or vagina. Various causes of postcoital/postmenopausal bleeding are enumerated in Table 9.8. Infectious etiologies such as *Chlamydia* and *Gonorrhea* are common causes of postcoital bleeding, which must be excluded and treated if required. Uterine or cervical polyps may also be a source of bleeding. Dysplastic or malignant lesions of the cervical or vaginal epithelium may cause irregular or postcoital bleeding. Therefore it is especially important to rule out the presence of cervical/vaginal malignancy in these cases.

## Case Study 6

Mrs XYZ, a 32-year-old, resident of ABC, G3P2A0L2 woman presented to the ANC clinic having 24 weeks amenorrhea with the complaints of vaginal bleeding and discharge since past few days. The patient gave history of being diagnosed with cervical cancer a year back. On per abdominal examination, abdomen was enlarged to 24-weeks gestation with a single live fetus in cephalic presentation. On per speculum examination, an irregular lesion was observed at the 3 O' clock position of the cervix. The lesion bled on touch. Before performing a per vaginal examination, the placental position was localized on ultrasound examination. On vaginal examination, uterus appeared soft, 24 weeks in size with a single live fetus. The cervix was long, uneffaced, closed and fixed. Vaginal fornices were free, but the vaginal wall was involved up to the upper-third. Per rectal examination was within normal limits.

### Q. What is the most likely diagnosis in the previously-mentioned case study?

**Ans.** The most likely diagnosis in the above-mentioned case study is Mrs XYZ, a 32-year-old, resident of ABC, G3P2A0L2 woman with complaints of 24 weeks amenorrhea, corresponding to 24 weeks gestation having a single live fetus in cephalic presentation with a diagnosed case of carcinoma cervix (FIGO stage IIA), also confirmed on clinical examination.

### Q. How should the diagnosis of cervical cancer be established in a pregnant patient with cervical cancer?

**Ans.** Pregnancy does not change the course of cervical cancer. The rate of cervical cancer in pregnant patients is similar to that in nonpregnant patients of the same age. Diagnosis usually requires the performance of a cone biopsy, which carries increased risks of hemorrhage and poor perinatal outcome in the first trimester. Conization must not be therefore performed before the second trimester of pregnancy. Also, it must be performed in patients in whom colposcopy findings are consistent with cancer; there is presence of biopsy proven microinvasive cancer or strong cytological evidence of invasive cancer. Following conization, there is no harm in delaying definitive treatment until fetal maturity is achieved in patients with cervical cancer.

### Q. What are the likely complications which can occur due to presence of cervical cancer in pregnant woman?

**Ans.** The following complications can occur due to the presence of carcinoma cervix in pregnant women:

- Preterm labor.
- PPROM.
- Irregular vaginal bleeding.
- Chronic vaginal discharge.
- Urinary tract infection.
- Fetal growth restriction.

### Q. What are the management options in a pregnant patient with cervical cancer?

**Ans.** Clinical stage of cervical cancer is the most important prognostic factor during pregnancy. Patients with cervical invasion between 3 mm and 5 mm and evidence of lymphovascular space invasion can be followed up to term and delivered after establishment of fetal pulmonary maturity. They may have cesarean delivery, immediately followed by modified radical hysterectomy and pelvic lymphadenectomy.

Patients having more than 5 mm cervical invasion should be treated as having a frankly invasive cancer. The recommended treatment option in these cases is classical cesarean delivery followed by radical hysterectomy and pelvic lymphadenectomy.

| **Table 9.8:** Various causes of postcoital bleeding | |
|---|---|
| *Region* | *Pathology* |
| Vulva | Vulval trauma, vaginitis and benign or malignant lesions of vulva |
| Vagina | Senile/atrophic vaginitis, vaginal tumors |
| Cervix | Cervical erosions, cervicitis, polyps, decubitus ulcers, malignancy |
| Uterus | Senile endometritis, tubercular endometritis, endometrial hyperplasia, polyps, endometrial cancer, DUB, metropathia hemorrhagica |
| Fallopian tube | Malignancy |
| Ovaries | Benign ovarian tumor, granulosa or theca cell tumors |
| Systemic diseases | Hypertension, blood dyscrasias |
| Medicines | Unopposed estrogen, cyclical HRT |
| Infections | *Chlamydia* and *Gonorrhea* infections |

*Abbreviations:* DUB, dysfunctional uterine bleeding; HRT, hormone replacement therapy

Stage III and IV disease must be treated with radiotherapy. If the fetus is viable, it must be delivered by classical cesarean birth and radiation therapy must be started postoperatively.

Most clinicians advocate cesarean delivery in cases with cervical cancer, because of the possibility of the recurrence of the disease at the site of episiotomy. Furthermore, vaginal delivery through a cervix with advanced cervical cancer is associated with an increased risk for hemorrhage, obstructed labor and infection.

### Q. How may the treatment for cervical cancer affect the patient's sexual life?

**Ans.** Removal of ovaries at the time of hysterectomy can result in an early menopause. The symptoms of the menopause can include hot flushes, dryness of skin and vagina, anxiety and loss of interest in sexual activity. Radiotherapy can cause cervical stenosis and fibrosis, which can result in pain and discomfort at the time of sexual intercourse.

### Q. Should hormone replacement therapy be used in women who have undergone treatment for cervical cancer?

**Ans.** Bothersome symptoms such as vasomotor symptoms, vaginal dryness or dyspareunia can result from treatment-induced early menopause. Hormone replacement therapy appears to be a safe treatment option for women with cervical cancer who experience troublesome symptoms following treatment.

# Carcinoma Endometrium

## Case Study 1

Mrs XYZ, a 55-year-old woman, resident of ABC, nulliparous, married since last 20 years, presented to the gynecological emergency with a severe episode of bleeding in the morning. She had attained menopause at the age of 48 years. The patient does not give any positive family history of cancer. She gives a history of undergoing treatment in the past which she was supposed to take on the first 5 days of the cycle. According to the patient, this was for treatment of her infertility. She also had been prescribed treatment for her excessive facial hair and advised to reduce her weight. She was unable to conceive despite of taking treatment. At the time of general physical examination her body mass index (BMI) was 27 (obese range) and blood pressure was 150/90 mm Hg.

### Q. What is the most likely diagnosis in the above-mentioned case study?

**Ans.** The above-mentioned case study corresponds to a case of abnormal uterine bleeding (AUB). The questions to be asked at the time of taking history and the parameters to be assessed at the time of examination in such a case are described in Tables 9.9 and 9.10 respectively. The most likely diagnosis in this case is Mrs XYZ, a 55-year-old woman, with an active married life of 20 years, resident of

ABC, nulliparous with chief complaint of having an episode of AUB, the cause of which must be established by doing several investigations. Since the patient is postmenopausal and appears to have risk factors associated with the development of endometrial cancer, investigations need to be done to rule out its presence.

### Q. In the previously mentioned case study what does the patient's history suggest? How is it significant regarding her current situation?

**Ans.** The history of the patient suggests that she most probably suffered from chronic anovulation as a result of polycystic ovarian disease. She was most probably prescribed clomiphene citrate for ovulation induction. Chronic anovulation is likely to cause unopposed endometrial stimulation with estrogen, resulting in development of endometrial hyperplasia and/or cancer in the long run. There are also other risk factors in the patient's history such as nulliparity, high BMI (obesity), high blood pressure and the patient belonging to perimenopausal age group, which point towards a high risk for development of endometrial malignancy.

### Q. What should be the next line of management in the above-mentioned case study?

**Ans.** The most serious concern in postmenopausal and perimenopausal women with AUB is endometrial carcinoma. Since the woman in the previously mentioned case study belongs to the perimenopausal age group, and also has numerous other factors associated with a high risk for development of endometrial cancer, investigations must be mainly directed towards ruling out endometrial cancer. This mainly involves the assessment of endometrial thickness using TVS and study of endometrial cytology using endometrial biopsy, aspiration, D&C or hysteroscopic guided D&C.

### Q. What is AUB and what are its likely causes?

**Ans.** AUB can be defined as any deviation in the normal frequency, duration or amount of menstrual blood loss in a woman belonging to the reproductive age group. It also includes any bleeding from the uterus other than the normal menstrual blood loss. The parameters for normal menstrual blood loss are shown in Table 9.11. AUB can occur due to several causes. AUB in young girls, who have not yet attained menarche, is usually due to sexual abuse and cancer. It is important to rule out pregnancy and its related complications in women of childbearing age. AUB can also occur after menopause. In these cases, unpredictable bleeding may occur 12 months or more after the cessation of periods. Of all the postmenopausal women presenting with AUB, 5–10% may have endometrial carcinoma. Other potential causes of bleeding include cervical cancer, cervicitis, atrophic vaginitis, endometrial atrophy, submucous fibroids, endometrial hyperplasia and endometrial polyps. The most important

| **Table 9.9:** Symptoms to be elicited at the time of taking history in a case of carcinoma endometrium/AUB |
|---|

*History of Presenting Complains*

*Abnormal perimenopausal and postmenopausal bleeding should always be taken seriously and properly investigated, no matter how minimal or nonpersistent.* Detailed history for assessing the nature of blood loss needs to be taken from the patient by elucidating the patient's clinical presentation. Some of these questions are described below.

*Nature of bleeding:* The clinician needs to ask questions to determine the pattern of bleeding: amount of bleeding; the time of bleeding (the days in the menstrual cycle during which the bleeding occurs); intermenstrual intervals (between the episodes of bleeding) and cycle regularity (whether the bleeding pattern is regular or irregular).

*Amount of bleeding*: Initially the clinician needs to establish whether the woman is having heavy, light or moderate amount of blood loss. Some questions which the clinician can ask in order to assess the amount of blood loss are as follows:

- Total number of pads or tampons used by the patient during the heaviest days of her bleeding. This can give a rough estimation of the amount of bleeding, though the number of pads used for the same amount of bleeding may vary from woman to woman depending on their hygienic preferences.
- How frequently does she require changing her pads during the day?
- Does she have to use double protection? (e.g. simultaneous use of a tampon and pad or use of double pads. For the purpose of calculating the amount of blood loss, it can be assumed that an average tampon holds 5 mL and the average pad holds 5–15 mL of blood).
- Does she have to get up in the night to change her protection?
- Is there any history of passage of blood clots? Presence of blood clots is usually indicative of heavy bleeding.
- Does she stain her bedding or clothes despite wearing tampons and pads?
- Does she ever experience "flooding" or sudden rushing out of a large quantity of blood?
- Does she have to stay at home or take time off work during the episode of bleeding?
- How long do her periods last?
- Is the amount of bleeding so much as to interfere with the patient's lifestyle?
- Is there constant pain in the lower abdomen during menstrual periods?
- Are the menstrual periods irregular?
- Does she experience tiredness, fatigue or shortness of breath (symptoms of anemia)?
- The type of sanitary protection being used by the patient is also important since the patient may be required to less frequently change the newer absorbent pads in comparison to the home-made cloth-based sanitary protection.

*Duration of bleeding:* Bleeding occurring for more than 7 days at a stretch can be considered as prolonged.

*Pattern of bleeding:* Sudden change in the bleeding pattern, for example, excessive bleeding at regular intervals, which suddenly becomes irregular must be regarded with caution. In these cases, investigations must be undertaken to discover the exact pathology.

*Smell:* Presence of a foul-smelling vaginal discharge points towards the presence of infection or a necrotic malignant growth. Malignant growths often undergo necrosis in the areas of reduced blood supply.

*Relation of bleeding to sexual intercourse:* Bleeding following sexual intercourse is usually related to the lesions of cervix or vagina. *If a woman presents with the history of postcoital bleeding, cervical cancer must be specifically ruled out.*

Other temporal associations of the bleeding episode whether postpartum, or post-pill, also need to be asked.

*History Based on Patient's Age*

Patient's age can provide important pointer towards the diagnosis of underlying pathology.
The endometrial cancer peaks in the age group of 55–70 years.

*Women of reproductive age group:* The most common cause of abnormal bleeding patterns in women belonging to the reproductive age group is pregnancy-related complications. Since pregnancy-related bleeding must be considered as the first differential diagnosis in the women of childbearing age who present with AUB, it is important to take history of the period of amenorrhea preceding the episode of blood loss or having a positive pregnancy test during that period. Potential causes of pregnancy-related bleeding include spontaneous miscarriage, ectopic pregnancy, placenta previa, abruptio placentae, trophoblastic disease, etc. Uterine leiomyomas are a common cause for menorrhagia in the women belonging to reproductive age group.

*Young patients:* The most common etiology in a young patient having irregular menses since menarche is anovulation. The following questions need to be asked in these patients:

- *Sexual activity/history of vaginal infection*
- *History of chronic anovulation* (e.g. that associated with PCOS): It is associated with unopposed estrogen stimulation. Presence of hirsutism or excessive growth of facial hair, obesity and acne point towards PCOS. Polycystic ovarian syndrome is associated with unopposed estrogen stimulation, elevated androgen levels, and insulin resistance and is a common cause of anovulation. Women with feminizing ovarian tumors are associated with unopposed estrogen production, which acts as a risk factor for endometrial cancer.

*(Contd...)*

*(Contd...)*

- *History of galactorrhea or secretion of milk from breasts:* Any patient complaining of a milky discharge from either breast (while not pregnant, postpartum or breastfeeding) needs estimation of prolactin levels to rule out the presence of a pituitary tumor. Galactorrhea could be related to underlying hyperprolactinemia, which can cause oligo-ovulation or eventual amenorrhea.
- *History of any eating disorder, stress, etc.:* It is important to elicit the history of any eating disorders/stress, etc. Hypothalamic suppression secondary to eating disorders, stress or excessive exercise may induce anovulation, which sometimes manifests as irregular and heavy menstrual bleeding or amenorrhea.
- *History of pain in the abdomen:* Pain in the abdomen could be indicative of underlying malignancy.
- *History of foul-smelling discharge per vaginum:* This could be related to the presence of sexually transmitted diseases or carcinoma cervix. Age is an important consideration in these cases because women in reproductive age groups are more likely to suffer from sexually transmitted diseases while diagnosis of cervical cancer is more likely in older women.
- *Presence of pressure symptoms:* This could be related to the presence of a large pelvic mass (uterine or adnexal mass) pressing upon the bladder or rectum resulting in pressure symptoms like increased urinary frequency and/or rectal symptoms such as constipation, tenesmus, etc.
- *Plans regarding future fertility and contraception:* It is important to take the patient's history regarding her plans for future fertility and childbearing in order to decide appropriate patient management, e.g. decision for hysterectomy must be avoided as far as possible in a young women desiring future fertility.
- *Symptoms suggestive of pregnancy:* Symptoms suggestive of pregnancy, e.g. morning sickness, breast changes, etc. also need to be enquired from the patient.
- *Previous Pap smears*: History of undergoing Pap smears in the past needs to be elicited. Previous normal Pap smears help in ruling out cervical malignancy.
- *History of genital trauma:* Genital trauma may result in bleeding from the vagina or rectum. It is especially important to rule out sexual abuse in young girls, presenting with bleeding who have yet not attained menarche.

### Past Treatment/Drug History

- *History of drug intake:* Intake of drugs such as anticoagulants (e.g. warfarin); hormones (e.g. unopposed estrogen, tamoxifen, etc.); selective serotonin reuptake inhibitors; antipsychotics; corticosteroids, etc. may typically cause bleeding. Thus, the patient should be asked if she had been prescribed any of the above-mentioned medicines in the past. Since herbal substances, such as ginseng, ginkgo and soy supplements, may also cause menstrual irregularities, history of intake of such products must also be taken.
- *History of contraceptive use (intrauterine device or hormones):* Commonly, an IUD causes increased uterine cramping and menstrual flow.
- *Use of unopposed estrogen without combination with progesterone (in form of oral contraceptive pills or HRT):* Use of unopposed estrogen (without combination of progesterone) may predispose the woman to develop endometrial hyperplasia or cancer in future.
- History of intake of drugs such as tamoxifen, usually administered for treatment of breast cancer.

### Menstrual History

The history of menstrual cycles before the occurrence of episode of abnormal bleeding, including features such as duration of bleeding, the cycle length, whether cycles were regular or irregular, whether there was pain during cycles, etc. needs to be enquired. The age of menarche and that at which menopause was attained also needs to be asked. Endometrial cancer is also more common in women who have had early menarche and late menopause. These factors are likely to result in a prolonged or unopposed exposure of the endometrium to estrogen, which may result in an increased risk for development of endometrial cancer.

### Obstetric History

Eliciting the patient's obstetric history is particularly important because certain pathological conditions (e.g. endometrial malignancy and uterine leiomyomas) are more likely to develop in nulliparous women. Since nulliparity acts as a risk factor for the development of both endometrial carcinoma and uterine leiomyomas, the two are frequently observed to coexist together. On the other hand, conditions like cervical malignancy are more likely to develop in multiparous women.

### Past Medical History

- *Past history of chronic illness:* The patient should be asked about the past history of any chronic medical illness like diabetes mellitus, hypertension, CAD, etc. and obesity. This is especially important because the triad of obesity, hypertension and diabetes is associated with an increased risk of endometrial cancer.
- *Symptoms of thyroid dysfunction:* The alteration of the hypothalamic-pituitary axis may result in either amenorrhea (hyperthyroidism) or menorrhagia (hypothyroidism).
- *Hepatic/renal failure:* History suggestive of systemic illnesses, including hepatic/renal failure needs to be asked. The disorders of these organs are likely to result in bleeding abnormalities.
- *History of excessive bruising or known bleeding/coagulation disorders:* AUB could be related to the presence of an underlying coagulation disorder.

### Family History

- Personal or family history of endometrial, ovarian or breast cancer is another predisposing factor for development of endometrial cancer.

*Abbreviations:* AUB, abnormal uterine bleeding; CAD, coronary artery disease; HRT, hormone replacement therapy; IUD, intrauterine device; PCOS, polycystic ovarian syndrome

**Table 9.10:** Various findings elicited at the time of clinical examination in a case of carcinoma endometrium/AUB

*General Physical Examination*

*Body mass index:* Obese women (with increased BMI) are more likely to be suffering from endometrial malignancies.

*Blood pressure:* Increased blood pressure could be related with an increased risk for endometrial cancer.

*Pallor:* Pallor could be related to anemia caused by excessive blood loss.

*Endocrinopathy:* The clinician must look for following signs in order to rule out the  presence of an endocrinopathy:

- Signs of hyperthyroidism and hypothyroidism.
- *Galactorrhea:* This could be related to increased prolactin production.

*Specific Systemic Examination*

At the time of systemic examination, efforts must be made to rule out the presence of any systemic anomaly (e.g. hypertension, diabetes, asthma, etc.), which could affect the patient's fitness for gynecological/surgical treatment of the diagnosed pathology.

*Per Speculum Examination*

Per speculum examination helps in identifying any trauma or bleeding causing lesions of vagina, cervix, etc. (e.g. cervical erosion, ulcer, growth, polyp, hypertrophy, etc.)

*Abdominal Examination*

Abdominal examination must be performed to detect the presence of hepatic and splenic enlargement or presence of any abdominal mass.

*Pelvic Examination*

A bimanual examination may reveal enlargement due to uterine fibroids, adenomyosis or endometrial carcinoma. An enlarged uniformly shaped uterus in a postmenopausal patient with bleeding suggests endometrial cancer until proven otherwise.

*Abbreviation:* BMI, body mass index

**Table 9.11:** Parameters for normal and abnormal menstrual blood loss

|  | Normal | Abnormal |
|---|---|---|
| Duration | 4–6 days | < 2 or > 7 days |
| Volume | 30 mL | < 30 mL or > 80 mL |
| Interval | 24–35 days | < 21 days or > 35 days |

thing to remember is that AUB could be a sign of a serious underlying health problem such as endometrial malignancy.

**Q. What is the prime responsibility of the clinician while evaluating AUB in women belonging to perimenopausal and menopausal groups?**

**Ans.** The prime responsibility of the clinician is to rule out the presence of endometrial malignancy in case of AUB, especially in women of perimenopausal and menopausal age groups. Presence of endometrial hyperplasia/malignancy must be ruled out in all postmenopausal women presenting with bleeding, especially those having risk factors for endometrial malignancy. Cervical cytology (Pap smear) is helpful in diagnosis of cervical malignancy, whereas endometrial studies are required to rule out endometrial malignancies. Various endometrial studies, which help in detecting underlying endometrial malignancy, include tests like EB, endometrial aspiration, dilatation and curettage, fractional curettage, etc. These would be described in details, later in the chapter.

**Q. What are the features indicative of presence of endometrial malignancy in a case presenting with AUB at the time of taking history?**

**Ans.** The pointers in the history of bleeding, indicative of underlying malignancy in case of AUB include the following:

- Sudden change in the bleeding pattern
- Irregular bleeding
- Intermenstrual bleeding
- Postcoital bleeding
- Dyspareunia, pelvic pain
- Lower extremity edema, which could be secondary to metastasis.

**Q. What is the most common type of endometrial cancer on histopathological diagnosis?**

**Ans.** Most cases of endometrial cancer are histologically of adenomatous type. The endometrioid type of adenocarcinoma accounts for about 80% of endometrial cancers. The endometrial cancers can be of different grades (G1, G2 and G3) based on the degree of cellular differentiation, anaplasia and glandular architecture, with higher grade of tumor associated with a worse prognosis.

**Q. What investigations must be performed in a woman with AUB?**

**Ans.** The aim of diagnosis in cases of AUB is to assess the nature and severity of bleeding. In case of severe acute bleeding, the aim of management is to stabilize the patient by maintaining the airway, breathing and circulation. In cases of severe bleeding, the emergency control of bleeding can be done through administration of conjugated estrogen. Once the bleeding has been controlled, steps must be taken to identify the underlying organic causes. The investigations which need to be undertaken are described next:

- *Complete blood count:* Estimation of the patient's hemoglobin levels with blood counts would help in determining the patient's degree of anemia. Chronic blood loss related to AUB may often result in the development of anemia.
- *Urine human chorionic gonadotropin levels:* Pregnancy remains the most common cause of AUB in patients of reproductive age group. Bleeding could be related to pregnancy complications including threatened abortion, incomplete abortion or ectopic pregnancy. Therefore, pregnancy should be the first diagnosis to be excluded in women of reproductive age group before instituting further testing or medications.
- *Study of coagulation factors:* Tests involving study of coagulation factors include prothrombin time, partial thromboplastin time, bleeding time, platelet count, assessment of Von Willebrand factor, etc. These tests are not routinely ordered because they are expensive and the bleeding disorders are rarely encountered. These tests are only ordered in cases of suspected coagulation disorders.
- *Thyroid function tests:* Though thyroid dysfunction can result in menorrhagia, thyroid function should not be routinely carried out on women with heavy menstrual bleeding. Thyroid testing should only be carried out when the patient shows signs and symptoms, suggestive of thyroid disease.
- *Liver function and/or renal function tests:* Dysfunction of either organ can alter coagulation factors and/or the metabolism of hormones resulting in abnormal bleeding patterns. Liver function tests are ordered when liver disease is suspected, such as in persons with alcoholism or hepatitis.
- *Hormone assays:* Measurement of luteinizing hormone (LH), follicle-stimulating hormone (FSH) and androgen levels help in diagnosing patients with suspected PCOS.
- *Ultrasound examination:* Pelvic ultrasound is the best noninvasive imaging investigation to assess uterine shape, size and contour; endometrial thickness and adnexal areas. Transabdominal sonography (TAS) helps in excluding pelvic masses, and various pregnancy-related complications. It helps in delineating the presence of an enlarged uterine cavity and/or presence of cystic/solid spaces within the uterine cavity. Transvaginal sonography (TVS) complemented by Doppler ultrasonography may be more informative than TAS. Transvaginal ultrasound is especially indicated in the women at high risk for endometrial cancer.

Measurement of endometrial thickness on transvaginal ultrasound has become a routine investigation in patients with AUB, especially those belonging to the postmenopausal age groups. If the endometrial thickness on TVS is more than or equal to 4 mm, an endometrial sample should be taken to exclude endometrial hyperplasia. Increased endometrial thickness on transvaginal ultrasound examination is an indication for further follow-up by saline infusion sonography (SIS) or endometrial sampling or hysteroscopic-guided EB. Histopathological examination is especially important in these cases to rule out endometrial hyperplasia, atypia and carcinoma. Endometrial sampling is not usually required in case the endometrial thickness is less than 4 mm.

- *Saline infusion sonography:* Saline infusion sonography employs the use of sterile saline solution as a negative contrast medium in conjunction with traditional transvaginal ultrasound.
- *Endometrial studies:* In case the endometrial thickness is more than 4 mm on transvaginal ultrasound examination, endometrial studies particularly endometrial sampling should be done in order to exclude endometrial hyperplasia. Endometrial sampling can be performed in an outpatient setting, most commonly using a pipelle device, without any requirement for anesthesia and is a noninvasive procedure.
- *Endometrial biopsy:* Endometrial biopsy is the most commonly used diagnostic test for AUB, which helps in providing histopathological examination of the endometrium.

### Q. What are the indications for endometrial biopsy?

**Ans.** Indications for endometrial biopsy are as follows:
- Endometrial thickness on TVS is greater than or equal to 4 mm (in postmenopausal women)
- Persistent intermenstrual bleeding
- AUB in a woman over 35 years of age
- AUB in postmenopausal women
- Treatment failure or ineffective treatment
- Patients having high risk factors for the development of endometrial cancer
- There is a pelvic mass and the uterus is larger than 10 weeks of gestation in size
- There is a pelvic mass and no facility for urgent ultrasound scan is available.

### Q. What is the significance of various histological findings on endometrial biopsy?

**Ans.** Histological examination of endometrial curettings is important because even if it does not reveal frank malignancy, it may show evidence of hyperplasia. Endometrial hyperplasia, especially that associated with atypia could act as a precursor of endometrial carcinoma in the long run. Some histological findings which can be observed on endometrial biopsy are as follows:

*Endometrial hyperplasia:* Chronic proliferation of the endometrium results in the development of hyperplasia (first simple hyperplasia, followed by atypical hyperplasia), leading to the development of endometrial carcinoma in future. Endometrial hyperplasia usually results from unopposed estrogen production, regardless of the etiology. If a woman takes unopposed estrogen (without progesterone), her relative risk of developing endometrial cancer is 2.3 compared to that of nonusers and increases to 9.5, if unopposed estrogen is taken for 10 years or longer.

Endometrial hyperplasia can be classified as simple (cystic) or complex (adenomatous), with or without cytological atypia.

*Simple endometrial hyperplasia:* This type of endometrial hyperplasia is associated with an increase in the number of glands and endometrial stroma. Some glands are cystically dilated. However, epithelium does not show any atypical features.

*Simple endometrial hyperplasia with atypia:* Endometrial hyperplasia with cytological atypia has high chance for progression into adenocarcinoma, if left untreated. These lesions must be regarded as precancerous lesions. Atypical lesions are distinguished from invasive cancer by the absence of stromal invasion.

*Complex endometrial hyperplasia—without atypia:* There is an increase in the number of glands which are aligned back-to-back. Glandular outlines are irregular. Complex proliferation of the epithelium occurs but without any associated atypical features. Some physicians treat complex hyperplasia with hormonal therapy (medroxyprogesterone 10–20 mg daily for up to 3 months).

*Complex endometrial hyperplasia—with atypia:* Besides the above-mentioned changes associated with complex endometrial hyperplasia, epithelium also shows features of atypia (hyperchromatism, mitotic figures, etc.).

### Q. How is endometrial sampling done?

**Ans.** For the details related to the Procedure of endometrial sampling aspiration, kindly refer to chapter 10.

### Q. When should hysteroscopy be performed in cases of AUB?

**Ans.** Hysteroscopy with biopsy can be regarded as the "gold standard" investigation for the diagnosis of AUB. Hysteroscopy allows for direct visualization of the endometrial cavity along with the facility for directed biopsy. Hysteroscopy with biopsy provides the most comprehensive evaluation of the endometrium and is recommended for use in any woman with equivocal or suspicious findings on biopsy or ultrasonography. Some of the indications for use of hysteroscopy are as follows:

- Women with erratic/irregular menstrual bleeding
- Medical therapy has failed to control the bleeding
- Transvaginal ultrasound suggestive of intrauterine pathology such as polyps or submucous fibroids.

### Q. How should AUB be treated?

**Ans.** There are medical, surgical and combined methods for treating AUB. The choice of approach depends on the patient's age (belonging to reproductive or perimenopausal age group), etiology and severity of bleeding, patient's fertility status, need for contraception and treatment options available at the care site. Besides using general measures like treatment of iron deficiency and maintenance of menstrual calendar, various medical and surgical modalities of treatment are described below:

- *Medical treatment:* Medical treatment (COCs, medroxyprogesterone acetate, etc.) is the option of choice in young women (< 20 years of age) presenting with atypical bleeding. In these cases, surgery is rarely indicated. Medical treatment with conjugated estrogen is also indicated in cases of acute, heavy and uncontrollable bleeding.
- *Surgical treatment:* Surgical options used for treatment of AUB can be of two types: uterine conservative surgery (endometrial ablation) and hysterectomy.
  - *Endometrial ablation:* Has been described later in the text
  - *Hysterectomy:* Hysterectomy can be performed by the following routes: abdominal, vaginal or laparoscopic.

### Q. Describe the staging of endometrial cancer.

**Ans.** Staging of endometrial cancer is described in the Table 9.12. Total extrafascial hysterectomy with bilateral salpingo-oophorectomy with pelvic and para-aortic lymph node dissection is the standard procedure used for staging endometrial cancer. If metastases are evident, cytoreduction may be performed. Surgery alone is curative for women who are at a low risk of disease persistence or recurrence. Women with intermediate or high-risk disease may require adjuvant therapy.

### Q. What are the treatment modalities of choice for endometrial cancer?

**Ans.** The treatment of endometrial cancer has been summarized in Tables 9.13 and 9.14. Indications for radiotherapy are tabulated in Table 9.15.

## Fibroid Uterus

### Case Study 1

Mrs XYZ, a 33-year-old P1+0 woman, resident of ABC, married since last 5 years, presented with complaints of excessive menstrual bleeding since last 6 months. Despite of heavy bleeding during the periods, the periods were otherwise regular. The patient was prescribed ibuprofen, but did not show any response to treatment. A D&C was done a month ago which showed benign pathology. Pelvic examination

**Table 9.12:** Staging of endometrial cancer

| Stage | Characteristics |
|---|---|
| Stage I* | Tumor confined to the corpus uteri |
| Stage IA* | No or less than half myometrial invasion |
| Stage IB* | Invasion equal to or more than half of the myometrium |
| Stage II* | Tumor invades cervical stroma, but does not extend beyond the uterus[†] |
| Stage III* | Local and/or regional spread of the tumor |
| Stage IIIA* | Tumor invades the serosa of corpus uteri and/or adnexa[§] |
| Stage IIIB* | Vaginal and/or parametrial involvement[§] |
| Stage IIIC* | Metastasis to pelvic and/or para-aortic lymph nodes[§] |
| Stage IIIC1* | Positive pelvic nodes |
| Stage IIIC2* | Positive para-aortic nodes with or without positive pelvic lymph nodes |
| Stage IV* | Tumor invades bladder and/or bowel mucosa and/or distant metastasis |
| Stage IVA* | Tumor invasion of the bladder and/or bowel mucosa |
| Stage IVB* | Distant metastasis including intra-abdominal metastasis and/or inguinal lymph nodes |

[*] Either G1, G2 or G3
[†] Endocervical glandular involvement only should be considered as stage I and no longer as stage II
[§] Positive cytology has to be reported separately without changing the stage

*Source:* FIGO Committee on Gynecologic Oncology. Revised FIGO staging for carcinoma of the vulva, cervix and endometrium. Int J Gynecol Obstet. 2009;105:103-4.

**Table 9.13:** Treatment of endometrial cancer

| | |
|---|---|
| Stage I and II tumors | Extrafascial total abdominal hysterectomy (TAH) and bilateral salpingo-oophorectomy with lymph node sampling. This may involve the resection of any enlarged nodes, and selective pelvic and para-aortic lymphadenectomy. The procedure also involves peritoneal cytology, thorough exploration of abdomen and pelvis and biopsy of extrauterine lesions. For further management in these patients, kindly refer to Table 9.14. |
| Stage II tumors | Radical hysterectomy with bilateral salpingo-oophorectomy with pelvic lymphadenectomy or use of the same standard surgical approach as described for stage I disease, followed by appropriate pelvic or extended field external and intravaginal irradiation. |
| Stage III tumors | TAH with bilateral salpingo-oophorectomy with selective lymphadenectomy, biopsies of suspicious areas, omental biopsy and debulking of tumor followed by radiotherapy. |
| Stage IV tumors | Palliative chemotherapy, radiotherapy and progestogens. |

**Table 9.14:** Surgical management in patients with stage I and II endometrial cancer following initial treatment

| Histopathological findings | Management option |
|---|---|
| • Grade 1, 2<br>• No or minimal myometrial invasion | Observation |
| • G2, superficial myometrial invasion<br>• G3, no myometrial invasion | Vaginal irradiation |
| • Deep myometrial invasion<br>• Cervical spread<br>• Positive lymph nodes | Pelvic radiotherapy and vaginal boost (extended field of positive para-aortic nodes) |
| • Adnexal spread<br>• Intraperitoneal disease<br>• Completely resected tumor | Whole abdominal radiation or chemotherapy |
| Positive peritoneal cytology | Observation or progestins |

**Table 9.15:** Indications of radiotherapy

*Postoperative vaginal irradiation*

- Stage IA G3 tumors
- Stage IB G1 and G2 tumors
- Stage IB G3 and stage IIA (G1 and G2) tumors

*External pelvic irradiation*

- Tumors in stage IIA (G3) and stage IIB (all grades), stage IIIA (all grades) or with lymphovascular space invasion
- Selected IVA patients
- All patients with positive lymph nodes
- Patients with documented para-aortic and common iliac lymph node involvement

revealed an irregularly enlarged uterus (about 6 weeks in size). The mass was contiguous with the cervix and could not be moved away from the cervix. An ultrasound examination was done, which showed presence of a submucous fibroid about 4 cm in diameter.

### Q. What is the most likely diagnosis in the above-mentioned case study?

**Ans.** The above-mentioned case study corresponds to a case of menorrhagia in which the cause was found to be the submucous fibroid leiomyona as diagnosed on transvaginal ultrasound examination. The questions to be asked at the time of taking history and the parameters to be assessed at the time of examination in such a case are described in Tables 9.16 and 9.17 respectively. The most likely diagnosis in this case is Mrs XYZ, a 33-year-old woman, with an active married life of 5 years, resident of ABC, P1+0 woman with chief complaint of having an episode of menorrhagia, the cause of which appears to be the submucous fibroids (as detected by transvaginal ultrasound examination). In case no investigations had been done in this case, the diagnosis would be a case of menorrhagia in which various investigations need to be performed to diagnose the underlying pathology.

### Q. What is menorrhagia?

**Ans.** Menorrhagia (Greek: meno—uterus; rhegnunai—to burst forth), is the medical terminology which describes the occurrence of heavy or prolonged bleeding during menstrual periods. The bleeding despite of being excessive or heavy occurs at regular intervals. Menorrhagia needs to be distinguished clinically from other common abnormal bleeding patterns including metrorrhagia (flow at irregular intervals), menometrorrhagia (frequent, excessive flow at irregular intervals), polymenorrhea (bleeding at intervals > 21 days) and dysfunctional uterine bleeding (DUB) (abnormal uterine bleeding without any obvious structural or systemic abnormality). Clinically, menorrhagia is defined as total blood loss exceeding 80 mL per cycle or menstrual period lasting longer than 7 days.

### Q. What are the various probable causes of menorrhagia?

**Ans.** Etiology of menorrhagia is divided into four categories, i.e. organic, endocrinologic, anatomic and iatrogenic (Table 9.18). In the previously mentioned case study, menorrhagia probably results due to uterine fibroids.

### Q. What are uterine myomas and what are the different types?

**Ans.** Myomas (fibromyomas, leiomyomas or fibroids) are well-circumscribed benign tumors developing from uterine myometrium, most commonly encountered among women of reproductive age group (30–45 years), with their prevalence ranging between 20% and 40%. A typical myoma is a pale, firm, rubbery, well-circumscribed mass distinct from neighboring tissues and has a whorled appearance due to presence of interlacing fibers of myometrial muscle, separated by varying amount of connective tissue fibers.

Fibroids can be classified as submucosal, intramural or subserosal based on their location within the uterine wall (Fig. 9.2). Of the different types of fibroids, the most common are intramural (interstitial) fibroids, which are present in nearly 75% cases, followed by submucous (15%) and subserous fibroids (10%).

*Submucosal fibroids:* Also known as subendometrial fibroids, these fibroids grow beneath the uterine endometrial lining. This type of fibroid is thought to be primarily responsible for producing prolonged, heavy menstrual bleeding. Submucosal fibroids are most likely to cause distortion of the endometrial cavity.

*Intramural fibroids:* These fibroids are the most common type and are located in the middle of myometrium. Intramural fibroids are also known as interstitial fibroids.

*Subserosal fibroids:* Also known as the pedunculated fibroids, these fibroids grow beneath the serosa, the outer uterine covering. Subserosal fibroids are those in which greater than 50% of the total volume protrudes out of the serosal surface. These types of fibroids are the least common type. Sometimes they may develop a pedicle and extrude out from the surface in form of pedunculated fibroids. Both submucous and subserosal fibroids can be pedunculated.

### Q. What investigations are required in the cases of uterine leiomyomas?

**Ans.** Investigations, which are required in a case of leiomyomas, are as follows:

*Complete blood count along with platelet count and a peripheral smear:* The complete blood count with platelet count must be conducted to rule out the presence of anemia.

*Imaging studies:* Nowadays, ultrasound examination (both transvaginal and transabdominal ultrasound) has become the investigation of choice for diagnosing myomas. Ultrasound examination helps in assessing the overall uterine shape,

**Table 9.16:** Symptoms to be elicited at the time of taking history in a case of uterine leiomyomas

*History of Presenting Complains*

- *Excessive or prolonged menstrual bleeding:* The main symptom attributable to leiomyomas is excessive or prolonged menstrual bleeding. Irregular bleeding is usually not a characteristic symptom of myomas. Therefore, in cases with irregular bleeding, endometrial disease must be ruled out. Every woman suffering from leiomyomas who has continuous or irregular bleeding should be subjected to endometrial aspiration to rule out the presence of endometrial cancer before her treatment is planned. Questions which need to be asked regarding the nature of bleeding, amount of bleeding, duration of bleeding, pattern of bleeding and timing of bleeding have already been described previously in the text.
- *Anemia:* Excessive bleeding, if remains untreated over a long period of time, can result in the development of anemia. Anemia can manifest itself by producing symptoms such as palpitations, lassitude, loss of weight, etc.
- *Pressure symptoms:* These may include symptoms such as backache (due to the pressure on spinal nerves); urinary symptoms, such as increased diurnal frequency and urgency (due to bladder irritability); bowel dysfunction (due to pressure on intestines); rectal tenesmus and constipation (due to pressure on rectum), etc.
- *Pain:* Fibroids are usually not painful. They may give rise to acute pain under exceptional circumstances such as torsion of pedunculated fibroids, degeneration, infection, associated endometriosis and/or expulsion of pedunculated submucous tumors through cervix. Red degeneration of fibroid (described later in the text) during pregnancy can also produce pain.
- *Infertility or pregnancy-related complications:* Besides abnormal bleeding patterns, uterine myomas can also cause infertility or give rise to certain problems during pregnancy. Presently, it is not yet known for sure whether infertility is the cause or the effect of leiomyomas.
- *Asymptomatic:* Despite of the above-mentioned symptoms, majority of the fibroids are asymptomatic.

*Other details:*

Other details which must be elicited while taking history include the following:

- *Patient's age:* As previously mentioned, patient's age can provide important pointer towards the diagnosis of underlying pathology. Uterine leiomyomas are typically more common among patients in the age group of 35–40 years.
- *Obstetric history:* Uterine fibroids are more common in nulliparous women in comparison to the multiparous women.
- *History of contraceptive use (intrauterine device or hormones):* Commonly, an IUD causes increased uterine cramping and menstrual flow.
- *Presence of any coagulation related disorder:* It is important to rule out the presence of any coagulation-related disorders by taking history suggestive of abnormal bleeding from any of the orifices.
- *Symptoms of thyroid dysfunction:* The alteration of the thyroid function may produce menstrual abnormalities like amenorrhea or oligomenorrhea (hypothyroidism) or menorrhagia (hyperthyroidism).
- *History of intake of any medications:* Intake of drugs like hormones or anticoagulants may typically cause bleeding.
- *Plans regarding future fertility and contraception:* These should be ascertained in order to decide appropriate patient management.
- History of undergoing Pap smears in the past.

*Risk Factors*

History related to risk factors, which can result in the development of fibroids, also needs to be taken :

- *Heredity:* Patients with a positive family history of fibroid, especially in the first degree relatives (mother or sister) are especially at an increased risk of developing fibroids.
- *Race:* Black women are more likely to have fibroids than the women of other racial groups.
- *High estrogen levels:* High estrogen levels predispose a woman to develop fibroids. Some factors which may be responsible for an increased risk of fibroids related to hyperestrogenism are as follows:
  - Exposure to OCPs at the age of 13–16 years is associated with a high risk for development of uterine fibroids.
  - Obesity increases the risk probably due to higher levels of endogenous estrogen.
  - Smoking reduces the risk of fibroids by decreasing the levels of endogenous estrogen.
  - Childbearing during the reproductive years (25–29) provides the greatest protection against myoma development by producing amenorrhea (thereby reduced estrogen levels) during pregnancy.
- There is a positive association between fibroids and the pelvic inflammatory disease.

*Abbreviations:* IUD, intrauterine device; OCPs, oral contraceptive pills

size and contour; endometrial thickness; adnexal areas and presence of hydronephrosis. It helps in detection of small, focal, irregular or eccentrically located endometrial lesions.

### Q. What is the management in cases of fibroid uterus?

**Ans.** In case the patient is diagnosed with fibroid uterus, the ultimate treatment depends on factors such as the number of fibroids, size of fibroids, the proximity of the fibroids to the endometrial cavity and severity of symptoms caused by them. The closer the fibroids are to the endometrial cavity, the more they are likely to be symptomatic.

The various treatment options, which can be used in a woman with fibroid uterus, are described in Flow chart 9.1. Various treatment options in a woman with fibroid uterus based on the patient's age and desire for future childbearing is described in Flow chart 9.2. If the woman has completed

**Table 9.17:** Various findings elicited at the time of clinical examination in a case of uterine leiomyomas

*General Physical Examination*

- *Signs of anemia:* Abnormal blood loss, if allowed to continue over a long period of time can result in the development of anemia.

*Specific Systemic Examination*

At the time of systemic examination, efforts must be made to rule out the presence of any systemic anomaly (e.g. hypertension, diabetes, asthma, etc.), which could affect the patient's fitness for gynecological/surgical treatment of the diagnosed pathology.

*Abdominal Examination*

- In case of a large fibroid, the mass may be palpable per abdomen. However, a leiomyoma has to attain the size of approximately 12–14 weeks before the abdominal swelling becomes palpable per abdominally. It may be difficult to detect the leiomyomas smaller than this on abdominal examination.
- In case of uterine fibroids, the mass usually appears to be arising from the pelvis, i.e. it may be difficult to get below the mass. The mass is usually well defined, having a firm consistency and a smooth surface. It is usually movable from side to side, but not from above downwards. If the fibroid has undergone cystic degeneration, it may appear soft and cystic in consistency, rather than hard.
- Presence of multiple fibroids can result in an irregular appearance of the mass.
- The mass is nearly always dull to percussion because the intestines usually lie behind and besides the mass. The mass is rarely tender on touch.
- In case of a single subserous leiomyoma with a long pedicle, it may be difficult to recognize its connection with the uterus. In such cases, it might be difficult to distinguish the fibroid from an ovarian tumor.

*Per Speculum Examination*

To look for any cervical erosion, ulcer, growth, polyp, hypertrophy, etc.

*Pelvic Examination*

- The method of conducting the pelvic and bimanual examination has been discussed in details in Chapter 8. Bimanual examination helps in assessment of uterine size, shape and contour.
- Presence of an enlarged, irregularly shaped, non-tender, mobile uterus with firm consistency is suggestive of fibroids in women aged 30–50 years. The mass may extend into one or more fornices.
- On bimanual examination, it is found that the tumor either replaces the uterus or is attached to the cervix. This is an important point because if the mass was lateral or moved apart from the cervix, the most likely diagnosis would have been presence of an adnexal mass.

**Table 9.18:** Causes of menorrhagia

| *Organic causes* | *Endocrinologic causes* | *Anatomic causes* | *Iatrogenic causes* |
|---|---|---|---|
| • Genitourinary infections<br>• Bleeding disorders<br>• Organ dysfunction: Hepatic or renal failure<br>• Sexual abuse resulting in bleeding from urethra or rectum<br>• Coagulation disorders like von Willebrand's disease; factor II, V, VII and IX deficiencies; prothrombin deficiency; idiopathic thrombocytopenic purpura and thromboasthenia | • Thyroid dysfunction: Hypothyroidism and hyperthyroidism<br>• Adrenal gland dysfunction<br>• Prolactin producing tumors of the pituitary gland<br>• PCOS<br>• Obesity<br>• Vasculature imbalance | • Uterine fibroids<br>• Endometrial polyps<br>• Endometrial hyperplasia<br>• Pregnancy complications (miscarriages)<br>• Adenomyosis<br>• Cancer (uterine, ovarian, cervical) | • IUDs (copper T 380 A/ParaGard)<br>• Steroid hormones: Medroxyprogesterone and other progestins (when stopped), prednisone<br>• Chemotherapy agents (paclitaxel, docetaxel, etc.)<br>• Medications (e.g. anticoagulants like aspirin, warfarin, heparin, etc.) |

*Abbreviations:* IUDs, intrauterine devices; PCOS, polycystic ovarian syndrome

her family and does not wish to preserve her uterus, hysterectomy can be done. Myomectomy is an option for women, who desire future pregnancy or wish to preserve their uterus. However, the women undergoing myomectomy should be counseled regarding the chances of occurrence of massive bleeding during myomectomy and the risk for conversion to hysterectomy at the time of surgery. Once the decision regarding myomectomy has been taken, the next step is deciding the route of myomectomy: hysteroscopic, laparoscopic or abdominal. Hysteroscopic myomectomy should be considered as first-line conservative surgical therapy for the management of symptomatic intracavitary or submucosal fibroids showing minimal myometrial involvement. Uterine artery embolization (UAE) may be

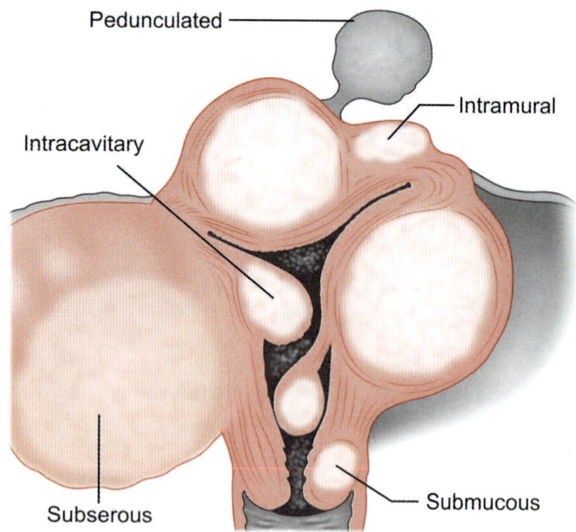



**Fig. 9.2:** Different types of leiomyomas

offered as an alternative to hysterectomy in selected women with symptomatic uterine fibroids who wish to preserve their uterus.

### Q. What would be the best treatment option in the previously-described case study?

**Ans.** Patient's age, desire for future fertility, and number, size and location of uterine myomas are important parameters for deciding the appropriate treatment option. Since the age of woman in the previously-mentioned case study is 33 years and she desires future fertility, myomectomy appears to be the best treatment option. The route for myomectomy needs to be determined based on many factors including the type of myomas, degree of myometrial invasion and number of myomas. The severity of the problem and its duration must also be taken into account. In this case the woman has a submucosal fibroid of size 4 cm on the ultrasound, having less than 50% myometrial invasion. Therefore the best option appears to be hysteroscopic resection.

**Flow chart 9.1:** Treatment options for a patient diagnosed with fibroid uterus

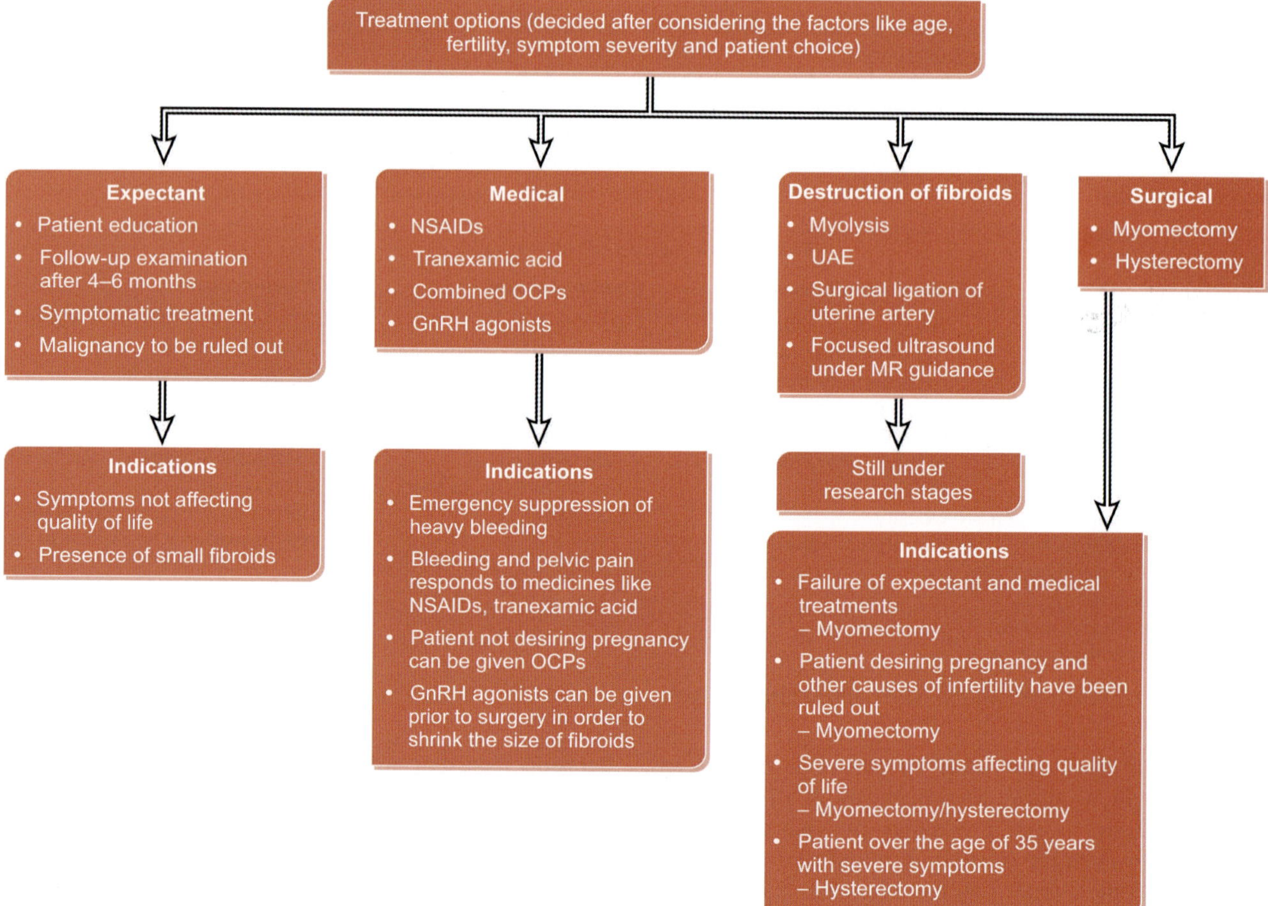



*Abbreviations:* NSAIDs, nonsteroidal anti-inflammatory drugs; OCPs, oral contraceptive pills; GnRH, gonadotropin releasing hormone; UAE, uterine artery embolization; MR, magnetic resonance.

**Flow chart 9.2:** Various treatment options in a woman with fibroid uterus based on the patient's age and desire for future childbearing

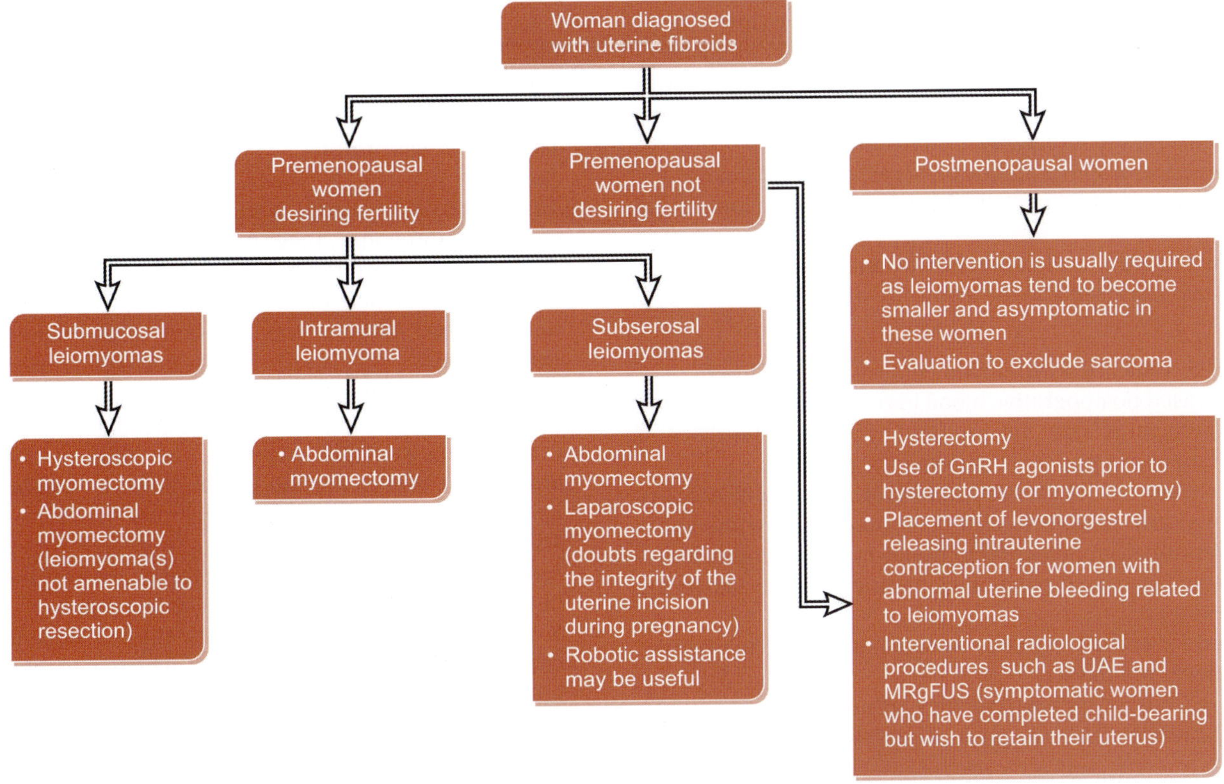


*Abbreviations:* UAE, uterine artery embolization; GnRH, gonadotropin-releasing hormone; MRgFUS, magnetic resonance-guided focused ultrasound surgery

| **Table 9.19:** Medical options available for treatment of menorrhagia |
| --- |

- *Antispasmodic agents:* NSAIDs, buscopan (menstruating days only)
- *Hemostatic agents:* Ethamsylate, tranexamic acid (menstruating days only)
- Combined oral contraceptive pills (day 5–25)
- Progestogens, [e.g. Norethisterone (Primolut N), dydrogesterone (Duphaston) and medroxyprogesterone (Provera)] (day 5–25)
- Hormone replacement therapy
- *Androgens:* Danazol, GnRH therapy (daily continuous therapy)
- Mirena (levonorgestrel intrauterine system)

*Abbreviations:* GnRH, gonadotropin-releasing hormone; NSAIDs, nonsteroidal anti-inflammatory drugs

### Q. What are the various medical therapeutic options for controlling menorrhagia?

**Ans.** Medical therapeutic options for control of menorrhagia in a patient with leiomyomas are described in Table 9.19.

### Q. What are the various surgical options to be used in cases of uterine leiomyomas?

**Ans.** Surgery forms the definite treatment modality for uterine leiomyomas. The three main surgical options, which can be used in the women with leiomyoma uterus include:

myomectomy, hysterectomy and more recently uterine artery embolization (UAE). Women should be informed that having a UAE or myomectomy would potentially allow them to retain their fertility.

### Q. Under what circumstances is surgery indicated?

**Ans.** Besides acting as a definitive cure for myomas, surgical management is also used in the following circumstances:

- Control of excessive uterine bleeding
- Control of pain and symptoms related to excessive pelvic pressure
- History of infertility or recurrent pregnancy loss with distortion of endometrial cavity or tubal occlusion
- Menorrhagia not responding to conservative or other medical treatment modalities
- There is a high clinical suspicion of malignancy
- Growth of fibroid continues even following menopause
- Menorrhagia results in severe iron deficiency anemia
- Recurrent pregnancy losses (all the other causes have been ruled out and uterine fibroids appear to be the most likely cause of recurrent miscarriages).
- Presence of large fibroids (greater than 3 cm in diameter)
- Severe bleeding, having a significant impact on a woman's quality of life, which is refractory to drug therapy.

### Q. When is myomectomy indicated?

**Ans.** Surgical removal of myomas from the uterine cavity is termed as myomectomy. Although myomectomy allows preservation of the uterus, present evidence indicates a higher risk of blood loss and greater operative time with myomectomy in comparison to hysterectomy. Some of the indications for myomectomy are as follows:

- Women with symptomatic myomas, desiring fertility
- Large myomas (especially the submucosal or intramural type)
- When in vitro fertilization (IVF) is indicated (especially if the myoma results in the distortion of the uterine cavity).

### Q. What are the major risks associated with myomectomy?

**Ans.** Risks associated with myomectomy are as follows:

- Increased postoperative blood loss
- Hysterectomy may be required during the surgery, if myomectomy appears dangerous or difficult
- Increased risk of uterine rupture at the time of delivery [can occur irrespective of the route for myomectomy (abdominal, laparoscopic or hysteroscopic myomectomy) due to excessive dissection of myometrial muscles during the surgery]
- Need for mandatory cesarean section in case the patient achieves pregnancy
- Increased risk for postoperative adhesions
- Recurrence of myoma postoperatively.

### Q. What is uterine artery embolization?

**Ans.** Uterine artery embolization is a relatively new, novel technique for treatment of uterine fibroids. It is a nonhysterectomy surgical technique, which helps in reducing the size of the uterine fibroids by shrinking them, without actually removing them. Besides uterine fibroids, the technique of embolization has been used to treat various other medical pathologies like inoperable cancers, brain aneurysms, arteriovenous shunts in the lung, etc.

In this technique, once the fibroids are visualized on X-ray, an embolizing agent [gelatin microspheres (trisacryl gelatin) or polyvinyl alcohol] is injected, which helps in blocking both the uterine arteries, thereby cutting off blood supply to the fibroids. In comparison to normal uterine cells, fibroid cells are much more sensitive to low oxygen saturation. Thus, due to the lack of sufficient blood supply, the fibroids become avascular and shrink, ultimately resulting in cell death, their degeneration and eventual absorption by the myometrium. The normal myometrium, on the other hand, receives new blood supply from vaginal and ovarian vasculature. As fibroids begin to undergo necrosis, any active bleeding commonly subsides. Uterine artery embolization can be an effective treatment for uterine fibroids, especially in women whose symptoms are sufficiently bothersome to warrant myomectomy or hysterectomy.

### Q. What could be the various complications associated with myomas?

**Ans.** Various complications related with uterine myomas include the following:

- Severe pain
- Infertility
- Toxic shock syndrome
- Anemia
- *Torsion:* Torsion of the pedicle of a subserous pedunculated leiomyoma may interfere first with venous, then with the arterial supply. This may result in an initial extravasation of blood followed by the eventual development of gangrene. Torsion is associated with extreme pain.
- *Ascites/Pseudo-Meigs syndrome:* Very mobile pedunculated subserous tumors may produce ascites by causing mechanical irritation of the peritoneum. Sometimes, ascites may be accompanied by a right-sided hydrothorax, resulting in the development of a condition known as Pseudo-Meigs syndrome.
- *Infection:* A submucous leiomyoma may sometimes become infected and ulcerated at its lower pole.
- *Secondary changes (degeneration):* Certain degenerative changes can occur in a fibroid, which can cause an interference with capsular circulation. As a result of the circulatory disturbances, the tumor becomes painful, tender, softened and enlarged. Some such degenerative changes taking place in the fibroids are described below:
  - *Atrophy:* Shrinkage of the fibroid can occur as a result of reduced blood supply to the fibroid, usually following menopause.
  - *Hyaline degeneration:* This is the most common type of degeneration in which the fibrous tissue cells are replaced by a homogeneous substance which stains pink with eosin. The bundles of muscle fibers become isolated and die off causing large areas of the tumor to become structureless. Eventually, the liquefaction of hyaline material occurs, leaving behind ragged cavities filled with colorless or blood-stained fluid.
  - *Calcification:* This type of degeneration may initially occur with the presence of fatty deposits within the leiomyomas. At a later stage in this process, there is deposition of phosphates and carbonates of calcium along the course of blood vessels. Calcification usually begins at the periphery of the fibroid and can be identified with the help of radiography.
  - *Myxomatous/cystic degeneration*
  - *Red/carneous degeneration:* This type of degeneration of uterine fibroid usually develops during pregnancy. It may be associated with constitutional symptoms like malaise, nausea, vomiting, fever and severe abdominal pain. The myoma may become soft and

necrotic in the center and is diffusely stained red or salmon pink in color. Though the pathogenesis of the condition is not yet clear, it is believed that the purple-red color of the myoma is probably due to the thrombosis of blood vessels supplying the tumor. The myoma may also develop a peculiar fishy odor due to infection by the coliform organisms. Although the patient may develop mild leukocytosis and a raised ESR, the condition is essentially an aseptic one. It needs to be differentiated from other conditions including appendicitis, twisted ovarian cyst, accidental hemorrhage, etc. Ultrasound examination usually helps in establishing the correct diagnosis. Red degeneration occurring during pregnancy must be managed conservatively. The patient must be advised bed rest and prescribed analgesics to relieve the pain. The acute symptoms subside gradually within the course of 3–10 days and pregnancy then proceeds uneventfully.

- *Sarcomatous change:* Occurrence of malignant changes in a leiomyoma is an extremely rare occurrence. A suspicion of malignancy must be kept in mind in case of sudden increase in the size of fibroid, sudden development of pain or tenderness in the myoma, systemic upset and pyrexia or postmenopausal bleeding.

### Q. What are the possible effects of fibroids on pregnancy?

**Ans.** Presence of fibroids during pregnancy can result in an increased risk of the following pregnancy-related complications, especially if the placenta implants over or is in close proximity to a myoma:

- Miscarriage
- First trimester bleeding
- Abruption (large fibroids, usually greater than 20 cm in diameter are more likely to cause abruption and abdominal pain)
- Prelabor rupture of membranes or preterm labor
- Intrauterine growth restriction
- Prolonged/obstructed labor
- Very large-sized uterine myomas can cause respiratory embarrassment and urinary retention.

Fibroids located in the lower uterine segment may be associated with an increased likelihood of the following complications:

- Fetal malpresentation (breech presentation)
- Cesarean section, cesarean hysterectomy
- Postpartum hemorrhage.

### Q. Is there any link between leiomyomas and cancer?

**Ans.** Fibroids are benign uterine growths. Furthermore, these fibroids usually do not turn malignant. The rate of malignancy in a fibroid uterus is about 0.5%. Also, the rate of occurrence of uterine leiomyosarcomas is extremely low. The average age of women who develop fibroids is 38 years. Although sarcomas can rarely occur in young women, the average age of a woman who develops a sarcoma is 63 years. So, in a young woman with fibroids, there is not much risk of malignancy.

### Q. What should you do if the patient's fibroid is observed to be increasing in size?

**Ans.** If the patient's fibroids are observed to be growing, she should be called for a repeat pelvic examination after every 1–3 months. If the fibroid suddenly becomes symptomatic or increases in size, then surgery may be considered. Since, the incidence of sarcomas is so low, it is not clinically justifiable to believe that a growing fibroid indicates malignancy. However, if the patient is postmenopausal, any growth in the uterus may be a cause for concern. In these cases, endometrial carcinoma must be ruled out first.

### Q. Can fibroids cause infertility?

**Ans.** The relationship between myomas and infertility is still controversial and has been a subject of extensive debate. Mere presence of myomas in an infertile patient should not be considered as a cause of her infertility. Firstly, she should be investigated for all the other common causes of infertility (including tubal factor, ovarian factor, male factor, etc.). Only after all the other common causes of infertility in a woman have been ruled out, presence of myomas may be considered as the cause for infertility in a woman.

# Genital Prolapse

## Case Study 1

Mrs XYZ, a 48-year-old para 5 woman, married since last 20 years, resident of ABC, presented with the complaints of something descending out of vaginal introitus since past 1 year. According to the patient the feeling worsens while coughing or standing. On per speculum examination, a grade II cystocele and a grade I rectocele were noticed. There was no enterocele. Both the cystocele and rectocele were observed to increase in size when the patient strained. On bimanual examination, uterus was normal sized, anteverted and mobile. There has been no history of urinary incontinence. Her previous menstrual history has also been normal. She has completed her family and has five children. All her children were delivered at home by a *dai* (untrained midwife). She works on the farm with her husband. Due to lack of social support, she had to resume her daily activities immediately following each delivery.

### Q. What is the most likely diagnosis in the above-mentioned case study?

**Ans.** The above-mentioned case study corresponds to a case of uterine prolapse. The questions to be asked at the time of taking history and the parameters to be assessed at the time of examination in such a case are described in Tables 9.20 and 9.21 respectively. The most likely diagnosis in this case is Mrs XYZ, a 48-year-old para 5 woman, married since last

| **Table 9.20:** Symptoms to be elicited at the time of taking history in a case of uterine prolapse |
|---|
| *History of Presenting Complains* |
| • Protrusion of tissue/some body parts: The patient may complain of experiencing an annoying protrusion at the vaginal introitus. The patient may complain about a "bearing down sensation" or the feeling that "everything is falling". <br> • There may be pelvic pain, heaviness or pressure. <br> • History of urinary symptoms such as increased frequency, urgency dysuria, and inability to empty the bladder until the mass is reduced with fingers. <br> • Sexual dysfunction, including dyspareunia, decreased libido and difficulty in achieving orgasm. <br> • Lower back pain: There may be feeling of discomfort and aching in the lower back. <br> • History of bowel complaints: There may be difficulty in defecation, or inability to evacuate completely unless the protruding mass is reduced with the fingers. Cystocele may be associated with voiding difficulties such as imperfect control of micturition and stress incontinence. <br> • Difficulty in walking. <br> • Rarely the prolapsed uterus may become ulcerated (decubitus ulcer) resulting in purulent discharge and bleeding. |
| Symptoms of prolapse are typically exacerbated by prolonged standing or walking and are relieved by lying down. As a result, the patients may feel better in the morning, with symptoms worsening throughout the day. |
| *Risk Factors* |
| The risk factors associated with the development of uterine prolapse, which need to be elicited at the time of taking history, are described as follows: <br> • Obstetrical trauma associated with multiple vaginal deliveries in the past is especially associated with development of prolapse in future. While uterine prolapse is usually more common in multiparous women compared to the nulliparous ones, prolapse may also be sometimes seen in unmarried or nulliparous women. <br> • Decreased estrogen levels (e.g. menopause) may be associated with loss of strength and elasticity of pelvic structures. <br> • Increased intra-abdominal pressure (e.g. obesity, chronic lung disease, asthma). <br> • History of smoking is particularly important. Not only does smoking act as a risk factor for the surgery, habitual smoking can have both direct and indirect effects in causing weakness of the pelvic connective tissues. |
| *Medical History* |
| • History of many medical conditions (e.g. obesity, chronic pulmonary disease, smoking, constipation, chronic lung disease and asthma) may result in prolapse by causing an increase in intra-abdominal pressure. <br> • Abnormalities in connective tissue (collagen), such as Marfan's disease, and Ehlers Danlos syndrome are associated with an increased risk of uterine prolapse. |
| *Obstetric History* |
| Previous obstetric history is particularly important in cases of pelvic prolapse because it may reveal the exact pathology responsible for development of prolapse. Some of the points in the history which need to be asked are as follows: <br> • *Route of delivery:* Vaginal delivery or delivery by cesarean route. <br> • *Vaginal delivery:* In case of vaginal delivery, the clinician needs to ask the following: <br> Whether untrained midwife, trained midwife or a doctor took delivery? <br> The untrained midwives tend to adopt certain techniques, which may serve as a risk factor for development of prolapse. Some of these techniques are as follows: <br> – Asking the patient to bear down before full dilation of the cervix. <br> – The untrained midwife does not make use of forceps or vacuum in the case of prolonged second stage of labor. <br> – The untrained midwife usually uses Crede's method of placental extraction, which involves giving vigorous downwards push on the uterus to expel the placenta. This method may weaken the ligaments and muscles, which support the genital tract. <br> – The untrained midwife may not stitch the lacerations or tears of the perineum, which occur during the childbirth. Unless sutured immediately, these tears and lacerations may cause the widening of the hiatus urogenitalis. <br> – Application of fundal pressure by the untrained midwife may also be responsible for development of prolapse. <br> – The untrained midwife may not empty the bladder before taking the delivery. <br> – The untrained midwife usually does not give an episiotomy, which is a surgical incision and prevents perineal muscles from stretching. As a result, the second stage of the labor may be prolonged resulting in undue stretching of the pelvic floor muscles. <br> • Number of previous pregnancies and interval between successive deliveries. Interval between successive pregnancies is especially important because rapid succession of the pregnancies prevents proper puerperal rehabilitation, thereby resulting in a tendency to develop prolapse. <br> • Whether delivery took place at home or hospital? Home delivery may force the women to resume the household activities soon after delivery without taking proper rest or doing pelvic floor exercises. This may further predispose the woman to develop prolapse in the long run. <br> • Whether squatting position was used during delivery? Squatting during delivery may cause excessive stretching of the pelvic floor muscles and ligaments. <br> • Did the women use the birthing ball to facilitate the process of normal vaginal delivery? Birthing ball facilitates fetal descent by causing gentle stretching of the muscles of pelvis. <br> • The woman must be asked about the weight at birth of each baby she has delivered. <br> Delivery of a large sized baby is likely to stretch the perineal muscles, resulting in patulous introitus and thereby prolapse. |

| **Table 9.21:** Various findings to be elicited at the time of doing clinical examination in a case of uterine prolapse |
|---|

### General Physical Examination

Usually no specific finding is observed on general physical examination in cases of uterine prolapse.

General physical examination may help in diagnosing serious complications related to uterine prolapse, including infection, urinary obstruction, hemorrhage, strangulation with uterine ischemia, urinary outflow obstruction with renal failure, etc.

### Specific Systemic Examination

*Per Abdominal Examination*

- Check for the tone of anterior abdominal wall (if poor tone, rectus sheath cannot be used for abdominal cervicopexy)

*Per Speculum Examination*

- The vaginal tissue must be evaluated for estrogen status on the per speculum examination. Some of the signs of reduced estrogen status include the following:
  - Loss of rugosity of the vaginal wall mucosa
  - Reduced vaginal and cervical secretions
  - Thinning and tearing of the perineal skin
  - Hypertrophy of cervix, decubitus ulcerations
  - Keratinization/pigmentation of cervicovaginal mucosa
- Examination of the pelvic organ prolapse begins by asking the woman to attempt the Valsalva maneuver* prior to placing a speculum in the vagina. Patients who are unable to adequately complete a Valsalva maneuver are asked to cough.
- To perform the evaluation and grading of prolapse, a standard Sim's speculum and an anterior vaginal wall retractor are used. The Sim's speculum is placed in the vaginal vault to visually examine the vagina and cervix. The speculum is then replaced into the posterior vaginal wall, allowing visualization of the anterior wall. The speculum is then everted in order to visualize the posterior wall. The point of maximal descent of the anterior, lateral and apical vaginal walls is noted in relation to the ischial spines and hymen. The level to which the cervix descends on staining can be described as "descends to 2 inches below the introitus", etc. The term "procidentia" should be reserved for the patients who have a total uterine prolapse with eversion of the entire vagina.
- *Measuring the uterocervical length (UCL):* The UCL is checked using a uterine sound in cases of uterine prolapse.

*Pelvic Examination*

- Firstly, the vaginal examination is carried out in the lithotomy position. The tone of pubococcygeus muscles on each side of the lower vaginal wall must be estimated. For this, two fingers are placed inside the vaginal introitus in such a way that each finger opposes the ipsilateral vaginal wall. The patient is then asked to contract these muscles as if she was attempting to stop the flow of urine during the act of voiding. Any protrusion felt on the vaginal fingers is noted. Following the evaluation of the lateral vaginal support system, the apex (cervix and apical vagina) is assessed. The examination is then repeated with the patient standing and in bearing down position in order to note the maximum descent of the prolapse.
  The prolapse can be exaggerated by having the patient strain during the examination or by having her stand or walk prior to examination. The patient is asked to strain as if she was attempting to defecate or she may also be asked to cough.
- Next, the strength and quality of pelvic floor contraction is assessed by asking the patient to tighten the levator muscles around the examining finger. The diameter of the vaginal introitus and length of perineal body must also be assessed.
- A bimanual examination must be performed in order to note the uterine size, mobility and adnexa. Bimanual examination also helps in ensuring that the pelvic organs are free and not restricted by adhesions or any pathology.
- Lastly, a rectal examination is performed in order to assess the tone of external sphincter muscles, to note the presence of any palpable pathology, presence of blood on the examining finger, presence of the rectocele, for differentiating between rectocele and enterocele, strength of the perineal body and for assessing the rectovaginal septum. The rectovaginal septum may feel to be unusually thin in between the examining fingers.
- The examiner needs to differentiate between rectocele and enterocele. For this, the index finger of the clinician's left hand is placed in the rectum with the tip directed upwards. Two fingers of the right hand are then placed in the vagina. The patient is asked to strain downwards. If a bulge is felt between the examining fingers in the space between the rectum and upper posterior vaginal wall, it is most likely to be an enterocele. On the other hand, if the bulge is felt on the tip of the index finger in the rectum, the bulge is most likely to be a rectocele. The thickness of the perineum can be assessed by feeling the distance between the anal orifice and posterior fourchette, with the finger in the rectum and the thumb pressing against the perineum. Observation of the small bowel peristalsis behind the vaginal wall is definitively indicative of enterocele. In general, the bulges at the apical segment of the posterior vaginal wall implicate enterocele, whereas the bulges in the posterior wall are most likely to be rectocele.

*Testing for Urinary Incontinence*

- In patients with significant degree of uterine prolapse, it is imperative to exclude the potential urinary incontinence. By definition, potential urinary incontinence must be present only when the prolapse is reduced. To test for potential urinary incontinence, the bladder is retrograde filled to maximum capacity (at least 300 mL) with sterile water or saline while replacing and elevating the prolapsed part digitally or with an appropriately fitted pessary. The patient is then asked to cough. If the patient leaks urine, the urinary incontinence is suspected and the patient must be evaluated by performing a complete urodynamic test.

*Check the Integrity of the Sacral Pathways*

- For this the bulbocavernous reflex and anal reflex are evaluated. Presence of both these reflexes suggests normal sacral pathways. The bulbocavernous reflex is elicited by tapping or stroking lateral to the clitoris and observing the contractions of bulbocavernous bilaterally. Innervation of the external anal sphincter is evaluated by stroking lateral to the anus and observing the relative contraction of the anus.

*Abbreviation:* UCL, uterocervical length

* The Valsalva maneuver is performed by asking the patient to forcibly exhale while keeping the mouth and nose closed.

20 years, resident of ABC, presenting with the complaints of something descending out of vaginal introitus since past 1 year. The diagnosis of uterine prolapse with grade II cystocele and grade I rectocele was confirmed on pelvic examination.

### Q. What is uterine prolapse?

**Ans.** Uterine prolapse is a descent or herniation of the uterus into or beyond the vagina. Uterine prolapse is best considered under the broader heading of "pelvic organ prolapse," which also includes cystocele, urethrocele, enterocele and rectocele. Anatomically, the vaginal vault has three compartments (Fig. 9.3): an anterior compartment (consisting of the anterior vaginal wall), a middle compartment (cervix) and a posterior compartment (posterior vaginal wall). Weakness of the anterior compartment results in cystocele and urethrocele, whereas that of the middle compartment in the descent of uterine vault and enterocele. The weakness of the posterior compartment results in rectocele. Uterine prolapse involves the middle compartment.

### Q. What would be the next step of the management in the above-mentioned case study?

**Ans.** In the above-mentioned case study, the prolapse significantly interfered with the patient's day-to-day functioning and prevented her from standing for prolonged periods. Therefore, it needs to be treated. Since the patient was over 40 years and did not want to preserve her uterus, a transvaginal hysterectomy was planned. The anesthetists promptly gave their clearance since the patient did not have any history of previous medical disorders. No other hazards to contraindicate surgery could be identified. In order to prevent the recurrence of prolapse, the surgical treatment for various types of defects must be performed together at the time of surgery. It is very important that the physician carefully inspects the vagina for other prolapses. At the time of hysterectomy in this patient, the following repairs were planned: anterior colporrhaphy, posterior colporrhaphy and a McCall's culdoplasty. McCall's culdoplasty was performed in this patient in order to obliterate the cul-de-sac and to prevent the future development of both vaginal vault prolapse and enterocele.

### Q. Describe the etiology and staging of uterine prolapse.

**Ans.** Uterine prolapse usually occurs in postmenopausal and multiparous women in whom the pelvic floor muscles and the ligaments that support the female genital tract have become slack and atonic. Injury to the pelvic floor muscles during repeated childbirths causing excessive stretching of the pelvic floor muscles and ligaments acts as a major risk factor for causing reduced tone of pelvic floor muscles. Reduced estrogen levels following menopause is another important cause for atonicity and reduced elasticity of the muscles of pelvic floor. Uterine prolapse can be classified into four stages based on Baden-Walker Halfway system as described in Table 9.22.

### Q. What are different levels of support for vaginal tissues?

**Ans.** Different levels of support for vaginal tissues are described in Table 9.23.

In the supine position, the upper vagina lies almost horizontal and superior to the levator plate. The uterus and vagina have two main support systems. Active support is provided by the levator ani (level III support). On the other hand, passive support is provided by the condensations of the endopelvic fascia (i.e. the uterosacral-cardinal ligament complex, the pubocervical fascia, and the rectovaginal septum) and their attachments to the pelvis and pelvic

**Table 9.22:** Baden-Walker Halfway system for evaluation of pelvic organ prolapse

| Stage | Definition |
| --- | --- |
| Stage 0 | Normal position for each respective site |
| Stage I | Descent of the uterus to any point in the vagina above the hymen |
| Stage II | Descent of the uterus up to the hymen |
| Stage III | Descent of the uterus halfway past the hymen |
| Stage IV | Total eversion or procidentia |

**Table 9.23:** Different levels of support for vaginal tissues

| Different levels of vaginal support | Support elements |
| --- | --- |
| Level I (for proximal 1/3rd of vagina) | Cardinal and the uterosacral ligaments |
| Level II (for middle 1/3rd of vagina) | Paravaginal fascia |
| Level III (for distal 1/3rd of vagina and the introitus) | Levator ani and perineal muscles |

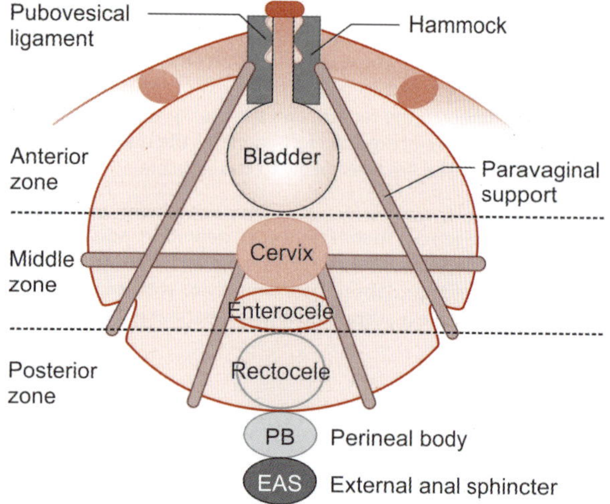


**Fig. 9.3:** Different pelvic compartments

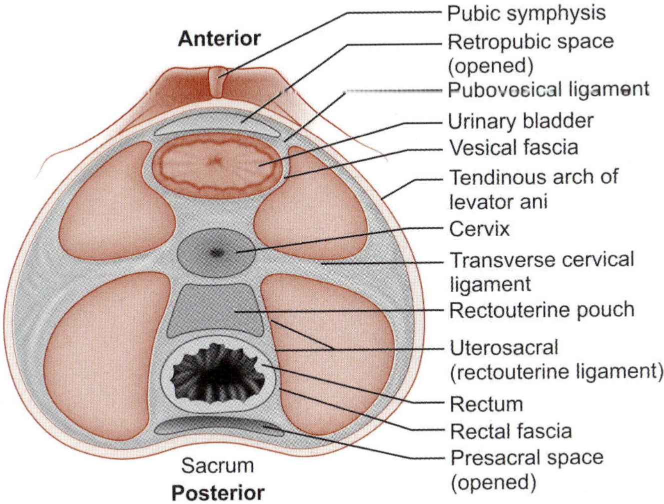


**Fig. 9.4:** Different ligamentous supports of the uterus

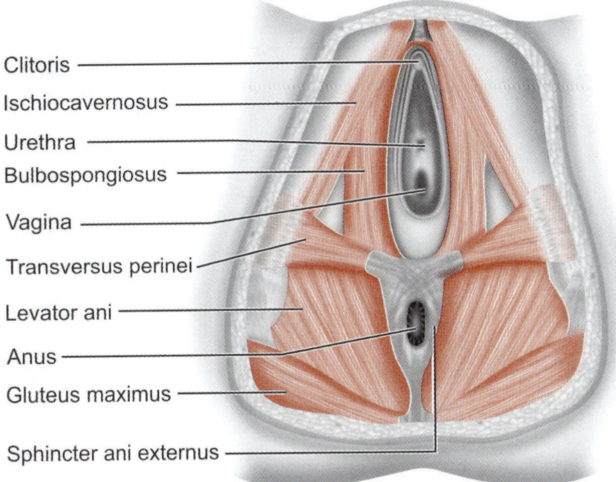


**Fig. 9.5:** Muscles of the pelvic floor including muscles of the pelvic diaphragm (levator ani muscle); muscles of the urogenital diaphragm (deep transverse perineal muscle); superficial muscles of the pelvic floor (superficial transverse perineal muscle, external anal sphincter and bulbospongiosus)

sidewalls through the arcus tendineus fascia pelvis (level I and level II support). Different ligamentous supports of the uterus are described in Figure 9.4.

When the tone of levator ani muscles decreases, the vagina drops from a horizontal to a semi vertical position. This causes widening of the genital hiatus thereby predisposing the prolapse of pelvic viscera.

### Q. Describe the muscles of the pelvic floor.

**Ans.** Muscles of pelvic floor (Fig. 9.5) can be grouped into three layers:
1. Muscles of the pelvic diaphragm (levator ani muscle)
2. Muscles of the urogenital diaphragm (deep transverse perineal muscle)
3. Superficial muscles of the pelvic floor (superficial transverse perineal muscle, external anal sphincter and bulbospongiosus)

*Levator ani muscle:* The levator ani muscle constitutes the pelvic diaphragm and supports the pelvic viscera. The levator ani muscle creates a hammock-like structure by extending from the left tendinous arch to the right tendinous arch. The muscle has openings through which the vagina, rectum and urethra traverse. Contraction of the levator muscles tends to pull the rectum and vagina inwards towards the pubic symphysis. This causes narrowing and kinking of both vagina and rectum. The origin of levator ani muscles is fixed on the anterior end because the muscle arises anteriorly either from the bone or from the fascia which is attached to the bone. As a result, the anterior attachment of the muscle largely remains immobile. On the other hand, the levator ani muscles posteriorly get inserted into the anococcygeal raphe or into the coccyx, both of which are movable. Thus, the contraction of levator ani muscles tends to pull the posterior attachment towards the pubic symphysis.

The pelvic diaphragm consists of two levator ani muscles, one on each side. Each levator ani muscle consists of three main divisions: Pubococcygeus, Iliococcygeus and Ischiococcygeus (Figs 9.6A and B). The pubococcygeus muscle originates from the posterior surface of the pubic bone. It passes backwards and lateral to the vagina and rectum to be inserted into the anococcygeal raphe and the coccyx. The inner fibers of this muscle which come to lie posterior to the rectum are known as the puborectalis portion of the muscle. These form a sling around the rectum and support it. Some of the inner fibers of puborectalis fuse with the outer vaginal wall as they pass lateral to it. Other fibers decussate between the vagina and rectum in the region of perineal body. The decussating fibers divide the space between the two levator ani muscles into an anterior portion (hiatus urogenitalis), through which pass the urethra and vagina and a posterior portion (hiatus rectalis), through which passes the rectum. The iliococcygeus is fan-shaped muscle, which arises from a broad origin along white line of pelvic fascia. It passes backwards and inwards to be inserted into the coccyx. The ischiococcygeus muscle takes its origin from the ischial spine and spreads out posteriorly to be inserted into the front of coccyx. The superior and inferior surfaces of the levator muscles are covered with tough fibrous tissue known as pelvic fascia, which separates the muscles from the cellular tissues of the parametrium above and from the fibrous and fatty tissues of ischiorectal fossa below. This fascia is composed of two components: pelvic component (also known as the endopelvic fascia) and the vaginal component (also known as periurethral fascia at the level of the urethra, and the perivesical fascia at the level of the bladder). The "pelvic component" fuses with the "vaginal

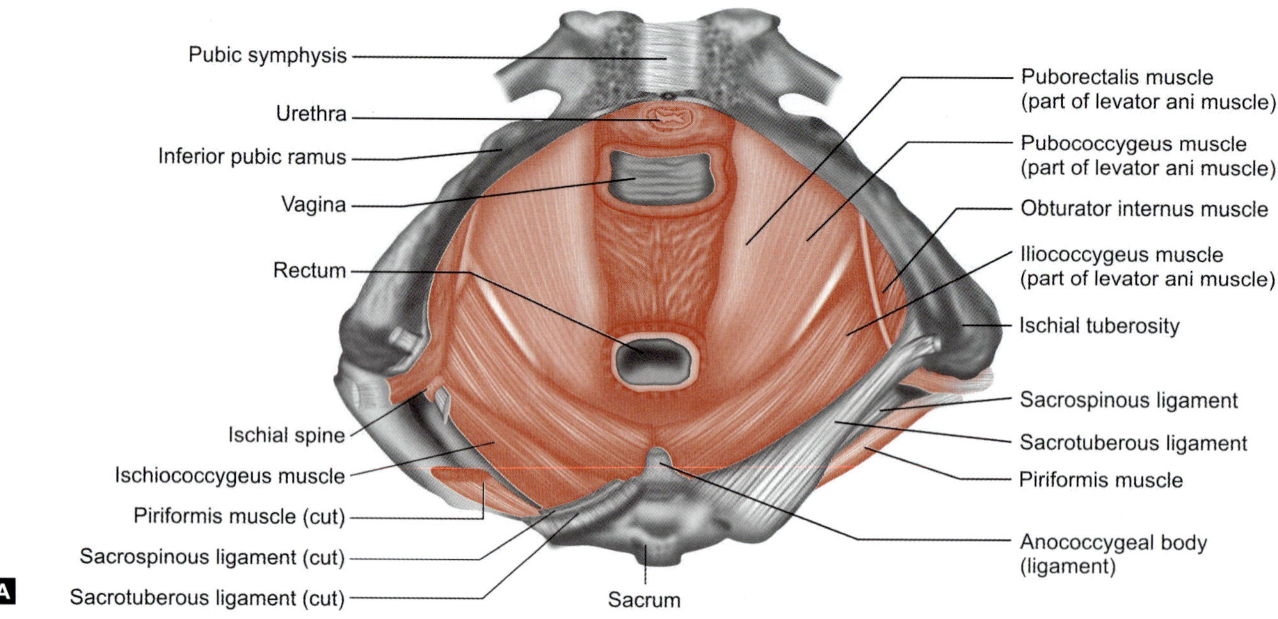

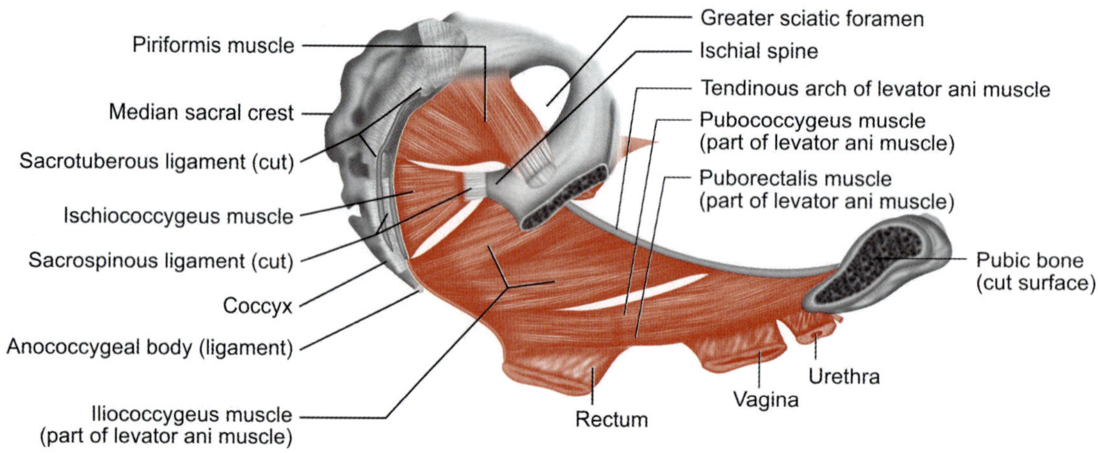

**Figs 9.6A and B:** Levator ani muscle: (A) Inferior view; (B) Lateral view

component" to get inserted into the tendinous arch. Within the two components of the levator fascia are present the various pelvic organs, such as the urethra, bladder, vagina and uterus to which it provides support.

### Q. Describe the perineal body.

**Ans.** The perineal body is also known as the central tendinous point of the perineum. It is a pyramid-shaped fibromuscular structure lying at the midpoint between the vagina and the anus. It lies at the level of the junction between the middle-third and lower one-third of the posterior vaginal wall. Perineal body assumes importance in providing support to the pelvic organs as it provides attachment to the following eight muscles of the pelvic floor: superficial and deep transverse perineal muscles, and the levator ani muscles of both the sides, bulbocavernosus anteriorly, and the external anal sphincter posteriorly (Fig. 9.7).

*The deep transverse perineal muscle:* The deep transverse perineal muscles of both the sides run transversely across the pelvic floor and lie within the urogenital diaphragm. They thus lie deep to the superficial transverse perineal muscles and are continuous with the sphincter urethrae muscle anteriorly. They originate from the medial surface of the ischiopubic ramus and get inserted into the midline raphe and the perineal body.

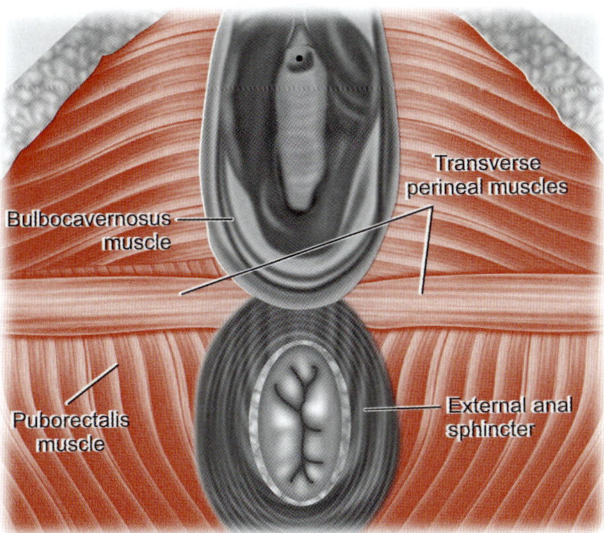



**Fig. 9.7:** Attachments of perineal body

*The superficial transverse perineal muscle:* These muscles arise from the upper and innermost part of the ischial tuberosity and run transversely across the pelvic floor, while lying superficial to the deep transverse perineal muscles. Running medially, they get inserted into the perineal body.

### Q. How can childbirth and labor result in the development of prolapse?

**Ans.** Perineal tears occurring at the time of delivery and parturition tend to either divide the decussating fibers of levator ani or cause damage to the perineal body. Both these factors can cause the hiatus urogenitalis to become patulous and result in the development of prolapse.

### Q. What should be the management in cases of prolapse?

**Ans.** The various laboratory investigations which may be required in cases of prolapse prior to the surgery are as follows:

- Hemoglobin: Estimation of hemoglobin levels gives an idea about the patient's anemic status.
- Urine examination: Urine analysis is important because it is essential to rule out UTI before undertaking surgery.
- Blood urea and creatinine levels: These tests of renal function may be indicated in cases with suspected urinary obstruction.
- Blood sugar.
- X-ray chest.
- Electrocardiography.
- Urine culture: Urine culture is specifically indicated in cases of suspected UTI.
- High vaginal swab: High vaginal swabs are indicated in cases of vaginitis.
- Cervical cultures are indicated for cases complicated by ulceration or purulent discharge.

- A Pap smear cytology may be indicated in cases of suspected carcinoma, although this is a rare occurrence.
- Imaging studies: A pelvic ultrasound examination may be useful in distinguishing prolapse from other pathologies, especially when other differential diagnoses are suspected on the basis of the history and physical examination. Ultrasound also serves as an important investigation modality for diagnosing hydronephrosis and for excluding presence of pelvic masses such as uterine fibroids, adnexal masses, etc.

### Q. What steps can be taken for prevention of prolapse?

**Ans.** Several steps, which can be taken to prevent the development of uterine prolapse, are as follows:

- Steps must be taken to minimize obstetrical trauma during vaginal delivery.
- The second stage of labor must be properly supervised and managed. Earlier it was thought that the routine use of episiotomy in primigravida would help in preventing undue stretching of the pelvic floor muscles and subsequently prolapse in the long run. However, in the light of present evidence, routine use of episiotomy and its role in preventing prolapse have largely been questioned.
- Low forceps delivery should be undertaken in cases of delayed second stage of labor.
- A perineal tear must be immediately and accurately sutured after delivery.
- The patient must be advised to maintain a reasonable time interval between pregnancies using family planning methods. This helps the pelvic muscles to recover their tone in between pregnancies.
- Antenatal physiotherapy, postnatal exercises, early postnatal ambulation and physiotherapy are highly beneficial in preventing prolapse. Adequate rest must be provided to the patient for first 6 months after delivery and there must be availability of home help for carrying out heavy domestic duties.
- The woman should be advised to maintain a healthy body weight. She should be instructed to exercise regularly for 20–30 minutes, three to five times per week. She should be especially advised to do Kegel exercises, which may be done up to four times a day.
- The woman must be advised to eat a healthy balanced diet containing appropriate amounts of protein, fat, carbohydrates and high amounts of dietary fiber (such as whole grain cereals, legumes and vegetables). A healthy, well-balanced diet can help to maintain weight and prevent constipation, which may serve as a predisposing factor for development of prolapse.
- The patient should be advised to stop smoking. This helps in reducing the risk of developing a chronic cough, which is likely to put extra strain on the pelvic muscles.
- Prophylactic hormone replacement therapy (HRT) in menopausal women can avoid or delay the occurrence of prolapse.

- The woman should be instructed to use correct weight lifting techniques in order to avoid undue straining of the pelvic floor muscles.

### Q. What are the indications for nonsurgical management?

**Ans.** Expectant management including the pelvic floor exercises (Kegel exercises) and pessaries are the current mainstays of nonsurgical management of patients with uterine prolapse. Nonsurgical management must be primarily used in cases with mild degree of uterovaginal prolapse with no or minimal symptoms. Since severe degree of prolapse may interfere with the functioning of urinary tract, such patients should not be managed expectantly.

Pessaries are a nonsurgical method for supporting the uterine and vaginal structures. A small pessary may help in maintaining normal uterine position. Pessaries are usually used for attaining temporary relief in cases with symptomatic prolapse. Some indications for using pessaries are as follows:

- A young woman planning a pregnancy in future.
- During early pregnancy, immediately after delivery and during lactation.
- Temporary use while clearing infection and decubitus ulcer prior to the actual surgery.
- Women unfit for surgery.
- Women who do not desire surgery.

### Q. What is the definite treatment for prolapse?

**Ans.** Surgery acts as a definitive treatment for prolapse. Surgery helps in providing relief against symptoms of prolapse and helps in restoring pelvic anatomy, sexual functioning and human physiologic functions (micturition and defecation). Since uterine prolapse is not a life-threatening condition, surgery is indicated only if the patient feels that her condition is severe enough that it warrants correction. Mild prolapse, which is rarely symptomatic, does not require surgical correction. Surgery is usually advised in women over 40 years unless it is contraindicated or is hazardous on account of some medical disorders.

Since the surgical treatment for various types of prolapse can be performed together at the time of surgery, it is very important that the physician carefully inspects the vagina for other prolapses. All forms of vaginal relaxation should be treated at the same time as the hysterectomy or uterine suspension. It is possible to have vaginal prolapse surgery without the need for hysterectomy or uterine suspension if there is no prolapsed uterus. The main challenge for the pelvic surgeon is to recreate normal pelvic anatomy while restoring normal physiological functioning as far as possible. Experienced surgeons can re-evaluate the anatomy intraoperatively, noting the strength and consistency of the various support structures (e.g. uterosacral ligaments). If these structures are found to be weak, it may be necessary to use other, stronger reattachment sites, such as the sacrospinous ligament or the presacral fascia, for the correction of the defect. In addition, the surgeon must make every attempt to prevent the possibility of recurrence of pelvic organ prolapse. Surgical options, which can be used in cases of prolapse, are enumerated in Table 9.24. The choice of surgery depends on numerous factors such as:

- Degree of prolapse
- Areas specific for prolapse
- Desire for future pregnancies
- Desire to maintain future sexual function
- Other medical conditions
- Preservation of vaginal function
- The woman's age and general health
- Patient's choice (i.e. surgery or no surgery)
- Medical condition and age
- Severity of symptoms
- Patient's suitability for surgery
- Presence of other pelvic conditions requiring simultaneous treatment, including urinary or fecal incontinence
- Presence or absence of urethral hypermobility
- History of previous pelvic surgery.

### Q. What are the principles of surgery for pelvic organ prolapse?

**Ans.** The principles of surgery for the treatment of pelvic organ prolapse are as follows:

- At the time of clinical examination when the patient is made to bear down, the site of primary damage appears first followed by the sites of secondary damage. The clinician must take special note of this site of primary damage. The primary site of damage should be identified first and over-repaired to reduce the chances of recurrence.
- The surgeon must repair all relaxations even if they are minor in order to prevent recurrence in the future. The strength of the various support structures should be evaluated.
- As far as possible, the surgeon must try to create a normal anatomy. Normal vaginal length should be maintained because a shortened vagina is likely to prolapse again.
- The vagina should be suspended in its normal posterior direction over the levator plate and rectum, pointing into the hollow of the sacrum, towards S3 and S4. The surgeon should avoid suspending the vaginal vault anteriorly to the abdominal wall.

---

**Table 9.24:** Surgical options which can be used in cases of prolapse

- Vaginal hysterectomy, posterior culdoplasty, colporrhaphy
- Vaginal hysterectomy, closure of enterocele sac, total colpectomy, colporrhaphy, colpocleisis
- Combined vaginal colporrhaphy and abdominal hysterectomy
- Moschcowitz culdoplasty, sacral colpopexy and suprapubic urethrocolpopexy
- Manchester operation
- Le Fort colpocleisis and colporrhaphy
- Vaginal repair and uterine suspension

- The cul-de-sac should be closed and rectocele repaired in all cases. A posterior colpoperineorrhaphy should be preferably performed in all cases where possible.
- When performed in properly selected patients, anterior colporrhaphy serves as an effective procedure for treating stress incontinence, which may be commonly associated with anterior cystocele.
- Removal of uterus helps in facilitating the repair of an enterocele. The choice of surgery for repair of enterocele and massive eversion of vagina include perineorrhaphy.
- A hysterectomy with colporrhaphy and colpopexy works for the patient with prolapse who wishes to preserve coital interest. Colpocleisis can be considered for patients in whom preservation of the sexual functioning is not important.

### Q. What is anterior colporrhaphy?

**Ans.** Anterior colporrhaphy operation is one of the most commonly performed surgeries to repair a cystocele and cystourethrocele. This surgery is usually performed under general or regional anesthesia. Anterior colporrhaphy comprises of the following steps: excision of a portion of relaxed anterior vaginal wall; mobilization of bladder; pushing the bladder upwards after cutting the vesicocervical ligament; and permanently supporting the bladder by tightening the pubocervical fascia.

### Q. What are indications for hysterectomy in cases of prolapse of uterus?

**Ans.** Indications for hysterectomy in case of prolapse of uterus are as follows:
- Removal of a nonfunctioning organ in postmenopausal women
- Uterine or cervical pathology (e.g. large fibroid uterus, endometriosis, pelvic inflammatory disease (PID), endometrial hyperplasia, carcinoma)
- Bulky uterus
- Patient desires removal of the uterus.

### Q. What is posterior repair?

**Ans.** Posterior repair comprises of colporrhaphy and colpoperineorrhaphy. While repairing the rectocele, most surgeons also perform a posterior colporrhaphy. This process involves nonspecific midline plication of the rectovaginal fascia after reducing the rectocele. The lax vaginal tissue over the rectocele is excised. The medial fibers of the levator ani are then pulled together, approximated and sutured over the top of rectum. This helps in restoring the caliber of the hiatus urogenitalis, and strengthening the perineal body. An adequate amount of perineum is also created which helps in separating the hiatus urogenitalis from the anal canal.

### Q. What is Manchester repair and what are its indications?

**Ans.** Manchester repair is performed in those cases where removal of the uterus is not required. Indications of Manchester operation are described as follows:

- Childbearing function is not required
- Malignancy of the endometrium has been ruled out by performing a dilatation and curettage
- Absence of UTI
- Presence of a small cystocele with only first or second degree prolapse
- Absence of an enterocele
- Symptoms of prolapse are largely due to cervical elongation. Patient requires preservation of the menstrual function.

*Procedure:* The procedure for Manchester repair (also called Fothergill operation) comprises of the following steps:
1. Anterior colporrhaphy is firstly performed.
2. The bladder is dissected from the cervix. A circular incision is given over the cervix.
3. The attachment of Mackenrodt ligaments to the cervix on each side are exposed, clamped and cut.
4. The vaginal incision is then extended posteriorly around the cervix.
5. The cervix is amputated and posterior lip of cervix is covered with a flap of mucosa.
6. The base of cardinal ligament is sutured over the anterior surface of cervix.
7. The raw area of the amputated cervix is then covered.
8. Colpoperineorrhaphy is ultimately performed to correct the posterior and perineal defects.

### Q. What are the uterine suspension procedures?

**Ans.** Vault prolapse is a delayed complication of both abdominal and vaginal hysterectomy when the supporting structures, i.e. paravaginal fascia and levator ani muscles become weak and deficient. Uterine suspension procedures involve putting the vaginal vault back into its normal position. Various types of uterine suspensions can be performed either via the abdominal or vaginal route. This may be done by reattaching the pelvic ligaments to the lower part of the uterus to hold it in place (e.g. sacrospinous colpopexy). Another technique uses special materials, which act like sling in order to support the uterus in its proper position (abdominal sacral colpopexy).

*Abdominal sacral colpopexy:* This procedure comprises of suspending the vault to the sacral promontory extraperitoneally using various grafts such as harvested fascia lata, abdominal fascia, dura mater, Marlex, Prolene, Goretex, Mersilene, or cadaveric fascia lata.

*Transvaginal sacrospinous ligament fixation:* In this method, the vaginal apex is attached, using permanent sutures, to the sacrospinous ligament.

### Q. What complications can occur in cases of prolapse of uterus?

**Ans.** Uterine prolapse, if not corrected, can interfere with bowel, bladder and sexual functions and result in the development of the following complications:

- Ulceration.
- Infection/urosepsis (including due to pessary use).
- Urinary incontinence.
- Constipation.
- Fistula.
- Postrenal failure.
- Decubitus ulceration.

# Dysfunctional Uterine Bleeding

## Case Study 1

Mrs XYZ, a 28-year-old, para 2 woman, married since last 6 years, resident of ABC, presented to the gynecological emergency with an episode of irregular menstrual bleeding since past 4 months. She had her last regular period, a week ago.

### Q. What is dysfunctional uterine bleeding?

**Ans.** Dysfunctional uterine bleeding, is defined as abnormal bleeding not caused by pelvic pathology, medications, pregnancy or systemic disease. In these cases, no obvious structural (pelvic, adnexal or extragenital) cause of bleeding can be demonstrated on clinical examination or laboratory evaluation. Bimanual examination of the uterus and adnexa remains normal. The development of DUB is related to an imbalance in the levels of hormones, estrogen and progesterone. Though DUB remains the most common cause of AUB, it is largely a diagnosis of exclusion. Diagnosis of DUB is made only after the other causes of AUB including, pregnancy, iatrogenic causes, systemic conditions, and obvious genital tract pathology have been ruled out.

### Q. What is the likely diagnosis in the above-mentioned case study?

**Ans.** The above-mentioned case study corresponds to a case of irregular menstrual bleeding. Case of AUB, due to endometrial malignancy has been discussed previously. The questions to be asked at the time of taking history and the parameters to be assessed at the time of examination in such a case are described in Tables 9.25 and 9.26 respectively. The most likely diagnosis in this case is Mrs XYZ, a 28-year-old, para 2 woman, married since last 6 years, resident of ABC, presenting with an episode of irregular menstrual bleeding since past 4 months. Diagnosis of DUB was made on the basis of the results of various investigations, which did not reveal

---

**Table 9.25:** Symptoms to be elicited at the time of taking history in a case of DUB

*History of Presenting Complains*

In the majority of women with true anovulatory bleeding, the cause of bleeding can be established by taking history itself. Characteristics of ovulatory and anovulatory menstrual cycles which can be determined by taking appropriate history are as follows:

*Anovulatory menstrual cycles*: Anovulatory bleeding is typically infrequent, irregular, and unpredictable that varies in amount, duration and character. It is usually not preceded by any pattern of premenstrual molimina. Also, the anovulatory cycles are painless.

*Ovulatory menstrual cycles:* Ovulatory cycles are regular, predicatable and associated with blood loss, which is normal and regular in amount, duration and character.

Detailed history to be taken in cases of AUB has been described previously. Important points in the patient's history, which may be particularly important in cases of DUB, include the following:

- Patient's age
- Time of last menstrual period and last normal menstrual period. The specific points, which need to be elicited, include the following:
  - *Intermenstrual intervals between the episodes of bleeding:* Number of days following which the bleeding occurs and cycle regularity.
  - *Volume of bleeding:* Heavy, light, or variable.
  - *Duration of the bleeding episode:* Normal or prolonged, consistent or variable.
  - *Temporal association of the bleeding episode:* Whether postcoital, postpartum, or post-pill.
- History of intake of any medications (especially hormonal agents, NSAIDs, or warfarin)
- History of any endocrine abnormalities (thyroid dysfunction)
- Symptoms of pregnancy (morning sickness, breast changes, etc.)
- Symptoms suggestive of coagulopathies
- History of use of hormonal contraceptive agents in the past
- History of trauma
- History of weight gain or loss, galactorrhea, hirsutism
- History of symptoms suggestive of premenstrual molimina (breast tenderness, edema, mood swings, etc.), and other symptoms like dyspareunia, dysmenorrhea, dyschezia, etc.
- Presence of underlying systemic illnesses (renal, hepatic failure, etc.)
- History of Pap smears, previously done must be enquired from the patient. The results of recently done Pap smear tests also need to be documented.

*Abbreviations:* AUB, abnormal uterine bleeding; DUB, dysfunctional uterine bleeding; NSAIDs, nonsteroidal anti-inflammatory drugs

**Table 9.26:** Various findings elicited at the time of clinical examination in a case of DUB

*General Physical Examination*

- Signs related to excessive blood loss (tachycardia, hypotension)
- Symptoms related to endocrinopathies, including polycystic ovary disease (such as obesity and hyperandrogenism: acne, hirsutism, deepening of voice), hyperprolactinemia, etc.
- Signs suggestive of hypothyroidism or hyperthyroidism
- *Breast examination:* Breast examination in cases of DUB should specifically aim at the following:
  - *Detection of a breast lump:* Detection of a tumorous mass could be an indicator of breast malignancy. History of treatment with tamoxifen (anticancer drug, commonly used in cases of breast malignancy) needs to be enquired in such patients. Abnormal bleeding in women under treatment with tamoxifen could be related to endometrial hyperplasia. This therefore warrants prompt investigation and careful follow-up of these patients.
  - *Presence of galactorrhea:* Hyperprolactinemia is an important cause of amenorrhea and infertility.

*Specific Systemic Examination*

*Pelvic Examination*

Pelvic examination is unnecessary and must not be done in young girls presenting with the history of menorrhagia, who are not sexually active. Pelvic examination may be particularly useful in women belonging to reproductive age group, presenting with DUB. The pelvic examination has been described in detail in Chapter 8. On vaginal and bimanual examination, the size, shape, position, and firmness of the uterus should also be examined.

*Per Speculum Examination*

This includes inspection of the vagina and cervix for presence of visible lesions [polyps, erosions, tears, malignancy, pregnancy-related complications (expulsion of products of conceptions) or infection]. Signs of excessive blood loss must be noted on per speculum examination.

*Abbreviation:* DUB, dysfunctional uterine bleeding

any pathological cause for abnormal bleeding. The cause of bleeding appeared to be due to hormonal imbalance. Therefore a provisional diagnosis of DUB was made.

### Q. What would be the next line of management in the above-mentioned case study?

**Ans.** The initial step is to stabilize the patient. Depending on the severity of her bleeding, she can be administered either oral or parenteral conjugated estrogen to control the initial episode of bleeding. On clinical examination, no significant cause of AUB could be found in this case. Once the bleeding episode has been controlled, the patient is to be prescribed oral progestogens (10 mg/day) for last 15 days of cycle. This, when administered over a period of 4–6 months would also help in regularizing the cycle. After the patient was stabilized the investigations mentioned in Table 9.27 were ordered to rule out the presence of any significant pathology.

### Q. What is the etiology of DUB?

**Ans.** Imbalance between the levels of various hormones involved in the menstrual cycle could be responsible for producing irregular bleeding related to DUB. Dysfunctional bleeding could be related to estrogen withdrawal, estrogen breakthrough, progesterone withdrawal and progesterone breakthrough. The etiology of this condition is purely hormonal. DUB can be of two types: anovulatory and ovulatory type. Anovulation represents a common cause of DUB.

*Anovulatory dysfunctional uterine bleeding:* Anovulatory bleeding can occur as a result of estrogen withdrawal or

**Table 9.27:** Laboratory investigations to be considered in case of dysfunctional uterine bleeding

| Test | Indication (to rule out) |
|---|---|
| Urine pregnancy test | Pregnancy |
| CBC with platelet count | Anemia and coagulation defects |
| PT/aPTT | Coagulation abnormalities |
| Ristocin cofactor assay | Von Willebrand's disease |
| Pap smear | Cervical cancer |
| Liver function and/or renal function tests | Hepatic and renal disease |
| TSH | Thyroid disease |
| Prolactin level | Pituitary adenoma |
| LH, FSH, and androgen levels | Polycystic ovary disease |
| Endometrial biopsy | To rule out endometrial cancer |
| Ultrasound examination | For the evaluation of endometrial thickness |

*Abbreviations:* CBC, complete blood count; FSH, follicle-stimulating hormone; LH, luteinizing hormone; PT, prothrombin time; aPTT, activated partial thromboplastin time; TSH, thyroid-stimulating hormone

estrogen breakthrough. This causes anovulatory bleeding, which is usually heavier than normal menstrual flow. The anovulatory woman is always in the follicular phase of the ovarian cycle and in the proliferative phase of endometrium cycle. In the absence of ovulation, there is no luteal or secretory phase and therefore, the corpus luteum fails to form, resulting in reduced progesterone secretion. Uninterrupted stimulation of the endometrium by estrogen results in its continued growth. The endometrial proliferation occurs to abnormal heights until it becomes fragile. Without the structural support by progesterone, focal areas of bleeding and breakdown occur, resulting in an irregular and prolonged bleeding. Anovulatory DUB may also occur in the following circumstances: puberty menorrhagia, bleeding in perimenopausal women, metropathia hemorrhagica, chronic illness or excessive exercise, extreme degree of weight loss, eating disorders, stress, polycystic ovarian disease and idiopathic chronic anovulation.

*Ovulatory dysfunctional bleeding:* Although less common than anovulatory bleeding, ovulatory DUB may also sometimes occur. Ovulatory dysfunctional bleeding may include menstrual abnormalities like polymenorrhea, oligomenorrhea, premenstrual spotting (Mittelschmerz syndrome), hypomenorrhea, and menorrhagia. Ovulatory DUB can occur due to the following abnormalities: shortened proliferative or secretory phase, corpus luteal insufficiency, persistent corpus luteum (Halban's disease), and irregular shedding.

### Q. What is puberty menorrhagia?

**Ans.** Immediately after menarche, the maturation of the hypothalamic-pituitary-ovarian axis may not be complete. In the first 18 months after menarche, the immature hypothalamic-pituitary axis may fail to respond to estrogen and progesterone, resulting in anovulation. As a result, puberty menorrhagia is an important cause of DUB primarily because nearly 80% of menstrual cycles are anovulatory in the first year following menarche. Menstrual cycles usually become ovulatory within 2 years following menarche. If no cause of menorrhagia can be found on the diagnostic work-up of an adolescent patient, she can be diagnosed as a case of DUB due to puberty menorrhagia.

### Q. What is metropathia hemorrhagica (Schroeder's disease)?

**Ans.** Though generally seen in postmenopausal women, this special type of menorrhagia may also be sometimes seen in the women under the age of 20 years. The bleeding is mainly of anovulatory type. The problem lies at the level of ovaries and is due to the disturbances of rhythmic gonadotropin secretion. There is slow and steady increase in estrogen levels with no inhibitory feedback effect on FSH secretion. Since there is no ovulation, the endometrium is primarily under the effect of estrogen. Also, there is prolonged absence of progesterone. Due to this, there are increased estrogen levels with amenorrhea for about 6–8 weeks. After a variable period of amenorrhea, there occurs relative or absolute estrogen deficiency. Relative deficiency sets in because estrogen levels, despite of being normal are not able to sustain the hyperplastic endometrium. Absolute estrogen deficiency eventually sets in

when high levels of estrogen start suppressing FSH levels. This in turn causes an absolute decrease in the level of estrogen secretion. As a result, the most common clinical presentation is a period of amenorrhea of about 8–10 weeks followed by an episode of heavy bleeding.

On macroscopic examination, there may be slight symmetrical enlargement of the uterus up to 8–10 weeks, the size of a pregnant uterus. There may be a mild degree of myohyperplasia with the thickness of uterine walls being about 25 mm. The ovary may show presence of single or multiple cystic changes. There could be the presence of estrogen-containing fluid in these cysts. The ovary may not be clinically palpable. There is no evidence of corpus luteum. The endometrium may become thick and polypoidal with thin slender polpi projecting into the uterine cavity. DUB due to metropathia hemorrhagica is completely painless.

### Q. What is Mittelschmerz syndrome?

**Ans.** Mittelschmerz syndrome (midcycle spotting) is a type of midcycle bleeding, which occurs just before or at the time of ovulation. It results from a physiological fall in estrogen levels, which occurs just prior to the LH surge.

### Q. How should the cases of DUB be managed?

**Ans.** Many cases of DUB may simply represent normal physiological variation of menstrual cycle and thereby resolve with clinical observation. In these cases, the patient must be instructed to maintain a menstrual calendar. The treatment of moderate to severe DUB or that uncontrolled by clinical observation mainly comprises of medical therapy. Endometrial ablation procedures can be used in patients who are unresponsive to medical therapy, those who have completed their families or those with severe DUB. For severe bleeding, intravenous estrogen therapy (2.5 mg) conjugated equine estrogen every 4 hours until bleeding subsides or for 24 hours can be very effective. When bleeding is less severe, but still quite heavy, treatment can be given with 1.25 mg conjugated estrogen or 2.0 mg micronized estrogen every 4–6 hours for 24 hours. This can be tapered to once a daily dose for another 7–10 days after bleeding has been controlled.

In cases of acute hemorrhage, if the endometrium is thickened, progestogens can also be administered. Norethisterone acetate is usually started in high dosage, administered in the dosage of 10 mg TDS, for 24–48 hours to stop the bleeding. This is gradually tapered down to a dose of 5 mg/day when the bleeding reduces and continued in a dose of 5 mg/day for further 20 days. The patient should be warned about the episode of withdrawal bleeding following the stoppage of therapy.

### Q. How is anovulatory DUB treated?

**Ans.** If anovulatory bleeding is not heavy or prolonged, no treatment is necessary. All cases of anovulatory DUB represent a progesterone-deficient state. In such patients with irregular cycles secondary to chronic anovulation or oligo-ovulation, progestins help to prevent the risks associated with prolonged unopposed estrogen stimulation of the endometrium. Thus progestins form the mainstay of treatment for anovulatory bleeding, once presence of any uterine pathology has been ruled out. Exogenous progestogens must be prescribed to help control anovulatory bleeding and also to protect against endometrial cancer; 5–10 mg of medroxyprogesterone acetate can be administered daily for the first 15–16 days of each month for 4–6 months. Depot medroxyprogesterone (150 mg) or progesterone in oil (100–200 mg) may be given intramuscularly every 3 monthly to achieve similar effects. Combined oral contraceptive pills (OCPs) can also be used if contraception is also desired. If pregnancy is desired, ovulation induction with clomiphene citrate may be required. The treatment strategy may vary depending on the age group of the woman experiencing anovulatory DUB.

### Q. How is ovulatory dysfunctional uterine bleeding treated?

**Ans.** Medical therapy for ovulatory DUB primarily includes nonsteroidal anti-inflammatory drugs (NSAIDs), OCPs, the levonorgestrel-releasing intrauterine system (Mirena), danazol and GnRH agonists. Oral contraceptive pills are also commonly used both for cycle regulation and contraception in patients with ovulatory DUB. While the medical therapies like NSAIDs and Mirena are commonly used, the use of androgens such as danazol and GnRHs is largely limited due to high costs and high incidence of side-effects.

In cases of moderately heavy DUB, OCPs may be given up to four times a day for 5–7 days or until bleeding stops, followed by the rest of the pills to be taken once a day until the pack is finished and withdrawal bleeding occurs. In patients with mild DUB, OCPs may be administered in the dose of one pill every day.

### Q. What is endometrial ablation?

**Ans.** Endometrial ablation involves surgical destruction of the endometrium. In this method, the endometrium is destroyed to the level of the basalis layer of myometrium, which is approximately 4–6 mm deep, depending upon the stage of the menstrual cycle. The procedure may help in controlling the amount of bleeding. The women whose bleeding does not respond to hormonal or pharmacological therapy and who want to conserve their uterus must be offered endometrial ablation. If endometrial ablation does not control heavy bleeding, further treatment or surgery may be required.

### Q. What are the indications for endometrial ablation?

**Ans.** Some indications for endometrial ablation are as follows:
- Ovulatory menorrhagia in premenopausal women
- Acute AUB in hemodynamically stable women in whom medical therapy is contraindicated or unsuccessful
- Women with chronic menorrhagia
- Woman does not desire future fertility
- Menorrhagia is related only to DUB and no other cause
- Menorrhagia is unresponsive to hormonal or pharmacological therapy
- Malignant disease of the cervix and/or endometrium has been ruled out
- Uterine size less than 10 weeks; submucous fibroids less than 5 cm
- Endometrium is normal with no risk of hyperplasia.

Women with anovulatory bleeding or those with high risk factors for endometrial malignancy may be at a high risk for developing endometrial hyperplasia and/or endometrial cancer following endometrial ablation. These women, therefore, must not be offered treatment with endometrial ablation techniques.

### Q. What are the various methods for endometrial ablation?

**Ans.** The methods of endometrial ablation help in treating DUB by destroying the endometrial lining. These methods for endometrial ablation are mainly of two types: First generation (hysteroscopic) methods and second generation (nonhysteroscopic) methods. Hysteroscopic methods include laser and electrosurgical resection [roller ball and transcervical resection of the endometrium (TCRE)]. Electrosurgical method that uses the wire loop to resect out the endometrial lining is called transcervical endometrial resection. The wire loop is around 6-mm long and is attached at an angle to a pencil-shaped handle. On the other hand, electrosurgical technique that uses the heated roller ball to burn away the endometrial tissue is called roller ball ablation. The roller ball is a ball about 2 mm wide that rotates freely on its handle. Some nonresectoscopic (second generation) technologies, which have been approved for use in the United States by the Food and Drug Administration (FDA) include using bipolar radiofrequency (NovaSure device); hot liquid-filled balloon (THERMACHOICE); cryotherapy (Her Option); circulating hot water (Hydro ThermAblator); microwave [microwave endometrial ablation (MEA)], etc. Nonresectoscopic endometrial ablation techniques are more widely practiced than resectoscopic ablation, since they require less specialized training and often have a shorter operative time.

### Q. What treatments for DUB are there for a young woman?

**Ans.** Teenagers and young women wishing to retain their fertility generally require medical treatment. The combined OCP is frequently an effective first choice for younger patients particularly when there is a need for contraception. Teenagers with heavy periods may be having anovulatory cycles; progestogens prescribed in the second half of the cycle may prove to be effective. Tranexamic acid, two or three tablets taken three or four times daily, on the days of heavy period is otherwise a sensible first choice. When pain accompanies the heavy loss, a nonsteroidal anti-inflammatory agent may be appropriate. Mefenamic acid 500 mg three times daily is a popular selection.

# Infertility

## Case Study 1

Mrs XYZ, a 28-year-old woman, married since last 5 years, resident of ABC, presented to the gynecology outpatient department along with her husband with the complaint of infertility. The couple has been practicing regular sexual intercourse since last 2 years. On general physical examination, there was no significant findings except that the patient's BMI was 27. There were no signs of hyperandrogenism (hirsutism), galactorrhea or thyroid dysfunction. The woman's menstrual history revealed that she has been having irregular menstrual cycles since last 3 years. The cycle duration ranges within 30–35 days. The cycles last for approximately 4–5 days. However, the woman has been observing a progressive decrease in the amount of menstrual blood flow over the past few months. The couple had previously visited an infertility specialist 6 months back who had ordered a semen analysis. The result of this investigation was within normal limits.

### Q. How can infertility be defined?

**Ans.** Infertility is defined as the inability to conceive even after trying with unprotected intercourse for a period of 1 year for couples in which the woman is under 35 years and 6 months of trying for couples in which the woman is over 35 years of age. Investigations may be started earlier in a women with irregular menstrual cycles or in presence of known risk factors for infertility, such as endometriosis, history of PID, reproductive tract malformations, etc. or having a male partner with known or suspected poor semen quality.

Infertility commonly results due to the disease of the reproductive system, in either a male or a female, which inhibits the ability to conceive and deliver a child.

### Q. What is the likely diagnosis in the above-mentioned case study?

**Ans.** The above-mentioned case study corresponds to an infertile couple (no cause could be established based on history and physical examination). The questions to be asked at the time of taking history and the parameters to be assessed at the time of examination in such a case are described in Tables 9.28 and 9.29 respectively. The most likely diagnosis in this case is Mrs XYZ, a 28-year-old woman, with an active married life of 5 years, resident of ABC, nulliparous woman with chief complaints of infertility since past 2 years. Some investigations would be required to delineate the exact cause of infertility in this case. Minimal investigations required to determine the cause of infertility in this case have been tabulated in Table 9.32.

### Q. What are the causes of infertility?

**Ans.** Infertility can be attributed to several factors enlisted in Table 9.33.

Some of the likely causes of male and female infertility are tabulated in Tables 9.34 and 9.35 respectively.

### Q. What is the desirable management in cases of infertility?

**Ans.** Evaluation of the couple is the starting point for treatment of infertility as it may suggest specific causes and appropriate treatment modalities. Patient evaluation should begin by taking a detailed history from both the partners. Sometimes simple reassurance and explanation about the physiology of menstrual cycle and importance of having regular intercourse is sufficient in achieving pregnancy. Although the history and physical examination is able to provide important information, specific diagnostic tests are also required to evaluate infertility. Once the cause of infertility has been identified, treatment must be aimed at correcting the underlying etiologies. Besides instituting corrective measures, the couple must be counseled to observe certain changes in lifestyle such as cessation of smoking, reducing excessive caffeine and alcohol consumption, and maintaining appropriate frequency of sexual intercourse (every 1–2 days around the anticipated time of ovulation).

### Q. What investigations must be done in case of an infertile couple?

**Ans.** Evaluation of infertile couples should be organized and thorough. Diagnostic tests should start from the simplest (e.g. semen analysis, pelvic ultrasonography, etc.) tests onto the more complex and invasive ones (e.g. laparoscopy). Also, the evaluation of fertility must first begin with tests for the assessment of male fertility. The semen analysis is the most commonly performed test of male infertility, which yields tremendous amount of information as to the potential causes of male infertility. The tests which are useful for the initial evaluation of an infertile couple are listed in Table 9.32.

### Q. What minimum investigations must be offered in the above-mentioned case study?

**Ans.** Since the causes of infertility can be multifactorial, a systematic approach typically is used and involves testing for male factor, ovulatory factor, uterotubal factor and peritoneal factor. Since the evaluation for male factor infertility has already been done in form of semen analysis, the next step should be towards evaluation of ovulatory factors. These must include tests such as serum progesterone level, serum basal FSH level, and clomiphene citrate challenge test (CCCT).

### Q. What advice must be given in this case?

**Ans.** Couples concerned about their fertility should be informed that about 84% of couples in the general population will conceive within 1 year if they do not use contraception and have regular sexual intercourse. Of those who do not conceive in the 1st year, about half will do so in the 2nd year (cumulative pregnancy rate of 92%). Regular sexual intercourse after every 2–3 days is likely to maximize the overall chances of natural conception, as spermatozoa survive in the female reproductive tract for up to 7 days after

**Table 9.28:** Symptoms to be elicited at the time of taking history in a case of infertility

Infertility is a problem that may involve both male and female partners; therefore the initial assessment must involve both the partners. The initial evaluation must include a detailed reproductive history and at least two semen analyses at a laboratory that is qualified to perform the testing. Diagnostic testing must not be performed if the couple has not attempted to conceive for at least 1 year, unless the woman is 35 years old or older, or there is a history of male factor infertility, endometriosis, tubal factor, exposure to DES, PID, or pelvic surgery. In many cases, attempts at alleviation of anxiety through reassurance and briefly explaining the physiology of reproduction are usually enough to lessen the couple's anxiety.

**History from the Female Partner**

*History of Presenting Complains*

- *Type of infertility:* A detailed medical history regarding the type of infertility (primary or secondary), its duration and if any treatment for this had been sought in the past needs to be elicited. Primary infertility implies that woman had never been able to conceive in the past. Secondary infertility implies that the woman had conceived in the past, (irrespective of the outcome of pregnancy, whether she progressed till term or had a miscarriage) but is presently not being able to conceive.
- *Patient's age:* It is important to know the woman's age because increasing age of the women (greater than 35 years) is associated with reduced fertility.
- *Duration of infertility:* Duration of the couple's attempts for becoming pregnant, whether or not they have ever had children or a positive pregnancy test together with same or a different partner in the past needs to be asked. Number and outcome of any previous pregnancies including ectopic pregnancy and/or miscarriages also needs to be determined.
- *Thyroid dysfunction or galactorrhea:* Symptoms suggestive of thyroid disease, pelvic or abdominal pain and galactorrhea must be asked. Thyroid dysfunction is commonly associated with menstrual abnormalities and reduced fertility. Galactorrhea or milk secretion from the breasts is often a manifestation of pineal gland tumor and may be associated with amenorrhea.
- *Previous history of Pap smears:* Previous history of abnormal Pap smears or undergoing treatment for cervical intraepithelial neoplasia could be responsible for producing cervical stenosis.
- *History of vaginal or cervical discharge:* This must be enquired. The infections could be at times responsible for producing infertility, e.g. infection with *Chlamydia* can cause PID and tubal blockage resulting in subsequent infertility.

*Sexual History*

- Sexual history must be taken in details in order to enquire about the frequency of sexual intercourse, use of lubricants (e.g. K-Y gel) that could be spermicidal, use of vaginal douches after intercourse and history of any sexual dysfunction. History of sexual dysfunction such as absence of orgasm or painful intercourse (dyspareunia) must be enquired. History related to the frequency of intercourse and presence of deep dyspareunia (suggestive of endometriosis) also needs to be enquired. Use of any form of contraception including natural methods, medical methods and surgical form of contraception (e.g. vasectomy, tubal ligation) needs to be asked.
- The patient should be explained about the period of fertility during her cycles. The optimal chances for pregnancy occur if the patient has intercourse in the 6 days before ovulation, with day 6 being the actual day of ovulation. Sometimes, simply advising the patients to adjust the timing of their intercourse can result in a significantly increased chance for pregnancy.

*Patient's Lifestyle*

Detailed history regarding the patient's lifestyle; consumption of alcohol, tobacco, use of recreational drugs of abuse (amount and frequency); occupation; and physical activities must be asked.

*Menstrual History*

- The age of attaining menarche and puberty must be asked. The woman should be questioned in details about her menstrual history and asked about the frequency, cycle length, patterns since menarche and history of dysmenorrhea. Regular menstrual cycles are usually ovulatory in nature, while irregular cycles may be anovulatory in nature.

*Obstetric History*

- The patient should be enquired about details regarding previous pregnancies (including miscarriages or medical terminations of pregnancy and previous history of live births), dead babies or stillborn children. She should also be asked if she has ever undergone evaluation regarding infertility issues and any medical or surgical management that had been instituted. The patient should be asked about outcome of each of the previous pregnancies; interval between successive pregnancies and presence of any other complications associated with any pregnancy. If the patient has ever experienced pregnancy losses, she should be asked about the duration of pregnancy at the time of miscarriage, hCG levels, if they were done, ultrasonographic data, if available, and the presence or absence of fetal heartbeat as documented on the ultrasound report.

*Past History*

- A previous history of pelvic infection, endometriosis, fibroids, cervical dysplasia, septic abortion, ruptured appendix, ectopic pregnancy, and gynecological surgery, e.g. abdominal myomectomy, adnexal surgery, surgery of cervix, fallopian tube, pelvis, abdomen, etc. raises the suspicion for tubal or peritoneal disease.
- Past or current episodes of sexually transmitted diseases or PIDs must also be enquired.
- The patient must be asked if she is currently receiving any medical treatment, the reason for treatment and if she has any history of allergies.
- She must be asked if she had been using intrauterine copper devices or any other form of contraception in the past.

*(Contd...)*

*(Contd...)*

<table>
<tr><td align="center">*Family History*</td></tr>
<tr><td>Family history of birth defects, mental retardation, early menopause or reproductive failure needs to be taken.</td></tr>
<tr><td align="center">**History from the Male Partner**</td></tr>
<tr><td>

- Determination of the period of infertility at the time of taking history is most important.
- The history should include several points specific to the patient's sexual functioning including history of impotence, erectile dysfunction, premature ejaculation, change in libido, precise nature of the dysfunction, for example, whether the problem is in attaining or sustaining an erection, or whether there is difficulty with penetration due to insufficient rigidity.
- The presence or absence of nocturnal and morning erections and their quality must be asked.
- The patient must be enquired if he is taking any treatment, both pharmacologic and nonpharmacologic, for his problem.
- Complaints of reduced libido may also be associated with depression, loss of interest in daily activities, a decline in erectile function, fatigue, etc. Thus, history related to these symptoms must also be elicited. Additionally, the time period since which these complaints have been present must be enquired from the patient.
- History related to the frequency of intercourse or use of any lubricants which may be toxic to sperms must be enquired.
- History of pain both during time of ejaculation and erection must be enquired. The time of pain onset, its localization to any specific organ and the quality of pain must also be asked.
- History of testicular trauma, previous sexual relationships, history of any previous pregnancy and the existence of offspring from previous partners must also be asked.
- History of undergoing previous treatment for infertility including semen analysis must also be asked.
- Any complaints specific to the genitourinary structures, such as complaints of a dull ache or fullness in the scrotum, or nonradiating pain on one side, dysuria, dyspareunia, etc. must also be asked.
- History of exposure to environmental toxins, such as excessive heat, radiation, and chemicals such as heavy metals, and glycol ethers or other organic solvents needs to be asked.

</td></tr>
<tr><td align="center">*Medical History*</td></tr>
<tr><td>

- History of treatment for malignancy (especially chemotherapy or radiotherapy), regardless of site, should be documented.
- History of medical disorders such as diabetes, chronic obstructive pulmonary disease, renal insufficiency, hemochromatosis, hepatic insufficiency, etc. which may contribute to male subfertility must be asked.
- History of systemic illness, particularly, a febrile illness, and any recent weight gain or loss in last 6 months must be asked.

</td></tr>
<tr><td align="center">*Surgical History*</td></tr>
<tr><td>

- History of any surgery related to genitourinary organs such as orchidopexy, repair of inguinal hernia, epispadias or hypospadias repair, prostate surgery, bladder reconstructions, bladder or testicular surgeries needs to be asked. The patient should be asked specifically if there is a history of a vasectomy.

</td></tr>
<tr><td align="center">*Treatment History*</td></tr>
<tr><td>

- The dose and duration of use of certain prescription drugs which can affect sperm count, motility, and morphology must be documented. Some of the drugs which can commonly affect semen parameters by reducing spermatogenesis include calcium-channel blockers, spironolactone, chemotherapy drugs, anabolic steroids, etc. The patient must also be asked about the ingestion of herbal drugs or drugs belonging to other alternative systems of medicine and other over-the-counter medications. Many times the patient may not disclose this history unless specifically enquired. Any of these substances may be responsible for affecting spermatogenesis.

</td></tr>
<tr><td align="center">*Social History*</td></tr>
<tr><td>

- Cigarette smoking, excessive alcohol consumption and consistent marijuana use are all known to be gonadotoxins. A careful history of the use of these agents and other illicit drugs use must be part of the complete male infertility evaluation. Cigarette smoking has been thought to cause changes in sperm morphology, production and motility while chronic alcohol use may contribute to infertility by causing erectile dysfunction and hypogonadism. Simply eliminating these agents can improve semen parameters in the absence of other physical findings.
- Certain occupations which result in exposure of male genital organs to high temperature such as men working in blast furnaces may be the reason behind the patient's infertility.

</td></tr>
<tr><td align="center">*Family History*</td></tr>
<tr><td>

- It is important to elicit the family history of birth defects or reproductive failure. The family history must include a discussion regarding the presence of testicular or other genitourinary malignancies specifically related to prostate or bladder in other family members.

</td></tr>
</table>

*Abbreviations:* DES, diethylstilbestrol; hCG, human chorionic gonadotropin; PID, pelvic inflammatory disease

insemination. In this case, the sexual history revealed that the couple had reasonable knowledge regarding the female reproductive cycle and had been having regular unprotected sexual intercourse. The main abnormality detected on the general physical examination was an increased BMI. Also the menstrual cycles were irregular. Both these things raised suspicion towards the likely ovulatory dysfunction in this patient. Keeping in mind the diagnosis of anovulatory cycles, the woman was advised the following investigations: pelvic ultrasound examination, serum progesterone levels 1 week

**Table 9.29:** Various findings elicited at the time of clinical examination in a case of infertility

*General Physical Examination*

General physical examination requires routine measurement of the patient's vital signs including pulse rate, blood pressure and temperature. Other important aspects of the general physical examination include measurement of the following parameters:

- *Body mass index:* Measurement of the patient's height and weight to calculate the BMI. Calculation of BMI is important because extremely low or extremely high BMI may be associated with reduced fertility. Moreover, abdominal obesity may be associated with insulin resistance.
- *Thyroid examination:* Note for thyroid enlargement, nodule or tenderness.
- *Eye examination:* Eye examination must be performed in order to establish the presence of exophthalmos, which may be associated with hyperthyroidism.
- *Stigmata of Turner's syndrome:* The presence of epicanthus, low set ears and hairline, and webbed neck can be associated with chromosomal abnormalities.
- *Breast examination:* A breast examination must be performed in order to evaluate breast development and to assess the breasts for the presence of abnormal masses or secretions, especially galactorrhea. This opportunity must be taken by the clinician to educate patients about breast self-examination during the early days of their menstrual cycles.
- *Signs of androgen excess:* Signs of androgen excess such as hirsutism, acne, deepening of the voice, hypertrichosis, etc. must be looked for. Androgen deficiency during early gestation may result in development of ambiguous genitalia. Androgen exposure in childhood may present as delayed pubertal development; while in adulthood as reduced sexual function, infertility, and ultimately, loss of secondary sexual characteristics.
- *Examination of extremities:* The extremities must be examined in order to rule out malformations, such as shortness of the fourth finger or cubitus valgus, which can be associated with chromosomal abnormalities and other congenital defects.
- *Examination of the skin:* The skin must be examined for the presence of acne, hypertrichosis and hirsutism.
- *Examination of the secondary sexual characteristics:* Failure of development of secondary sexual characteristics must always prompt a workup for hypopituitarism. Loss of axillary and pubic hair and atrophy of the external genitalia should lead the physician to suspect hypopituitarism in a previously menstruating young woman who develops amenorrhea. Tanner stages of development of breasts and pubic hair is shown in Figures 9.8, 9.9 and Tables 9.30 and 9.31 respectively.

**Examination of Female Partner**

*Specific Systemic Examination*

*Abdominal Examination*

The abdominal examination should be done to detect the presence of abnormal masses in the abdomen. Masses felt in the hypogastrium could be arising from the pelvic region.

*Per Speculum Examination*
- A thorough gynecologic examination has already been described in Chapter 8.
- The distribution of hair pattern on the external genitalia should be particularly noted.
- The inspection of the vaginal mucosa may indicate a deficiency of estrogens or the presence of infection.
- Cervical stenosis can be diagnosed during a speculum examination. Complete cervical stenosis is confirmed by the inability to pass a 1–2 mm probe into the uterine cavity.

*Bimanual Examination*
- Bimanual examination should be performed to establish the direction of the cervix and the size and position of the uterus.
- The clinician should look for presence of any mass, tenderness or nodularity in adnexa or cul-de-sac. Various pelvic pathologies such as fibroids, adnexal masses, tenderness or pelvic nodules indicative of infection or endometriosis can be detected on bimanual examination. Many uterine defects related to infertility such as absence of the vagina and uterus, presence of vaginal septum, etc. can be detected during the pelvic examination.
- Tenderness or masses in the adnexae or posterior cul-de-sac (pouch of Douglas) is suggestive of chronic PID or endometriosis. Palpable tender nodules in the posterior cul-de-sac, uterosacral ligaments, or rectovaginal septum are additional signs of endometriosis.

**Examination of Male Partner**

The patient should be examined for age-appropriate development of male secondary sex characteristics, gynecomastia, or hirsutism. The structures of male external genitalia which must be evaluated include the penis, scrotum, testes, epididymis, spermatic cord and vas deferens. The clinician must examine the external genitalia for the presence of following abnormalities:

- The scrotum must be carefully and thoroughly palpated, and the presence of all scrotal structures should be confirmed, along with their size and consistency.
- Presence of congenital abnormalities of the genital tract, e.g. hypospadias, cryptorchidism (undescended testes), absence of the vas deferens (unilateral or bilateral), etc. must be assessed.
- Testicular size, presence of tenderness on palpation of testicles and presence of any associated mass must be assessed. If any mass is palpated, it must be verified whether the mass is arising from the testicles or is separate from it.

*(Contd...)*

*(Contd...)*

- Urethra must be assessed for presence of any stenosis, diverticulum, etc.
- Presence of an inguinal hernia or varicocele: A varicocele can be exaggerated during physical examination by asking the patient to perform the Valsalva maneuver while standing. The varicocele normally disappears when the patient lies down. A long-standing varicocele may result in testicular atrophy. If the varicocele is large, it may be visible during inspection resulting in "bag of worms" appearance.
- The complete physical examination should also include a digital rectal examination.

*Abbreviations:* BMI, body mass index; PID, pelvic inflammatory disease

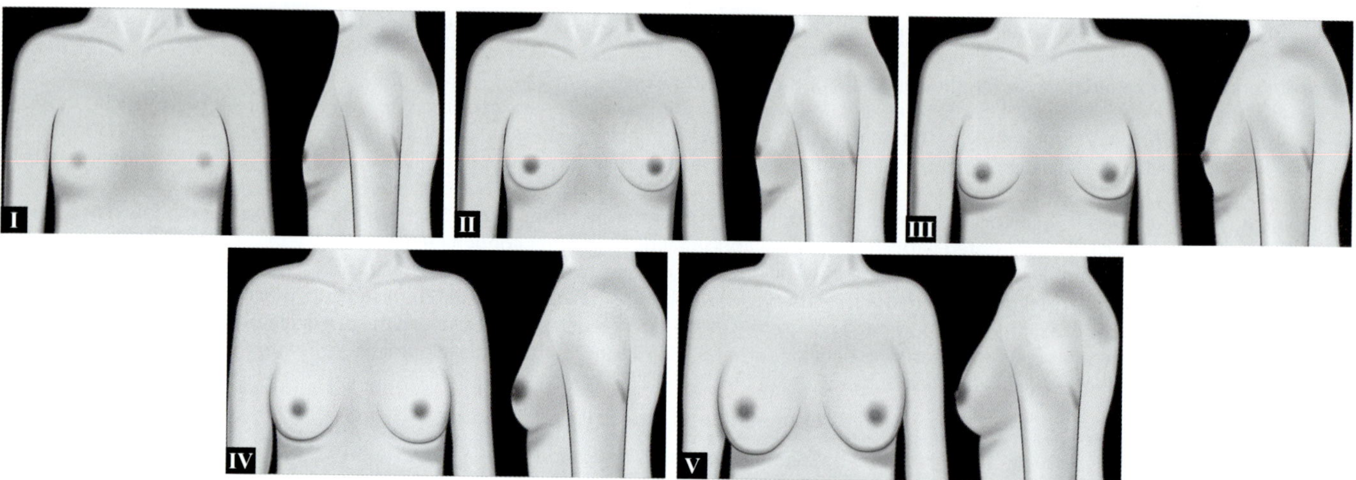

**Fig. 9.8:** Tanner stages of breast development

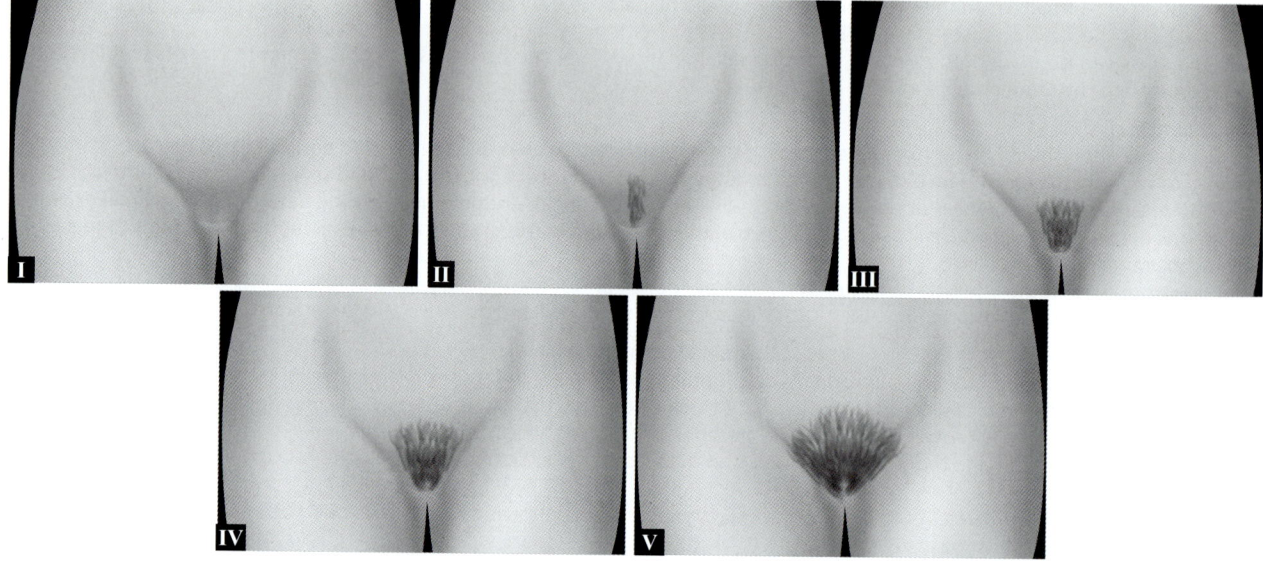

**Fig. 9.9:** Tanner stages of pubic hair development

**Table 9.30:** Tanner stages of breast development

| Stage | Characteristics |
|---|---|
| Stage 1 | Elevation of papilla |
| Stage 2 | Elevation of breast and papilla as a small mound, increased areolar diameter (median age: 9.8 years) |
| Stage 3 | Further enlargement without the separation of breast and areola (median age: 11.2 years) |
| Stage 4 | Secondary mound of areola and papilla above the breast (median age: 12.1 years) |
| Stage 5 | Recession of areola to the contour of breast (median age: 14.6 years) |

**Table 9.31:** Tanner stages of pubic hair development

| Stage | Characteristics |
|---|---|
| Stage 1 | No pubic hair, prepubertal |
| Stage 2 | Sparse, long pigmented hair mainly along labia majora (median age: 10.5 years) |
| Stage 3 | Dark, coarse curled hair, sparsely spread over the mons (median age: 11.4 years) |
| Stage 4 | Adult-type, abundant hair, but limited to the mons (median age: 12.0 years) |
| Stage 5 | Adult type spread in quantity and distribution (median age: 13.6 years) i.e. spread occurs to the medial aspect of thighs |

**Table 9.32:** Work-up of an infertile couple

*Minimal investigations (required in most couples)*

- Semen analysis to assess male factors
- Menstrual history, assessment of LH surge in urine prior to ovulation, and/or luteal phase progesterone level to assess ovulatory function and endometrial receptivity
- Hysterosalpingography to assess tubal patency and the uterine cavity
- Day 3 serum FSH and estradiol levels to assess ovarian reserve.

*Additional tests required in select couples*

- Pelvic ultrasound to assess for uterine myomas and ovarian cysts.
- Laparoscopy to diagnose endometriosis or other pelvic pathology.
- *Additional tests for assessment of ovarian reserve in women over 35 years of age:* Clomiphene citrate challenge test, ultrasound for early follicular antral follicle count, day 3 serum inhibin B level, or anti-Müllerian hormone measurement
- Assessment of thyroid function.

*Abbreviations:* FSH, follicle-stimulating hormone; LH, luteinizing hormone

**Table 9.33:** Causes of infertility (both male and female factors)

| Causes of infertility | Percentage of cases |
|---|---|
| • Male causes | 35% |
| • Female causes:<br>  – Tubal and pelvic pathology<br>  – Ovulatory dysfunction | 50%<br>    35%<br>    15% |
| • Unusual causes | 5% |
| • Unexplained causes | 10% |

**Table 9.34:** Various causes of female infertility

*Cervical Factor Infertility*

- Abnormalities of the mucus-sperm interaction
- Narrowing of the cervical canal due to cervical stenosis

*Uterine Factor Infertility*

- *Congenital defects:* Abnormalities in the development of the Müllerian ducts may result in a spectrum of congenital/Müllerian duct abnormalities varying from total absence of the uterus and vagina (Mayer-Rokitansky-Küster-Hauser syndrome) to minor defects such as arcuate uterus and vaginal septa (transverse or longitudinal).
- *Acquired causes:* These may include the following:
  - Drug-induced uterine malformations: e.g. diethylstilbestrol
  - Asherman's syndrome, endometritis: Endometritis or inflammation of the uterine cavity due to infections such as tuberculosis.
  - Leiomyomas

*Causes of Ovulatory Dysfunction*

Classification of various ovulatory disorders as devised by WHO is described in Table 9.36.

*Tubal Obstruction*

- Pelvic inflammatory disease: PID is typically associated with gonorrheal and Chlamydial infection.
- Formation of scar tissue and adhesions due to infections (especially *Chlamydia* and gonorrhea), endometriosis, pelvic tuberculosis, and salpingitis isthmica nodosa (i.e. diverticulosis of the fallopian tube) or abdominal or gynecological surgery

*Abbreviations:* DES, diethylstilbestrol; PID, pelvic inflammatory disease; WHO, World Health Organization

| **Table 9.35:** Causes of male infertility |
|---|
| • Hypothalamic pituitary disease (secondary hypogonadism)<br>  – *Congenital disorders:* Kallmann's syndrome, Laurence-Moon-Biedl syndrome, Prader-Willi syndrome, lower oculocerebral syndrome, familial cerebellar ataxia, etc.<br>  – Acquired diseases<br>    - Tumors: Pituitary macroadenomas (macroprolactinomas and nonfunctioning adenomas)<br>    - Infiltrative diseases: Sarcoidosis, histiocytosis, tuberculosis, fungal infections, transfusion siderosis, hemochromatosis, etc.<br>    - Vascular lesions: Pituitary infarction and carotid aneurysm<br>    - Hormonal: Hyperprolactinemia, estrogen excess, glucocorticoid excess and androgen excess<br>    - Drugs: Opioid-like or other central nervous system-activating drugs, including many psychotropic drugs, GnRH analogs (agonists and antagonists), etc.<br>    - Systemic illness: Any serious systemic illness or chronic nutritional deficiency |
| • Testicular disease<br>  – Congenital or developmental disorders of the testes: These include Klinefelter's syndrome, Y chromosome microdeletions, cryptorchidism, varicoceles, and other less common disorders<br>    - Defective androgen receptor or synthesis: Men with congenital androgen insensitivity due to androgen receptor or postreceptor abnormalities and those with 5-alpha-reductase deficiency are nearly always infertile<br>    - Disorders of the estrogen receptor or estrogen synthesis<br>    - Inactivating mutation in FSH receptor gene<br>    - Myotonic dystrophy<br>  – Acquired disorders of the testes<br>    - Drugs: Cyclophosphamide, chlorambucil, antiandrogens (flutamide, cyproterone, spironolactone), ketoconazole, cimetidine, etc.<br>    - Radiation<br>    - Environmental factors: Environmental toxins such as lead, cadmium, and mercury, and exposure of testes to high temperature (e.g. workers in blast furnace)<br>    - Antisperm antibodies<br>    - Systemic disorders: Chronic renal insufficiency, cirrhosis, or malnutrition |
| • Post-testicular defects (disorders of sperm transport)<br>  – Abnormalities of the epididymis: Absence, dysfunction, or obstruction of the epididymis.<br>  – Abnormalities of the vas: Bilateral obstruction, ligation, or altered peristalsis of the vas deferens results in infertility, infection (gonorrhea, *Chlamydia*, tuberculosis) resulting in the development of obstruction.<br>  – Defective ejaculation: Spinal cord disease or trauma, sympathectomy, or autonomic disease (e.g. diabetes mellitus), erectile dysfunction, mechanical obstruction (condoms and diaphragm use), premature ejaculation, infrequency of intercourse, etc. |
| • Idiopathic: Failure to conceive with an apparently normal female partner despite of having repeatedly normal semen analyses |

*Abbreviations:* FSH, follicle-stimulating hormone; GnRH, gonadotropin-releasing hormone

| **Table 9.36:** WHO classification of ovulatory disorders | | |
|---|---|---|
| *WHO class* | *Pathology* | *Causes* |
| WHO class 1: Hypogonadotropic hypogonadal anovulation | Low or low-normal levels of serum FSH and low serum estradiol concentrations | Excessive exercise or low body weight |
| WHO class 2: Normogonadotropic normoestrogenic anovulation | Normal levels of gonadotropins and estrogens. However, FSH secretion during the follicular phase of the cycle is subnormal | Women with polycystic ovarian syndrome |
| WHO class 3: Hypergonadotropic hypoestrogenic anovulation | High to normal levels of gonadotropins and low levels of estrogen | Women with primary gonadal failure (previously called premature ovarian failure) or gonadal dysgenesis |
| Hyperprolactinemic anovulation | Inhibition of gonadotropin and estrogen secretion due to hyperprolactinemia; gonadotropin concentrations in this condition are usually normal or decreased | Prolactinoma (microadenomas, macroadenomas) |

*Abbreviations:* FSH, follicle-stimulating hormone; WHO, World Health Organization

before the expected time of menses, serum LH:FSH ratio, fasting insulin levels and serum testosterone levels. In view of the raised BMI, the woman was advised lifestyle changes in order to reduce her weight. She was advised to indulge in brisk walking for 30 minutes every day. She was also referred to the nutrition specialist to help her devise a proper dietary plan in order to bring her weight under control.

**Q. On the basis of the results of various investigations, a diagnosis of PCOS was established in this case. What should be next step of management in this case?**

**Ans.** Since the ultrasound examination revealed findings suggestive of polycystic ovarian disease, she was started on clomiphene citrate in the dosage of 50 mg/day for first 5 days of the menstrual cycle. However, even after a course of 6 months, there was no ovulation. Keeping in view the increased BMI and insulin resistance, she was also simultaneously administered metformin, 500 mg OD, which was soon increased to 500 mg BID. Ultrasound examination for follicular monitoring in this case revealed evidence of ovulation.

**Q. What is the most important test for investigating the infertile couple?**

**Ans.** Semen analysis is the most important test to be performed while evaluation of an infertile couple. A comprehensive semen analysis must be performed in a certified andrology laboratory. Male patient should be instructed well in advance that they must provide a semen sample after a period of abstinence of 2–5 days. This sample is collected through masturbation, and must be collected into a container, which is nontoxic to the sperms. Ideally, the specimen must be collected at the same andrology laboratory, which would conduct the test. If the sample is collected at home, it should be transported to the laboratory within 30 minutes to ensure the accuracy of results. The primary values that are evaluated at the time of semen analysis include volume of the ejaculate, sperm motility, total sperm concentration, sperm morphology, motility and viability. The odds of male infertility increase with the number of major semen parameters (sperm concentration, mobility and morphology) in the subfertile range. Normal parameters for semen analysis are described by WHO in Table 9.37. Spermatogenesis takes approximately 72 days. Therefore, the sperm analysis must be repeated after 3 months if any of the parameters appear abnormal or as soon as possible in case of gross sperm deficiency.

**Q. What tests must be performed for evaluation of the female partner?**

**Ans.** A complete evaluation of the female reproductive tract must involve cervical, uterine, endometrial, tubal, peritoneal and ovarian factors. Since thyroid disease and hyperprolactinemia can cause menstrual abnormalities and infertility, serum thyroid-stimulating hormone (TSH) and prolactin levels must be checked first before instituting further investigations.

**Table 9.37:** Parameters for semen analysis: lower reference limits (95% CI) in fertile men (World Health Organization, 5th Edition, 2010)

| Parameter | Normal range |
| --- | --- |
| Volume | 1.5 mL (1.4 mL–1.7 mL) |
| Sperm concentration | 15 (12–16) million/mL or greater |
| Total sperm number | 39 (33–46) million spermatozoa per ejaculate or more |
| Motility | 32%, forward progression; 40% total motility (progressive + nonprogressive motility) |
| Morphology | Normal sperms (> 4%) using "strict" Tygerberg method |
| Vitality | 58 (55–63)% or more live |

- *Evaluation of cervical factor:* These include the following tests:
  - *Postcoital test (Sims or Huhner's test):* This test has been described in details in Chapter 10.
- *Tests for uterine factor:* The commonly used investigations include hysterosalpingogram (HSG), pelvic ultrasonography and endometrial biopsy. For details of these tests, refer to Chapter 10.

  Operative procedures such as laparoscopy and hysteroscopy are often necessary for confirmation of the final diagnosis. Screening tests for *Chlamydia trachomatis* are also performed.
- *Tests for ovarian factors:* These include tests for checking ovarian reserve such as determination of day 3 FSH levels, clomiphene citrate challenge test, astral follicle count and measurement of anti-Müllerian hormone levels. Measurement of serum progesterone levels serves as the simplest, most common and reliable test of ovulatory function. A serum progesterone concentration of less than 3 ng/mL implies anovulation.
- *Tests for tubal and peritoneal factors:* These include HSG, SIS and laparoscopy.

**Q. What is a hysterosalpingogram?**

**Ans:** The HSG is the most frequently used diagnostic tool for evaluation of the endometrial cavity as well as the tubal pathology. If performed meticulously under fluoroscopic guidance, HSG helps in providing accurate information about the endocervical canal; endometrial cavity; cornual ostium; patency of the fallopian tubes and status of the fimbriae. Tubal patency is indicated by spillage of dye into the endometrial cavity. HSG is able to accurately define the shape and size of the uterine cavity. It can help diagnose uterine developmental anomalies, (e.g. unicornuate uterus, septate uterus, bicornuate uterus and uterus didelphys), submucous myomas, adnexal masses, intrauterine adhesions and endometrial polyps. The procedure of hysterosalpingography has been described in details in Chapter 10.

### Q. How is laparoscopic examination useful in cases of infertility?

**Ans.** Gynecological laparoscopy is used for diagnosis as well as treatment of pelvic pathology.

- During laparoscopic examination, a laparoscope is used for visualizing the pelvic area, uterine surface, anterior and posterior cul-de-sac, fallopian tubes and ovaries.
- Gynecological laparoscopy is commonly used for diagnosing and treating endometriosis, PID, ectopic pregnancy and removal of adhesions and scar tissue.
- Laparoscopy can be used for monitoring the effects of ovulation induction medicines on the ovaries, and taking biopsies from ovarian cysts.
- Injection of a dye solution through the cannula inserted inside the cervix permits evaluation of tubal patency (chromotubation). Currently, laparoscopy has become the gold standard method for detection of tubal patency.
- In suspected cases of endometriosis or pelvic adhesions, diagnostic laparoscopy and chromotubation is preferred. Ablation of implants and lysis of adhesions can also be performed at the time of laparoscopy.

### Q. What is basal body temperature charting?

**Ans.** Basal body temperature (BBT) charts can be used for predicting ovulation. This test has been described in details in Chapter 10.

### Q. What treatment should be instituted in the case of male infertility?

**Ans.** In most cases of male factor infertility due to oligo-spermia, intrauterine insemination (IUI) is the treatment of choice if more than 2 million sperms are recovered after the sperm wash. Men with hypogonadotropic hypogonadism should be offered treatment with gonadotropin drugs because these are effective in improving fertility. Patients with ejaculatory sexual dysfunction may benefit from a prescription for phosphodiesterase type 5 inhibitors, e.g. sildenafil.

Where appropriate expertise is available, men with obstructive azoospermia should be offered surgical correction of epididymal blockage because it is likely to restore patency of the duct and improve fertility. Other options which can be considered as an alternative to surgery include surgical sperm recovery and IVF.

### Q. What kind of treatment should be instituted in the cases of cervical factor infertility?

**Ans.** Chronic cervicitis may be treated with antibiotics. The easiest and most successful treatment option for infertility related to cervical factors is artificial IUI in conjunction with ovulation inducing agents. In case of unsuccessful attempts at IUI, IVF must be used as the next option.

### Q. What is artificial intrauterine insemination?

**Ans.** Artificial insemination can be performed by depositing the sperms at the level of internal cervical os (cervical insemination) or inside the endometrial cavity (IUI). Since cervical insemination is associated with low success rate in comparison with IUI, the latter is more commonly used. IUI may be performed either during a natural cycle (unstimulated IUI) or following ovulation induction with clomiphene citrate or gonadotropins (stimulated IUI). The average pregnancy rate achieved after a natural-cycle IUI is 8%. Artificial insemination can be of two types: (1) homologous and (2) heterologous. While the homologous insemination refers to the use of sperm from the patient's partner, heterologous insemination refers to the use of frozen donor sperms that have been quarantined for at least 6 months.

### Q. What are the indications for intrauterine insemination?

**Ans.** Indications for IUI are as follows:

- Unexplained infertility
- Cervical factor infertility
- Failure to conceive after ovulation induction treatment
- Immunological causes (antisperm antibodies)
- Couples with minimal to mild endometriosis
- Mild-moderate male factor infertility and other causes of male infertility such as ejaculatory failure and retrograde ejaculation.

### Q. What is the mode of treatment of uterine factor infertility?

**Ans.** Surgical treatment for uterine factor infertility involves lysis of uterine septae and uterine synechiae, and surgical treatment of uterine anomalies (e.g. bicornuate uterus, etc.). Uterine synechiae and septae are corrected using operative hysteroscopy. Treatment of fibroids may be required if they are associated with AUB or if they are thought to be the cause of infertility. Treatment of myomas has been previously described in the text. Women having an irreparable uterine defect may require a gestational carrier (surrogate mother). Treatment of infertility in women with luteal phase defect is best dealt with help of ovulation inducing agents rather than with progesterone.

### Q. What should be the mode of treatment in case of tubal factors of infertility?

**Ans.** The treatment of tubal-factor infertility has undergone tremendous changes, especially during the last few decades with the widespread use of tubal microsurgery and assisted reproductive techniques.

### Q. How is the ovarian factor infertility treated?

**Ans.** In case of patients with ovulatory dysfunction, the most appropriate treatment option is to begin with ovulation inducing drugs. The treatment can be started imme-diately before other potential causes of infertility have been investigated. Women with ovulatory disorders due to hyperprolactinemia should be offered treatment with dopamine agonists such as bromocriptine. In cases where anovulation is the only obstacle to overcome, most couples would conceive promptly on using ovulation induction agents. In these cases, the various ovulation induction agents which can be used include clomiphene citrate, human menopausal gonadotropin (hMG), hCG, recombinant FSH, and recombinant LH.

The standard dose of clomiphene citrate is 50 mg PO once a day for 5 days, starting on the day 3–5 of the menstrual cycle or after progestin-induced bleeding. The response to clomiphene citrate is monitored using pelvic ultrasonography starting on the day 12 of the menstrual cycle. The follicle should develop to a diameter of 23–24 mm before a spontaneous LH surge occurs.

Human menopausal gonadotropin and its derivatives are indicated for ovulation induction in patients with primary amenorrhea and/or infertility, who did not respond to ovulation induction with clomiphene citrate. hMG (Menopur) contains 75 U of FSH and 75 U of LH per mL.

### Q. What is in vitro fertilization?

**Ans.** In vitro fertilization consists of retrieving preovulatory oocytes from the ovary and fertilizing them with sperms in the laboratory, with subsequent embryo transfer within the endometrial cavity. The procedure of IVF comprises of the following steps:

- *Ovarian stimulation:* In order to increase the number of ovarian follicles which get recruited, selected and finally get transformed into a dominant follicle, several ovarian stimulation protocols may be used. These include clomiphene citrate protocol; use of clomiphene citrate with hMG; use of hMG only; use of GnRH agonists (GnRHa) and GnRH antagonists.
- *Follicular aspiration:* Oocytes are aspirated from the ovary 35–36 hours following administration of a stimulating protocol. Initially all aspirations were performed under laparoscopic guidance. However now, follicular aspirations are commonly performed under ultrasonographic guidance, both transabdominal as well as transvaginal. The transvaginal route for follicular aspiration has now become the preferred procedure in most IVF programs.
- *Oocyte classification:* Following their aspiration, the oocytes are graded according to the appearance of the corona-cumulus complex.
- *Sperm preparation and oocyte insemination:* The procedure of sperm preparation involves the removal of certain components of the ejaculate (i.e. seminal fluid, excess cellular debris, leukocytes, morphologically abnormal sperms, etc.) along with the retention of the motile fraction of sperms. A final number of 200,000 motile sperms in a small volume of media with a layer of mineral oil on top is added to the oocytes.
- *Embryo culture:* The inseminated oocytes are incubated in an atmosphere of 5% carbon dioxide in air with 98% humidity. Presence of two pronuclei and the extrusion of a second polar body are the criteria which ascertain fertilization, and should occur approximately 18 hours following insemination. The fertilized embryos are transferred into growth media and placed in the incubator. No further evaluation is performed over the next 24 hours. A 4–8 cell stage, pre-embryo is observed approximately 36–48 hours after insemination.
- *Embryo transfer:* The procedure of embryo transfer into the endometrial cavity is performed within 72 hours after oocyte insemination, when the embryo has become approximately 8–16 cells in size. The transfer is usually performed transcervically under guidance of transabdominal ultrasound.

### Q. What is intracytoplasmic sperm injection?

**Ans.** Intracytoplasmic sperm injection (ICSI) is an assisted reproductive technology procedure involving the direct injection of a sperm into an oocyte. ICSI has revolutionized the treatment of severe male factor infertility because only a single live sperm is required, which is injected directly into the ovum. ICSI is commonly used in cases of male factor infertility such as obstructive azoospermia (due to congenital absence of the vas deferens). ICSI nowadays is also commonly being used as part of an IVF cycle. The procedure of ICSI is as follows:

The sperm can be obtained through masturbation, epididymal aspiration, testicular biopsy, or needle puncture of the testes. The sperm is paralyzed by stroking the distal portion of its tail. The oocyte is stripped from the cumulus using a solution of hyaluronidase. To inject the sperm, first the oocyte is stabilized with a micropipette, then the sperm is loaded, tail first, into a microneedle. The oocyte membrane is pierced with the microneedle and the oolemma is entered. The spermatozoon is released inside the oolemma, and the microinjected oocyte is kept in the incubator.

### Q. What are the indications for ICSI?

**Ans.** Indications for ICSI are as follows:
- Severe deficits in semen quality
- Obstructive azoospermia
- Nonobstructive azoospermia
- Failure of previous IVF treatment cycles.

### Q. What is polycystic ovarian syndrome? How is it diagnosed?

**Ans.** Polycystic ovarian syndrome is the most common cause of hyperandrogenic chronic anovulation. According to ESHRE and ASRM, Rotterdam, 2003, for the diagnosis of PCOS, at least two of the following three criteria must be present:
1. Oligo/anovulation
2. Clinical or biochemical signs of hyperandrogenism
3. Ultrasound findings suggestive of PCOS (Fig. 9.10):
   - Presence of multiple small cysts of the size 0.5–1 mm, (usually more than 10 in number) along the periphery of the ovary, giving rise to the "necklace appearance" on the ultrasound.

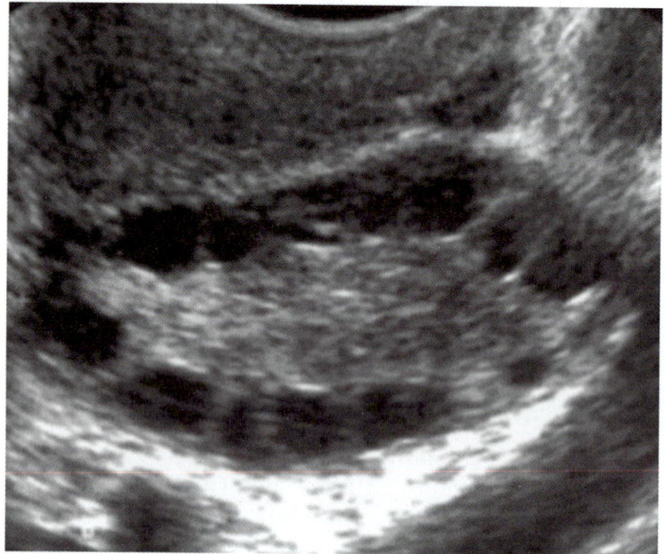

**Fig. 9.10:** Transvaginal sonography showing a row of intermediate sized subcapsular follicles present peripherally in both the ovaries suggestive of polycystic ovarian disease

– Hyperplasia of the stroma results in an increase in the ovarian volume to more than 8 mL or 9 cm³.

### Q. What is the gross appearance and ultrasound appearance of ovaries in these cases?

**Ans.** Grossly, the ovaries of most women with PCOS are bilaterally enlarged and globular and have a thickened capsule. Due to the presence of a smooth glistening capsule, the ovaries often have an "oyster shell" appearance. The tunica albuginea is often thickened diffusely and many cysts of 3–7 mm in diameter are present in the periphery on cut section. Ultrasound appearance of ovaries in case of PCOS is described in the previous question.

### Q. How is PCOS treated?

**Ans.** Some commonly used treatment options for PCOS include ovulation-inducing medicines such as clomiphene citrate, insulin sensitizing agents (such as glucophage and metformin), dietary changes (low glycemic diet) and surgery (ovarian drilling). The primary treatment for PCOS is weight loss through diet and exercise. Modest weight loss helps in lowering the androgen levels, improving hirsutism, normalization of menstrual cycles, resumption of ovulation and reduction of insulin resistance. However it may take months, before these results become apparent.

Besides facilitating fertility, the aims of treatment in women with PCOS are to control hirsutism, to prevent endometrial hyperplasia from unopposed acyclic estrogen secretion, and to prevent the long-term consequences of insulin resistance. The treatment must be individualized according to the needs and desires of each patient. Use of OCPs or cyclic progestational agents can help to maintain a normal endometrium and also reduce the increased risk of endometrial hyperplasia and carcinoma.

For the woman with PCOS who wants to conceive, clomiphene citrate is used initially because of its high success rate and relative simplicity and inexpensiveness. Clomiphene citrate is able to induce ovulation in nearly 80% of the individuals and 40% are able to conceive. Other possible therapeutic approaches for ovulation induction include the use of insulin-sensitizing agents, gonadotropins (perhaps preceded by GnRH analogs), FSH alone, pulsatile GnRH and wedge resection of the ovaries at laparotomy.

Women with PCOS who have not responded to clomiphene citrate can be offered laparoscopic ovarian drilling because it is as effective as gonadotropin treatment and is not associated with an increased risk of multiple pregnancy. This procedure involves creation of approximately 4–20 holes, having a size of 3 mm diameter and 3 mm depth to be made in each ovary, preferably on the antimesenteric side.

# Abnormal Vaginal Discharge

## Case Study 1

Mrs XYZ, a 23-year-old unmarried woman, resident of ABC, presented to the gynecological OPD with the complaints of vaginal discharge since last 4–5 days. She described the discharge as being white in color and curd-like in consistency. It was associated with significant itching and discomfort, which greatly interfered with her normal routine and disturbed her sleep. The patient does not give history of ever having any sexual partner or indulging in any kind of sexual activity. There is no past medical history of diabetes or any other medical disorder in the past. The patient does give history of taking a 7-day course of the antibiotic erythromycin, which was prescribed to her by a general practitioner for throat infection, a few days back.

### Q. What is the likely diagnosis in the above-mentioned case study?

**Ans.** The questions to be asked at the time of taking history and the parameters to be assessed at the time of examination in such a case are described in Tables 9.38 and 9.39 respectively. The most likely diagnosis in this case is Mrs XYZ, resident of ABC, a 23-year-old unmarried woman presenting with the complaints of vaginal discharge since last 4–5 days. The patient's symptomatic history is typically indicative of candidal vulvovaginitis. The predisposing factor, which led to the development of vaginitis, in this case is most likely to be exposure to antibiotics. However certain investigations (microscopic examination) need to be done to confirm the exact pathology.

### Q. What are the different causes for abnormal vaginal discharge?

**Ans.** Different causes for vaginal discharge in various age groups are described in Table 9.40.

**Table 9.38:** Symptoms to be elicited at the time of taking history in a case of abnormal vaginal discharge

*History of Presenting Complains*

- *Vaginal discharge:* Appearance of vaginal discharge is a prominent symptom of vaginitis. Since some amount of discharge may be due to physiological causes, it is important to enquire the patient about change in the volume, color, or odor of vaginal discharge, if also observed previously.
- The amount of discharge
- Color of vaginal discharge
- Duration of symptoms
- Presence of any odor with the discharge
- Association of the discharge with menstrual cycles
- *Site of symptoms:* The site commonly involved (e.g. presence of ulcers on vulva or vagina) needs to be asked.
- *History of constitutional symptoms:* History of constitutional symptoms such as fever, pelvic or abdominal pain and malaise may be associated with PID.
- *History of vulvar/vaginal irritation and itching:* History of any vaginal pruritus or discomfort in association with the vaginal discharge needs to be asked. While there is usually no vulvar/vaginal irritation in cases of bacterial vaginosis, vaginal irritation or pruritus is characteristically present in cases of trichomoniasis or VVC. Asking the time when the patient experiences discomfort is also important. History of pruritus and discomfort especially at night is typically suggestive of pinworm infection.
- *History of urinary symptoms:* History of urinary symptoms such as increased frequency of urination, urgency and dysuria needs to be enquired. This is important because such symptoms may be frequently associated with vaginitis.
- *Estrogen status:* Since atrophic vaginitis is a common cause of vaginitis in a hypoestrogenic woman, the clinician needs to take the history related to estrogen status. In order to establish the estrogen status of a woman, it is important to know if she is menopausal or otherwise hypoestrogenic (e.g. taking antiestrogenic drugs).
- *Hygiene practices:* It is important to ask the patient about certain hygiene practices, which may have an important role in the etiopathogenesis of her problem. Some of these habits include:
  - Habits such as vaginal douching at least once a week are associated with an increased risk of bacterial vaginosis, suggesting that daily habits may play an important role in the development of bacterial vaginosis.
  - Regular use of irritants such as soaps, baths, spermicides, perfumes, douches and creams can also cause vulvovaginitis.
  - Tight fitting, synthetic, nylon undergarments can increase moisture, exacerbating the condition. The patient should be asked to wear loose fitting cotton undergarments.
  - Wiping the anus from posterior to anterior while using the toilet paper is likely to increase the risk for developing vaginitis.
- History of symptoms suggestive of malignancy: In women belonging to perimenopausal and postmenopausal age groups, malignancy (vulval, vaginal, endometrial or cervical) is a common cause of vaginal discharge. Thus, in these women, it is important to enquire about vaginal bleeding or spotting, watery discharge and postmenopausal or postcoital bleeding. Vaginal intraepithelial neoplasia can present with vaginal discharge and/or postcoital spotting. Vulvar intraepithelial neoplasia may cause vulvar pruritus. Fallopian tube cancer, though a rare type of cancer, may present with a serosanguineous vaginal discharge and pelvic pain.
- *Dysuria and dyspareunia:* History of dysuria and dyspareunia may be commonly associated with vulvovaginitis. However, both these conditions could be related to numerous other causes, which need to be ruled out. For example, the exact time of dysuria in relation to the flow of urine needs to be asked. Dysuria related to vaginitis is usually external and produces pain and burning sensation when urine touches the vulva. On the other hand, internal dysuria, defined as pain inside the urethra, is usually a sign of cystitis.

*Sexual History*

A detailed history related to the patient's sexual practices needs to be taken. History suggestive of a recent change in sexual partner is associated with an increased risk of acquiring sexually transmitted infections such as *Trichomonas vaginalis*, or cervicitis related to *N. gonorrhoeae* or *C. trachomatis*. Previous history of any STDs needs to be enquired. The other questions which need to be asked include the following:

- Current and previous sexual partners
- History of having protected or unprotected intercourse
- Frequent change of sexual partners in past 3 months
- History of having multiple sexual contacts
- Similar symptoms (e.g. dysuria, dyspareunia, etc.) in the partner
- Use of any oral contraceptives, or IUCDs in the past
- Presence of positive pregnancy test in the patient
- The gender of the woman's sexual partner needs to be asked. Women having sexual intercourse with other women are at an increased risk of bacterial vaginosis.

*Past Medical History*

- Any history of experiencing similar symptoms in the past
- Use of any antibiotics in recent past (act as a predisposing factor for development of candidal vulvovaginitis)
- History of a systemic disease that could affect the vulvovaginal area (e.g. HSV and Behçet's disease can cause vulvovaginal ulcers).
- Women with diabetes or HIV infections are prone to develop VVC.

*Abbreviations:* HIV, human immunodeficiency virus; HSV, herpes simplex virus; IUCDs, intrauterine contraceptive devices; PID, pelvic inflammatory disease; STDs, sexually transmitted diseases, VVC, vulvovaginal candidiasis

| **Table 9.39:** Various findings elicited at the time of clinical examination in a case of abnormal vaginal discharge |
|---|
| *General Physical Examination* |
| • Presence of lesions over external genitalia or presence of foreign bodies and signs of cervical inflammation. |
| *Specific Systemic Examination* |
| *Per Speculum Examination*<br>On per speculum examination, the following features need to be observed:<br>• Identification of the site of discharge: A per speculum examination can help to identify the anatomic site of involvement (vulva, vagina or cervix).<br>• *Thickness of vaginal mucosa:* Vaginal mucosa may be thin and friable with loss of folds in cases of atrophic vaginitis.<br>• *Signs of vaginal mucosal inflammation:* Presence of erythema, petechial spots or ecchymoses on vaginal mucosal surface, could be related to VVC or trichomoniasis.<br>• *Type of vaginal discharge:* The pooled vaginal discharge should be assessed for color, consistency, volume, odor and adherence to the vaginal walls. While bacterial vaginosis is typically characterized by absence of inflammation, both trichomonal and candidal infection may be associated with vulvar and vaginal erythema, edema and excoriation. Punctate hemorrhages may be visible on the vagina and cervix.<br>• *Presence of any lesions:* The external genitalia must be examined for the presence of inflammation, lesions (ulcers, nodules, etc.) or masses. There may be presence of lesions over external genitalia or foreign bodies and signs of cervical inflammation. |
| *Bimanual Pelvic Examination*<br>• The clinician must assess the patient for presence of uterine or tubo-ovarian tenderness on vaginal examination. Cervical tenderness could be indicative of PID. The technique of bimanual examination has been explained in Chapter 8. |

*Abbreviations:* PID, pelvic inflammatory disease; VVC, vulvovaginal candidiasis.

| **Table 9.40:** Different causes of abnormal vaginal discharge | | |
|---|---|---|
| *Premenarchal* | *Childbearing age* | *Postmenarchal* |
| • Vaginal foreign body<br>• Secondary to sexual abuse<br>• Poor perineal hygiene (wiping the anus from posterior to anterior)<br>• Chemical irritants (e.g. bubble baths, lotions)<br>• Vaginal foreign bodies<br>• Pinworm infection<br>• Skin conditions—Eczema, psoriasis, seborrhea | • Sexually transmitted diseases of the lower genital tract (Chlamydial infection, herpes simplex virus, gonorrheal infection)<br>• Bacterial vaginosis, *Trichomonas* species, *Candida* species and gonorrhea (many of these are associated with sexual abuse)<br>• Chemical irritants | • Atrophic vaginitis<br>• Cervicitis, cervical cancer, vulvar, vaginal, or sometimes even endometrial cancer |

Vaginal discharge could be either physiological or pathological. Nonpathological increase in the quantity of vaginal secretions is referred to as leukorrhea. In these cases, there is no increase in the number of leukocytes or infiltration by pathological organisms. Nonpurulent vaginal discharge could be due to excessive cervical secretions (e.g. chronic cervicitis, cervical erosions, mucus polyps, ectropion, etc.) or due to excessive vaginal secretions (pregnancy, congested, prolapsed ovaries, chronic PID). Purulent or abnormal vaginal discharge may be due to infections, ulcerated growths of vagina, etc. Some common causes of pathological vaginal discharge are described in Table 9.41.

**Q. How does one differentiate between the pathological causes and physiological causes of vaginal discharge?**

**Ans.** The most important challenge for the clinician is to differentiate between the pathological and physiological causes of discharge (Table 9.42). Healthy women belonging to the reproductive age groups may normally produce some amount of physiological vaginal discharge. A normal vaginal discharge consists of 1–4 mL of fluid that is white or transparent and odorless. This physiologic discharge is formed by sloughing epithelial cells, normal bacteria and vaginal transudate.

**Q. How can you differentiate between different kinds of vulvovaginitis which can cause vaginal discharge?**

**Ans.** Vulvovaginitis can be considered as one of the most common causes for pathological vaginal discharge, irritation and itching in women. Vulvovaginitis commonly results due to inflammation of the vagina and vulva or changes in the normal vaginal flora and is most often caused by bacterial, fungal or parasitic infection. Nearly 90% of cases of vaginitis are secondary to bacterial vaginosis, vulvovaginal candidiasis (VVC) and trichomoniasis. The characteristic features of different types of vaginitis are summarized in Table 9.43.

**Q. What is the pathophysiology of vulvovaginitis?**

**Ans.** The normal vaginal epithelium undergoes cornification under the influence of estrogen. This thickening of the vaginal

**Table 9.41:** Causes of pathological vaginal discharge

| Infective discharge | Other causes for discharge |
|---|---|
| • Vulvovaginal candidiasis<br>• Vaginitis caused by *Trichomonas vaginalis, Chlamydia trachomatis*<br>• Sexually transmitted disease *(Neisseria gonorrhoeae)*<br>• Bacterial vaginosis<br>• Acute pelvic inflammatory disease<br>• Postoperative pelvic infection<br>• Postabortal/postpartum sepsis<br><br>*Less common causes*<br>• Human papillomavirus<br>• Primary syphilis<br>• *Mycoplasma genitalium*<br>• *Ureaplasma urealyticum*<br>• *Escherichia coli* | • Retained tampon or condom<br>• Chemical irritation<br>• Allergic responses<br>• Ectropion<br>• Endocervical polyp<br>• Intrauterine device<br><br>*Less common causes*<br>• Atrophic changes<br>• Physical trauma<br>• Vault granulation tissue<br>• Vesicovaginal fistula<br>• Rectovaginal fistula<br>• Neoplasia (cervical, vulvar, vaginal or endometrial) |

**Table 9.42:** Differentiating between physiological and pathological causes of vaginal discharge

| Physiological vaginal discharge | Pathological vaginal discharge |
|---|---|
| • Does not usually cause any discomfort to the patient (except for hygiene problems) | • Usually causes significant distress and irritation to the patient |
| • Translucent to whitish in color | • May vary in color from dirty-white to yellowish-green |
| • Is not associated with itching | • May be associated with itching |
| • Not foul smelling | • May be foul smelling |
| • Amount of discharge may vary in different phases of menstrual cycle | • Amount of discharge does not vary in different phases of menstrual cycle |
| • Discharge is usually not adherent to the vaginal walls | • Discharge is usually adherent to the vaginal walls and pools up in the dependent areas of vagina |

epithelium helps in protecting women against infection. Normal vaginal epithelium is inhabited by the bacteria, *Lactobacillus acidophilus*, which produces hydrogen peroxide. This is not only toxic to the pathogens present in the vagina; it also helps in maintaining the healthy vaginal pH between 3.8 and 4.2. Vaginitis occurs either due to alteration of vaginal flora by the introduction of pathogens or due to the changes in the vaginal environment that allow pathogens to proliferate. Vaginal pH may increase with age, phase of menstrual cycle, sexual activity, hormone therapy, contraception choice, pregnancy, presence of necrotic tissue or foreign bodies and use of hygienic products or antibiotics. This change in vaginal pH may encourage the growth of pathogenic microorganisms. Changes in the vaginal environment, such as an increase in glycogen production in pregnancy or altered estrogen and progesterone levels from the use of oral contraceptives, may also encourage the growth and development of *Candida albicans*.

### Q. What is Amsel's criteria?

**Ans.** Amsel's diagnostic criteria for bacterial vaginosis comprises of the following parameters:
- Thin, homogeneous discharge
- Positive "Whiff test"

- Presence of "clue cells" on microscopic examination
- Vaginal pH greater than 4.5

Amsel's criterion helps in establishing the diagnosis of bacterial vaginosis in nearly 90% of affected women. Three of the previously-mentioned four criteria must be met in order to establish the accurate diagnosis of bacterial vaginosis. Of the various criteria mentioned, presence of clue cells on microscopic examination is a highly significant criterion.

### Q. What are the various treatment options which can be used in cases with symptomatic bacterial vaginosis?

**Ans.** Commonly used treatment options for both pregnant and nonpregnant women are tabulated in the Table 9.44. While previously, some clinicians avoided the use of metronidazole in the first trimester because of its potential to cross the placenta, the CDC no longer discourages the use of metronidazole in the first trimester.

### Q. What are the likely risk factors for the development of vulvovaginal candidiasis?

**Ans.** Severe factors are thought to be associated with an increased risk for uncomplicated VVC. Some such factors, which are associated with an increased risk of this infection, include the following:

**Table 9.43:** Features of the most common causes of vaginitis

| Basis of diagnosis | Bacterial vaginosis | Vulvovaginal candidiasis | Trichomoniasis |
|---|---|---|---|
| Causative agent | Caused due to the alteration of normal vaginal flora resulting in the proliferation of organisms which are normally not present | Caused by the yeast *Candida albicans* | Caused by the motile protozoa *Trichomonas vaginalis* |
| Signs and symptoms | Thin, grayish to off-white colored discharge; unpleasant "fishy" odor, with odor especially increasing after sexual intercourse. The discharge is usually homogeneous and adheres to vaginal walls. | Thick, white (curd like) discharge with no odor | Copious, malodorous yellow-green colored discharge, pruritis and vaginal irritation, dysuria, no symptoms in 20-50% of affected women. |
| Physical examination | Normal appearance of vaginal tissues; grayish-white colored discharge may be adherent to the vaginal walls. | Vulvar and vaginal erythema, edema and fissures. Thick, white discharge that adheres to vaginal walls | Vulvar and vaginal edema and erythema, "strawberry cervix" in upto 25% of affected women. These may be frothy, purulent discharge. |
| Vaginal pH (normal ≤ 4.5) | Elevated (> 4.5) | Normal | Elevated (> 4.5) |
| Microscopic examination of wet-mount and potassium hydroxide (KOH) preparations of vaginal discharge | "Clue cells" (vaginal epithelial cells coated with coccobacilli): few lactobacilli, occasional motile, curved rods, belonging to *Mobiluncus* species | Pseudohyphae, mycelial tangles or budding yeast cells | Motile trichomonads, many Polymorphonuclear cells |
| "Whiff" test (Normal = no odor) | Positive | Negative | Can be positive |
| Additional tests | Amsel's criteria is positive in nearly 90% of affected women with bacterial vaginosis | KOH microscopy, gram stain, culture | Deoxyribonucleic acid (DNA) probe tests: sensitivity of 90% and specificity of 99.8% Culture: sensitivity of 98% and specificity of 100% |

**Table 9.44:** Treatment options for women with bacterial vaginosis

| Pregnant women | Nonpregnant women |
|---|---|
| • Metronidazole 500 mg orally twice daily for 7 days<br>• Metronidazole 250 mg orally three times daily for 7 days<br>• Clindamycin 300 mg orally twice daily for 7 days<br>• Intravaginal preparations of metronidazole and clindamycin are avoided by some experts during pregnancy | • Metronidazole 500 mg twice daily orally for 7 days<br>• Metronidazole gel 0.75% (5 g) once daily vaginally for 5 days<br>• Clindamycin 2% vaginal cream once daily at bedtime for 7 days<br>• Clindamycin 300 mg twice per day orally for 7 days<br>• Clindamycin 100 mg vaginal suppositories at bedtime for 3 days<br>• Clindamycin bioadhesive cream (Clindesse) 2% as a single vaginal dose of 5 g of cream containing 100 mg of clindamycin phosphate |

- Women using OCPs or an IUCD for contraception
- Diabetes mellitus
- Antibiotic use
- Immunodeficiency or use of immunosuppressive agents
- Use of tightfitting synthetic undergarments
- Pregnancy
- Previous episode of VVC

This infection is more likely to occur during pregnancy probably because high levels of estrogen or glycogen in the vaginal secretions during pregnancy are likely to increase a woman's risk of developing VVC.

### Q. What is atrophic vaginitis?

**Ans.** Atrophic vaginitis is one of the most common causes for vaginal discharge in the postmenopausal women. After menopause, vaginal atrophy can result due to falling estrogen levels. Dyspareunia is a common complication of atrophic vaginitis. Per speculum examination in women with vaginal atrophy may show loss of vaginal rugosity and thinning of the vaginal epithelium. This condition can be treated using topical formulations of conjugated estrogens (Premarin) in the dosage of 2–4 g intravaginally qHS (every night at bedtime).

**Q. What are the general principles involved in the evaluation of a woman with leukorrhea?**

**Ans.** General principles involved in the evaluation of a woman with leukorrhea are as follows:

- Obtaining a history and performing a physical examination
- Testing for the three most common disorders causing vaginitis in premenopausal women: bacterial vaginosis, VVC, and trichomoniasis
- If tests for evaluation of these three common causes of vaginal discharge are negative, then evaluation for less common and rare causes of vaginitis, including tests for sexually transmitted diseases need to be done.

**Q. What should be offered for severe pruritus to a woman with vulvovaginal candidiasis?**

**Ans.** A mildly sedating antihistamine at bedtime may help in relieving the nocturnal irritation and scratching (e.g. chlorpheniramine 4 mg orally).

**Q. What investigations must be carried out in the cases of leukorrhea?**

**Ans.** In a patient presenting with vaginal discharge, the following investigations need to be carried out:

*Pregnancy test*: Pregnancy test must be done to rule out pregnancy because certain treatment medicines might be contraindicated during pregnancy.

*Microscopic examination:* If the findings of the history and/or physical examination suggest that the patient has vaginitis, a sample of the vaginal discharge should be obtained for gross and microscopic examination. Microscopic examination of normal vaginal discharge mainly shows squamous epithelial cells, polymorphonuclear leukocytes, and microorganisms related to the *Lactobacillus* species. Pathological vaginal discharge could be associated with the presence of candidal buds or hyphae in case of candidal infection or presence of motile trichomonads in case of infection with *Trichomonas vaginalis*. Clue cells (epithelial cells studded with adherent coccobacilli) may be observed in cases of bacterial vaginosis. Presence of a large number of polymorphonuclear cells without any evidence of candidal species, trichomonads, or clue cells is highly suggestive of cervicitis.

*KOH preparation:* The slide is prepared by placing a drop of vaginal secretion on a slide with a drop of 10–20% KOH and using a coverslip to protect the microscope lens. A coverslip is placed on the slide and air or flame dried before examination is carried out under the microscope. KOH by dissolving the nonfungal elements is useful for detection of candidal hyphae, mycelial tangles and spores. This test is particularly useful in diagnosis of candidal vaginitis. Following the examination of the slide, the KOH Whiff test is performed.

*KOH Whiff test:* Smelling (whiffing) the slide immediately after applying KOH is useful for detecting the fishy (amine) odor of bacterial vaginosis. The odor results from the liberation of amines and organic acids produced from the alkalization of anaerobic bacteria. A positive Whiff test/amine test is suggestive of bacterial vaginosis.

*Nitrazine pH paper:* Nitrazine pH paper is used to evaluate the pH of vaginal discharge sample, which is collected at the time of per speculum examination. The normal vaginal pH ranges between 3.8 and 4.2. The clinician must remember that both blood and cervical mucus are alkaline in nature and their presence may alter the pH of a vaginal sample. The pH level is also high in cases with atrophic vaginitis. A pH greater than 4.5 is found in 80–90% of patients with bacterial vaginosis and frequently in patients with trichomoniasis. VVC is normally associated with a pH of less than 4.5.

*Vaginal culture:* Vaginal culture may help to diagnose the exact etiology in case of a bacterial or fungal infection. If the microscopic examination for candidal species is negative, vaginal culture for *Candida* species must be done because microscopic examination is not sufficiently sensitive to exclude the diagnosis of *Candida* organisms in symptomatic patients.

*Cervical culture:* In a woman with purulent vaginal discharge, culture of cervical secretions is important for establishing the diagnosis of cervicitis, typically due to *N. gonorrhoeae* or *C. trachomatis.*

**Q. What treatment should be instituted in cases of leukorrhea?**

**Ans.** Normal physiological vaginal discharge usually requires no treatment. Discharge associated with infections should respond to the specific treatment. If infections like gonorrhea, Chlamydia or trichomoniasis, are suspected, the woman's sexual partner/s must also be tested and treated.

*Patient education:* Both the women belonging to premenarchal and the childbearing age groups must be given the following advice:

- Patient must be advised to wipe thoroughly and anteriorly to posteriorly while using toilet paper.
- The importance of wearing loosefitting, cotton undergarments must be particularly stressed.
- The patient must be advised to avoid using vaginal irritants such as bubble baths and creams. A sitz bath with baking soda may also be helpful.
- The patient must be advised to thoroughly dry up her perineum and avoid unnecessary prolonged exposure to moisture (e.g. wearing a wet bathing suit for prolonged periods of time).

*Therapeutic options:* Treatment should be specifically aimed at treatment of specific bacterial, parasitic or fungal infection. Treatment of various causes of vaginal discharge has been summarized in Table 9.45.

Topical antifungal therapy for vaginitis has been described in Table 9.46.

**Table 9.45:** Treatment summary of various causes of vaginal discharge

| Treatment regimens | Bacterial vaginosis | Vulvovaginal candidiasis | Trichomoniasis |
|---|---|---|---|
| Acute regimens | Metronidazole (Flagyl), 500 mg orally twice daily for 7 days, forms the first-line treatment. Clindamycin phosphate vaginal cream (2%): application of one full applicator (5 g) intravaginally each night for 7 days or metronidazole gel 0.75% (Metrogel-vaginal): application of one full applicator (5 g) intravaginally twice daily for 5 days | Topical antifungal agents (Table 9.46) or fluconazole 150 mg orally, single dose | Metronidazole 2 g orally in a single dose |
| Alternative regimens | Metronidazole, 2 g orally in a single dose or clindamycin (Cleocin), 300 mg orally twice daily for 7 days or metronidazole 375 mg TID, orally for 7 days | Boric acid powder in size-0 gelatin capsules intravaginally once or twice daily for 2 weeks | Metronidazole, 200 mg orally thrice daily for 7 days |
| Pregnancy | Metronidazole, 250 mg orally three times daily for 7 days (recommended regimen) | Only topical azole agents such as clotrimazole, miconazole, tercona-zole, and tioconazole intravaginally for 7–10 days | Metronidazole, 2 g orally in a single dose (usually not recommended in first trimester) |
| Recurrence | Retreat with an alternative regimen | For four or more episodes of symptomatic vulvovaginal candidiasis annually: initial acute intravaginal regimen for 10–14 days followed immediately by maintenance regimen for at least 6 months (e.g. ketoconazole, 100 mg orally once daily) | Metronidazole, 2 g orally once daily for 3–5 days (Note that treatment of sexual partners increases cure rate) |

**Table 9.46:** Topical antifungal therapy for vaginitis

| Antifungal drug | Intravaginal cream preparation |
|---|---|
| Butoconazole | 2% cream: Application of 5 g/day intravaginally for 3 days |
| Clotrimazole | 1% cream: Application of 5 g/day intravaginally for 7–14 days |
| Miconazole | 2% cream: Application of 5 g/day intravaginally for 7 days |
| Tioconazole | 5% ointment: Application of 5 g intravaginally in a single application |
| Terconazole | 0.4% cream: Application of 5 g/day intravaginally for 7 days<br>0.8% cream: Application of 5 g/day intravaginally for 3 days |
| **Antifungal drug** | **Intravaginal suppository** |
| Clotrimazole | • 100 mg vaginal tablet, one tablet per day intravaginally for 7 days<br>• 500 mg vaginal tablet, one tablet administered intravaginally in a single dose application<br>• Clotrimazole 100 mg vaginal tablet, two tablets per day intravaginally for 3 days |
| Miconazole | 200-mg vaginal suppository per day for 3 days or 100 mg vaginal suppository per day for 7 days |
| Nystatin | 100,000 unit vaginal tablet (Mycostatin), one tablet per day intravaginally for 14 days |
| Terconazole | 80 mg vaginal suppository, one suppository per day for 3 days |

# Genitourinary Fistula

## Case Study 1

Mrs XYZ, a 38-year-old, P4+2 woman, with married life of 8 years, resident of ABC, presented to the gynecology clinic with the complaints of leakage of urine since past 4–5 years. Last childbirth was a difficult vaginal delivery as described by the patient due to cephalopelvic disproportion and obstructed labor. The delivery was taken by an untrained midwife and occurred after nearly 2 days of labor; the baby was born dead. The general physical examination during the present visit was within normal limits. Per vaginal examination revealed a small punched out lesion at the anterior vaginal wall, about 1 inch in size at 12 O' clock position. Constant dribbling of urine was observed through this.

**Q. What is the most likely diagnosis in the above mentioned case study?**

**Ans.** The above-mentioned case study corresponds to urogenital fistula (UGF) (based on history and physical examination) occurring as a result of cephalopelvic disproportion and obstructed labor. The questions to be asked at the time of taking history and the parameters to be assessed at the time of examination in such a case are described in Tables 9.47 and 9.48 respectively. The most likely diagnosis in this case is Mrs XYZ, a 38-year-old woman, with an active married life of 8 years, resident of ABC, P4+2 woman with chief complaints of leakage of urine since past 4–5 years. Diagnosis of UGF on the anterior vaginal wall was established at the time of clinical examination. A methylene blue dye test is required to confirm the diagnosis and help the surgeon plan the repair process.

**Q. What are urogenital fistulas and how can they be classified?**

**Ans.** Urogenital fistulas can be defined as abnormal communication tracts (between the genital tract and the urinary tract or the alimentary tract or both. It can be lined by epithelium, fibrous or granulation tissue or malignant tissues depending upon the cause. UGFs can be classified as follows (Fig. 9.11):

- Urethrovaginal fistula
- Vesical fistula [vesicovaginal fistula (VVF) or vesico-cervical fistula]
- Ureterovaginal fistula
- Rectovaginal fistula

Vesicovaginal fistula is an abnormal fistulous tract extending between the bladder and the vagina that allows the continuous involuntary discharge of urine into the vaginal vault.

**Q. What are the likely factors which can result in the development of urogenital prolapse?**

**Ans.** Various risk factors for the development of urogenital prolapse are enumerated next:

- Most common cause for development of urogenital prolapse in developing countries is obstructed labor. Other obstetric causes include difficult forceps applications or cesarean delivery

---

**Table 9.48:** Various findings elicited at the time of clinical examination in a case of genitourinary fistula

*General Physical Examination*

No specific finding may be observed at the time of general physical examination. The patient may appear depressed. Presence of UGF may often result in the symptoms of depression

*Specific Systemic Examination*

*Per Speculum Examination*

Evaluation of the fluid collection noted upon examination of the vaginal vault must be performed to rule out presence of urine or vaginal discharge. Once the diagnosis of urine is made, the clinician needs to identify its source.

*Pelvic Examination*

Bimanual pelvic examination may give information regarding the fixity and the extent of scarring of the surrounding tissues.

*Abbreviation:* UGF, urogenital fistula

---

**Table 9.47:** Symptoms to be elicited at the time of taking history in a case of genitourinary fistula

*History of Presenting Complains*

- The uncontrolled continuous leakage of urine into the vagina is the hallmark symptom of patients with UGFs.
- Patients may complain of urinary incontinence or an increase in vaginal discharge.
- Constant wetness in the genital areas can lead to the excoriation of the vagina, vulva, perineum and thighs.
- Presence of recurrent cystitis or pyelonephritis, abnormal urinary stream and hematuria following surgery may point towards an underlying UGF.

*Obstetric History*

Previous history of obstructed labor, cephalopelvic disproportion, difficult forceps delivery could act as the risk factor for development of UGF.

*Surgical History*

- History of undergoing any gynecological surgery (especially surgery for extensive endometriosis, pelvic inflammatory disease, cancer cervix, etc.) in the past.
- History of injury to any organ (e.g. ureter, bladder, etc.) at the time of surgery
- History of receiving radiation therapy in the past.

*Abbreviation:* UGF, urogenital fistula

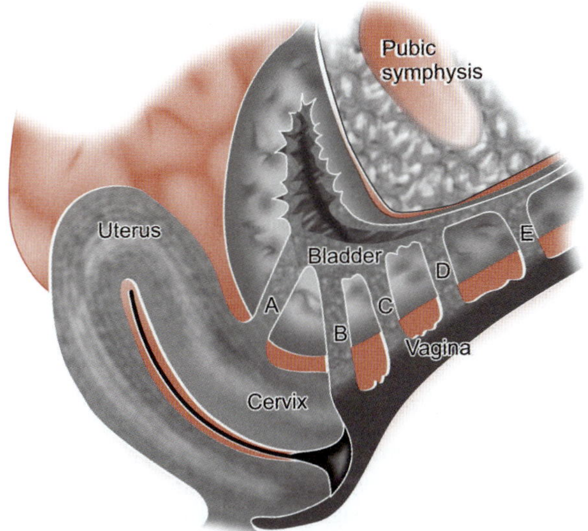


**Fig. 9.11:** Types of genitourinary fistulas. (A) Uterovesical fistula; (B) Cervicovesical fistula; (C) Midvaginal vesicovaginal fistula (VVF); (D) VVF involving the bladder neck; (E) Urethrovaginal fistula

- The majority of UGFs in developed countries are a result of gynecological surgery (pelvic surgery, surgery for gynecological malignancy, hysterectomy, urologic and gastrointestinal surgery)
- Radiotherapy and surgery for malignant gynecologic disease is also responsible for a minority of cases.

### Q. What is the mechanism of development of fistula in the above-mentioned case study?

**Ans.** Obstructed labor and CPD results in prolonged impaction of the fetal presenting part in the pelvis. This may result in tissue edema, hypoxia, necrosis and sloughing off of the soft tissues of the vagina, bladder base and urethra. This is likely to result in the development of UGF.

### Q. What investigations are required in these cases?

**Ans.** The following investigations need to be done in these cases:

- Complete blood count
- *Urine investigations:* This includes urine routine, and microscopy, and urine culture and sensitivity.
- *Renal function tests:* This includes estimation of serum urea, uric acid, creatinine and electrolytes.
- *Cystoscopy:* With the vagina filled with water or isotonic sodium chloride solution, the infusion of gas through the urethra with help of a cystoscope produces air bubbles in the vaginal fluid at the site of a UGF (Flat tire sign).
- Cystoscopy with indigocarmine excretion test (5 mL IV) helps in visualizing the efflux of dye from each ureteric orifice individually.
- *Methylene blue three-swab test:* This test has been described in details in Chapter 10.
- *Ultrasonography:* Sonography of the kidney, ureter and bladder must be performed.
- *Descending pyelography*
- *Methylene blue dye test:* The bladder can be filled with sterile milk or methylene blue in retrograde fashion using a small transurethral catheter to identify the site of leakage.

### Q. When is cystoscopy indicated?

**Ans.** Cystoscopy is indicated in case of multiple fistulae to determine their location and relation to the trigone and ureteric orifices.

### Q. What is the mode of management in these cases?

**Ans.** Management in these cases can include the following:

### Conservative Management

Conservative management can be considered for small fistulas (< 1 cm), and comprises of using an indwelling catheter to ensure continuous drainage of urine and administration of antibiotic therapy.

### Surgical Management

In case of established, larger fistulas, surgical repair is required.

*Steps of surgery:* The vaginal approach for surgery includes the following procedures:

- *Latzko's partial colpocleisis procedure:* This involves denuding the vaginal epithelium all around the edge of the fistula and then approximating the wide raw surfaces with rows of absorbable sutures (Figs 9.12A to C). The vesical edges of the fistula are not denuded. The posterior vaginal wall becomes the posterior bladder wall and re-epithelializes with transitional epithelium.
- *Chassar Moir flap-splitting technique:* This technique is described in Figures 9.13A to E and involves widely separating the vagina and bladder all around by the flap-splitting method and separately suturing the bladder and vagina in two layers. Absence of tension on the suture lines promotes tissue healing.
- In case of extensive fibrosis, application of omental grafts or interpositioning of maritus or gracilis muscle graft between the bladder and vaginal muscles promotes healing.

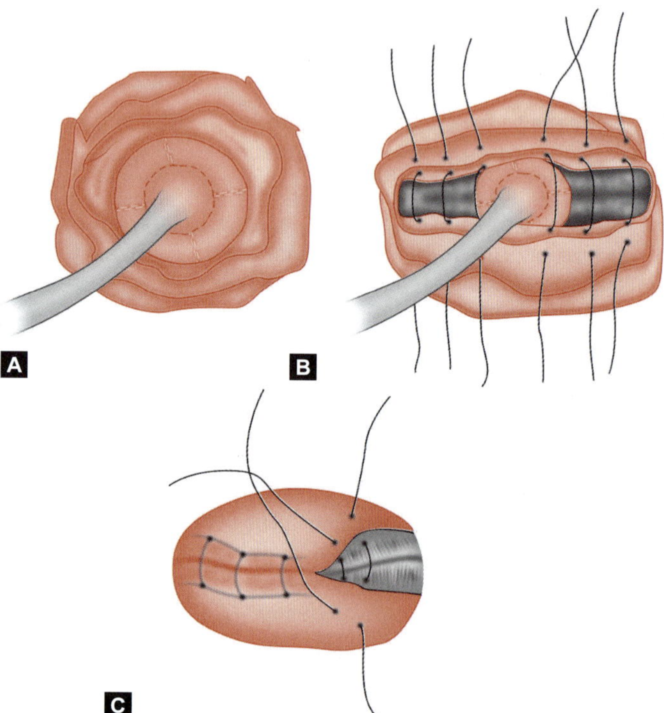

**Figs 9.12A to C:** Steps of Latzko's partial colpocleisis

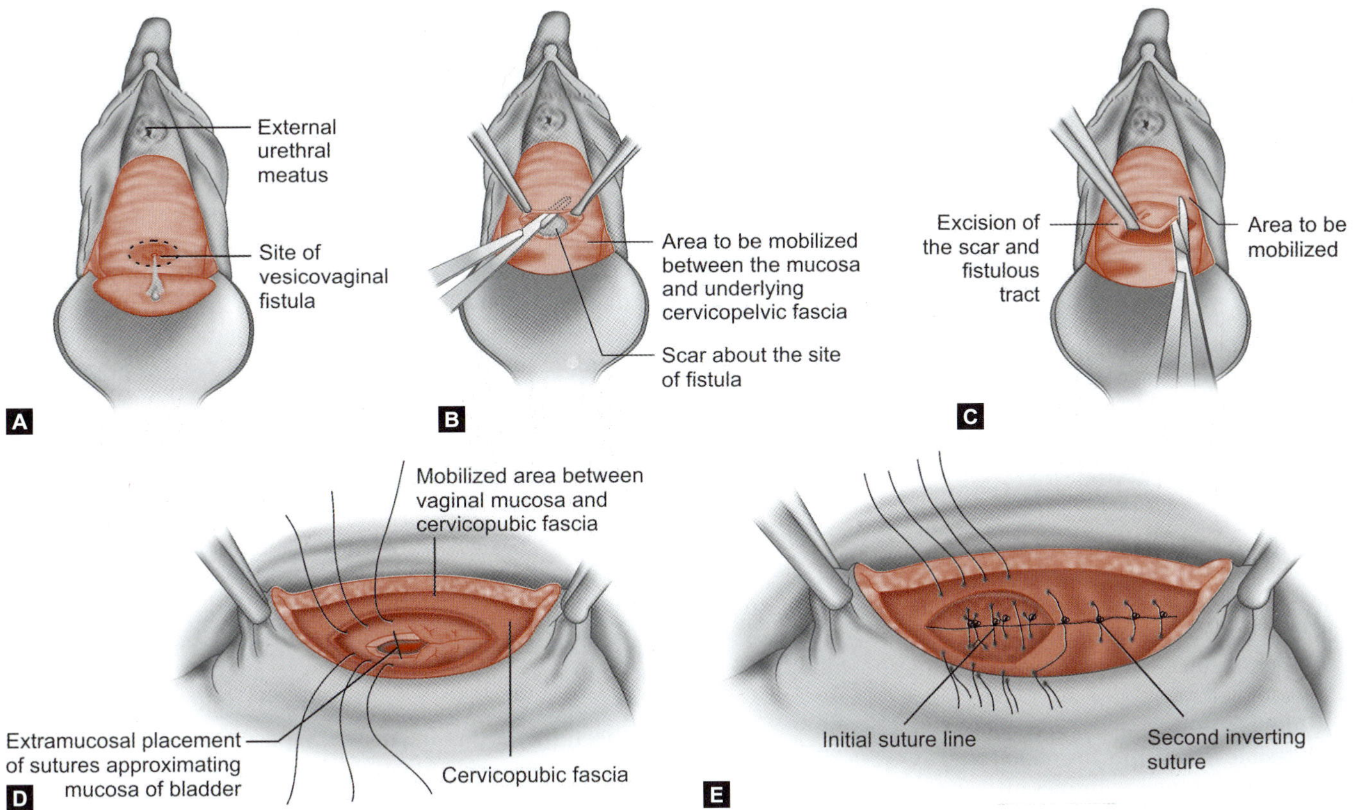



**Figs 9.13A to E:** Flap-splitting technique. (A) Vesicovaginal fistula located on the posterior wall of the bladder; (B) An incision is made about the fistula opening, which is extended into a transverse vaginal incision. The vagina is dissected from the bladder to allow mobilization of tissues and subsequently reduced tension on the suture lines; (C) The fistula scar is excised converting the opening into fresh injury; (D) Closure is performed; (E) The initial suture line is inverted with similar suture. Each suture line inverting the previous sutures line is placed 3–4 mm lateral to the initially closed suture line with the initial suture layer of 4-0 delayed absorbable sutures placed in an extramucosal fashion

- At the time of surgery, routine excision of the fistula tract is not mandatory.
- Successful fistula repair requires adequate dissection and mobilization of tissues, meticulous hemostasis and reapproximation under minimal tension.
- Urinary diversion procedures (e.g. implantation of ureters into the sigmoid colon, creating an ileal loop bladder or a rectal bladder) can be considered in cases where there is extensive loss of bladder tissue, previous failed attempts at fistula closure or fistula formation due to radiation injury.

### Q. If the first attempt at the fistula repair fails, when should the second attempt be undertaken?

**Ans.** If the first attempt at the fistula repair fails, the second must be undertaken only after a period of 3 months.

### Q. What is the best route for performing surgery in these cases?

**Ans.** Vaginal route is the best route for the repair of genitourinary fistula.

### Q. How long does it take following the surgery for the healing to occur?

**Ans.** Healing usually occurs within 6 months to a year following the surgery. Contraception is usually recommended after 6 months for a period of 2 years before another pregnancy is planned. The future delivery must be by a cesarean section. This helps in preventing the risk of recurrence of fistula in future pregnancies.

### Q. What is the appropriate timing for surgery in these cases?

**Ans.** A waiting period for an 8-week to 12-week interval is required for the healing of the tissues from postpartum changes to occur. This delay ensures better tissue healing, reduced rate of infection, better healing and reduced hemorrhage at the time of surgery and postoperative period.

### Q. What are other precautions which must be observed in the preoperative period?

**Ans.** Prior to undertaking surgery, urine sample must be collected by catheterization and must be submitted for culture and sensitivity. Any infection must be treated prior to surgery.

### Q. What steps must be taken in the postoperative period in these patients?

**Ans.** Following steps must be taken in the postoperative period in these patients:

- *Bladder drainage:* Continuous bladder drainage postoperatively is vital for successful UGF repair
- *Antibiotics:* Treatment with antibiotics helps in eradication of infection
- *Acidification of urine:* This helps in reducing the risk of complications such as cystitis, mucus production and formation of bladder calculi. Vitamin C in the dosage of 500 mg orally 3 times per day may be used to acidify urine
- *Pelvic rest:* Pelvic and speculum examinations of the vagina must be avoided during the first 4–6 weeks postoperatively because during this time, the tissue is fragile and delicate. Sexual intercourse and tampon use must also be prohibited.

### Q. What are the various complications associated with the surgical repair of urogenital fistulas?

**Ans.** The various complications which can occur are as follows:

- Risks of infection, hemorrhage, thromboembolism and even death
- Injury to other organs, particularly the ureters
- Possible new fistula formation
- Sexual dysfunction or dissatisfaction, new-onset incontinence, and/or worsening of the previously present incontinence
- Requirement for cesarean delivery during subsequent pregnancies.

### Q. What is urinary incontinence? What are the two different types?

**Ans.** Urinary incontinence can be defined as an involuntary loss of urine which is a social or hygienic problem and can be demonstrated with objective means. There are two main types of urinary incontinence: stress incontinence and urge incontinence. Stress urinary incontinence (SUI) can be defined as involuntary leakage of urine during conditions causing an increase in intra-abdominal pressure (exertion, sneezing, coughing or exercise), which cause the intravesical pressure to rise higher than that which the urethral closure mechanisms can withstand (in the absence of detrusor contractions).

Urge urinary incontinence, on the other hand, can be defined as involuntary leakage of urine accompanied by or immediately preceded by urgency. The corresponding urodynamic term is detrusor overactivity, which is evident in form of involuntary detrusor contractions at the time of filling cystometry.

### Q. How is urinary incontinence different from leakage of urine due to UGF?

**Ans.** In case of UGF, the leakage of urine occurs constantly. On the other hand in cases of incontinence, the leakage of urine does not occur continuously. It may be precipitated by stress, e.g. exertion, sneezing, coughing or exercise, etc. (stress incontinence) or may be immediately preceded by urgency (urge incontinence).

### Q. How should the testing for stress incontinence be done?

**Ans.** Stress testing should be performed with a full bladder, with the patient in both lithotomy and standing positions. In either case, the clinician must directly visualize the urethra. The patient then is asked to cough forcefully and repetitively or to perform a strong Valsalva maneuver. Loss of urine directly observed from the urethral meatus, coincident with the peak of increase in intra-abdominal pressure is strongly suggestive of stress incontinence.

# Abdominal Lump

## OVARIAN CANCER

### Case Study 1

Mrs XYZ, a 60-year-old, para 2 woman, resident of ABC, having an active married life of 33 years presented to the gynecology OPD with the complaints of a lump in the abdomen, which has been increasing in size since past 6 months. There also has been anorexia, bloating sensation, vague pain in the left iliac fossa, fatigue, weakness and increased frequency of micturition since last 1 month. Patient has experienced severe weight loss of nearly 10 kg over past 6 months. There was no significant personal history or family history of cancers. The woman has been menopausal since last 10 years and never had any gynecological problems in the past. On per abdominal examination, a small mass of the size of a lemon was palpable in the left iliac fossa. The mass appeared fixed with restricted mobility. The abdomen was soft and nontender with no evidence of ascites. Vaginal examination revealed the presence of a solid, nodular, irregular-shaped, fixed mass of size of a lemon arising from left ovary. An ultrasound examination revealed an ovarian mass of size 6 cm having mixed echogenicity, thick wall and papillary projections. CA 125 levels were performed which were found to be elevated (> 35 IU/L).

### Q. What is the likely diagnosis in the above-mentioned case study?

**Ans.** The above-mentioned case study corresponds to a case of abdominal lump (as confirmed on history and clinical examination). The questions to be asked at the time of taking history and the parameters to be assessed at the time of examination in such a case are described in Tables 9.49 and 9.50 respectively. The most likely diagnosis in this case is Mrs XYZ, a 60-year-old, para 2 woman, resident of ABC, having an active married life of 33 years, presented with chief complaints of an abdominal lump, which has been increasing in size since past 6 months. Diagnosis of the origin of mass

| **Table 9.49:** Symptoms to be elicited at the time of taking history in a case of carcinoma ovary |
|---|

### History of Presenting Complains

- Acute or subacute presentation: The clinical presentation in case of an epithelial ovarian carcinoma may be either acute or subacute. Acute presentation could be as follows:
  - *Pleural effusion:* Shortness of breath
  - *Bowel obstruction:* Severe nausea and vomiting
  - *Venous thromboembolism*

  Subacute presentation could be as follows:
  - *Adnexal mass:* Discovered on a routine pelvic examination or an imaging study performed for another indication
  - *Pelvic and abdominal symptoms:* Bloating, urinary urgency or frequency, difficulty in eating or early satiety, pelvic or abdominal pain
- Late onset of symptoms: Most women with early-stage cancer of the ovary do not have any symptoms for a long time. This is an important cause for late diagnosis of ovarian cancer.
- Nonspecific symptoms: A few symptoms which do develop are quite nonspecific and may be indicative of other gastrointestinal pathologies. Some of the symptoms which could be suggestive of ovarian cancer and need to be elicited while taking the history include the following:
  - Abdominal bloating/distension: Quite often ovarian malignancy may present as a large intra-abdominal mass and ascites. Both these could be responsible for producing abdominal distension and bloating.
  - Pelvic pain and/or dyspareunia
  - Loss of appetite or early satiety
  - Pressure symptoms such as increased urinary urgency and frequency could result due to an ovarian tumor placed in the uterovesical pouch. On the other hand, a tumor impacted in the POD may cause constipation.
  - Nausea, vague indigestion, constipation or diarrhea
  - Feeling of tiredness, unexplained loss of weight, anemia and cachexia
  - Rapidly increasing abdominal swelling and dyspnea due to development of ascites
  - Pain: Normally the benign ovarian tumors cause no abdominal pain and are comfortably placed in the abdominal cavity which is distensible. Large intra-abdominal tumors, on the other hand, may cause abdominal discomfort and difficulty in walking. Acute abdominal pain may develop if the ovarian tumor undergoes torsion, rupture or hemorrhage.
- Rare symptoms: Rarely there may be abnormal vaginal bleeding (postmenopausal bleeding or menorrhagia). Presence of estrogen secreting granulosa cell tumors may produce menometrorrhagia and episodes of dysfunctional uterine bleeding. However, women with postmenopausal bleeding should be assessed for uterine pathology before proceeding with an evaluation for ovarian cancer. In case of abnormal uterine bleeding and/or presence of an adnexal/ uterine mass, endometrial sampling should be performed.
- Rectal bleeding: This may be sometimes present in some women with epithelial ovarian cancer (EOC). However, it is unlikely that this would be present as the only presenting symptom and deserves further evaluation for an EOC only if other clinical features suggestive of an ovarian malignancy are present (e.g. adnexal mass, hereditary ovarian cancer syndrome, etc.)
- Presence of ascites, omental metastases or bowel metastases in the late stages of the disease may produce symptoms such as abdominal distension, bloating, constipation, nausea, early satiety, etc.
- Presence of lump in the abdomen: This could be related to the presence of ovarian malignancy per se or development of omental cake due to infiltration of the omentum by malignant cells.

### Risk Factors For Ovarian Cancer

Some factors are known to affect a woman's chance of developing ovarian cancer—these need to be elicited at the time of taking history and are described below:

- *Age:* Ovarian cancer is more common in the women belonging to the age group between 50 years and 70 years, with the peak incidence of the disease occurring at the age of 62 years.
- *Lifestyle factors*
- *Body mass index:* Having an increased body mass index (overweight or obese) may be associated with an increased risk of developing ovarian cancer.
- *Diet:* Eating a diet, high in animal fats and low in fresh fruits and vegetables, may increase the woman's risk of developing ovarian cancer.

### Personal History

- Women who previously had cancer of the breast, uterus, colon, or rectum are at a higher risk of developing ovarian cancer in future.
- Previous history of endometriosis/polycystic ovarian syndrome also acts as a risk factor.

### Family History

- Family history of ovarian cancer can be considered as one of the most important risk factors for the development of ovarian cancer. Women who have a mother, daughter, or sister with ovarian cancer are at an increased risk of developing the disease. This risk is even higher in women who have two or more first-degree relatives with ovarian cancer.
- Women with hereditary ovarian cancer syndromes have a lifetime probability of 25–50% for developing ovarian cancer in future. Some of the hereditary ovarian syndromes include:
  - The Lynch II syndrome: Cancers of the colon, breast, endometrium, and ovary with hereditary nonpolyposis colorectal cancer.
  - Breast-ovarian cancer syndrome: Usually occurs in association with a BRCA1 or BRCA2 mutation.

*(Contd...)*

*(Contd...)*

<table>
<tr><td>

*Menstrual History*

- Patients with a history of early menarche (before the age of 12 years) and late menopause (after the age of 52 years) are associated with an increased risk for ovarian cancer.
- *History of menstrual cycles:* It is important to take the history regarding menstrual cycles in the woman because most ovarian tumors, even bilateral ones, do not affect the menstrual cycles. The only tumors causing menorrhagia are granulosa cell tumors and theca cell tumors because both these types of ovarian tumors are associated with increased estrogen secretion. On the other hand, masculinizing tumors may cause amenorrhea and virilization. Postmenopausal bleeding may occur in cases of benign Brenner tumors and feminizing tumors of the ovary.

</td></tr>
<tr><td>

*Obstetric History*

- Women with a history of nulliparity or low parity are at an increased risk for development of ovarian cancer. On the other hand, multiparity and the history of breastfeeding act as a protective factor in the development of ovarian cancers.
- History of using oral contraceptive pills or tubal ligation or hysterectomy also acts as a protective factor.

</td></tr>
</table>

*Abbreviations: EOC, epithelial ovarian cancer; POD, pouch of Douglas*

**Table 9.50:**  Various findings elicited at the time of clinical examination in case of carcinoma ovary

*General Physical Examination*

Features suggestive of advanced stage of the malignant disease on general physical examination include:
- Anemia
- Unexplained weight loss
- Unilateral nonpitting edema of the leg
- Pleural effusion
- Hepatic enlargement
- Lymph node enlargement (especially the supraclavicular nodes)

*Specific Systemic Examination*

*Abdominal Examination*

- The method of examination of an intra-abdominal swelling has been detailed in Chapter 8. The movement of abdominal wall over the swelling can be observed when the patient takes a deep inspiration. On abdominal palpation, the upper and lateral limits of the tumor can be defined. However, in most of the cases it is impossible to identify the lower pole of the tumor except in case of a small cyst with a long pedicle. Small cysts are generally movable from side-to-side, but large, especially the malignant ones may be fixed. The consistency of the cystic tumor is tense and cystic and a fluid thrill can be elicited. All patients with a possible ovarian cyst should be examined carefully for the presence of ascites because the presence of the ascites is a strong indicator that the tumor is malignant.
- In some cases even benign tumors may be associated with ascites, e.g. Meigs syndrome associated with fibroma, Brenner tumor and occasionally granulosa cell tumor.

*Ascites*

Abdominal distension due to ascites is a common feature associated with malignant ovarian growth. In most of the cases, ascites can be differentiated from large ovarian growths on abdominal examination (Chapter 8). With a large ovarian cyst, the percussion note over the tumor is dull, whereas both the flanks are resonant. In cases of ascites, the note is dull over the flanks, while the abdomen in the midline is resonant. The physical signs of shifting dullness and fluid thrill may be obtained. A sample of ascitic fluid must be taken to look for malignant cells.

*Pelvic Examination*

- Detailed description of pelvic examination has been done in Chapter 8. Pelvic examination helps in assessment of the adnexa for presence of any lumps or mass. Presence of a solid, irregular, fixed pelvic mass on pelvic examination is highly suggestive of an ovarian malignancy. In addition, if there is presence of an upper abdominal mass or ascites, the diagnosis of ovarian cancer is almost certain. As a general rule, under normal circumstances ovaries must become nonpalpable in women who are at least 1 year past menopause. Presence of any palpable pelvic mass in these patients should arouse the suspicion of malignancy.
- The method of conducting pelvic examination has been described in details in Chapter 8. The physical signs on bimanual examination vary according to the size of the ovarian tumor. With small tumors, the uterus can be palpated without difficulty and the ovarian mass be outlined bimanually. A large ovarian cyst usually displaces uterus to the opposite side and it may get difficult to outline the uterus with larger sized cysts.
- The ovarian mass needs to be differentiated from uterine mass on bimanual examination. The cardinal sign which helps in distinguishing a mobile ovarian tumor from a uterine tumor is that when the ovarian tumor is raised up by the abdominal hand, the cervix remains stationary to the vaginal fingers. However, in case of a mass of uterine origin, rising up of tumor by abdominal hand results in simultaneous movement of the vaginal fornices.
- In all cases, the POD should be examined carefully for presence of any nodules. The vaginal examination may reveal fixed nodules in the POD. A common site for metastasis is the POD and these deposits are often palpable on vaginal examination. Presence of hard nodules in the POD is a strong indicator of malignancy.

*Abbreviation: POD, pouch of Douglas*

and its exact nature (whether benign or malignant) can be confirmed on by various investigations, particularly imaging studies. In this case diagnosis of an ovarian mass (with a suspicion for malignancy) was confirmed by ultrasound examination, which had already been done in this case. Though the various findings on history, clinical examination and ultrasound examination were suggestive of malignancy, the exact diagnosis of the type of cancer and its stage can be established by exploratory laparotomy.

**Q. What are the various causes for an abdominal lump?**
**Ans.** There can be various causes for presence of an abdominal lump in a patient presenting to the gynecological OPD. Some of these causes are listed in Table 9.51.

**Q. If an abdominal lump is of ovarian origin, what are the different types of ovarian masses, which can be encountered?**
**Ans.** Ovarian cysts are the most common ovarian masses encountered among women belonging to the reproductive age group. Ovarian cysts can be either neoplastic or non-neoplastic in nature. Ovarian neoplasms (tumors) can be benign or malignant in nature. Most ovarian tumors (80–85%) are benign and occur in the women between 20 years and 44 years.

Non-neoplastic cysts of ovary are extremely common and can occur at any age (early reproductive age until perimenopause). These cysts are also known as functional cysts and include follicular cysts, corpus luteum cysts and theca lutein cysts. Histological classification of various neoplastic ovarian growths is shown in Table 9.52.

**Q. What are the features suggestive of malignant ovarian growth based on the findings of history and clinical examination from the above-mentioned case history?**
**Ans.** The features suggestive of malignancy in the above-mentioned case study are as follows:
- *Rapidity of growth:* A rapidly growing tumor is highly suggestive of malignancy, while a slow growing tumor is

---

**Table 9.51:** Causes for an abdominal lump

*Pelvic Masses*
- Adenomyosis
- Endometrial hyperplasia and cancer
- Bladder cancer
- Ovarian masses (benign and malignant)
- Ectopic pregnancy
- Uterine fibroids (especially pedunculated subserous fibroids)

*Extrapelvic Masses*
- Distended bladder (hypogastric region)
- Cholecystitis (right hypochondriac region)
- Colon cancer (iliac, hypogastric and umbilical regions)
- Bowel obstruction (iliac, hypogastric and umbilical regions)
- Diverticulitis (iliac, hypogastric and umbilical regions)
- Gallbladder tumor (right hypochondriac region)
- Hydronephrosis (lumbar regions)
- Cancer of the kidneys (lumbar regions)

---

**Table 9.52:** Histological classification of neoplastic ovarian growth

*I. Common epithelial tumors*

A. *Serous Tumors*
  1. Benign
    a. Cystadenoma and papillary cystadenoma
    b. Surface papilloma
    c. Adenofibroma and cystadenofibroma
  2. Of borderline malignancy (carcinomas of low malignant potential)
    a. Cystadenoma and papillary cystadenoma
    b. Surface papilloma
    c. Adenofibroma and cystadenofibroma
  3. Malignant
    a. Adenocarcinoma, papillary adenocarcinoma and papillary cystadenocarcinoma
    b. Surface papillary carcinoma
    c. Malignant adenofibroma and cystadenofibroma

B. *Mucinous Tumors*
  1. Benign
    a. Cystadenoma
    b. Adenofibroma and cystadenofibroma
  2. Of borderline malignancy (carcinomas of low malignant potential)
    a. Cystadenoma
    b. Adenofibroma and cystadenofibroma
  3. Malignant
    a. Adenocarcinoma and cystadenocarcinoma
    b. Malignant adenofibroma and cystadenofibroma

C. *Endometrioid Tumors*
  1. Benign
    a. Adenoma and cystadenoma
    b. Adenofibroma and cystadenofibroma
  2. Of borderline malignancy (carcinomas of low malignant potential)
    a. Adenoma and cystadenoma
    b. Adenofibroma and cystadenofibroma
  3. Malignant
    a. Carcinoma
      i. Adenocarcinoma
      ii. Adenoacanthoma
      iii. Malignant adenofibroma and cystadenofibroma
    b. Endometrioid stromal sarcomas
    c. Mesodermal (Müllerian) mixed tumors, homologous and heterologous

D. *Clear Cell (Mesonephroid) Tumors*
  1. Benign
  2. Of borderline malignancy (carcinomas of low malignant potential)
  3. Malignant: Carcinoma and adenocarcinoma

E. *Brenner Tumors*
  1. Benign
  2. Of borderline malignancy (proliferating)
  3. Malignant

F. *Mixed Epithelial Tumors*
  1. Benign
  2. Of borderline malignancy
  3. Malignant

*(Contd...)*

*(Contd...)*

| |
|---|
| G.  *Undifferentiated Carcinoma* |
| H.  *Unclassified Epithelial Tumors* |
| **II.  Sex cord stromal tumors** |
| A.  *Granulosa-Stromal Cell Tumors* |
|     1.  Granulosa cell tumor |
|     2.  Tumors in the thecoma-fibroma group |
|         a.  Thecoma |
|         b.  Fibroma |
|         c.  Unclassified |
| B.  *Androblastomas, Sertoli-Leydig Cell Tumors* |
|     1.  Well-differentiated |
|         a.  Tubular androblastoma, Sertoli cell tumor (tubular adenoma of Pick) |
|         b.  Tubular androblastoma with lipid storage, Sertoli cell tumor with lipid storage (folliculome lipidique of Lecene) |
|         c.  Sertoli-Leydig cell tumor (tubular adenoma with Leydig cells) |
|         d.  Leydig cell tumor, hilus cell tumor |
|     2.  Of intermediate differentiation |
|     3.  Poorly differentiated (sarcomatoid) |
|     4.  With heterologous elements |
| C.  *Gynandroblastoma* |
| D.  *Unclassified* |
| **III.  Germ cell tumors** |
| A.  *Dysgerminoma* |
| B.  *Endodermal sinus tumor* |
| C.  *Embryonal carcinoma* |
| D.  *Polyembryoma* |
| E.  *Choriocarcinoma* |
| F.  *Teratomas* |
|     1.  Immature |
|     2.  Mature |
|         a.  Solid |
|         b.  Cystic |
|            i.  Dermoid cyst (mature cystic teratoma) |
|           ii.  Dermoid cyst with malignant transformation |
|     3.  Monodermal and highly specialized |
|         a.  Struma ovarii |
|         b.  Carcinoid |
|         c.  Struma ovarii and carcinoid |
|         d.  Others |
| G.  *Mixed Forms* |
| **IV.  Lipid (lipoid) cell tumors** |
| **V.  Gonadoblastoma** |
|   A.  Pure |
|   B.  Mixed with dysgerminoma or other form of germ cell tumor |
| **VI.  Soft tissue tumors not specific to ovary** |
| **VII.  Unclassified tumors** |
| **VIII.  Secondary (Metastatic) tumors** |
| **IX.  Tumor-like conditions** |

(Contd...)

*(Contd...)*

| |
|---|
| A.  Pregnancy luteoma |
| B.  Hyperplasia of ovarian stroma and hyperthecosis |
| C.  Massive edema |
| D.  Solitary follicle cyst and corpus luteum cyst |
| E.  Multiple follicle cysts (polycystic ovaries) |
| F.  Multiple luteinized follicle cysts and/or corpora lutea |
| G.  Endometriosis |
| H.  Surface-epithelial inclusion cysts (germinal inclusion cysts) |
| I.  Simple cysts |
| J.  Inflammatory lesions |
| K.  Parovarian cysts |

more likely to be benign. A tumor which has been rapidly increasing in size over the past 6 months is suggestive of malignancy.

- *Consistency of the mass:* In this case, the growth appeared solid, nodular and had irregular margins on vaginal examination. This is more likely to be malignant. On the other hand, growths which are smooth, cystic and have regular margins are more likely to be benign.
- *Fixation of the tumors:* Malignant tumors are more likely to be adherent to the underlying structures and have a restricted mobility in comparison to the benign masses which are not adherent to the underlying structures and have a greater mobility.
- *Presence of ascites:* Presence of free fluid in the abdominal cavity is usually indicative of peritoneal metastasis or at least the fact that the tumor has perforated the ovarian capsule. However, in this case no ascitic fluid was present on per abdominal examination.
- *Cancer cachexia:* Cachexia, associated with severe degrees of weight loss, muscle wasting, weakness and fatigue typically occurs with malignant growths. A benign tumor is usually not painful unless there is an underlying complication. A malignant tumor, on the other hand, is associated with pain in the abdomen.

**Q. What would be the most appropriate management in the above-described case study?**

**Ans.** In the above-mentioned case study, after taking into consideration the patient's age and findings of ultrasound examination, the suspicion of malignancy must be definitely ruled out by the clinician. The best modality of diagnosis in patient with suspected ovarian cancer is surgical staging on exploratory laparotomy.

**Q. What investigations must be done in cases of suspected ovarian malignancy?**

**Ans.** The following blood tests can be done:

- Complete blood count (CBC) with platelet count, kidney and liver function tests, determination of CA 125 levels.
- Imaging tests such as transvaginal sonography, CT, MRI examination, positron emission tomography, etc.

Once the ovarian malignancy has been diagnosed or suspected, a preoperative evaluation must be done in order to evaluate the extent of malignancy prior to undertaking surgery. The preoperative evaluation helps in excluding other primary cancers (e.g. gastrointestinal malignancy), which could be metastatic to the ovary. The preoperative evaluation in case of ovarian malignancy comprises of the following investigations:

- Chest X-ray, colonoscopy and barium enema, intravenous pyelography, cervical cytology, etc.
- *Exploratory laparotomy:* Sometimes cancer of the ovary cannot be diagnosed before an exploratory laparotomy is carried out. The staging of ovarian cancer is done at the time of exploratory laparotomy. Surgical staging helps in estimating the spread of cancer. Staging of the ovarian cancer is particularly important because subsequent treatment depends upon the stage of the disease.

**Q. The surgical staging revealed papillary cystadeno-carcinoma stage IA (grade I). What would be the next step of management?**

**Ans.** Total abdominal hysterectomy with bilateral salpingo-oophorectomy was performed in this case. Removal of both the ovaries is unlikely to cause any problem in this case as she has completed her family and is postmenopausal. However, she needs to be periodically monitored with routine pelvic examinations and determination of serum CA 125 levels every 3–4 months for the first 2 years and then 6-monthly for 5 years.

**Q. Describe the staging system for ovarian cancer.**

**Ans.** The FIGO system is used for cancer staging based on the findings of exploratory laparotomy and is as follows:

*Stage I:* Cancer growth is limited to the ovaries. This stage is divided into three subgroups:

1. Stage IA: The growth is limited to one ovary. There is no ascites containing malignant cells; no tumor is present on the external surface; and capsule is intact.
2. Stage IB: The growth is limited to both the ovaries. There is no ascites containing malignant cells; no tumor is present on the external surface; and capsule is intact.
3. Stage IC: The cancer is either at stage IA or 1B, but with tumor on the surface of one or both the ovaries; or with capsule ruptured or with ascites present containing malignant cells or with positive peritoneal washings.

*Stage II:* Growth involves one or both ovaries with pelvic extension. There are three subgroups:

1. Stage IIA: The cancer has spread to the uterus and/or fallopian tubes.
2. Stage IIB: There is extension to other pelvic tissues, such as the rectum or bladder.
3. Stage IIC: The cancer is either at stage IIA or IIB, with tumor on the surface of one or both ovaries; or with capsule ruptured; or with ascites present, containing malignant cells or with positive peritoneal washings.

*Stage III:* Tumor involves one or both the ovaries, with peritoneal implants outside the pelvis and/or positive retroperitoneal or inguinal nodes. Superficial liver metastasis equals stage III. Tumor is limited to the true pelvis, but with histologically proven extension to small bowel or omentum. There are three subgroups:

1. Stage IIIA: Tumor grossly limited to true pelvis with negative nodes but with histologically confirmed seeding of abdominal/peritoneal surfaces.
2. Stage IIIB: Tumor of one or both ovaries with histologically confirmed implants of abdominal peritoneal surfaces, none exceeding 2 cm in diameter. Nodes are negative.
3. Stage IIIC: Abdominal implants greater than 2 cm in diameter and/or positive retroperitoneal or inguinal lymph nodes.

*Stage IV:* Growth involving one or both ovaries with distant metastasis. If pleural effusion is present, there must be positive cytological test results to allot a case to stage IV. Parenchymal liver metastasis equals stage IV.

**Q. What definitive therapy must be instituted in cases of ovarian cancer?**

**Ans.** The treatment of a patient with ovarian cancer is as follows:

*Stage IA (Grade I):* Primary treatment for stage I epithelial ovarian cancer (EOC) is surgical, i.e. a total abdominal hysterectomy with bilateral salpingo-oophorectomy and surgical staging. The uterus and contralateral ovary can be preserved in woman with stage IA, grade I disease who desire to preserve their fertility. However, such women must be periodically monitored with routine pelvic examinations and determination of serum CA 125 levels.

*Stage IA and IB (Grade II and III) and Stage IC:* Treatment options in this case include additional chemotherapy or radiotherapy besides surgery as described above. Chemotherapy is the more commonly used option and the treatment is usually administered in the form of either cisplatin or carboplatin or combination therapy including either of these drugs with paclitaxel for three to four cycles.

*Stage II, III and IV:* Debulking surgery or cytoreductive surgery is performed in these cases. This involves an initial exploratory procedure with the removal of as much disease as possible (both tumor and the associated metastatic disease). Postoperative chemotherapy and radiotherapy in advanced cases may help improve the survival and quality of life.

**Q. How useful is the measurement of CA 125 levels for diagnosing ovarian cancer?**

**Ans.** Carcinoma antigen (CA) 125 is a surface glycoprotein found on the surface of ovarian cancer cells and on some normal tissues. A high CA 125 level could be a sign of cancer or other conditions. Estimation of CA 125 levels is associated with low specificity because it can also be raised in presence of benign conditions like endometriosis, tuberculosis, leiomyomas, liver or kidney disease, PID, etc. Therefore, the CA 125 test should not be used as a stand alone test to diagnose ovarian cancer. This test is approved by the Food and Drug Administration for monitoring a woman's response to ovarian cancer treatment and for detecting its return after treatment. Values of CA 125 greater than 35 IU/mL are found in over 80% of cases with nonmucinous EOCs.

### Q. What is the role of ultrasound examination in evaluation of an ovarian tumor?

**Ans.** Ultrasonography (both transabdominal and trans-vaginal) is accurate in differentiating tumors of the ovary from other types of tumors of the pelvis, in more than 90% of the patients. Discrimination between benign and malignant lesions of the ovary can be made on the basis of ultrasonic patterns.

Anechoic lesions have a high likelihood of being benign. As the percentage of echogenic material in the cyst increases, the likelihood of malignancy also increases. In general, benign lesions are likely to be unilateral, unilocular and thin walled with no papillae or solid areas. Septae, if present in benign masses are also thin. In contrast, malignant lesions are often multilocular with thick walls, thick septae and mixed echogenicity due to the presence of solid areas.

Doppler flow studies of the ovarian artery may also help in differentiating between benign and malignant growths. Normally a high resistance pattern (resistive index > 0.70) is indicative of a benign growth. In malignant tumors due to increased blood supply, the resistance index is usually low (< 0.4) and there is a high peak velocity.

Other signs suggestive of malignancy include presence of irregular solid parts within the mass, indefinite margins, papillary projections extending from inner wall of the cyst, presence of ascites, hydronephrosis, pleural effusion, matted bowel loops, omental implants, other evidence of peritoneal disseminated disease and lymphadenopathy. Size of tumor may also give clues regarding the nature of the mass. Larger tumors, usually greater than 8 cm in size have been thought to be associated with higher risk of malignancy in comparison to the smaller ones.

### Q. Should ovaries be palpable in a normal menopausal patient?

**Ans.** Normally it takes 3–5 years after the menopause for the ovaries to atrophy. Therefore in postmenopausal women, ovaries must not be palpable. There is no such thing as physiologic enlargement of the postmenopausal ovary. Since there are no follicles or corpus luteum in postmenopausal ovary, no such cysts can arise. Therefore, palpable ovary in postmenopausal women must be considered as a significant finding. The patient without delay should be subjected to an advanced imaging examination (Ultrasound, CT, MRI, etc.). In cases of positive findings during this examination, the findings should be confirmed on laparotomy. The enlarged ovaries should be removed without a biopsy in postmenopausal woman.

### Q. What are the potential benefits of cytoreduction in women with epithelial ovarian cancer?

**Ans.** Potential benefits of cytoreduction in women with epithelial ovarian cancer are as follows:
- Removal of bulky disease helps in rapidly improving the disease-related symptoms (e.g. abdominal pain, increased abdominal girth, dyspnea, early satiety, etc.) and the quality of life.
- Removal of tumor bulk may help improve host immune competence by reducing the production of immunosuppressive cytokines e.g. interleukin-10, vascular endothelial growth factor, which are normally produced by the tumor tissue.
- Reduction of tumor bulk helps in reducing the tumor burden (which now becomes well-perfused and therefore mitotically active), thereby maximizing the effect of chemotherapeutic agents.

### Q. What are the various indications for chemotherapy?

**Ans.** Various indications for chemotherapy are as follows:
- Early stage ovarian (stage IB or IC) cancer (after surgery in order to reduce the chance of the cancer recurrence): Adjuvant chemotherapy
- Moderate or high grade ovarian cancer (after surgery)
- Neoadjuvant chemotherapy before surgery in advanced stage ovarian cancer
- Stage IV cancer with distant metastasis

Presently platinum and taxane-based combination therapy has been recommended as the first-line treatment for EOC. The use of carboplatin is associated with reduced toxicity in comparison with cisplatin. Therefore recent trend is to replace cisplatin with carboplatin and use it in combination with taxane, paclitaxel.

### Q. What is the pattern of spread of an ovarian malignancy?

**Ans.** The most common pattern of spread of EOC is through the exfoliation of the cancer cells that implant along the surfaces of the peritoneal cavity. Exfoliation of the cancer cells that implant along the surfaces of the peritoneal cavity tends to follow the circulatory path of the peritoneal fluid. As a result, metastases are typically seen on the posterior cul-de-sac, paracolic gutters, right hemidiaphragm, liver capsule and peritoneal surfaces of the intestine, their mesenteries and the omentum.

Other less common modes of spread of ovarian cancer include lymphatic and hematogenous spread. Lymphatic spread can lead to the involvement of pelvic and para-aortic group of lymph nodes. Lymphatic spread above the diaphragm can result in the involvement of supraclavicular lymph nodes. Hematogenous spread can occur to organs like lungs and liver.

# Endometriosis

## Case Study 1

Mrs XYZ, a 25-year-old nulliparous patient, with an active married life of 3 years, resident of ABC, presented with complaints of chronic pelvic pain (CPP) since last 2 years. The pain is mainly present in the lower back and abdomen and typically exacerbates at the time of menstrual periods. During this time, the pain becomes severe enough to interfere with the quality of life. The patient gives history of experiencing mild-to-moderate pain at the time of sexual intercourse. The patient also gives history of experiencing primary infertility. On bimanual pelvic examination, localized areas of tenderness were felt in the pelvic region. However, no nodularity or thickness of uterosacral ligaments, cul-de-sac or rectovaginal septum was felt.

### Q. What is the most likely diagnosis in the above-mentioned case study?

**Ans.** The above-mentioned case study corresponds to a case of CPP with primary infertility. The questions to be asked at the time of taking history and the parameters to be assessed at the time of examination in such a case are described in Tables 9.53 and 9.54 respectively. The most likely diagnosis in this case is Mrs XYZ, a 25-year-old nulliparous woman, with an active married life of 3 years, resident of ABC, with chief complaints of CPP since past 2 years. Diagnosis of endometriosis is suspected on the basis of history and clinical examination. However, it needs to be confirmed by performing various investigations (imaging studies and laparoscopy).

### Q. What is the next step of management in the above-mentioned case study?

**Ans.** In this patient, the history points towards the likelihood of endometriosis as the likely diagnosis. However, since the main complaint of the patient is infertility rather than CPP, she must undergo a thorough basic evaluation for other causes of infertility before diagnostic laparoscopy is undertaken.

### Q. What is endometriosis?

**Ans.** Endometriosis is one of the most common causes of CPP in women belonging to the reproductive age groups and may be associated with infertility in nearly 30–40% cases. Endometriosis is characterized by occurrence of endometrial stroma and glands outside the uterus in the pelvic cavity, including all the reproductive organs as well as on the bladder, bowel, intestines, colon, appendix and rectum (Fig. 9.14). In normal women, endometrial glands and stroma are largely limited to the uterus. Common sites for endometriotic lesions include uterine scars, uterosacral ligaments and pelvic side walls. The ectopic endometrial tissue, both the glands and the stroma, are capable of responding to cyclical hormonal stimulation and has the tendency to invade the normal surrounding tissues. Endometriosis is a disease, which is largely encountered in the women belonging to the reproductive age group. It is a leading cause of disability in women of reproductive age, responsible for causing dysmenorrhea, pelvic pain and subfertility.

### Q. Describe the various lesions of endometriosis.

**Ans.** The common sites for the occurrence of endometriosis include the ovaries, the pouch of Douglas, uterosacral ligaments and serosal surface of the uterus, bladder, sigmoid colon, appendix, cecum, uterine scars, etc. The ovary is the most common site for endometriosis. Lesions can vary in size from spots to large endometriomas. The classic lesion is a chocolate cyst of the ovary that contains old blood that has undergone hemolysis. On gross microscopic examination, the tunica albuginea appears to be thickened. Red vascular lesions may be well marked on the under surface of the ovary.

Endometriotic lesions can also involve the uterine serosa and the anterior surface of the bladder. Involvement of uterine serosa and formation of dense adhesions can lead to fixed retroversion of the uterus. Posteriorly, the disease may cause obliteration of the cul-de-sac and form dense adhesions between the posterior vaginal wall or cervix and the anterior rectum. Deep endometriotic nodules can also cause infiltration of the uterosacral ligaments and rectovaginal septum. Through contiguous spread, endometriosis may invade the rectovaginal septum and the anterior rectal wall, the ileum, appendix and cecum may also be involved, resulting in intestinal obstruction.

In the beginning, the endometriotic lesions appear as red colored, papular vesicles. With the passage of time, these lesions progressively change their appearance from dark-red to bluish-black appearance. Scarring in the surrounding tissues may give it a puckered appearance. Old inactive lesions of endometriosis may appear as powder burnt areas.

### Q. What are the likely causes of infertility in a patient with endometriosis and how must be such patients managed?

**Ans.** The possible mechanisms for infertility in patients with endometriosis are as follows:
- Deformity of pelvic organs
- Alteration of peritoneal environment
- Increase in macrophages
- Reduced sperm motility
- Phagocytosis of spermatozoa
- Interference with oocyte pickup.

In case of minimal/mild lesions of endometriosis diagnosed at the time of laparoscopic examination, excision or ablation of the implants should be performed, followed by timed intercourse with or without controlled ovarian hyperstimulation (COH) for 3–6 months. If the patient fails to conceive, IUI after 2–3 cycles of COH may be followed by IVF. For moderate-to-severe disease, surgical excision of the lesions followed by treatment by IUI or IVF is recommended. Resection of endometriomas has not been shown to

| **Table 9.53:** Symptoms to be elicited at the time of taking history in a case of endometriosis |
|---|
| *History of Presenting Complains* |
| The following characteristics related to pain need to be enquired: <br><br> • *The exact area of pain localization:* The pain may be localized to the pelvis, lower back, perineal region or the lower abdomen. <br> • *The severity and duration of pain:* The clinician needs to assess whether the pain is acute or chronic in nature and whether it is mild or severe in intensity. A significant number of women with endometriosis remain asymptomatic. Though the endometriotic lesions commonly cause CPP, at times, there may be acute exacerbations of pelvic pain caused by chemical peritonitis due to leakage of old blood from an endometriotic cyst. <br> • The aggravating or relieving factors for pain must be enquired. <br> • Timing during the day when the pain occurs or increases in intensity. <br> • *Correlation of pain with menstrual cycles:* Chronic pelvic pain due to endometriosis is commonly associated with dysmenorrhea and low back pain that worsens during menses. The diagnosis of endometriosis should be considered especially if a patient develops dysmenorrhea after years of pain-free menstrual cycles. Pain due to endometriosis typically commences prior to menses. <br> • *Details related to the menstrual cycle:* The details related to menstrual cycle (e.g. cycle length, duration of menstrual flow, etc.) also need to be elicited because increased exposure to menstruation (i.e. shorter cycle length, longer duration of flow and nulliparity), acts as a risk factor for the development of endometriosis. <br> • *Nature of pain:* The patient needs to be asked if the pain follows any cyclic pattern and whether it remains same all the time. Cyclic pain is the pain that accompanies bleeding at the time of menstruation. Cyclical pain associated with hormonal changes taking place during the menstrual cycle is likely to result from endometriosis or adenomyosis, while a nonhormonal pattern of pain may be more indicative of a musculoskeletal pathology or other conditions such as adhesions, IBS, or interstitial cystitis. <br> • The effect the pain has on the patient's quality of life needs to be assessed. <br> • Relation of pain to the bowel movements or urination needs to be asked. <br> • The clinician needs to take history regarding any correlation between the symptoms of pain and the sexual intercourse. Relation of pain with deep penetration during intercourse or dyspareunia needs to be asked. |
| • A woman presenting with a combination of dysmenorrhea, CPP and dyspareunia is most likely to be suffering from endometriosis. |
| Other questions which need to be asked at the time of taking history include: <br><br> • The patient's age <br> • Any previous history of STD or PID <br> • Symptoms indicative of malignancy such as unexplained weight loss, hematochezia, perimenopausal irregular bleeding, postmenopausal vaginal bleeding, or postcoital bleeding, should prompt an investigation to rule out malignancy. |
| *Obstetric History* |
| • In a nulliparous woman with infertility, pain may be due to endometriosis, pelvic adhesions or PID. <br> • History of using OCPs or any other methods of birth control need to be asked. |
| *Surgical History* |
| • Prior history of abdominal surgery increases the woman's risk for developing pelvic adhesions. |
| *Psychosocial History* |
| • It is important to investigate all contributing factors related to the pain including psychological, social and environmental causes. |
| *Previous Treatment History* |
| • The patient needs to be asked if she has ever undergone an assessment or treatment for pain in the past. <br> • The patient needs to be asked if she has been taking any medicines. <br> • She also needs to be asked if she has ever suffered from psychiatric disorders like depression or anxiety. |

*Abbreviations:* CPP, chronic pelvic pain; OCPs, oral contraceptive pills; PID, pelvic inflammatory disease; STD, sexually transmitted disease; IBS, irritable bowel syndrome

improve fertility potential and must be only performed for gynecological indications, such as pelvic pain.

### Q. What are main considerations which must be kept in mind before evaluating a case of chronic pelvic pain?

**Ans.** The main issue in evaluating patient with CPP is distinguishing between gynecologic and nongynecologic causes of the pain. This would enable the clinician to institute the most appropriate course of further investigations and management. A definite diagnosis and the cause of the pain cannot always be elicited clinically. If the gynecological cause of pain cannot be established with surety, the clinician can make use of the hormonal suppression test to distinguish between the gynecological and nongynecological causes of pain. The hormonal suppression test is a functional study that provides a practical means of making this distinction and uses progestogens to create a hypoestrogenic environment. If the pain emanates from a gynecologic source or is exacerbated by

**Table 9.54:** Various findings elicited at the time of clinical examination in a case of endometriosis

*General Physical Examination*

- Altered vital signs such as elevated temperature, hypotension and tachycardia could be indicative of presence of underlying intra-abdominal pathology.
- Constant low-grade fever is commonly present in inflammatory conditions such as diverticulitis and appendicitis. Higher temperature may be associated with conditions such as advanced stages of PID, pyelonephritis or advanced peritonitis.
- Evaluation of the patient's pulse and blood pressure may help in assessment of hypovolemia. Reduced blood pressure (hypotension) and tachycardia may indicate the underlying hypovolemia. If hypovolemia is present, an intravenous access must be established prior to completion of the examination.
- *Evaluation of the patient's posture:* Evaluation of the patient's posture may point towards underlying musculoskeletal pathology.
- The back must be examined posteriorly for presence of structural deformities such as scoliosis, kyphosis, lordosis, etc. and symmetry of the shoulders, gluteal folds and knee creases also needs to be assessed. Asymmetry may be indicative of underlying musculoskeletal disease.
- The clinician must also evaluate the mobility of spine by asking the patient to bend in forward and sideways direction at the waist. Limitation in forward flexion may be indicative of underlying orthopedic or musculoskeletal disease

*Specific Systemic Examination*

*Abdominal Examination*
- Both abdominal and pelvic examinations must proceed slowly and gently because both the abdominal and pelvic components of the examination may be painful.
- The abdominal examination can help to identify areas of tenderness and the presence of masses or other anatomical findings which may help in reaching the accurate diagnosis.
- The abdomen must be inspected for the presence of previous surgical scar marks. Presence of previous surgical scars increases the possibility of postoperative adhesions, which could be an important cause of pelvic pain.
- Anterior abdominal wall must also be inspected for the signs of hernia. Hernias involving the anterior abdominal wall or pelvic floor may be associated with CPP.
- Palpation of the abdomen must systematically explore each abdominal quadrant and begin away from the area of indicated pain.
- Superficial palpation of the anterior abdominal wall by the clinician may reveal sites of tenderness or knotty muscles which may reflect nerve entrapment or myofascial pain syndromes.
- Deep palpation of the lower abdomen may identify pathology originating from the pelvic viscera.
- Following inspection and palpation, auscultation must be done. Presence of high-pitched bowel sounds is characteristic of bowel obstruction.
- *Carnett's sign for patients with pelvic pain:* This sign helps in distinguishing whether the pain is due to an intra-abdominal pathology or pathology in the anterior abdominal wall. In this test while the clinician places a finger on the painful, tender area of the patient's abdomen, the patient is instructed to raise her head and shoulders while tensing the anterior abdominal wall muscles. A positive test occurs when the pain increases during this maneuver and is typical of anterior abdominal wall pathology and indicates myofascial cause of the pain. On the other hand, tenderness originating from inside the abdominal cavity usually decreases with this maneuver.

*Pelvic Examination*
Detailed description of the method for conducting the pelvic examination has been described in Chapter 8. The pelvic examination should commence with inspection of the external genitalia.

*Per Speculum Examination*
Vagina and vulva must be inspected for presence of generalized changes and any local lesions. Findings of purulent vaginal discharge or cervicitis may be indicative of PID.
- Presence of bluish-black puckered spots, which are tender to touch, may be noted on per speculum examination. This feature of endometriosis is pathognomonic of endometriosis.
- Bleeding through the vagina could be due to pregnancy-related complications, benign or malignant reproductive tract neoplasia or acute vaginal trauma. Cervical motion tenderness is commonly associated with peritoneal irritation and may be seen with PID, appendicitis and diverticulitis.

*Bimanual Pelvic Examination*
Tenderness upon pelvic examination is best detected at the time of menses when the endometrial implants are likely to be the largest and most tender.
- Since the pelvic examination must be performed slowly and gently, it should begin with a single-digit of one-hand. A moistened cotton swab should be used to elicit point tenderness in the vulva and vagina. Following the single-digit examination, a bimanual examination should be performed.
- During the pelvic examination, it is important to determine whether any manipulations reproduce the pain especially upon the palpation of the uterus or rectum. The bimanual examination may reveal the following findings:
  - Nodularity and thickening of the uterosacral ligaments and the cul-de-sac may be present in cases of moderate to severe endometriosis. Women with minimal or mild endometriosis may have focal tenderness of the uterosacral ligaments or cul-de-sac without palpable nodules.
  - Pain with deep palpation of the vaginal fornices may be observed with endometritis and cervical motion tenderness may be noted with PID.
  - The uterus may be fixed in retroversion, owing to adhesions. Besides endometriosis, immobility of the uterus could be related to PID, malignancy or adhesive disease from prior surgeries. Evaluation of adnexa may reveal masses or tenderness.
  - A bluish nodule may be seen in the vagina due to infiltration from the posterior vaginal wall.
  - Myofascial tenderness involving the puborectalis and coccygeus muscles may be noted by firmly sweeping the index finger across these muscles.
  - Tenderness of urethra and bladder are potential indicators of urethral diverticulum or interstitial cystitis respectively. The patient should be checked for point tenderness along the bladder or other musculoskeletal structures.
  - The size of the uterus must be assessed on pelvic examination. While an irregularly enlarged uterus is indicative of leiomyomas, a regularly enlarged uterus with softening could indicate adenomyosis or pregnancy.
  - Adnexal tenderness with or without enlargement may indicate ovarian endometriosis.

*Rectovaginal Examination*
This should include the palpation of rectovaginal septum. A rectal examination may show rectal or posterior uterine masses, presence of nodules in the uterosacral ligaments, cul-de-sac or rectovaginal septum and/or pelvic floor point tenderness. The rectovaginal nodule suggestive of DIE may be easily palpated on rectovaginal examination, especially during menstruation when it becomes tender and more prominent.

*Abbreviations:* DIE, deep infiltrating endometriosis; PID, pelvic inflammatory disease

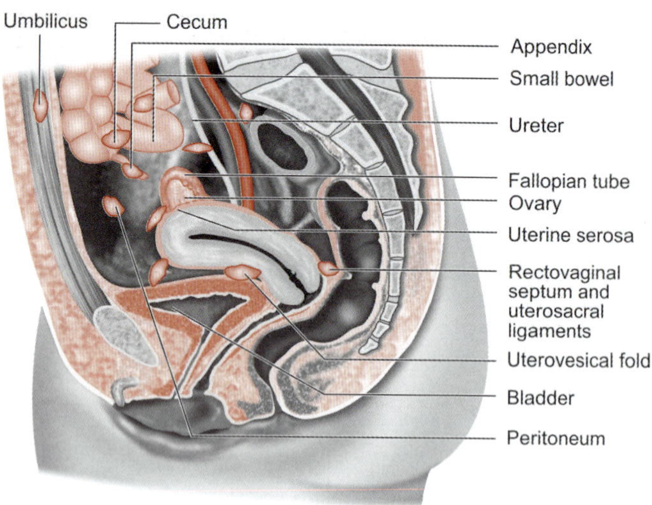


**Fig. 9.14:** Common sites of endometriotic lesions

| **Table 9.55:** Appearance of lesions of endometriosis |
| --- |
| • Brown/black (Powder burn/gunmetal lesions)<br>• Clear (atypical) nodules<br>• Peritoneal windows<br>• Classic blue-black blisters<br>• Flame-like blisters<br>• White plaques<br>• Macroscopically normal peritoneum may have microscopic endometrial glands |

normal menstrual physiology, the symptoms should improve significantly with hormone suppression.

### Q. Which investigations help in establishing the diagnosis of endometriosis?

**Ans.** Various investigations which help in establishing the diagnosis of endometriosis are as follows:

*Ultrasound examination:* Ultrasound examination (both transabdominal and transvaginal) is the most commonly used investigation, which may help in revealing the pelvic pathology responsible for producing pain. Imaging investigations such as CT and MRI may be helpful in some cases where sonographic findings are equivocal or nondiagnostic. Doppler ultrasound may be used for diagnosis of pelvic congestion.

*Diagnostic laparoscopy:* Diagnostic laparoscopy remains the gold standard for diagnosis of pelvic pathology. Laparoscopy detects small nodules of endometriosis which may remain undetected clinically. Laparoscopy can also detect pelvic adhesions and small inflammatory pelvic masses. Varied appearance of the lesions of endometrosis as observed on laparoscopic examination is described in Table 9.55. Therapeutic treatment such as adhesiolysis and cauterization of endometriotic lesions can be applied in the same sitting.

### Q. How is endometriosis treated?

**Ans.** Treatment for endometriosis may be expectant, or either medical or surgical. Each modality of treatment is associated with its own specific advantages and disadvantages, which are described in Table 9.56. Perhaps the strongest reason for beginning with surgical treatment is the apparently lower recurrence rate compared with medical treatment. One of the main criteria which helps the clinician decide next step in management is the patient's main presenting complaint, i.e. whether the patient's main complaint is infertility or pelvic pain.

The likelihood of subsequent conception can be significantly increased by undertaking surgery in infertile patients. Since medical treatment has not been shown to help these patients conceive, surgical treatment is usually preferred in patients desiring fertility. Furthermore, pregnancy is contraindicated in patients receiving medical treatment and is in fact unlikely, because the drugs that are used may interfere with ovulation and endometrial implantation. On the other hand, both medical and surgical approaches have been used successfully for reducing the pain associated with endometriosis. Algorithm for treatment of patients with endometriosis is described in Flow chart 9.3.

### Q. What kind of treatment must be instituted for mild-to-moderate cases?

**Ans.** For patients with mild disease, hormonal treatment (e.g. GnRH analogs, danazol and medroxyprogesterone) has been shown to be effective in reducing pain, but has no impact on fertility. However, for severe endometriosis, the efficacy of hormonal treatment has not yet been established. Since no pharmacologic method appears to restore fertility, medical treatment should be reserved for use in patients with

| **Table 9.56:** Advantages and disadvantages associated with different treatment modalities | | |
| --- | --- | --- |
| *Treatment* | *Advantages* | *Disadvantages* |
| Surgical therapy | • Beneficial for infertility<br>• Possibly better long-term results<br>• Definitive diagnosis and treatment<br>• Associated with a much lower rate of recurrence | • Expensive<br>• Invasive |
| Medical therapy | • It is associated with reduced initial cost and is effective for providing relief from pain. | • Adverse effects are commonly present; it is unlikely to improve fertility and is associated with a high recurrence rate. |

**Flow chart 9.3:** Algorithm for treatment of patients with endometriosis

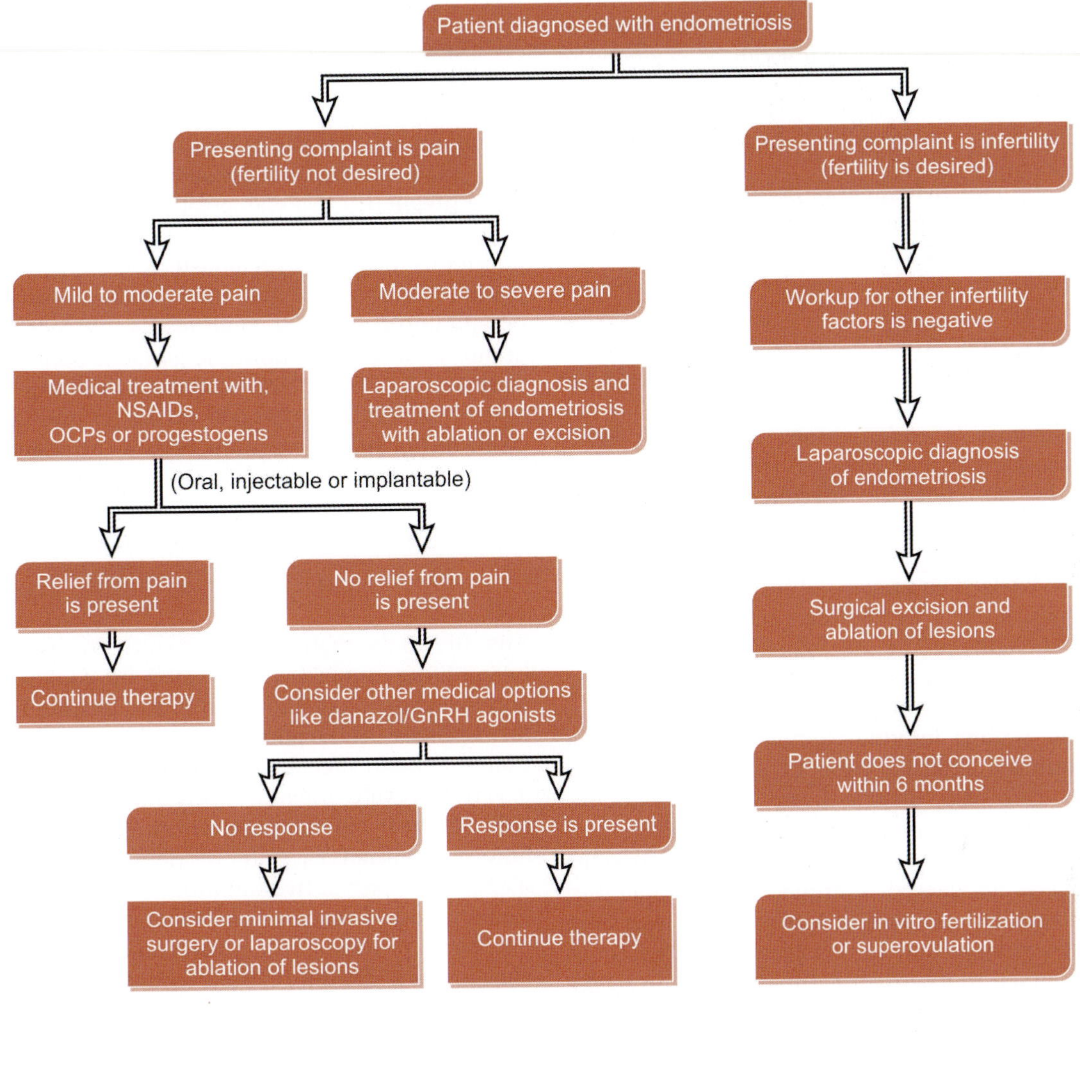


**Table 9.57:** Adverse effects caused by danazol

| *Cause of side effect* | *Side effects caused* |
| --- | --- |
| Estrogen deficiency | Headache, flushing, sweating, atrophic vaginitis and breast atrophy |
| Androgenic effect | Acne, edema, hirsutism, deepening of the voice and weight gain |

pain or dyspareunia. Medical treatment comprises of oral analgesic agents such as NSAIDs, progesterone therapy, oral contraceptive agents, GnRH agonists, danazol and Mirena IUCD.

## Q. Describe the drug, danazol.

**Ans.** Danazol, a synthetic androgen is the derivative of ethinyl testosterone, which has been shown to be highly effective in relieving the symptoms of endometriosis by inhibiting pituitary gonadotropins (FSH and LH). This may result in the development of a relative hypoestrogenic state. Endometrial atrophy is the most likely mechanism, which provides relief from pain due to endometriosis. Danazol acts by inhibiting the midcycle FSH and LH surges and preventing steroidogenesis in the corpus luteum. It can be considered as a highly effective drug for treatment of endometriosis. However, its use may be associated with numerous side effects (Table 9.57), which may largely preclude its use.

Danazol therapy is started when the patient is menstruating, usually on the 1st day of the menses. The initial dosage should be 800 mg per day, given in two divided oral doses. Patients with less severe symptoms may be given 200–400 mg/day, in two divided oral doses. Treatment is usually administered for 6 months, but can be extended to 9 months in responsive patients with severe disease.

### Q. What is the role of laparoscopic surgery in cases of endometriosis?

**Ans.** Laparoscopy can help in establishing the diagnosis of endometriosis by identifying the lesions such as endometriotic nodules or lesions having blue-black or a powder-burned appearance. However, the lesions can be red, white, or nonpigmented. Peritoneal defects and adhesions are also indicative of endometriosis. Laparoscopy can also detect presence of blood or endometriotic deposits in cul-de-sac and its obliteration.

Besides diagnosis of endometriotic lesions at various locations, laparoscopy can also help in treating the patient. Powder-burn lesions over the uterine surface may be amenable to laser obliteration. Some of the endometrial lesions are cystic or nodular and can be excised. Laparoscopic surgery can also be used for excision of adhesions.

Until recently, surgery in infertile patients with limited disease was thought to be no better than expectant management. However, according to the recent evidence, laparoscopic surgery has been found to significantly improve the fertility rate among infertile women with minimal or mild endometriosis. Infertile patients with documented endometriosis can also benefit from the reproductive techniques such as superovulation, IVF, etc.

The usefulness of conservative surgery for pain relief is unclear, but it appears that immediate postoperative efficacy is at least as high as that with medical treatment and long-term outcomes may be considerably higher. Since laparoscopy is much more expensive in comparison to the medical treatment, some physicians advocate that the overall costs can be reduced by making aggressive use of empiric medical treatment before surgery is considered. Definitive surgery, which includes hysterectomy and oophorectomy, is reserved for use in women with intractable pain who no longer desire pregnancy.

In summary, surgical treatment improves pregnancy rate and is the preferred initial treatment for infertility caused by endometriosis. Surgery also appears to provide better long-term pain relief than medical treatment.

### Q. Can endometriomas undergo malignant transformation?

**Ans.** While majority of endometriomas are benign, they may sometimes serve as precursors to epithelial ovarian cancers, most commonly endometrioid adenocarcinoma or clear cell carcinoma. Despite the apparent link between endometriosis and certain types of ovarian cancers, the risk of malignant transformation is quite low, and endometriosis cannot be considered to be a premalignant condition.

# Molar Gestation

## Case Study 1

Mrs XYZ, a 20-year-old nulliparous woman, married since last one and half years, resident of ABC, presented with the complaints of bleeding per vaginum at 9 weeks of gestation. Per vaginal examination revealed a bulky soft uterus and the urine pregnancy test was positive. Ultrasound examination showed an ill-defined gestational sac with absent cardiac pulsations and a few small cisterns in region of placenta. A possible diagnosis of missed abortion was made. However, possibility of a partial mole also could not be ruled out. Serum beta human chorionic gonadotropin (β-hCG) levels were found to be 125,000 mIU/mL at the time of initial visit and it increased to 138,000 mIU/mL after 48 hours. The suspicion of molar gestation became stronger and suction evacuation was performed. The evacuated products were sent for histopathological examination, which confirmed the diagnosis of partial hydatidiform mole (PHM).

### Q. What is the most likely diagnosis in the above-mentioned case study?

**Ans.** The above-mentioned case study corresponds to partial hydatidiform mole (as confirmed by clinical examination and investigations). The questions to be asked at the time of taking history or the parameters to be assessed at the time of examination in such a case are described in Tables 9.58 and 9.59 respectively. The most likely diagnosis in this case is Mrs XYZ, a 20-year-old nulliparous woman, with an active married life of one and half year years, resident of ABC, with a confirmed diagnosis of partial hydatidiform mole on histopathological examination. If the result of histopathological analysis had not been provided, the provisional diagnosis of missed abortion or hydatidiform mole would be made.

### Q. What is hydatidiform mole?

**Ans.** Hydatidiform mole belongs to a spectrum of disease known as gestational trophoblastic disease (GTD), resulting from overproduction of the chorionic tissue, which is normally supposed to develop into the placenta. H. mole can be considered as a neoplasm of trophoblastic tissue and involves both syncytiotrophoblast and cytotrophoblast. H. moles are nonviable and genetically abnormal conceptions, showing excessive expression of paternal genes. In this condition, the placental tissues develop into an abnormal mass. There also occurs edema or hydropic degeneration of the connective tissue stroma of the villi, leading to their distension and formation of vesicles. Disappearance of blood vessels from the villi is often responsible for avascularity of the villi, resulting in an early death of the embryo. Often, there is no fetal mass at all. These changes are accompanied with excessive secretion of hormones such as hCG, chorionic thyrotrophin and progesterone. On the other hand, estrogen

| **Table 9.58:** Symptoms to be elicited at the time of taking history in a case of hydatidiform mole |
|---|
| *History of Presenting Complains* |

Clinical features commonly observed in cases with molar gestation are as follows:
- *Irregular vaginal bleeding:* There may be history suggestive of vaginal bleeding early in pregnancy. Bleeding occurs due to the separation of molar tissue from decidua. Vaginal bleeding is the most common clinical presentation of molar pregnancy. Presence of "prune juice" discharge (brownish-watery discharge) is a characteristic feature suggestive of molar gestation. If the bleeding is concealed, there may also be associated uterine tenderness and enlargement.
- Passage of grape-like tissue is strongly suggestive of the diagnosis of H. mole.
- *Hyperemesis:* Excessive nausea and vomiting in cases of H. mole may be related to high serum levels of β-hCG.
- *Exaggeration of the normal early pregnancy symptoms and signs:* This could be related to excessive β-hCG production.
- *Excessive uterine enlargement:* The second most common symptom of molar gestation is excessive uterine enlargement in relation to the gestational age.
- *Abdominal pain:* There may be dull-aching abdominal pain due to rapid distension of the uterus by the mole or by concealed hemorrhage. This pain may become colicky in nature when the patient starts expelling.
- *Early failed pregnancy*: Initially, the symptoms may be suggestive of early pregnancy; however, the uterus is often larger than the period of gestation. The fetal movements and heart tones are usually absent.
- *Symptoms of hyperthyroidism:* There may be symptoms suggestive of hyperthyroidism including tachycardia, restlessness, nervousness, heat intolerance, unexplained weight loss, diarrhea, tremors in hands, etc.
- *Preeclampsia:* Hydatidiform mole may be associated with early appearance of preeclampsia (usually by the first or early second trimester of pregnancy).
- *Respiratory symptoms:* Metastasis to the lungs (in cases of malignant moles) may result in symptoms like dyspnea, cough, hemoptysis, chest pain, etc.

***Risk Factors***
Factors which may be associated with an increased risk for CHM and need to be elicited while taking history are described as follows:
- *Race and ethnicity:* Though the exact reasons are not known, Asian populations are affected more in comparison to other ethnic groups.
- *Maternal age:* Mothers in extremes of age groups, i.e. either too young (< 20 years) or too old (older than 40 years) are usually affected. The risk of development of H. mole in women older than 40 years is about five times more than that in younger women.
- *Blood group:* Hydatidiform mole has been typically found to be associated with individuals having AB blood group. On the other hand, a woman with blood group A, partnered with a man, also having blood group A is at the lowest risk.

***Nutritional History***
Inadequate diet deficient in proteins, folic acid and vitamin A, and containing excessive amounts of fats has also been found to be associated with H. mole. Therefore, a detailed dietary history needs to be elicited in these patients.

*Abbreviations:* CHM, complete hydatidiform mole; hCG, human chorionic gonadotropin

| **Table 9.59:** Various findings elicited at the time of clinical examination in a case of hydatidiform mole |
|---|
| *General Physical Examination* |

- *Signs suggestive of preeclampsia:* Signs suggestive of preeclampsia such as high blood pressure, proteinuria, and swelling in ankles, feet and legs, may be observed.
- *Signs suggestive of hyperthyroidism:* Signs including warm, moist skin, heat intolerance, restlessness, tremors in hands, etc. may be observed.
- *Signs suggestive of early pregnancy:* These may include signs like amenorrhea, positive pregnancy test, breast changes suggestive of pregnancy, etc.
- *Extreme pallor:* The patient may appear extremely pale. The pallor may be disproportionate to the amount of blood loss due to concealed hemorrhage.

*Specific Systemic Examination*

*Abdominal Examination*
- On the abdominal examination the uterine size is usually abnormal in relation to the period of gestation. In most of the cases of CHM the uterine size may be larger than the period of gestation, whereas in cases of PHM the uterine size may be smaller in relation to the period of gestation.
- The uterus may appear doughy in consistency due to lack of fetal parts and amniotic fluid.
- Fetal movements and fetal heart sounds are absent.
- Fetal parts are usually not palpable.
- External ballottement is absent.

*Vaginal Examination*
- There may be some vaginal bleeding or passage of grape like vesicles.
- Internal ballottement cannot be elicited due to lack of fetus.
- Unilateral or bilateral enlargement of the ovaries in form of theca lutein cysts may be palpable.

**Table 9.60:** Classification of gestational trophoblastic disease

*Benign forms (90%)*

- Complete hydatidiform mole
- Partial hydatidiform mole

*Malignant forms (10%)*

- Invasive mole
- Choriocarcinoma
- Placental site trophoblastic tumor
- Epithelioid trophoblastic tumor

production is often on the lower side. However, sometimes, partial moles may show presence of fetal tissue.

Gestational trophoblastic disease represents a spectrum of premalignant and malignant diseases (Table 9.60) including potentially benign hydatidiform mole entities like complete hydatidiform mole (CHM) and PHM, and potentially malignant entities which are collectively known as gestational trophoblastic neoplasia (GTN). This may include entities such as invasive mole, choriocarcinoma and placental site trophoblastic tumor (PSTT). GTN is characterized by persistence of GTD, most commonly defined as a persistent elevation of β-hCG (even after 8–10 months following suction evacuation).

**Q. What is the difference between CHM and PHM?**
**Ans.** The difference between CHM and PHM is listed in Table 9.61.

**Q. Besides hydatidiform mole, which other condition may be associated with early appearance of preeclampsia?**
**Ans.** Early appearance of preeclampsia (prior to 20 weeks) is strongly suggestive of either H. mole or twin gestation, because occurrence of preeclampsia is extremely rare during this time period in normal pregnancies.

**Q. What should be the next step of management in the patient described in the above-mentioned case presentation?**
**Ans.** The patient now needs to be investigated to rule out the presence of persistent GTD. For this, serial determination of β-hCG levels needs to be done. Measurement of three

consecutive negative levels help in ensuring that complete sustained remission has been achieved. Following evacuation, serial assays of serum and urine β-hCG levels should be carried out on 2-weekly basis for at least 8 weeks.

In benign disease, β-hCG concentrations spontaneously return to normal by 8 weeks following evacuation of molar pregnancy. In these cases, regular follow-up in form of pelvic examination and urine β-hCG titers at monthly interval needs to be carried for a period of 6 months. However, women who have the persistent form of GTN may show plateauing or rising β-hCG titers, which usually remain elevated beyond 8 weeks. Such patients should have monthly follow-up in form of pelvic examination and urine β-hCG titers for at least 2 years.

**Q. In this case the results of serial serum β-hCG levels are tabulated in the Table 9.62. What do these results suggest?**
**Ans.** Serum β-hCG levels appear to be declining and have almost reached nonpregnant levels by 8–10 weeks. This pattern is highly suggestive of a nonpersistent disease pattern. In normal circumstances, serum β-hCG levels after nontrophoblastic abortions should fall to undetectable level by 3 weeks. Serum β-hCG levels after trophoblastic abortions should fall to a nondetectable level by 8-10 weeks.

**Q. What are initial investigations which must be done in cases of molar gestation?**
**Ans.** Ultrasound examination helps in establishing the diagnosis prior to evacuation; however the definitive

**Table 9.62:** Postevacuation serum β-human chorionic gonadotropin (β-hCG) level determination

| Time duration | Serum β-hCG levels |
|---|---|
| After 4 weeks | 543 mIU/mL |
| After 6 weeks | 58.73 mIU/mL |
| After 8 weeks | 11.67 mIU/mL |
| After 10 weeks | 3.16 mIU/mL |

*Abbreviation:* hCG, human chorionic gonadotropin

**Table 9.61:** Comparison between complete and partial mole

| Parameter under consideration | Complete mole | Partial mole |
|---|---|---|
| Cytogenetic studies | 46XX karyotype | Triploid karyotype 69XXY |
| Pathophysiology | Duplication of the haploid sperm following fertilization of an "empty" ovum or dispermic fertilization of an "empty" ovum | These contain two sets of paternal haploid genes and one set of maternal haploid genes. They usually occur following dispermic fertilization of an ovum |
| Histopathological analysis | There is no evidence of fetal tissue | There may be an evidence of fetal tissue or red blood vessels |
| Invasive potential and propensity for malignant transformation | Persistent trophoblastic disease following uterine evacuation may develop in about 15% cases with a complete mole | Persistent trophoblastic disease may develop in less than 5% cases of partial mole |

diagnosis is made only following the histological examination of the products of conception. Other investigations which must be done are as follows:

*Complete blood count, blood grouping and crossmatching:* Determination of hematocrit and hemoglobin levels help in estimating the degree of anemia. Blood grouping and cross-matching is required as blood transfusion may be required in case of severe maternal anemia.

*Platelet count and coagulation profile:* Measurement of platelet count and various coagulation parameters (bleeding time, clotting time, etc.) help in detecting the presence of any underlying coagulopathy.

*β-hCG levels:* Beta human chorionic gonadotropin is secreted by active trophoblastic tissues of the placenta and is detected in the blood 7–9 days following ovulation. In normal gestation a concentration of 100 mIU/mL is reached 2 days after the date of an expected menses. Peak levels of hCG (approximately 100,000 mIU/mL) are attained by 10 weeks of gestation. Normal serum β-hCG levels during pregnancy depending on the period of gestation are tabulated in Table 9.63.

Estimation of β-hCG levels may be helpful in diagnosing molar pregnancies. In molar gestation, β-hCG levels in both serum and urine are raised. While in normal pregnancy, urine pregnancy test is positive in dilutions up to 1/100; in cases of molar gestation, this test is positive in high dilution: positive test in a dilution of 1/200 is highly suggestive, whereas a positive test in a dilution of 1/500 is surely diagnostic of molar gestation. Serum β-hCG levels greater than two multiples of the median are also indicative of molar gestation. In cases of complete mole, serum β-hCG levels may be more than 100,000 mIU/mL.

**Table 9.63:** Measurement of serum β-hCG levels in normal pregnancy

| Period of gestation (from the date of conception) | Period of gestation (from last menstrual period) | Serum β-hCG levels (IU/L) |
|---|---|---|
| 7 days | 3 weeks | 0–5 |
| 14 days | 28 days | 3–426 |
| 21 days | 35 days | 18–7,340 |
| 28 days | 42 days | 1,080–56,500 |
| 35–42 days | 49–56 days | 7,650–229,000 |
| 43–64 days | 57–78 days | 25,700–288,200 |
| 65–78 days | 79–92 days | 13,300–253,000 |
| 17–24 weeks | Second trimester | 4,060–65,400 |
| After several days postpartum | – | Nonpregnant levels |

*Abbreviation:* hCG, human chorionic gonadotropin

*Ultrasound of the pelvis:* Sonography is the imaging investigation of choice to confirm the diagnosis of H. mole. Sonographic examination is not only helpful in establishing the initial diagnosis, it also helps in assessing the response to treatment regimens; determining the degree of invasion in malignant forms of GTN; determining the disease recurrence in malignant forms of GTN and evaluation of liver metastasis. Sonographic examination may reveal marked swelling of the villi showing resemblance to the molar tissue. There may be presence of vesicles, cysts, fetal remains and an abnormal placenta. Both transabdominal and transvaginal imaging must be performed using transducers with the highest ultrasound frequency possible. In cases of CHM, on ultrasound examination, there may be presence of numerous anechoic cysts, sized 1–30 mm with intervening hyperechoic material. Ultrasound may also show the presence of theca lutein cysts in the ovaries. Characteristic vesicular pattern, also known as "snowstorm appearance" may be present due to generalized swelling of the chorionic villi and presence of many small cystic spaces. In cases of PHM, the ultrasound findings include: a large placenta, cystic spaces within the placenta, an empty gestational sac, or the sac containing amorphous echoes or growth retarded fetus.

*Doppler ultrasonography:* Presence of cystic vascular spaces showing high-velocity, low-impedance flow on Doppler ultrasound is characteristic of invasive disease. Doppler ultrasonography also has a role in monitoring the response of the disease following chemotherapy. Regression of cystic vascular masses following chemotherapy is indicative of successful treatment.

*Chest X-ray:* The lungs are the most common site for metastasis in case of malignant GTD and may show the presence of distinct nodules or cannon ball appearance. Other radiographic patterns which can be produced on the X-ray include an alveolar or snowstorm pattern, pleural effusion and an embolic pattern caused by pulmonary arterial occlusion. Metastasis to lungs is often associated with symptoms like dyspnea, cough, hemoptysis, chest pain, etc. A suspicion of pulmonary metastasis on chest X-ray must be followed by a CT or MRI examination of both head and abdomen.

*Histopathological examination:* The diagnosis of H. mole is confirmed by histological examination. Therefore, all products of conception from nonviable pregnancies must be submitted for routine pathological evaluation to exclude presence of trophoblastic neoplasia.

### Q. What advice regarding contraception should be given in the patient in previously described case study?

**Ans.** Women with molar pregnancy should be advised to avoid pregnancy until hCG levels have been normal for 6 months following evacuation of a molar pregnancy and for 1 year following chemotherapy for GTN. There has been some controversy regarding the use of OCPs as a method of contraception following evacuation, until the serum β-hCG levels have returned to normal. Some studies suggest that the use of combined OCP may increase the risk of malignancy in women whose β-hCG titers remain high, whereas other studies have shown no risk. While some centers continue to prescribe OCPs as a method of contraception, most centers from the UK recommend that these women must not take the pills until their hormone concentrations have returned to normal. If the woman had started taking OCPs before the diagnosis of GTD had been made, she should be counseled regarding a small, but an increased risk of developing GTN in case she chooses to remain on oral contraception.

The small potential risk of using emergency hormonal contraception (comprising of progesterone), in women with raised β-hCG levels, is outweighed by the potential risk of pregnancy to the woman. An IUCD is inadvisable as it may cause bleeding, which may be confused with the presence of persistent disease. Also insertion of IUCD before the normalization of hCG levels may be associated with the risk of uterine perforation. Surgical methods or barrier contraception proves useful in these cases. Also, presently there is no evidence regarding any adverse effect of single-agent progestogens on GTN.

### Q. What are the management options in case of H. mole?

**Ans.** The two main treatment options in case of H. mole are suction evacuation and hysterectomy.

### Suction Evacuation

In case of benign disease, treatment is by suction evacuation. In case of complete absence of fetal parts, evacuation of the uterine contents is carried out by means of suction evacuation, irrespective of the uterine size. Due to the lack of fetal parts, a suction catheter, up to a maximum size of 12 mm, is usually sufficient to evacuate all complete molar pregnancies. A uterus of size up to 20 weeks can be readily evacuated. In case of partial mole with presence of fetal parts, medical method of evacuation (oxytocic agents) can be used.

Prior to suction evacuation, an intravenous line must be set up. Blood should be cross-matched and kept available. Cervical dilatation is usually not required as the cervix is soft and readily permits the entry of a suction cannula. Prolonged cervical preparation with prostaglandins is not usually required and should be avoided wherever possible to reduce the risk of embolization of trophoblastic cells. Passage of the uterine sound prior to the evacuation is avoided as this may cause uterine perforation. The tip of the suction cannula must be inserted just beyond the internal os. If the uterus is larger than 12 weeks in size, one hand must be placed on the fundus and the uterus should be massaged with the other in order to stimulate uterine contractions, thereby reducing the risk of uterine perforation. Routine curettage following suction evacuation is not recommended.

*Follow-up with β-hCG levels following suction evacuation:* Patients with both complete and partial molar pregnancy should be monitored with serial β-hCG measurements after evacuation to ensure that complete sustained remission has been achieved. Serial assays of serum and urine β-hCG levels should be carried out on 2-weekly basis until three negative levels are obtained. In benign disease, hCG concentrations spontaneously return to normal by 8 weeks following evacuation of molar pregnancy. In these cases, regular follow-up in form of pelvic examination and urine β-hCG titers at monthly interval needs to be done for a period of 6 months. However, women who have the malignant form of trophoblastic disease may show β-hCG titers, which either plateau or rise and remain elevated beyond 8 weeks. Such patients should have monthly follow-up in form of pelvic examination and urine β-hCG titers for at least 2 years. A chest X-ray is indicated to rule out metastatic disease if the β-hCG levels rise.

### Hysterectomy with Mole in Situ

Hysterectomy may serve as an option in the following cases:
- Elderly multiparous women (age > 40 years) who do not wish to become pregnant in the future
- Those women with H. mole desiring sterilization
- Those with severe infection or uncontrolled bleeding
- Patients with nonmetastatic persistent disease who have completed childbearing or are not concerned about preserving fertility.

### Q. When should chemotherapy be instituted following evacuation?

**Ans.** Women who undergo chemotherapy following evacuation are advised not to conceive for 1 year after completion of treatment. Some indications for chemotherapy [as recommended by Society of Obstetricians and Gynaecologists of Canada, (2002)], following evacuation of molar gestation are as follows:
- An abnormal-hCG regression pattern (a 10% or greater rise in hCG levels or plateauing of hCG levels comprising of three stable values over 2 weeks)
- Histological diagnosis of choriocarcinoma or placental site trophoblastic tumor
- The presence of metastases in brain, liver, gastrointestinal tract, lungs, or vulvar or vaginal walls
- High hCG levels (> 20,000 mIU/mL more than 4 weeks postevacuation).
- Persistently elevated hCG levels 6 months postevacuation.

### Q. How should the persistent disease be treated?

**Ans.** Following the evacuation of molar gestation, if the β-hCG level does not normalize within 8–10 weeks, the disease is classified as persistent. Any woman experiencing persistent or irregular vaginal bleeding following a pregnancy event (miscarriage, therapeutic termination of pregnancy

**Flow chart 9.4:** Management of persistent disease

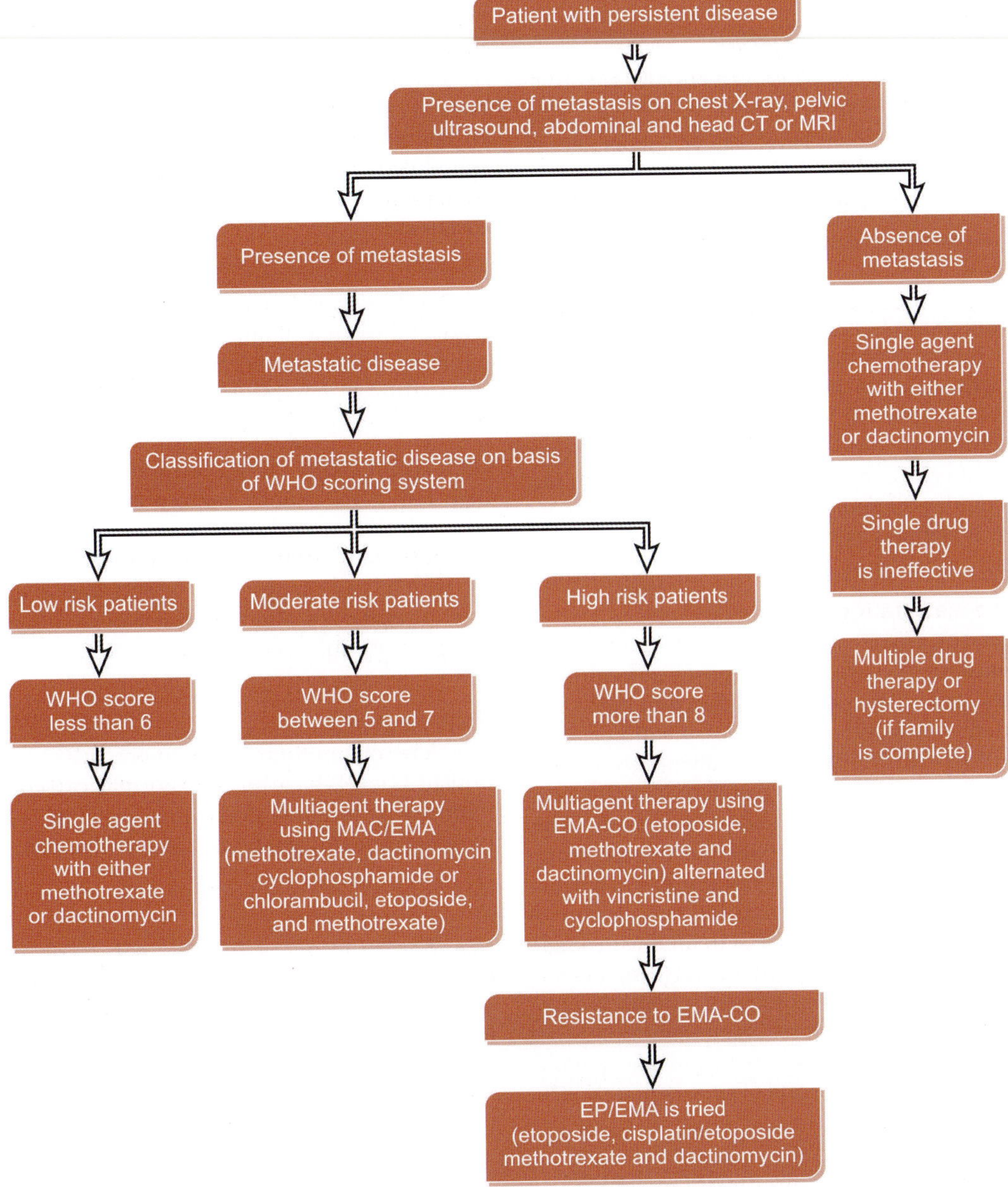


or following the baby's delivery) is at risk of developing persistent GTN. The management plan for the treatment of persistent disease is shown in Flow chart 9.4. In these cases it is important to measure β-hCG levels. In these cases, chest X-ray and CT scan of brain, chest, abdomen and pelvis also need to be done. If metastasis is detected on these investigations, the disease is classified as metastatic. If no metastasis is detected, the disease is classified as nonmetastatic.

### Q. Describe the FIGO staging of malignant disease

**Ans.** The FIGO staging of malignant disease is shown in Table 9.64.

### Q. How should the nonmetastatic disease be treated?

**Ans.** In most of the cases, nonmetastatic disease can be treated with a single chemotherapeutic drug (methotrexate or dactinomycin). Methotrexate is the drug which is most commonly used. Women who develop resistance to methotrexate are treated with a combination of intravenous dactinomycin and etoposide. If single drug chemotherapy is ineffective, hysterectomy or multidrug chemotherapy can be tried. Methotrexate can be administered in the dosage of 0.4 mg/kg (maximum 25 mg) intravenously or intramuscularly daily for 5 days per treatment course. Another commonly used

**Table 9.64:** FIGO staging of GTN

| Stage | Description |
| --- | --- |
| Stage I | Disease confined to the uterus |
| Stage II | GTN extends outside the uterus but is limited to the genital structures (adnexa, vagina, broad ligament) |
| Stage III | GTN extends to the lungs with or without genital tract involvement |
| Stage IV | All other metastatic sites |

*Abbreviation:* GTN, gestational trophoblastic neoplasia

regimen of methotrexate is administration of methotrexate in the dose of 1 mg/kg intramuscularly given on days 1, 3, 5 and 7 along with calcium leucovorin rescue in dose of 0.1 mg/kg on days 2, 4, 6 and 8, 30 hours following injection of methotrexate. Courses are repeated every 14 days dependent on toxicity, i.e. first course on day 1; second course on day 15; third course on day 29 and so on. An adequate response to chemotherapy is defined as fall in the-hCG levels by 1 log after a course of chemotherapy.

#### Q. How should the metastatic disease be treated?

**Ans.** Consultation with a gynecologic oncologist is required for treatment of metastatic diseases. For purposes of treatment, patients with metastatic disease are classified into high- risk, moderate-risk and low-risk groups. The classification system adopted by the WHO and FIGO for classifying gestational trophoblastic tumors and treatment protocols has become the most widely used prognostic scoring system. This classification system is shown in Table 9.65. The low-risk group will have a score of 0–6; the moderate-risk group has a score between 5 and 7; and the high-risk group will have a score of 7 or higher. Low-risk metastatic disease is treated with single or multiple drug chemotherapy. Moderate-risk metastatic disease is usually treated with multiagent chemotherapy. High-risk metastatic disease requires aggressive multidrug chemotherapy. Low-risk disease has cure rate of nearly 100%, whereas high-risk disease has cure rate of approximately 95%.

*Low-risk metastatic disease (WHO Score: Less than 6):* Women belonging to low risk, i.e. scoring six or less on the classification system must receive IM methotrexate. Methotrexate is administered intramuscularly, alternating daily with folinic acid for 1 week followed by 6 rest days. Women who develop resistance to methotrexate are treated with a combination of IV dactinomycin and etoposide. The dosage and treatment schedule for methotrexate and dactinomycin is same as that for patients with nonmetastatic disease and has already been discussed.

*Moderate-risk patients (WHO Score: 5 to 7):* Traditionally, moderate-risk patients (WHO score of 5–7) have been treated with multi-agent chemotherapy. The most commonly used combination chemotherapy include: MAC based combination (methotrexate, dactinomycin, cyclophosphamide or chlorambucil) or EMA (etoposide, methotrexate and dactinomycin).

*High-risk patients (WHO Score: 8 or Greater):* Women with high-risk GTN usually require combination chemotherapy with selective use of surgery and radiotherapy. The standard chemotherapy regimen in high-risk group is EMA/CO in which the drugs like etoposide, dactinomycin and methotrexate are alternated at weekly intervals with drugs like cyclophosphamide and vincristine.

#### Q. How should the patient be followed-up after chemotherapy?

**Ans.** After chemotherapy treatment, hCG is measured weekly until hCG levels have become normal for 3 consecutive weeks, followed by monthly determination of hCG levels until they have become normal for 24 consecutive months (2 years).

#### Q. What are the various complications, which can occur as a result of molar gestation?

**Ans.** Benign forms of H. mole can result in complications like uterine infection, sepsis, hemorrhagic shock and preeclampsia, which may occur during early pregnancy. Recurrence of molar gestation may occur in 1–2% cases. Excessive vaginal bleeding can be associated with molar pregnancy. Gestational trophoblastic disease does not impair

**Table 9.65:** The classification system by the WHO and FIGO for classifying gestational trophoblastic tumors and treatment protocols

| Risk factor | Risk score | | | |
| --- | --- | --- | --- | --- |
| | 0 | 1 | 2 | 4 |
| Age (years) | < 40 | ≥ 40 | – | – |
| Antecedent pregnancy | Mole | Abortion | Term | – |
| Interval (end of antecedent pregnancy to chemotherapy) in months | < 4 | 4–6 | 7–13 | > 13 |
| Human chorionic gonadotropin (IU/L) | $< 10^3$ | $10^3–10^4$ | $10^4–10^5$ | $> 10^5$ |
| Number of metastasis | 0 | 1–4 | 5–8 | > 8 |
| Site of metastasis | Lung | Spleen, kidney | Gastrointestinal tract | Brain, liver |
| Largest tumor mass | – | 3–5 cm | > 5 cm | – |
| Previous chemotherapy | – | – | Single drug | ≥ 2 drugs |

fertility or predispose to prenatal or perinatal complications (e.g. congenital malformations, spontaneous abortions, etc.). The most important complication related to GTD is the development of GTN, which include conditions like invasive mole, choriocarcinoma and Placental site trophoblastic tumor. All of these may metastasize and are potentially fatal if left untreated.

## FURTHER READINGS


1. ACOG Committee on Gynecologic Practice. The role of the generalist obstetrician-gynecologist in the early detection of ovarian cancer. Gynecol Oncol. 2002;87(3):237-9.
2. ACOG Committee on Practice Bulletins-Gynecology. ACOG Practice Bulletin No. 51. Chronic pelvic pain. Obstet Gynecol. 2004;103(3):589-605.
3. American Academy of Family Physicians summary of policy recommendations for periodic health examination. AAFP Policy Action. 1997;1-14.
4. Soper JT, Mutch DG, Schink JC, American College of Obstetricians and Gynecologists. Diagnosis and treatment of gestational trophoblastic disease: ACOG Practice Bulletin No. 53. Gynecol Oncol. 2004;93(3):575-85.
5. American College of Obstetricians and Gynecologists Committee on Gynecologic Practice. ACOG Committee Opinion No. 420, November 2008: hormone therapy and heart disease. Obstet Gynecol. 2008;112(5):1189-92.
6. American College of Obstetricians and Gynecologists Women's Health Care physicians. Executive summary. Hormone therapy. Obstet Gynecol. 2004;104(4 suppl):1S-4S.
7. American College of Obstetricians and Gynecologists. ACOG Committee Opinion. Number 310, April 2005. Endometriosis in adolescents. Obstet Gynecol. 2005;105:921-7.
8. American College of Obstetricians and Gynecologists. ACOG practice bulletin, clinical management guidelines for obstetrician-gynecologists, number 65, August 2005: management of endometrial cancer. Obstet Gynecol. 2005;106(2):413-25.
9. American College of Obstetricians and Gynecologists. ACOG practice bulletin. Clinical Management Guidelines for Obstetrician-Gynecologists. Number 61, April 2005. Human papillomavirus. Obstet Gynecol. 2005;105(4):905-18.
10. American College of Obstetricians and Gynecologists. Amenorrhea. ACOG Technical Bulletin 128. Washington, DC: ACOG; 1989.
11. American College of Obstetricians and Gynecologists. Endometriosis. ACOG technical bulletin no. 184. Washington, DC: ACOG; 1993.
12. American Society for Reproductive Medicine (ASRM). (2004). Frequently asked questions about infertility. [online] Available from www. asrm.org/Patients/faqs.html#Q2 [Accessed November, 2014].
13. American Urological Association (AUA) and American Society for Reproductive Medicine (ASRM). (2001). Report on optimal evaluation of the infertile male. [online] Available from www. auanet.org/timssnet/products/ guidelines/main_reports/ optimalevaluation. pdf [Accessed November, 2014].
14. CDC. 1998 guidelines for treatment of sexually transmitted diseases. MMWR Morb Mortal Wkly Rep. 1998;47:1-111.
15. Committee on Practice Bulletins—Gynecology. Practice bulletin no. 128: diagnosis of abnormal uterine bleeding in reproductive-aged women. Obstet Gynecol. 2012;120: 197-206.
16. FIGO Oncology Committee. FIGO staging for gestational trophoblastic neoplasia 2000. FIGO Oncology Committee. Int J Gynecol Obstet. 2002;77(3):285-7.
17. National Institute for Clinical Excellence (2003). Guidance on the use of paclitaxel in the treatment of ovarian cancer. [online] Available from www.nice.org.uk/nicemedia/ live/11486/32539/32539/.pdf. [Accessed November, 2014].
18. National Institute for clinical excellence (2004). Guidance on cancer services: Improving supportive and palliative care for adults with cancer—The manual. [online] Available from www.nice.org.uk/nicemedia/pdf/(sgspmanual.pdf [Accessed November, 2014].
19. North American Menopause Society. Estrogen and progestogen use in postmenopausal women: 2010 position statement of The North American Menopause Society. Menopause. 2010;17(2):242-55.
20. North American Menopause Society. The 2012 hormone therapy position statement of: The North American Menopause Society. Menopause. 2012;19(3):257-71.
21. Royal College of Obstetricians and Gynaecologists. Guideline No. 41: The initial management of chronic pelvic pain. London, UK: RCOG Press; 2005.
22. Royal College of Obstetricians and Gynaecologists. The Management of Tubal Pregnancy. Guideline No. 21. London: RCOG Press; 2004.
23. Royal College of Obstetricians and Gynaecologists. The Management of Gestational Trophoblastic Neoplasia. Guideline No. 38. London: RCOG Press; 2004.
24. Royal College of Obstetricians and Gynecologists (2010). The management of gestational trophoblastic neoplasia. Green-top Guideline No. 38. [online] Available from www.rcog. org. uk/files/rcog-corp/GT38ManagementGestational0210.pdf. [Accessed November, 2014].
25. Royal College of Obstetricians and Gynecologists. The initial management of menorrhagia: Evidence-based guidelines No. 1. London, UK: RCOG Press; 1998.
26. Sekharan PK. The management of gestational trophoblastic neoplasia FOGSI – ICOG consensus statement. SOGC Practice Guidelines. Gestational Trophoblastic Disease. J Obstet Gynaecol Can. 2002;24(5):434-9.
27. The Endocrine Society®. (2006). The Endocrine Society Position Statement. [online] Available from www.endo-society. org/advocacy/ policy/upload/BH_position_Statement_ final_10_25_06_w_Header.pdf. [Accessed November, 2014].
28. The Practice Committee of the American Society for Reproductive Medicine. Current evaluation of amenorrhea. Fertil Steril. 2004;82(Suppl 1):S33-9.
29. World Health Organization. WHO Laboratory Manual for the Examination of Human Semen and Semen-Cervical Mucus Interaction, 3rd edition. Cambridge: Cambridge University Press; 1992.
30. World Health Organization. WHO Laboratory Manual for the Examination of Human Semen and Sperm Cervical Mucus Interaction, 4th Edition. Cambridge, United Kingdom: Cambridge University Press; 1999.

# Operation Theater Procedures: Gynecology



## Cervical Biopsy

Cervical biopsy is a procedure, which is performed to obtain a sample of cervical tissue especially in cases of suspected malignancy or premalignancy. The various types of biopsies which can be performed are as follows:

- *Simple punch biopsy:* The biopsy sample is taken from the cervical lesion using a punch biopsy forceps. The cervical tissue is obtained from the junction of healthy and unhealthy tissues. The tissue obtained is stored in formalin and the histopathological diagnosis is established.
- *Biopsy after Schiller's test:* In this test, the cervix is painted with Schiller's iodine solution, which allows the cancer cells to remain unstained, while the healthy tissue takes up the iodine stain. Biopsy is taken from the junction of stained and the unstained areas. Diagnostic accuracy considerably improves after Schiller's test.
- *Four-quadrant biopsy:* Four-quadrant biopsy is taken from all the four quadrants and sent for histopathological examination. A four-quadrant biopsy may be especially required in cases where the lesion is not clearly defined.
- *Colposcopic-directed biopsy:* The biopsy is directed under colposcopic guidance.
- *Cone biopsy.*

All these various types of biopsies can be performed as an OPD procedure, except for the cone biopsy, which is performed in an operation theater.

### Cone Biopsy

*Introduction*

Cone biopsy serves as both a diagnostic and therapeutic procedure. It also helps in ruling out advanced cancer of the cervix. The procedure involves the removal of the entire area of abnormality (Fig. 10.1). It is also capable of providing tissue for histopathological examination. For nulliparous women, shallow cone is preferred, whereas in case of multiparous women, narrow cone is suitable.

*Indications*

Indications for cone biopsy are as follows:
- The area of the abnormality is large, or its inner margin has receded into the cervical canal.
- The limits of the lesion cannot be visualized by colposcopy.
- The squamocolumnar junction is not completely observable on colposcopy.
- There is discrepancy between the findings of cytology and colposcopy.

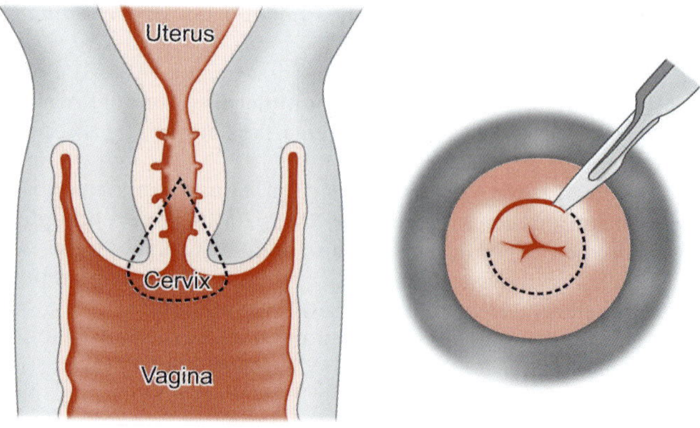


**Fig. 10.1:** Cone biopsy

- There is a suspicion of microinvasion based on the results of biopsy, colposcopy or cytology.
- The findings of endocervical curettage are positive for cervical intraepithelial neoplasia (CIN 2, CIN 3 or carcinoma in situ).
- Colposcopist is unable to rule out invasive cancer.

### Procedure

- The cone biopsy may be performed in an operation theater under general or regional anesthesia.
- This method involves obtaining a wide cone of excision including the entire outer margin of the lesion and the entire endocervical lining. It may include cold knife conization as well as loop electrical excision procedure (LEEP). It can be performed using a surgical knife or a carbon dioxide laser.
- In case a shallow cone is taken, the endocervical canal must be curetted out later to rule out carcinoma.
- Raw area of the cone can be left alone or covered with Strumdorf sutures.

### Postprocedural Advice

- Antibiotics and painkillers can be prescribed.
- Sterile vulval pad must be used for 2–3 days following the procedure. The patient must be asked to report immediately to the healthcare provider if she develops excessive bleeding or discharge or pain and fever with chills.
- A repeat Pap smear must be done after 3–6 months.

### Complications

The procedure of cone biopsy can result in the following complications:

- Primary or secondary hemorrhage.
- Infection.
- Cervical stenosis.
- Cervical incompetence.
- Infertility.

# Cryosurgery

## Introduction

Cryosurgery is a locally destructive OPD procedure in which the dysplastic cells are destroyed using freezing agents [$CO_2$ (–60°C) or nitrous oxide (–80°C)]. The optimal temperature required for effective tissue destruction must be in the range of –20°C to –30°C. Cryosurgery or cryocauterization is performed using a hand-held instrument with an attachment for a cryoprobe. Different sizes of cryoprobes, which carry nitrous oxide gas, are available. The cryoprobe is pushed out at a high pressure over the surface of cervix. On contact with the cervical tissue, an ice ball is formed over the surface epithelium.

## Indications

Indications of the procedure are as follows:

- Cervical erosion.
- Small cervical polyps.
- Chronic cervicitis.
- Benign cervical lesions presenting with irregular bleeding or chronic vaginal discharge.
- CIN 1.

## Contraindications

Various contraindications for performing cryosurgery are as follows:

- Pregnancy.
- Severe PID.
- Endometriosis.
- Active hemorrhage.

## Procedure

### Preprocedural Preparation

- No specific preparation is required prior to the procedure.
- The procedure is usually done post menses.
- The patient is placed in a lithotomy position.
- A Pap smear or colposcopic examination may be done at the same setting.

### Actual Procedure

- The cryosurgery equipment comprises of a gas tank containing nitrous oxide and a "green gun" which activates the probe. The gas cools the probe to a temperature 95° F below zero. The correct size of the cryocautery probe is then selected and attached. For detailed description of the cryomachine, kindly refer to Chapter 13.
- The cryoprobe is used, usually without any anesthesia or analgesia and causes destruction of the cells by crystallization of intercellular fluid.
- The probe is fixed on the surface of cervix and the "freeze" started (Fig. 10.2). Cervix and probe freeze together forming an ice ball.
- The freeze lasts for about 3 minutes followed by thawing for another 5 minutes. This is described as the "freeze-thaw-freeze" technique in which an ice ball is achieved 5 mm beyond edge of the probe. The cryoprobe is applied over the area of abnormality for over 9 minutes and destroys the tissue up to the depth of about 4–5 mm.
- The time required for the procedure is related to the pressure of gas. The higher the pressure of gas, faster is the rate of ice ball formation.

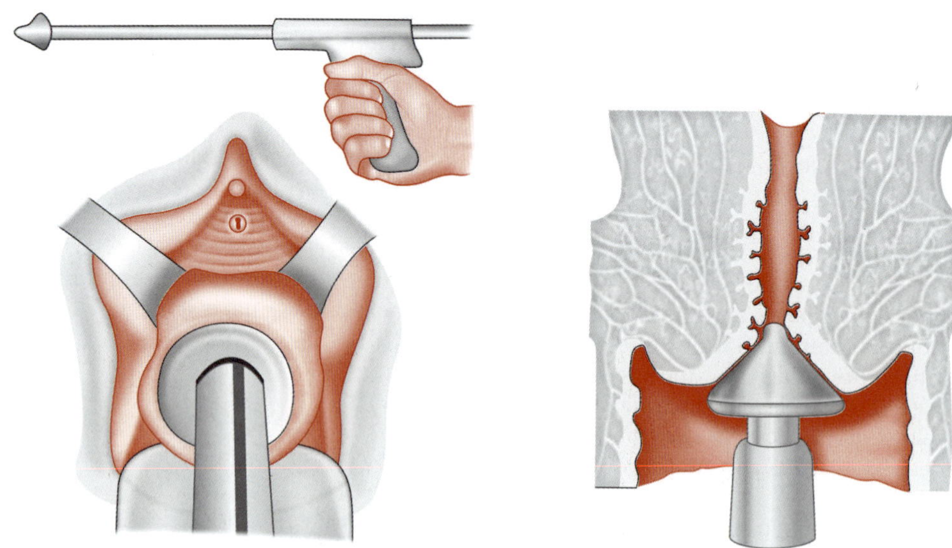

**Fig. 10.2:** Application of cryoprobe over the surface of cervix

*Postprocedural Care*

- Patient is advised rest for 2 days.
- Antibiotics are prescribed.
- Plenty of fluids may be advised.
- Abstinence for about 15 days.

*Follow-Up Advice*

- Regular Pap smears must be advised at 3 or 6 months post-procedure in high-risk cases. In cases of premalignancy, both Pap smear and colposcopy may be required.
- *Patient education:* The patient must be educated on various aspects of her disease so that she can visit her healthcare provider in case she experiences symptoms such as irregular vaginal bleeding, excessive vaginal discharge or severe lower abdominal pain.

## Complications

Overall, cryosurgery is a relatively safe procedure with few complications. Some of the complications which can rarely occur are mentioned next:
- Severe pain
- Heavy watery discharge for about 4–6 weeks
- Urinary/vaginal infection
- Irregular bleeding

## Tests for Tubal Patency

Various tests for tubal patency include Rubin's test, laparoscopic chromopertubation, hysterosalpingogram, etc.

These tests help in determining if the fallopian tubes are open or blocked in cases of infertility.

## RUBIN'S TEST

This test was previously used for testing of tubal patency. It is rarely used in the present times. It involves the following steps:
- Patient is placed in the lithotomy position under mild sedation
- Rubin's cervical insufflation cannula is inserted through the cervical os and carbon dioxide gas is injected under pressure into the uterine cavity
- Presence of hissing sound due to the escape of gas from the fimbrial ostia into the peritoneal cavity is indicative of tubal patency.

## HYSTEROSALPINGOGRAPHY

As described in Chapter 9, hysterosalpingography (HSG) is the most frequently used diagnostic tool for evaluation of the endometrial cavity as well as the tubal pathology (Figs 10.3A to H). Hysterosalpingography is a radiological procedure commonly used in gynecology.

## Indications

Indications for performing HSG are as follows:
- *Infertility:* In cases of infertility, HSG serves as a reliable, noninvasive, cost-effective test for ruling out tubal occlusion. In comparison to laparoscopy, HSG is less invasive, does not require general anesthesia, and is

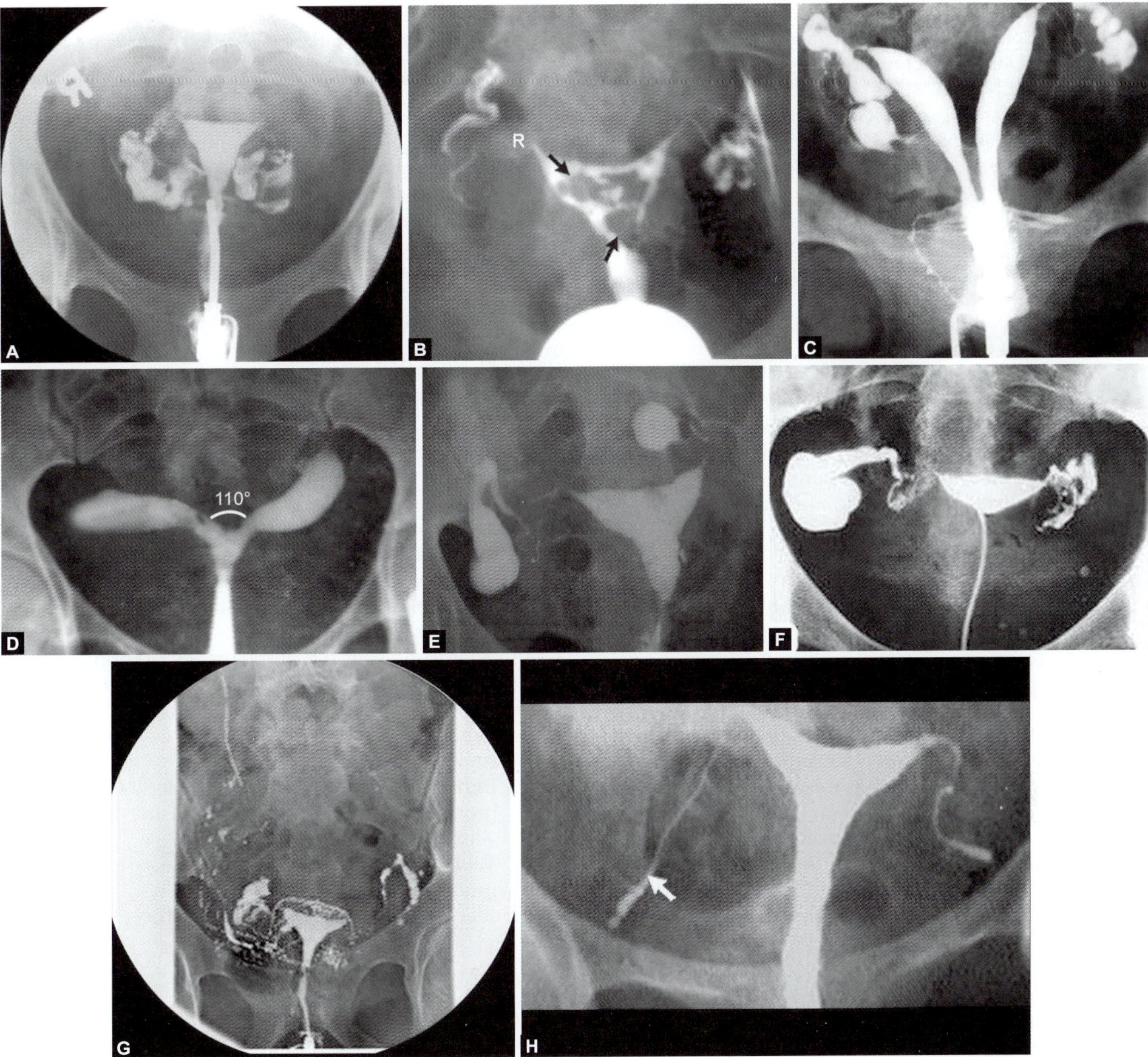

**Figs 10.3A to H:** Use of hysterosalpingography (HSG) for diagnosis of various abnormalities. (A) Normal HSG showing smooth triangular uterine cavity, with the dye spilling from the ends of both tubes; (B) HSG revealing irregular filling defects in the endometrium suggestive of endometrial adhesions (arrows represent adhesions). The patient was diagnosed to be suffering from Asherman's syndrome on hysteroscopy on which resection of the intrauterine adhesions was done; (C) HSG showing presence of uterine septum, which was confirmed on hysteroscopy; (D) HSG showing a single cervical canal and a possible duplication of the uterine horns. It was difficult to differentiate between bicornuate uterus and septate uterus on ultrasound alone. Since an angle of greater than 105° was found to be separating the two uterine horns, the diagnosis of bicornuate uterus was made, which was confirmed on laparoscopy; (E) Bilateral cornual block; (F) HSG showing right-sided hydrosalpinx; (G) HSG showing venous intravasation; (H) Lead pipe-like appearance of tubes in a case of tuberculosis (indicated by an arrow)

able to reveal the internal structure of the uterus and tubes. Also, HSG is associated with a much lower rate of complications, such as injury to the bowel or blood vessels.

- *Genital tuberculosis:* HSG is contraindicated in an established case of genital tuberculosis due to the risk of spread of infection. HSG findings in case of tuberculosis are as follows:
    - Bilateral cornual block with extravasation of the dye
    - Lymphatic or vascular intravasation of the dye
    - A rigid, nonperistaltic, lead-pipe like appearance of tubes
    - Beading and variations in the filling density of the fallopian tubes
    - Calcification of tubes
    - Jagged fluffiness of the tubal outline
- Diagnosis of congenital anomalies of uterus, e.g. bicornuate uterus, septate uterus, arcuate uterus, etc.
- Diagnosis of intrauterine adhesions
- Diagnosis of uterine tumors: Submucosal polyps, fibroids, adenomyosis, etc.
- Localization of IUCD
- Diagnosis of cervical incompetence
- Assessment of uterine scar integrity in patients with previous history of cesarean delivery.

## Contraindications

Some contraindications for performing HSG are as follows:

- Presence of acute comorbid disorders: Women who are known to have comorbid disorders (such as PID, lower genital tract infection, previous ectopic pregnancy or endometriosis) should not be offered HSG as a screening test for tubal occlusion. Women who are thought to have comorbidities should be offered laparoscopy with dye instillation so that tubal and other pelvic pathology can be assessed at the same time
- Pregnancy
- During the phase of menstrual periods/premenstrual phase of menstrual cycles
- Known sensitivity to contrast medium
- Suspected genital tuberculosis
- Irregular uterine bleeding (evaluate the cause of bleeding first).

## Normal Findings

Normal uterine cavity is symmetrical and triangular in shape, with each side being approximately about 4 cm. It is widest at the level of cornual orifices near the fundus. The cervix is about 2.5 cm long. If the fallopian tubes are patent, the contrast medium would be seen spilling out of the abdominal ostia and smearing the adjacent bowel. If the tube is blocked, the site of block can be visualized on the fluoroscopic image.

A hydrosalpinx would appear as a large confined mass of dye without the peritoneal spill.

## Timing

The HSG should be performed postmenstrually during the early follicular phase, usually after the end of menstrual bleeding and before the occurrence of ovulation, during the 2–5 days interval period immediately following the end of menses. At this time, the endometrium is thin and the HSG can help delineate the minor defects. Additionally, performance of HSG before the occurrence of ovulation eliminates the possibility of accidental irradiation to the fetus in case of an undiagnosed pregnancy.

## Procedure

*Preprocedural preparation:* This involves the following steps:

- No specific patient preparation is required prior to the procedure. Patient reassurance and explanation of the procedure are mainly required.
- 5–10 mg of diazepam can be administered intravenously in case of an anxious patient.
- Atropine, 0.6 mg can be administered intramuscularly to prevent vasovagal attacks.
- In order to prevent the development of cornual spasm during the procedure, the following medicines can be administered prior to the procedure:
    - Sublingual trinitrate.
    - Amyl nitrate inhalation
    - Intramuscular injection of atropine is unreliable in providing relief against cornual spasm
    - Glucagon.
    - Tablet isoxsuprine, 20 mg, 1 hour prior to the procedure.
- Bladder must be emptied prior to the procedure.

## Steps of the Procedure

The procedure of HSG involves the following steps:

- The procedure is performed in the radiology room with an image intensifier.
- The patient is made to lie on the examination table either in lithotomy position, with her feet held up with stirrups or in dorsal position with her knees bent.
- The posterior vaginal wall is retracted using a Sims speculum and the anterior lip of cervix is held with a tenaculum.
- The procedure is performed after observing strict aseptic precautions. The cervix is cleansed with a povidone-iodine solution (betadine).
- After cleaning the cervix, an injection catheter/cannula, attached to a syringe prefilled with the dye up to the tip, is inserted through the cervix inside the uterine cavity. This helps in avoiding air in the catheter from forming

air bubbles inside the uterine cavity. The most common type of cannula used in the cases of primary infertility is Rubin's cannula. Leech Wilkinson's cannula can also be sometimes used. For detailed description of both these cannulas, kindly refer to Chapter 13.

- A uterine sound is passed to determine the direction and size of uterine cavity.
- Following the injection of dye, the speculum and tenaculum are removed and the patient is carefully situated underneath the fluoroscopy device so that her pelvis lies over the X-ray plate.
- The contrast material is inserted through the catheter into the uterine cavity. In normal cases, it passes through the uterine cavity into the fallopian tubes, finally into the peritoneal cavity and fluoroscopic images are taken. The first fluoroscopic image is taken at the time of uterine filling before the contrast opacification becomes too dense. This helps in visualizing the small filling defects and deformities in the uterus. The second X-ray image is taken when the uterus and fallopian tubes are delineated and the peritoneal spill has just started occurring from the fimbrial end. The third X-ray image is taken 10–15 minutes later to show the pattern of peritoneal spill. All the X-ray images are taken in the anterior-posterior view, except for the cases where the integrity of previous cesarean scar needs to be tested, wherein the lateral view is taken. The X-ray images can help in determining whether the fallopian tubes are patent or blocked and whether the blockage is located at the proximal or at the distal end of the fallopian tube.
- Initially oil-based dye, lipoidal was used as the contrast media for performing HSG. However, now water-soluble contrast material (conray 280 or 420 or urograffin) is generally being preferred as it helps in preventing the development of possible complications such as oil embolism, oil granuloma, peritoneal irritation, etc., which were more commonly associated with oil-based dyes.

## Postprocedural Care

- When the procedure is complete, the catheter is removed. Since the injection of dye can sometimes cause cramping, the woman is asked to remain lying on the table for a few minutes following the completion of the procedure in order to let her recover from this cramping.
- The patient must be assured that the minimal amount of bleeding and/or vaginal discharge is a normal phenomenon.
- The patient should be asked to inform her day-care provider in case the pain, swelling, infection, headache, dizziness or fever persists.

## Complications

Hysterosalpingogram is usually not associated with any major complications. Some complications which can rarely occur are as follows:

- *Infection:* If the procedure is performed maintaining strict asepsis, infection rarely occurs. However, routine prophylactic treatment with doxycycline 100 mg twice a day for 5 days, beginning 1–2 days before HSG is usually justified because of the potential drastic consequences of a postprocedural infection. Antibiotic prophylaxis is especially indicated when the tubal disease is highly suspected or HSG reveals distal tubal obstruction because in these cases the risk for acute salpingitis is increased and treatment can prevent clinical infection.
- *Pain and collapse or vasovagal attack:* This can be avoided by injecting atropine half-an-hour prior to the procedure.
- *Allergy:* Allergic reaction to the dye can occur.
- Vaginal bleeding.
- Uterine perforation.
- Intravasation of the dye.

## SALINE INFUSION SONOGRAPHY/ SONOSALPINGOGRAPHY

### Introduction

Saline infusion sonography (SIS) or sonosalpingography (SION) test provides a simple and inexpensive method for evaluation of the uterine cavity and for assessing tubal patency. In this test, about 200 mL of physiological saline solution is injected into the uterine cavity via a Foley's catheter. The bulb of the catheter is inflated so that it lies above the internal os, thereby preventing leakage. In case the fallopian tubes are patent, the saline solution flows along the tubes and emerges out at the fimbrial end. The procedure is well-tolerated by patients and can be performed in the OPD. In comparison to HSG, SIS helps in eliminating the risks associated with the use of dye and radiation required by the HSG. SIS helps in diagnosing intracavitary uterine abnormalities and tubal patency.

### Timing

The SIS should be performed during days 6–12 of the menstrual cycle prior to the occurrence of ovulation. Thin uterine endometrium during this phase allows better detection of intrauterine lesions. In addition, this ensures that an undiagnosed pregnancy is not disrupted.

### Indications

- *Confirmation of the tubal patency:* SIS can be performed as a part of investigation for evaluation of cases of infertility. While the SIS can confirm tubal patency, it does not provide information about the contour of the tubes. Thus, if a patient has a history of endometriosis or other tubal disease, laparoscopy is preferred.

- *Cases of DUB:* In these cases, SIS helps in evaluation of endometrium and for diagnosing endometrial polyps.
- *Imaging the uterine cavity:* SIS serves as an alternative to hysteroscopy for evaluation of the uterine cavity. The advantage of SIS over hysteroscopy is that this technique also helps in scanning the ovaries, pelvis and peritoneal cavity, while imaging the uterine cavity.
- *Differentiating between endometrial polyps and submucosal myomas:* SIS helps in differentiating between focal lesions (polyps and submucosal myomas) and global endometrial thickening (Figs 10.4A and B). SIS can be used as a second-line diagnostic procedure in women with AUB when findings from transvaginal ultrasound are nonconclusive.
- Amenorrhea due to Asherman's syndrome.
- *Recurrent pregnancy loss:* Especially those suspected to be due to uterine anomalies.

### Procedure

The procedure of SIS involves the following steps:
- The patient is asked to empty her bladder.
- A speculum is used to expose the cervix, which is cleansed with a betadine swab.
- A catheter is then inserted inside the uterine cavity. Various catheters may be used, including: 5-F urinary catheter, with or without an occlusive balloon; pediatric feeding tubes; insemination catheters, etc.
- It is important to flush the catheter with sterile saline solution before inserting it inside the uterine cavity in order to prevent the introduction of echogenic air bubbles.
- Advancement of the catheter inside the uterine cavity can be assisted by grasping the end of the catheter 2–3 cm from the tip with a ring forceps and gently feeding it through the cervical os so as to position the tip beyond the endocervical canal.
- After correct placement of the catheter, the speculum is carefully removed while the catheter is left in place. Following the correct placement of the catheter, sterile saline solution is instilled inside the uterine cavity. Only about 2–5 mL of sterile solution is required to produce an adequate distention.
- While the sterile saline solution is being instilled inside the uterine cavity, a covered transvaginal probe is inserted into the vagina and continuous scanning in the sagittal and coronal or transverse planes is performed.

### Complications

Saline infusion sonography is associated with minor side effects like pelvic discomfort (cramping or menstrual like pain). Complications like severe pain and infection can occur, but are relatively rare.

There is a theoretical possibility of propulsion of cancer cells from the uterine cavity into the peritoneal cavity. This can be prevented by using low pressure infusion in women at risk for cancer.

## Tests for Ovarian Function

These include the following tests:
- Ferning/cervical mucus change
- Endometrial biopsy

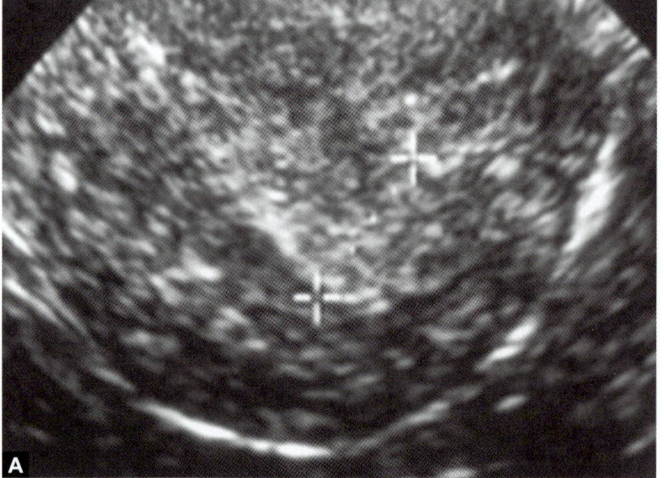

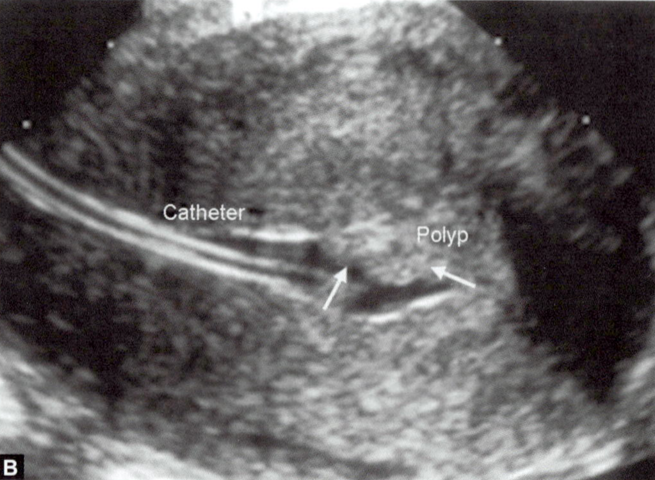


**Figs 10.4A and B:** (A) Presence of thickened endometrium on TVS in a patient with AUB; (B) In the same patient whose TVS has been shown on the right, saline infusion sonography revealed presence of an endometrial polyp

- Basal body temperature.
- Serial ultrasound scans for detection of dominant follicle.
- Serum progesterone levels: Serum progesterone levels greater than 10 ng/mL on the day 21 of the cycles is indicative of ovulation.
- Laparoscopic examination for the visualization of corpus luteum and ovaries.

## ENDOMETRIAL BIOPSY

### Introduction

This test comprises of curetting small pieces of endometrium from the uterine cavity with the help of an endometrial biopsy curette. The endometrial lining constantly changes in response to the various hormones secreted during the different phases of the menstrual cycle. The endometrial biopsy helps in analyzing the histopathological characteristics of endometrium in the various phases of menstrual cycle. During the follicular phase of the menstrual cycle, the endometrium exhibits a proliferative pattern. The growth is stimulated by rising levels of estrogen derived from the dominant ovarian follicle. Progesterone secreted by the corpus luteum causes secretory transformation of the endometrium. The endometrium in anovulatory women is always in the follicular phase.

### Timing

Endometrial biopsy is usually performed 1–2 days prior to the onset of menstruation in case of regular periods or the first day of menses in case of irregular periods.

Pathologists date the endometrium by estimating the number of days that have passed since ovulation. Ovulation can be detected by measuring LH surge or by observing the signs of follicular collapse on ultrasound examination. Agreement between the histological and sampling dates by 2 days is considered as normal. If there is a discrepancy of more than 2 days, the endometrium is considered to be out of phase. This is known as luteal phase deficiency.

Besides evaluating whether the maturity of the secretory endometrium is in phase (i.e. consistent with menstrual cycle date) or out of phase (i.e. luteal phase defect), this test is also an indirect indicator of ovulation (secretory phase). However, this test is not considered as a gold standard investigation for either of these indications because it is associated with several disadvantages such as being invasive, expensive, uncomfortable, inaccurate, etc.

Endometrial biopsy was once considered as the basic element in the evaluation of infertility for establishing the diagnosis of luteal phase. However, this is no longer the situation because endometrial dating cannot guide the clinical management of women with reproductive failure and/or infertility. Therefore, presently this investigation has no place in the diagnostic evaluation of infertility.

Ovulation can be instead monitored by serial ultrasound scanning.

### Indications

- Confirmation of ovulation.
- Endometrial tuberculosis.
- Endometrial hyperplasia.
- Suspected cases of malignancy.

### Procedure

Endometrial biopsy is performed without any prior cervical dilatation and comprises of the following steps:

- Firstly, the patient is placed in the lithotomy position and then a bimanual examination is conducted in order to assess the uterus (size, position, presence of masses, etc.). Cervical os is cleaned with the help of betadine solution.
- A uterine sound is then inserted gently through the cervical os until the sound passes easily to the fundus. The distance from the fundus to the external cervical os can be measured with the help of gradations on the uterine sound and is usually equal to 6–8 cm. This helps in assessing the position and size of the uterine cavity and minimizing the risk of perforation.
- When the position and size of the uterine cavity have been assessed, the EB curette (Chapter 13) is inserted gently inside the uterine cavity until any significant resistance is felt (Fig. 10.5A). The EB curette is a narrow metal cannula having serrated edges with side openings on one end and a syringe can be attached for suction at the other end.
- While inside the uterine cavity, the cannula is rotated several times in order to scrape off the endometrial lining (Figs 10.5B and C).
- This procedure should be repeated at least four times and the device rotated by 360° to ensure adequate coverage of the area.
- The cervix is then visualized with help of a Sims' speculum and a tenaculum (which is applied over the anterior lip of cervix). These endometrial scrapings are then sucked into the syringe.
- When adequate amount of endometrial curettings have been obtained, the curette is removed and samples are sent for microscopic examination.
- One set of sample is sent in normal saline for assessment of acid-fast bacilli (AFB). Other set of sample is sent in acetone for assessment of histopathology. In cases of suspected genital tuberculosis, the endometrium must be subjected to culture. Nowadays, PCR test is preferred for detection of tuberculosis.

### Contraindications

Endometrial biopsy should not be performed in the presence of a normal or ectopic pregnancy.

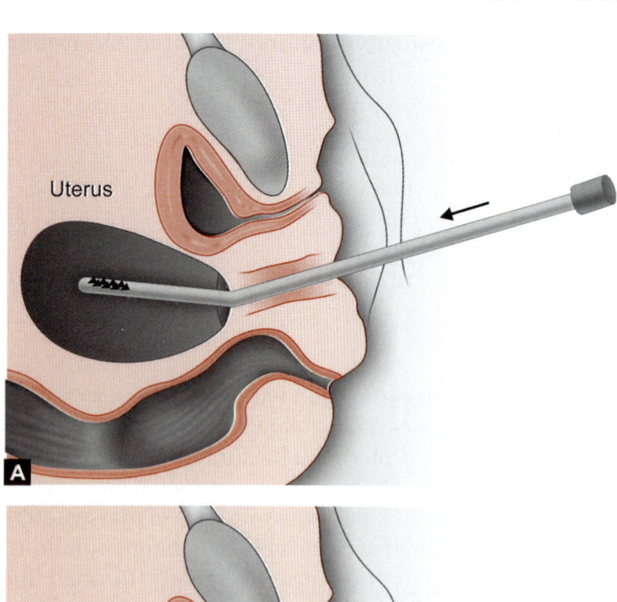



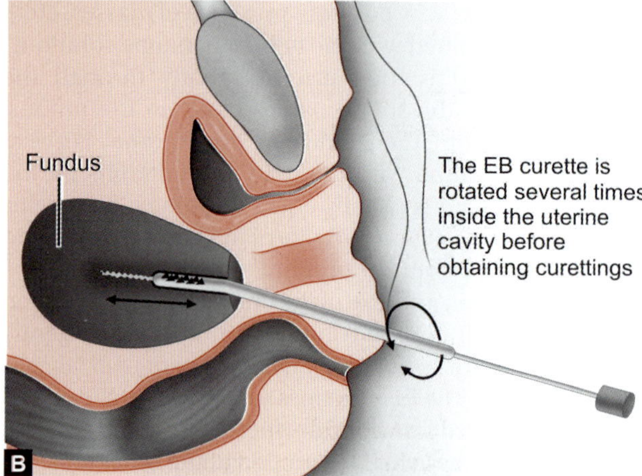



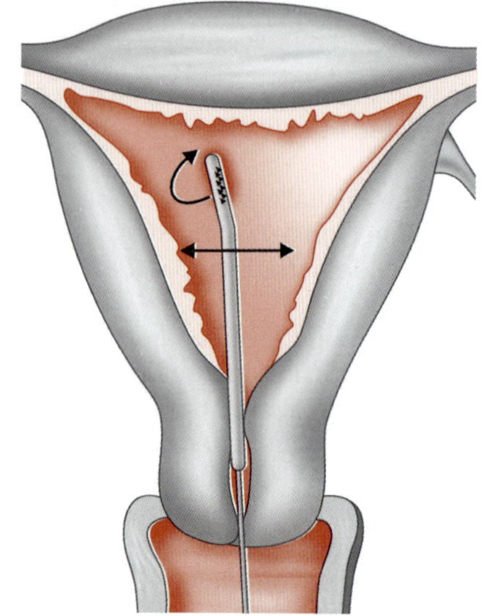



**Figs 10.5A to C:** (A) Placement of the EB curette inside the uterine cavity; (B) Before obtaining the endometrial curettings, the EB curette is rotated several times inside the uterus; (C) Transverse section of endometrial cavity showing the EB curette

## Complications

Though EB is largely a safe procedure, it can be associated with certain complications which are as follows:

- Prolonged bleeding.
- Infection, bacteremia, sepsis and acute bacterial endocarditis.
- Uterine perforation.
- Intraoperative and postoperative cramping.

Bacteremia can occur after endometrial sampling (antibiotic prophylaxis must be given to the patients at risk of endocarditis).

## FERNING

In normal women, at the beginning of the menstrual cycle, cervical mucus is scanty, viscous and very cellular. This mucus does not allow the sperms to pass into the uterine cavity. Mucus secretion from the cervix increases during the midfollicular phase and reaches its maximum approximately 24–48 hours before ovulation. Just prior to ovulation, the mucus becomes thin, watery, alkaline, stretchable, acellular, and elastic in appearance due to increase in the concentration of salt and water in the mucus under the influence of estrogen. In this type of cervical mucus pattern, multiple microchannels are formed so that the spermatozoa can travel through the mucus into the uterine cavity and the mucus also acts as a filter for abnormal spermatozoa and cellular debris present in the semen. Furthermore, during this phase, the mucus assumes a fern-like pattern when allowed to dry on a slide under the microscope and also shows a Spinnbarkeit phenomenon (Figs 10.6A and B). Following ovulation, under the effect of progesterone, the cervical mucus changes its character. During this stage, the mucus becomes opaque, viscid and may become hostile, resistant and impenetrable to sperms (Fig. 10.7). Also during this phase, the ferning pattern and the Spinnbarkeit phenomenon disappears.

## BASAL BODY TEMPERATURE METHOD

Basal body temperature (BBT) charts can be used for predicting ovulation. In this method, the woman is asked to measure her oral temperature with an oral glass or mercury thermometer, the first thing when she wakes up in the morning or after at least 3 hours of uninterrupted sleep. She should measure her temperature throughout the entire duration of her menstrual cycle for at least three menstrual cycles. The temperatures are then plotted on a graph paper.

Basal body temperature varies between 97.0°F and 98.0°F during the follicular phase of the cycle and rises by 0.4–0.8°F over the average preovulatory temperature during the luteal phase. The thermogenic shift in BBT occurs when serum progesterone levels rise above 5 ng/mL, usually occurring for up to 4 days following ovulation. In a normal ovulating woman, there occurs a rise in body temperature by 0.5–1.0°F immediately following ovulation under the thermogenic effect of progesterone (Fig. 10.8). This increase in temperature remains sustained throughout the luteal phase. The temperature again falls to baseline just before or after the onset of menses. This biphasic pattern is evident in ovulatory women. Besides providing an evidence for ovulation, BBT recording can also help in determining the approximate time of ovulation. BBT recording can also reveal an abnormally long follicular phase or a short luteal phase. Treatment of these may help in improving fertility. Though an easy, noninvasive and cost-effective procedure, taking the temperature daily can become cumbersome. BBT serves as a useful method for couples who are reluctant or unable to pursue more formal and costly evaluations.

# Cytologic Screening: Pap Smear

## Introduction

Nowadays, cytological screening in the form of Pap smear has become the investigation of choice for detection of precancerous lesions of the cervix. The widespread introduction of the Pap test for cervical cancer screening has resulted in significantly reducing the incidence and mortality of cervical cancer in developed countries. Presence of

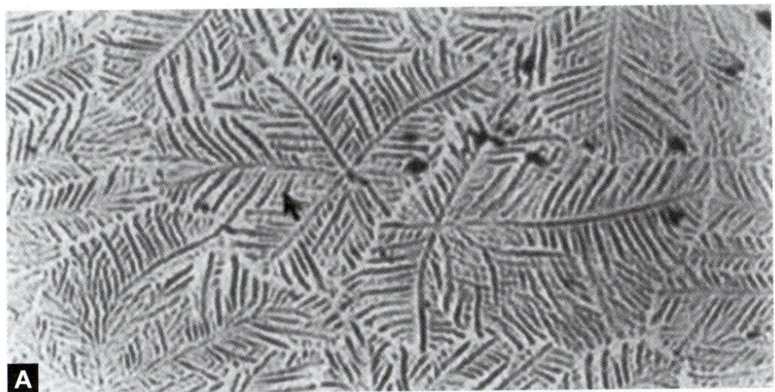

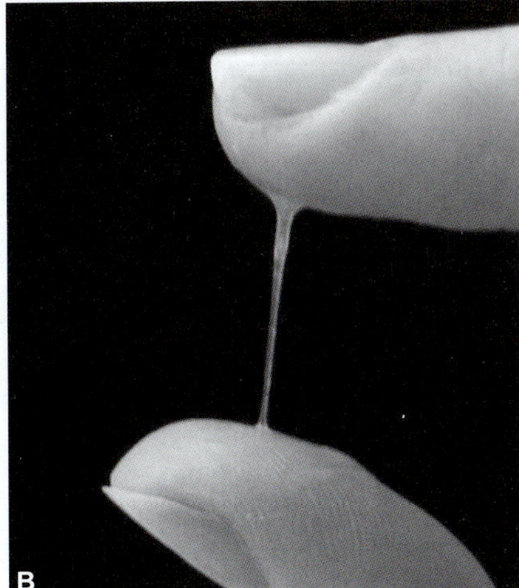

**Figs 10.6A and B:** Estrogen-dominant cervical mucus: (A) Ferning pattern; (B) Spinnbarkeit test

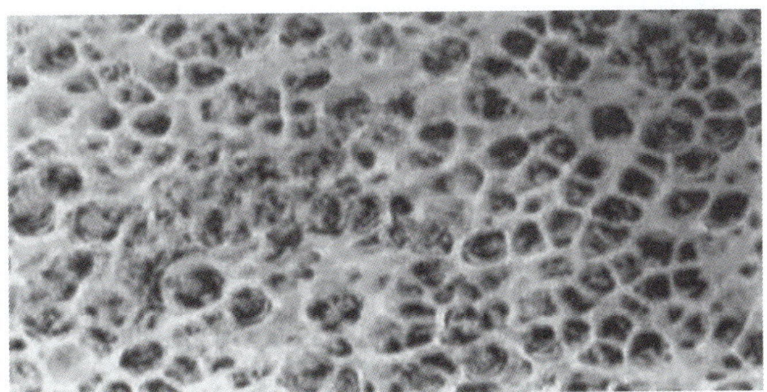

**Fig. 10.7:** Progesterone dominant cervical mucus

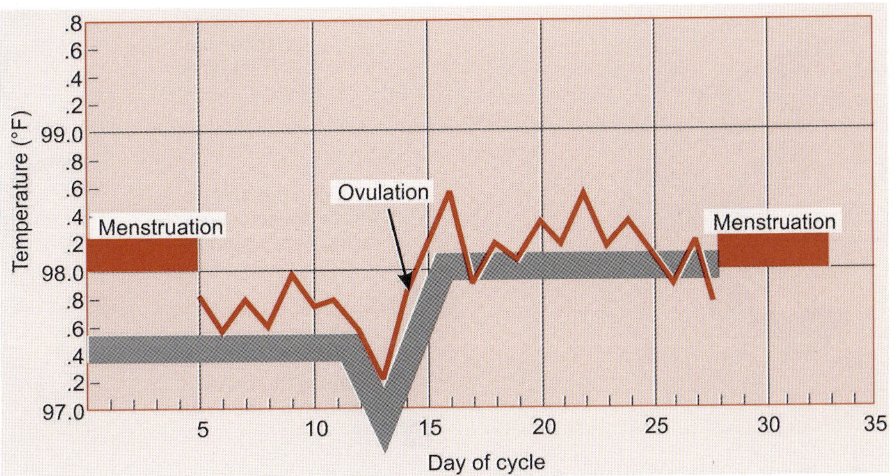


**Fig. 10.8:** Basal body temperature method

abnormal results on Pap test or symptoms of cervical cancer may mandate further testing in the form of colposcopy, colposcopic-directed biopsy and endocervical curettage, which can help in confirming if abnormal cells are dysplastic or cancerous.

Since Pap smear is associated with a negative reporting rate of 30%, it is important to repeat Pap smear annually for three consecutive years. If still, the Pap smear continues to remain negative, it should be repeated at 3–5 yearly intervals up to the age of 65 years. After the age of 65 years, Pap smear is not required, because the incidence of CIN drops to 1%.

### Prerequisites before Taking a Pap Smear

- No vaginal douching should be done 48 hours prior to the test.
- Vaginal creams should not be used for 1 week before the test.
- There should be abstinence from sexual intercourse 24 hours prior to the test.

### Procedure

- Figure 10.9 shows the Pap smear kit, while Figures 10.10A and B demonstrate the procedure for taking a Pap smear. The patient is made to lie in a dorsal position and adequate light must be used to visualize the cervix and vagina properly.
- A Cusco's speculum must be used to expose the cervix.
- No lubricant should be used on the Cusco's speculum.
- After exposing the cervix, an endocervical brush or cotton tipped swab must be placed inside the endocervix and rotated firmly against the canal in order to take an endocervical sample, which is then placed on the glass slide.

- Next, the Ayre's spatula must be placed against the cervix with the longer protrusion in the cervical canal.
- The spatula must be rotated clockwise for 360° against the cervix. This would help in scraping the entire transformation zone.
- If it appears that the entire transformation zone has not been adequately sampled, the spatula must be rotated several times.
- The sample from the spatula is placed onto the glass slide by rotating the spatula against the slide in a clockwise manner.
- The slide must be immediately fixed with the help of a spray fixative, which is held at a distance of about 9–12 inches.

### Qualities of a Good Smear

The smear should be thick enough, but not transparent. Too thin smear may result in formation of artifacts upon drying.

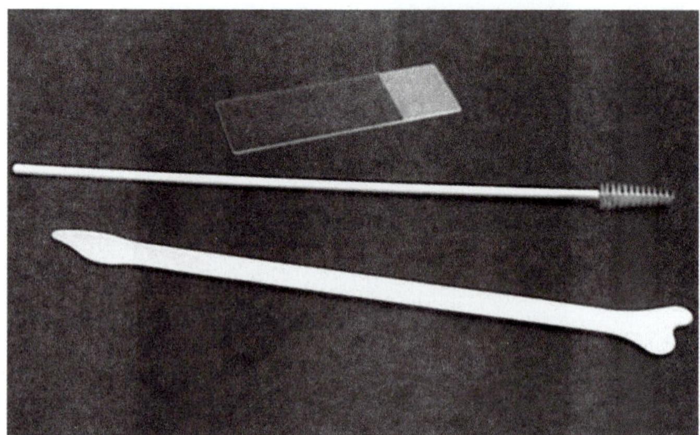

**Fig. 10.9:** Pap smear kit

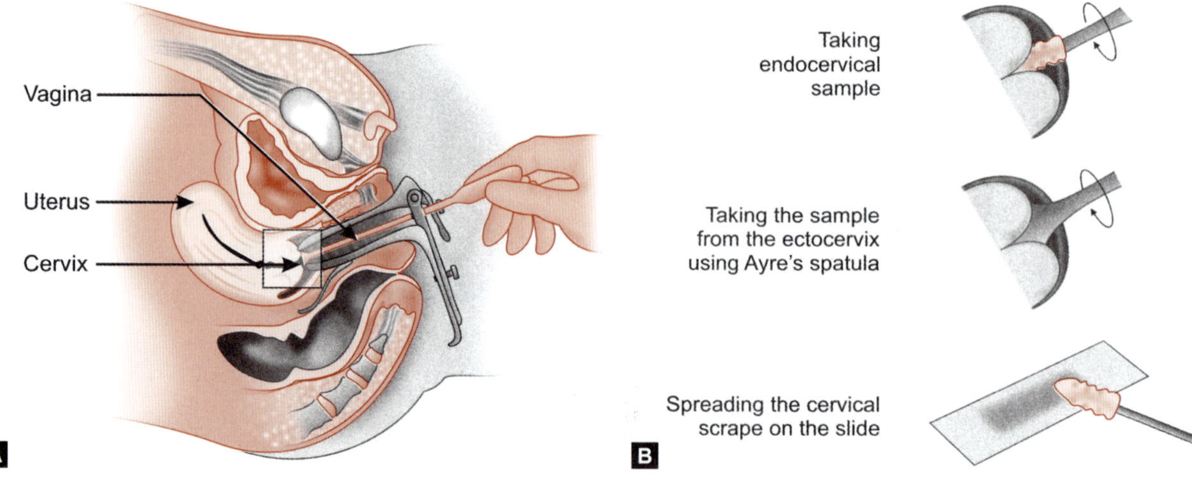


**Figs 10.10A and B:** (A) Placing the Cusko's speculum in the cervix; (B) Taking a Pap smear

Also, a thin smear might contain too few cells, which might not allow adequate sampling. On the other hand, if the smear is too thick, the Papanicolaou stain will not penetrate.

## Frequency of Doing Pap Smear

The recommendations for Pap smear testing as described by the American Cancer Society, American Society for Colposcopy and Cervical Pathology, and American Society for Clinical Pathology, which have been introduced in 2012 are summarized in Table 10.1.

## Types of Cell Changes in Pap Smear

According to the WHO, cervical dysplasia has been categorized into mild, moderate or severe and a separate category called "carcinoma in situ" (CIS). The term "cervical intraepithelial neoplasia" was introduced by Richart (1968). CIN 1 represents mild to moderate dysplasia; CIN 2 is an intermediate grade and CIN 3, severe dysplasia or CIS. However, according to the most recent classification that is the Bethesda System, all cervical epithelial precursor lesions have been divided into two groups: LSIL and HSIL. LSIL corresponds to CIN 1 and HSIL includes CIN 2 and CIN 3.

## Risks Associated with Pap Smear

The risks of cervical cancer screening include the occurrence of false-negative as well as false-positive test results. False-negative test results imply that screening test results may appear to be normal even though cervical cancer is present. This may delay the patient from seeking medical care even if she has symptoms suggestive of cancer. False-positive test results occur when screening test results appear to be abnormal even though no cancer is present. This can cause unnecessary patient anxiety. A false-positive test may be followed by more invasive tests and procedures such as colposcopy, cryotherapy or LEEP, which are associated with their own risks. Also, the long-term effects of these procedures on fertility and pregnancy are not known.

## Liquid-Based Cytology in Cervical Screening

Liquid-based cytology is a new way of sampling and preparing cervical cells (Fig. 10.11). While the conventional "Pap smear" involves direct preparation of the slide from the cervical scrape obtained, the procedure of "ThinPrep" involves making a suspension of cells from the sample, which is then used to produce a thin layer of cells on a slide. In this technique, the sample is taken using a plastic spatula, which could either be an endocervical brush or a cervical broom, also known as the cervex. Using this technique, the cells collected from the cervix are placed in a preservative fluid, which is then sent to the laboratory rather than being directly spread onto a slide. At the laboratory, the sample is treated to remove unwanted material (blood, mucus and inflammatory material) and then a thin layer of the cell suspension is placed on the slide for inspection.

Though this method was thought to offer several advantages over the conventional Pap smear, according to the latest recommendations by the "Screening for cervical cancer: US Preventive Services Task Force" (2012), liquid-based

**Table 10.1:** Latest screening guidelines for the prevention and early detection of cervical cancer

| Population | Recommended Screening Method | Comments |
|---|---|---|
| Aged less than 21 years | No screening | |
| Aged 21–29 years | Cytology alone every 3 years | |
| Aged 30–65 years | *Preferred screening method*: HPV and cytology co-testing every 5 years. In case of nonavailability of HPV testing, cytology alone is indicated every 3 years | Screening by HPV testing alone is not recommended |
| Aged more than 65 years | No screening is necessary after adequate negative prior screening results | Routine age-based screening must be continued for at least 20 years in women with a history of CIN 2, CIN 3 or adenocarcinoma in situ |
| After total hysterectomy | No screening is necessary in women without a history of CIN 2, CIN 3, adenocarcinoma in situ, or cancer in the past 20 years | |
| After HPV vaccination | The same age-specific recommendations as unvaccinated women need to be followed in these cases | |

*Abbreviations:* CIN, cervical intraepithelial neoplasia; HPV, human papillomavirus
*Source:* Saslow D, Solomon D, Lawson HW, Killackey M, Kulasingam SL, Cain J, et al. American Cancer Society, American Society for Colposcopy and Cervical Pathology, and American Society for Clinical Pathology screening guidelines for the prevention and early detection of cervical cancer. CA Cancer J Clin. 2012;62(3):147-72.

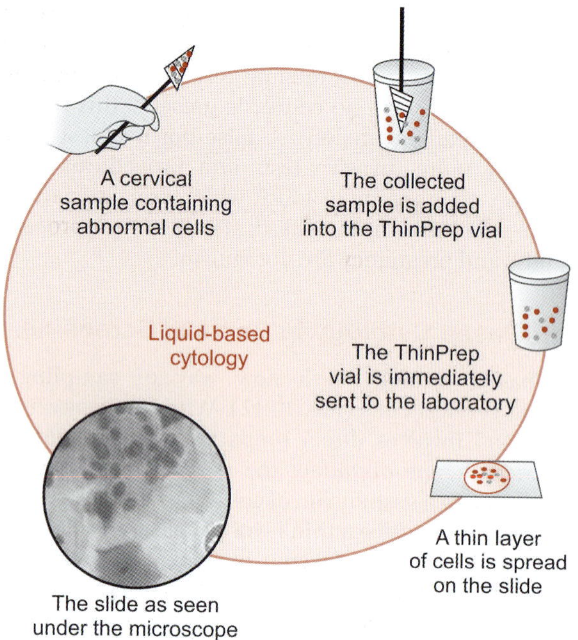



**Fig. 10.11:** Liquid-based cytology

testing has not been shown to significantly improve the accuracy of testing in comparison to the conventional cytology testing using a Pap smear.

# Colposcopy

## Introduction

If abnormal cells are found in a smear test or liquid-based cytology, the patient may be referred for a colposcopic examination and/or a colposcopic-directed biopsy. While the Pap smear detects abnormal cells, colposcopy helps in locating the abnormal lesions. A colposcope is like a small microscope with a light and enables the clinician to perform a thorough examination of the cervix. Colposcopy is an office-based procedure during which the cervix is examined under illumination and magnification before and after application of dilute acetic acid and Lugol's iodine. The characteristic features of malignancy and premalignancy on colposcopic examination include changes such as acetowhite areas, abnormal vascular patterns, mosaic pattern, punctation and failure to uptake iodine stain. Endocervical sampling may accompany colposcopy, particularly in nonpregnant women where the cytology shows atypical glandular cells or adenocarcinoma in situ. Satisfactory colposcopy requires visualization of the entire squamocolumnar junction and transformation zone for the presence of any visible lesions. Both a regular white light and a green light are used during colposcopy. The green filter enhances visualization of blood

vessels by making them appear darker in contrast to the surrounding epithelium.

## Indications

The indications for colposcopy are as follows:
- Epithelial cell abnormalities as detected on cervical cytology
- Presence of high-risk human papillomavirus DNA
- Suspicious cervical lesions
- History of in utero diethylstilbestrol exposure
- Sexual partners of patients with genital tract neoplasia
- Vulval and vaginal intraepithelial neoplasia
- Unexplained vaginal bleeding/postcoital bleeding
- Positive screening test by cervicography/spectroscopy.

## Advantages

The colposcopic examination helps in the following:
- When abnormal cells have been detected on the Pap smear, location and extent of abnormal lesions on the cervix can be assessed with the help of colposcopy.
- Biopsy can be taken from the areas of abnormality.
- Conservative surgery (e.g. conization) can be performed under colposcopic guidance.
- Colposcopic examination can also be performed during follow-up examination of cases that have undergone conservative therapy.

## Procedure

- The patient is placed in the lithotomy position.
- Under all aseptic precautions, a speculum is inserted inside the vagina.
- The colposcope is brought into the position. The perineum, vulva, vagina and cervix must be examined for presence of lesions using the colposcope's white light and then green light.
- The entire cervix must be viewed both under the low- and high-power magnification. Higher-power magnification helps in visualization of small details and features.
- Cervix is visualized after the application of both dilute 5% acetic acid and Lugol's iodine in order to enhance any abnormal epithelial findings. Both acetic acid and Lugol's iodine are applied onto the cervix with the help of a cotton swab and allowed to remain there for at least 30 seconds.
- Under white light, the cervix is visualized for acetowhite changes. The location of the squamocolumnar junction, transformation zone, abnormal and atypical vessels and areas of acetowhite changes are recorded. On application of Lugol's iodine, the areas of abnormalities, such as those with squamous metaplasia, leukoplakia as well as neoplastic tissue do not take up iodine stain and become yellowish in appearance, whereas the normal

glycogen-containing cervical cells turn deep brown. A scoring system such as "the Reid's Colposcopic Index" may be used to help the colposcopist in classifying the colposcopic appearance.
- The cervix is reexamined under the green light, which helps in accentuating the margins of the acetowhite areas and in identifying the abnormal blood vessels.

### Colposcopic-Directed Punch Biopsy

Following identification of the biopsy site, the cervical punch biopsy forceps are used to obtain the specimen under colposcopic visualization. Specimens are firstly obtained from the most inferior aspect of the cervix to avoid bleeding from the biopsy site and obscuring other biopsy sites. Monsel's paste or silver nitrate can be used to achieve hemostasis after cervical punch biopsy.

# Dilatation and Curettage

## Introduction

Some surgeons may choose to perform dilatation and curettage (D&C) as the initial procedure in women presenting with AUB. This may include the women who cannot tolerate an office biopsy, those with heavy bleeding (D&C serves as both a therapeutic and diagnostic procedure in these cases) and women who are at a high risk of developing endometrial cancer (e.g. those with Lynch syndrome). Women having insufficient endometrial cells with EB may undergo repeat sampling with an office biopsy or may undergo D&C. Evaluation with D&C may be required in case of persistent or recurrent bleeding, even after office EB reveals benign findings. D&C helps in an extensive sampling of the uterine cavity and has the advantage of being both a diagnostic and a therapeutic procedure.

## Indications

### Routine Indications

Indications for D&C are as follows:
- When an adequate sample cannot be obtained on EB.
- Cervical os is stenotic.
- Medical treatment fails to control severe bleeding.
- Persistent or recurrent bleeding between 20 years and 40 years of age and the clinical suspicion of malignancy is high.
- Diagnosis of endometrial polyps, intrauterine mucous fibroids, areas of endometritis, hyperplasia or cancer or lost IUDs.
- Bleeding recurs following a negative report on endometrial biopsy/aspiration.

### Diagnostic Indications

- Detection of ovulation in case of primary and secondary infertility.
- Diagnosis of tubercular endometritis.
- Diagnosis of endometrial hyperplasia or carcinoma: Not only does D&C help in detecting the site of malignancy, but also gives an idea regarding the spread of malignancy. The sample obtained on D&C is larger than the one obtained by an EB.
- Diagnosis of DUB.
- Diagnosis of causes of primary or secondary amenorrhea.
- Diagnosis of AUB.

### Therapeutic Indications

- Excision of endometrial polyps.
- Excision of intrauterine synecheiae.
- Dysfunctional uterine bleeding (To arrest excessive bleeding; D&C may be therapeutic in nearly 50% cases).
- Removal of IUCD embedded inside the uterine cavity.

## Contraindications

- Suspected cases of pregnancy
- Lower genital tract infection
- Pelvic inflammatory disease.

## Timing of the Procedure

- When D&C is performed for the detection of ovulation, it must be performed in the premenstrual phase (5–7 days prior to the menses).
- When D&C is performed for arresting hemorrhage, it must be done during the episode of bleeding.

## Procedure

The procedure of D&C involves obtaining scrapings from the endometrium and the cervix and is usually performed under general anesthesia.

### Preprocedural Preparation

This comprises of the following steps:
- Patient is placed in lithotomy position.
- The part is cleaned and draped, following which a vaginal examination is performed.
- The procedure is performed observing strict aseptic precautions.
- External os is swabbed with antiseptic solution.

### Steps of Actual Procedure

- Uterine sound is passed in order to measure the uterocervical length.

- This procedure involves the gradual dilatation of the cervix to less than 8 cm under general anesthesia.
- This is followed up by the use of small sharp curette for systematic, thorough, gentle sampling of all parts of the uterine cavity in a systematic manner (anterior wall, right lateral wall, posterior wall, left lateral wall and fundus. In suspected cases of tuberculosis, special care is taken to curette out the cornual regions.

### Disadvantages

The main disadvantages associated with the procedure are as follows:
- Small lesions can be missed
- It is associated with a low sensitivity rate (65%) for detection of intrauterine pathology.

### Complications

Complications of D&C are as follows:
- Uterine perforation.
- Cervical damage due to use of large dilators, resulting in the development of cervical incompetence in future.
- Postoperative infection or intrauterine adhesions.

### Advantages

Advantages of D&C are as follows:
- Diagnosis of organic disease, e.g. tuberculosis.
- Diagnosis of uterine pathology, e.g. endometritis, polyp, carcinoma, fibroids, etc.
- Diagnosing the type of endometrial histopathology: hyperplastic, proliferative, secretory, irregular ripening, irregular shedding, atrophic endometrium, etc.
- Therapeutic effect (controversial).
- Arrest of severe or persistent bleeding, particularly that associated with hyperplastic endometrium.

### FRACTIONAL CURETTAGE

This method involves histological study of the endocervical scrapings before dilating the cervix followed by cervical D&C from the uterine isthmus, body of the uterus and fundus separately so that the extent of endometrial lesion (especially malignancy) can be evaluated. Nowadays, two samples are sent for histopathological analysis: endocervical and endometrial samples. Previously, six samples were obtained: endocervical canal, each of the four uterine walls and fundus.

## Endometrial Aspiration

### Introduction

Endometrial aspiration or aspiration cytology from the uterine cavity is effective in screening women who may be at a high risk for the development of endometrial cancer. Endometrial aspiration can be done as an outpatient procedure without anesthesia. It can be done with the help of devices like, Pipelle curette, Sharman curette, Gravlee jet washer, Isaacs cell® sampler, Vabra® aspirator, etc. The diagnostic accuracy of this procedure is 92–98% when compared with subsequent D&C. Endometrial aspiration is often combined with endocervical curettage to rule out cervical pathology.

### Procedure

*Preprocedure preparation:* This comprises of the following steps:
- The patient should be nil orally
- The bladder must be emptied
- Patient must be put in a lithotomy position
- Per vaginal examination is done for assessing uterine size and direction.

### Actual Procedure

- A Sims' or Cusco's speculum is inserted to retract the posterior vaginal wall.
- Anterior lip of the cervix is held with a vulsellum or a tenaculum.
- A uterine sound is inserted to measure the uterocervical length.
- A Pipelle® catheter is inserted inside the uterine cavity (Figs 10.12A and B).
- The endometrial tissue is obtained by suction through the syringe attached to the Pipelle® catheter.
- The tissue is sent for histopathological examination and microbiology for acid fast bacillus culture.

### Postprocedural Advice

- Antibiotics
- Painkillers
- Rest for 24–48 hours.

### Complications

Complications can rarely occur and include perforation, hemorrhage and infection.

## Female Sterilization

### Introduction

In today's time, surgical sterilization for both men and women has become a popular and well-established method of contraception.

Tubal sterilization is a method of permanent sterilization, which causes sterility by blocking a woman's fallopian tubes. As a result of the blockage of tubes, the sperm and ovum cannot fertilize each other, thereby preventing the occurrence

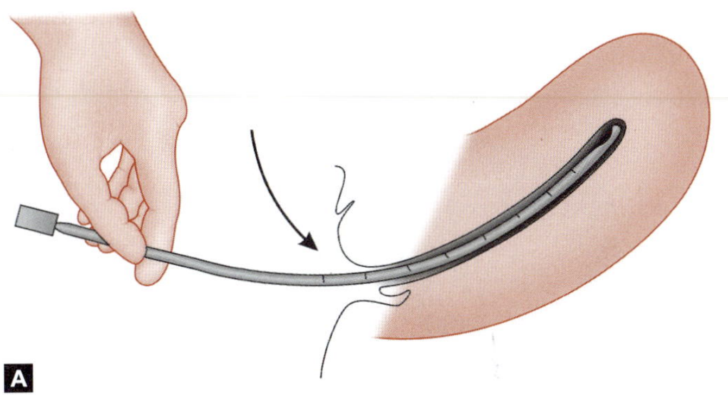 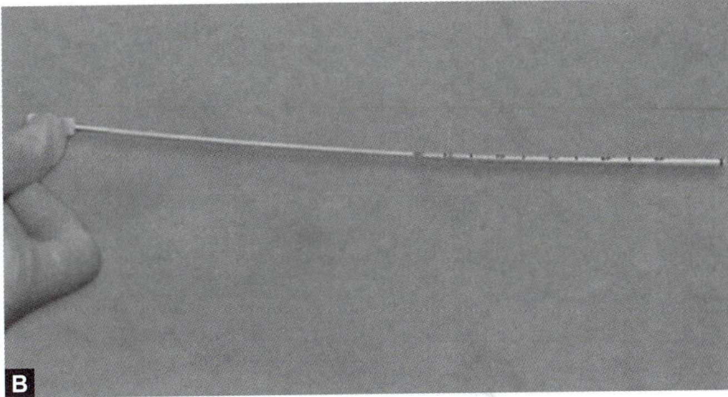

**Figs 10.12A and B:** (A) Diagram showing endometrial aspiration; (B) Pipelle® endometrial sampler for doing endometrial aspiration.

of pregnancy. Tubal sterilization is a surgical procedure involving occlusion of the tubes.

This can be achieved either by resection of a tubal segment or blocking the fallopian tube using rings or clips. This can be achieved by any of the following three routes: abdominal tubectomy, vaginal tubectomy or laparoscopic sterilization.

## Indications

Tubal sterilization is indicated for women, who want a permanent method of contraception and are free of any gynecologic pathology that would otherwise dictate an alternative procedure. Tubal sterilization is also indicated for women, in whom pregnancy could represent a significant clinical and medical risk.

## Surgery

### Preoperative Preparation

- A preoperative workup comprises of adequate history taking, general physical examination, urine analysis and hematocrit with a complete blood count.
- *Preoperative counseling:* Counseling is essential prior to the procedure. Patients, especially those who are young, require preoperative patient counseling. Myths and misinformation related to the procedure need to be removed. The risk of surgery failure and ectopic pregnancy needs to be explained to the patient. Tubal ligation is not a temporary method of contraception and must be considered as an irreversible procedure.
- *Written and informed consent:* After adequate counseling of the patient, written and informed consent is essential.
- *Confirming that the patient is nonpregnant:* This is usually done by performing a urine β-hCG test. Under normal circumstances, the test usually becomes positive approximately 1 week after conception. The test can detect hCG levels as low as 20 mIU/mL. The test should be ideally performed on the day of surgery. The procedure of sterilization should preferably be done in the first few

days of the menstrual cycle to be totally sure that the patient is not pregnant.
- *Anesthesia:* Majority of tubal ligation procedures are performed using general, local or regional anesthesia.

### Actual Steps of Surgery

*Incision:* In puerperal cases, where the uterus is felt per abdomen, the incision is made approximately 1 inch below the fundus. In interval ligations, the incision is made two finger breadths above the pubic symphysis. This incision could be midline, paramedian or transverse.

*Delivery of the tubes:* In case of laparotomy or minilaparotomy, the index finger is introduced through the incision and is passed across the posterior surface of the uterus and then to the posterior leaf of the broad ligament from where the tube is hooked out. The tube is identified by the fimbrial end and the mesosalpinx containing uteroovarian anastamosing vessels.

*Tubal ligation:* Tubal ligation is then performed by one of the techniques described next:
- *Pomeroy's technique:* Only Pomeroy's technique has been described in detail because this is the most commonly used technique in clinical practice.
- Modified Pomeroy's
- Parkland
- Uchida
- Fimbriectomy
- Madlener's technique.

*Pomeroy's technique:* This technique involves the following steps (Figs 10.13A to D):
- The mid portion of the oviduct is grasped with a Babcock clamp, creating a loop, which is tied with no. 1 plain catgut or no. 0 chromic catgut sutures.
- Segment of the tube having a length of about 1.2–1.5 cm, distal to the ligature is excised.
- The surgeon must then inspect the segment of the loop that has been removed to ensure that the wall has not been partially resected.

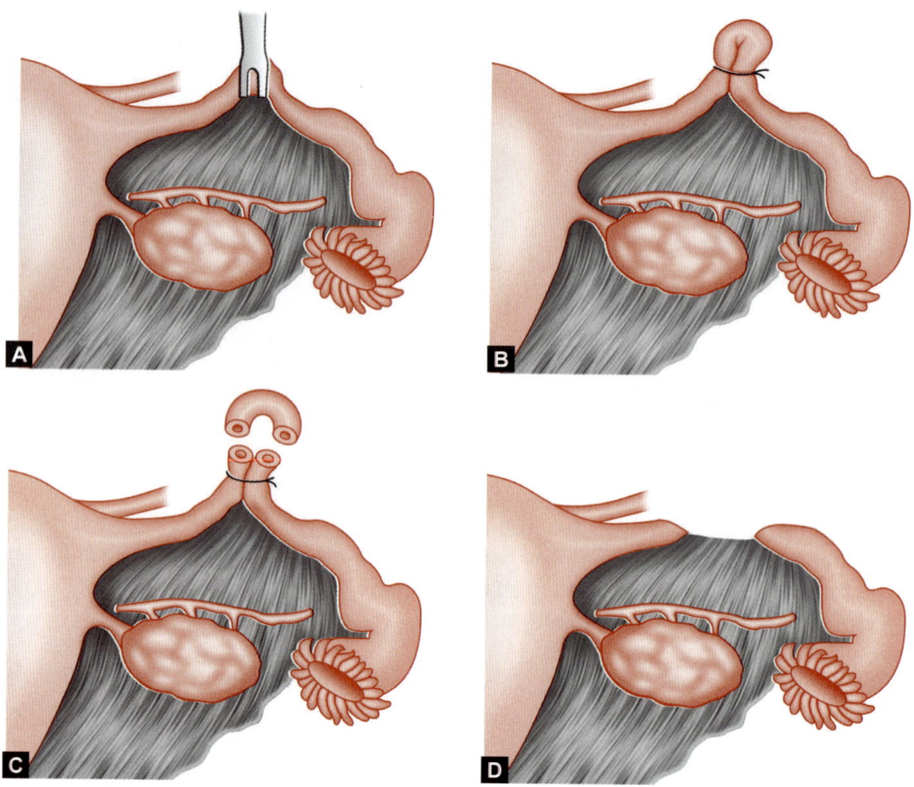

**Figs 10.13A to D:** Pomeroy's technique of tubal sterilization. (A) The fallopian tube is grasped with Babcock clamp; (B) A loop is created, which is tied with no. 1 plain catgut sutures; (C) Excision of the loop; (D) Several months later, the ends of the tube get fibrosed, retracting from one another

- The same procedure is then repeated on the other side.
- Specimens are then submitted for histopathological examination.
- The rationale for this technique is based on the principle that over a period of time, the cut ends of the tube become independently sealed off, thereby retracting from one another. This occurs due to prompt absorption of the suture ligature with subsequent separation of the cut ends of the tube, which then become sealed by spontaneous reperitonealization and fibrosis. This technique is highly successful and the failure rate varies between 0.1 to 0.5%.

*Modified Pomeroy's technique:* Many modifications of the Pomeroy's technique have been described. These modifications aim at reducing the failure rate associated with Pomeroy's technique. The most commonly performed modification involves doubly ligating each loop.

### Timing of Tubal Ligation

*Tubal sterilization following normal vaginal delivery:* Tubal sterilization following completion of a vaginal delivery is usually performed 24–48 hours after delivery. The optimal time of surgery is within 6 hours. Nevertheless, it must be performed within 48 hours. The main advantage of choosing this timing is that at this point of time the surgery is technically simple, because the uterine fundus is at the level of umbilicus. As a result, the fallopian tubes are readily accessible through a small periumbilical abdominal incision. Moreover, if the surgery is performed during this period, postoperative and postpartum convalescence periods would coincide, so hospitalization is minimally increased. In comparison with interval sterilization, subumbilical minilaparotomy, following delivery in the early puerperium is convenient, simple and cost-effective. However, if maternal or infant complications exist, sterilization should be delayed.

*Tubal sterilization following cesarean delivery:* Bilateral tube ligation may be performed after closure of the uterine incision during cesarean delivery.

*Interval ligation:* The operation can be performed beyond 6 weeks following delivery or abortion. Ideal time for undertaking surgery is the postmenstrual phase during the early proliferative phase.

*Postabortal ligation:* Sterilization can be performed along with the medical termination of pregnancy or even following spontaneous abortion under antibiotic coverage, provided anemia and infection have been ruled out.

### Types of Surgical Approaches

*Minilaparotomy:* As the name suggests, minilaparotomy involves giving a small incision about half to three-fourths inches in size. The size of the incision is usually smaller than 5 cm and is usually given in the suprapubic area. The procedure is usually performed under local anesthesia with sedation. The operation can be performed either as an interval procedure, few months after delivery or within the first 48 hours after delivery. It consists of the following steps:

- After giving the incision, the skin is stretched with the help of Allis forceps.
- Dissection is carried down up to the level of the fascia, which is opened transversely.
- The peritoneum is exposed, which can be entered sharply.
- Once the uterus is visualized, it is manipulated and retracted, in order to visualize the fallopian tubes, which are then grasped with a Babcock clamp.
- The position of Babcock clamps is progressively shifted, until the fimbriated end can be identified. This step is important because it helps in differentiating the fallopian tube from round ligament. One of the major causes of failure of sterilization is the inadvertent ligation of the round ligament, which is mistakenly identified as the fallopian tube.
- After performing tubal ligation on both sides, the minilaparotomy incision is closed in layers. The various methods of tubal ligation have previously been described. In our setup, the Pomeroy's technique of tubal ligation is most commonly used.
- Patient is usually discharged within 24–48 hours of surgery.

*Laparoscopy:* Tubal ligation using laparoscopic approach has been practiced since 1970s. Presently, it has become the most commonly used approach for tubal ligation. The major advantage of laparoscopic sterilization procedure is that it is a minimally invasive technique, involves use of small incision, reduced duration of hospital stay, rapid recovery and the ability to inspect the pelvis and upper abdomen at the time of surgery. However, the major disadvantage of the procedure is the complications associated with general anesthesia and those associated with laparoscopic surgery (risks of injury to vessel/viscera with needle insufflation/trocar entry, etc.).

Laparoscopic tubal ligation can be carried out using techniques, such as electrodessication of tubes using electrosurgery or mechanical blockage of tubes using Falope rings or Filshie clips. In our setup, the most commonly employed technique for tubal ligation under laparoscopic approach is the use of Falope rings.

### Postoperative Care

The postoperative care comprises of the following steps:

- A discharge card containing detailed notes and postoperative findings and dates for follow-up visit must be given to each patient at the time of discharge.
- After undergoing tubal sterilization, the patient must be instructed to come for a follow-up visit at 1–2 weeks postoperatively. This visit should involve examination of the surgical site and removal of nonabsorbable sutures.
- The patient should be instructed to report immediately in case of any missed period, in order to rule out the possibility of pregnancy.
- All women who have undergone sterilization must be explained in details, regarding the signs and symptoms of intrauterine as well as ectopic pregnancy and instructed to seek immediate medical attention, if such signs and symptoms occur.
- The woman must also be instructed to notify her healthcare provider, in case she develops fever (38°C or 100.4°F), increasing or persistent abdominal pain, or bleeding, or purulent discharge from the incision site.

## Complications

The procedure of tubal sterilization may be associated with certain complications, such as:

- *Effects of anesthesia:* Though the procedure is usually performed under local anesthesia, sometimes the procedure may also be performed under general anesthesia. In these cases, the woman is at risk of complications inherent to general anesthesia.
- *Pain:* After undergoing laparoscopic sterilization, the woman may experience some degree of chest and shoulder pain due to pneumoperitoneum, which has been created prior to the insertion of trocar. Mild analgesics are usually sufficient to control this pain.
- *Bleeding and/or infection:* The laparoscopic procedure may be associated with complications such as infection and bleeding. The procedure of minilaparotomy can be associated with complications, such as wound infections, hematoma and severe infection, such as pelvic inflammatory diseases. However, with the observation of strict asepsis the chances of infection are highly reduced. Therefore, the use of prophylactic antibiotics prior to the procedure is usually not recommended.
- *Injury to the body organs:* There is a risk of causing injury to the body organs such as gastrointestinal and genitourinary tract and major vessels, especially when the procedure is performed under laparoscopic guidance.
- *Failure of the procedure:* Although sterilization is highly effective and considered the definitive form of pregnancy prevention, it has a failure rate of 0.1–0.8% during the first

year. At least one-third of these are ectopic pregnancies. Causes of failure of the procedure may be as follows:

- Conception had occurred prior to the procedure of ligation.
- *Misidentification of the oviduct:* This could be in the form of ligation of the round ligament instead of the oviduct.
- *Incomplete occlusion of the fallopian tubes:* This could be in the form of improperly placed Falope rings.

- *Ectopic pregnancy:* The failure of the procedure of tubal sterilization is associated with high likelihood of ectopic pregnancy, in comparison to the intrauterine pregnancy.
- *Mortality:* The risk of death from tubal sterilization is 1–2 cases per 100,000 procedures; most of these are due to complications of general anesthesia. The most common cause of death during laparoscopic bilateral tubal ligation appears to be hypoventilation related to anesthesia. Cardiopulmonary arrest and hypoventilation are reported as the leading cause of death in most cases.
- *Unintended laparotomy:* Unintended laparotomy occurs with 1–2% of laparoscopic procedures; most of these conversions can be attributed to the technical inability to complete the laparoscopic procedure.
- *Patient regret:* Sterilization is intended to be permanent, but patient regret can commonly occur. Poststerilization regret is a complex condition often caused by unpredictable life events.
- *Post-tubal ligation syndrome:* Proposed in 1951, this syndrome is a constellation of symptoms, including pelvic discomfort, ovarian cystic changes and menorrhagia. These are likely to occur as a result of disruption of the utero ovarian blood supply, with resultant disturbances of ovulatory function after bilateral tubal ligation.

# Three Swab Test

## Introduction

Three-swab test is done for diagnosing the location of fistula in cases where there is leakage of urine from the vagina. Different types of vaginal fistulae, which can occur, include, urethrovaginal fistula, vesicovaginal fistula and ureterovaginal fistula.

## Procedure

- The vaginal cavity is packed with three sterile swabs: one high up in the posterior fornix, one in the center and one near the vaginal introitus.
- A catheter is introduced into the bladder through the urethra.
- Approximately, 50–100 mL of methylene blue dye is injected into the bladder via the catheter.
- The patient is asked to walk around for about half-an-hour.

- The swabs are then removed one-by-one and examined.
- If the lowermost swab gets stained, the leakage is from urethra. Staining of the middle swab points towards a vesicovaginal fistula. If none of the swabs get stained, but the upper-most swab gets wet from urine, leakage is probably from the ureter, pointing towards a ureterovaginal fistula.

### Advantages

This is a simple, nonexpensive and a noninvasive test for diagnosing the location of fistula. Minimal complications are likely to occur with this test.

# Test for Cervical Factor Infertility

## Postcoital Test

### Introduction

Postcoital test (PCT; Sims' or Huhner's test) aims at identifying the cervical factor infertility by testing the characteristics of the cervical mucus and sperm-mucus interaction. This test also gives an indirect evidence of any abnormalities in the sperms, especially in cases where a semen sample cannot be made available otherwise. The male factor infertility is analyzed by studying the sperm count, analyzing the sperm mobility, and detecting the presence of pus cells or antisperm antibodies. The most common cause for a "negative" PCT is improper timing. While of historical interest, this test is no longer routinely performed in the standard infertility workup because it has been found to be associated with poor predictive value. Furthermore, infertility due to cervical factors can be easily overcome by performing intrauterine inseminations.

### Procedure

- The couple is advised to have intercourse in the early hours of morning and present to the clinic as soon as possible in the morning, preferably within 1–2 hours of having a sexual intercourse, up to a maximum of 6 hours. Ideally, the male partner must have abstained from ejaculation at least 48 hours prior to the test.
- The aspirated mucus is grossly assessed for characteristics such as spinnbarkeit, ferning and presence of any motile sperms. Presence of sperms in the cervical fluid indicates that the coitus had been effective. Absence of sperms from both cervix and vagina suggests that effective intercourse had not occurred. Presence of sperms in the vagina, but their absence from the cervix suggests cervical factor infertility. Normal cervical mucus shows a ferning pattern and a spinnbarkeit of 6–8 cm. Abnormal cervical mucus may not stretch more than 2–3 cm and does not show any fern-like pattern on drying up.

- The mucus, which is aspirated from the cervical canal, is also spread over the glass slide and then examined under the microscope. Normally, there are 10–50 motile sperms per high power field. Presence of less than 10 motile sperms is considered abnormal and requires the performance of a proper semen analysis. However, many researchers consider presence of a single motile sperm in most fields as a "positive" or normal test result. Normally, the sperms show progressive mobility. Presence of a jerky or rotatory mobility could be due to presence of antisperm antibodies. No pus cells or bacteria are observed in a normal sample.
- A normal PCT implies that the cervical mucus is favorable and the sperm count and function is normal. It also helps in ruling out the cervical and male factor infertility. This allows a higher chance of spontaneous natural conception. Abnormal PCT points to cervical factor infertility, most commonly due to the immunological causes, related to the presence of antisperm antibodies.

### Advantages

The advantages of PCT are as follows:
- A cheap, simple, easy, noninvasive and a nonexpensive test, which helps in checking many factors (both the cervical factor and the male factor).
- Also analyzes male factor when the semen sample is unavailable.
- This test may result in the occurrence of pregnancy in some cases.

### Disadvantages

The disadvantages of PCT are as follows:
- Stressful test due to the requirement of on-demand sexual activity.
- No longer used due to the availability of more contemporary treatment options like intrauterine insemination.
- May result in false negative results if the test is improperly timed.

# Hysteroscopy

## Introduction

Hysteroscopy is a minimally invasive procedure, involving the direct inspection of the cervical canal and endometrial cavity through a rigid, flexible or a contact hysteroscope. The procedure allows for the diagnosis of intrauterine pathology and serves as a method for surgical intervention (operative hysteroscopy). Hysteroscopy has the benefit of allowing direct visualization of the uterus, thereby avoiding or reducing iatrogenic trauma to delicate reproductive tissues. Not only does hysteroscopy allow direct observation of the intrauterine/endometrial pathology (presence of submucous fibroids, endometrial cancer, etc.), it also acts as a way of sampling the endometrium under direct visualization. While performing hysteroscopy, solutions such as Hyskon (previously used) and glycine and sorbitol (used nowadays) are used for intrauterine instillation. Hysteroscopy is useful in numerous diagnostic as well as operative procedures, which are listed below.

## Indications

### Diagnostic Indications

- Diagnosis of causes of infertility (abnormalities on HSG such as filling defects, adhesions, Asherman's syndrome, etc. can be confirmed by hysteroscopy).
- Diagnosis of causes of abnormal bleeding such as menorrhagia, irregular bleeding, AUB, postmenopausal bleeding, etc.
- Diagnosis of congenital uterine abnormalities (e.g. septate uterus, T-shaped uterus, etc.).
- Diagnosis of lost or misplaced IUDs.

### Operative Indications

The indications of operative hysteroscopy are as follows:
- Treatment of AUB [endometrial ablation, transcervical resection of endometrium (TCRE)].
- *Polypectomy:* Removal of endometrial polyps.
- *Adhesiolysis:* Hysteroscopic resection of adhesions is achieved either using microscissors or thermal energy modalities. This method is also used in case of presence of intrauterine adhesions (e.g. Asherman's syndrome).
- Myomectomy for submucosal fibroids.
- Treatment of congenital uterine malformations or Müllerian abnormalities: metroplasty for incision of uterine septum.
- Removal of misplaced/embedded IUCD.
- Sterilization (use of electrocoagulation or tubal plugs to block the cornual ends of the tubes).
- Targeted endometrial biopsy (suspected cases of tuberculosis, endometrial cancer).
- Hysteroscopy allows access to the uterotubal junction for entry into the fallopian tube: this is useful for tubal occlusion procedures for sterilization and for falloposcopy.
- Management of cornual and interstitial tubal blockage: tubal cannulation can be useful in cases of cornual or interstitial blocks.
  Hysteroscopy allows for direct visualization of the endometrial cavity along with the facility for directed biopsy.

Therefore, it serves as a better option in comparison to D&C alone. However, there are the following disadvantages associated with the use of hysteroscopy: it is a more invasive procedure, is associated with significant financial cost, as well as more physical discomfort in comparison to EB or D&C. Also, hysteroscopy may not be always available, especially in the primary setup.

## Surgery

### Preoperative Preparation

- Hysteroscopy is best done in the immediate postmenstrual phase when the endometrium is relatively thin, which facilitates intracavitary viewing.
- Paracervical block using 1% lidocaine is usually sufficient for diagnostic hysteroscopy procedures. Operative hysteroscopic interventions are usually performed under general endotracheal anesthesia.
- Informed consent must be taken from the patient.
- Prior to diagnostic/operative hysteroscopy, a detailed patient history, physical examination and discussion regarding the choice of procedure and the type of anesthesia to be used needs to be performed.
- In order to reduce the pain and discomfort associated with the procedure, mild sedatives or NSAIDs (ibuprofen, 600–800 mg) can be administered prior to the procedure.
- Patients with high-risk cardiac conditions may be offered an antibiotic prophylaxis prior to the procedure.
- For the procedure, the patient is placed in a standard lithotomy position with legs apart in order to maximize the vaginal access.
- The perineum and vagina are gently swabbed with povidone-iodine or another suitable antiseptic solution.

### Actual Steps of Surgery

The steps of diagnostic hysteroscopy are as follows:
- The posterior vaginal wall is retracted using Sims' speculum.
- The anterior edge of cervix is grasped with the help of a single-toothed tenaculum.
- Most diagnostic hysteroscopic procedures using a 5-mm diagnostic sheath can be performed without cervical canal dilatation. Insertion of diagnostic sheaths with a larger diameter may require prior cervical dilatation.
- Surgeon then selects a suitable telescope and checks its eyepiece for proper clarity. If required, the lens is cleansed with the help of a saline or water-soaked sponge.
- The light generator is switched on and the fiberoptic cable is attached to the telescope.
- The telescope is inserted into the diagnostic sheath.
- The selected distention medium is flushed through the sheath to expel any air.
- Before introducing the hysteroscope, the irrigation system is connected and the fluid let in so that it starts filling the tubing and the uterus gets distended prior to insertion of the hysteroscope.
- The hysteroscope is engaged into the external cervical os, following which it is gently advanced inside the endocervical canal into the uterine cavity.
- As the hysteroscope engages into the external os, the flow of distention medium must be started.
- The hysteroscope is gently moved forwards, and the panoramic view of all the uterine walls and tubal ostia is visualized. If a therapeutic procedure is required (e.g. removal of a polyp/biopsy, etc.), it can be done during this stage.
- The scope is withdrawn from the cervical os after finishing the procedure.

### Postoperative Care

- Following the procedure, especially operative hysteroscopy, the patient must be observed for at least 6–12 hours for the signs of any potential complications.
  Presence of bowel injury could be associated with signs and symptoms such as worsening of postoperative pain, fever, nausea, abdominal distention, etc. On the other hand, signs, such as diminished urinary output, fever and abdominal distention, could be suggestive of bladder or urethral trauma and/or infection. Tachycardia and/or hypotension could be suggestive of continuing third-space hemorrhage.
- In case of diagnostic hysteroscopy performed under local anesthesia, the patient can be discharged home, 1 hour after the procedure.
- Activity is restricted for a few days (depending on the type of procedure performed).
- Abstinence is advised for about 2 weeks.
- Painkillers and antibiotics may be prescribed following the procedure.
- Patient must be asked to report to the healthcare provider in case she experiences excessive pain, bleeding, fever, discharge, dizziness or abdominal bloating.

## Complications

Various complications which can occur during the intraoperative period are as follows:
- *Traumatic injury:* Intraoperative complications which can occur during the procedure include traumatic injury to the cervix and rarely uterus as well. At times, injury to the bowel and bladder can also occur.
- *Perforation:* A possible problem associated with the procedure is uterine perforation which commonly occurs when either the hysteroscope itself or one of its operative instruments breach the uterine wall. A small perforation may be symptomless and heal on its own. A large perforation, however, can cause considerable bleeding and damage to other organs.

- *Poor visibility of the operative field:* Inability to properly visualize the operative field may commonly be associated with deep insertion of a hysteroscope or overdilatation of cervix.
- *Intraoperative and postoperative bleeding:* A common complication associated with the procedure is the occurrence of bleeding during and after the procedure.
- *Infection:* Infection rarely occurs if the procedure is performed using strict aseptic precautions.
- *Gas embolism:* Gas embolism is a rare, but devastating complication of hysteroscopy.
- *Electrical and laser injuries:* Uterine perforation caused by either laser fiber or electrode is likely to be more serious than the injury caused by mechanical devices, such as scissors, because thermal injury is likely to inflict greater damage to the surrounding tissues.
- *Complications caused by the distention media:* The use of insufflation media can result in serious and even fatal complications due to embolism or fluid overload with electrolyte imbalances. Fluid overload can occur with the use of distention media such as normal saline.
- *Hematometra:* Hematometra may occur due to the development of intrauterine adhesions in the area of active endometrium, which continues to undergo active cyclical bleeding. Patients may present with cyclical pain and the condition may be diagnosed on TVS. Drainage may be performed by a repeat hysteroscopy.
- *Uterine rupture:* Uterine rupture during pregnancy has been reported in cases where women have become pregnant following endoscopic procedures such as myoma or septum resection.
- *Operator inexperience:* The most likely complications with hysteroscopy commonly occur in the presence of operator inexperience. If the surgeon is properly acquainted with hysteroscopic techniques, the rate of complications would be much less.

# Marsupialization of Bartholin's Cyst

## Introduction

Bartholin's glands are also known as greater vestibular glands. These are two glands, each of which is located to the left and right of the vaginal introitus, slightly towards the posterior side. These glands secrete mucus, which helps in lubricating the vagina. Though the presence of Bartholin's glands may remain unnoticed, sometimes, these glands may become infected, resulting in pain and swelling. These glands may develop into a cyst-like structure as a result of inflammation and blockage of the ducts of the Bartholin's gland. Though the cysts may not be painful, it may result in extreme discomfort and swelling. Blockage of the ducts of Bartholin's glands result in the accumulation of secretions inside the cyst, which may subsequently get infected resulting in abscess formation.

The diagnosis of Bartholin's cyst is confirmed on clinical examination.

## Procedure

Permanent resolution of the cyst is done either using marsupialization or incision and drainage with Word's catheter placement. Placement of Word's catheter helps in creating a new epithelialized tract for gland drainage after emptying the cyst cavity through the procedure of incision and drainage. Marsupialization requires greater degree of analgesia, larger incision, placement of sutures and longer procedural time. It may be the preferred procedure in case of recurrence of cysts with previously placed Word's catheter. With the introduction of Word's catheter, use of marsupialization has declined. The procedure of marsupialization is described as follows:

### Preprocedural Preparation

- The patient is asked to pass urine and then administered anesthesia (regional or general).
- Parts are cleaned and draped.
- Patient is placed in lithotomy position and the bladder is catheterized.
- Labial stitches are applied.

### Actual Procedure

- The steps of the procedure are illustrated in Figures 10.14A to F.
- A vertical incision about 2–3 cm in size is made on the vestibule near the medial edge of labia minora and approximately 1 cm lateral and parallel to the hymenal ring at the mucocutaneous junction, following which the escaping fluid or pus is drained out.
- The cyst wall is then incised with a scalpel and the incision extended with scissors.
- Allis clamps are then placed on the four edges in order to grasp the edges of the cyst wall. The edges of the cyst wall are then everted out, excised and sutured to the adjacent skin edges with interrupted delayed absorbable sutures, such that an open space remains.
- A wick can be left inside the cavity.

### Postprocedural Care

- A perineal pad can be applied over the perineum.
- No packing or drainage is usually required.
- Hot sitz baths are advised from the second postoperative day.
- Laxatives and stool softeners are administered from the third postoperative day.
- Antibiotic therapy is based on the results of culture and sensitivity.
- Sexual intercourse should be resumed after 4 weeks of surgery.

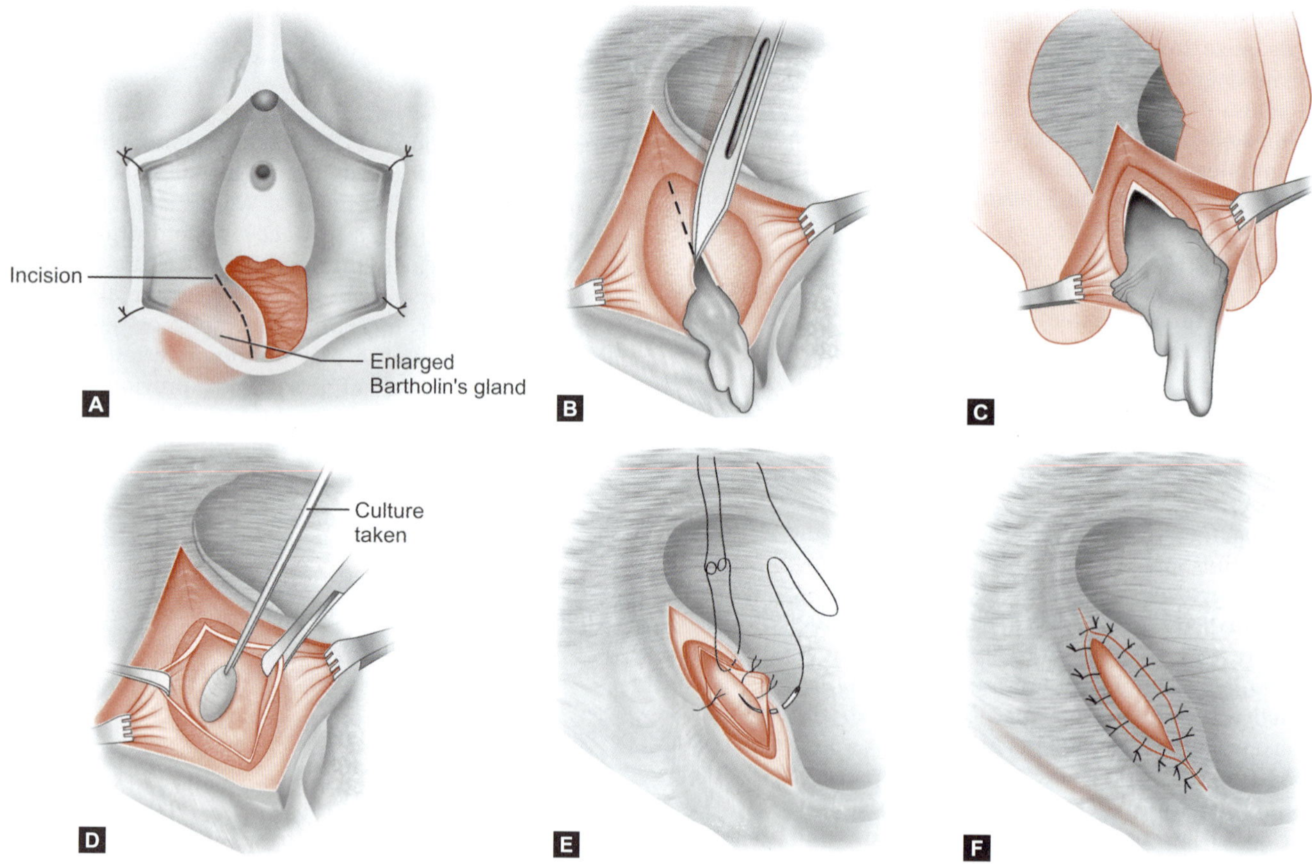

**Figs 10.14A to F:** Procedure of marsupialization. (A) Administration of an incision over an enlarged Bartholin's gland; (B) Drainage of the Bartholin's cyst/abscess; (C) The contents of the abscess are evacuated; (D) The edges of the abscess are held with Allis forceps and a swab is used for taking the sample for culture and sensitivity; (E) Marsupialization: the walls of the abscess is sutured with 3-0 synthetic absorbable sutures to the skin of introitus laterally and to the vaginal mucosa medially; (F) The process of marsupialization is complete

# Hysterectomy

## ABDOMINAL HYSTERECTOMY

### Introduction

Abdominal hysterectomy is a commonly performed gynecological procedure utilized for removal of the uterus (with or without removal of ovaries) in cases of benign and malignant gynecological diseases. Depending on the route through which the hysterectomy is performed, it can be classified as abdominal hysterectomy (performed through an abdominal incision), vaginal hysterectomy (performed through vaginal incision) or as a laparoscopic procedure [laparoscopic hysterectomy (LH)] or laparoscopic assisted vaginal hysterectomy (LAVH).

### Indications

Hysterectomy is commonly performed for the following indications:

- *Fibroid uterus:* Especially in cases of symptomatic fibroids
- *Malignancies of the genital tract:* These may include endometrial cancer; cancer of the cervix or severe cervical dysplasia (CIN grade III) and cancer of the ovary
- *Endometriosis:* A hysterectomy may be recommended when medication and minimal invasive surgery fails to cure endometriosis
- Persistent vaginal bleeding
- *Uterine prolapse:* Moderate or severe prolapse of the uterus
- *Complications during childbirth:* Hysterectomy may be performed as an emergency procedure to control atonic primary PPH.

### Surgical Management

*Preoperative Preparation*

- A complete history and physical examination.
- *Routine preoperative investigations:* Investigations such as complete blood count with platelet count, fasting blood

glucose, kidney function test and liver function test must be performed. Other preoperative investigations include tests such as endometrial biopsy or aspiration, Pap smear and ultrasound examination.

- *Informed consent:* Written informed consent must be obtained from the patient prior to the surgery.
- *Nil per orally:* The patient should not take either food or water by mouth for at least 6 hours prior to the time of scheduled surgery.
- *Analgesics and antibiotics:* Painkillers, mild sedatives and antibiotics may be prescribed before the procedure.
- *Part preparation:* The abdomen and genital area may be shaved and prepared for the surgery.
- *Bowel preparation:* An enema may be administered to the patient 6–10 hours prior to the surgery.
- *Anesthesia:* Abdominal hysterectomy can be performed under spinal or general anesthesia.
- *Patient position:* The patient is put in approximately 15° Trendelenburg position for the surgery.
- *Cleaning and draping:* Under all aseptic precautions, the lower abdominal area, the genital area and upper parts of the thighs are cleaned and draped using sterile aseptic technique.
- *Foley's catheter:* The bladder is catheterized with the help of Foley's catheter.

### Steps of Surgery

The procedure of abdominal hysterectomy is illustrated in Figures 10.15 to 10.26.

Abdominal closure is the final concluding step of abdominal hysterectomy. Prior to closing the abdomen, all the stumps must be inspected for hemostasis.

### Postoperative Care

- The patient must be closely observed for the signs of hemorrhage for the first few hours following the surgery.
- Intravenous and oral pain-killer medications can provide relief from postoperative pain. Patient controlled analgesia can be utilized for adequate control of pain.
- Foley's catheter may be removed in the morning following surgery or the patient may remain catheterized for 1–2 days to help her pass urine.
- Intravenous fluids are administered for the first 24 hours following surgery.
- Lifting of heavy weights or vaginal sexual intercourse must be discouraged for at least 4–6 weeks until the vaginal cuff heals completely.

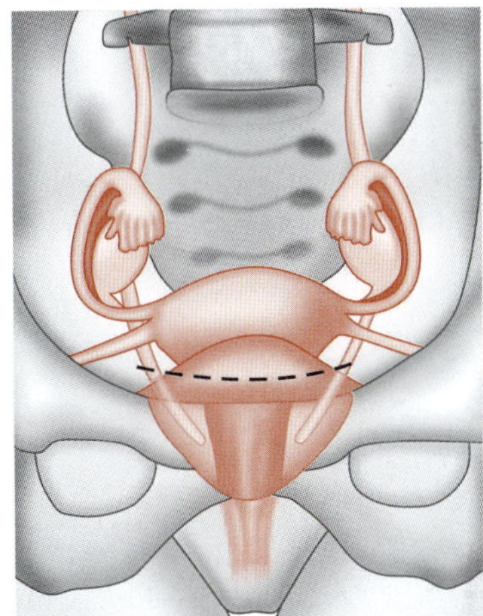

**Fig. 10.15:** Opening the abdomen using a Pfannenstiel transverse abdominal incision

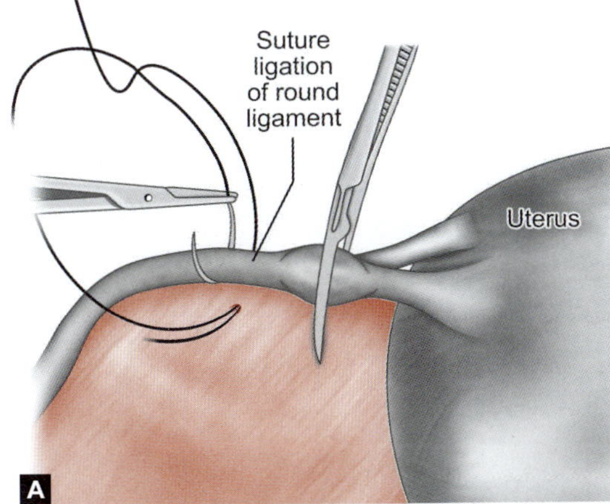


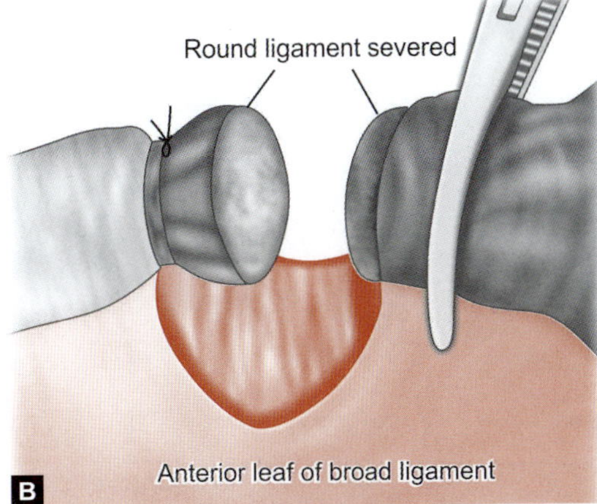


**Figs 10.16A and B:** Clamping, ligating and transecting the round ligaments, and incising the anterior leaf of broad ligament

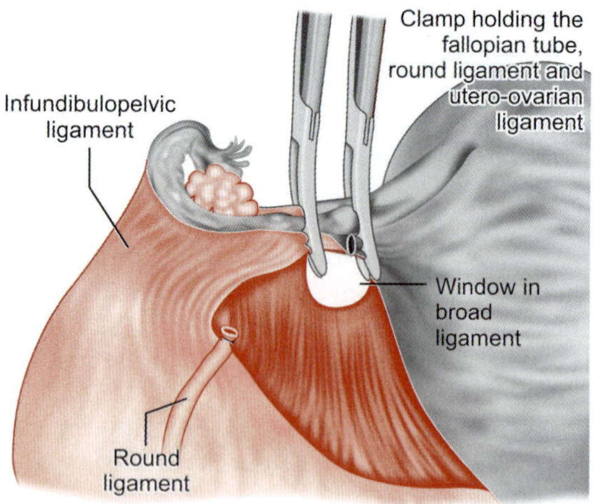


**Fig. 10.17:** Clamping, cutting and ligation of the fallopian tubes and utero-ovarian ligaments in case the tubes and ovaries are to be preserved

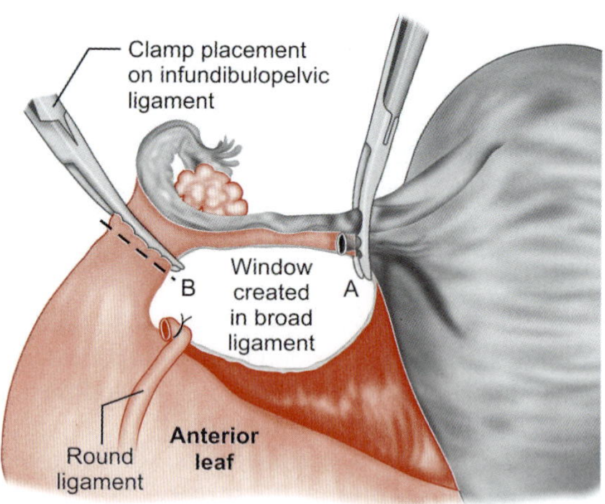


**Fig. 10.18:** Clamping, cutting and ligating the infundibulopelvic ligaments, in case the tubes and ovaries have to be removed

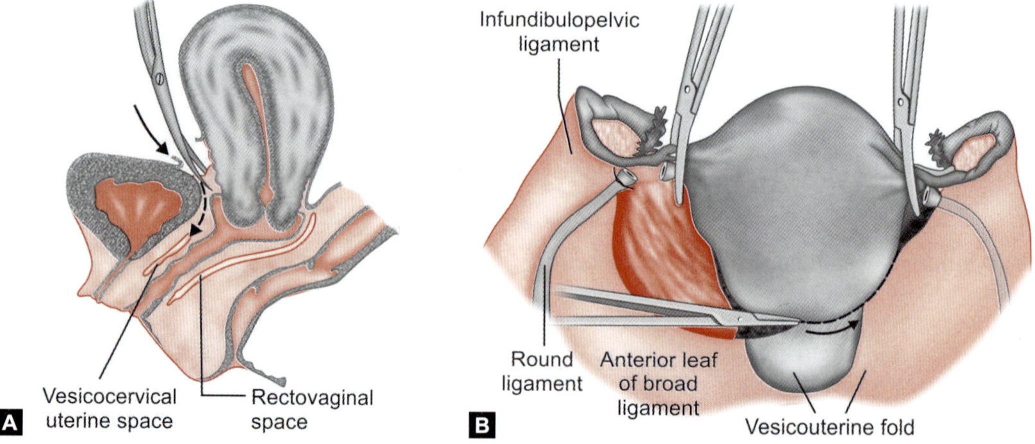


**Figs 10.19A and B:** Identification and incision of the vesicouterine fold of peritoneum, which is extended over the anterior leaf of broad ligament

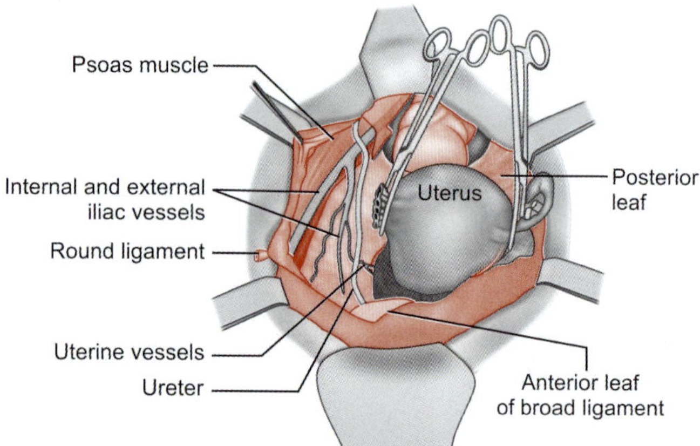


**Fig. 10.20:** Identification of the ureter as it crosses the common iliac vessels by following the external iliac artery cephalad to the bifurcation

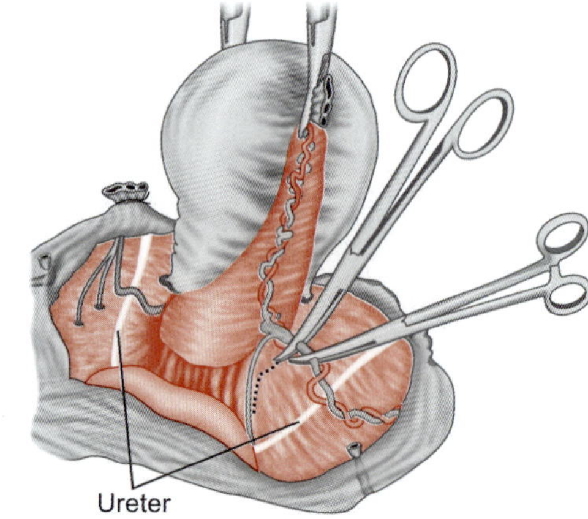


**Fig. 10.21:** Clamping, cutting and ligating the uterine vessels after skeletonizing the vessels

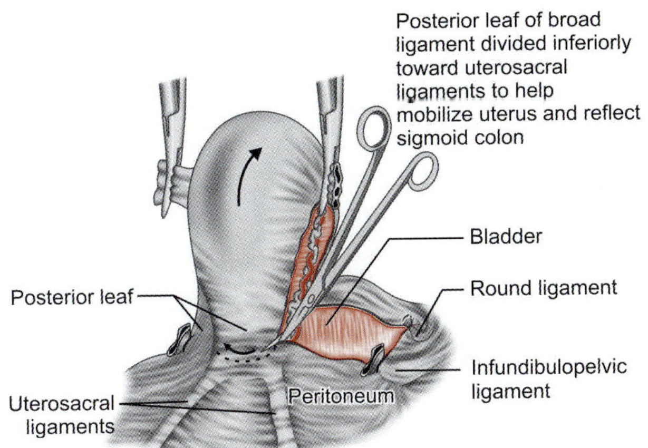



**Fig. 10.22:** The posterior leaf of broad ligament is then incised to the point where the uterosacral ligaments join the cervix and the rectum is mobilized from the posterior cervix

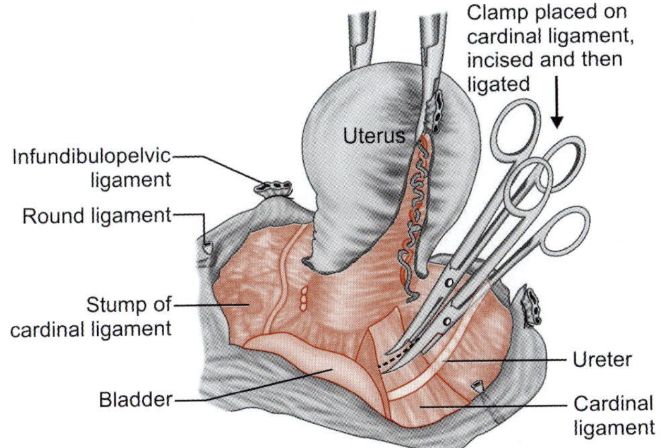



**Fig. 10.23:** Diagrammatic representation of clamping, cutting and ligating the Mackenrodt's and uterosacral ligaments

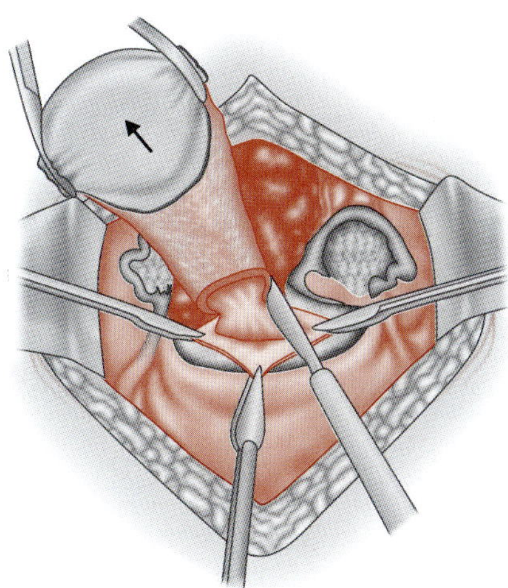

**Fig. 10.24:** Clamping and cutting of the vaginal angles

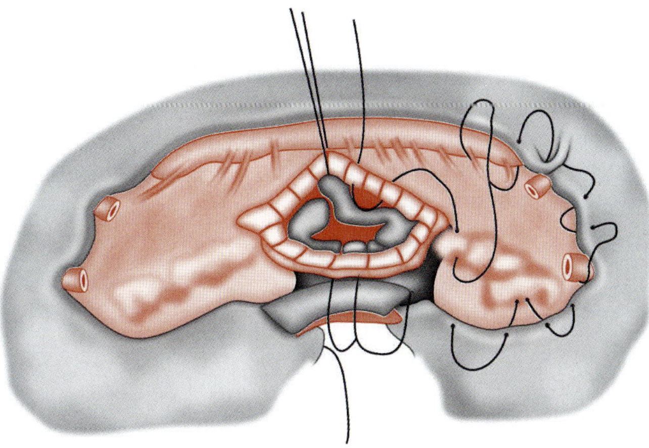

**Fig. 10.25:** Vaginal cuff is left open with running locking stitch sutures placed along the cut edge of vaginal mucosa

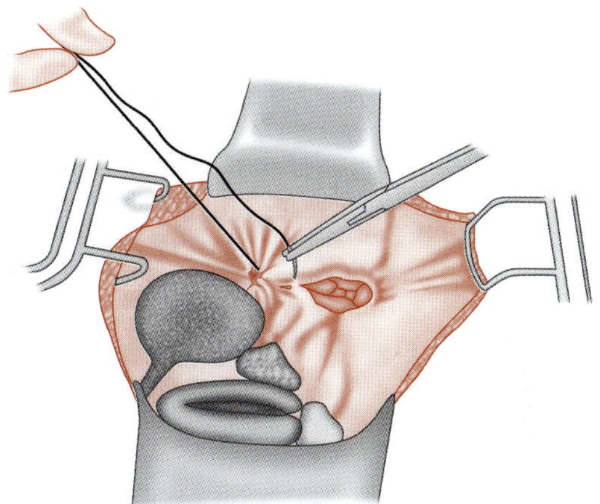

**Fig. 10.26:** Reperitonization of the pelvis

- Skin sutures are removed on 7th to 10th postoperative day.

## COMPLICATIONS

### Immediate Postoperative Period

- *Hemorrhage:* Primary and reactionary, immediately following surgery or secondary hemorrhage after 24 hours of surgery
- Injury to adjacent structures such as bladder, intestines and ureter
- Anesthetic complications
- *Shock:* Hypovolemic shock
- *Urinary complications:* These may include complications such as retention, cystitis, anuria and incontinence such as overflow, stress or true incontinence

- *Pyrexia:* Pyrexia more than 100.8°F, commonly due to infection
- *Hematoma:* Cuff or rectus sheath hematoma
- Wound dehiscence
- Paralytic ileus and intestinal obstruction
- *Venous complications:* Phlebitis, deep vein thrombosis and pulmonary embolism.

### Remote

- Vault granulation, vault prolapse
- Prolapse of fallopian tubes
- Incisional hernia
- Postoperative adhesion formation
- High mortality rate
- Early surgical menopause in case of salpingo-oophorectomy.

## VAGINAL HYSTERECTOMY

### Introduction

Vaginal hysterectomy is based on the same principle as that of abdominal hysterectomy, it is just that the uterus is removed through the vaginal route rather than the abdominal route and the various steps as described previously with abdominal route are now performed vaginally. The main advantages of the vaginal hysterectomy are that there is no visible scar, healing is faster in comparison to abdominal hysterectomy and there is an overall reduced rate of morbidity and mortality.

### Indications

When the hysterectomy is performed for uterovaginal prolapse, the vaginal route is more commonly used. However, the absence of prolapse is not a contraindication for vaginal route. Only in cases where the vaginal route is not possible, should a surgeon consider LAVH or abdominal route.

### Surgical Management

*Preoperative Preparation*

Preoperative preparation is same as that with abdominal hysterectomy described previously.

*Steps of Surgery*

The steps of surgery are described in Figures 10.27 to 10.37.

*Postoperative Care*

Postoperative care is same as that for abdominal hysterectomy described previously.

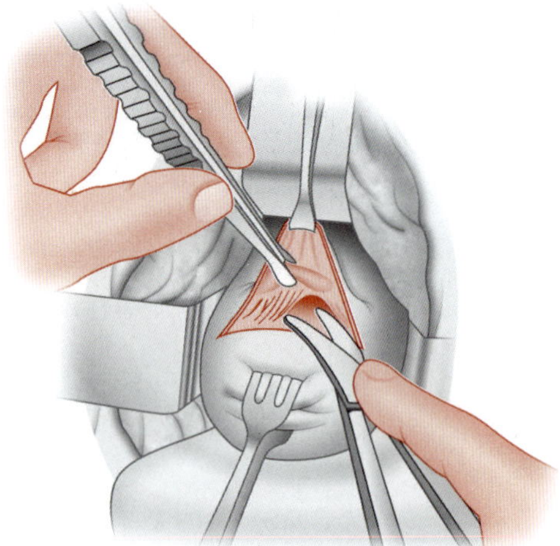

**Fig. 10.27:** Sharp dissection of the vaginal mucosa after making a circumferential incision in the vaginal epithelium at the junction of the cervix just below the bladder sulcus

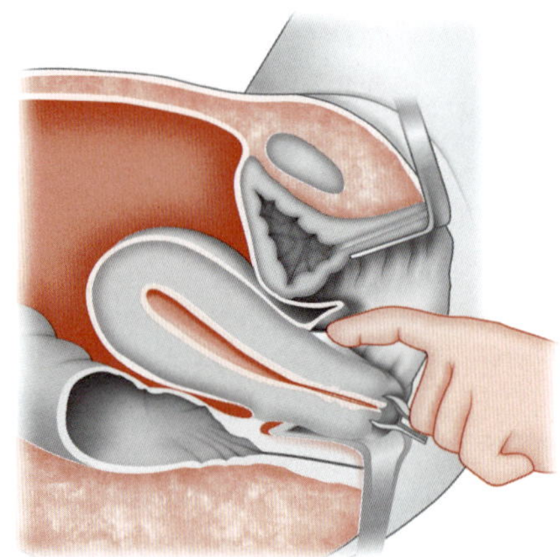

**Fig. 10.28:** Identification of the vesicouterine fold

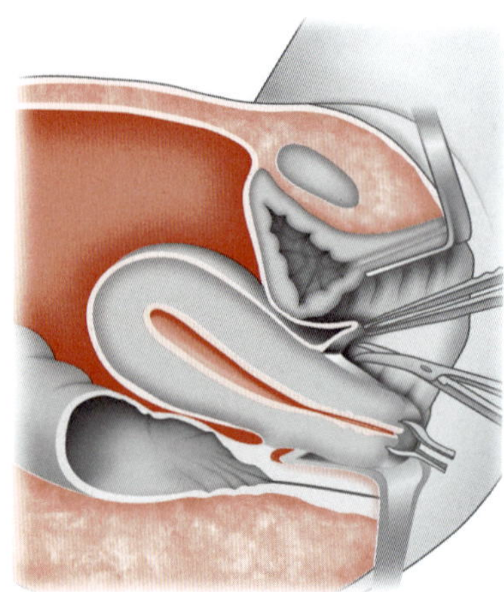

**Fig. 10.29:** Incision of the vesicouterine fold

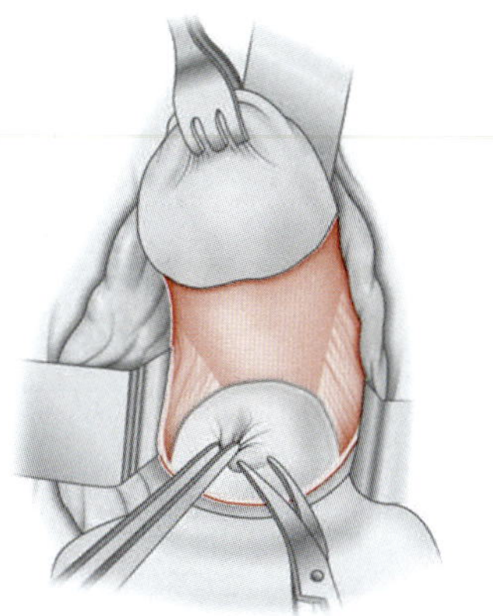

**Fig. 10.30:** Entry into the Cul-de-sac after identifying and incising the pouch of Douglas

## Complications

Postoperative complications are same as that with abdominal hysterectomy, described previously.

- The main disadvantages associated with vaginal hysterectomy are that there is less room for the surgeon to visualize and operate. Therefore, the procedure can only be used for smaller sized uterus and there is a higher chance for causing injury to the adjoining organs.
- Vaginal hysterectomy, however, cannot be performed in presence of certain complications, such as uterus greater than 12 weeks in size; invasive cancer of the cervix or inaccessible cervix; vesicovaginal fistula or rectovaginal fistula and uterine pathology such as endometriosis with severe adhesions or presence of large uterine myomas, adenomyosis, etc.

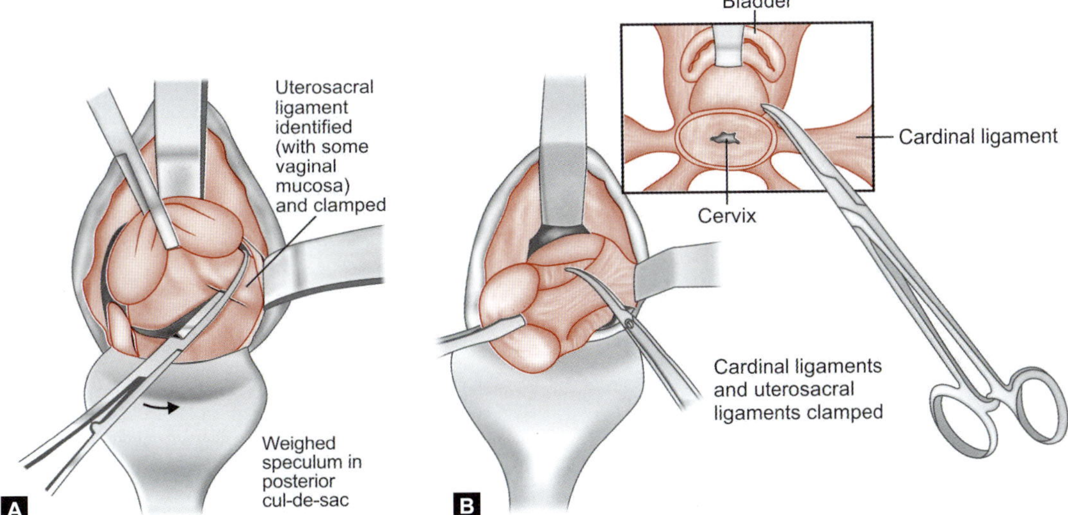


**Figs 10.31A and B:** With the retraction of lateral vaginal wall and countertraction on the cervix, first the uterosacral ligaments and then the cardinal ligaments are identified, clamped, cut and suture ligated

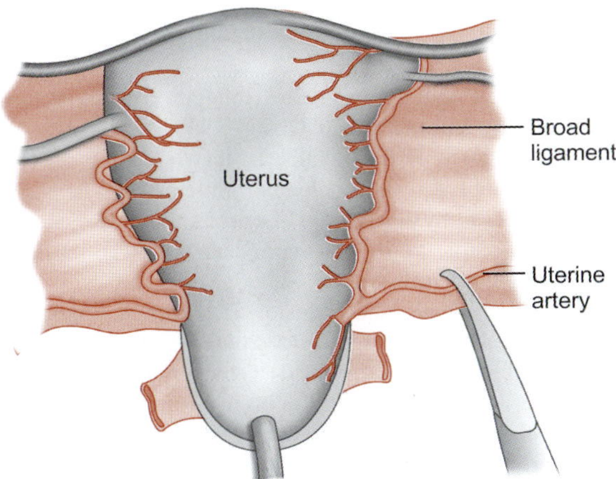


**Fig. 10.32:** The uterine vessels are identified, clamped, cut and suture ligated

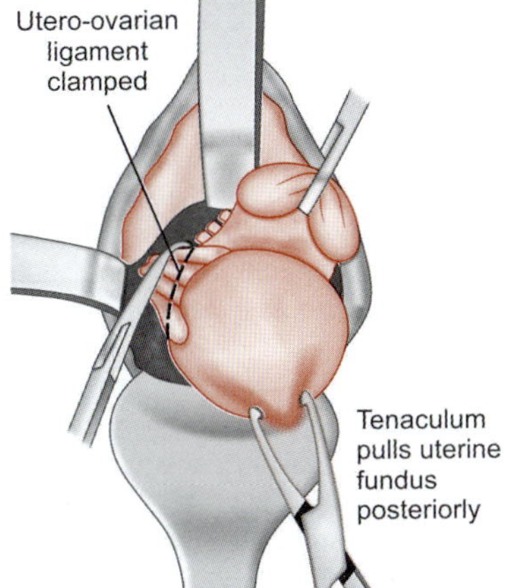


**Fig. 10.33:** A tenaculum is placed onto the uterine fundus in a successive fashion in order to deliver the fundus posteriorly

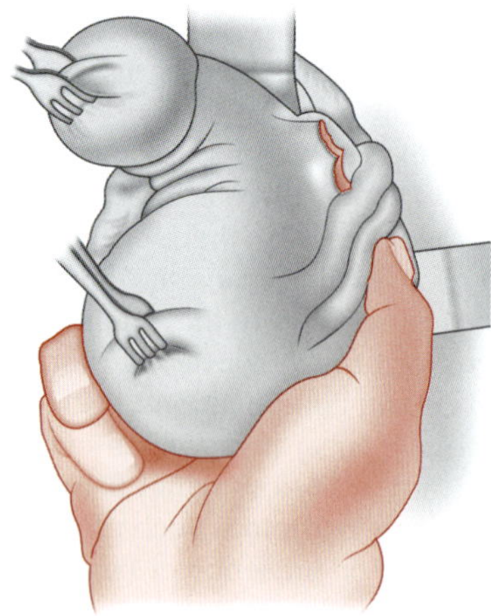

**Fig. 10.34:** Transection of the utero-ovarian and round ligaments in cases where the fallopian tubes and ovaries need to be retained.

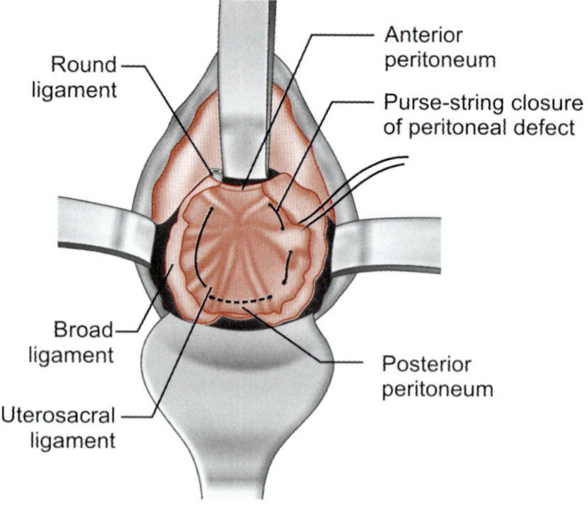



**Fig. 10.36:** If the peritoneal closure is performed, the peritoneum is reapproximated in a purse-string fashion using continuous absorbable sutures

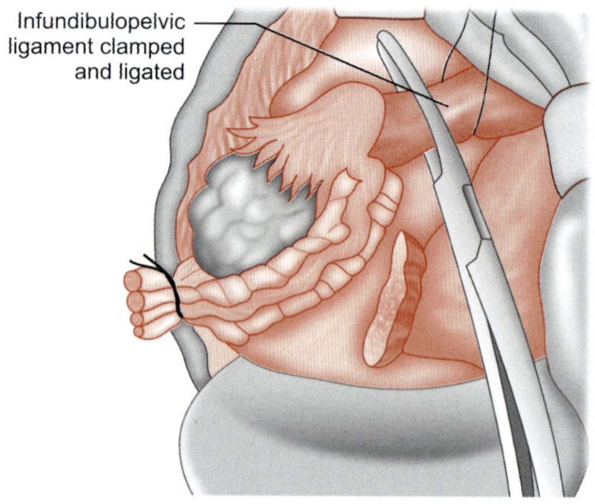



**Fig. 10.35:** If the ovaries have to be removed, a Heaney's clamp is placed across the infundibulopelvic ligaments which are then ligated and transected to remove the tubes and ovary

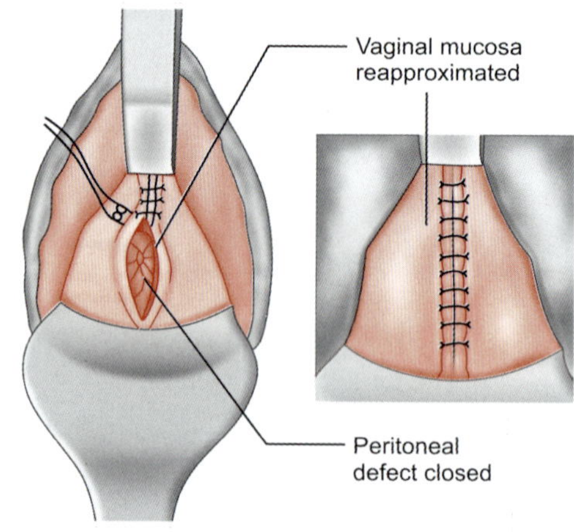



**Fig. 10.37:** The vaginal mucosa can be reapproximated in a vertical or horizontal manner using either interrupted or continuous sutures

## FURTHER READINGS

1. ACOG Committee Opinion. Evaluation and management of abnormal cervical cytology and histology in the adolescent. Number 330, April 2006. Obstet Gynecol. 2006;107(4):963-8.
2. American College of Obstetricians and Gynecologists. ACOG Practice Bulletin number 66, September 2005. Management of abnormal cervical cytology and histology. Obstet Gynecol. 2005;106(3):645-64.
3. ACOG committee opinion. New Pap test screening techniques. Number 206, August 1998. Committee on Gynecologic Practice. American College of Obstetricians and Gynecologists. Int J Gynaecol Obstet. 1998;63(3):312-4.
4. ACOG committee opinion. Recommendations on frequency of Pap test screening. Number 152—March 1995. Committee on Gynecologic Practice. American College of Obstetricians and Gynecologists. Int J Gynaecol Obstet. 1995;49(2):210-1.
5. Royal College of Obstetricians and Gynaecologists (RCOG), British Society for Gynecological Endoscopy. Best practice in outpatient hysteroscopy. London, UK: Royal College of Obstetricians and Gynaecologists (RCOG); 2011. p. 22 (Green-top guideline; no. 59).
6. Simpson WL, Beitia LG, Mester J. Hysterosalingography: a reemerging study. Radiographics. 2006;26:419-31.
7. Society of Obstetricians and Gynaecologists of Canada. Diagnosis of endometrial cancer in women with abnormal vaginal bleeding. SOGC Clinical Practice Guideline 86. J Soc Obstet Gynaecol Can. 2000;22(1):102-4.

# 11
## CHAPTER

# Contraception



## Introduction

The goal of family planning is to enable couples and individuals to freely choose how many children to have and when to have them. This can be best done if the clinician provides them with a full range of safe and effective contraceptive methods and gives them sufficient information to ensure they are able to make informed choices. Contraceptive methods may be of two types: temporary or permanent. Contraception may be required for following indications: postponement of first pregnancy, birth spacing, and control and prevention of pregnancy. Various contraceptive methods are based on three general strategies: (1) prevention of ovulation, (2) prevention of fertilization or (3) prevention of implantation. Various methods for contraception are described in Table 11.1. Various temporary methods of contraception include barrier methods, hormonal contraception (combined hormonal contraception and progestogen-only contraception), IUCDs and emergency (postcoital) contraception. Permanent methods of contraception include sterilization, which in women can be done using tubal ligation and in men using vasectomy. The WHO eligibility criteria for the use of various contraceptive methods have been described in Table 11.2.

Before the prescription of a particular method of contraception to a patient certain questions, which need to be asked at the time of taking history or the parameters to be assessed at the time of examination such cases are described in Tables 11.3 and 11.4 respectively.

**Table 11.1:** Various methods of contraception

*Temporary methods*
- Natural regulation of fertility
- Barrier methods
- Hormonal contraception
  1. Combined hormonal contraception (combined oral contraceptive pills)
     a. Monophasic pills (each tablet containing a fixed amount of estrogen and progestogen).
     b. Biphasic pills (each tablet containing a fixed amount of estrogen, while the amount of progestogen increases in the luteal phase of the cycle).
     c. Triphasic pills (the amount of estrogen may be fixed or variable, while the amount of progestogen increases over three equally divided phases of the cycle).
  2. Progestogen-only contraception:
     a. Progestogen-only pill
     b. Injections (Depo-Provera)
     c. Implants (Norplant I and II)
     d. Patches
     e. Vaginal rings
- Intrauterine contraceptive devices
- Emergency (postcoital) contraception

*Permanent methods*
- Female sterilization (tubal ligation)
- Vasectomy

*Abbreviation:* COCPs, Combined oral contraceptive pills

**Table 11.2:** World Health Organization eligibility criteria for the use of various contraceptive methods

| Category | Description |
|---|---|
| 1 | A condition where there is no restriction for the use of the contraceptive method |
| 2 | A condition where the advantages of using the method generally outweigh the theoretical or proven risks |
| 3 | A condition where the theoretical or proven risks usually outweigh the advantages of using the method |
| 4 | A condition that represents an unacceptable health risk if the contraceptive method is used |

# Natural Family Planning Methods

These methods aim at controlling childbirth by instructing the couple to abstain from sexual intercourse during the fertile period of menstrual cycle. Some of these methods are as follows:

## Calendar/Rhythm Method

In this method the fertile period is calculated by subtracting 18 days from the shortest cycle and 10 days from the longest cycle. This would give the first and the last day of the fertile period respectively. The couple must be instructed to abstain from sexual relations during this period. For example, if the shortest cycle is of 25 days and the longest cycle is of 35 days, then she should perceive the period of her maximum fertility to be starting from day 7 (25 – 18 = 7) through day 25 (35 – 10

= 25). In order to avoid pregnancy, she should abstain from having sexual intercourse between day 7 to day 25.

## Basal Body Temperature Method

This method is based on the fact that basal body temperature (BBT) increases by 0.2–0.5°C following ovulation due to thermogenic effect of hormone progesterone (Fig. 11.1). Since the increase in temperature under thermogenic effect of progesterone is about 0.4–0.8°F, a specially designed thermometer must be used for taking the temperature. The couple must be instructed that the safest way to use BBT for avoiding pregnancy is to avoid intercourse or use a barrier method during at least the first half of the menstrual cycle until 3 days after there has been a rise in BBT.

## Ovulation Method (Cervical Mucus or Billings Method)

This method is based on the fact that during the proliferative phase (prior to ovulation), the cervical mucus increases in amount, becomes clearer in color, wetter, stretchy and slippery. Under the effect of estrogens, cervical mucus becomes thin, watery, clear and profuse. It has a high content of sodium chloride in it due to which it forms a characteristic pattern of ferning when dried on a glass slide. It has great elasticity and is able to withstand stretching up to 10 cm. This is also known as the spinnbarkeit or the thread test, which is an evidence of estrogenic activity. Following ovulation, with the beginning of luteal phase, under the effect of progesterone the nature of cervical mucus changes again. There is a loss of

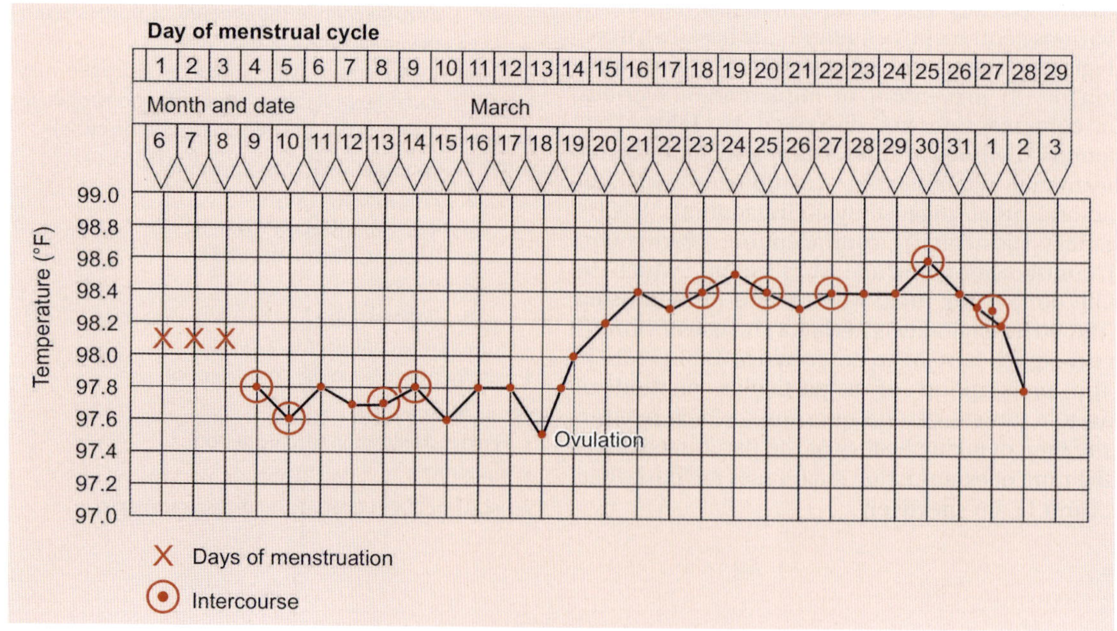



**Fig. 11.1:** Basal body temperature method

| **Table 11.3:** Indicators to be elicited at the time of taking history before prescribing a particular contraceptive agent |
| --- |

*History of Presenting Complaints*

*Type of Contraception Required*
- Before prescription of a particular method of contraception to the patient, the clinician must tell the woman about the various types of available contraceptive agents.
- The women must be counseled that there is no perfect method of contraception available. The clinician must present the advantages and disadvantages related to various methods and then help the woman make a choice about the type of contraceptive method she wants by balancing the advantages of each method against their disadvantages and decide the method she prefers to use.

Factors to be considered before prescribing a particular contraceptive agent include the following:
- *Efficacy:* The failure rate of different types of contraceptive agents vary. While some contraceptive agents are highly effective, (e.g. IUCDs, POI, implants, COCP, etc.), the others may not be that effective (e.g. barrier method, natural methods of family control, etc.). Reliability of a contraceptive method can be described in terms of its failure rate.
- *Convenience:* The contraceptive agent prescribed to the patient should be such that that the patient finds it convenient to use it. Reduced patient convenience may be associated with high rate of noncompliance, which is likely to result in high failure rate for even a very effective form of contraception. For example, COCPs are associated with a failure rate of 0.1 per 100 women years of use (considering the perfect use). However, if the woman does not find this method appropriate, misses the pills and fails to take them regularly, the failure rate may become very high.
- *Duration of contraceptive protection required:* It is also important to know the time duration for which woman wants contraceptive protection. If she wants to postpone her pregnancy for a few years, a contraceptive device which offers protection for few years, e.g. IUCD, implants, POI, etc. may be used.
- *Reversibility and time to return of fertility:* With some contraceptive agents, the return of fertility is almost immediate upon discontinuation (e.g. removal of an IUCD is associated with an immediate return of fertility). On the other hand, with some agents return of fertility may not be immediate even after discontinuation of that agent. For example, return of fertility may not be immediate after discontinuation of COCP.
- *Effect on uterine bleeding:* Effect of a particular contraceptive agent on uterine bleeding also needs to be considered before prescription. While some contraceptive methods may have no effect on the duration and amount of menstrual bleeding, some methods may increase (e.g. copper-containing IUCD) it or some methods may reduce it (e.g. COCPs, Mirena®, etc.). Therefore, a multiparous woman suffering from menorrhagia, looking for a long-term contraceptive method must be prescribed Mirena® rather than copper-containing IUCD. Mirena® insertion is likely to provide protection from menorrhagia as well as the contraceptive effect lasts for about 5 years.
- *Type and frequency of side effects and adverse events:* The choice of contraceptive agent is often based upon the kind of advantages and disadvantages it provides. For example, use of estrogen helps in maintaining the bone density. At the same time use of estrogen could be associated with side effects such as nausea, breast tenderness, bloating, headache and risks such as venous thromboembolism. Progestin-only contraceptives can be an option in those women who need to avoid using estrogen. Progestin-only contraceptives, however, can be associated with an increased risk of break through bleeding.
- *Cost:* A couple's socioeconomic condition must also be kept in mind before prescribing a particular contraceptive agent.
- *Accessibility:* Some women may prefer to use a contraceptive agent, which is available over-the-counter rather than the one available on doctor's prescription.
- *Noncontraceptive benefits:* Some contraceptive methods can provide certain noncontraceptive benefits, e.g. COCPs besides their contraceptive effects can also provide reduction in dysmenorrhea, menorrhagia, ectopic pregnancy, premenstrual syndrome, menstrual molimina and dysmenorrhea, risk of benign breast disease, development of new ovarian cysts, etc.
- *Medical contraindications:* It is important for the clinician to elicit the patient's past medical history in details. History of certain medical disorders and conditions may act as a risk factor to the use of some contraceptive agents. This has been discussed in details under the heading of past medical history.

*Patient Targeted History*

The following questions would guide the clinician in helping the patient choose the most suitable form of contraception:
- *Patient's age and parity:* Taking the history related to the patient's age and parity is particularly important in these cases. Prescription of oral contraceptive agents to a woman above the age of 35 years must be done with caution and under medical supervision. In case of woman below the age of 20 years seeking contraceptive device, it is important to counsel the patient to correctly use appropriate contraception to ensure that she does not conceive because she may not be physically or mentally mature enough to produce a healthy baby. History regarding parity is also important because some forms of contraception may be safer in multiparous women (e.g. IUCDs must be preferably avoided in unmarried and nulliparous women because of the risk of PID and subsequent tubal infertility.

*(Contd...)*

*(Contd...)*

- *Patient's contraceptive goals:* How long the patient wants to postpone her pregnancy and what is the reason for her postponement? Does she ever plan to get pregnant in future? If she does plan to get pregnant in future, for approximately how long does she want to wait? The patient should be asked if she is looking for a temporary or a permanent option for contraception. If she has completed her family and does not wish to have more children in future, a permanent method of contraception (male or female sterilization procedure) can be suggested to her. In case she wants to just temporarily postpone her pregnancy, a temporary method of contraception can be suggested. In case of a temporary method of contraception, the effects last until the time the couple keeps using the method. The fertility returns immediately or within a few months of the discontinuation of the temporary method.

- *Present sexual activity:* Is she currently sexually active? Taking the history related to her frequency of sexual intercourse would help the clinician in deciding the strength of effectiveness of the contraceptive agent to be prescribed.

- *Use of any contraceptive method in the past:* The clinician needs to enquire if the woman has tried any form of contraception in the past. If she has tried some method in the past, what was the method she had tried? What was the reason of using that particular contraceptive method? Was there anything, which she liked or disliked about that method? It is important for the clinician to know if the patient is aware about various methods of contraception. Is there any method in particular which she would want to try? How regular does the patient consider herself for taking a pill every day, in case she is prescribed birth control pills?

- *Spontaneity of use:* The patient must be enquired about the importance of spontaneity of use.

- *Protection from sexually transmitted diseases:* There are some contraceptive methods (e.g. Condoms), which can also provide protection against the STD, while the others (e.g. COCPs, etc.) may provide no protection. Contraceptive agents such as IUCD may increase the risk of transmitting the STD. If the patient appears to be at a high risk of acquiring STD, she must be prescribed a contraceptive agent, which may help provide her some protection.

*Past Medical History*

- *Past medical illness:* It is important to take history related to the presence of any medical disorder in the past (e.g. hypertension, diabetes, liver diseases, thromboembolism, etc.). In the presence of any of these medical disorders, prescription of COCPs is best avoided.

- *Past gynecological history:* Taking history related to the presence of any gynecological disorder in the past is also important. In case of the history of pelvic organ prolapse, cystocele, rectocele, etc. barrier contraception such as diaphragm should preferably be avoided because accurate fitting of the diaphragm may not be possible in these cases. Use of intrauterine contraceptive agents may not be advisable in cases with fibroid uterus due to irregular uterine cavity. IUCDs should also not be used in presence of congenital malformations such as bicornuate uterus, septate uterus, etc.

- *Past history of allergies:* In case the patient gives history of allergy to latex or rubber, use of condoms/diaphragms, etc. is best avoided.

*Obstetric History*

- *Number of previous childbirths and spacing between them:* Taking a detailed obstetric history is also very important in these cases. The number of children woman has; their ages and health status needs to be asked. It is important to enquire about the time since the last childbirth because keeping birth spacing of about 3 years between the children is likely to be beneficial both for the mother and the baby.

- *Breastfeeding:* Taking the history of breastfeeding is important. Some contraceptive agents, e.g. COCPs must not be prescribed in the breastfeeding mothers because they are likely to cause suppression of the breast milk. They may also increase the risk of thromboembolism in the postpartum period.

- *Requirement for a permanent method of contraception:* History of previous two cesarean births is likely to increase the woman's surgical risk at the time of next delivery. Such women should be preferably offered a permanent method of contraception (e.g. tubal sterilization of the woman or vasectomy of the male partner). If the woman gives the history of genetic defect in her previous children, she should undergo genetic counseling and suggested to consider a permanent method of contraception.

*Menstrual History*

The details which may be particularly important in these cases include the following:

- *Regularity of menstrual cycles:* In a woman having irregular menstrual cycles, the success rate of natural family planning methods is likely to be less.

- *Amount of bleeding:* The type of contraception prescribed to a patient may differ based on the amount and duration of bleeding. For example use of copper IUCD is likely to increase the amount of bleeding. Therefore, a woman already having heavy bleeding during periods must not be prescribed copper-containing IUCDs because this may further increase the bleeding, resulting in anemia. Increased patient discomfort may also result in noncompliance.

- *Dysmenorrhea:* Taking the history of dysmenorrhea is particularly important. Some contraceptive agents such as COCPs may help in reducing dysmenorrhea by making the cycles anovulatory. Some contraceptive agents like copper-containing IUCDs may further worsen menstrual pain by causing uterine cramping.

*Abbreviations:* COCPs, Combined oral contraceptive pills; IUCDs, intrauterine contraceptive devices; PID, pelvic inflammatory disease; POI, progestogen-only injectable; STD, sexually transmitted disease

**Table 11.4:** Various findings to be elicited at the time of clinical examination before prescription of a particular method of contraception

*General Physical Examination*

- *Measurement of blood pressure:* The physical examination should include a blood pressure measurement in case of prescription of COCPs. Prescription of COCPs should be preferably avoided in hypertensive women.
- *Pallor:* Assessment of woman for signs of anemia is important because some types of contraceptive methods may be associated with an increased blood flow (e.g. IUCDs) thereby worsening anemia, while others may help in reducing the blood and making the menstrual cycles lighter (e.g. COCPs, Mirena®, etc.) thereby improving anemia.

*Specific Systemic Examination*

*Per Speculum Examination*
- *Signs of infection:* Per speculum examination is specifically required prior to the insertion of an IUCD. The cervix should be carefully inspected for any signs of infection such as mucopurulent discharge or pelvic tenderness.

*Pelvic Examination*
A pelvic examination is not mandatory before prescription of COCPs. A pelvic examination must be performed prior to the insertion of IUCD to determine the position and the size of uterus.

*Abbreviations:* COCPs, Combined oral contraceptive pills; IUCDs, intrauterine contraceptive devices

elasticity, ferning pattern and the spinnbarkeit. The mucus becomes thick, tenacious and viscous, and breaks easily when put under tension. This property is known as tacking.

Sexual intercourse is considered safe during the dry days immediately following the menses until the cervical mucus starts appearing. Thereafter the couple is advised to abstain until the fourth day after the "peak mucus day".

This method is safe and there are no side effects. However, this method is associated with high failure rate of approximately 20–25 pregnancies per 100 women years of use. The high failure rate associated with this method commonly results due to irregular ovulation or irregular menstrual cycles.

## Coitus Interruptus (Withdrawal)

This is a method in which the man takes his penis out of the woman's vagina just before he ejaculates. Ejaculation may or may not take place afterwards.

## Symptothermal Method

This method includes the combination of calendar method, BBT and cervical mucus method.

## SIDE EFFECTS

Fertility awareness methods are natural and safe and there are no side effects. Still there are some disadvantages associated with the use of these methods. Some of the disadvantages associated with the use of these methods are as follows:

- These methods require a learning period, careful record keeping, periodic abstinence and partner's cooperation.
- They do not provide protection against HIV infection and other STDs.
- *High failure rate:* Perfect use is associated with a failure rate of 2%, whereas typical use is associated with a failure rate of 20%. These methods are associated with high failure rate of approximately 20–25 pregnancies per 100 women years of use.
- The high failure rate associated with these methods commonly results due to irregular ovulation or irregular menstrual cycles.

# Barrier Method of Contraception

These methods are moderately effective, but one of the most commonly used methods of contraception. These methods aim at creating a type of barrier, which prevents the sperm from meeting the ovum. Barrier contraceptives are associated with a failure rate of 9–30 per 100 women years of use (combined rate of various forms of barrier contraception). Some of the commonly used barrier methods of contraception include male condom, female condom, diaphragm, cervical cap, vaginal sponge and spermicides. Latex condoms provide protection against STDs. Condoms also provide limited protection against HPV that can cause genital warts, thereby lowering the risk for development of cervical dysplasia and cancer. Condoms are not associated with any medical side effects, are inexpensive and easily accessible. They are associated with a pregnancy rate of 10–14 per 100 women years of use. Use of spermicides along with other forms of barrier contraception is likely to reduce the pregnancy rate. Spermicides do not require a prescription, may be discontinued at any time and are safe. While using spermicides, douching should not be allowed for at least 6 hours after coitus.

## MALE CONDOM

A male condom is a thin sheath made of latex or other materials (Fig. 11.2). The man puts the condom on his erected penis, while the condom holds the semen. After having sexual intercourse, the man must carefully take off the condom so that it does not leak. Each condom can be used only once.

## Application of a Male Condom

The man must ensure correct application of condom to ensure its maximum efficacy. While putting on a condom, the rolled up ring must be on the outside and not on the inside. Various precautions, which must be observed to ensure maximal effectiveness of condoms are as follows:
- It must be used with every act of coitus.
- It must be applied before penis has any contact with the vagina.

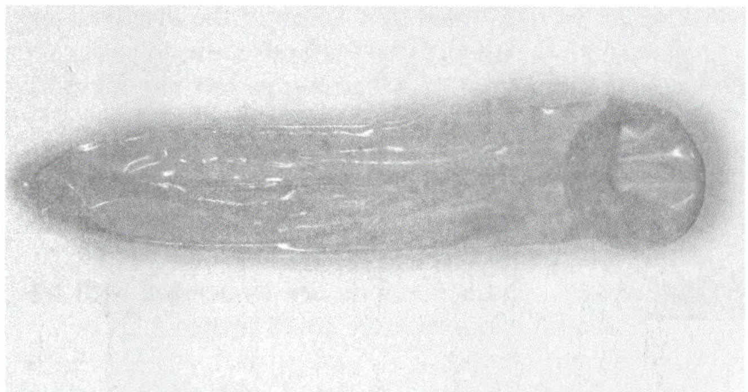

**Fig. 11.2:** An unrolled-up male condom made up of latex

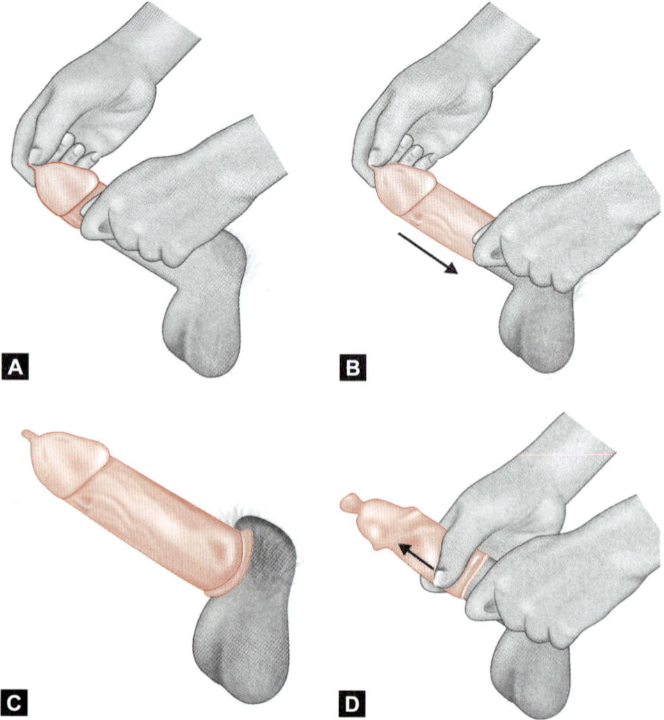

**Figs 11.3A to D:** Application of male condom

- Withdrawal must occur with the penis still erect.
- The base of the condom must be held at the time of withdrawal to prevent it from slipping out. The man puts the condom on his erected penis, while the condom holds the semen. The process of application of male condom is described in Figures 11.3A to D. After having sexual intercourse, the man must carefully take off the condom so that it does not leak. Each condom can be used only once. In order to improve the contraceptive effect of condoms, spermicides can be used alongside either in form of intravaginal application or in form of condom lubricated with a spermicide.

## FEMALE CONDOM

Female condom comprises of strong, soft, transparent polyurethane sheath, which is inserted in the vagina before sexual intercourse (Fig. 11.4). It is approximately 15 cm in length and 7 cm in diameter. It has two flexible rings, the inner ring and an outer one. The inner ring at the closed end of the condom eases insertion into the vagina, covering the cervix and holding the condom in place. The outer ring, which is larger than the inner one, stays outside the vagina and covers part of the perineum and labia during intercourse. Female condom is available under the brand names of Reality®, Femidom®, Dominique®, etc.

Similar to the male condom, female condom also helps to prevent pregnancy and STDs as it is impermeable to HIV, cytomegalovirus and hepatitis B virus. The pregnancy rate with a female condom is higher than that with a male condom. Female condoms may be expensive or limited in their availability and may be difficult to insert.

### Application of a Female Condom

The female condom is inserted in the vagina just before sexual intercourse. The female condom is made of polyurethane sheath and comprises of a polyurethane ring at each end.

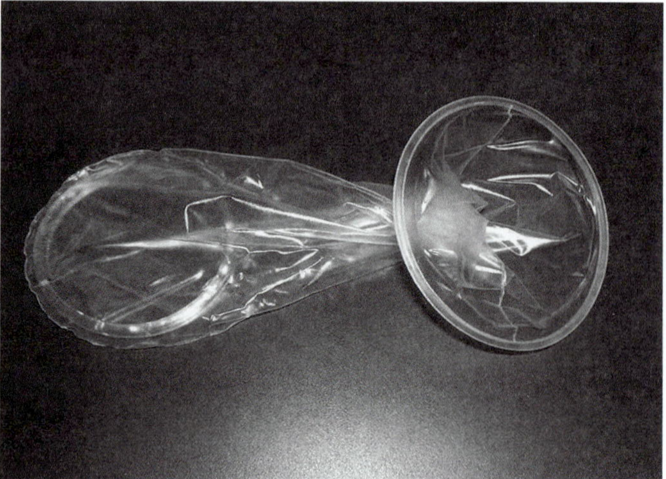

**Fig. 11.4:** Female condom

The open ring remains outside the vagina whereas the closed external ring is fitted behind the symphysis and beneath the cervix like a diaphragm. The method of application of female condom is described in Figures 11.5A to F. Before inserting the condom through the vagina, the inner ring of the condom must be squeezed with the help of thumb and middle finger so that it becomes long and narrow. The inner ring must be then gently guided with help of fingers through the vaginal opening as far as possible towards the cervical opening. The outer ring should remain on the outside of the vagina, covering the vulva partially. At the time of sexual intercourse, the erect penis must be directed into the condom so that it does not slip into the vagina outside the condom. At the time of insertion, the woman can be sitting, squatting or be lying down.

The condom must be inserted straight and not be twisted inside the vagina. The female condom must be lubricated well prior to use. Female condoms can be safely used with water or silicone-based lubricants. Male and female condoms must not be used together because they are likely to slip, tear or become displaced. Since the female condoms cover part of the vulva, they also provide protection against human papillomavirus and herpes.

## DIAPHRAGM

A diaphragm is a shallow rubber dome with a firm flexible rim (Fig. 11.6). It is often used in combination with contraceptive jelly, spermicide, etc. Though it is available in many sizes ranging from 50 mm to 105 mm, the most commonly used size in clinical practice is 75 mm. It is an immediately effective and reversible method of contraception, which can be inserted up to 6 hours before intercourse. It should remain in place for at least 6 hours after the intercourse. However, it must not be left inside the vagina for more than 24 hours.

Different types of cervical diaphragms are available. It is made either of latex or silicone. Various types of cervical diaphragms include latex arcing spring, coil spring, flat spring and silicone wide seal rim.

## Application of Cervical Diaphragm

The application of a cervical diaphragm involves the following steps: The ring of the diaphragm is lubricated and then folded so that the two sides of ring are touching each other. The vulva is opened with one hand; the other hand is used to gently guide the folded diaphragm inside the vagina and to direct its placement towards the posterior fornix so that the dome of the diaphragm covers the cervical opening. The anterior rim of the diaphragm must be directly behind the pubic bone.

When the diaphragm is properly fitted, the patient should not be able to feel anything. The patient should be instructed to use spermicidal jelly inside the cup of diaphragm in order to improve its contraceptive efficacy. The cervical diaphragm should not have any holes or tear. After use, it must be removed, washed with soap and water, rinsed, dried and stored in an airtight container.

## CERVICAL CAP

A cervical cap is a soft, deep rubber cup with a firm, round rim that fits snugly over the cervix (Fig. 11.7). The cap provides effective contraception for 48 hours. The cervical cap acts as a

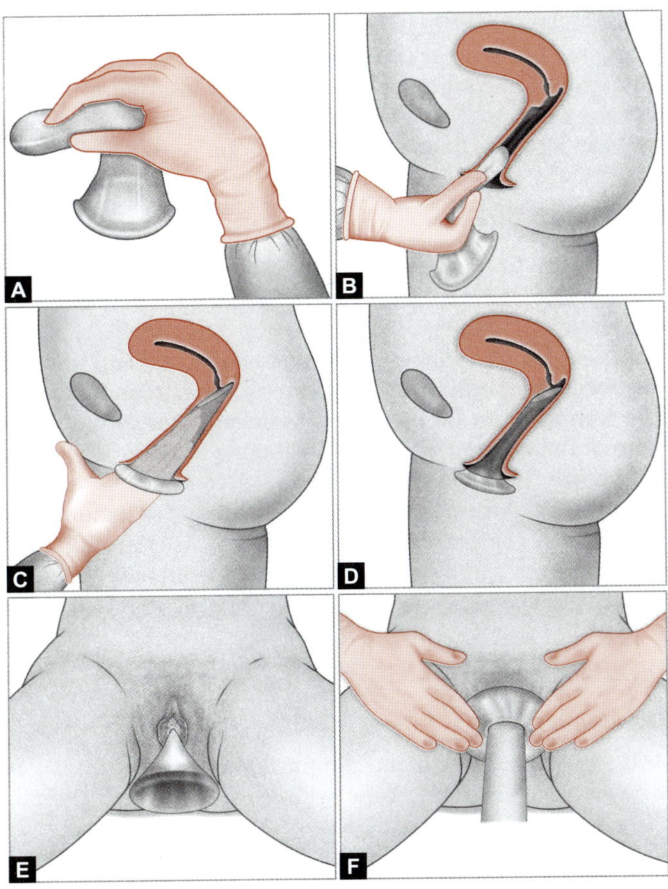

**Figs 11.5A to F:** Method of application of female condom

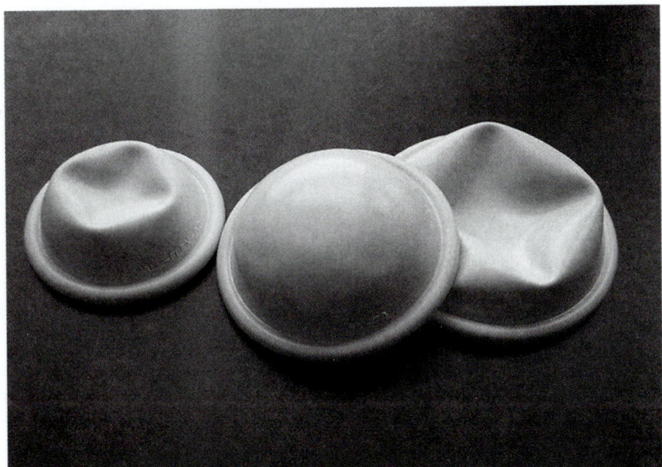

**Fig. 11.6:** Cervical diaphragm

physical barrier between the sperm and egg by fitting snugly over the cervix. It must be inserted at least 15 minutes prior to intercourse and must be kept in place for a minimum of 6–8 hours but can be left in place for up to 48 hours, following which, it should be removed. Pregnancy rate have been found to vary between 11% and 32%. A health care professional may be required to fit the cervical cap for a young girl.

Prior to insertion, the health care provider must perform a pelvic examination to determine size of the cap that would be right for her. The health care provider can then teach her how to insert and remove the cap. Prior to insertion, hands must be thoroughly washed. Also, after each time of use, the cap must be washed with soap and water, rinsed and dried and then stored in a case.

## CONTRACEPTIVE SPONGE

Sponge is a safe, nonhormonal form of contraception, which provides protection for nearly 24 hours. The contraceptive sponge is marketed under the brand name of Today's sponge® (Fig. 11.8) in the United States.

### *Mechanism of Action*

Besides acting as a physical barrier, it also contains a spermicidal agent (nonoxynol-9). The sponges provide contraceptive action by two ways. One is by preventing the sperms from moving inside the cervix. Second is the presence of spermicide in the sponge, which causes immobilization of the sperms. Success rate with the use of Today's sponge® have been found to vary between 77% and 91%.

### *Method of Use*

Prior to insertion, the sponge must be soaked in water so that it gets completely wet. This causes activation of the

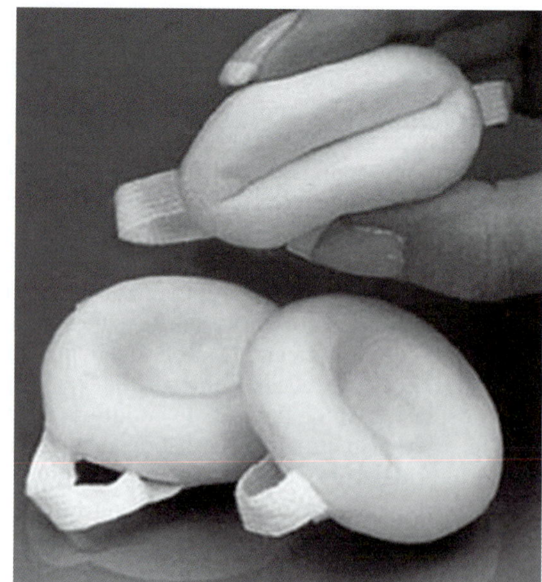

**Fig. 11.8:** Today's sponge

spermicidal agent. Then it is inserted inside the vagina so that it covers the cervix. It can be inserted up to 24 hours before the sexual intercourse. It should remain inserted for about 6 hours following sexual intercourse. However, it should not be worn for more than 30 hours in one go.

## SPERMICIDES

Two basic components of spermicides include active spermicidal agents such as surfactants (Nonoxynol-9, Octoxynol-9, Menfegol, etc.) and the base (carrier) agent such as foams, jellies, creams, foaming tablet, melting suppositories, aerosols, soluble films or vaginal suppositories. The woman must be instructed to insert the recommended dose of the spermicide deep into vagina to cover the cervix completely, just before having sexual intercourse.

A second dose of spermicide may be required if more than 1 hour passes before she has sexual intercourse. An additional application of spermicides is needed for each additional act of intercourse.

## SIDE EFFECTS OF BARRIER CONTRACEPTION

### *Condoms*

*Male condoms*: Some of the complications include:
- Condoms can interrupt with sexual activity, thereby interfering with sexual pleasure.
- Condoms may sometimes tear or leak and can cause an allergic reaction.

*Female condoms*: May be expensive or limited in their availability and may be difficult to insert.

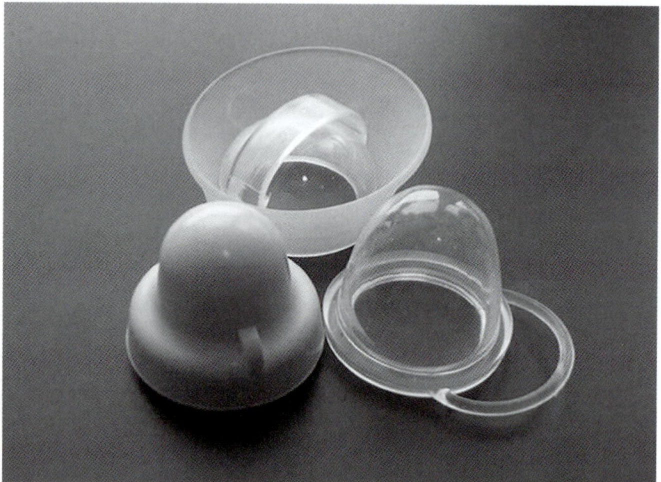

**Fig. 11.7:** Cervical cap

## Diaphragm

Some of the complications associated with the use of diaphragm include:

- The diaphragm is not an appropriate method if the man or woman has allergy to rubber, latex or spermicide, or if the woman has frequent urinary tract or bladder infections and/or anatomical abnormalities.
- May be difficult to insert and remove.
- May cause irritation in the vagina.

## Cervical Cap

Some complications associated with the use of cervical cap include:

- Toxic shock syndrome.
- Unpleasant odor.
- Discomfort and awareness of the cap during coitus.
- Accidental dislodgment.

## Spermicides

Some complications associated with the use of spermicidal agents include:

- May cause irritation in the vagina or on the penis, or an allergic reaction.
- They cause interruption of sexual activity
- They do not provide protection against STDs.

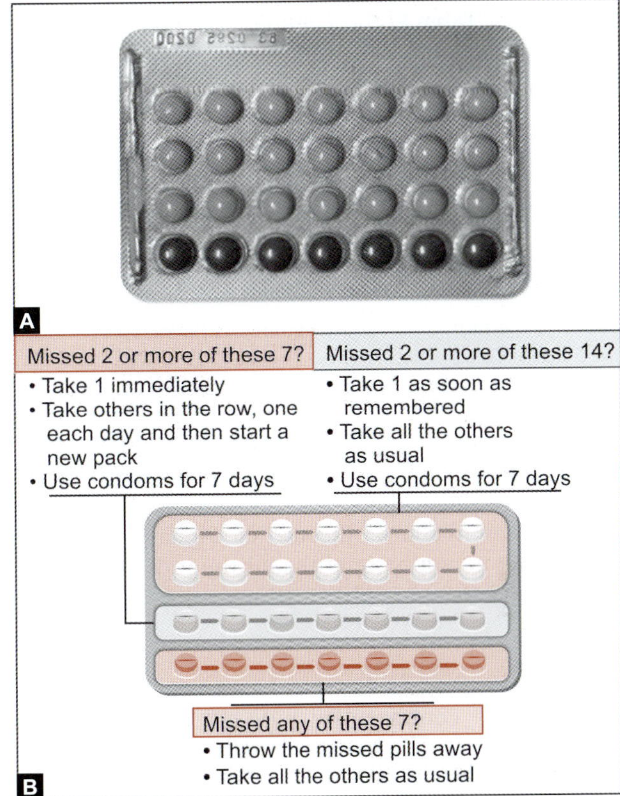


**Figs 11.9A and B:** Pack of combined oral pills

# Hormonal Method of Contraception

There are two main types of hormonal contraception, one being the combined hormonal contraception (containing both estrogen and progestogen), commonly available as COCPs, and the other being formulations containing progestogen only. Besides being available in form of pills, combined hormonal contraceptives can also be available in form of patch or ring. While the pill is used on a daily basis, patch can be used on a weekly basis, and a ring can be used on a monthly basis.

# Combined Oral Contraception Pills

Three types of COCPs formulations are available: (1) monophasic pills, (2) biphasic pills and (3) triphasic pills. Monophasic pills are COCPs laving the same amount of estrogen and progestin in each achive pill in a pack. Most COCPs are contained in a compact package of 21 active pills and 7 inactive pills (Figs 11.9A and B). However, some 21-day packages may not contain any inactive pills. Side effects of oral contraceptive pills are related to the amount of estrogen present in them. The newer COCPs contain lower amounts of estrogen along with the latest third generation progestogen.

The newer progestogens have a higher efficacy and a better side effects profile.

Most COCPs available in the market contain a combination of ethinyl estradiol in the dosage of 20–30 μg along with an orally active progestogen, which is 19-norsteroid (levonorgestrel). The two COCPs available free of cost in India are Mala D and Mala N. While Mala D contains 0.5 mg of D-norgestrel, Mala N contains 1 mg norethisterone. Composition of some commonly available COCPs is described in Table 11.5.

Use of COCPs is a highly effective method of reversible contraception with the failure rate being approximately 0.1 per 100 women years of use. However, COCPs do not provide any protection against STDs or HIB infection. Normal menstrual cycles are likely to occur in 99% of the women within 6 months of stopping the pills. The use of COCPs provides a protective effect against the development of ovarian and endometrial cancer, and probably even colorectal cancer. There is no evidence that the COCPs cause teratogenic effects if taken inadvertently during pregnancy. Normal menstrual cycles are likely to occur in 99% of the women within 6 months of stopping the pills. However, return of fertility may be slightly late due to delayed return of ovulation.

**Table 11.5:** Composition of some commonly available monophasic combined oral contraceptive pills

| Commercial name | Composition | | Pack presentation |
|---|---|---|---|
| | *Estrogen* | *Progestin* | |
| Mala N® (Govt. of India) | Ethinyl estradiol (30 µg) | Norethisterone (1.0 mg) | 21 active pills + 7 iron tablets |
| Mala D® (Govt. of India) | Ethinyl estradiol (30 µg) | D-Norgestrol (0.5 mg) | 21 active pills + 7 iron tablets |
| Novelon® (Schering-Plough) | Ethinyl estradiol (30 µg) | Desogestrel (0.15 mg) | Pack of 21 pills |
| Femelon® (Schering-Plough) | Ethinyl estradiol (20 µg) | Desogestrel (0.15 mg) | Pack of 21 pills |
| Loette® (Wyeth) | Ethinyl estradiol (20 µg) | Levonorgestrel (0.1 mg) | Pack of 21 pills |
| Yasmin® (Schering) | Ethinyl estradiol (30 µg) | Drospirenone (3 mg) | Pack of 21 pills |

*Phasic pills:* In order to reduce side effects and increase compliance associated with the use of COCs, pills containing different amount of hormones over 2 weeks (biphasic pills) or 3 weeks (triphasic pills) were introduced. The available evidence does not favor the use of triphasic or biphasic pills over the monophasic ones and the present trend is to continue using the monophasic variety.

## Mechanism of Action

Combined oral contraceptive pills act through following mechanisms:
- Prevention of ovulation.
- Thickening of mucus at the cervix so that sperms cannot pass through.
- Changing the environment of the uterus and fallopian tubes to prevent fertilization and/or implantation.

## Preprescription Assessment

The following need to be done before the prescription of COCPs:
- *Patient assessment:* Before prescription of COCPs, a thorough history should be taken as described previously.
- Adequate counseling prior to initiation of COCPs may help to improve compliance and adherence.

## Prescription

Conventionally, the COCPs must be started during the first 5 days of the menstrual cycle. Once a woman has started taking a COCP, it is important for her to be consistent and take the pill regularly at the same time each day. Women who use a 21-day preparation need to take the pills for 21 days followed by a 7-day pill-free interval. She should be cautioned not to exceed the 7-day pill-free interval between packs. Most clinicians now recommend start taking the pills from the first day of menses. This assures immediate protection.

Another method for starting the COCPs is the quick-start method. In this method, the patient is asked to take the pill immediately on the same day. This method is associated with a better patient compliance. However, in these cases pregnancy must be ruled out first before starting the pills. A backup method must be used during the first week.

### Missing the Pill

*One pill is missed:* If the woman forgets to take one tablet in a 21-day period, she should take the missed pill as soon as possible. The next pill is taken as usual.

*Two pills are missed:* If two pills are missed during the first 2 weeks, the woman must be instructed to take two pills daily for the next 2 days and then finish the pack as usual. It is unlikely that a backup method may be required, but nevertheless it is usually advised for 7 days.

If two pills are missed during the third week, a backup method of contraception must be immediately used for next 7 days. In case the woman is a day 1 starter, she must be asked to start a new pack.

*Three or more pills are missed:* If the woman is a day 1 starter, she should start a new pack immediately. A backup method must be used for 7 days. Backup method of contraception (e.g. condoms, foam, etc.) may also be required in case the woman exceeds the pill-free interval of 7 days; misses more than one tablet in a cycle; experiences a serious adverse effect or requires protection from STDs.

*Vomiting or diarrhea:* If the patient experiences vomiting or diarrhea after taking the pill, it should be dealt with as if the patient has missed taking a pill.

## Follow-Up

Follow-up visit after 6 weeks is required to check patient compliance and well-being.

## Contraindications

Contraindications to the use of oral contraceptive pills are as follows:
- History of cardiac disease/hypertension.
- Smoker over the age of 35 years.

- History of diabetes (alteration of carbohydrate tolerance)
- Chronic liver disease.
- Breast cancer/thyroid disease.
- Patient on enzyme-inducing drug (e.g. rifampicin).
- Lactating woman.
- Monilial vaginitis.

## Side Effects

*Minor side effects:* These include clinical features such as irregular bleeding, breast tenderness, nausea, weight gain and mood changes.

*Major risks:* These include side effects such as venous thromboembolism, myocardial infarction, stroke, gallbladder disease, breast cancer, cervical cancer, etc.

The patient should be counseled to report any adverse effects related to the use of COCPs, which can be remembered with the mnemonic ACHES:

- A—Abdominal pain (severe).
- C—Chest pain (severe), cough, shortness of breath or sharp pain upon breathing.
- H—Headache (severe), dizziness, weakness or numbness (especially one-sided).
- E—Eye problems (complete loss of or blurring of vision).
- S—Severe leg pain (calf or thigh).

# Progestogen-Only Contraception

Progestogen-only containing contraceptive methods is available in various formulations:

- *Progestogen-only pill (POP) or minipill:* The POPs may contain 350 μg of norethisterone or 75 μg of norgestrel or 30 μg of levonorgestrel.
- Subdermal contraceptive implants (Norplant I, II and Implanon).
- Progestogen-only injectables (POIs), e.g. depot-medroxyprogesterone acetate (DMPA).
- Intrauterine system (Mirena and Progestasert).
- Injectable contraceptives.

## Progestogen-Only Pill

Progestogen-only pills have lower effectiveness than COCPs (pregnancy rate of 2–3 per 100 women years of use). Cerazette® is an estrogen-free, progestogen-only oral contraceptive pill containing 75 μg of desogestrel.

## Mechanism of Action

Progestogen-only pill acts through the following mechanisms:

- Inhibition of follicular development and ovulation.
- Thickening of cervical mucus, thereby reducing sperm viability and penetration.
- Making the endometrium unfavorable to implantation.

### Prescription

Progestogen-only pills must be started within 5–7 days of menstruation. Unlike the COCPs, these pills must be taken on a continuous basis without any breaks between packets. These must be consumed in accordance with a strict time schedule every day (within 3 hours vs 12 hours for COCPs). A backup method should be used for 2 days if a woman is more than 3 hours late taking a dose.

Backup contraception should be considered during the first month when the woman first starts taking minipills and then at mid-cycle every month thereafter (the time when ovulation is likely to occur).

### Side Effects

Use of POPs is associated with the following side effects:

- Irregular bleeding, spotting, break through bleeding, etc.
- Depression, headache, migraine.
- Weight gain and ectopic pregnancy.
- Mastalgia (breast tenderness).
- Mood swings.
- Abdominal cramps.

Unlike the COCPs, minipills are not associated with an increased risk of complications such as deep vein thrombosis or heart disease. Minipills are recommended over COCPs in women who are breastfeeding because they do not affect milk production.

## Progestogen-Only Injectables

These comprise of delivering certain hormonal drugs in form of deep intramuscular injections into the muscles of arms or buttocks. Two types of injectable contraceptives are available: progestogen-only formulations and combined formulations. The POIs contain only the hormone, progestogen. Two main types of POIs are DMPA and norethisterone enanthate (NET-EN). Combined formulations (e.g. Mesigyna, Cyclofem, etc.) on the other hand, contain both progestogen and estrogen.

Injectable contraceptives provide women with safe, highly effective and reversible contraceptive protection with the failure rate being 0.1–0.4%. They overcome the inconvenience of daily compliance required with POPs or COCP. This is a suitable method for women in whom estrogens present health risks. POIs can be used by breastfeeding women at 6 weeks postpartum without adverse effects on nursing infants. Fertility is not impaired after discontinuation of DMPA or NET-EN, although its return may be delayed. They do not provide protection against HIV and STDs.

*Mechanism of action:* The mechanism of action of injectable progestogens is similar to that of POPs as described previously.

### Prescription

The medicine must be injected into the thigh, buttocks or deltoid muscle four times a year (every 11–13 weeks) and provides pregnancy protection starting a week after the first injection. The injection site should not be massaged afterwards, since this may accelerate absorption of the drug. Since DMPA is an aqueous suspension, a DMPA vial must be shaken vigorously, before it is loaded into the syringe, to resuspend any active ingredient at the bottom of the vial. The syringe should then be checked to ensure that it contains the correct dosage. Any leakage from the syringe should be checked and kept under control.

### Complications

Various complications associated with the use of POIs are as follows:

- *Menstrual irregularities:* Disruptions of the menstrual cycle include abnormalities such as amenorrhea, prolonged menses, spotting between periods, and heavy or prolonged bleeding.
- *Other side effects:* These include adverse effects such as weight gain, headache, dizziness and low bone mass.

# Subdermal Implants

Contraceptive implant is a method of birth control, where the device is inserted under the skin. Pregnancy rate varies from 0.2 to 1.3 per 100 women years. Return of fertility with the use of subdermal implants is almost immediate following the removal of capsules. It does not harm the quality and quantity of the breast milk and can be used by nursing mothers starting 6 weeks after childbirth. However, these capsules do not provide protection against STDs. Available subdermal implants are as follows:

- Norplant I and Jadelle (Norplant II)
- Implanon®
- Sino-implant II marketed as Zarin, Femplant and Trust.

These implants ensure slow, sustained release of progestogens. It is long-acting form of contraception, which is associated with minimal side effects.

### Norplant I

This contains six silastic capsules made-up of siloxane of the size 34 mm × 2.4 mm with each containing about 36 mg of levonorgestrel (Fig. 11.10). Its effects last for approximately 5 years. The implants release 85 mg of levonorgestrel per day in the first 3 months; 50 mg/day for next 18 months and then gradually levels to about 30 mg/day.

### Norplant II

This comprises of two rods, each containing about 75 mg of levonorgestrel. Each rod is 0.25 cm in diameter and 4.3 cm long. Initially, the progestin is released at 80 μg/day in the first month. This gradually decreases to 50 μg/day by 9

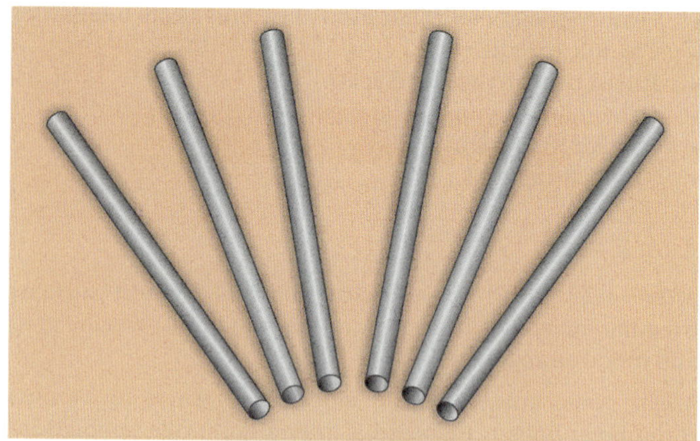

**Fig. 11.10:** Norplant I

months. Thereafter, this reduces to 25–30 μg/day. Norplant II is supposed to provide protection for 3–5 years.

### Implanon/Nexplanon

This is the only type of contraceptive implant available in the USA. It was originally marketed under the brand name Implanon but was consequently amended and marketed as Nexplanon. It is a single rod having dimensions 4 cm by 2 mm, containing 68 mg of a progestogen, etonogestrel (the 3-keto derivative of desogestrel) and usually remains effective for a period of 3 years. Approximately 30 μg of hormone is released daily.

### Levonorgestrel-Implant (Sino-Implant)

Sino-implant comprises of two rods, with each rod containing 75 mg levonorgestrel. The main difference from Norplant II (Jadelle) is that it can be left in place for up to 4 years, whereas Norplant II can be left in place for up to 5 years.

## Mechanism of Action

Mechanism of action of subdermal implants is as follows:
- Thickening of cervical mucus making it difficult for sperm to pass through.
- Inhibition of ovulation.

## Insertion of Implants

The implants are inserted on first day of the menstrual cycle. Following application of a local anesthetic over the upper arm, a needle-like applicator is used to insert the Norplant capsules under the skin (Fig. 11.11). They are inserted subdermally on the medial aspect of upper arm. Since the capsules are nonbiodegradable, they need removal at the end of use or earlier if the side effects are intolerable. Both insertion and

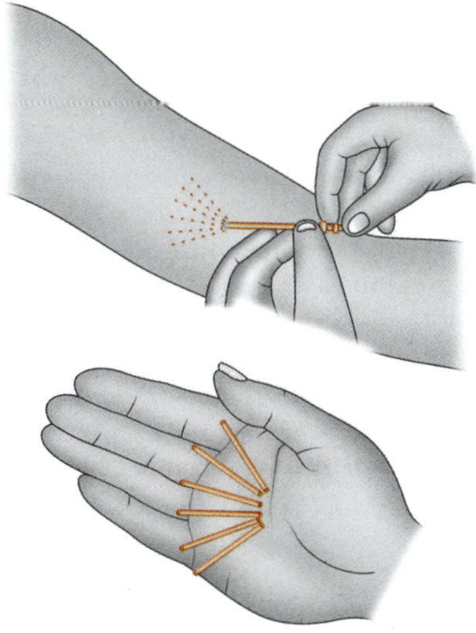

**Fig. 11.11:** Subdermal insertion of Norplant I

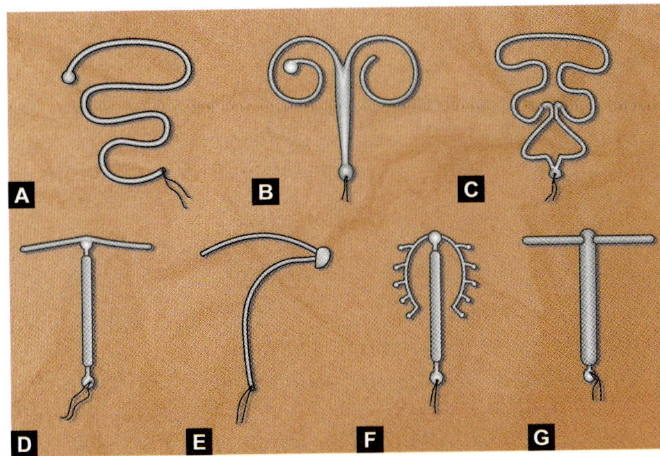

**Figs 11.12A to G:** Different types of intrauterine contraceptive devices. (A) Lippes-Loop; (B) Saf-T-Coil; (C) Dana-Super; (D) Copper-T (Gyne-T); (E) Copper-7 (Gravigard); (F) Multiload; (G) Progesterone intrauterine device (IUD)

removal of these implants requires local anesthesia and a small incision.

## Side Effects

- Side effects profile is similar to those related to POIs, described previously.
- The main disadvantage associated with this form of contraception is that the woman cannot start or stop using this method on her own. Capsules must be inserted and removed in by a specially trained practitioner.
- Some amount of discomfort may be present for several hours following insertion.
- Removal is sometimes painful and often more difficult than insertion.
- Ectopic pregnancy can occur in approximately 1.3% patients.
- This is an expensive form of contraception.

# Intrauterine Contraceptive Devices

Intrauterine contraceptive devices are flexible plastic devices made up of polyethylene, which are inserted inside the uterine cavity for the purpose of contraception. Each device has a nylon thread, which protrudes out through the cervical canal into the vagina, where it can be felt by the patient or the doctor. IUCD is a highly effective method of contraception with the pregnancy rate being 2–6 per 100 women years. Though IUCD is commonly inserted in multiparous women, nulliparity is not a contraindication for IUCD use. It can be successfully used in carefully selected nulliparous women.

Initially, biologically inert devices such as Lippes loop and saf-T-coil were introduced, which have now been withdrawn from the market. Newer devices are medicated and contain substances such as copper, progestogens, etc. Copper carrying devices include copper-T-200, copper-7, multiload, copper-250, copper-T-380, copper-T-220 and nova T. Their effective life varies from 3 years to 5 years (Figs 11.12A to G). IUDs containing progestogen include Progestasert, Levonova and Mirena®. Mirena® is a type of progestogen containing IUCD, having 52 mg of levonorgestrel, which is released at the rate of 20 µg/day. The effects of Mirena® last for about 5 years. It is sometimes also known as levonorgestrel-intrauterine system (LNG-IUS).

## Mechanism of Action

The possible mechanisms of action of IUD are as follows:
- Copper IUCD acts as a foreign body in the uterine cavity, which makes migration of spermatozoa difficult.
- Increased release of prostaglandins provokes uterine contractility. This causes the fertilized egg to be rapidly propelled along the fallopian tube so that it reaches the uterine cavity before the development of chorionic villi and thus is unable to implant.
- Leukocytic infiltration of the endometrium.
- Presence of copper results in certain enzymatic and metabolic changes in the endometrial tissues, which may inhibit implantation of the fertilized ovum.

## Contraindications

Contraindications to the use of IUCDs are as follows:
- Suspected pregnancy.
- Pelvic inflammatory disease.
- Menorrhagia and dysmenorrhea.

- Severe anemia.
- Previous history of ectopic pregnancy.
- Scarred uterus.
- Uncontrolled diabetes (increased risk of pelvic infection)
- Heart disease (increased risk of infection).
- Congenital uterine anomalies (septate uterus/bicornuate uterus).

## Side Effects

The following complications can be associated with the use of IUCD:

- *Difficulties at the time of insertion:* Immediate difficulties at the time of insertion include vasovagal attack, difficulty in insertion of the copper device and presence of uterine cramps.
- *Bleeding:* Irregular menstrual bleeding, spotting, menorrhagia, etc. are the most common side effects of IUCDs in the first month after insertion. Use of NSAIDs or tranexamic acid may be helpful.
- *Pain or dysmenorrhea:* Pain may be a physiological response to the presence of the device, but the possibility of infection, malposition of the device (including perforation) and pregnancy should be excluded. The LNG-IUS has been associated with a reduction in menstrual pain.
- *Systemic hormonal side effects:* These may be typically associated with the LNG-IUS
- *Functional ovarian cysts:* They may occur in up to 30% of LNG-IUS users and usually resolve spontaneously.
- *Uterine perforation:* Uterine perforation is a rare, but serious complication of IUCD insertion, occurring at a rate of 0.6–1.6 per 1,000 insertions. This may occur either at the time of insertion or at a later stage due to the embedment of the device into the myometrium and its subsequent migration into the intra-abdominal cavity. If the IUCD strings are not seen in the cervical os, the device may have been expelled or may have perforated the uterine wall. If the IUCD strings cannot be found, ultrasound is the preferred method to identify the location of the IUCD. If the device is not identified within the uterus or the pelvis, a plain X-ray of the abdomen should be performed to determine whether the device has perforated the uterine wall.
- *Infection:* Infection at the time of insertion can result in the development of PID in the long run. To prevent the occurrence of vaginal infection, IUCD users should continue to use condoms for protection against STDs.
- Actinomyosis infection also occurs commonly.
- *Expulsion:* Expulsion of the IUCD is most common in the first year of use (2–10% of users).
- *Ectopic pregnancy:* Ectopic pregnancy can sometime occur with IUCD in situ.

## INSERTION OF INTRAUTERINE CONTRACEPTIVE DEVICE

### Prior to Insertion

The following steps must be taken prior to the insertion of IUCDs:

- *Informed consent:* Prior to insertion, informed consent should be obtained and the patient should be aware of the potential side effects, benefits and alternative methods of contraception. It should be emphasized to the patient that the IUCD does not provide protection against STIs or HIV.
- *Per speculum and pelvic examination:* A per speculum and pelvic examination must be performed prior to the procedure.

### Insertion

Various parts of a copper IUCD are shown in Figure 11.13, whereas the method for insertion is shown in Figure 11.14. The procedure of copper IUCD insertion comprises of the following steps:

- Under all aseptic precautions, the posterior vaginal wall is retracted with Sims speculum and the anterior lip of cervix is grasped with Volsellum or Allis forceps.
- Length of the uterine cavity is determined with help of an uterine sound.
- The copper device with an insertion tube is available in presterilized packs. The IUCD is mounted into the insertion tube and the flange on the insertion tube is adjusted according to the length of the uterine cavity.
- The insertion tube is then passed into the uterine cavity through the cervix.
- As the solid white rod plunger is put inside the insertion tube, the IUCD recoils within the uterine cavity.

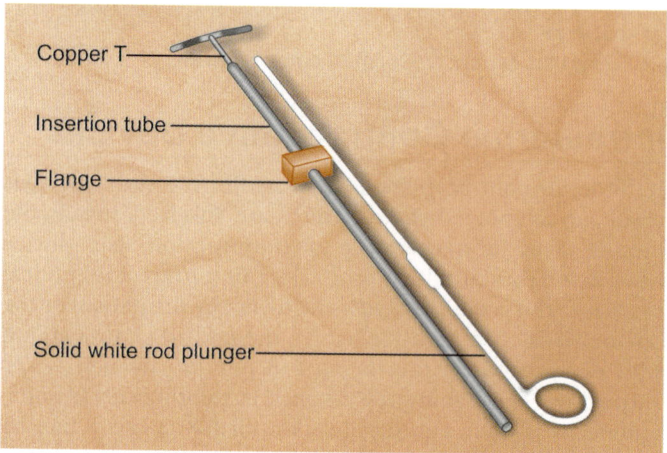


**Fig. 11.13:** Parts of a copper device

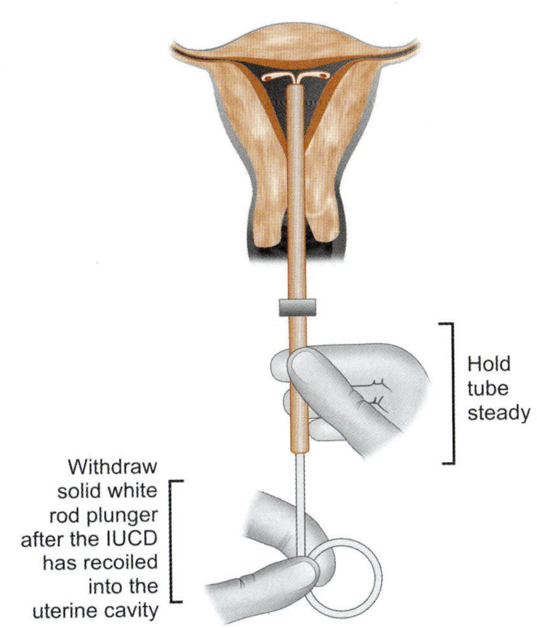



**Fig. 11.14:** Method of insertion of intrauterine contraceptive device (IUCD)

- After withdrawing the plunger, insertion tube is removed and the nylon thread is cut to the required length. The speculum and the forceps are then removed.

## Postinsertion

- The patient is instructed to examine herself and feel for the thread every week.
- A follow-up visit should be scheduled 6 weeks postinsertion for the exclusion of presence of infection, an assessment of any abnormal bleeding, and evaluation of the patient and partner satisfaction.

An IUCD user should be instructed to contact her health care provider if any of the following occur: IUCD's thread cannot be felt; she or her partner can feel the lower end of the IUCD; she experiences persistent abdominal pain, fever, dyspareunia and/or unusual vaginal discharge, etc.

## Emergency Contraception

Emergency contraception (EC) also known as "postcoital contraception" or the "morning-after pill" is a method of contraception, which is used after intercourse and before the potential time of implantation. EC provides women with a safe means of preventing pregnancy following unprotected sexual intercourse or potential contraceptive failure. EC is a backup method for occasional use and should not be used as a regular method of birth control. EC prevents pregnancy and does not interrupt previously established pregnancy. ECs are not a good option for providing long-term contraception and do not protect against STDs. ECs do not increase the risk of ectopic pregnancy, nor do they affect future fertility. Presence of pregnancy (either confirmed or suspected) is a contraindication for the use of EC because it would not be effective in these cases. The various methods for EC are as follows:

1. *Hormonal methods:* This involves the use of emergency contraceptive pills. The various hormonal preparations, which can be used, are:
   - *One containing only the progestin levonorgestrel:* The regimen consists of two doses of 750 µg levonorgestrel taken orally 12 hours apart.
   - *The other containing a combination of ethinyl estradiol and levonorgestrel (Yuzpe method):* This method comprises of the oral administration of two doses of 100 µg ethinyl estradiol and 500 µg levonorgestrel taken 12 hours apart.
2. *Postcoital insertion of a copper-containing IUCD:* The advantage of using copper-containing IUCD is that it is a highly effective method, which can be used up to 5 days of unprotected intercourse. The advantage of using copper-containing IUCD is that it provides continuing contraception even after the initial event.
3. *Antiprogestins:* Drugs such as ulipristal acetate (a selective progesterone receptor modulator) and mifepristone are both antiprogestins and are highly effective for use as EC. They are more effective than progestins due to their ability to delay ovulation as well as inhibition of implantation. Gestrinone also appears to be as effective as mifepristone as an emergency contraceptive agent. In the US, ulipristal acetate is available under the brand name of Ella® which is administered in form of a single oral dose to be taken no later then 120 hours (5 days) after unprotected intercourse.
4. *Investigational drugs:* Some drugs, which have a potential to be used for EC and are still under the investigational stage include prostaglandin inhibitors (e.g. COX-1 and COX-2 inhibitors).

## Indications

Indications for the use of EC are as follows:
- Unwanted pregnancy.
- Failure to use a contraceptive method.
- Condom breakage or leakage.
- Dislodgment of a diaphragm or cervical cap.
- Two or more missed birth control pills.
- Injection of Depo-Provera injection is late by 1 week or more.
- Sexual assault when the woman is not using reliable contraception.

### Preprescription Assessment

A pelvic examination is not a prerequisite to providing EC. There should be no history of recent PID and vaginal or cervical infection. Hormonal EC should be considered for any woman wishing to avoid pregnancy who presents within 5 days of unprotected or inadequately protected sexual intercourse. Although they have generally been used only up to 72 hours after intercourse, both hormonal methods of EC are effective when taken between 72 hours and 120 hours after unprotected intercourse. A postcoital IUCD insertion can be considered up to 7 days after unprotected intercourse. IUCDs containing at least 380 mm² of copper have the lowest failure rate and should be the first-line choice, particularly if the woman intends to continue the IUCD as long-term contraception.

### Prescription

Various options for EC are described in Table 11.6.

The levonorgestrel EC regimen is more effective and causes fewer side effects than the Yuzpe regimen. Moreover, its use does not require a prescription. One double dose of levonorgestrel EC (1.5 mg) is as effective as the regular two-dose levonorgestrel regimen (0.75 mg each dose), with no difference in side effects.

A barrier method such as the condom can be used for the remainder of the current menstrual cycle, and a regular contraceptive method can be initiated at the beginning of the next cycle if the woman desires.

### Side Effects

- The common side effects of hormonal EC are gastrointestinal and mainly include nausea, vomiting, dizziness and fatigue. Antiemetics such as meclizine can be used for controlling these side effects.
- Less common side effects of hormonal methods include headache, bloating, abdominal cramps and spotting or bleeding.
- Possible complications of postcoital IUCD insertion include pelvic pain, abnormal bleeding, pelvic infection, perforation and expulsion.

# Permanent Methods of Contraception

In today's time, surgical sterilization for both men and women has become a popular and well-established method of permanent contraception. Tubal sterilization is a method of permanent sterilization, which causes sterility by blocking a woman's Fallopian tubes. Occlusion of the Fallopian tubes has been considered as the most popular method of female sterilization all over the world. As a result of the blockage of tubes, the sperm and ovum cannot fertilize each other, thereby preventing the occurrence of pregnancy. In the tubal sterilization procedures, the isthmic portion of the Fallopian tube is the most commonly preferred site of occlusion because of the relative ease of reanastomosis at this site, should the reversal be required in future. Both laparoscopic sterilization and minilaparotomy approach are associated with a very-low risk of complications, when performed according to the accepted medical standards. Although the procedure of tubal sterilization is practically irreversible, in dire circumstances the reversal can be attempted using microsurgical techniques. Female sterilization technique has been described in details in Chapter 10.

### Male Method of Sterilization (Vasectomy)

Detailed discussion related to male method of permanent sterilization or vasectomy is beyond the scope of this chapter because this chapter is mainly devoted to female methods of contraception.

| Table 11.6: Various options for emergency contraception | | | |
|---|---|---|---|
| *Drug* | *Dosage* | *Duration of provision of emergency contraception* | *Efficacy (pregnancy prevention rate)* |
| Leveonorgestrel | 0.75 mg given twice, 12 hours apart or given as a single dosage of 1.5 mg | Up to 72 hours of unprotected intercourse | 60–95% |
| Yuzpe regimen | 100–120 µg of ethinyl estradiol + 500–600 µg levororgestrel in each dose given twice, 12 hours apart | Up to 72 hours of unprotected intercourse | 50–90% |
| Mifepristone* | 600 mg single dose | | 99–100% |
| Ulipristal (EllaOne) | Single oral dosage of 30 mg | Provision of emergency contraception up to 72–120 hours of unprotected intercourse | 98–99% |
| Copper IUCD | | Provision of emergency contraception up to 120 hours of unprotected intercourse | At least 99% |

*Note available for emergency contraception in the united states
*Abbreviation:* IUCD, intrauterine contraceptive device

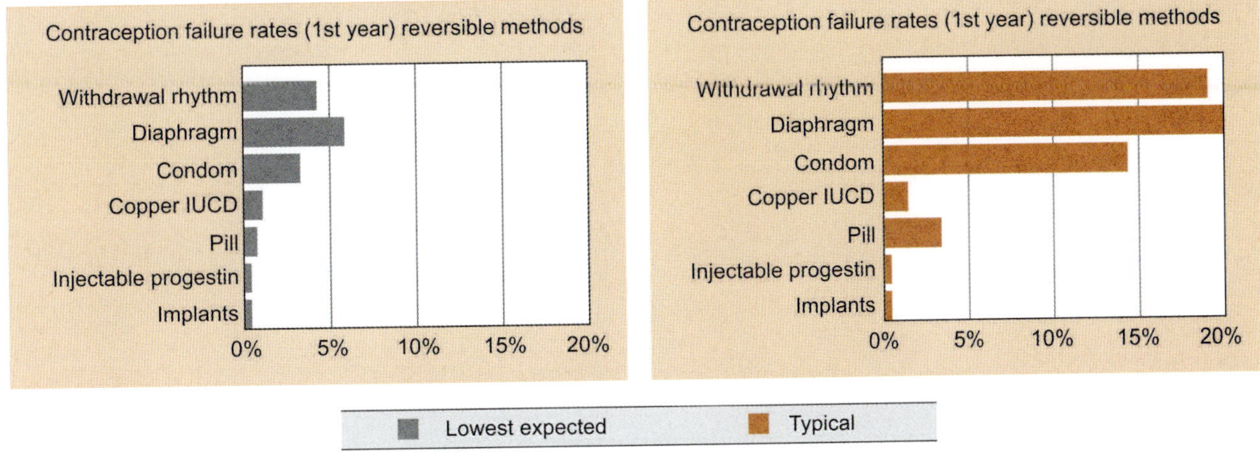



**Fig. 11.15:** Failure rates associated with various methods of contraception

## Failure Rate

Of the various methods of contraception available, some of the most effective methods of contraception include IUCDs, injectable hormones, hormonal implants and permanent sterilization. This is followed by some relatively less effective options such as oral contraceptive pills, hormonal patches and rings. Some of the less effective options include barrier methods (male and female condom, cervical cap, diaphragm, etc.) and natural methods of contraception such as withdrawal method. The prescription of a contraceptive device must be individualized. The type of contraception, which must be prescribed to a particular patient, is the one that provides effective contraception, acceptable cycle control and is associated with least side effects. Failure rate associated with various methods of contraception are illustrated in Figure 11.15. Efficacy of a contraceptive method is calculated with help of pearl's index. Pregnancy failure rate per hundred women years of use (HWY) is calculated with help of the following formula:

$$\text{Pregnancy failure rate /(HWY)} = \frac{\text{No. of accidental pregnancies} \times 1200}{\text{No. of patients observed x months of use}}$$

## FURTHER READINGS

1. ACOG Committee on Practice Bulletins- Gynecology. ACOG practice bulletin. No. 73: Use of hormonal contraception in women with coexisting medical conditions. Obstet Gynecol. 2006;107(6):1453-72.

2. ACOG Practice Bulletin No. 110: Noncontraceptive uses of hormonal contraceptives. Obstet Gynecol. 2010;115(1):206-18.

3. Committee On Adolescence. Emergency contraception. Pediatrics. 2012;130(6):1174-82.

4. American College of Obstetricians and Gynecologists Committee on Gynecologic Practice. ACOG committee opinion. No. 337: Noncontraceptive uses of the levonorgestrel intrauterine system. Obstet Gynecol. 2006;107(6):1479-82.

5. American College of Obstetricians and Gynecologists. ACOG practice bulletin no. 112: Emergency contraception. Obstet Gynecol. 2010;115(5):1100-9.

6. Centers for Disease Control and Prevention. U.S. Medical Eligibility Criteria for Contraceptive Use. (2010). Classification for emergency contraception. [Online] Available from www.cdc.gov/mmwr/pdf/rr/rr59e0528.pdf [Accessed November, 2013].

# Imaging, Instruments, Specimens and Drugs

- Imaging in Obstetrics and Gynecology
- Instruments in Obstetrics and Gynecology
- Specimens in Obstetrics and Gynecology
- Drugs in Obstetrics and Gynecology

# Imaging in Obstetrics and Gynecology

## CHAPTER OUTLINE

- Obstetric Ultrasound
- Gynecological Ultrasound
- Diagnostic Radiology in Obstetrics
- X-rays in Gynecology

## Obstetric Ultrasound

### PREGNANCY SCANNING

#### Gestational Sac at Four Weeks and Three Days of Pregnancy

Ultrasound examination in the first trimester is crucial for establishing intrauterine pregnancy, gestational age, early pregnancy failure, and to exclude other causes of bleeding such as ectopic and molar pregnancy, missed abortion, incomplete abortion, etc. Figure 12.1 shows intrauterine gestational sac at 4 weeks and 3 days of gestation. During normal pregnancy, at the time of transvaginal sonography (TVS), the gestational sac appears first by 4.5–5 weeks; the yolk sac by 5–5.5 weeks; the fetal pole by 5.5–6 weeks and fetal

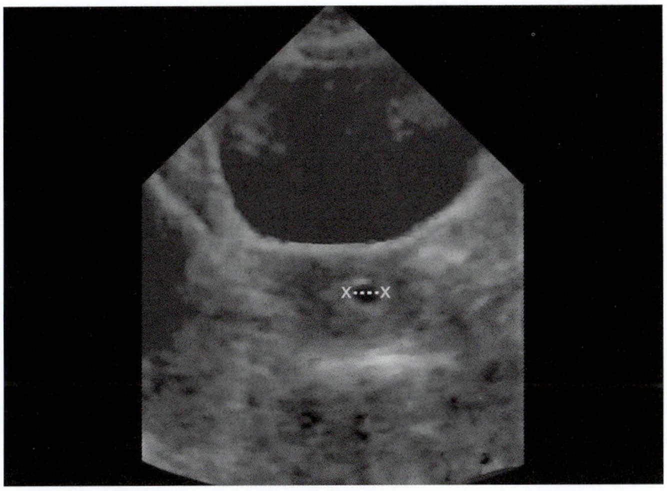

**Fig. 12.1:** Intrauterine gestational sac at 4 weeks and 3 days of gestation

heartbeat by 6 weeks. All these findings are likely to appear 1 week later on the transabdominal scan.

#### Gestational Sac at Five Weeks of Pregnancy

Transvaginal ultrasound is most useful in the first trimester and is of great help especially in fat women and in those with retroverted uterus, in whom transabdominal ultrasound may not be able to visualize pelvic details clearly. Double-rimmed gestational sac can be considered as a sign of intrauterine pregnancy during early weeks of gestation (4–6 weeks) in cases where the embryo or yolk sac has yet not made its appearance. In cases of normal intrauterine pregnancy, hyperechogenic ring of decidua capsularis is surrounded by another hyperechogenic ring (decidua parietalis). The gestational sac appears double rimmed because these two layers of decidua are separated by an anechoic space and fluid within the uterine cavity (Fig. 12.2).

#### Yolk Sac

In a normal intrauterine pregnancy, the yolk sac normally appears by 5–6 weeks of gestation (Fig. 12.3) whereas the embryo appears at about 6 weeks of gestation. The yolk sac appears as a round sonolucent structure surrounded by a bright rim. Yolk sac does not increase to a size more than 6 mm in case of a normal pregnancy. The pregnancy may be considered to be abnormal if no yolk sac appears at the gestational sac size of 10 mm or no fetal pole is seen at the gestational sac size of 18 mm.

#### Fetal Heart at Nine Weeks of Gestation

Fetal heart can be observed on ultrasound by 6–7 weeks of gestation. A detailed four-chamber view (with or without Doppler) can help in delineation of various cardiac defects

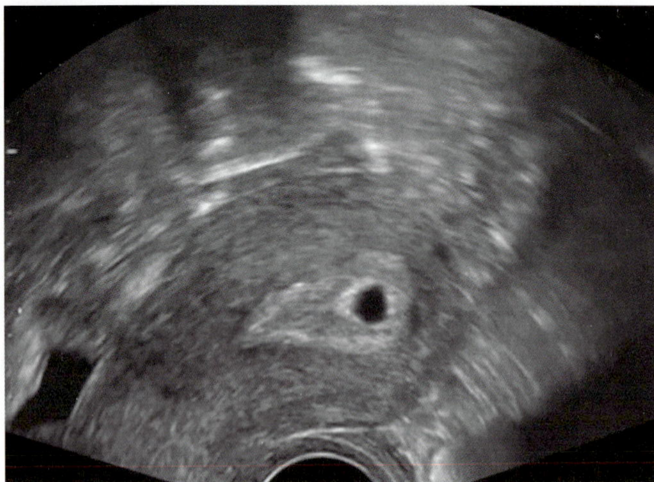

**Fig. 12.2:** Transvaginal scan demonstrating an intrauterine pregnancy at 5 weeks of gestation showing a double-rimmed gestational sac

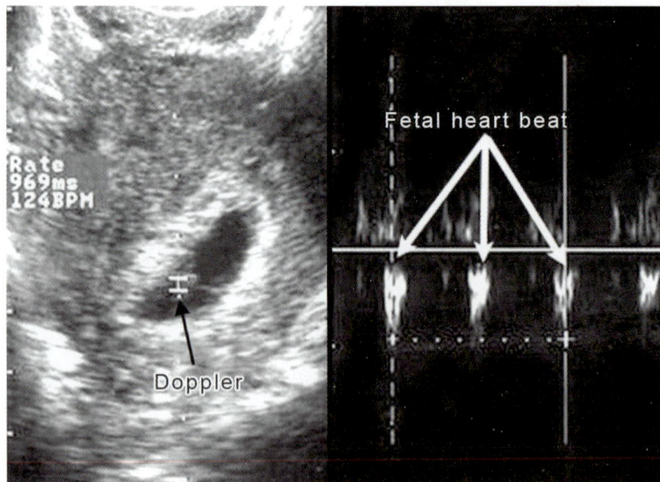



**Fig. 12.4:** Fetal heart at 9 weeks of gestation as observed on Doppler examination

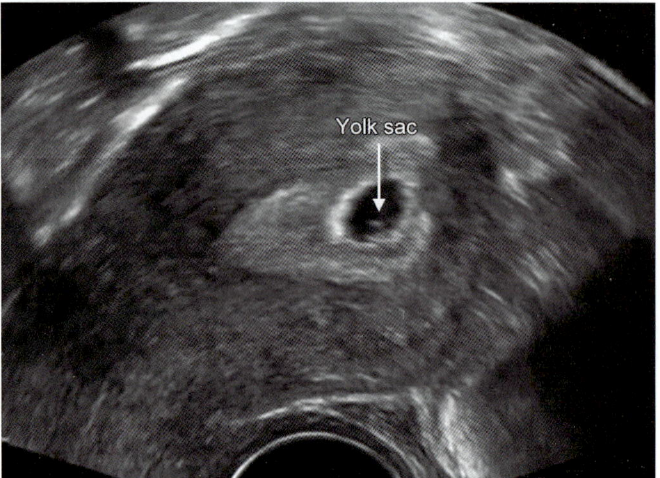



**Fig. 12.3:** Appearance of yolk sac (shown by arrow) on transvaginal sonography at 6 weeks of gestation

(Fig. 12.4). In most of the cases, by the time the embryo measures 2 mm, fetal heart activity may be clearly seen and is as high as 85 beats per minute (BPM), which may increase to 100–175 BPM by 5–9 weeks of gestation. If the fetal pole measures 5 mm or more with no heartbeat, diagnosis of miscarriage is usually made.

### Fetal Spine

Figures 12.5A and B demonstrate the longitudinal and coronal views of fetal spine respectively. Neural tube defects of the central nervous system can be considered as one of the most common congenital malformation. Most scans, aimed towards diagnosing the neural congenital anomalies, are done around mid-gestation (at about 20 weeks of pregnancy).

Longitudinal section of the fetal spine must be performed because it helps in revealing various spinal malformations such as vertebral anomalies and sacral agenesis. Longitudinal section of the spine (at about 14 weeks) demonstrates three ossification centers (one inside the body and one at the junction between the lamina and pedicle on each side). These appear as three parallel lines depending upon the orientation of ultrasound beams. Attempts must also be made to demonstrate the intactness of the skin overlying the spine. Presence of a mass bulging out must also be observed.

### Fetal Abdomen and Heart

The fetal heart can be visualized and it appears to be rhythmically contracting on real-time ultrasound examination. Size, location and arrangement of stomach and diaphragm can also be determined. Fetal abdomen shows presence of stomach bubble. Diaphragm can be visualized as a thin line separating the chest from abdomen. Fetal heart, stomach and diaphragm can be visualized in Figure 12.6.

### Placenta

Figure 12.7 demonstrates an anteriorly placed placenta in fundal region. Placenta is recognized by the presence of chorionic plate. The above-mentioned figure shows a grade 0 placenta. Grading of placenta is as follows:
- *Grade 0 placenta (first and second trimester):* It has uniform echogenicity with a smooth chorionic plate without indentations.
- *Grade I placenta (mid-second trimester to early third trimester):* The chorionic plate shows subtle indentations. There are small diffuse calcifications randomly dispersed throughout the placenta.

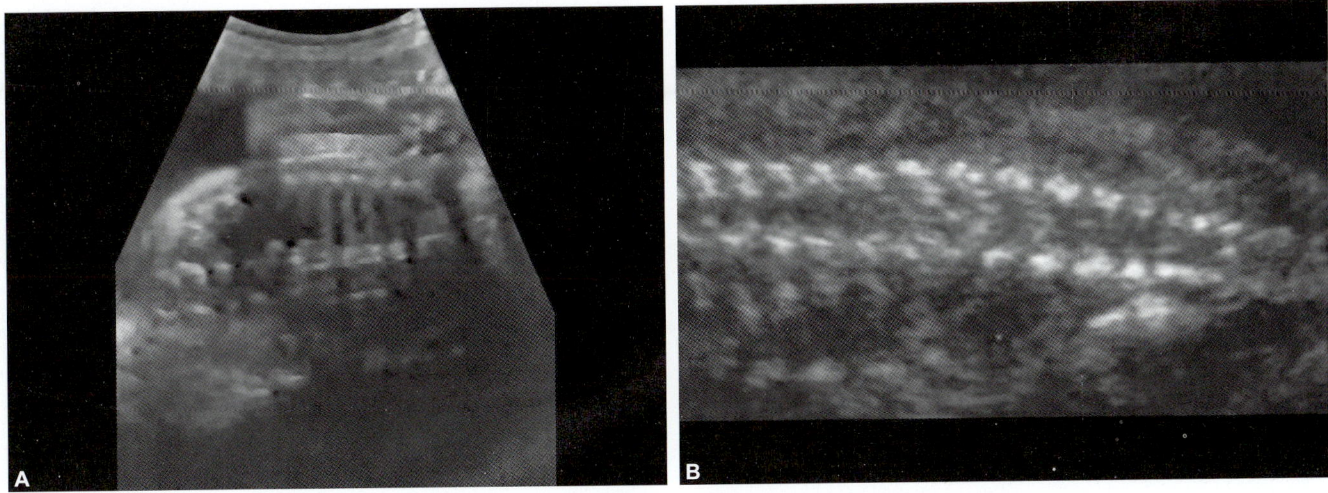

**Figs 12.5A and B:**  (A) Fetal spine in longitudinal section; (B) Coronal view of fetal spine

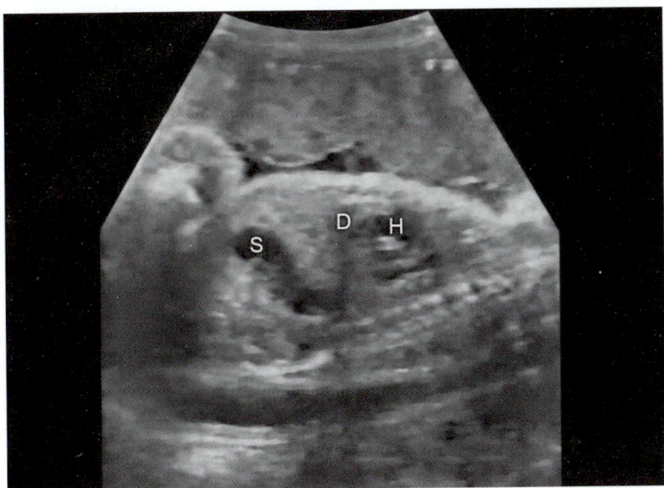

**Fig. 12.6:**  Visualization of fetal heart (H), stomach (S) and diaphragm (D) on transvaginal ultrasound examination

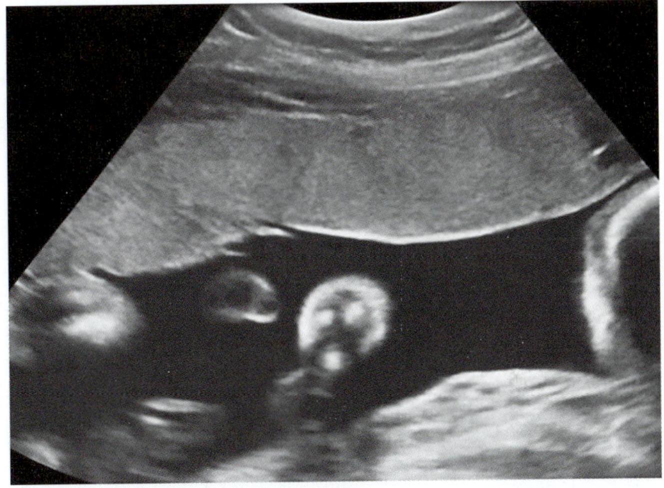

**Fig. 12.7:**  Grade 0 placenta on the ultrasound, placed in the fundal region

- *Grade II placenta (late third trimester):* The indentations throughout the chorionic plate become larger and calcifications also become more prominent.
- *Grade III placenta (39 weeks to postdated):* Complete indentations of the chorionic plate reaching all the way to the basilar plate are present. This results in the formation of cotyledons with a significant increase in the number of calcifications.

## Measurement of Fetal Heart Rate

M-mode is a type of ultrasound, which records moving echoes from the heart (Fig. 12.8). The depth of echo-producing interface is displayed along one axis and time is displayed along the second axis. This information is then interpreted in the form of fetal heart rate. The fetal heart rate at term usually varies between 120 BPM and 160 BPM.

## Four-Chamber View of Fetal Heart

Detailed assessment of the four chambers of fetal heart is usually performed routinely on ultrasound examination in the second trimester (Fig. 12.9). In the fetuses at risk of congenital heart disease (previous history of heart disease in a parent or sibling or presence of noncardiac structural defect), this view may be particularly required. The four-chambered view is obtained in a horizontal section, just above the level of diaphragm.

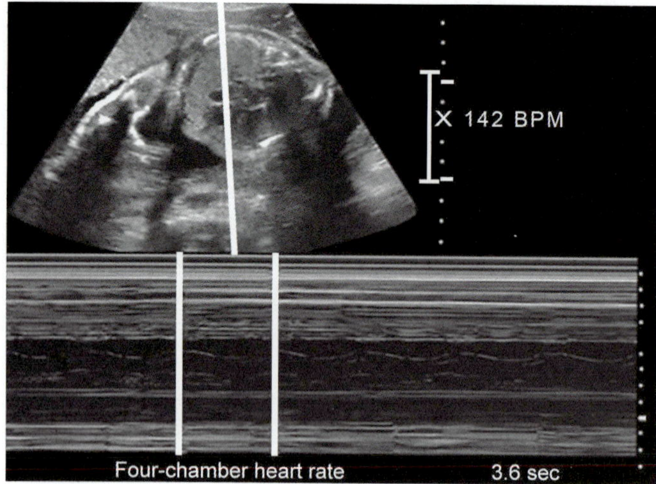

**Fig. 12.8:** Measurement of fetal heart rate using M-mode ultrasound

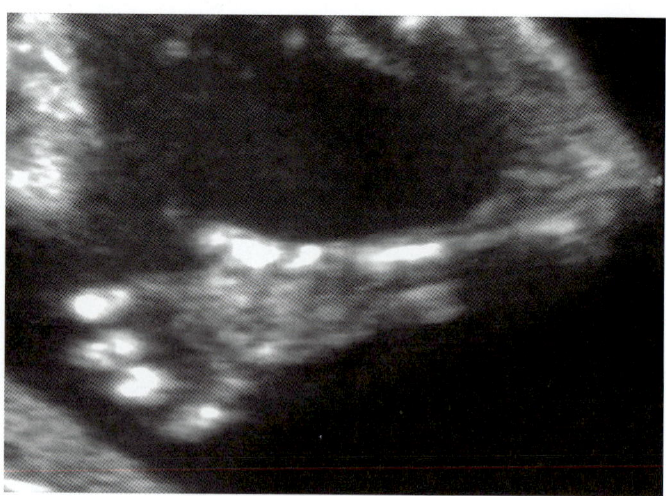

**Fig. 12.10:** Two-dimensional ultrasound scan showing fetal hand and elbow

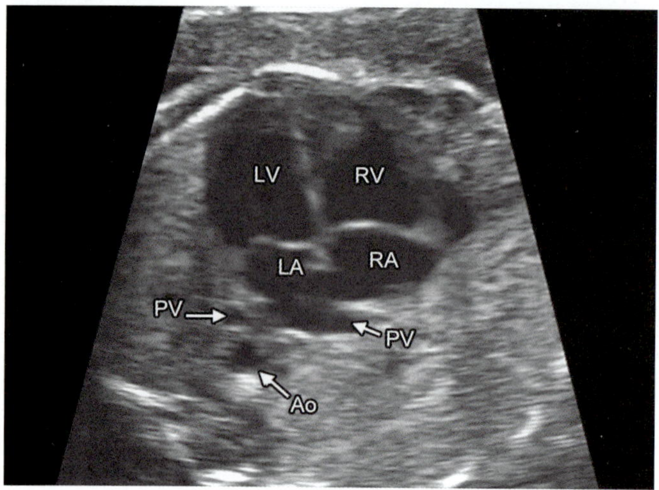

**Fig. 12.9:** Four-chamber view of fetal heart
*Abbreviations:* Ao, Aorta; LA, Left atrium; LV, Left ventricle; PV, Pulmonary vein; RA, Right atrium; RV, Right ventricle

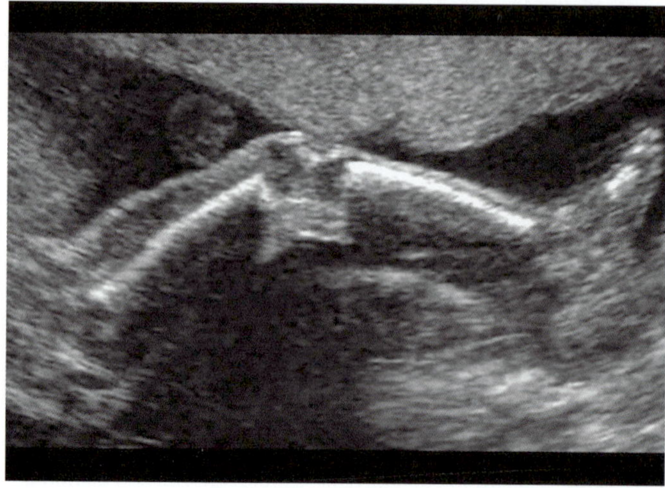

**Fig. 12.11:** Two-dimensional ultrasound scan showing lower limb

## Two-Dimensional Scan Showing Fetal Hands and Elbow

Figure 12.10 illustrates a two-dimensional ultrasound image showing fetal arm with fingers and wrist extended and the elbow slightly flexed. Second trimester ultrasound assessment of fetal fingers at 18–20 weeks of gestation helps in evaluation of various types of congenital anomalies in fetal fingers. Three-dimensional ultrasound of fetal hand in these cases is not essential, but it does enable the parents to identify and understand the lesion, and also enables exploration of future surgical plan by the plastic surgeons.

## Two-Dimensional Scan Showing Fetal Lower Limb

Figure 12.11 shows two-dimensional ultrasound scan demonstrating left lower limb of a 24 weeks of fetus with the hip and knee semi-extended and feet showing presence of five toes. Toes of the feet are examined for presence of abnormalities similar to those found in fingers.

## Term-Fetuses on Two-Dimensional Sonography Scan

Figure 12.12 shows a term-fetus at 40 weeks of gestation in a normal pregnancy. At this time all the organ systems are

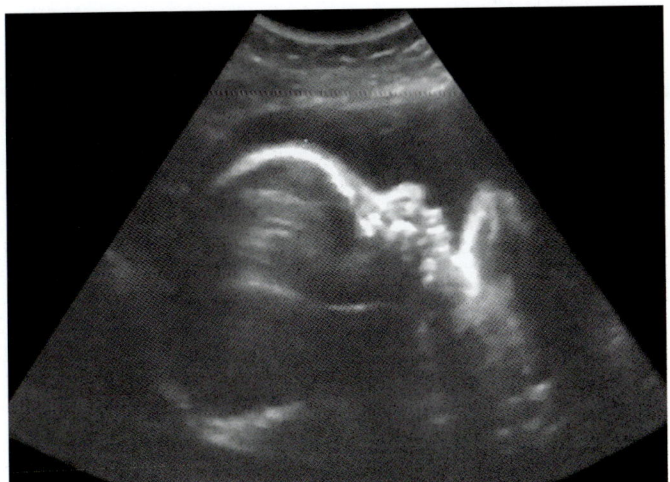

**Fig. 12.12:** Fetus at term as observed on two-dimensional ultrasound scan

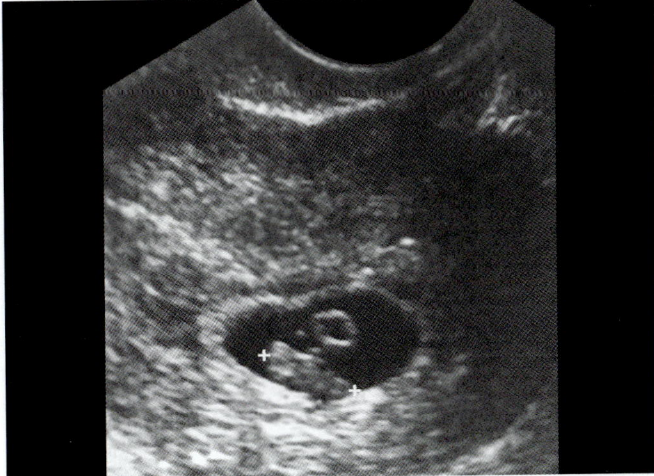

**Fig. 12.13A:** Ultrasound measurement of the crown-rump length

mature enough to facilitate its survival in the extrauterine environment. During this time the fetal weight varies between 2.7 kg and 4.0 kg and fetal length between 50 and 55 cm. The placenta has attained grade 3 maturity and the amount of amniotic fluid appears normal.

## FETAL BIOMETRY

### Crown-Rump Length

*Measurement of the crown-rump length (Figs 12.13A and B):* Crown-rump length (CRL) is an ultrasonic measurement, which is made earliest in pregnancy, when the gestational age is between 7 weeks and 13 weeks. It gives the most accurate measurement of the gestational age. CRL is the longest length of the fetus excluding the limbs and the yolk sac. CRL is about 1 mm at 5 weeks and 4 mm at 6 weeks of normal gestation.

Crown-rump length helps in measuring the length of human embryo starting from the top of head (crown) to the lowest part of the buttocks (rump). Measurement of CRL can help the clinician give an accurate assessment of the woman's expected date of delivery through estimation of her gestational age. Early in pregnancy, the accuracy of determining gestational age though CRL measurement is within ± 4 days but later in pregnancy due to different growth rate of the fetus, the accuracy of determining gestational age with help of CRL decreases considerably.

### Biparietal Diameter

*Measuring the biparietal diameter (Figs 12.14A and B):* Biparietal diameter is the distance between the two sides of the head. It can be measured at the level of the plane defined by the frontal horns of the lateral ventricles and the cavum septum pellucidum anteriorly, falx cerebri in the midline, the thalami symmetrically positioned on either side of the

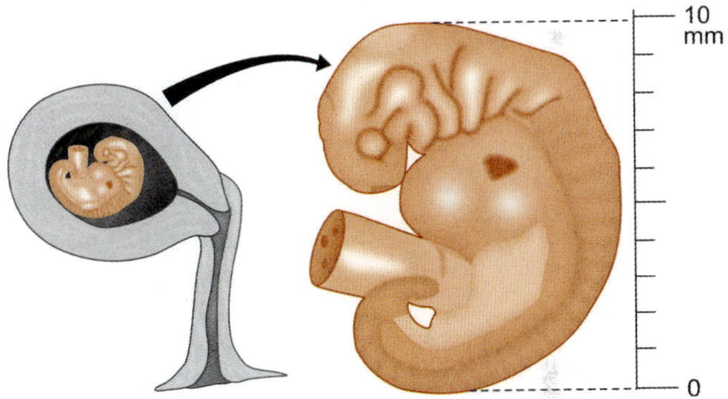

**Fig. 12.13B:** Diagrammatic measurement of the crown-rump length

falx in the center, and occipital horns of the lateral ventricles, Sylvian fissure, cisterna magna and the insula posteriorly. Septum pellucidum can be visualized at one third of the fronto-occipital distance. The measurement is taken from outer table of the proximal skull to the inner table of the distal skull with the cavum septum pellucidum perpendicular to the ultrasound beam.

Biparietal diameter is usually measured after 13 weeks of pregnancy for dating of pregnancy. It increases from about 2.4 cm at 13 weeks to about 9.5 cm at term. A clinician maintaining a chart showing serial measurements of BPD is able to efficiently monitor the fetal growth. The BPD remains the standard against which other parameters of gestational age assessment are compared. At 20 weeks of gestation, accuracy of BPD is within 1 week.

### Abdominal Circumference

*Measuring the fetal abdominal circumference (Figs 12.15A and B):* Abdominal circumference is a measure of fetal abdominal girth. The abdominal circumference is measured in an axial

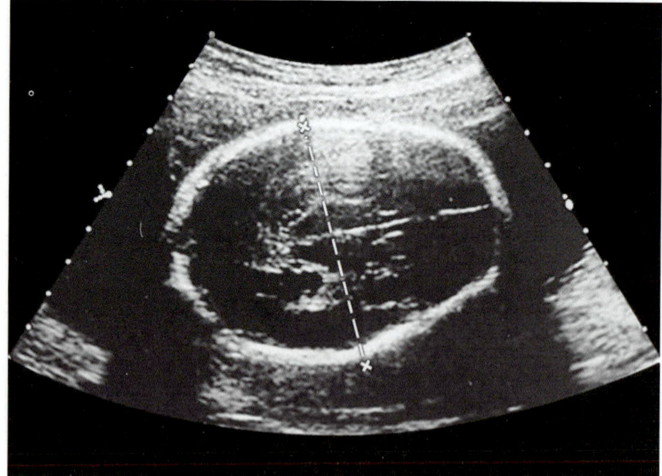

**Fig. 12.14A:** Measuring the biparietal diameter

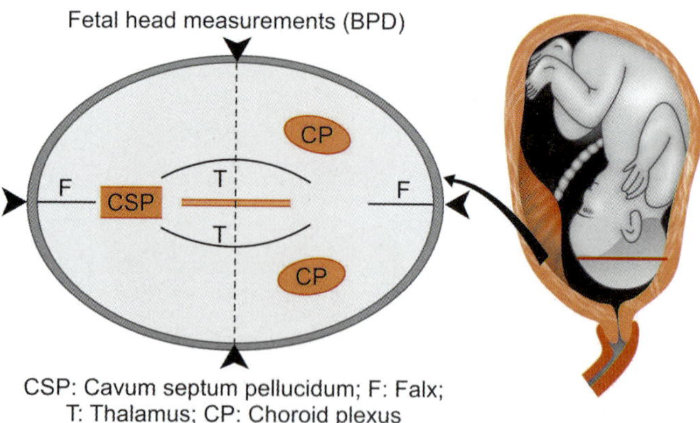



CSP: Cavum septum pellucidum; F: Falx;
T: Thalamus; CP: Choroid plexus

**Fig. 12.14B:** Diagram showing measurement of biparietal diameter

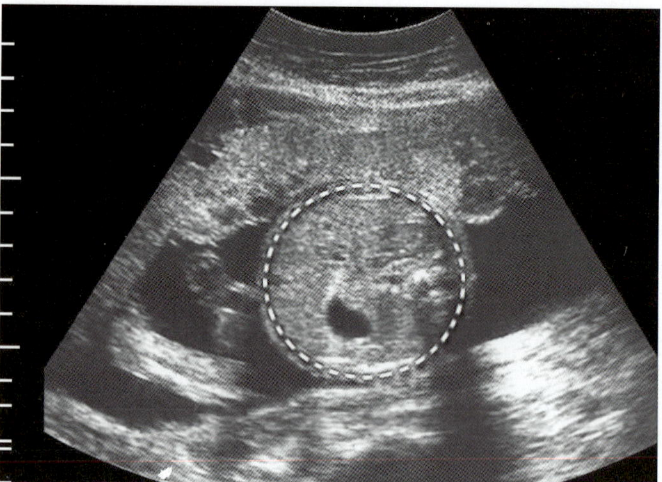

**Fig. 12.15A:** Ultrasound measurement of abdominal circumference

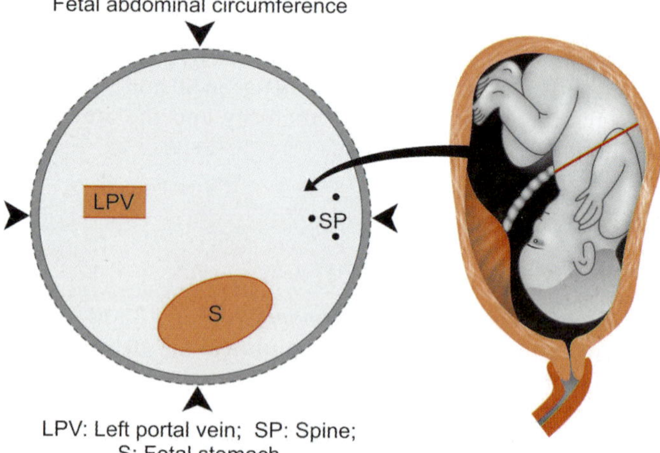



LPV: Left portal vein;  SP: Spine;
S: Fetal stomach

**Fig. 12.15B:** Diagrammatic method for the measurement of
abdominal circumference

plane at the level of the stomach and the bifurcation of the main portal vein into the right and left branches.

While measuring the abdominal circumference, the radiologist must be careful about keeping the section as round as possible and not letting it get deformed by the pressure from the probe.

### Fetal Femur

Femur length is the length of femoral diaphysis, the longest bone in the body and represents the longitudinal growth of the fetus. Femur appears as an echogenic structure on ultrasound examination (Fig. 12.16).

*Measuring the femoral length (Figs 12.17A and B):* At the time of measuring femur length, the femoral diaphysis should be horizontal showing a homogeneous echogenicity.

Femur length is measured from the origin of the shaft to the distal end of the shaft, i.e. from greater trochanter to the lateral femoral condyle. The femoral head and distal femoral epiphysis, which present after 32 weeks are not included

in the measurements. Femur length increases from about 1.5 cm at 14 weeks to about 7.8 cm at term.

## DOPPLER ULTRASOUND

### Doppler Blood Flow Indices

The most commonly used Doppler blood flow indices for pregnancy assessment are as follows (Fig. 12.18):

$$\text{Systolic/diastolic (S/D) ratio:} \frac{\text{Peak systolic blood flow}}{\text{End diastolic velocity}}$$

$$\text{Pulsatility index (PI):} \frac{\text{Peak systolic velocity–end diastolic velocity}}{\text{Mean systolic velocity}}$$

$$\text{Resistance index (RI):} \frac{\text{Peak systolic velocity–end diastolic velocity}}{\text{Peak systolic velocity}}$$

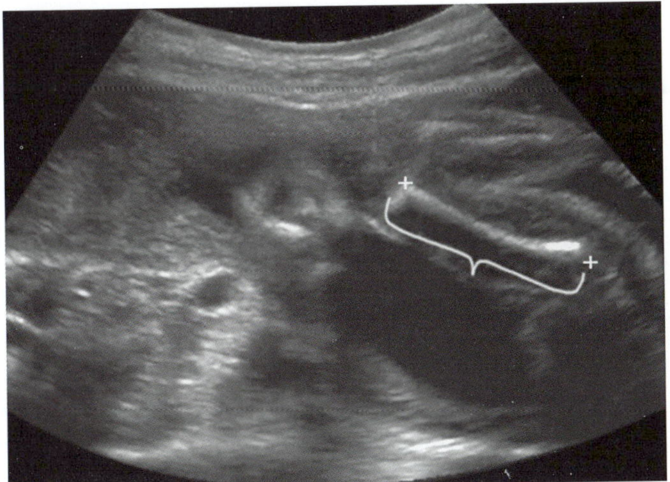

**Fig. 12.16:** Fetal femur on transvaginal sonography

## Normal Blood Flow within the Ovary

On Doppler ultrasound examination of ovaries, perifollicular vascularity can be observed around a preovulatory follicle (Fig. 12.19). Several follicles in various stages of development can be observed. It may be difficult to visualize the complete path of vascular flow around the larger follicles due to the tortuosity of the ovarian vessels and its branches.

## Normal Uterine Perfusion

During a normal pregnancy, there is an increase in the uterine size and vascularity, particularly in the third trimester (Fig. 12.20). The increased uterine vascularity is related to dilatation of uterine vessels and increase in terminal vascular branches. In normal pregnancy, the perfusion of the entire uterofetoplacental circulation is supplied by the uterine vessels.

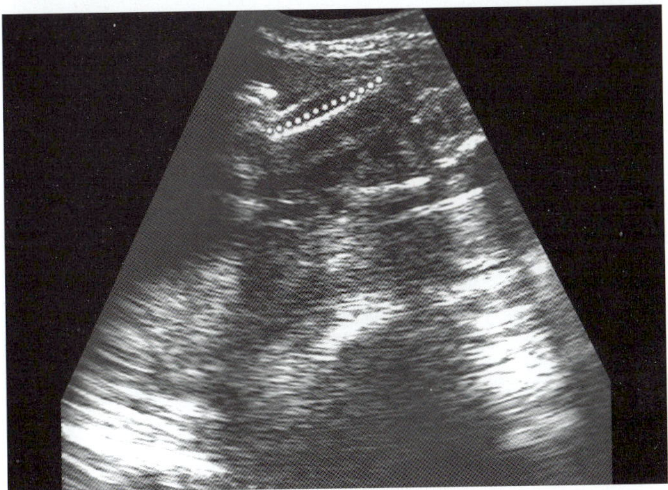

**Fig. 12.17A:** Measurement of femur length

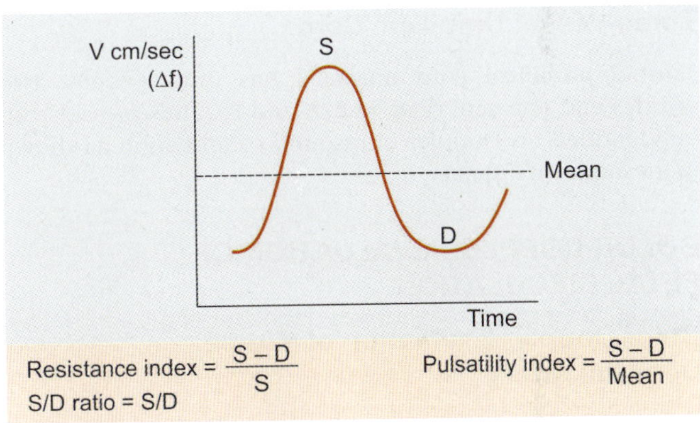



**Fig. 12.18:** Description of various Doppler indices

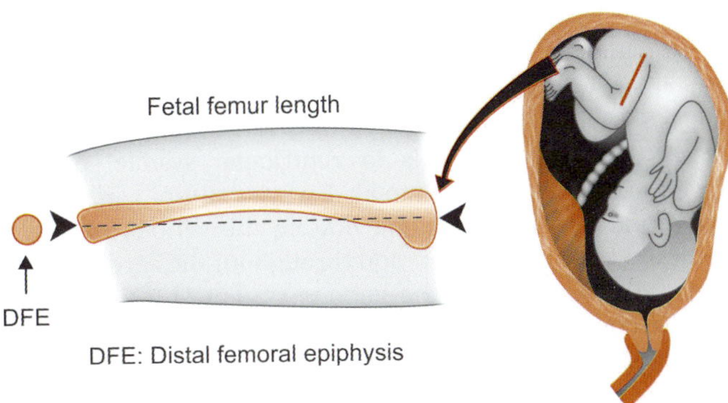



**Fig. 12.17B:** Diagrammatic method for the measurement of femur length

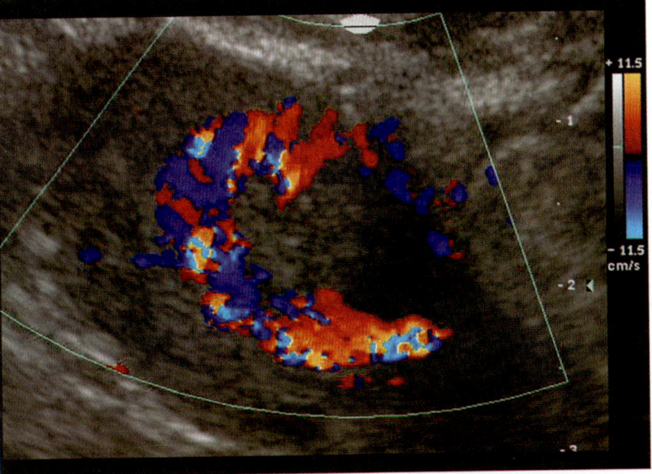



**Fig. 12.19:** Blood flow within the ovary with recently ovulated follicles as visualized on color Doppler ultrasound

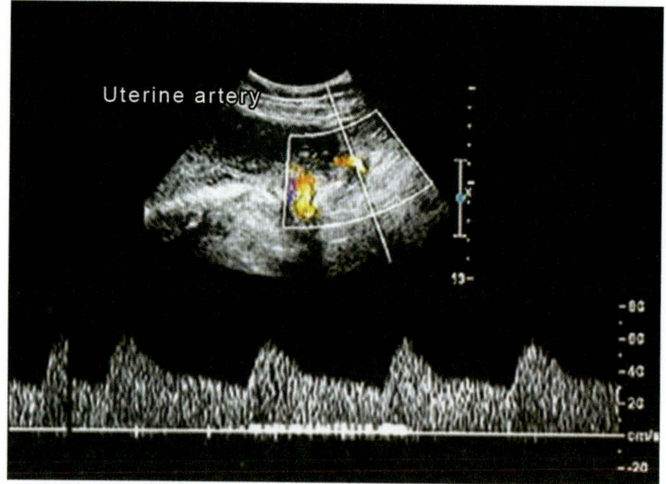

**Fig. 12.20:** Uterine artery Doppler in normal pregnancy

## Three-Vessel Umbilical Cord

Normal umbilical cord normally has three vessels: two arteries and one vein (Figs 12.21A and B). These vessels can be identified on Doppler ultrasound examination as shown in the adjacent figures.

## COLOR DOPPLER EVALUATION OF FETAL CIRCULATION

### Color Doppler Evaluation of Middle Cerebral Artery

Color Doppler evaluation of fetal middle cerebral artery (MCA) is shown in Figures 12.22A and B. Middle cerebral artery is a major lateral branch of the circle of Willis, which is most accessible to ultrasound imaging and carries nearly 80% of cerebral blood. On Doppler imaging, MCA can be seen to be running anterolaterally at the borderline between the anterior and the middle cerebral fossae.

### Blood Flow in Ductus Venosus

The ductus venosus (DV) is a very important part of fetal venous circulation. This vessel acts as a shunt and helps in directly connecting the umbilical vein to the inferior vena cava. The fetus receives oxygenated blood from the mother through placenta in the form of umbilical veins. As this oxygenated blood bypasses DV, some of the oxygenated blood goes to the liver, but most of it bypasses the liver and empties directly into the inferior vena cava, which enters the right atrium. This highly oxygenated and nutrient-rich umbilical venous blood is eventually supplied to the fetal brain and myocardium instead of the fetal liver. Normal blood flow through DV has been shown in Figure 12.23 and comprises of the following waves: S wave (related to peak systolic velocity);

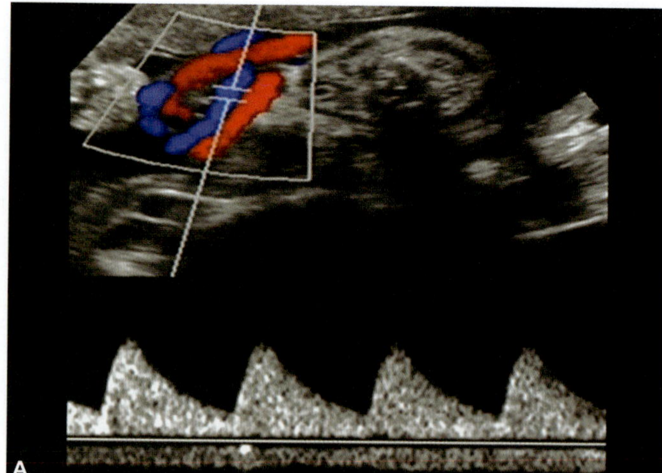

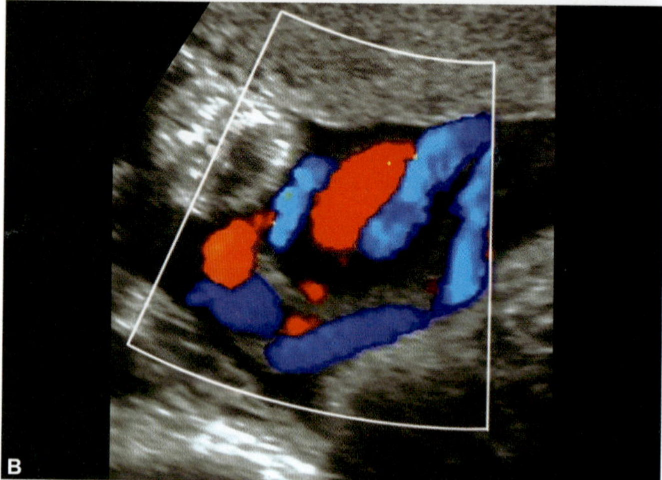

**Figs 12.21A and B:** Three-vessel umbilical cord

D wave (related to ventricular diastole) and A wave (related to atrial contraction) (Fig. 12.24).

## Normal Doppler Analysis of Venous Blood Flow

The typical waveform for the blood flow in the venous vessels consists of three phases related to cardiac cycle (Fig. 12.24). Peak S wave corresponds to ventricular systole, peak D wave to early diastole and peak A wave to atrial contraction. In normal fetuses, the blood flow in the venous system is always in the forward direction throughout the cardiac cycle. Forward blood flow in the venous system is a function of cardiac compliance, contractibility and afterload. A decline in forward velocities in venous system results in increased Doppler indices and suggests impaired preload handling. Absence or even reversal of the A wave is the hallmark of the advancing circulatory deterioration since this documents the inability of the heart to accommodate venous return.

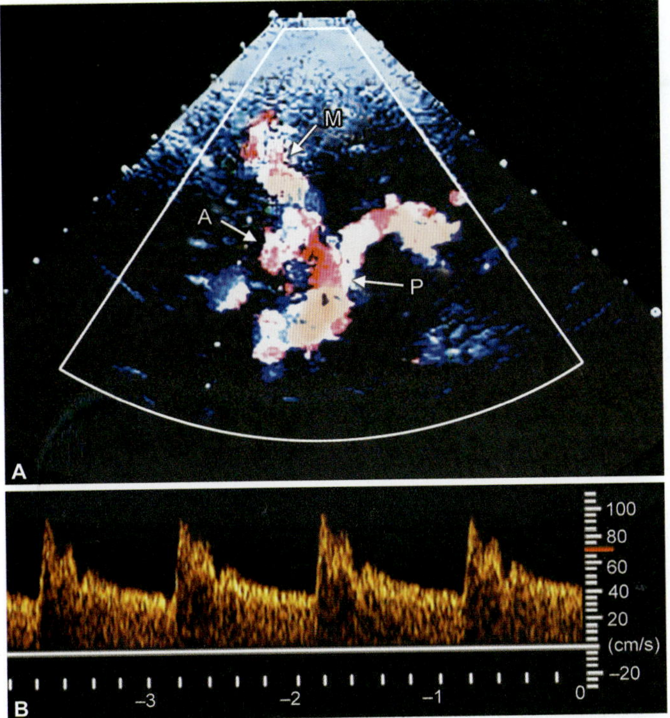

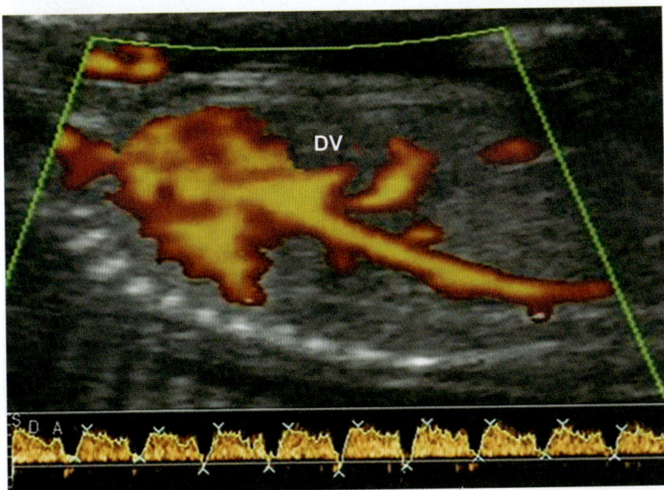

**Figs 12.22A and B:** (A) Color Doppler evaluation of middle cerebral artery (MCA) showing circle of Willis; (B) Doppler velocity waveforms in MCA (A, Anterior cerebral artery; M, Middle cerebral artery; P, Posterior cerebral artery)

**Fig. 12.23:** Normal blood flow in the ductus venosus (DV)

## Reversed Blood Flow in Ductus Venosus

Abnormal blood flow in the DV is associated with either absence of A wave or reversal of blood flow in the A wave (as shown in Figures 12.25A and B). Abnormal DV flow could

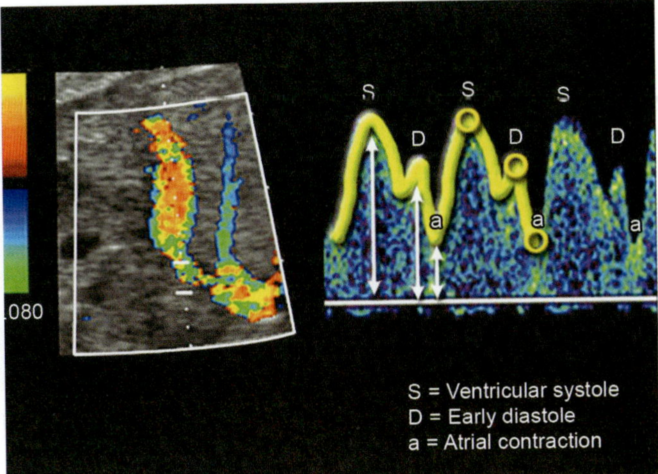


**Fig. 12.24:** Doppler analysis of venous blood flow

be indicative of intrauterine growth restriction (IUGR) or cardiac abnormality or underlying Down's syndrome. During the periods of fetal hypoxia, a compensatory mechanism occurs, causing transient dilatation of the ductus, which is supposed to increase oxygenated blood flowing through it during these periods of hypoxia or reduced umbilical flow.

## Color Doppler Evaluation of Umbilical Artery

The assessment of umbilical blood flow provides information regarding blood perfusion of the fetoplacental unit. The deoxygenated blood from the fetus is delivered by two umbilical arteries whereas the oxygenated blood moves to the fetus via umbilical vein. These vessels are connected to the mother via the placenta and to the fetus via the umbilical cord. In a normal pregnancy, the impedance to the blood flow in umbilical vessels continuously decreases throughout the gestation. The blood flow during the diastole is often absent in the first trimester. The diastolic component becomes evident with advancing gestational age. Characteristic umbilical blood flow has saw-toothed appearance of pulsatile arterial flow in one direction and continuous umbilical venous blood flow in the other (Figs 12.26A and B).

## Color Doppler Evaluation of Uterine Artery

Uterine artery Doppler helps in evaluating the uteroplacental perfusion (Fig. 12.27). Doppler ultrasound of the uterine arteries is a noninvasive method for assessing the resistance of vessels supplying the placenta. In normal pregnancies, due to the trophoblastic invasion of spiral vessels, there is an increase in blood flow velocity and a decrease in resistance to flow.

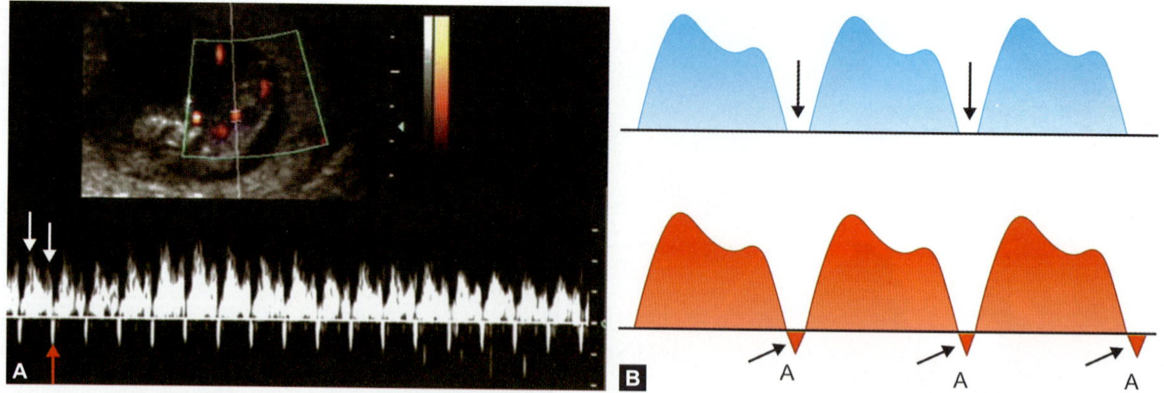

**Figs 12.25A and B:** Reversed blood flow in the ductus venosus (arrow pointing in upward direction)

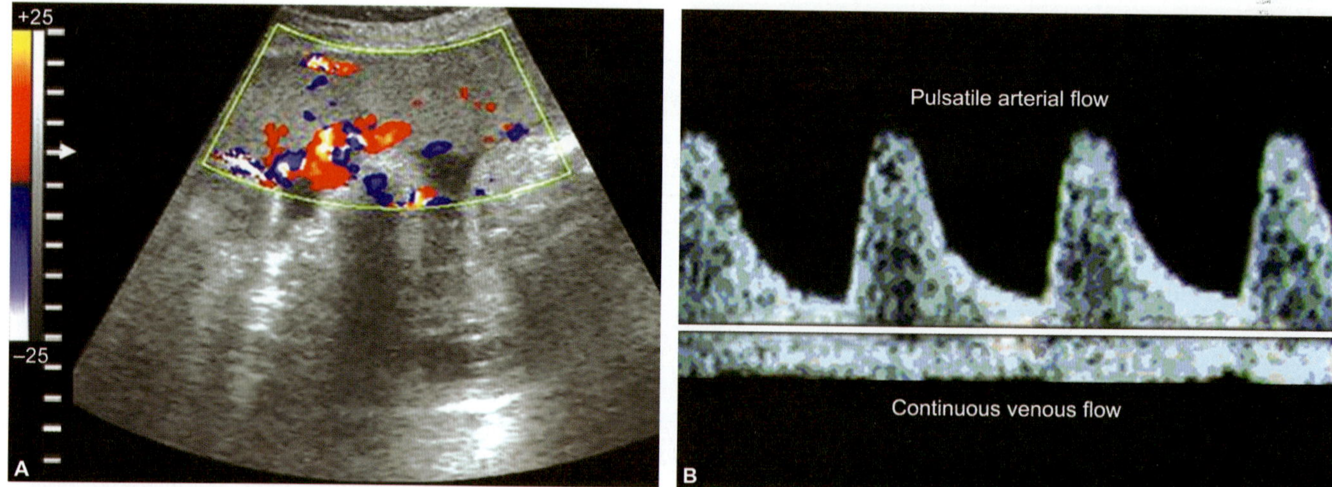


**Figs 12.26A and B:** (A) Umbilical artery circulation on color Doppler ultrasonography; (B) Umbilical artery Doppler ultrasound waveforms

## *Uterine Artery Blood Flow Patterns*

The normal uterine artery waveform (Fig. 12.28A) comprises of two components:

1. *A pulsatile component:* Formed by the interaction of an outgoing wave and reflected wave. The outgoing wave upon reaching the uteroplacental vascular bed is reflected back to the heart.

2. *A steady waveform:* Due to a fall in the resistance of uterine vessels during pregnancy, there occurs increased diastolic flow resulting in a steady waveform pattern.

In pregnancies complicated by hypertensive disorders, IUGR, etc., there is increased resistance to blood flow in the uterine blood vessels. Initially, the Doppler ultrasound of the uterine artery shows increased resistance to flow (decreased mean velocity) and reduced diastolic blood flow. This results in an elevated PI and RI. With an increase in vascular resistance, there occurs an early diastolic notch (Fig. 12.28B).

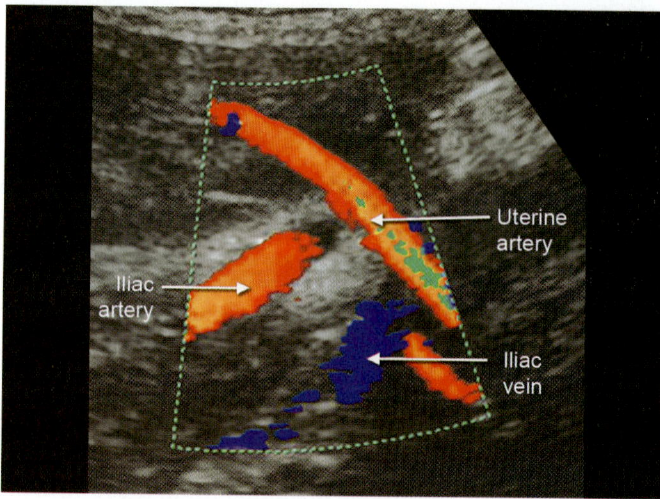


**Fig. 12.27:** Uterine artery Doppler analysis

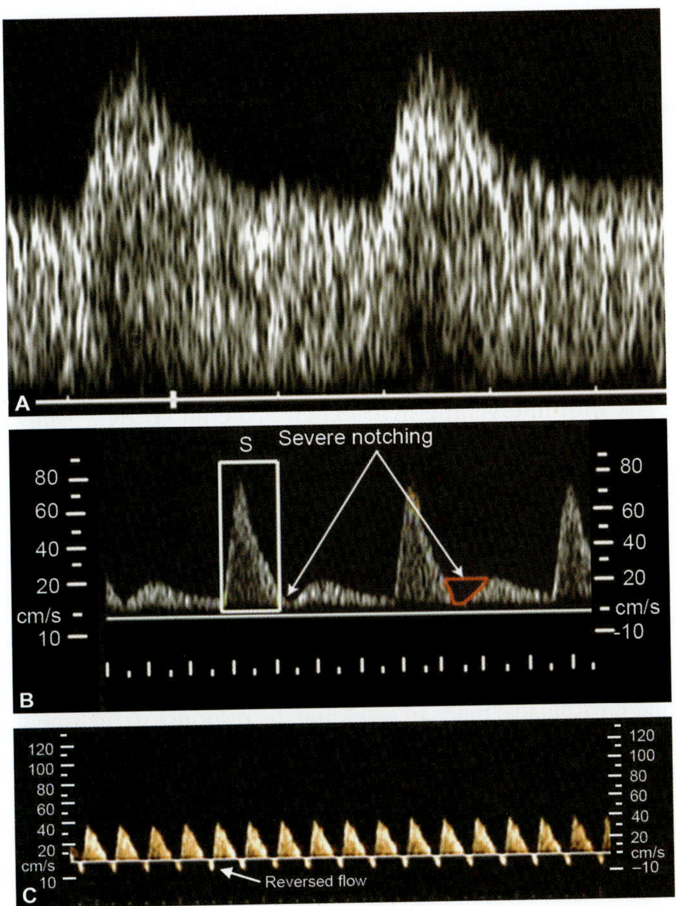

**Figs 12.28A to C:** Uterine artery blood flow patterns: (A) Normal uterine artery blood flow; (B) Diastolic notching in the uterine vessels; (C) Reversed flow on uterine artery Doppler

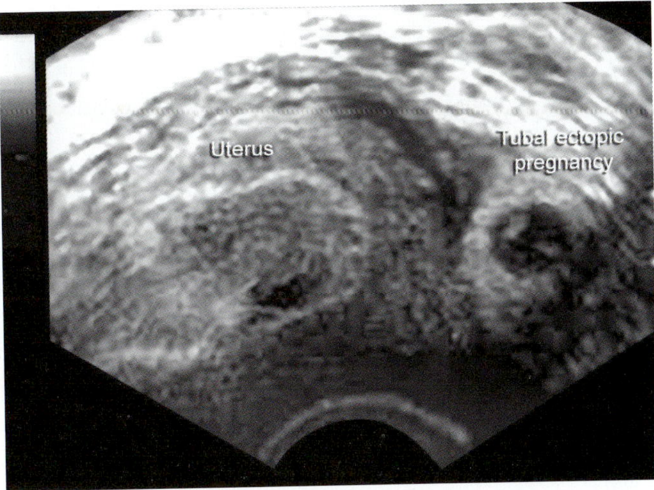


**Fig. 12.29A:** Ectopic pregnancy in left tube

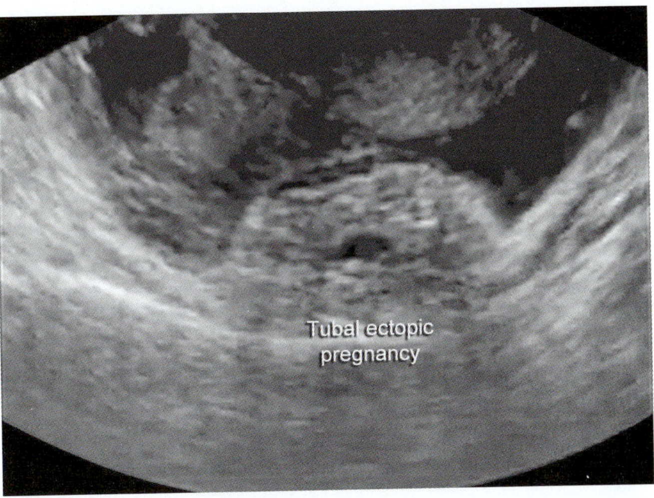


**Fig. 12.29B:** Bagel's sign

With further worsening of situation, the blood flow in the diastole stops completely (absent end diastolic flow) or blood starts flowing in reverse direction (Fig. 12.28C). Reversed end diastolic velocity is an ominous finding warranting close monitoring and mandates immediate delivery depending on the clinical situation of the patient.

## ULTRASOUND FOR DIAGNOSIS OF ECTOPIC PREGNANCY

Figures 12.29A to E illustrate the use of ultrasound for diagnosis of ectopic pregnancy. Ectopic pregnancy can have multiple presentations on ultrasonography. Most common type of presentation is empty uterus with or without presence of free fluid in the pouch of Douglas (POD) and a complex tubal adnexal mass (Fig. 12.29A). Other signs of a definite ectopic pregnancy on ultrasound include presence of a thick, bright echogenic, ring-like structure, which is located outside the uterus, having

a gestational sac containing an obvious fetal pole or yolk sac or both. This usually appears as an intact, well-defined tubal ring (Doughnut or Bagel's sign as shown in Figure 12.29B). Ectopic pregnancy must be ruled out in all cases presenting with abdominal pain or vaginal bleeding with positive pregnancy test and absence of intrauterine gestational sac on ultrasound examination.

Figure 12.29C shows presence of free fluid in the POD, which is suggestive of a tubal ectopic pregnancy. This forms the basis of the diagnostic test "culdocentesis" in which aspiration of blood/blood clots from the POD is indicative of ectopic pregnancy.

Figure 12.29D represents a tubal gestational sac, which was about 10–12 weeks in size and fetal heart rate could be observed on ultrasound examination. Severe adnexal tenderness with probe palpation was also observed, which is also suggestive of ectopic pregnancy.

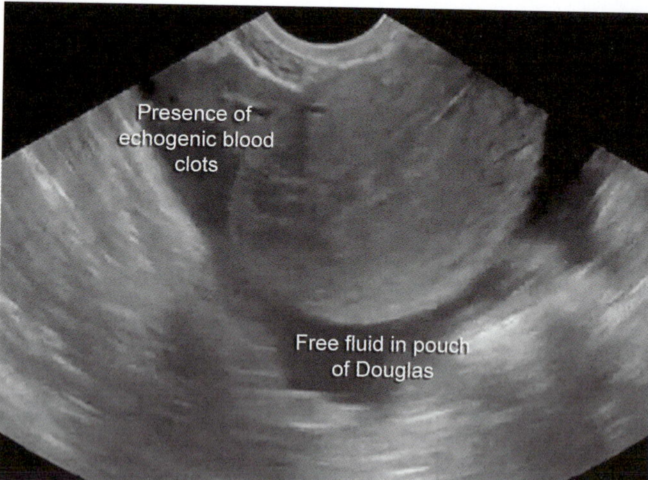



**Fig. 12.29C:** Free fluid in the pouch of Douglas

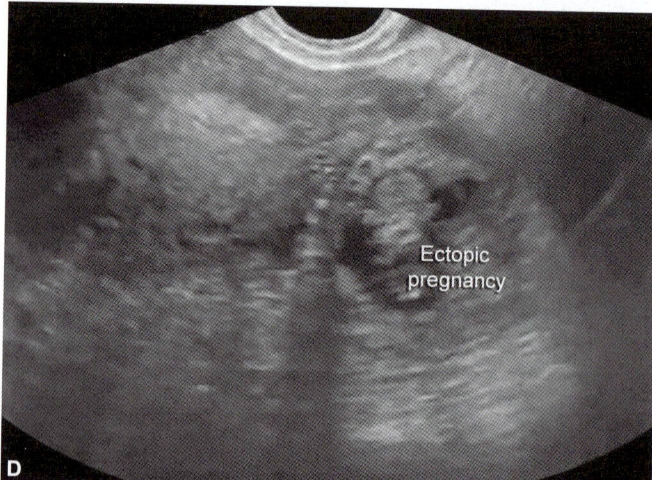



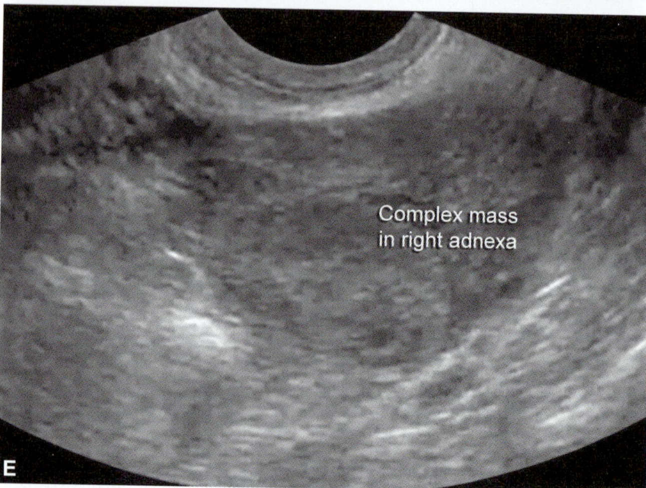



**Figs 12.29D and E:** (D) Left-sided ectopic pregnancy; (E) Complex right adnexal mass

In Figure 12.29E, no definite gestational sac could be identified. Hematosalpinx (presence of free fluid or blood in the fallopian tubes) probably resulted in an echogenic complex mass in this case. An empty uterus or a pseudogestational sac on TVS images in patients with a serum β-hCG level greater than the discriminatory cut-off value is also considered to be an ectopic pregnancy until proven otherwise.

## ULTRASOUND FOR THE DIAGNOSIS OF HYDATIDIFORM MOLE

Figure 12.30 shows an ultrasound picture in case of a molar pregnancy in which there is presence of numerous anechoic cysts with intervening hyperechoic material giving a "snow storm appearance". In a typical sonographic appearance of complete hydatidiform mole in the second and third trimesters, there may be presence of an enlarged uterine endometrial cavity containing homogeneously hyperechoic endometrial mass with innumerable anechoic cysts sized 1–30 mm. Ultrasound may also show presence of theca lutein cysts in the ovaries. Sonography is the imaging investigation of choice to confirm the diagnosis of H. mole. Sonographic examination is not only helpful in establishing the initial diagnosis, it also helps in assessing the response to treatment regimes; determining the degree of invasion in malignant forms of gestational trophoblastic neoplasia (GTN); determining the disease recurrence in malignant forms of GTN and evaluation of liver metastasis.

Figure 12.31 shows MRI examination in a 25-year-old woman who presented at 10 weeks of gestation with elevated levels of β-hCG and no visible gestational sac on ultrasound examination. On sagittal T2-weighted MRI, there was presence of high-signal intensity heterogeneous material filling the uterine cavity. Histopathological examination of the evacuated materials confirmed the presence of complete

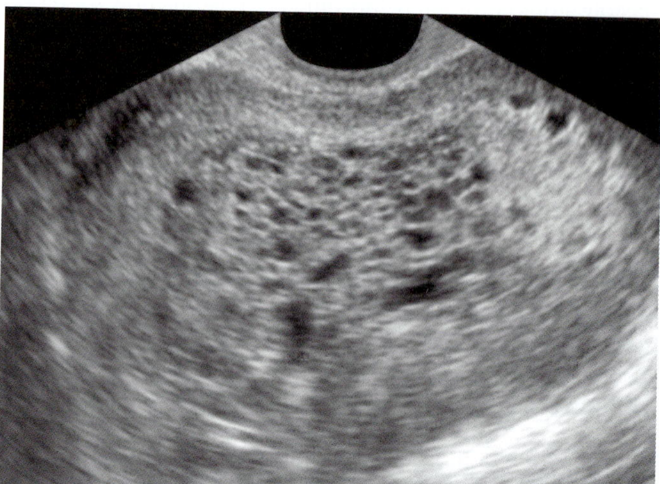

**Fig. 12.30:** Ultrasound showing hydatidiform mole

molar pregnancy. At present, MRI plays no role in the diagnosis of H. mole. Presently, it is not an essential investigation for management of nonmetastatic molar gestation. However, it is beneficial in diagnosing the metastatic disease.

Magnetic resonance imaging is also used for characterizing the degree of myometrial and/or parametrial invasion and for assessing the response to chemotherapy.

## DIAGNOSIS OF MISCARRIAGE USING ULTRASOUND

### Inevitable Abortion

Figure 12.32A demonstrates the ultrasound findings in case of inevitable abortion. There is a loss of definition of gestational sac, resulting in a smaller diameter of gestational sac. There are no central echoes in the gestational sac which are normally indicative of a healthy pregnancy. Fetal cardiac activity is normally absent.

### Missed Abortion

Figure 12.32B demonstrates the ultrasound findings in case of missed abortion. There was absence of the growth of the fetal pole over a 5 days observation period. The fetal heart rate was also absent.

### Anembryonic Pregnancy

Figure 12.32C shows an anembryonic pregnancy where there is large gestational sac having a size 3 × 2 cm. The gestational sac was empty without having presence of yolk sac or fetal pole. The pregnancy may be deemed abnormal if no yolk sac appears at the gestational sac size of 10 mm or no fetal pole is seen at the gestational sac size of 18 mm. If the gestational sac has an irregular or scalloped appearance, that is also abnormal.

### Complete Abortion

Figure 12.32D shows an ultrasound image in case of a complete abortion, where the gestational sac and products of conception (POCs) have been completely expelled out. As a result, the triple line uterine endometrium with an empty uterine cavity can be seen on TVS.

## ULTRASOUND FOR DIAGNOSIS OF MULTIFETAL GESTATION

### Twin Gestation

Presence of multiple fetuses/gestational sacs (Fig. 12.33A) and/or multiple placentas on ultrasound examination is the most diagnostic feature of multifetal gestation.

In the same patient when an ultrasound examination was performed at 30 weeks of gestation, two fetal heads were identified suggestive of twin gestation (Fig. 12.33B).

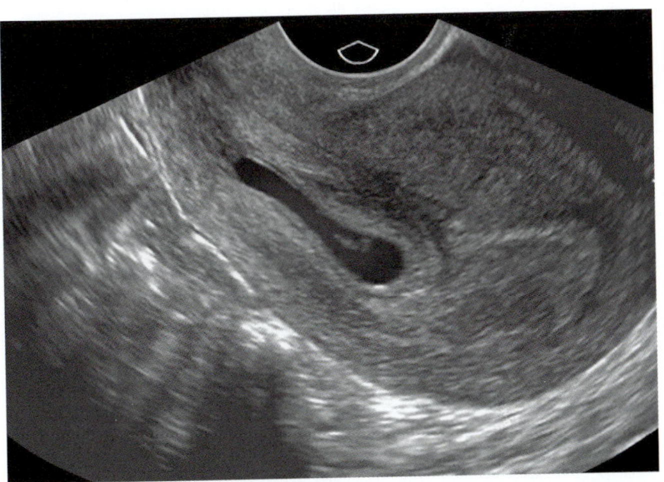

**Fig. 12.32A:** Inevitable abortion

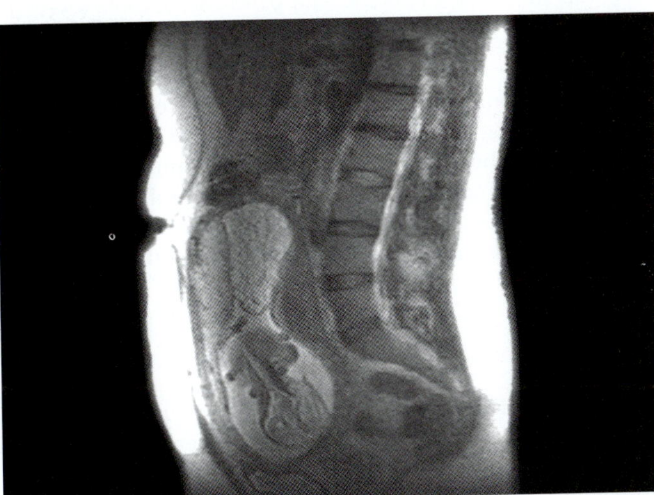

**Fig. 12.31:** Magnetic resonance imaging showing hydatidiform mole

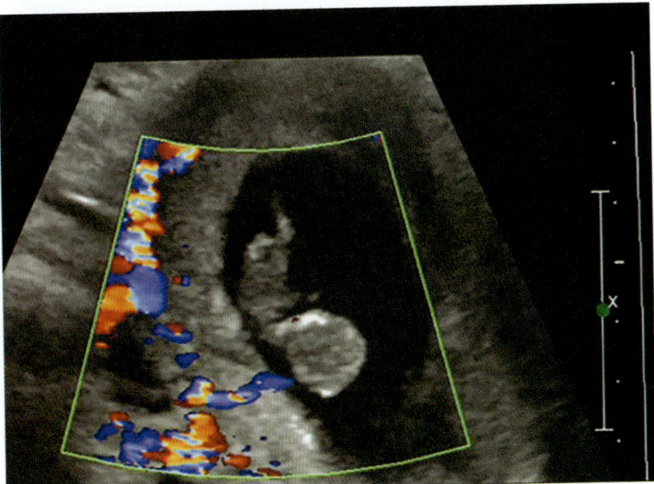

**Fig. 12.32B:** Missed abortion

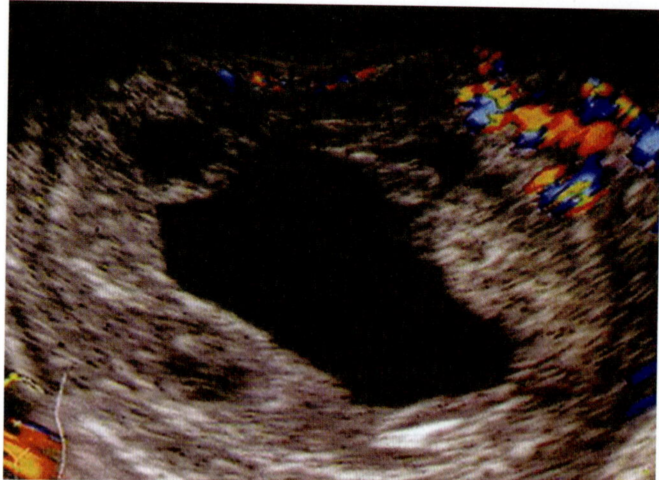

**Fig. 12.32C:** Anembryonic pregnancy as observed on color Doppler ultrasound

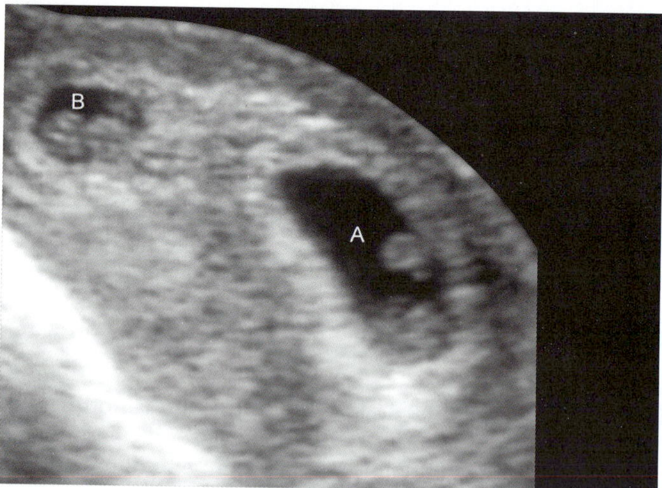

**Fig. 12.33A:** Presence of two gestational sacs with A = 7.6 weeks and B = 5.7 weeks

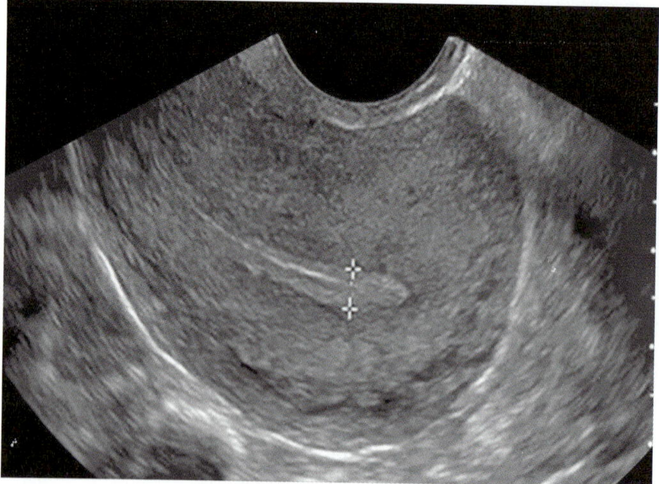

**Fig. 12.32D:** Complete abortion

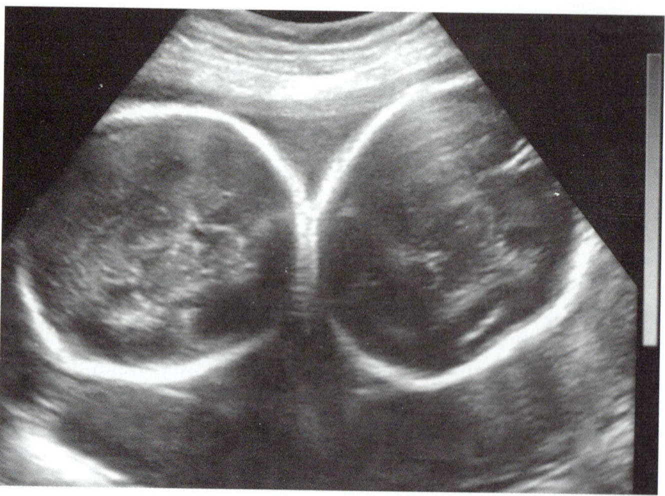

**Fig. 12.33B:** Ultrasound of the same patient at 30 weeks, showing two fetal heads

*Triplets*

Figures 12.34A and B show triplets at 7 weeks of gestation. Three separate gestational sacs, each having an embryo can be observed. The three fetuses share a common placenta as observed on Doppler ultrasound examination.

# Gynecological Ultrasound

## NORMAL ANATOMY ON TVS

### Anatomy in the Proliferative Phase

In the proliferative phase on TVS, there is presence of a well-defined "three-line sign", which is formed by the central hyperechoic reflection representing the endometrial cavity and the additional hyperechoic reflections representing the thin developing layer of the endometrium on either side (Fig. 12.35A). The outer lines represent the interface between endometrium and myometrium. There is minimal or absent posterior acoustic enhancement. The ovary may show presence of a dominant follicle with several other follicles in different stages of development (Fig. 12.35B).

### Anatomy in the Luteal Phase

In the immediate pre- and postovulatory period (2 days postovulation), an additional inner hyperechogenicity of variable thickness, which corresponds to a relatively high fluid content of these inner functional layers, can be seen with TVS. A small amount of fluid (1–2 mL) can be seen in some

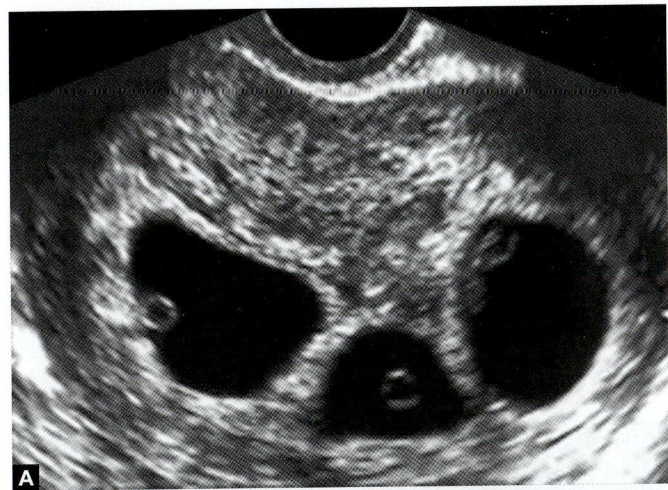

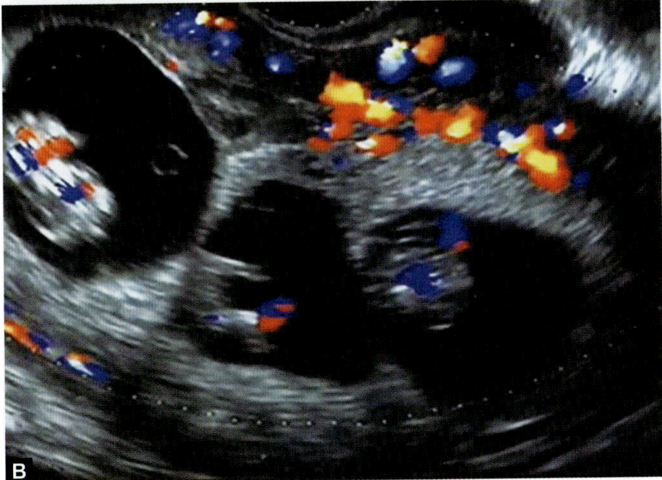

**Figs 12.34A and B:** Triplets at 7 weeks of gestation: (A) Transvaginal ultrasound; (B) Color Doppler ultrasound

individuals within the lumen of the endometrium resulting in the halo sign. The total double layer thickness in the luteal phase ranges from 4 mm to 12 mm with an average of 7.5 mm. The luteal phase endometrium tends to be hyperechoic and maximum in thickness (Fig. 12.36A). There is presence of posterior acoustic enhancement and "three-line sign" is also absent. In this phase, corpus luteum appears as an echogenic structure within the ovary with prominent peripheral vascularization (Figs 12.36B and C).

## NORMAL ANATOMY ON TAS

### Normal Uterus

Figure 12.37A shows sagittal section of the uterus showing hyperechogenic endometrium. Figure 12.37B shows transverse section of the uterus on transabdominal scan.

### Normal Ovary

Figure 12.38 shows normal ovary as visualized on transabdominal scan. Multiple follicles of different sizes in various stages of development can be visualized. Since the image was captured in early proliferative phase, when the ovulation was not about to occur immediately, the dominant follicle was not visualized.

## EVALUATION OF ENDOMETRIAL THICKNESS

### Thin Endometrium

*Ultrasound showing thin endometrium in menopausal women:* Menopause is defined by the WHO as the permanent cessation of menstruation resulting from the loss of ovarian follicular activity. The most serious concern in

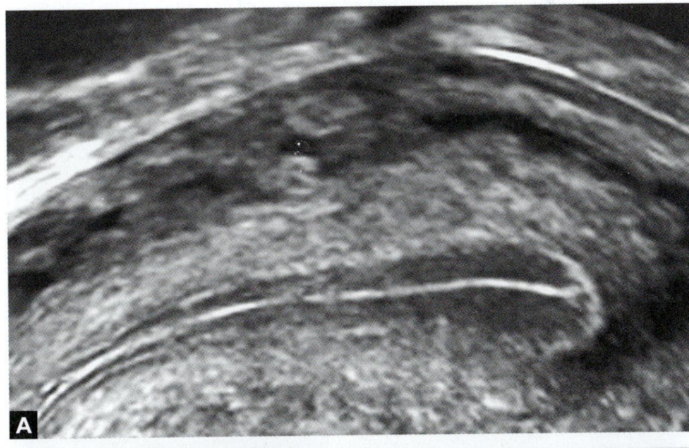

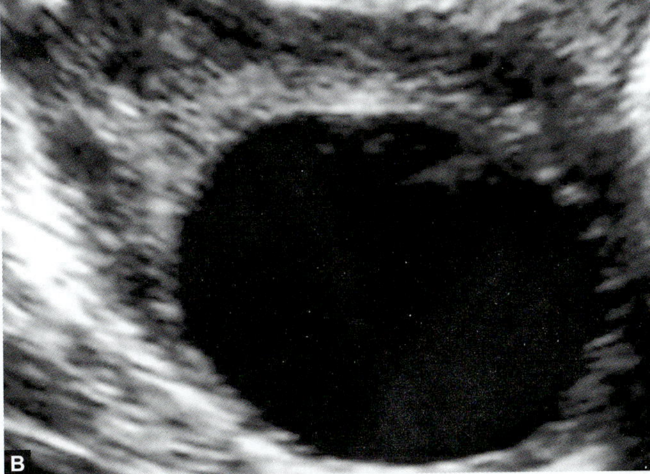

**Figs 12.35A and B:** (A) Transvaginal sonography of the uterus in the proliferative phase, showing presence of a well-defined "three-line sign"; (B) Ovary showing presence of a dominant follicle

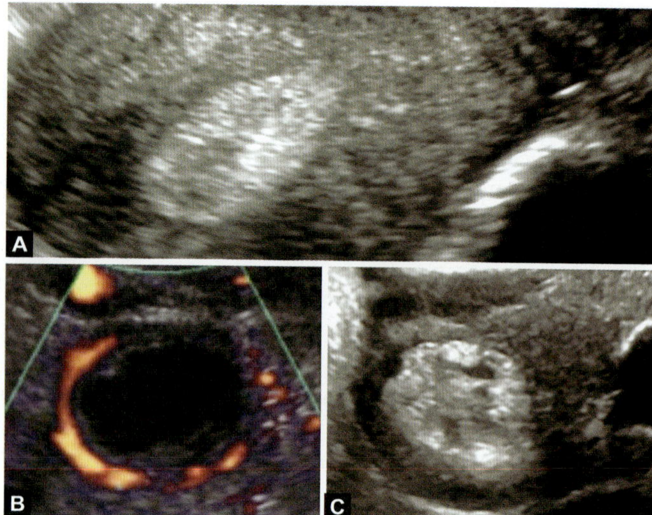

**Figs 12.36A to C:** (A) Transvaginal sonography in the luteal phase showing uniformly hyperechogenic endometrium; (B and C) Two small pictures in the bottom half show corpus luteum, which appears as an echogenic structure within the ovary with prominent peripheral vascularization

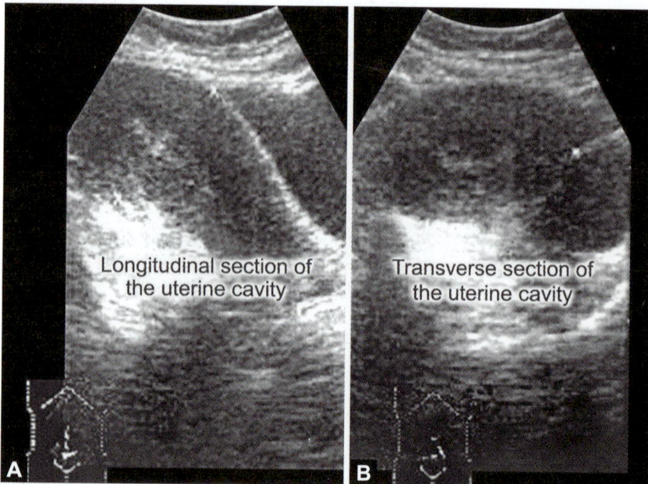



**Figs 12.37A and B:** Normal uterus as visualized on transabdominal scan: (A) Longitudinal section; (B) Transverse section

postmenopausal and perimenopausal women with abnormal postmenopausal bleeding (PMB) is endometrial carcinoma. The first line of management in these patients is performance of a transvaginal ultrasound to evaluate the endometrial thickness. In normal postmenopausal women (Fig. 12.39), there is a thin hyperechogenic endometrium and empty ovaries with absence of any follicle. Endometrial biopsy is usually not required in these cases. Follow-up may be done to evaluate any further bleeding.

*Ultrasound showing an increased endometrial thickness:* Figure 12.40 displays an ultrasound showing an increased

endometrial thickness. In this case, the patient has presented with a history of PMB. The most commonly used noninvasive investigation for diagnosis of cases of PMB is ultrasonography. According to ACOG (2009) recommendations, postmenopausal cases of AUB with endometrial thickness greater than 4 mm require additional evaluation with investigations such as saline infusion sonography (SIS), hysteroscopy or EB. In premenopausal patients with AUB, no further evaluation is recommended for a normal appearing endometrium with thickness less than or equal to 10 mm.

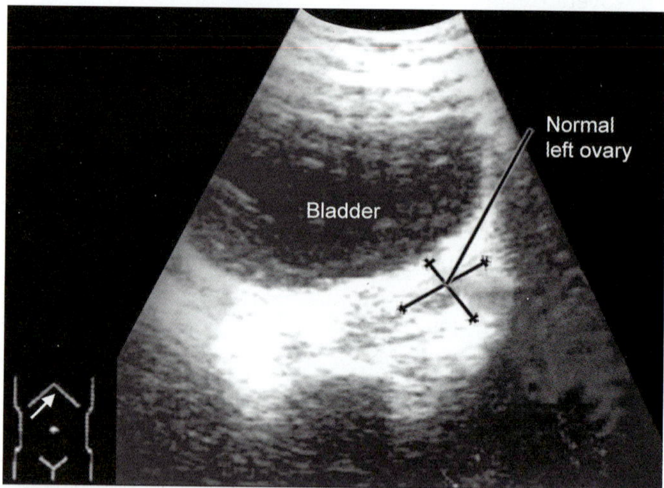



**Fig. 12.38:** Normal ovary as visualized on the transabdominal scan

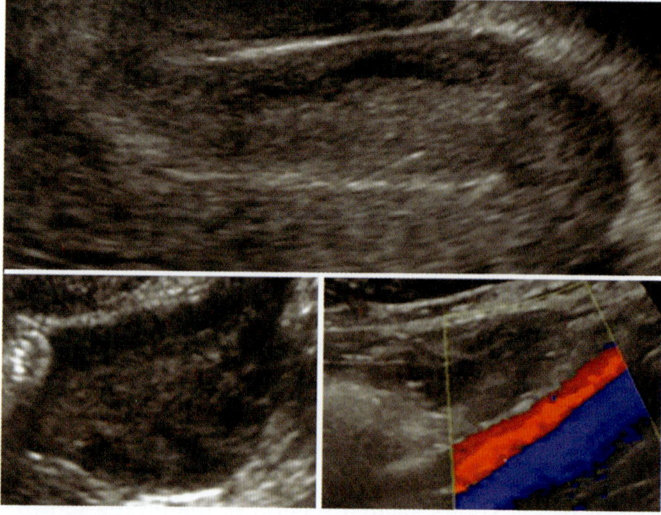

**Fig. 12.39:** A patient presenting with postmenopausal bleeding in which TVS shows presence of thin hyperechogenic endometrium. Color Doppler demonstrates the presence of iliac vessels adjacent to the ovary with no growing follicle

# FIBROIDS

## Intramural Fibroid

Ultrasound examination can help in assessing the size, location and number of uterine fibroids. Preoperative finding on sonography can guide the clinician while performing surgery, hysteroscopy, laparoscopy, etc. Nowadays, ultrasound examination (both transvaginal and transabdominal ultrasound) has become the investigation of choice for diagnosing myomas. The advantages of ultrasound imaging include good patient tolerance, noninvasive nature of the investigation, relatively low cost, easy availability and high accuracy rate. Ultrasound examination helps in assessing the overall uterine shape, size and contour; endometrial thickness; adnexal areas and presence of hydronephrosis. Figure 12.41A shows a transvaginal ultrasound scan revealing a well-defined hyperechoic area surrounded by an anechoic capsule located within the myometrium, diagnosed as an intramural fibroid.

## Pedunculated Subserosal Fibroid

Figure 12.41B shows a transvaginal ultrasound scan illustrating a well-defined mass measuring about 3.74 cm in diameter. The mass is located separately from the uterine fundus and is connected with help of a pedicle. Subserosal fibroids may sometimes develop a pedicle and extrude out from the serosal surface in the form of pedunculated fibroids. Both submucous and subserosal fibroids can be pedunculated. Long pedunculated fibroids may sometimes undergo torsion.

## Submucous Fibroid

Transvaginal ultrasound scan in Figure 12.41C shows a submucous fibroid protruding inside the endometrial cavity.

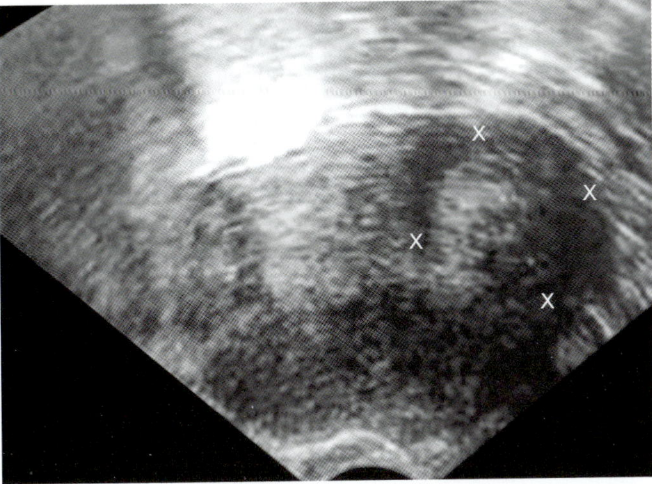

**Fig. 12.41A:** Intramural fibroid

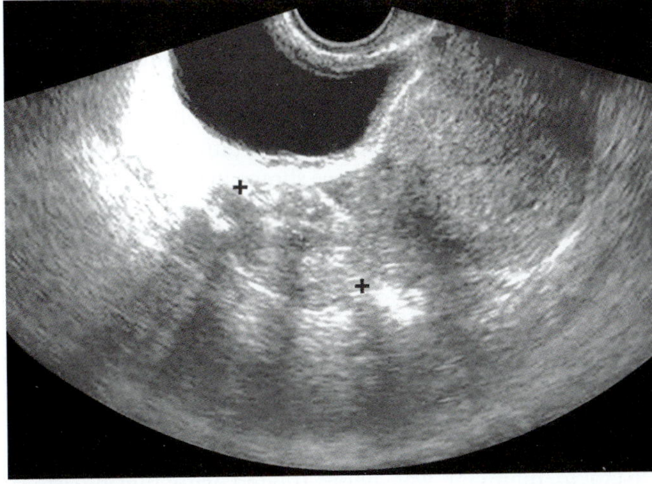

**Fig. 12.41B:** Pedunculated fibroid having a diameter of 3.74 cm

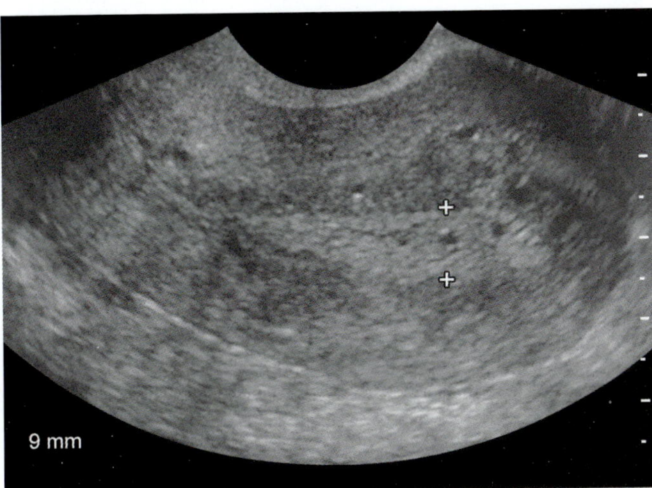

**Fig. 12.40:** Transvaginal sonography in a patient with postmenopausal bleeding showing an endometrial thickness of 9 mm

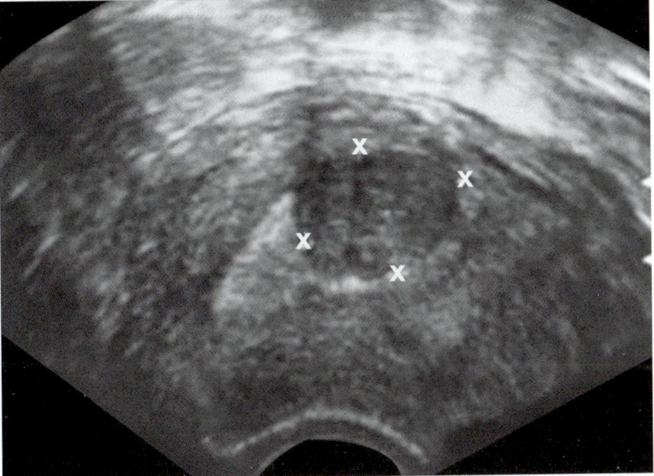

**Fig. 12.41C:** Submucous fibroid protruding inside the endometrial cavity

The characteristic symptom of a submucosal leiomyoma is menorrhagia. The duration of menstrual period may be normal or prolonged and the blood loss is usually heaviest on 2nd and 3rd day. The nearer the leiomyomas are to the endometrial cavity, the more likely are they to produce menorrhagia. It may be sometimes very difficult to differentiate between submucous myomas and endometrial polyps on ultrasound examination. In these cases, other investigations such as SIS and hysteroscopy may help in arriving at the correct diagnosis. Hysteroscopic myomectomy appears to be the best treatment option in these cases.

## Magnetic Resonance Imaging for Diagnosis of Fibroids

Presently, the ultrasound examination forms the most commonly used investigation modality for initial evaluation. Though MRI is an investigation which helps in accurately establishing the definitive diagnosis of myomas, the high cost associated with its use, prevents its widespread use in clinical practice. MRI was performed in cases demonstrated in Figures 12.42A and B because the diagnosis was not clear on ultrasound examination. In this case, no definitive diagnosis could be established on transvaginal ultrasound. The likely differential diagnoses in the case shown in Figure 12.42A were adenomyosis, fibroid uterus and endometrial cancer. MRI established the diagnosis of intramural fibroid.

Though the use of MRI is not routinely recommended, it is useful for mapping the size and location of leiomyomas and in accurately identifying adenomyosis, if present. Other pelvic pathology such as ovarian neoplasms can also be identified on MRI.

MRI was performed in the case shown in Figure 12.42B because the patient with a large submucosal fibroid about 18 cm in diameter was being treated with uterine artery embolization (UAE). Proper delineation of myometrium, junctional zone and endometrium was essential in this case in order to evaluate tumor regression as a result of UAE.

## ADENOMYOSIS

## Ultrasound Examination

Upon ultrasound examination, adenomyosis may present with heterogeneous myometrial echotexture, ill-defined, anechoic areas of thickened myometrium consisting of blood-filled, irregular cystic spaces, or as an area of hyperechoic myometrium with several cysts (hypoechoic lacunae) (Figs 12.43A and B). Other features suggestive of adenomyosis include asymmetrical uterine enlargement, indistinct endometrial-myometrial border and subendometrial halo thickening.

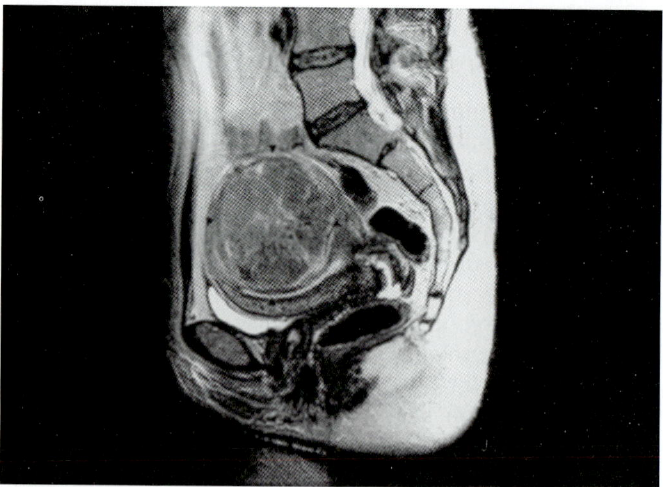

**Fig. 12.42A:** T1-weighted magnetic resonance image showing an intramural fibroid of size 8 cm

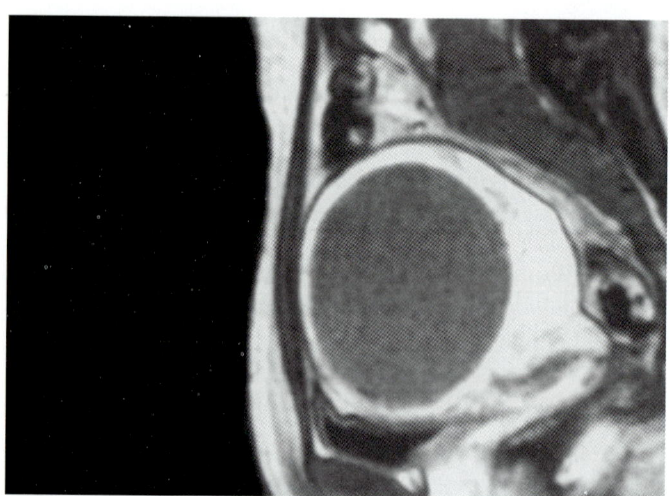

**Fig. 12.42B:** MRI of a 33-year-old woman with large submucosal fibroid. Enhanced T1-weighted magnetic resonance image obtained 4 months after uterine artery embolization shows that uterine fibroid decreased to 8 cm in maximum diameter (46% tumor volume reduction) and was not enhancing. Muscular layer of the uterus is enhanced

## MRI Examination

Magnetic resonance imaging is superior to ultrasound for diagnosis of adenomyosis (Fig. 12.43C). The presence of heterotopic endometrial glands and stroma in the myometrium appear as bright foci within the myometrium on T2-weighted MRIs. Adjacent smooth muscle hyperplasia may present as areas of reduced signal intensity on MRI. Though MRI is superior to ultrasound for the diagnosis of adenomyosis, the diagnosis of adenomyosis can only be confirmed by pathological examination.

## PELVIC INFLAMMATORY DISEASE

### Hydrosalpinx

Figure 12.44 shows an ultrasound scan of a 28-year-old patient presenting with infertility. Ultrasound revealed presence of bilateral tubular, cystic mass with multiple internal echoes. This mass was suggestive of hydrosalpinx. In order to establish a definitive diagnosis, a hysterosalpingography (HSG) was performed.

### Chronic Hydrosalpinx

Figure 12.45 shows appearance of hydrosalpinx on Doppler ultrasound examination. There is presence of

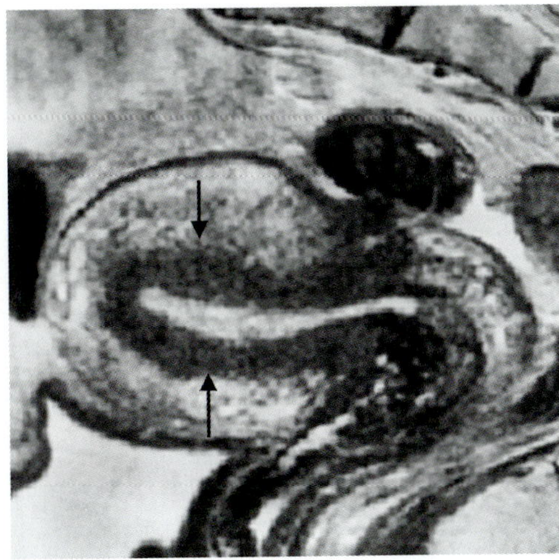

**Fig. 12.43C:** Sagittal T2-weighted MRI showing diffuse, even thickening of the junctional zone (as depicted by arrows), which is consistent with the diagnosis of diffuse adenomyosis

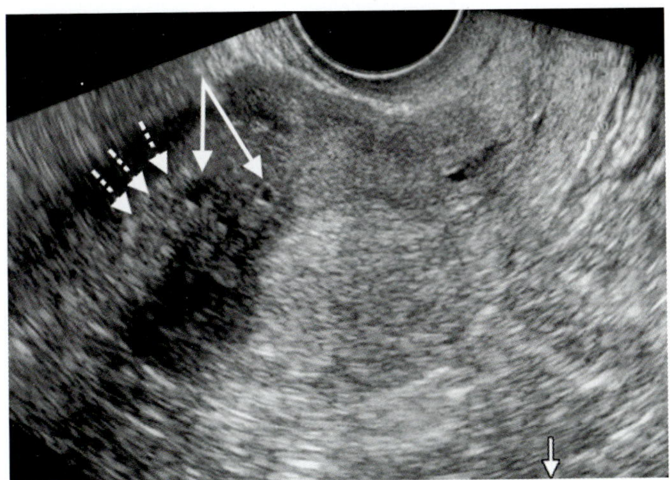

**Fig. 12.43A:** Ultrasound showing features suggestive of adenomyosis

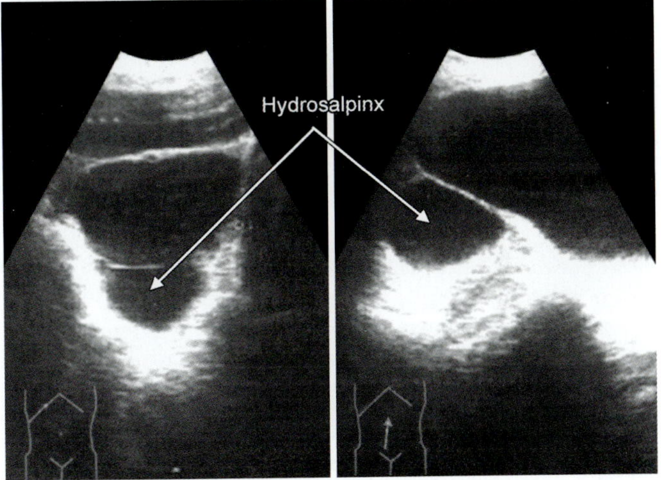


**Fig. 12.44:** Transabdominal sonography revealing the presence of bilateral masses with multiple internal echoes suggestive of hydrosalpinx

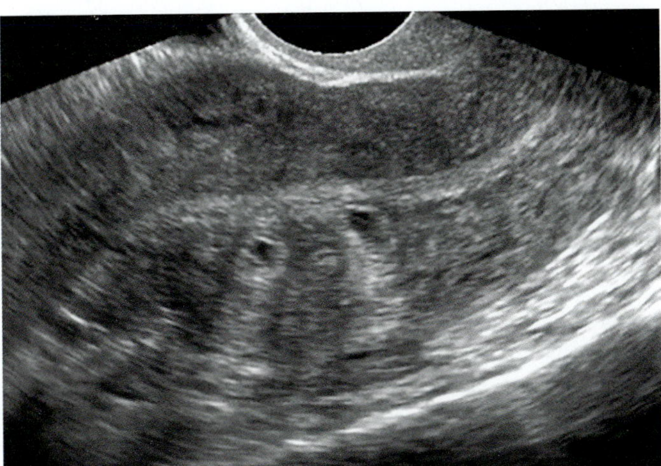

**Fig. 12.43B:** Transvaginal ultrasound in longitudinal plane suggestive of adenomyosis

a dilated fallopian tube with thin-walled incomplete septations. Presence of peripheral vascularization and poor vascularization of septa on Doppler sonography is highly indicative of a hydrosalpinx. Formation of peritoneal adhesions secondary to PID can compromise the motility of the fallopian tubes.

Furthermore, obstruction of the distal end of the fallopian tubes due to adhesions results in accumulation of the normally secreted tubal fluid, creating distention of the tube. This subsequently causes damage to the epithelial cilia and may result in development of hydrosalpinx.

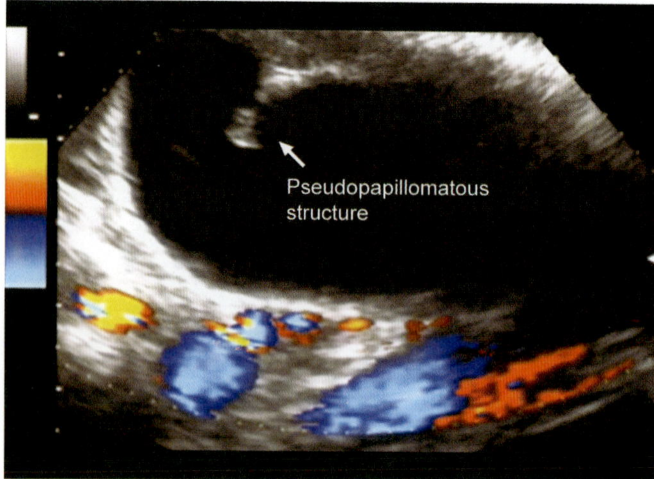



**Fig. 12.45:** Appearance of chronic hydrosalpinx on Doppler ultrasound examination

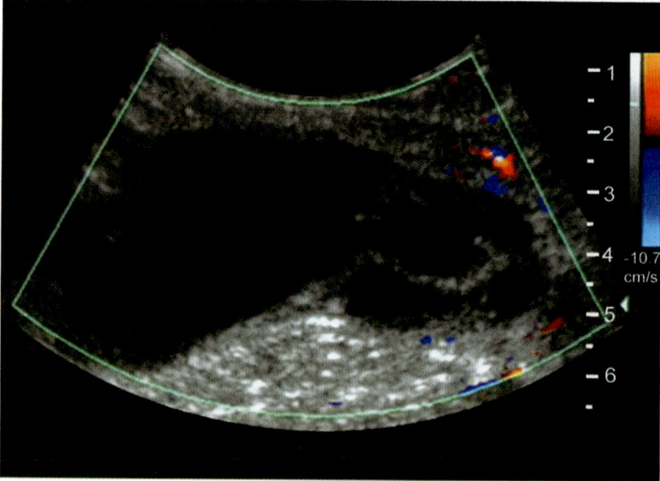

**Fig. 12.47:** Retort-shaped tubal mass suggestive of hydrosalpinx

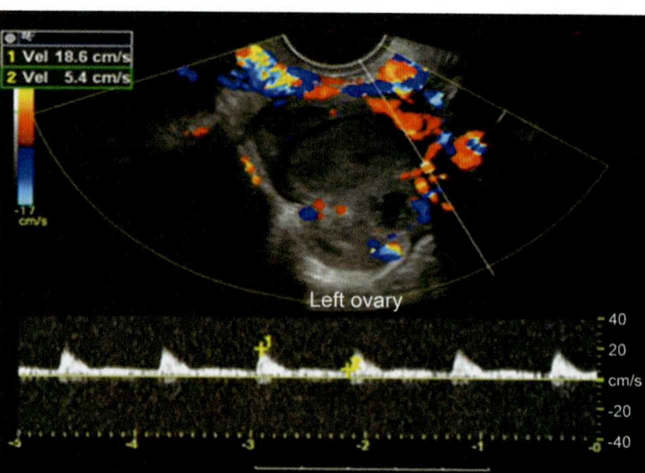



**Fig. 12.46:** Tubo-ovarian mass as visualized on color Doppler

## Color Doppler Ultrasound in Case of Tubo-Ovarian Abscess

Tubo-ovarian abscess (TOA) appears as a complex cystic-solid adnexal mass with thick irregular walls and septations. On color flow Doppler, there is prominent vascular perfusion with low-moderate vascular impedance (Fig. 12.46). For evaluation of cases of TOA, transvaginal rather than transabdominal approach is preferable. There may be presence of thickened fluid-filled fallopian tubes. However, absence of such finding also does not reduce the possibility of PID and treatment should be started if there are clinical features suggestive of PID. Ultrasound examination is actually useful in those patients in whom there may be a possibility of pelvic TOA.

## Retort-Shaped Tubal Mass Suggestive of Hydrosalpinx

Presence of a retort-shaped mass arising from the fallopian tubes on TVS is suggestive of hydrosalpinx (Fig. 12.47). The major clinical significance of a hydrosalpinx is its adverse effect on fertility, thereby resulting in a reduced pregnancy rate. A hydrosalpinx, although sterile, can be re-infected at a later date leading to formation of a pyosalpinx.

## OVARIAN NEOPLASMS

### Mucinous Cystadenoma

Ultrasonography (both transabdominal and transvaginal) is accurate in differentiating tumors of the ovary from other types of tumors of the pelvis, in more than 90% of the patients. Figure 12.48A displays a transabdominal sonography (TAS) scan showing a multiloculated mass with presence of cystic areas along with a few brightly echogenic areas. In this case, differential diagnosis of mucinous cystadenoma and dermoid cyst were established based on the findings of sonography. Laparoscopic examination and histopathology confirmed the diagnosis of a mucinous cystadenoma.

### Functional Cyst

Transvaginal sonography in Figure 12.48B shows a small cyst, which was less than 5 cm in diameter and diagnosed as a functional cyst. Functional cysts usually appear as anechoic, small masses on ultrasound examination. The mass was found to be decreasing in size on repeated sonographic examination. It eventually disappeared on its own within 3–4 months' time.

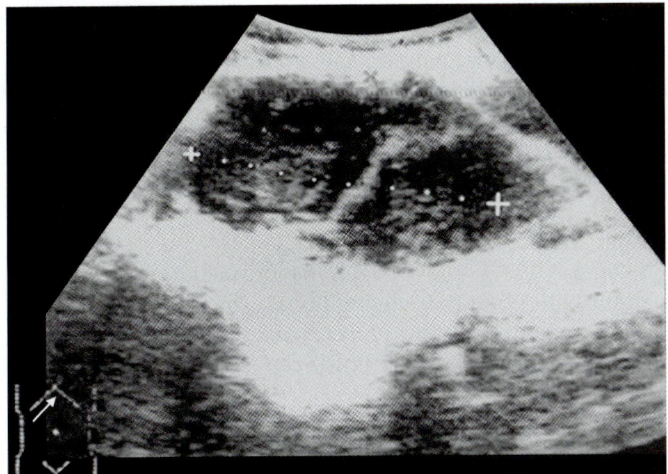

**Fig. 12.48A:** Transabdominal sonography showing a multiloculated mass with presence of cystic areas along with a few brightly echogenic areas

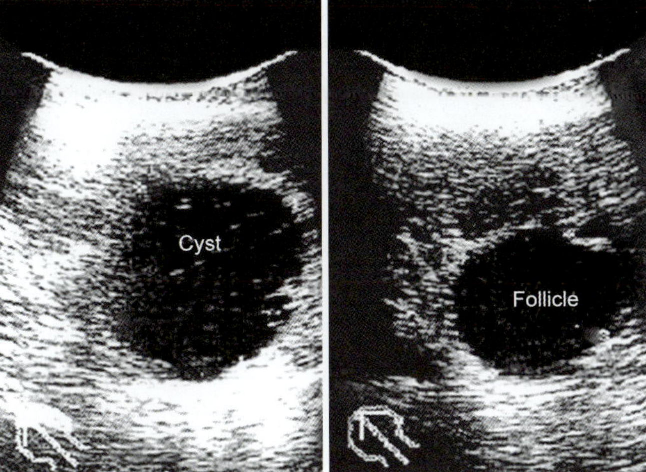



**Fig. 12.48B:** Transvaginal sonography revealing the presence of an ovarian cyst (with multiple internal echoes) on the right side. On the left side, the ovary is normal with presence of a dominant follicle.

Discrimination between benign and malignant lesions of the ovary can be made on the basis of ultrasonic patterns. Though sonography cannot definitely rule out malignancy, anechoic or almost anechoic lesions have a high likelihood of being benign. As the percentage of echogenic material in the cysts increases, the likelihood of malignancy also increases.

## Serous Cystadenocarcinoma

In general, benign lesions are likely to be unilateral, unilocular and thin walled with no papillae or solid areas. Septae, if present in benign masses, are also thin. In contrast, malignant lesions are often multilocular with thick walls, thick septae and mixed echogenicity due to the presence of solid areas. Doppler flow studies of the ovarian artery may also help in differentiating between benign and malignant growths. TAS scan in Figure 12.48C shows presence of a large thin-walled cyst of right ovarian origin with multiple septa and numerous internal echoes. The ultrasound features such as presence of a multilocular mass with numerous internal echoes in this mass were indicative of a malignancy. Findings on clinical examination such as presence of solid mass with irregular margins also pointed towards malignancy. The suspicion of malignancy was confirmed on biopsy, which revealed the diagnosis of serous cystadenocarcinoma.

## Ovarian Cystadenocarcinoma

Transvaginal scan in a 52-year-old patient, who presented with the complaints of anorexia, bloating sensation, vague pain in the left iliac fossa, fatigue, weakness, increased frequency of micturition and history of severe weight loss since 1 month, shown in Figure 12.49A. This scan demonstrated presence of a multiseptated complex adnexal

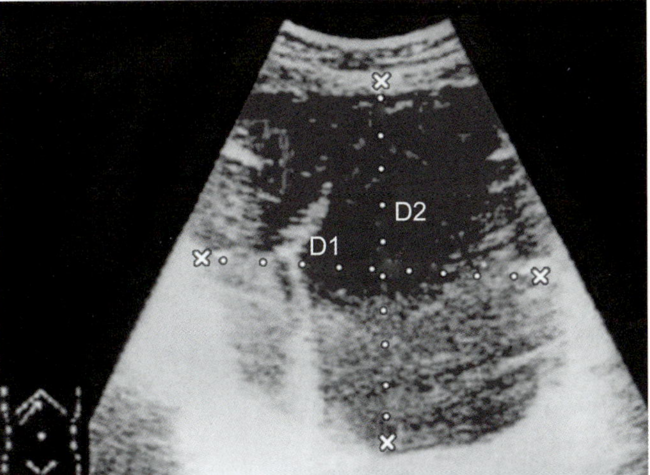



**Fig. 12.48C:** Transabdominal sonography showing presence of a large thin-walled cyst of right ovarian origin with multiple septa and numerous internal echoes

mass having heterogeneous solid areas. These features were highly suggestive of a malignancy. For establishing the diagnosis of ovarian cancer, the investigations which are most commonly performed include ultrasonography, CT and MRI. Biopsy of the tumor tissue and examination of the ascitic fluid may also be performed to reach a definitive diagnosis.

Color Doppler ultrasound in the patient described in Figure 12.49A showed increased blood flow (Fig. 12.49B). Biopsy revealed presence of an ovarian cystadenocarcinoma. Presence of low pulsatile index (< 1) and low resistance index (< 0.4) on Doppler ultrasound is suggestive of high blood flow within the mass. This is indicative of a malignant growth.

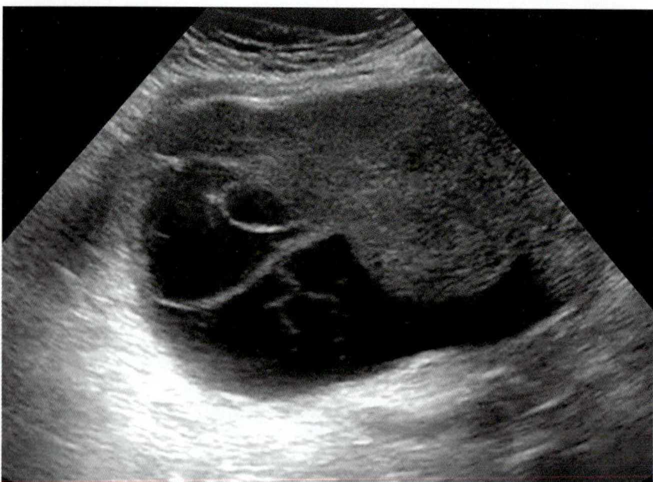

**Fig. 12.49A:** Transvaginal scan in a 52-year-old patient with complaints of anorexia, bloating sensation, vague pain in the left iliac fossa, fatigue, weakness, increased frequency of micturition and history of severe weight loss since 1 month

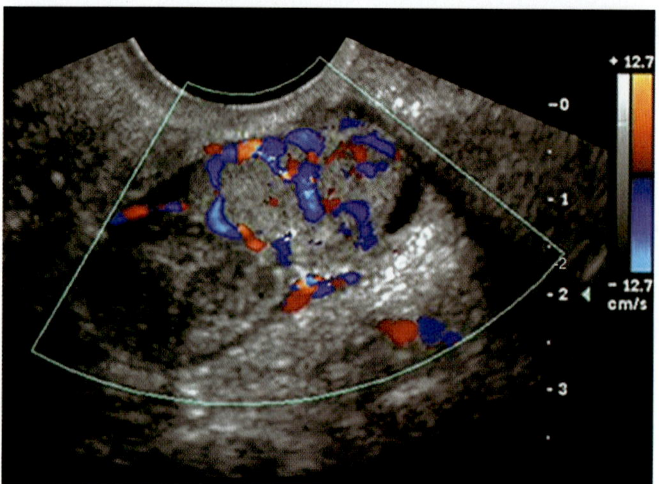

**Fig. 12.49B:** Transvaginal sonography color Doppler in the same patient

## ENDOMETRIAL CANCER

### Measurement of Endometrial Thickness

Measurement of endometrial thickness on transvaginal ultrasound has become a routine investigation in patients with abnormal uterine bleeding, especially those belonging to the perimenopausal age groups. Transvaginal ultrasound in Figure 12.40 showed an endometrial thickness of 9 mm. In this case, since the endometrial thickness on TVS is greater than or equal to 4 mm, an endometrial sampling/biopsy was performed to exclude endometrial hyperplasia. Biopsy revealed the presence of endometrial adenocarcinoma.

## Doppler Ultrasound

Prior to biopsy, Doppler ultrasound was performed in the previously mentioned patient (Fig. 12.40). It revealed endometrial hyperplasia with prominent peripheral vascular signals (Fig. 12.50). Increased blood flow and reduced resistance index on Doppler ultrasound is indicative of increased vascularization of the mass, which is a hallmark of malignant growth.

Figure 12.51 shows Doppler ultrasound in another patient with endometrial carcinoma. There were prominent peripheral and central vascular signals on ultrasound, which revealed presence of an advanced stage III endometrial adenocarcinoma.

A 58-year-old postmenopausal patient presented with irregular bleeding and abdominal pain since 1 month. Color Doppler ultrasound examination in this patient revealed thick heterogeneous endometrium with proliferation of

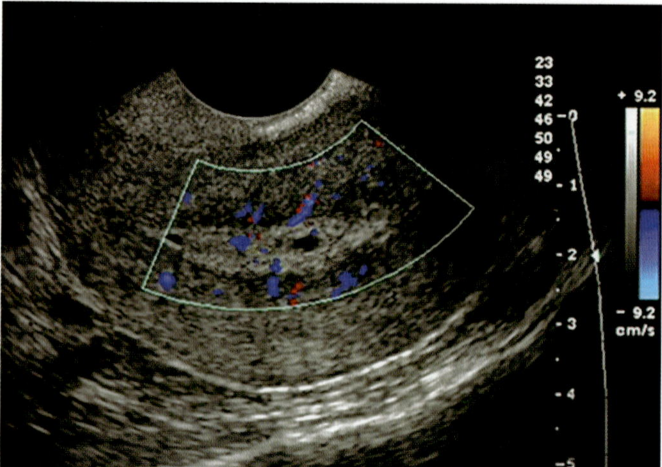

**Fig. 12.50:** Doppler ultrasound in the same patient as described in Figure 12.40

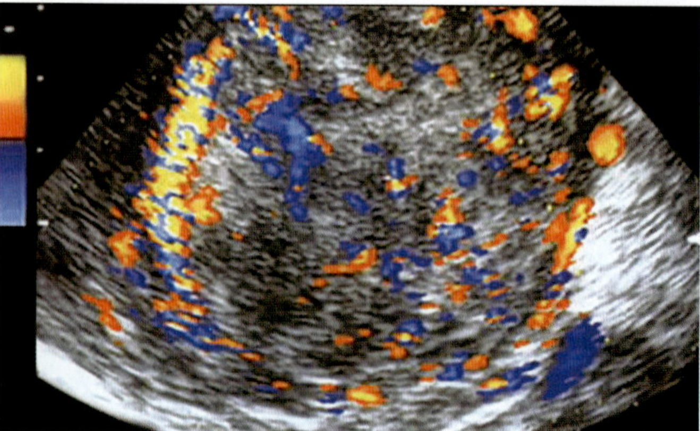

**Fig. 12.51:** Doppler ultrasound in a patient with endometrial carcinoma

blood vessels (Fig. 12.52A). A diagnosis of advanced stage endometrial cancer was made. In order to further assess the spread of endometrial cancer to distant body organs, an MRI examination was performed.

## MRI Examination

In order to further assess the spread of endometrial cancer to distant body organs in the case shown in Figure 12.52A, an MRI examination (shown in Figure 12.52B) was performed.

T1-weighted images on MRI examination revealed a large tumor of low signal intensity, expanding within the uterine cavity. There was no spread to distant body organs. On the basis of findings of clinical and radiological examination, the disease was classified as stage III endometrial cancer.

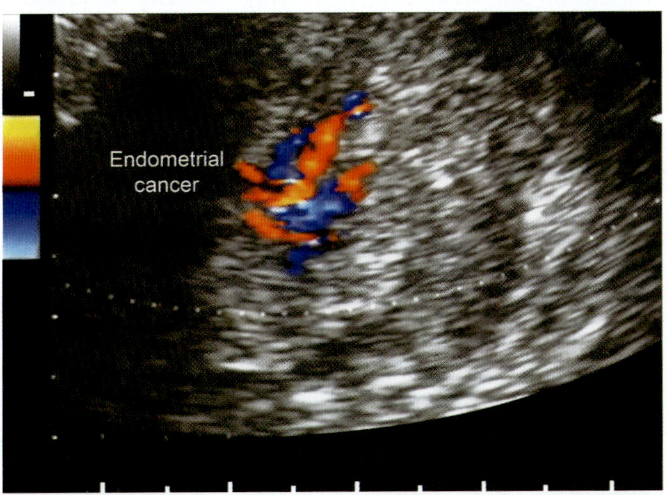


**Fig. 12.52A:** Color Doppler examination in a 58-year-old postmenopausal patient presenting with irregular bleeding and abdominal pain since 1 month

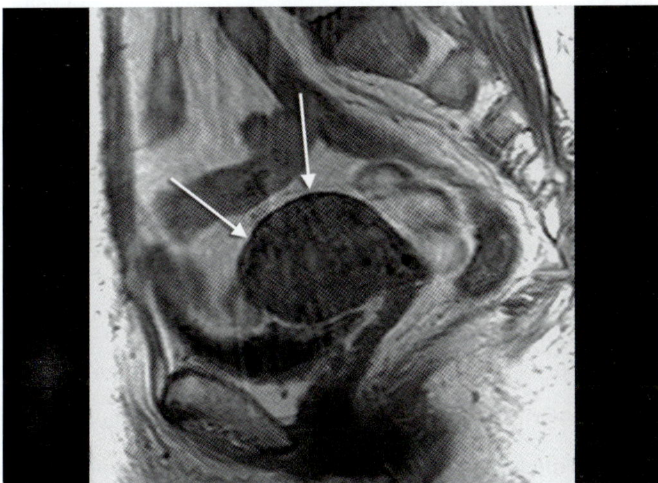

**Fig. 12.52B:** Magnetic resonance imaging scan showing endometrial adenocarcinoma in the same patient as described in Figure 12.52A

## CERVICAL CANCER

### Case 1

*Transabdominal sonography:* Transabdominal sonography in a 52-year-old postmenopausal patient with the history of abnormal vaginal bleeding revealed presence of a heterogeneous cervical mass (Fig. 12.53A). Diagnosis of cervical cancer is usually established with the help of symptoms such as abnormal vaginal bleeding and offensive vaginal discharge or leukorrhea.

Abnormal vaginal bleeding may manifest as irregular vaginal bleeding, postcoital bleeding, bleeding in between periods, etc.

*Doppler examination:* In the same patient as described in Figure 12.53A, a color Doppler examination was performed, which showed presence of randomly distributed irregular vessels in the mass arising from the posterior aspect of the cervix (Fig. 12.53B). This was highly suggestive of a malignancy.

*CT examination:* CT examination as shown in Figure 12.53C was performed, which revealed the diagnosis of stage I cervical malignancy. The tumor was limited to the cervix. No lymph node involvement or spread to adjacent organs was observed on the CT examination. CT examination in this patient showed a large lobulated cervical mass with central hypoattenuation.

### Case 2

Figure 12.54A shows TVS of cervix in another patient, 47 years old, who presented with severe suprapubic pain. TVS showed presence of a solid cervical mass measuring 3 × 2 × 2.5 cm. Biopsy of the cervical lesion helps in establishing the diagnosis in this case.

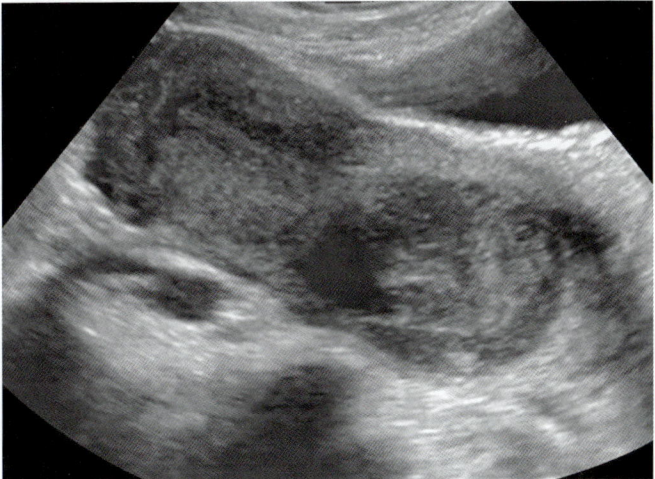

**Fig. 12.53A:** Transabdominal sonography showing solid heterogeneous cervical mass

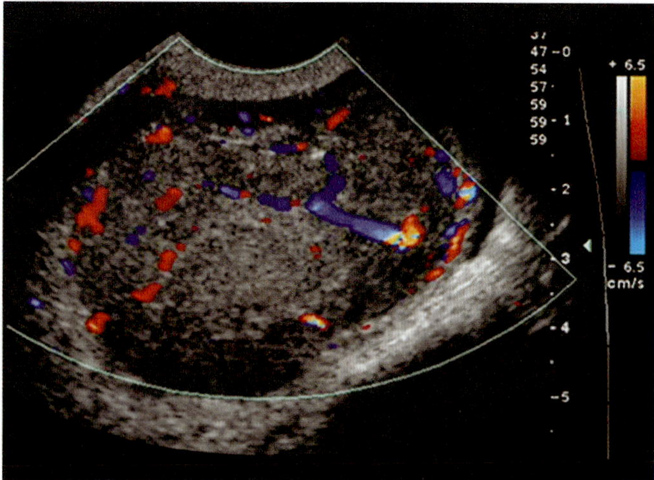

**Fig. 12.53B:** Color Doppler of the same patient as shown in Figure 12.53A

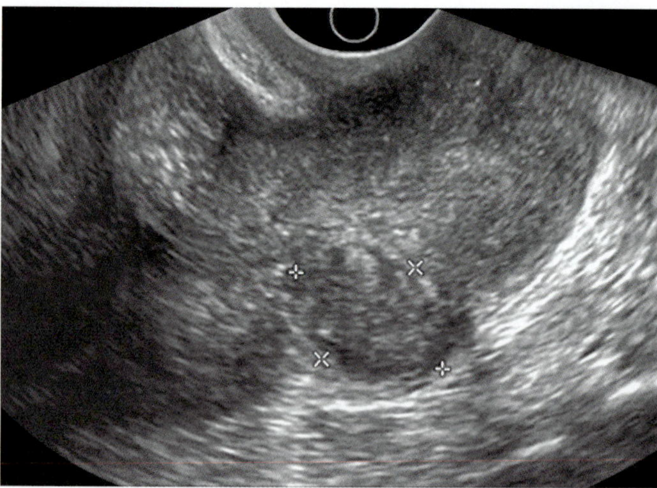

**Fig. 12.54A:** Transvaginal sonography of cervix of a 47-year-old patient with severe suprapubic pain

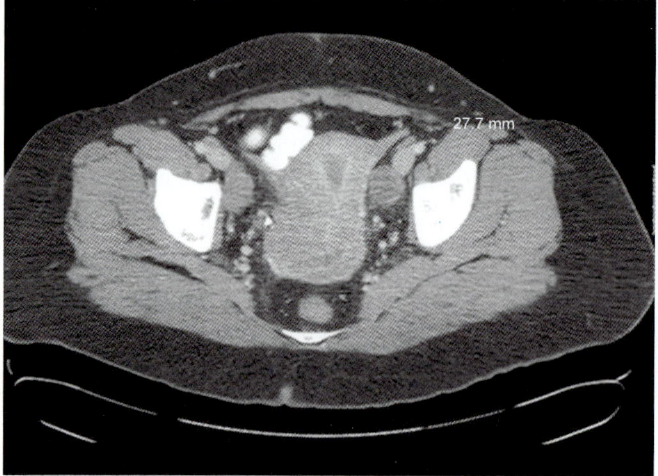

**Fig. 12.53C:** Computed tomography scan of the same patient as shown in Figure 12.53A

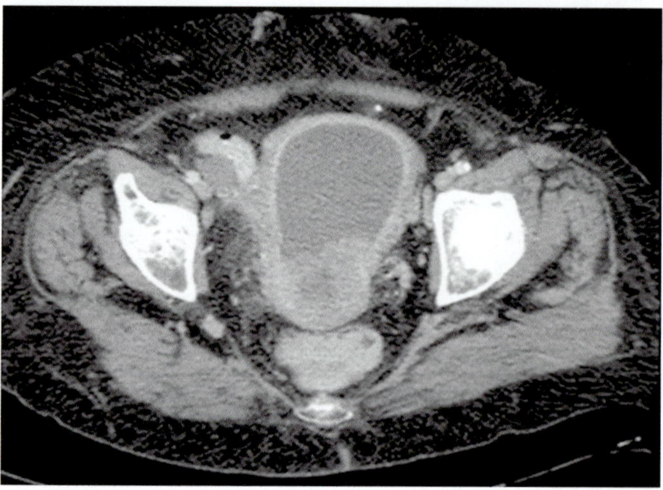

**Fig. 12.54B:** CT scan of the same patient as shown in Figure 12.54A

Figure 12.54B shows CT scan of the same patient as in Figure 12.54A, showing spread of the cancer. CT scan is one of the most commonly used imaging modalities for evaluation of metastasis and lymph node involvement in cases of cervical carcinoma. CT scan also provides a high resolution image of the pelvic anatomy, especially when used with a contrast medium.

## Diagnostic Radiology in Obstetrics

Irradiation of the pelvic area is contraindicated during pregnancy because of the risk of irradiation of maternal and fetal gonads as well as the whole body of pelvis. Nowadays, ultrasound has replaced X-ray for examination of the pregnant uterus and its contents. However, in some remote rural area where facilities for ultrasound may not be available, diagnostic radiology may be rarely used. Fetal shadow demonstrated on an X-ray may serve as a definite evidence of pregnancy. This fetus can be visualized as early as 16 weeks of gestation on X-ray examination. However, in modern obstetrics, diagnostic radiology is no longer used for confirmation of pregnancy or the fetal lie and position. Previously, before the advent of ultrasonography, X-ray was also used for the estimation of fetal maturity based on the ossification of various fetal bones.

### Intrauterine Fetal Death

Intrauterine fetal death can be defined as the diagnosis of the stillborn infant (with the period of gestation being > 28 weeks and fetal weight > 500 g).

Fetal deaths may be divided into two:

1. *Antepartum intrauterine death (IUD):* Fetal deaths occurring in the antenatal period and
2. *Intrapartum IUD:* Fetal deaths occurring during labor. Definitive diagnosis is made by observing the lack of fetal cardiac motion during a 10-minute period of careful examination with real-time ultrasound. Various radiological signs of fetal death are as follows:

   - *Spalding sign:* This is characterized by the irregular overlapping of the cranial bones and inwards collapse of the vault of skull. Nowadays, a sonographic examination is preferred to demonstrate this diagnostic feature of intrauterine fetal demise (Fig. 12.55). This sign usually occurs due to the liquefaction of the fetal brain and is usually evident 4–15 days after death.
   - Other signs of fetal death may include:
     - *Ball sign:* Attitude of extreme hyperflexion or hyperextension of the fetal spine and back and crowding of ribs due to the loss of tone of the muscles and ligaments of the back. As a result, the fetal back may be rolled up like a ball. This sign usually develops 4 weeks after fetal death.
     - *Helix sign:* Presence of gas shadows in the umbilical vessels.
     - *Robert's sign:* Appearance of gas shadows in the heart and great vessels.
     - *Dual halo sign:* This is seen around the cranial vault due to the elevation of pericranial fat as a result of underlying fluid accumulation. It is usually observed 2 days after the fetal death.

# X-rays in Gynecology

## HYSTEROSALPINGOGRAPHY

Hysterosalpingography has been described in details in Chapter 10. Kindly refer to Chapter 10 for details related to this topic.

## DIAGNOSIS OF PERFORATION CAUSED BY INTRAUTERINE DEVICES

Uterine perforation is a rare, but serious complication of IUCD insertion, occurring at a rate of 0.6–1.6 per 1,000 insertions. This may occur either at the time of insertion or at a later stage due to the embedment of the device into the myometrium and its subsequent migration into the intra-abdominal cavity. If the IUCD strings are not seen in the cervical os, the device may have been expelled out or may have perforated the uterine wall. In these cases, an ultrasound examination is the investigation of choice to check for the presence of copper device within the uterine cavity.

Ultrasound examination, both two-dimensional and three-dimensional, can demonstrate the presence of copper device within the uterine cavity. While the copper device is seen in the form of a bright echogenic shadow on two-dimensional ultrasound, three-dimensional images are able to properly delineate the device (Figs 12.56A to C).

Figure 12.56D is X-ray of the lower abdomen showing the presence of copper device outside the uterine cavity. Being a radiopaque structure due to the presence of impregnated barium sulfate, it can be easily identified on radiological examination. If the IUCD strings cannot be found, ultrasound

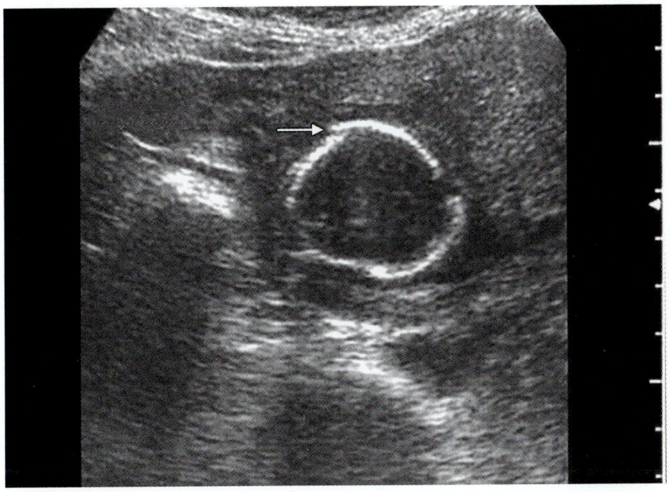

**Fig. 12.55:** Spalding sign: showing overlapping of the fetal skull bones (indicated by arrow)

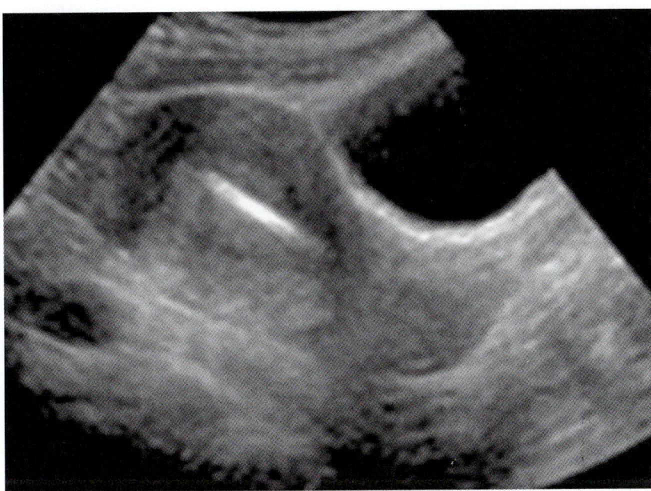

**Fig. 12.56A:** Two-dimensional ultrasound showing presence of copper device in the uterine cavity

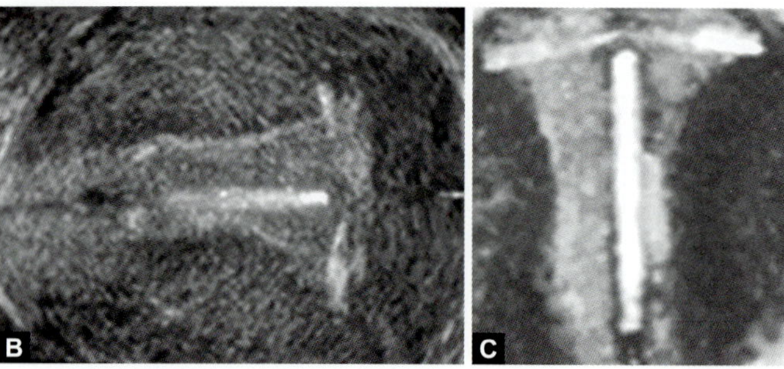

**Figs 12.56B and C:** Three-dimensional ultrasound showing the presence of an intrauterine copper device

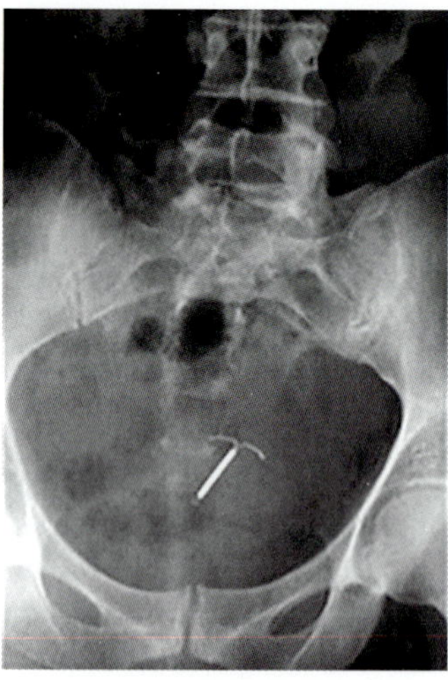

**Fig. 12.56D:** X-ray showing intrauterine device inside the abdominal cavity, confirming the diagnosis of uterine perforation

is the preferred method to identify the location of the IUCD. If the device is not identified within the uterus or the pelvis, a plain X-ray of the abdomen should be performed to determine whether the device has perforated the uterine wall.

## FURTHER READINGS


1. Alfrevic Z, Neilson JP. Doppler ultrasound in high risk pregnancies: systematic review with metaanalysis. Am J Obstet Gynecol. 1995;172(5):1379-87.
2. ACOG Committee on Practice Bulletins. ACOG Practice Bulletin No. 58. Ultrasonography in pregnancy. Obstet Gynecol. 2004;104(6):1449-58.
3. American College of Obstetricians and Gynecologists: Guidelines for diagnostic imaging during pregnancy. Committee Opinion No. 299. [online] Available from www.acog. org/-/media/Committee-Opinions/Committee-on-Obstetric-Practice/co299.pdf?dmc=1&ts=20141104T0432068221. [Accessed November, 2014].
4. American College of Obstetricians and Gynecologists. ACOG Practice Bulletin No. 27: Clinical Management Guidelines for Obstetrician-Gynecologists. Prenatal diagnosis of fetal chromosomal abnormalities. Obstet Gynecol. 2001;97 (5 Pt 1):suppl 1-12.
5. American College of Obstetricians and Gynecologists. ACOG Practice Bulletin No. 101: Ultrasonography in pregnancy. Obstet Gynecol. 2009;113(2 Pt 1):451-61.

# 13
## CHAPTER

# Instruments in Obstetrics and Gynecology

## CHAPTER OUTLINE

# Sims' Speculum (Fig. 13.1)

## DESCRIPTION

This speculum designed by Marion Sims, is a non-self-retaining vaginal speculum used in vaginal examination and operations to retract posterior vaginal wall (sometimes lateral or anterior wall) and view vagina and cervix. The main disadvantage of using this speculum is that an assistant is required to hold the speculum. Moreover, while using this speculum, one cannot visualize the cervix without retracting the anterior vaginal wall.

## USES

- *Gynecological uses*
  - Routine gynecological examination to visualize vagina and cervix
    - Inspection of cervix for growth, erosion and discharge
    - Inspection of vagina for vaginitis, cystocele, rectocele, enterocele and VVF
  - To collect discharge from posterior fornix (specimen for cytology, staining, culture, performance of a three swab test.
  - Hysterosalpingography
  - Performance of gynecological operations.
- Minor procedures on the cervix
  - Cervical biopsy, conization of cervix
  - Cervical tear stitching
  - Polypectomy
  - Dilatation of cervix.
- Procedures on the uterus
  - Dilatation and curettage (D&C)
  - Endometrial biopsy (EB)
  - Intrauterine contraceptive device insertion.
- Major gynecological operations
  - Vaginal hysterectomy
  - Fothergill's repair

  - Anterior colporrhaphy and posterior colpoperineorrhaphy
  - Vesicovaginal fistula repair.
- Diagnostic procedure
  - Hysteroscopy
  - Hysterosalpingography, sonosalpingography
  - Tubal insufflation.
- *Obstetric uses*
  - Routine per speculum examination (for diagnosing discharge, leaking, bleeding, etc.)
  - Manual vacuum aspiration (MVA), dilatation and evacuation (D&E), first trimester medical termination of pregnancy (MTP)
  - Application of cervical cerclage (McDonald stitch, Shirodkar stitch)
  - Diagnosis and repair of cervical tear.

# Sims' Anterior Vaginal Wall Retractor (Fig. 13.2)

## DESCRIPTION

This is a long instrument having a shaft and oval fenestrated ends. It is used along with the Sims' speculum to retract the anterior vaginal wall.

## USES

- The Sims' anterior vaginal retractor is commonly used along with Sims' speculum, to visualize cervix by retracting the anterior vaginal wall for various obstetric and gynecological indications (as described with Sims' speculum).
- It may be sometimes used in cases of postpartum hemorrhage just after delivery as a blunt curette to remove products of conceptions (POCs) and membranes.

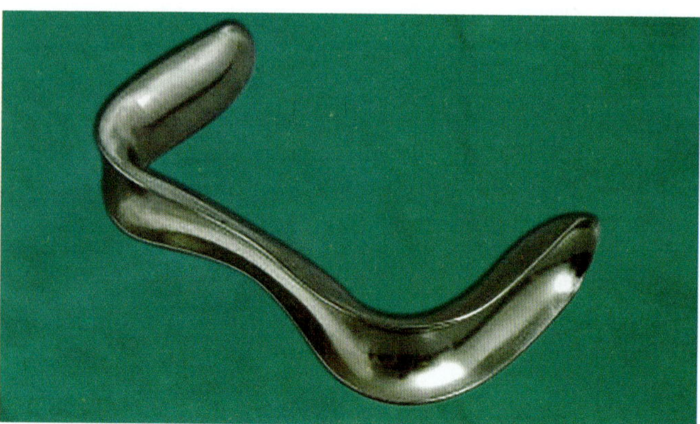

**Fig. 13.1:** Sims' speculum

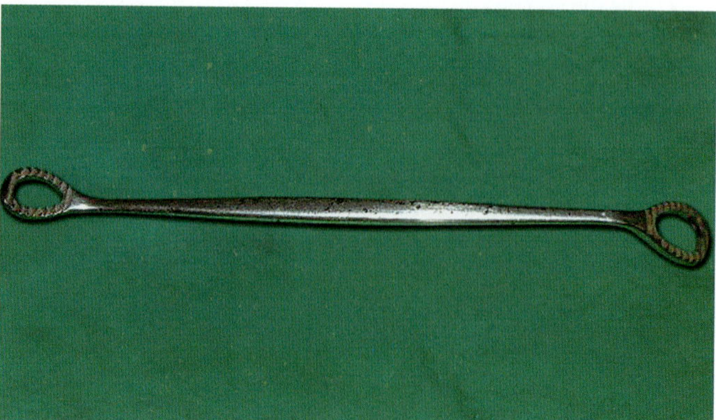

**Fig. 13.2:** Sims' anterior vaginal wall retractor

# Cusco's Speculum (Fig. 13.3)

## DESCRIPTION

It is a self-retaining vaginal speculum. This speculum is ideal for visualizing cervix and performing minor operations on cervix. Since it is self-retaining, no assistant is required. Moreover, it can be used even in those patients who cannot be put in the lithotomy position. The main disadvantage associated with its use is that it provides limited view of vagina because anterior and posterior walls cannot be visualized.

Prior to insertion, labia minora are gently separated and urethra is identified and the speculum is inserted with closed blades in vagina. When speculum is inserted completely it is angled approximately 30° downwards to reach the cervix. As speculum is opened ectocervix is visualized. The fixation screw is tightened depending on the amount of exposure needed. While removing the speculum, the fixation screw is unscrewed and blades are closed.

## USES

- Routine per speculum examination in gynecology
- Colposcopy
- Endometrial biopsy
- Cervical punch biopsy
- Pap smear
- Insertion and removal of IUCD
- Intrauterine insemination.

# Auvard's Weighted Self-Retaining Posterior Vaginal Speculum (Fig. 13.4)

## DESCRIPTION

It is self-retaining vaginal speculum with a heavy metal ball at one end. A groove or a channel is provided on the handle for collection and drainage of samples (e.g. blood/vaginal discharge, etc.). The speculum is inserted in such a way that weight of pendulum exerts a constant pull over the opening in which it is inserted. The speculum is self-retaining because the angle between the blades and the handle is less than 90°.

This speculum provides advantages of both Sims and Cusco's speculum in combination. It is self-retaining as well as provides good view of vagina. However, the prolonged use of this instrument may cause postoperative perineal pain and it can be only used when surgery is performed under anesthesia.

## USES

- Vaginal hysterectomy
- Anterior colporrhaphy
- Kelly's repair
- Fothergill's/modified Fothergill's repair
- Vesicovaginal fistula repair
- Schauta's radical vaginal hysterectomy.

# Soonawala's Self-Retaining Vaginal Speculum (Fig. 13.5)

## DESCRIPTION

This is another self-retaining vaginal speculum, which is sometimes used.

## USES

- Vaginal hysterectomy
- Vaginal tubal sterilization
- Vesicovaginal fistula repair
- Fothergill's repair/modified Fothergill's repair
- Schauta's radical vaginal hysterectomy.

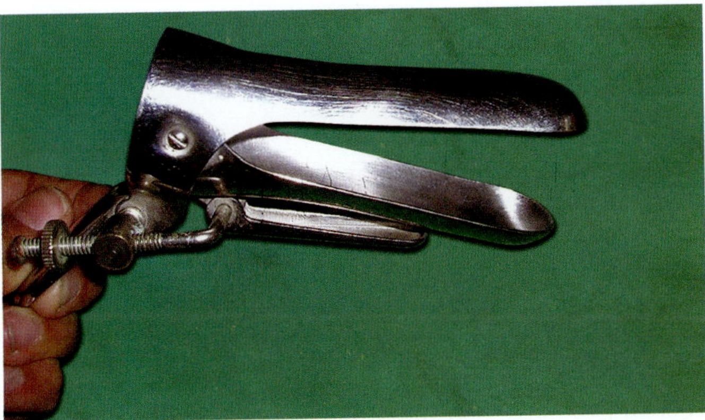

**Fig. 13.3:** Cusco's speculum

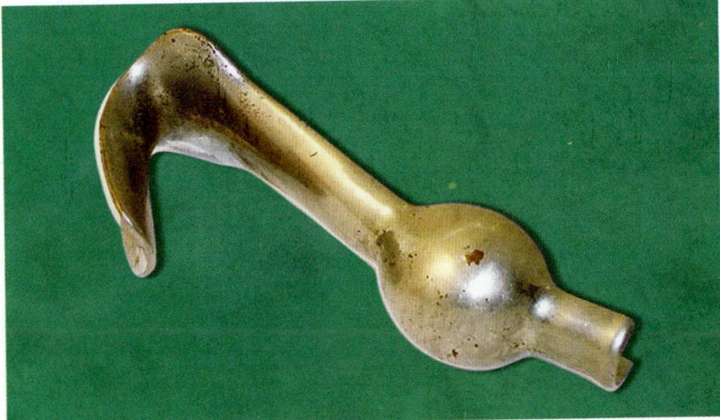

**Fie. 13.4:** Auvard's weighted self-retaining posterior vaginal speculum

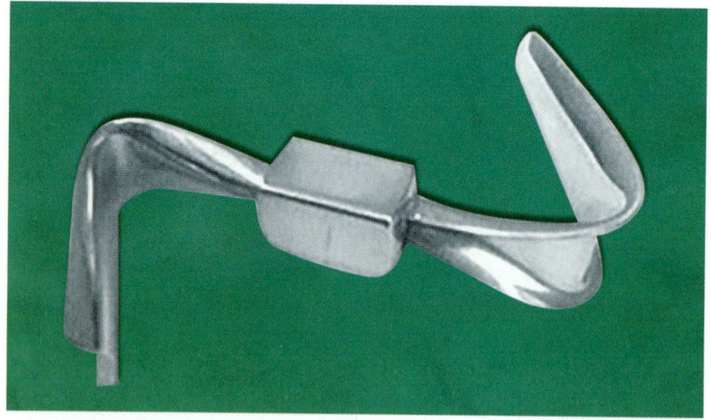

**Fig. 13.5:** Soonawala's self-retaining vaginal speculum

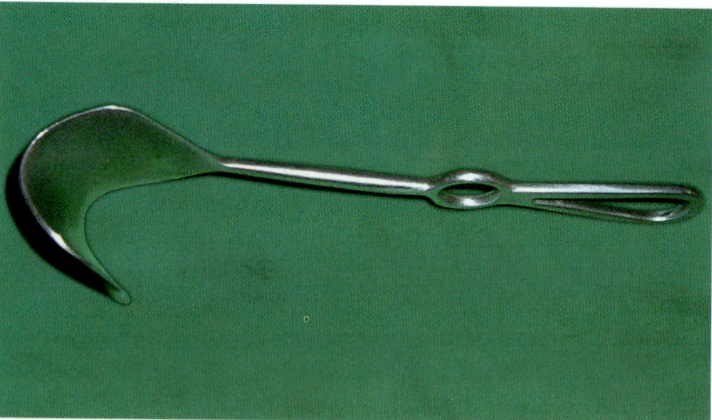

**Fig. 13.7:** Doyen's retractor

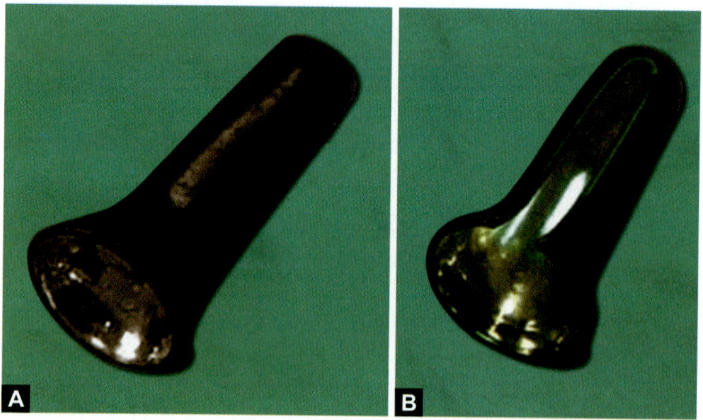

**Figs 13.6A and B:** Fergusson's tubular vaginal speculum. (A) Fergusson's mirror vaginal speculum; (B) Fergusson's fenestrated vaginal speculum

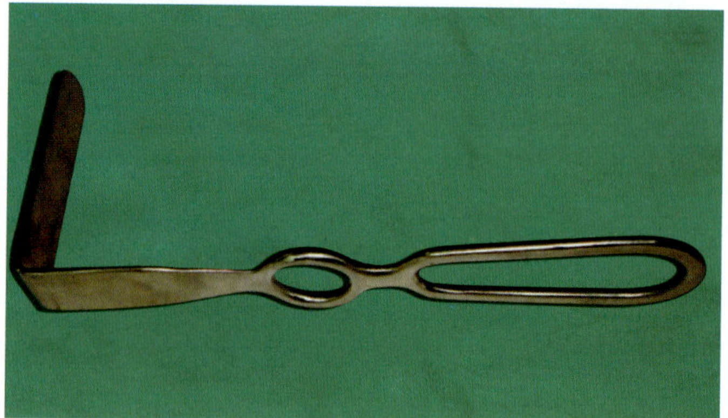

**Fig. 13.8:** Landon bladder retractor

# Fergusson's Tubular Vaginal Speculum (Figs 13.6A and B)

## DESCRIPTION

It is a cylindrical shaped cannula having a mirrored surface on the inner portion of its wall. Such speculums are nowadays less commonly employed in the clinical practice because they are associated with a limited field of vision. Moreover, its insertion may be associated with much pain.

# Doyen's Retractor (Fig. 13.7)

## DESCRIPTION

Doyen's retractor is a non-self-retaining, strong, heavy abdominal retractor having a large curved blade with inward turning margin. The solid blade compresses the cut edges of abdominal wall, thereby reducing blood loss from the injured vessels.

## USES

- *Gynecological surgery*
  - Abdominal hysterectomy
  - Wertheim's hysterectomy
  - Tuboplasty
  - Sling operation
  - Purandare's cervicopexy
  - Exploratory laparotomy for ovarian tumor
  - Myomectomy.
- *Obstetric surgery*
  - Cesarean section
  - Cesarean hysterectomy
  - Exploratory laparotomy for ruptured tubal ectopic pregnancy.

# Landon Bladder Retractor (Fig. 13.8)

## DESCRIPTION

It is an L-shaped instrument having a flat blade, which is at right angle to the handle. Present in between the blade and handle is a fenestration for gripping the instrument.

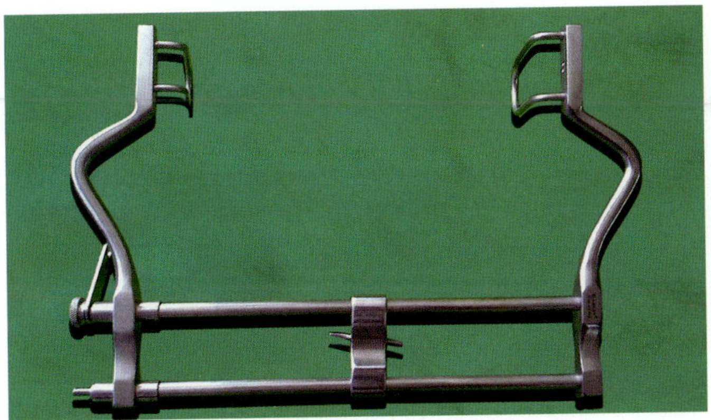

**Fig. 13.9:** Self-retaining abdominal retractors

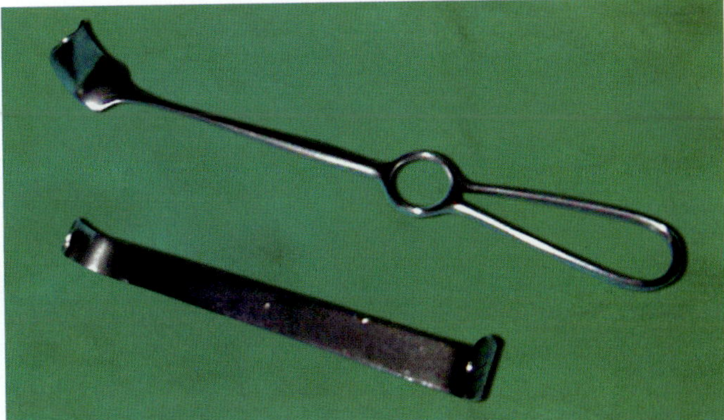

**Fig. 13.10:** Right angle retractor

## USES

- To retract the bladder away from cervix and uterus during vaginal hysterectomy. It is introduced into anterior pouch after the uterovesical fold of peritoneum has been opened.
- *Vaginal surgery:* The instrument is used for the retraction of lateral and anterior vaginal walls during any vaginal operation.

# Self-Retaining Abdominal Retractors (Fig. 13.9)

## DESCRIPTION

The self-retaining abdominal retractors have movable blades, the position of which can be fixed by screw locks. As a result, these retractors help in holding the abdominal wall muscles apart in three or four directions. When such retractors are used, an assistant is not required to hold the retractors in place. As a result, the assistant is free to participate in surgery. Moreover, application of correct and uniform amount of traction is possible throughout the operation. However, the main disadvantage associated with its use is that if used for extended period of time it can cause bruising of tissues, compression of nerve, even necrosis of rectus muscles.

## USES

- Prolonged and difficult surgeries
- To retract abdominal wall during tubal ligation
- To retract bladder and posterior vaginal wall during hysterectomy.

# Right Angle Retractor (Fig. 13.10)

## DESCRIPTION

This is the single-bladed right angle retractor, which is used for retracting different layers of abdominal wall or organs at the time of surgery.

Adequate retraction ensures that no damage would be caused to the underline organs and tissues at the time of dissection.

Double-bladed right angle retractors are also available, which enable the retraction of the underline organs and tissues at both the ends.

## USES

- To retract abdominal wall during tubal ligation
- To retract bladder and posterior vaginal wall during hysterectomy
- To retract bladder during abdominal hysterectomy.

# Tongue Depressor (Figs 13.11A and B)

## DESCRIPTION

Tongue depressor is a flat, thin, blade-like instrument either made of wood or metal, which is used for depressing the tongue in order to examine the mouth and throat.

## USE

- To examine oral cavity.

# Flushing Curette (Fig. 13.12)

## DESCRIPTION

This instrument has a long, hollow shaft ending in a small spoon-shaped scoop, which is used for scraping the uterine cavity for flushing out of the fetal brain matter at the time of craniotomy, a fetal destructive procedure. The instrument is rarely used nowadays for fetal destructive procedures.

## USES

- Flushing the uterine cavity (rarely used nowadays in obstetrics)

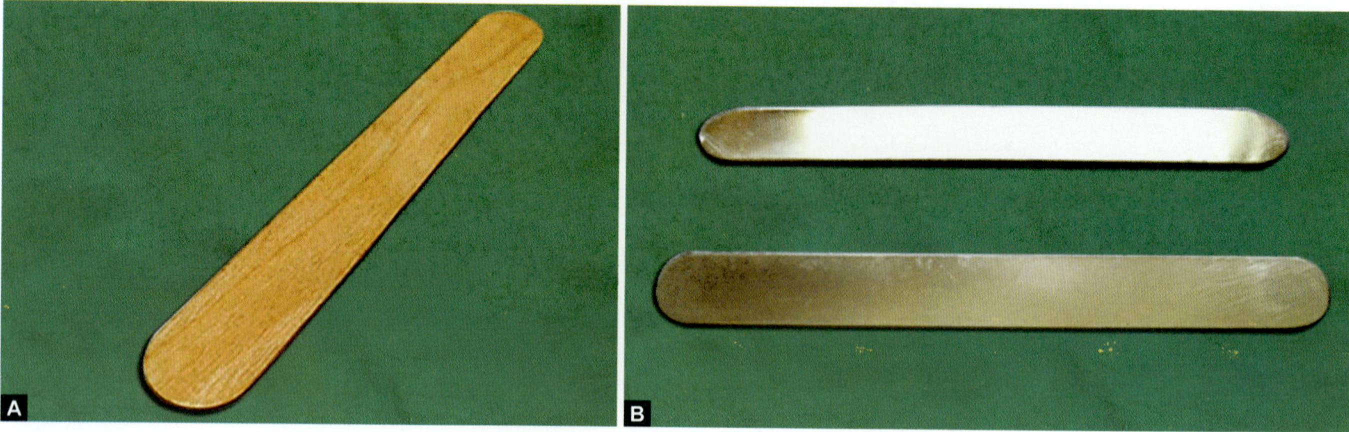

**Figs 13.11A and B:** Tongue depressor: (A) Wooden; (B) Metallic

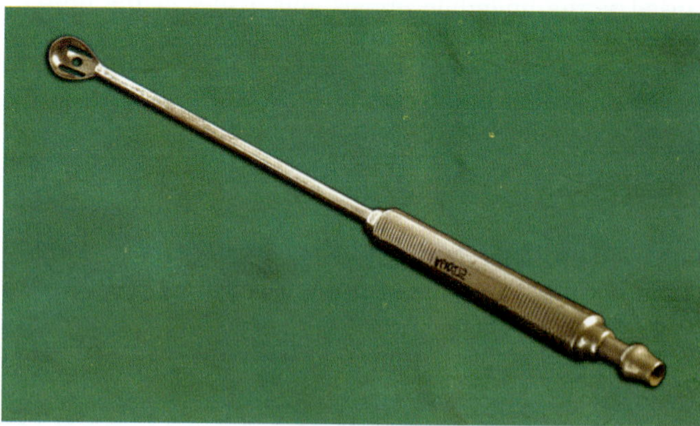

**Fig. 13.12:** Flushing curette

- Curetting the endometrial cavity for operations such as D&E, suction evacuation, D&C for indications such as MTP, incomplete/missed miscarriage, etc.
- Detection of endometrial pathology such as tuberculosis, endometrial cancer, proliferative or secretory phase endometrium, luteal phase defects, etc.

# Towel Clip (Figs 13.13A and B)

## DESCRIPTION

It is an instrument which is about 4–5" in length, light and strong, which is used for retracting surgical drapes from the site of surgery.

## USES

- For draping
- Can be used for hemostasis.

# Allis Tissue-Holding Forceps (Fig. 13.14)

## DESCRIPTION

Allis forceps is a commonly used instrument having sharp serrated edges/teeth, which are used for forcefully grasping or retracting tough tissues such as fascia as well as soft tissue (e.g. breast tissue, bowel tissue, etc.).

## USES

- *Gynecological surgeries:* To hold the edges of vagina
  - In anterior colporrhaphy, enterocele repair, colpoperineorrhaphy
  - In vaginal hysterectomy, abdominal hysterectomy
  - Fothergill's repair
  - Repair of vesicovaginal/rectovaginal fistula
  - To hold the cervix
  - Abdominal hysterectomy
  - To hold the lips of pediatric cervix
  - To hold the uterus
  - Vaginal and abdominal hysterectomy, myomectomy, utriculoplasty
  - Marchetti test for detection of stress urinary incontinence.
- *Obstetric indications*
  - In lower segment cesarean section (LSCS) to hold angles of uterine incision and to hold the rectus sheath while opening and closing abdominal wall
  - For correction of acute inversion of uterus.

# Needle Holder (Fig. 13.15)

## DESCRIPTION

As the name suggests, a needle holder is used for grasping the needle at the time of surgery. The inner surface of the tip

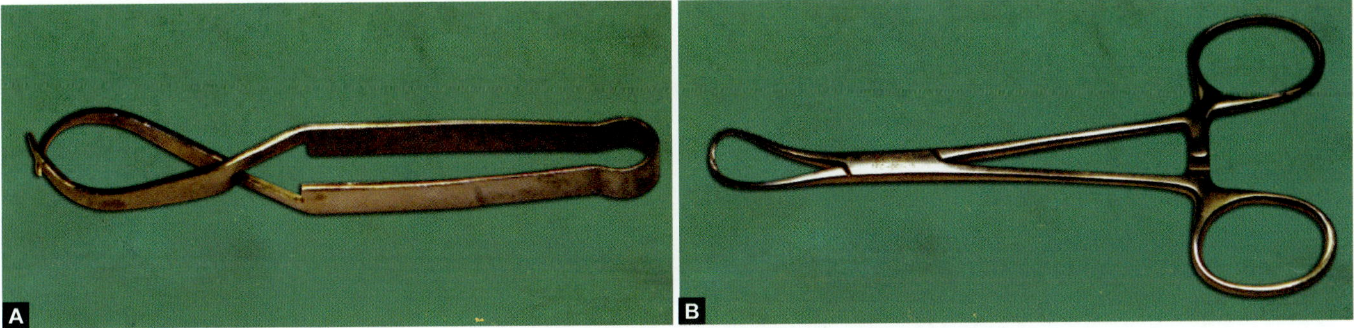

**Figs 13.13A and B:** Towel clips. (A) Jone's clip; (B) Mayo towel clip

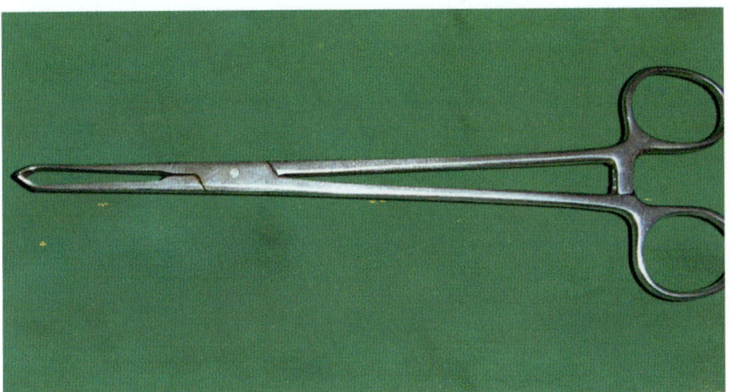

**Fig. 13.14:** Allis tissue-holding forceps

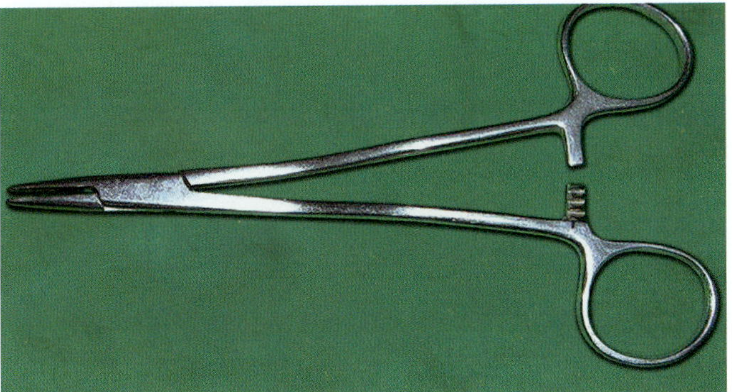

**Fig. 13.15:** Needle holder

has serrations and a small groove for the proper grasping of the curved needle. The joint of the equipment is close to the tip to help apply maximum pressure as a result of the lever effect.

## USE

- To hold needle during suturing.

# Artery Forceps (Figs 13.16A and B)

## DESCRIPTION

Artery forceps are primarily hemostatic forceps, which help in producing hemostasis by application of pressure through the lever action of the equipment. It can be used for grasping the tissues at the time of surgery. It can also be used for holding the stay sutures. Artery forceps can be of two types: curved and straight. The curved forceps is commonly used as a hemostat, wheresas the straight one is commonly used for holding the stay sutures.

## USES

- For hemostasis
- Holding structures like peritoneum, rectus sheath, vessels, muscles, etc. during any operative procedure
- For suture removal
- Can be used for clamping placenta after delivery of baby.

# Sponge-Holding Forceps (Fig. 13.17)

## DESCRIPTION

As the name suggests, the sponge-holding forceps is used for holding sponges during various surgical procedures. The instrument has elongated tips having smooth/serrated round edges. Many surgeons prefer to use these forceps because it causes minimal trauma to the tissues.

## USES

- *General indications*
  - Painting and preparing parts preoperatively
  - Swabbing out cavities like vagina and pelvic cavity

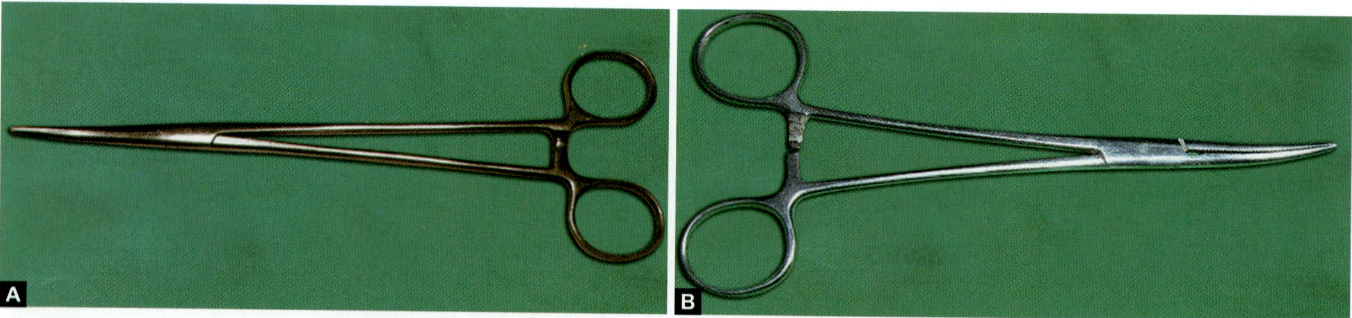

**Figs 13.16A and B:** Artery forceps. (A) Straight; (B) Curved artery forceps

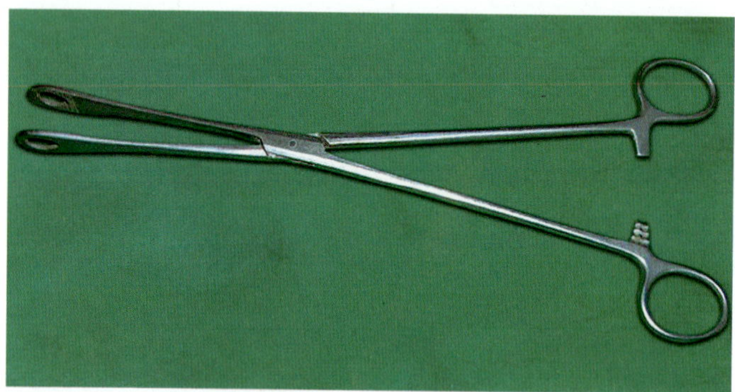

**Fig. 13.17:** Sponge-holding forcep

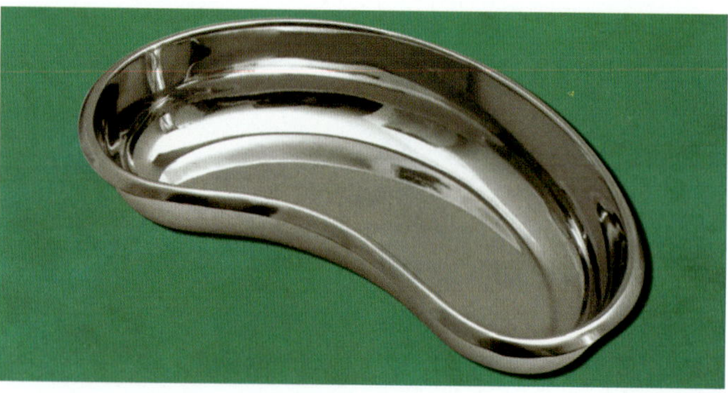

**Fig. 13.18:** Kidney tray

- *Gynecological indications*
  - For applying pressure over deep bleeding points during pelvic surgery
  - To check hemostasis of stumps during vaginal hysterectomy
  - For packing away omentum and intestines out of pelvis in gynecological operations
- *Obstetric indications*
  - To hold lips of pregnant cervix during tightening of os
  - For diagnosis and repair of cervical tears
  - Swab out blood from the uterine cavity.

# Kidney Tray (Fig. 13.18)

## DESCRIPTION

Kidney tray is a shallow basin having a kidney-shaped base and sloping walls. It is commonly used in the wards for receiving soiled dressings and other medical waste. Reusable kidney trays are made up of metal while the disposable ones are made up of paper pulp or plastic.

## USES

- To collect and hold urine
- To hold swabs for painting before any operation
- To collect placenta after delivery of baby
- To collect blood in ruptured ectopic pregnancy
- To collect vomitus.

# Kocher's Clamp (Figs 13.19A and B)

## DESCRIPTION

Kocher's clamps are clamps where the blades have teeth at one end. Presence of teeth ensures that the tissue the clamp is holding does not slip away. Due to the presence of teeth, the instrument can securely catch and hold the bleeders during hysterectomy, at the same time minimal amount of surrounding tissue is caught.

## USES

- *Gynecological indications*
  - To clamp the uterosacral ligaments, uterine blood vessels and the cornual structures or the infundibulopelvic ligaments in vaginal hysterectomy
  - To hold the uterus during abdominal hysterectomy
  - Oophorectomy for ovarian cysts or tumors
  - Removal of pedunculated leiomyomatous polyps
- Salpingectomy for tubal ectopic gestation

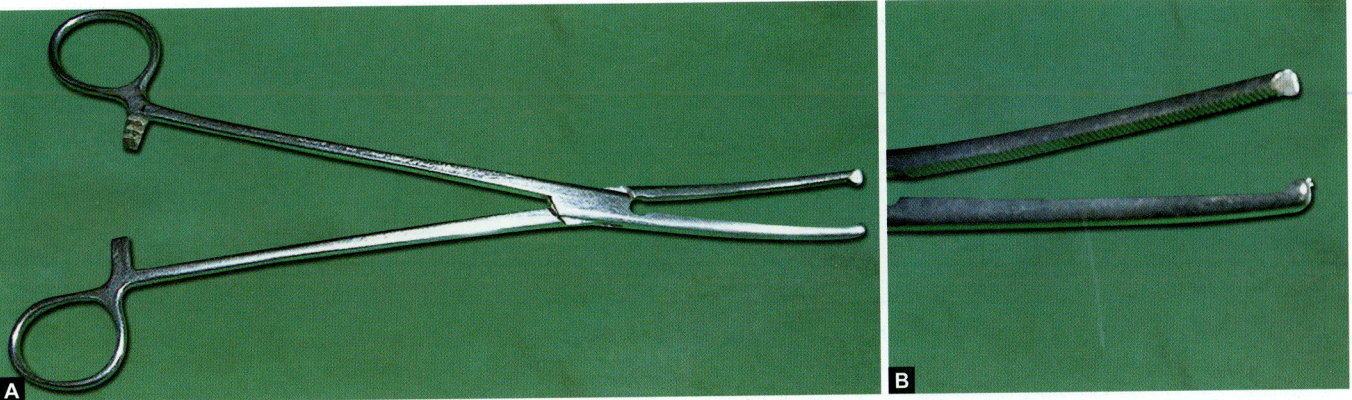

**Figs 13.19A and B:** Kocher's clamp: (A) The instrument; (B) Tip of Kocher's clamp

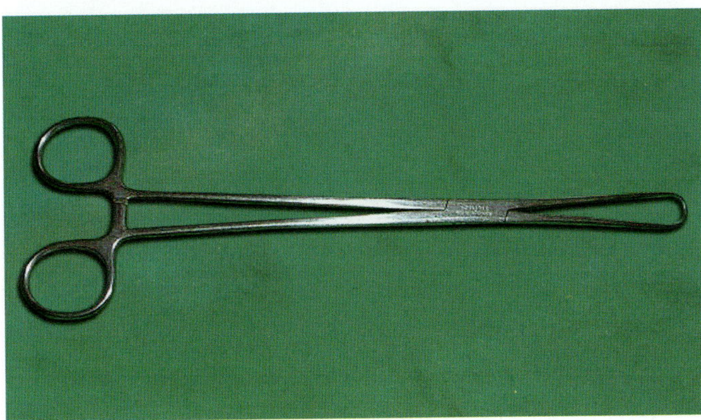

**Fig. 13.20:** Square-jaw single-tooth tenaculum

- *Obstetric indications*
  - Cesarean hysterectomy
  - Clamping the umbilical cord of the newborn
  - Artificial low rupture of membranes.

# Square-Jaw Single-Tooth Tenaculum (Fig. 13.20)

## DESCRIPTION

Tenaculum is an instrument having slender pointed hook at one end and is used for seizing and holding various body structures at the time of surgery.

## USES

- To hold the lips of nulliparous cervix
- To hold cervical stump in subtotal hysterectomy
- For steadying the cervix and uterus at the time of insertion of an intrauterine device.

## SPECIAL USES

- Hysterosalpingography
- Hysteroscopy
- Chromopertubation test
- Rubin's test.

# Straight Babcock Forceps (Figs 13.21A and B)

## DESCRIPTION

The instrument has loop-like triangular blades, which are semicircular in sagittal cross-section, at one end. Since the instrument is atraumatic, it is used for holding tubular structures such as the fallopian tube, appendix, intestine, ureter, etc. without compressing it.

## USES

To hold tubular structures like:
- Fallopian tubes in tubal sterilization, ruptured tubal ectopic pregnancy
- Round ligament
- Ureters in Wertheim's hysterectomy
- Vas in vasectomy
- To catch hold of the soft tissues such as appendix along with mesoappendix at the time of appendicectomy.

# Green Armytage Forceps (Fig. 13.22)

## DESCRIPTION

This instrument is primarily used for hemostasis because tip of the instrument has triangular-shaped wide areas which help in compressing the tissues it holds.

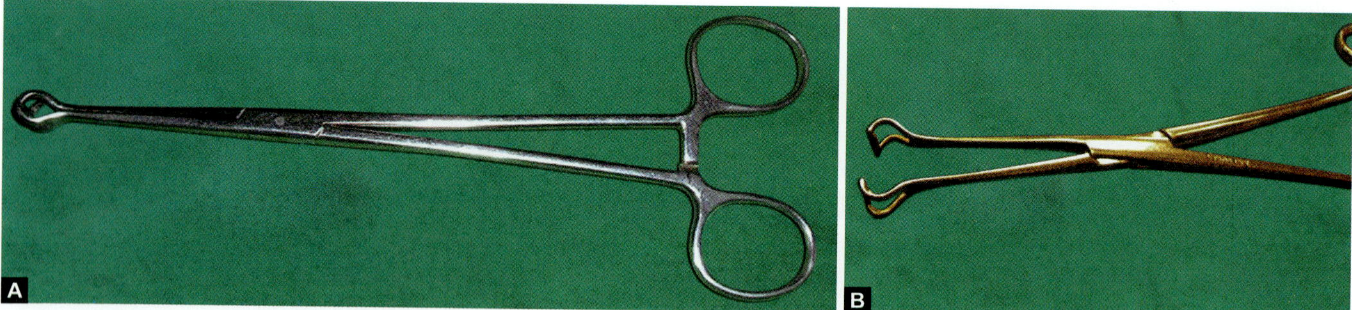

**Figs 13.21A and B:** Straight Babcock forceps. (A) The whole instrument; (B) Tip of Babcock forceps

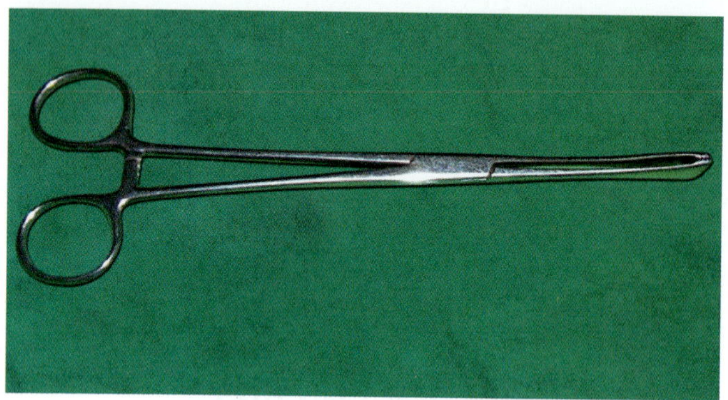

**Fig. 13.22:** Green armytage forceps

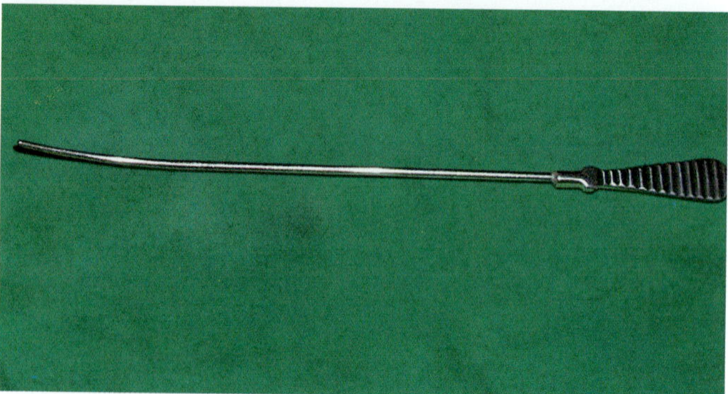

**Fig. 13.23:** Bladder sound

## USES

- To achieve hemostasis by compressing the bleeding uterine vessels during LSCS
- To lift uterine edges during suturing of uterus: for this purpose four forceps are used, two for holding the uterine angles and two for holding the upper and lower edges of the incision respectively
- To trace and repair cervical tears after vaginal delivery.

## Bladder Sound (Fig. 13.23)

### DESCRIPTION

Bladder sound is a long instrument having a gentle curve (unlike the uterine sound which is angled). Also, the instrument has no markings on it, unlike the uterine sound and is shorter in length in comparison to the uterine sound. Previously, this instrument was used for exploring the interior of a bladder because of united availability of noninvasive procedures such as radiography and ultrasonography. Nowadays, it has largely become an obsolete instrument.

### USES

- To define the limits of bladder during surgery (e.g. cystocele repair)
- To confirm a suspected bladder injury during vaginal hysterectomy
- To determine length and direction of vesicovaginal fistulae
- To sound a calculus or foreign body in the bladder
- To differentiate bladder or urethral diverticulum from anterior vaginal wall cyst.

## Simpson's Olive Pointed Graduated Metallic Uterine Sound (Fig. 13.24)

### DESCRIPTION

It is a long angulated instrument, about 30 cm long with handle at one end and a rounded blunt tip at the other end. It has graduations in inches or centimeters marked on it and is bent at an angle (at about 7 cm from the tip, which is the normal uterocervical length). The angle accommodates for flexion of uterus and prevents perforation as the instrument fits into the cavity of an anteverted or retroverted uterus. The tip of the instrument is blunt so that it does not cause injury when introduced inside the uterine cavity. The main disadvantage associated with this instrument is that it can cause uterine perforation in case the direction or size of the uterus is misjudged. Perforation is usually suspected when instrument travels deeper than the measured uterine length.

Uterine sounding must not be done in cases of suspected or confirmed pregnancy or infection.

## USES

- It helps to confirm the direction of uterus, i.e. anteverted or retroverted.
- It measures uterine cavity and cervical length, i.e. uterocervical length.
- It is used to diagnose cervical stenosis and congenital malformations, e.g. bicornuate uterus.
- Used as first dilator prior to operations on uterus and cervix, i.e. D&C, suction evacuation, etc.
- It helps to break the adhesions in Asherman's syndrome (therapeutic use).
- It helps to differentiate between chronic uterine inversion and a fibroid polyp.
- Diagnosis of uterine perforation: In cases of misplaced IUCD, uterine sound can be inserted and X-ray of pelvis is taken in AP and lateral view. Position of IUCD in relation to the uterine sound helps in detecting whether uterine perforation is present or not.

# Rubin's Cannula (Figs 13.25A and B)

## DESCRIPTION

This instrument was commonly used in the past for determining the patency of fallopian tubes. It is hardly used

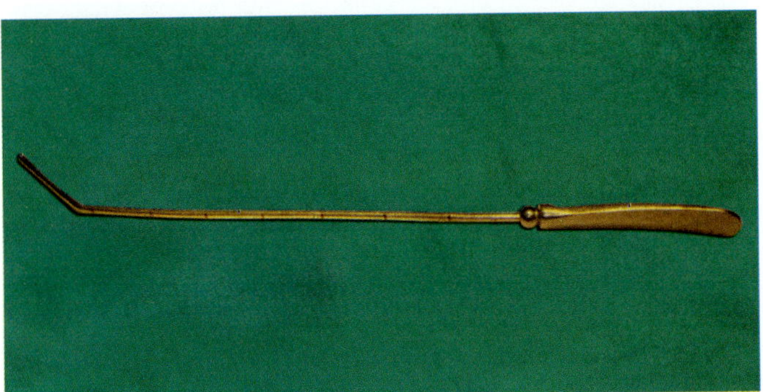

**Fig. 13.24:** Simpson's Olive pointed graduated metallic uterine sound

nowadays due to the introduction of advanced techniques such as ultrasound ( e.g. SIS) and laparoscopy (laparoscopic chromopertubation). This is a metal cannula having a rubber guard at one end. Position of this guard can be adjusted based on uterocervical length.

## USES

- It helps in detection of tubal patency in cases of suspected tubal factor infertility. For details related to Rubin's test, kindly refer to Chapter 10.
- Confirmation of tubal patency after tuboplasty.

# Leech Wilkinson/Colwin's Cannula (Figs 13.26A and B)

## DESCRIPTION

This instrument was commonly used in the past for determining the patency of fallopian tubes. It is hardly used nowadays due to the introduction of advanced techniques such as ultrasound (e.g. SIS) and laparoscopy (laparoscopic chromopertubation). This is a metal cannula with a conical tip having screw-like serrations. This helps in screwing the cannula inside the cervical canal to prevent the leakage of the dye.

## USES

- Hysterosalpingography
- Chromopertubation test in laparoscopy
- Hydrotubation.

# Plain Forceps (Fig. 13.27)

## DESCRIPTION

Forceps are hand-held, hinged instruments used for grasping and holding intricate objects, which are too small to be held with fingers (e.g. tissues at the time of surgery). There are two types of forceps: plain and toothed forceps. Plain forceps have smooth ends, which help in grasping smooth and delicate tissues such as peritoneum, fat, etc.

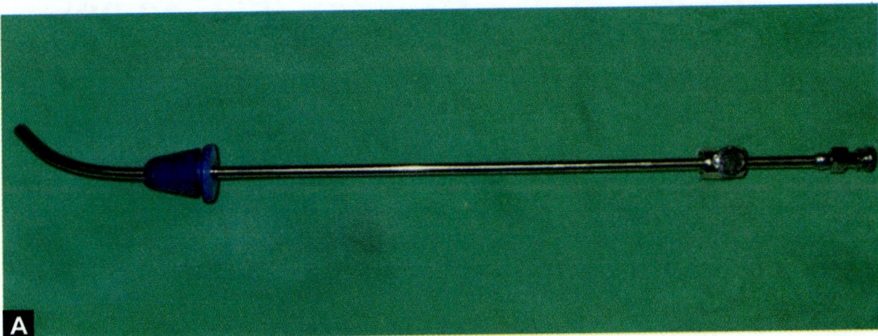
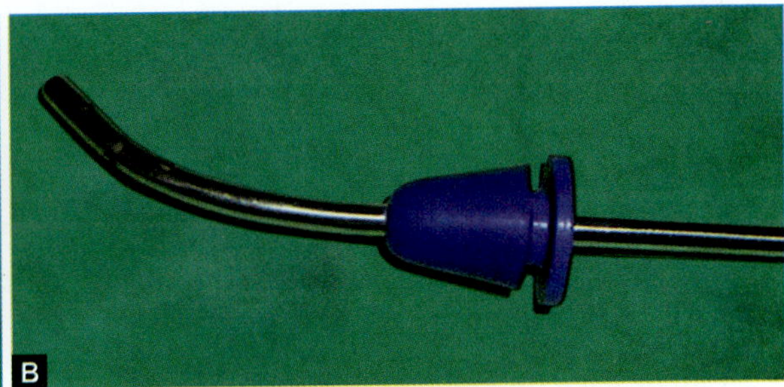

**Figs 13.25A and B:** Rubin's cannula. (A) The complete equipment; (B) The tip of Rubin's cannula

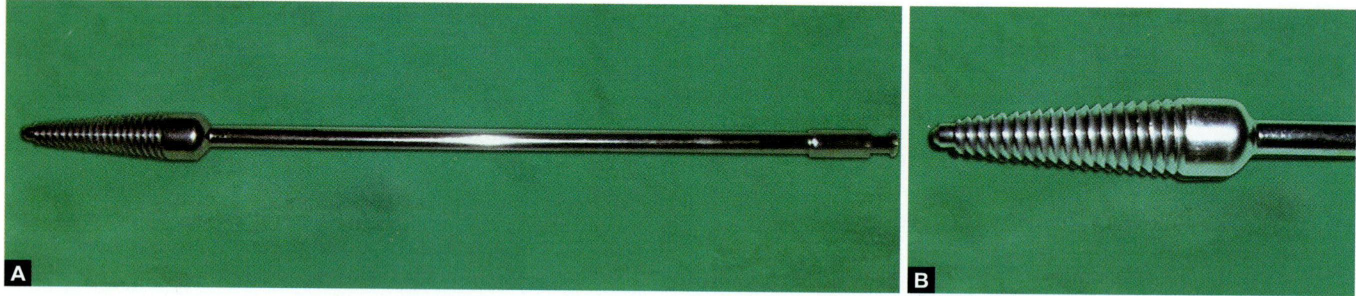

**Figs 13.26A and B:** Leech Wilkinson's cannula: (A) The whole equipment; (B) Tip of Leech Wilkinson's cannula

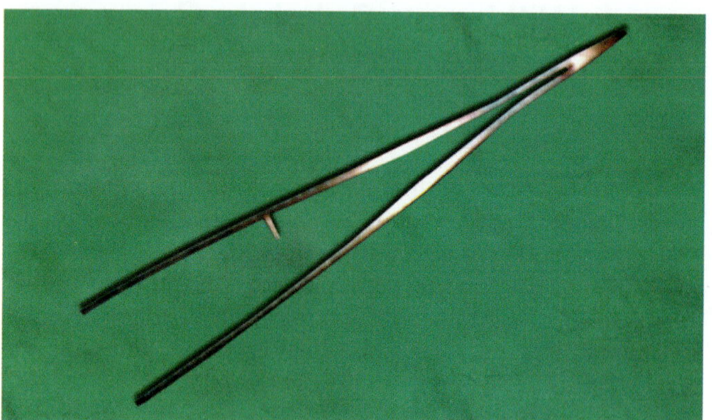

**Fig. 13.27:** Plain forceps

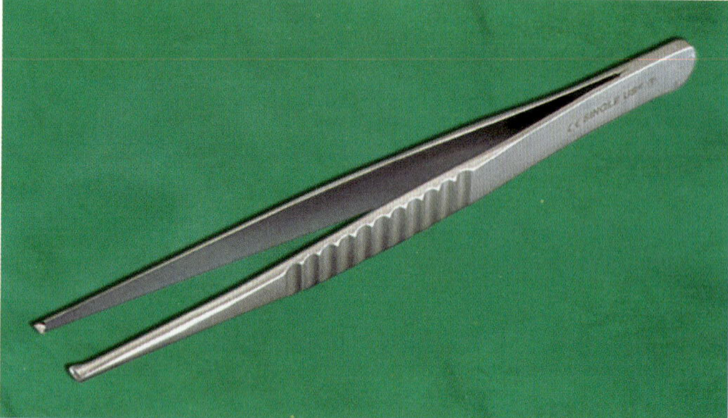

**Fig. 13.28:** Toothed forceps

## USES

- To hold thin delicate structures such as peritoneum, muscles, vessels, thin fascia, intestinal wall, bladder wall, etc.
- During suture removal
- Packing abdominal cavity during abdominal operations.

# Toothed Forceps (Fig. 13.28)

## DESCRIPTION

Toothed forceps have toothed ends, which helps in grasping tough tissues (e.g. rectus sheath, skin, etc.).

## USES

- To hold tough structures like:
  - Tendon
  - Fascia
  - Skin
  - Rectus sheath
  - Uterine wall, etc.
- Can be used for hemostasis.

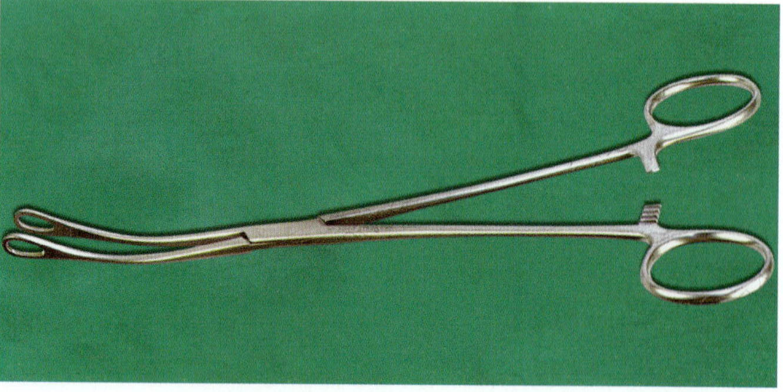

**Fig. 13.29:** Uterine polyp forceps

# Uterine Polyp Forceps (Fig. 13.29)

## DESCRIPTION

This is a curved grasping forceps having serrated rounded edges.

## USE

- Retrieval of polyps from the uterine cavity.

# Cheatle Forceps (Fig. 13.30)

## DESCRIPTION

It is a large heavy metallic, curved forceps having serrations for better grip. The instrument has no lock. The instrument is kept sterilized by keeping it dipped in a bottle containing savlon, cidex, etc. or by autoclaving it.

## USE

- Picking and transferring sterilized linen or instruments from one tray to other.

# Hegar's Dilator (Fig. 13.31)

## DESCRIPTION

Hegar's dilators are curved double-ended dilators with conical tips used for rapidly dilating the endocervical canal and internal os. Each double-ended dilator has two sizes with a difference of 0.5 mm. Different sizes are denoted by numbers, which vary depending on the diameter of the shaft, e.g. 2/2.5: one end of the dilator has a diameter of 2 mm while the other end has a diameter of 2.5 mm. Hegar's dilators may be single-ended or double-ended. Single-ended ones are available in a set of 25 sizes ranging in size from 2 mm upwards to 26 mm. On the other hand, double-ended ones are available as a set of 12 dilators ranging in size from 0.5 mm to 23/24 mm. The presence of a slight angle at the ends makes the instrument less traumatic. The increasing sizes of dilators make cervical canal patulous by gradually stretching the muscle and fibrous tissue of the cervix.

Complications associated with the use of this dilator are few and rare. The most important complication which can occur as a result of using this dilator is uterine perforation. Uterine perforation occurs mainly in soft uterus, i.e. pregnant uterus, in atrophic postmenopausal or scarred uterus and can also occur in malignant uterus.

## USES

- For the rapid dilatation:
  - Prior to endometrial curettage
  - Prior to suction aspiration for first trimester MTP
  - Prior to suction evacuation of mole
- Removal of endometrial polyp, placental polyp, leiomyomatous polyp
- Hysteroscopy
- Amputation of cervix, Fothergill's operation, following cervical conization
- Cervical stenosis
- Application of intrauterine radiotherapy
- Primary dysmenorrhea
- Diagnosis of incompetent os.

# Fenton/Pratt's Dilator (Fig. 13.32)

## DESCRIPTION

Fenton's dilators are similar to Hegar's dilators except that Fenton's dilators are more sinuous than the Hegar's dilators. Therefore they are more suitably curved for the uterocervical canal. As a result, dilatations are easier and there are fewer failures. However, the risk of perforation is also higher in

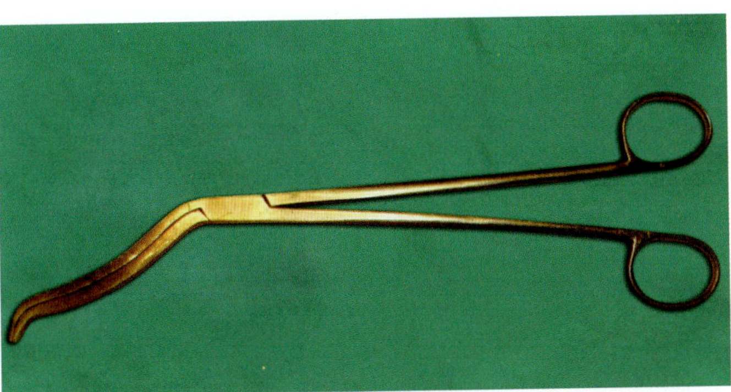

**Fig. 13.30:** Cheatle forceps

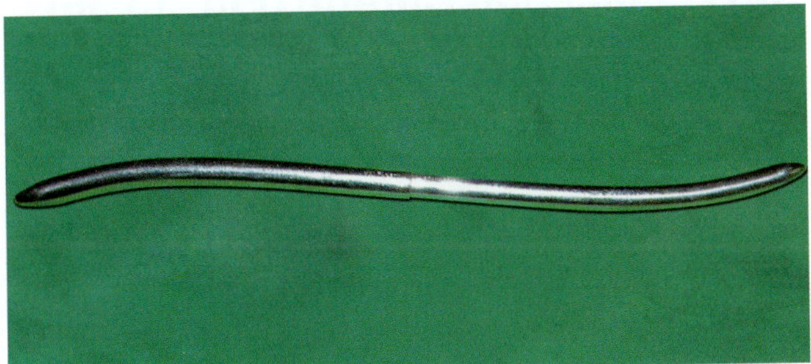

**Fig. 13.31:** Hegar's double-ended dilator

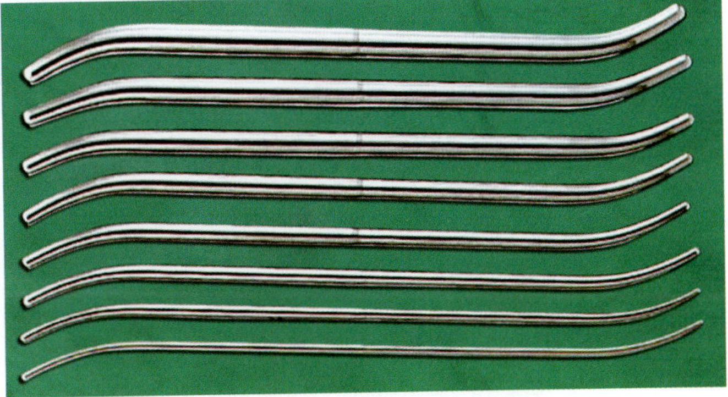

**Fig. 13.32:** Fenton/Pratt's dilator

comparison to the Hegar's dilators due to an increased curvature. They are available in a set of 12 dilators ranging from 3 mm to 26 mm.

## USE

- Same as that of Hegar's dilator.

# Hawkin Ambler Dilator (Fig. 13.33)

### DESCRIPTION

These dilators have a rounded base with the size of instrument imprinted on it. The markings on the instrument indicate the circumference in mm. The base is wider than the tip by 3 mm. Therefore, if the size is 4/7, it implies that the circumference of the tip is 4 mm and that of the base is 7 mm. The complete set ranges in size from 3/6 to 18/21 arranged according to the increasing circumference.

### USE

- Same as that of Hegar's dilators.

# Purandare MTP Dilators (Fig. 13.34)

### DESCRIPTION

This is a cervical dilator having a guard and a long tapering end. The guard is at a distance of 1.5 inches from the tip and helps in preventing insertion beyond that length, thereby protecting against perforation.

### USE

- Same as that of Hegar's dilators.

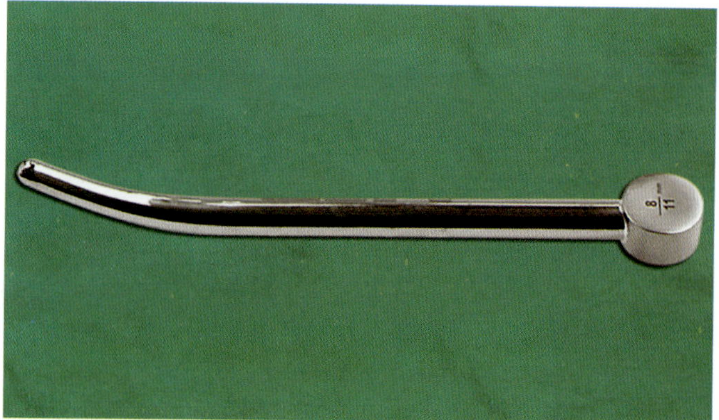

**Fig. 13.33:** Hawkin Ambler dilator

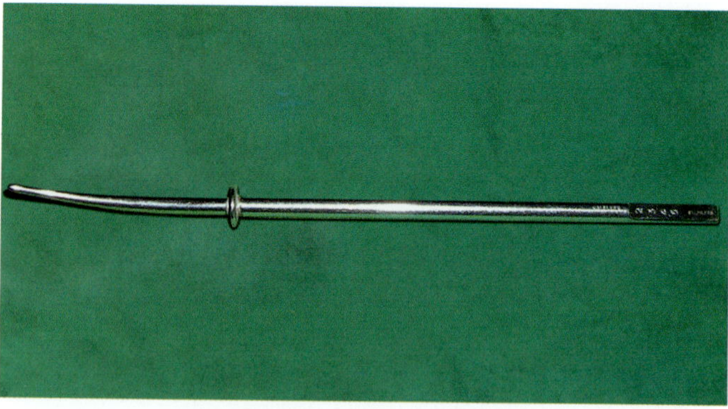

**Fig. 13.34:** Purandare MTP dilator

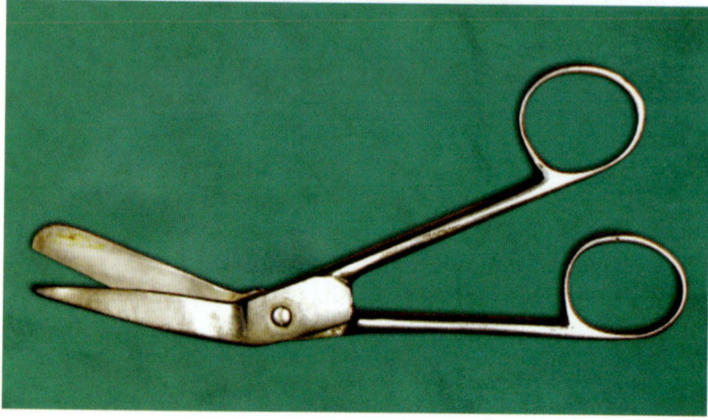

**Fig. 13.35:** Episiotomy scissors

# Episiotomy Scissors (Fig. 13.35)

### DESCRIPTION

These scissors have angulated blades with blunt tip, which helps in avoiding damage to the various tissue structures.

### USE

- This is used for giving episiotomy during crowning of the fetal head at the time of normal vaginal delivery.

# Cuzzi Placental Curette (Fig. 13.36)

### DESCRIPTION

This instrument has a blunt serrated scoop like end, which helps in scooping out residual tissues and blood clots from the uterine cavity.

### USES

- Check curettage for incomplete abortion and retention of the placenta in second trimester.

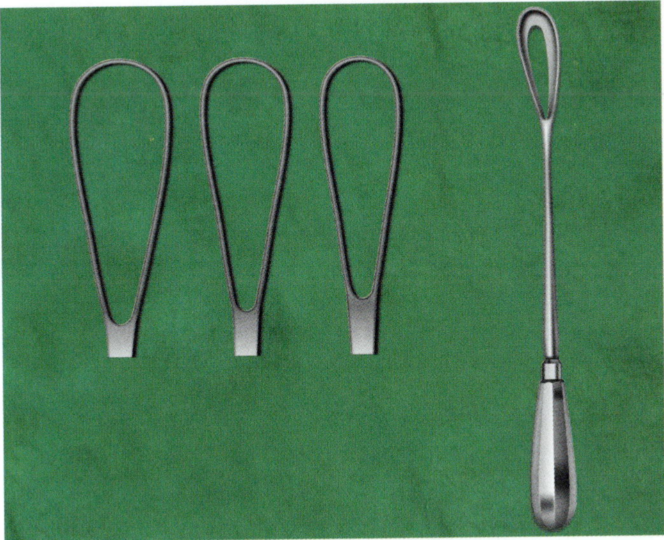

**Fig. 13.36:** Cuzzi placental curette

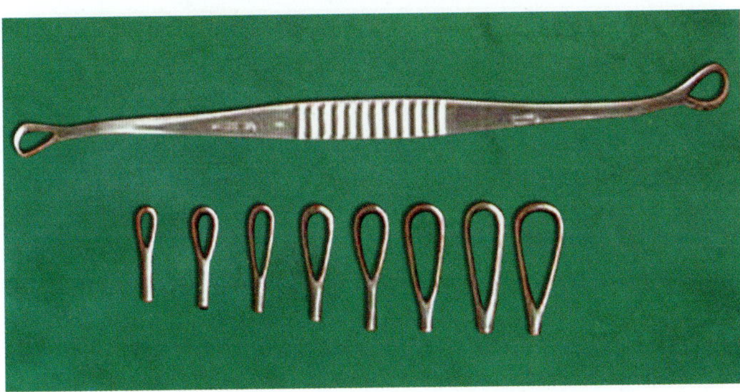

**Fig. 13.37:** Sharp and blunt uterine curette

- Removal of retained segments or bits of placenta after delivery of a viable fetus.

# Sharp and Blunt Uterine Curette (Fig. 13.37)

## DESCRIPTION

This instrument is used for scraping the endometrial cavity and has a sharp and blunt curette respectively at the two ends. The sharp curette is used for gynecological indications whereas the blunt curette is used in the pregnant uterus for performing check curettage.

## USES

- *Gynecological use*
  - Diagnostic
    - Primary or secondary infertility for detection of ovulation

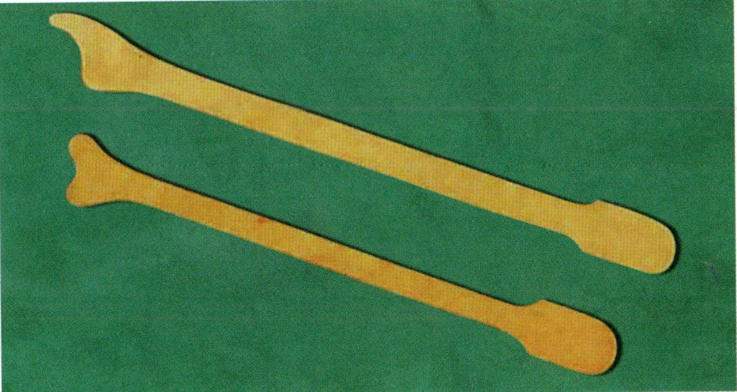

**Fig. 13.38:** Ayre's wooden spatula

- Tuberculous endometritis
    - Abnormal uterine bleeding
    - Endometrial hyperplasia/endometrial carcinoma
    - Carcinoma cervix
    - Secondary amenorrhea
    - Postmenopausal bleeding
  - Therapeutic
    - Dysfunctional uterine bleeding
    - Asherman's syndrome
    - To remove embedded intrauterine device
- *Obstetrical use*
  - Medical termination of pregnancy, check curettage
  - Blunt curettage in incomplete abortions.

# Ayre's Wooden Spatula (Fig. 13.38)

## DESCRIPTION

This is a wooden spatula made of birch wood. It is used for sampling ectocervix and posterior fornix in cervical cancer screening procedure.

It is about 15–20 cm in length and has smooth bifurcated edges, which can fit into the ectocervix.

## USES

- Pap smear (For details related to Pap smear, kindly refer to Chapter 10)
- To take surface biopsy in obvious cases of carcinoma cervix
- Hormonal cytology
- Cervicovaginal smear
- Buccal smear.

# Cytobrush (Fig. 13.39)

## DESCRIPTION

Cytobrush comprises of a stick-like structure made up of inert plastic material having gentle bristles of the brush at one end.

Presence of brush-like bristles on the endocervical brush help in collection of a large sample.

## USE

- Collection of aspirate from the endocervical canal (at the time of collection of Pap smear or otherwise).

# Rubber Catheter (Fig. 13.40)

## DESCRIPTION

Plain or simple red rubber catheter is a non-self-retaining catheter. It comes in various sizes and consists of a tube made of red rubber. Blunt end of tube is rounded with subterminal opening for drainage, whereas the other end is expanded.

## USES

- Single urethral catheterization
- To administer oxygen as an alternative to oxytube or oxygen set.

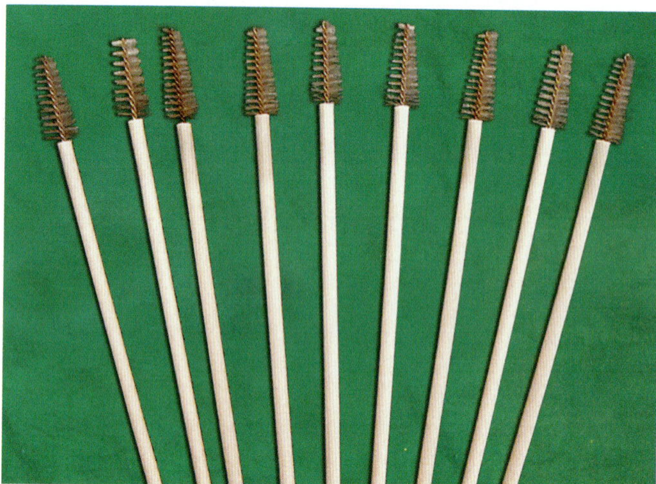

**Fig. 13.39:** Cytobrush

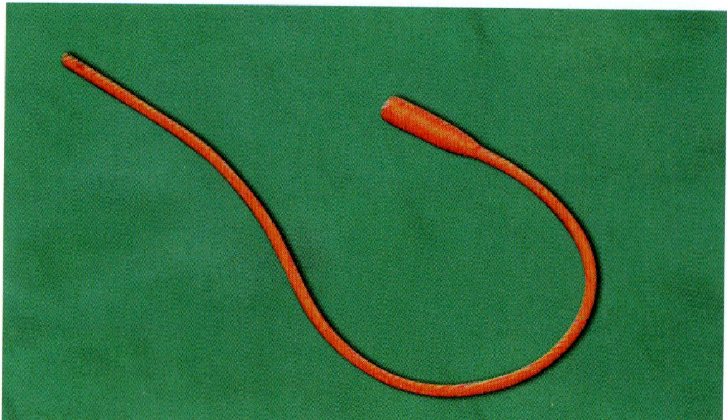

**Fig. 13.40:** Rubber catheter

- As tourniquet during myomectomy operation
- As a tourniquet for drawing blood samples
- To collect urine sample for culture sensitivity in cases of chronic urinary tract infections
- Performance of three swab test in cases of urinary fistula.

# Metal Catheter (Fig. 13.41)

## DESCRIPTION

It is a metal catheter for urine drainage. The tip has a curve and there are two eyes near the tip.

## USE

- A metal catheter is used for bladder drainage in cases where the rubber catheter cannot be passed.

# Foley's Catheter (Fig. 13.42)

## DESCRIPTION

This is a self-retaining catheter, made up of latex having silicon coating. The tip of the catheter has a subterminal opening for drainage. Beyond this is a balloon which is inflated with saline or plain water. Capacity of bulb is mentioned in catheters. There can be 2–3 channels. A two-channeled catheter is generally used in clinical practice: the main channel is for drainage, while the other channel is for inflating bulb. Foley's catheter is available in a variety of sizes marked by numbers according to French scale.

## USES

*Gynecological Indications*

- Gynecological operations
  - Hysterectomy
  - Wertheim's hysterectomy

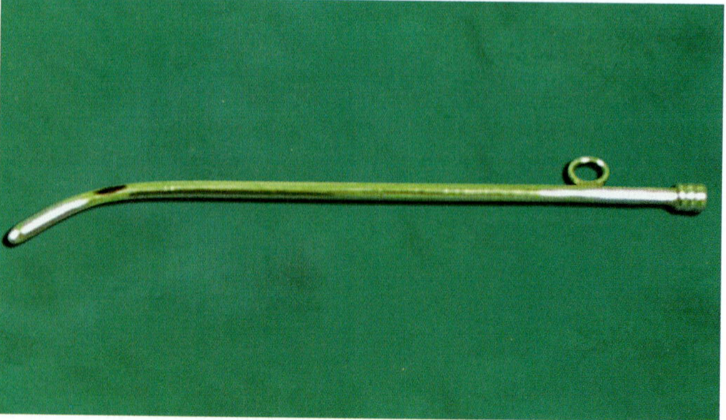

**Fig. 13.41:** Metal catheter

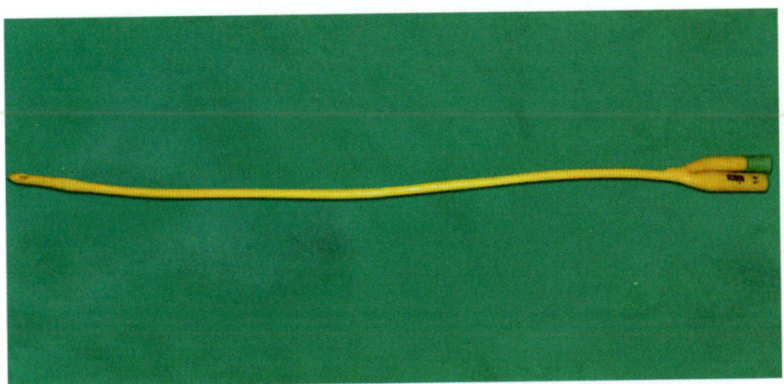

**Fig. 13.42:** Foley's catheter

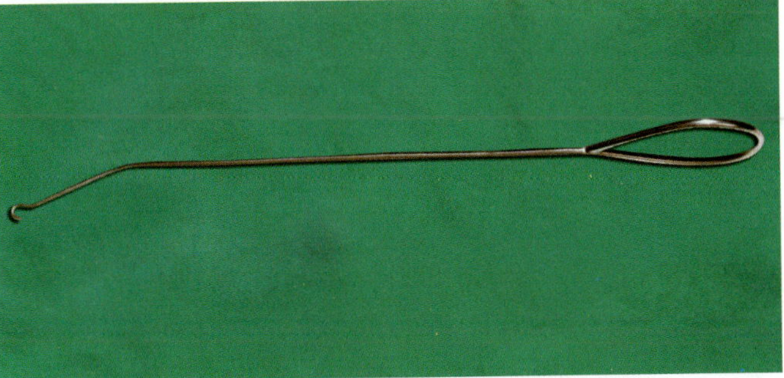

**Fig. 13.43:** IUCD removing hook

- Laparotomy
- Vaginoplasty
- Fothergill's repair
- VVF repair
- Repair of bladder injury
- Acute/chronic retention of urine
- Incontinence of urine
- Unconscious patients
- To measure residual urine
- Saline infusion sonography, hysterosalpingography (to push dye)
- Cystourethrography
- Neurogenic bladder.

*Obstetrical Indications*

- Retention of urine in retroverted gravid uterus
- Obstetric surgeries
  - Cesarean section
  - Cesarean hysterectomy
- During labor to void urine before ventouse/forceps application
- APH/PPH/ectopic pregnancy
- Second trimester MTP for extra-amniotic instillation of ethacridine lactate
- Eclampsia
- Obstructed labor.

# IUCD Removing Hook (Fig. 13.43)

## DESCRIPTION

This is a long, angled instrument, having a hook at the end. It may look similar to a uterine sound. It is differentiated from uterine sound by not having graduations (like in a uterine sound) and having a hook at tip to remove IUCD.

## USES

- Removal of an embedded IUCD from the uterine cavity
- Removal of tubal prosthesis from the uterine cavity.

# Vacuum Extractor (Figs 13.44A to C)

For more details related to a vacuum extractor, kindly refer to Chapter 6.

# Vulsellum (Fig. 13.45)

## DESCRIPTION

This is a long instrument with gentle curve used for grasping the cervix (most commonly the anterior lip of cervix). The tip of the blades have 3–4 teeth for holding and steadying the cervix while performing various procedures such as D&C, first trimester MTP, etc. Since the teeth of the instrument are sharp, it is not used at the time of pregnancy because it can cause cervical tears and lacerations, as the cervix is soft during this time. At this time, the sponge-holding forceps must be used for grasping the cervix.

## USES

- To hold the anterior lip of cervix at the time of:
  - Endometrial biopsy
  - IUCD insertion
  - Intrauterine insemination
  - Vaginal hysterectomy
  - Cauterization of cervix and cervical biopsy
- Posterior lip held in:
  - Colpopuncture for suspected rupture of ectopic pregnancy
  - Culdoscopy
  - Posterior colpotomy.

# Uterine Manipulator (Figs 13.46A and B)

## DESCRIPTION

Uterine manipulator is an instrument used for anteverting the uterus and for positioning the uterus as required

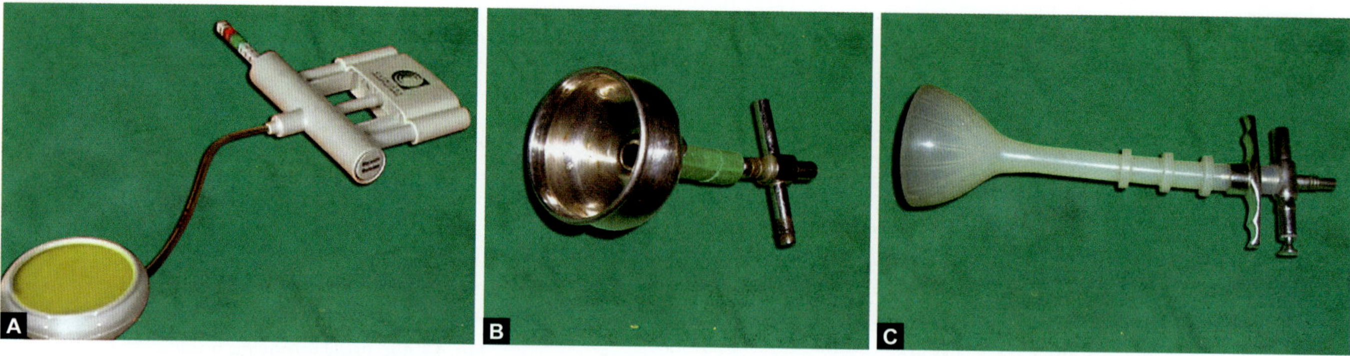

**Figs 13.44A to C:** (A) Vacuum extractor equipment; (B) Metallic cup; (C) Silastic cup

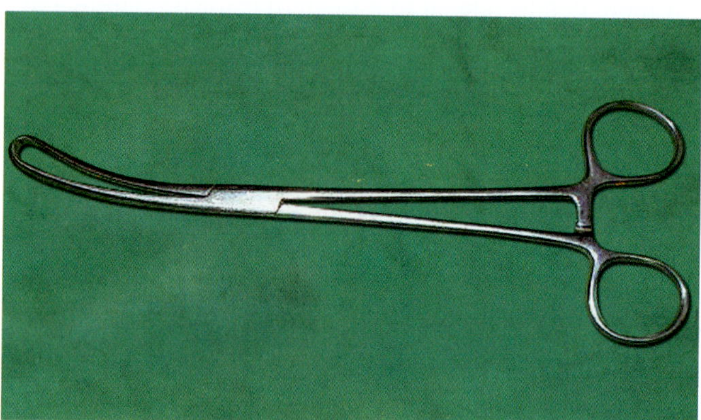

**Fig. 13.45:** Vulsellum

(depending on the type of operative procedure). Uterine manipulator could be specifically designed for laparoscopic surgeries (Fig. 13.46A) or could be a Hulka uterine manipulator as shown in Figure 13.46B. Presence of a trigger handle control in a laparoscopic uterine manipulator offers easy, precise positioning. Stainless steel cannula, present in most of the manipulator devices provides the required strength for confident control. Chances of uterine perforation are less due to the blunt tip of this cannula.

## USES

- It is used to elevate and manipulate position of uterus for the following:
    - Tubal ligation laparoscopic sterilization, minilaparotomy
    - Diagnostic laparoscopy
    - Visualization of pelvic structures by laparoscopy.

# Dartigue Uterus-Holding Forceps (Fig. 13.47)

## DESCRIPTION

This is an instrument where the blades are curved in opposite direction and are in a shape of question mark. The blades are usually covered with rubber caps so as to prevent trauma to the uterus. The space between the blades decreases the uterine compression so it cannot occlude the isthmus and is therefore not suitable for chromopertubation in tuboplasty operations.

## USES

- To hold and steady the uterus at the time of various surgeries (e.g. Shirodkar's sling procedure, Purandare's surgery, Khanna's sling surgery, etc.)
- To lift and hold the uterus at the time of salpingectomy for tubal pregnancy
- Repair of VVF and rectovaginal fistula

# Drew-Smythe Catheter (Fig. 13.48)

## DESCRIPTION

This is a "S-shaped" sinusoidal double curved instrument (made of either metal or rubber) having a double tube. There is an inlet and outlet in this catheter.

## USES

- High amniotomy
- To drain a hydrocephalic head through a spina bifida, in case of a breech delivered up to the head.

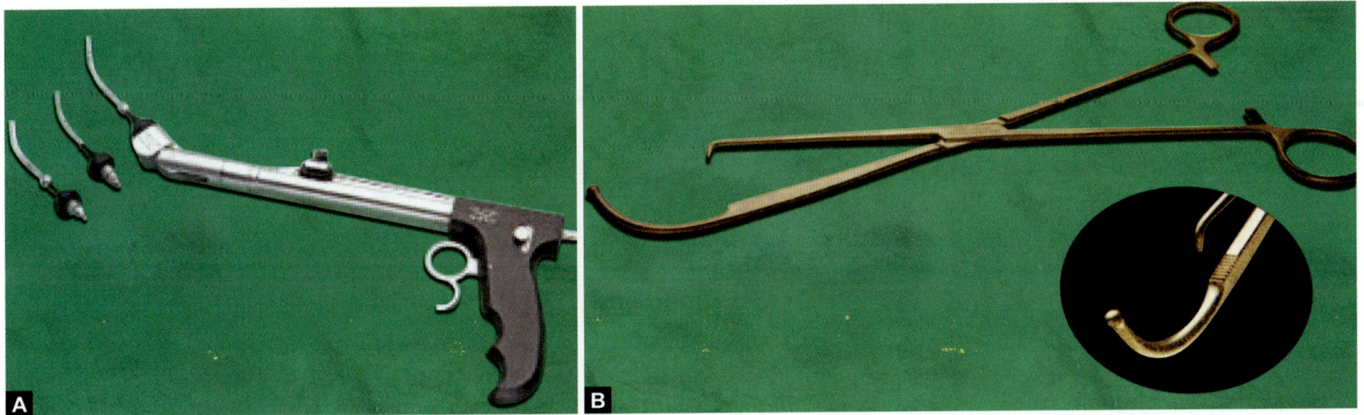

**Figs 13.46A and B:** Uterine manipulator. (A) Laparoscopic uterine manipulator; (B) Hulka uterine manipulator

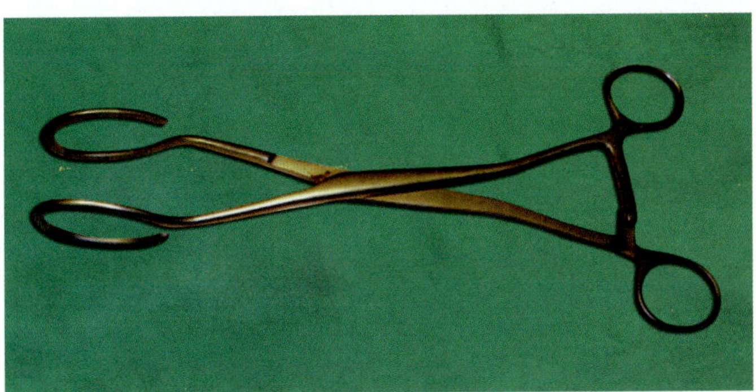

**Fig. 13.47:** Dartigue uterus-holding forceps

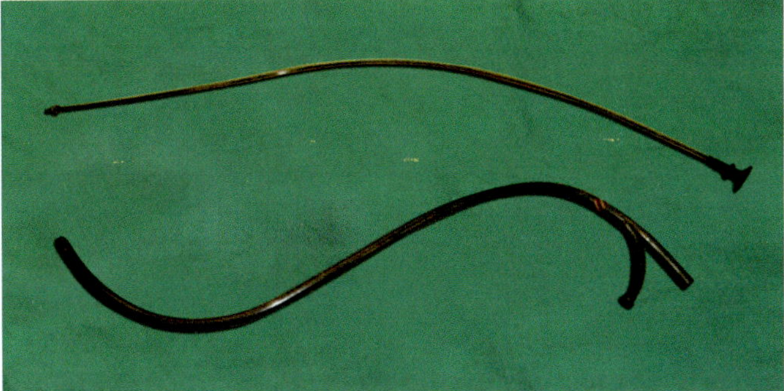

**Fig. 13.48:** Drew-Smythe catheter

# Uterine Packing Forceps (Fig. 13.49)

## DESCRIPTION

This is an "S-shaped" forceps with curvatures corresponding to the axis of birth canal (both uterus and vagina). Blades are blunt and curved, having transverse serrations on its inner surface. Handle of the instrument is slightly curved posteriorly.

## USES

*Uses in obstetrics:* These are as follows:
- *For packing the uterine cavity:* In atonic PPH and postabortal hemorrhage
- *For packing vagina:* To control bleeding in cases of traumatic PPH.

*Uses in gynecology:* These are as follows:
- To control oozing from vault after vaginal hysterectomy
- To control secondary hemorrhage from operative sites, e.g. vault, cervix, vagina
- To control bleeding after hysteroscopy

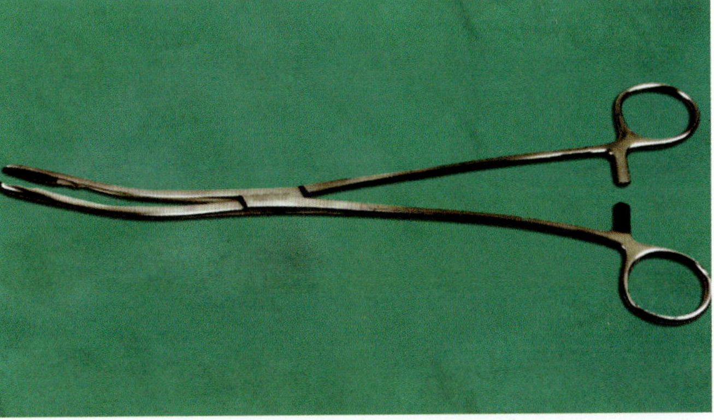

**Fig. 13.49:** Uterine packing forceps

- To control bleeding after polypectomy and cervical biopsy.

# Obstetric Forceps

Various types of obstetric forceps have been described in details in Chapter 6.

# Veress Needle (Fig. 13.50)

## DESCRIPTION

The Veress needle is available in three sizes depending upon its length: 80 mm, 100 mm and 120 mm. It has an inner blunt tip, which retracts on meeting resistance (like upon entering the skin and rectus sheath). This allows the outer sharp bevel to pierce. After entering the peritoneal cavity, this resistance is lost. At this time, the inner round tip comes out with spring action. This helps in preventing damage to the internal structures. The indicators of the successful entry of the needle inside the peritoneal cavity are:

- Drop of saline gets sucked
- Nothing comes out following the aspiration of syringe.

## USE

- Veress needle is used for creating a pneumoperitoneum, which can be considered as the first step of most laparoscopic surgeries. This helps in separating the internal organs and tissues from the abdominal wall so that the trocar can be inserted safely without causing any injury to the surrounding structures.

# Trocar and Cannula (Fig. 13.51)

## DESCRIPTION

Trocar is an instrument which is put inside the encasing outer sheath or the cannula, both of which are then inserted together inside the abdominal cavity for laparoscopy. This is also known as the port because it serves as the port of entry for the laparoscopic telescope and other instruments. It is numbered as per the outer diameter. 10 mm port is used for operative telescope, whereas 7 mm port is used for band application during tubal ligation. 5 mm port is used for the introduction of hand instruments, e.g. grasper.

## USE

- Introduction of operative telescope and other instruments at the time of laparoscopic surgery.

# Suction Cannula (Figs 13.52A and B)

## DESCRIPTION

Karman's cannula is a long tubular structure made of plastic or metal. Depending upon the constituent material it is made up of, the cannula could be either rigid or flexible. A plastic cannula is preferred because it is less traumatic, transparent and disposable. It is available in sizes varying from 4 mm to 12 mm. The number of cannula corresponds to diameter of cannula. At the distal end, there is a double whistle. Superior overhanging edge acts as a curette. The proximal end fixes into syringe.

## USES

- It is used for suction evacuation of the contents of the uterine cavity at the time of MTP
- Removal of the residual products of conception in cases of incomplete miscarriage
- Suction evacuation of inevitable abortion in first trimester
- Suction evacuation of vesicular mole.

# Doyen's Myoma Screw (Fig. 13.53)

## DESCRIPTION

This is an instrument having a ring-shaped handle used for gripping. The other end of the instrument has a corkscrew-like arrangement and a pointed tip.

## USE

- To hold, steady and apply traction on a fibroid during abdominal/vaginal myomectomy.

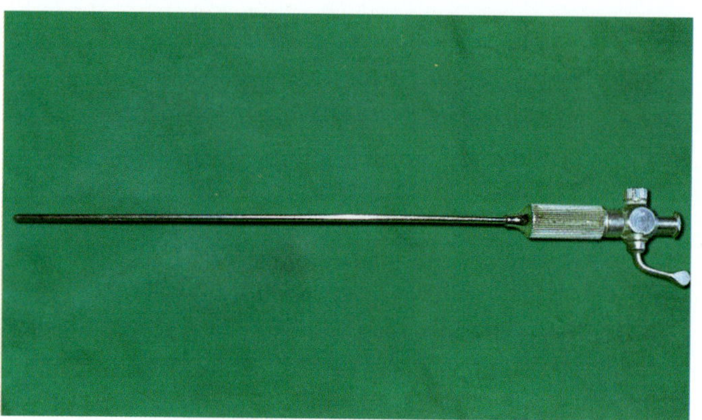

**Fig. 13.50:** Veress needle

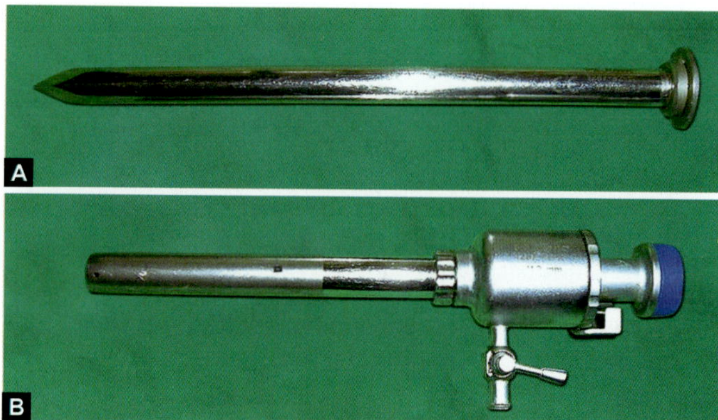

**Figs 13.51A and B:** (A) Trocar; (B) Cannula

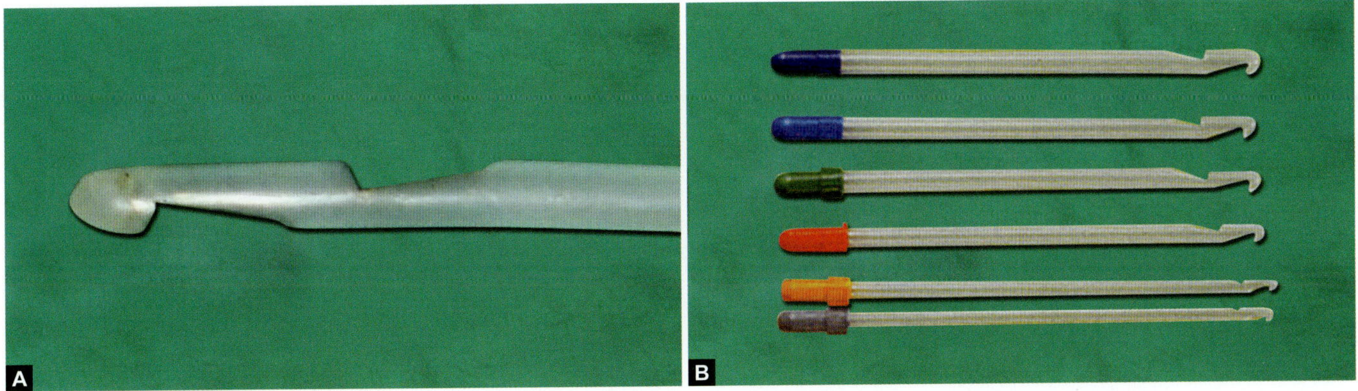

**Figs 13.52A and B:** (A) Suction cannula (From the region of tip); (B) Karman's cannula in varying sizes

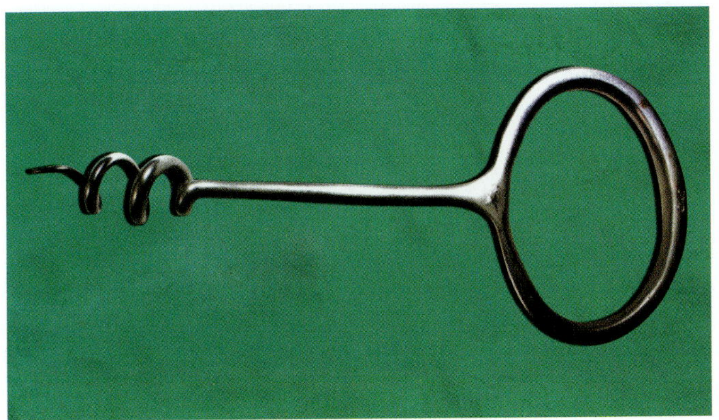

**Fig. 13.53:** Doyen's myoma screw

**Fig. 13.54:** Shirodkar uterus-holding forceps

# Shirodkar Uterus-Holding Forceps (Fig. 13.54)

## DESCRIPTION

This is an instrument where the blades have curved transverse bars at tip with distance in between. The gap between the transverse bars help in making it atraumatic. The bars help in occluding the isthmic region and cervical canal. The handles of the instrument provide firm grip, which allows manipulation of uterus.

## USE

- For holding and steadying the uterus during various surgeries.

# Simpson Perforator (Fig. 13.55)

## DESCRIPTION

This instrument, in the front has two blades having triangular tips with outer cutting edges. There is a transverse bar locking system between the ends of the handles, which locks the blades in closed position. To open the blades of the instrument, the bar has to be pushed in.

Proximal to the handles is a shoulder guard to prevent the blades from going too deep inside the skull, when the instrument is forcefully thrusted inside the skull. Long shanks of the instrument help in providing length to it. This is especially important if the head is very high and floating.

## USE

- It is used at the time of craniotomy to enter fetal skull and collapse it by draining brain matter for the following indications:

*Dead Baby*

- Vertex: Failed forceps/ventouse in cells of cephalopelvic disproportion
- Malposition: Brow, mentoposterior face, after-coming head of breech
- Interlocking head of twins.

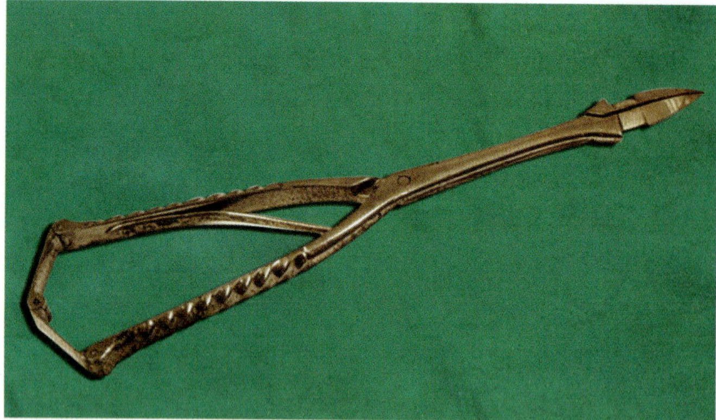

**Fig.13.55:** Simpson perforator

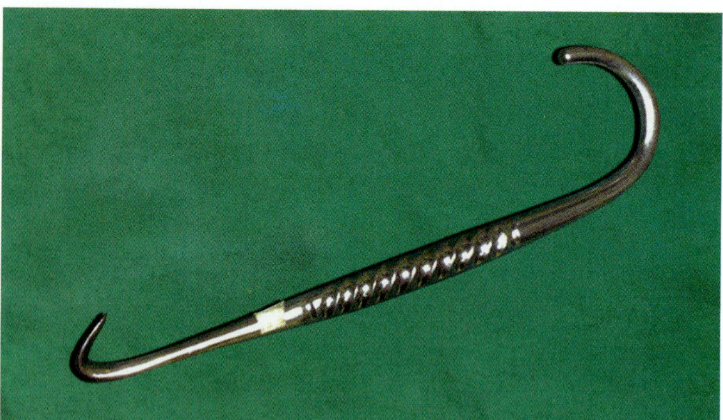

**Fig. 13.57:** Breech hook with crochet

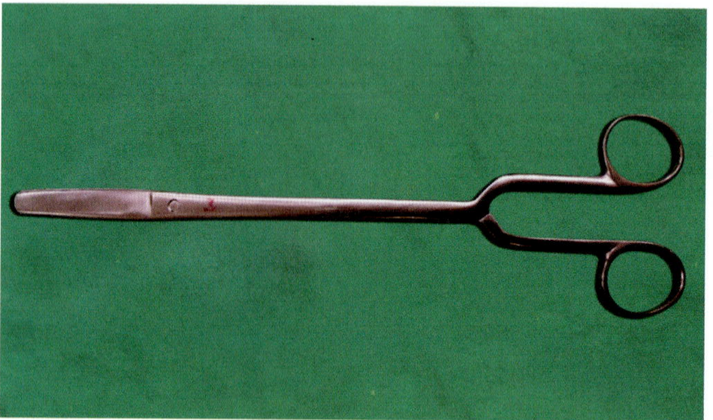

**Fig. 13.56:** Embrotomy scissors

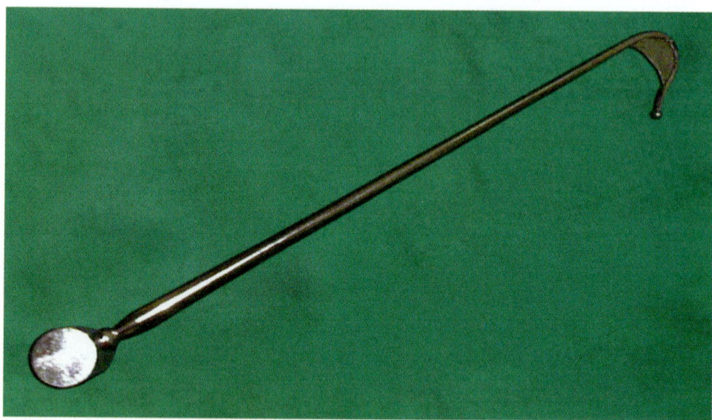

**Fig. 13.58:** Decapitation hook with knife

*Live baby*

Hydrocephalus.

For detailed description of craniotomy kindly refer to Chapter 7.

# Embryotomy Scissors (Fig. 13.56)

## DESCRIPTION

This is a long scissors with the hinge very close to the tip of the instrument. The presence of fulcrum (hinge) near the armload and far away from the effort arm offers it a great mechanical advantage. This makes it possible for the scissors to cut the bones like clavicle and vertebra.

## USE

- Opening fetal thorax or abdomen at the time of evisceration for removing the viscera piecemeal.

For detailed description of various destructive procedures, kindly refer to Chapter 7.

# Hook with Crochet (Fig. 13.57)

## DESCRIPTION

This is an instrument having two parts: Crochet, which is acutely bent and hook, which is wider and gradually bent.

## USES

- Crochet is used for hooking down a decapitated head through the mouth or hole in skull.
- Hook is used for applying traction on groin in case of impacted breech of a dead fetus.

# Ramsbotham's Decapitation Hook with Knife (Fig. 13.58)

## DESCRIPTION

This instrument has a blade at one end and the handle at the other. The blade is hooked with inner serrations.

## USE

- Decapitating the head of a dead baby especially in cases of arm prolapse.

## Auvard-Zweifel Combined Cranioclast and Cephalotribe (Fig. 13.59)

### DESCRIPTION

The instrument has a central blade, which is pushed through perforated skull and screwed in foramen magnum. The instrument also comprises of two side blades, which are introduced and screwed together with the central blade to obtain a firm grip on the head in order to crush the skull vault.

### USES

- Crushing the vault and base of fetal skull after craniotomy

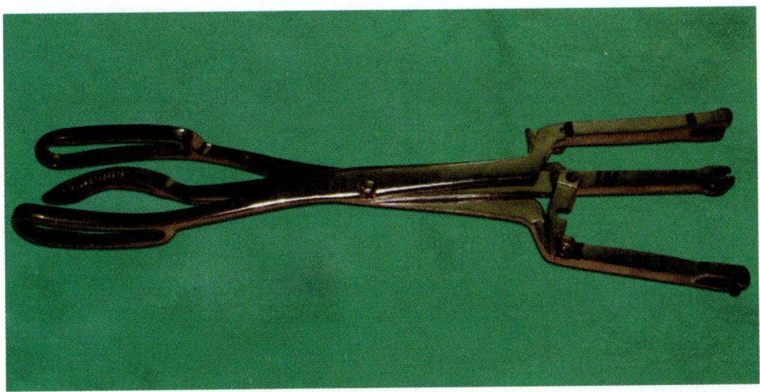

**Fig. 13.59:** Auvard-Zweifel combined cranioclast and cephalotribe

- *Cephalotripsy:* Completely crushing the perforated head before extraction
- *Cranioclasm:* Avulsion of the bones of cranial vault prior to extraction.

For detailed description of these procedures, kindly refer to Chapter 7.

## Willett Scalp Traction Forceps (Figs 13.60A and B)

### DESCRIPTION

This is a type of vulsellum forceps used for applying scalp traction. This instrument has no role in modern obstetries except in cases of dead baby.

### USES

- To control bleeding due to degree 1 or 2 placenta previa: Application of traction over the fetal head produces placental site tamponade.
- Application of traction on fetal head after craniotomy to hasten delivery.
- Application of scalp traction to deliver dead fetal head during cesarean section.
- Scalp traction to prevent recurrence of cord prolapse after replacement of the prolapsed cord above the level of dead fetal head.

## Martin Pelvimeter (Fig. 13.61)

### DESCRIPTION

This is an instrument previously employed to assess the size of the female pelvis in relation to childbirth to determine

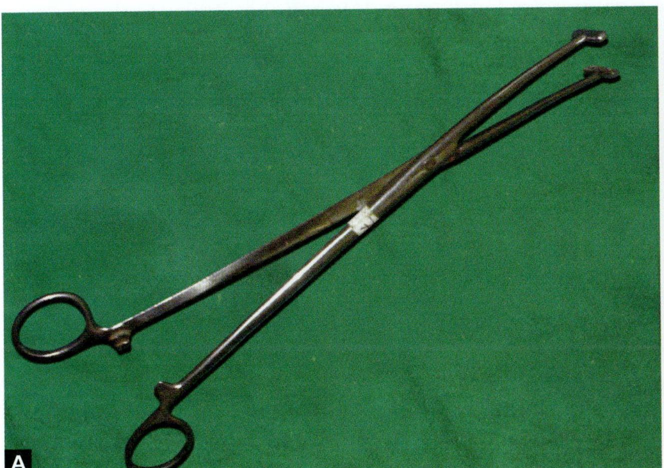

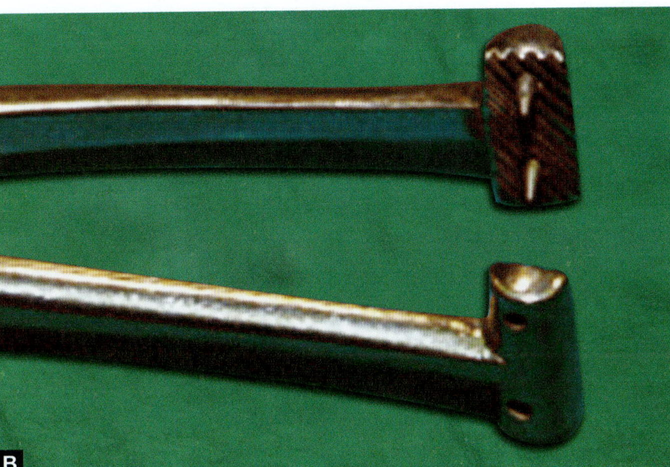

**Figs 13.60A and B:** Willett scalp traction forceps

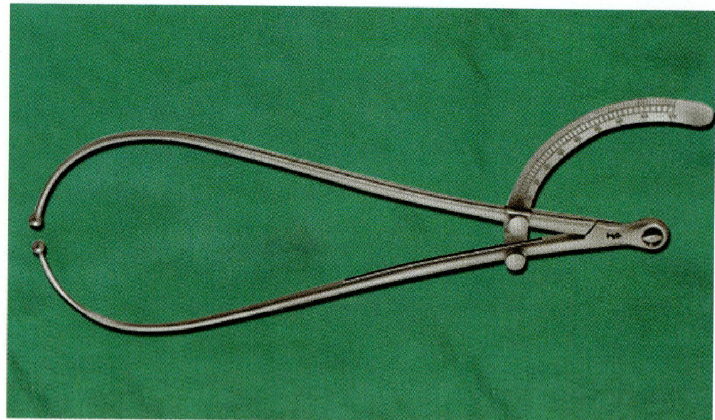

**Fig. 13.61:** Martin pelvimeter

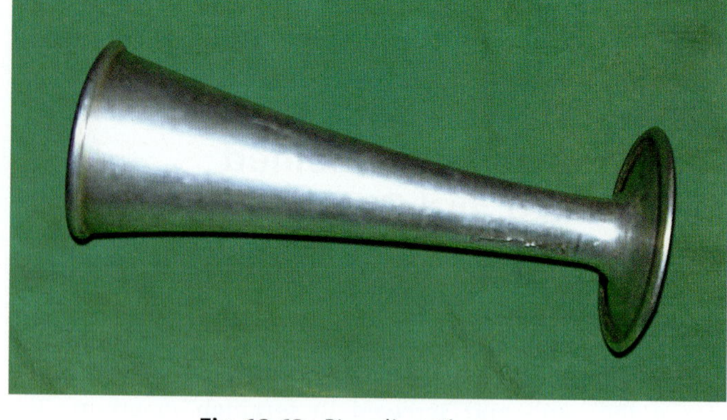

**Fig. 13.63:** Pinard's stethoscope

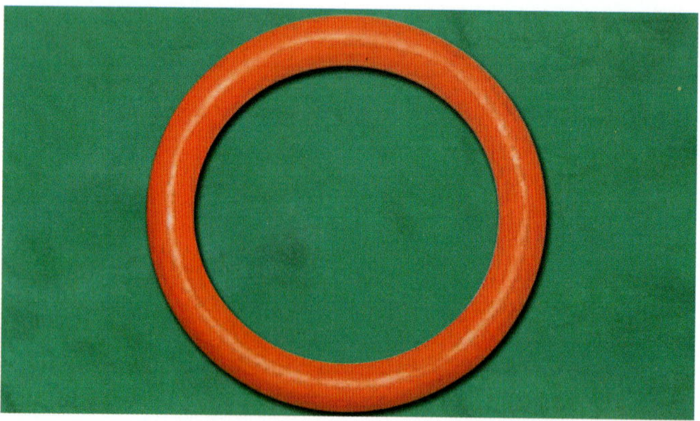

**Fig. 13.62:** Rubber ring pessary

whether natural vaginal delivery would be possible or not. The device has two bulbed arms, which help in grasping the entire pelvic width. There is a ruler, graduated in centimeters and inches, which is present at the hinge.

## USE

- The instrument was used in past for external pelvimetry. Various diameters such as external conjugate, intercristal, intertuberous, interspinous diameters were measured in the past using this instrument.

# Rubber Ring Pessary (Fig. 13.62)

## DESCRIPTION

It is a donut-shaped instrument made up of red rubber. It is sometimes employed as a conservative measure in cases of uterovaginal prolapse. A ring pessary helps to supports the uterus by resting on the two levator ani muscles acting as shelves.

## USE

For following indications in cases of uterocervical descent:
- Pregnancy up to 12–14 weeks
- During lactation
- When further child bearing is intended in near future
- When surgery is contraindicated in a patient
- If patient refuses surgery for prolapse
- As a therapeutic test to confirm whether the symptoms are due to prolapse
- To promote healing of the decubitus ulcer prior to surgery.

# Pinard's Stethoscope (Fig. 13.63)

## DESCRIPTION

It is an instrument previously used for auscultation of fetal heart rate. It is a hollow tool made up of either wood or metal and is about 8 inches long. Tapering rim of the device is applied to the clinician's ear and other wide side is pressed upon maternal abdomen. It functions similar to the trumpet by amplifying the sound.

## USE

- Auscultation of the fetal heart rate. This instrument is nowadays not commonly used in clinical settings due to the availability of advanced techniques for measurement of fetal heart rate.

# Stethoscope (Fig. 13.64)

## DESCRIPTION

It is a medical device commonly used for the auscultation of various body sounds in an adult.

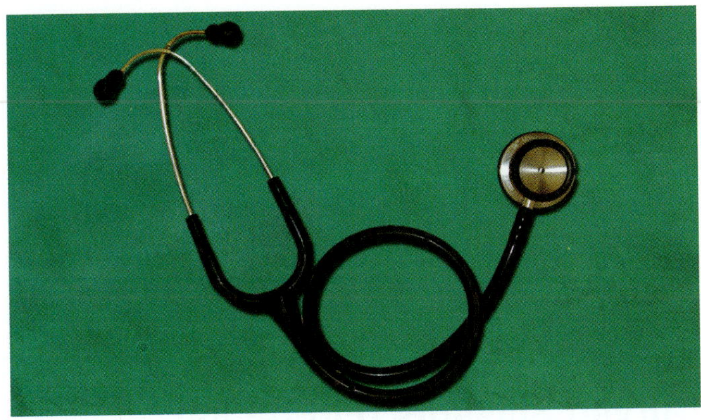

**Fig. 13.64:** Stethoscope

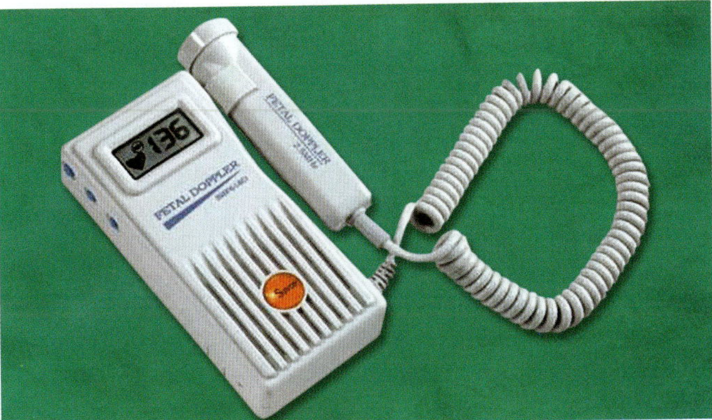

**Fig. 13.65:** Digital fetal doppler

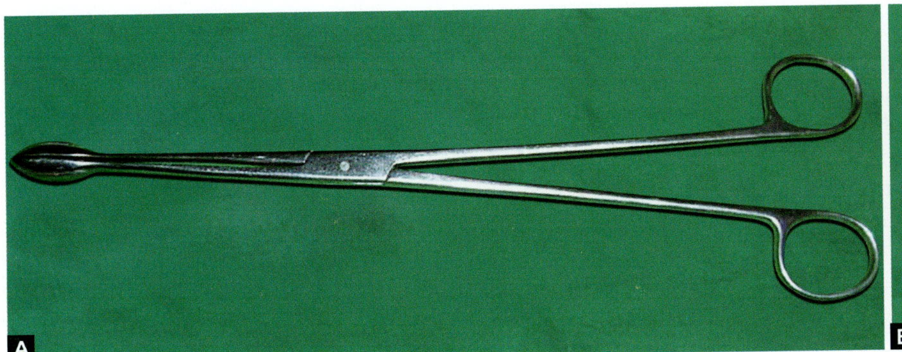

**Figs 13.66A and B:** Haywood Smiths ovum forceps

## USES

- The sounds commonly heard using a stethoscope include heart sounds and sounds in the lungs.
- It is also used for listening to the sounds of intestines and blood flow through the veins and arteries.
- In combination with a sphygmomanometer, it is used for the measurement of blood pressure.

# Digital Fetal Doppler (Fig. 13.65)

## DESCRIPTION

This is a battery-operated device which can be used at the time of obstetric examination in the antenatal ward or in the labor room for evaluation of fetal heart rate.

## USE

- Detection and measurement of fetal heart rate.

# Haywood Smiths Ovum Forceps (Figs 13.66A and B)

## DESCRIPTION

It is a forceps where the blades are spoon-shaped, fenestrated and have blunt ends. Due to these features, these forceps can hold good amount of tissues. The lock is absent in these forceps. Therefore anything held in blades is firmly caught but not nipped and so there is no crushing of tissues. Ovum forceps is differentiated from sponge-holding forceps by following points:

- It has no lock
- It has no serrations
- Catch lock is absent so there are less chances of injury to intra-abdominal structures.

## USES

- Evacuation of POCs in abortion and vesicular mole
- Evacuation of POCs in secondary PPH.

# Laminaria Tent (Fig. 13.67)

## DESCRIPTION

It is made up of hygroscopic material derived from the stems of seaweed called *Laminaria japonica*. It has a hygroscopic nature, i.e. it swells up by absorbing fluid and therefore acts as a slow dilator of cervix. Stem is about 5.5–6 cm in size. It is available in three sizes: small, medium and large depending upon the stem diameter. A string is looped through one end and tied to the gauze for easy removal. It is sterilized by dipping in absolute alcohol. The use of laminaria tents help in slow dilatation of cervix. Since the cervical os gets gradually dilatated, there are minimal chances of injury and development of incompetence.

## USES

- Two or three tents can be introduced side by side if required into the cervical canal. Tents swell up 3–5 times of their size after absorbing secretions of cervical canal in 12–24 hours and help in gradually dilating the cervix.
- First and second trimester pregnancy termination.
- Expulsion of POCs in missed abortion, incomplete abortion.
- Induction of labor.

# Bard Parker's Knife (Figs 13.68A to E)

## DESCRIPTION

This instrument is commonly known as surgeon's knife. It has a straight handle with a notch. Scalpel is usually held with a pencil grip and its movement is directed by thumb and index finger. Different sizes of blades can be attached with different sizes of handles. Larger sizes of blades are used for larger tissues and incisions. Smaller sizes of blades are used for finer and deeper incisions. The No. 10 scalpel blade is the

most commonly used size. Acute angle of No. 11 blade is used for giving stab incisions for inserting drains and for draining abscesses, e.g. Bartholin's abscess.

## USES

- For opening the abdomen by incising skin and subcutaneous tissue
- For cutting pedicles
- For sharp dissection
- For finer incision, i.e. incision of tough walled abscess.

# Curved Scissors (Fig. 13.69)

## DESCRIPTION

Scissors are instruments used for blunt and sharp dissection and for cutting sutures and pedicles. They may be of different types. Shown next in the picture is a curved scissors. This scissor is curved at acute angle along its long axis in horizontal plane.

## USES

- It is used for cutting obliquely directed tissue structures at the time of surgery
- Used for cutting sutures.

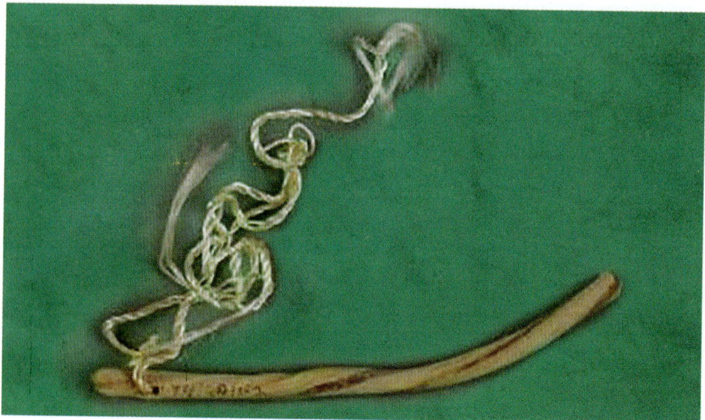

**Fig. 13.67:** Laminaria tent

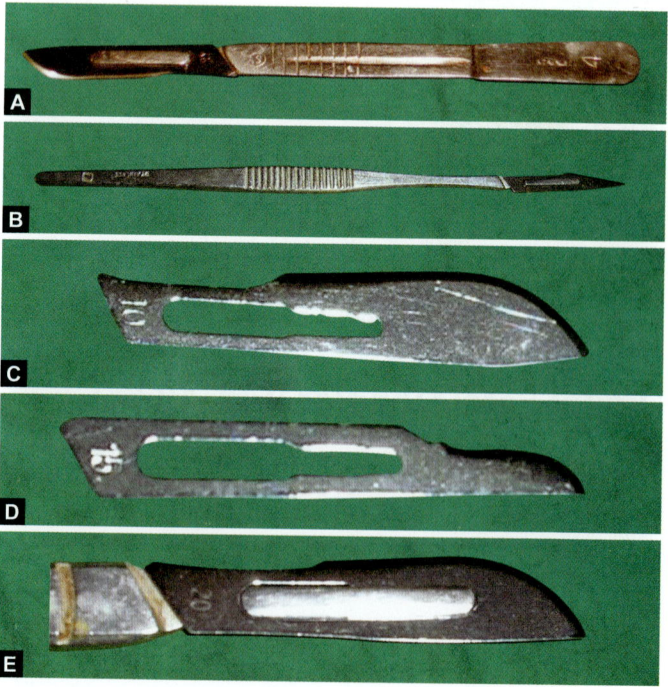

**Figs 13.68A to E:** (A) No. 4 Bard Parker knife for big blades; (B) No. 7 Bard Parker knife for small blades; (C) No. 10 blade for small incisions; (D) No. 15 blade for stab incisions; (E) No. 20 blade for skin incisions in case of LSCS, laparotomy

# Mayo's Scissors (Fig. 13.70)

## DESCRIPTION

Mayo's scissors are sturdy scissors and also known as the tissue scissors. It has blunt ends which cause little damage while separating the tissues. It has no ratchet and operating end is sharp.

## USES

- Used for tough tissue dissection such as rectus fascia, parametrial tissues, vaginal cuff, etc.
- They are heavy and accurate for gentle dissection particularly "separate and cut" technique.

# Metzenbaum Scissors (Fig. 13.71)

## DESCRIPTION

This scissor is similar to Mayo's scissors. However, it is more delicate than the Mayo's scissors.

## USES

- For cutting thinner tissues such as peritoneum, adhesions, vaginal epithelium, etc.
- They are used for retroperitoneal dissection and for developing tissue planes in distorted and adherent tissue.

# Umbilical Cord Clamp (Fig. 13.72)

## DESCRIPTION

It is a disposable clamp made of plastic. Inner surface of the clamp has transverse serrations for tight grip on the cord. Open end of the clamp can be locked after clamping the cord by applying pressure. The clamp automatically sheds off when the cord dries and falls off.

## USES

This instrument is mainly used for clamping the umbilical cord at the time of baby's delivery.

- Delayed cord clamping helps in transferring about 80 mL of the blood to the fetus.

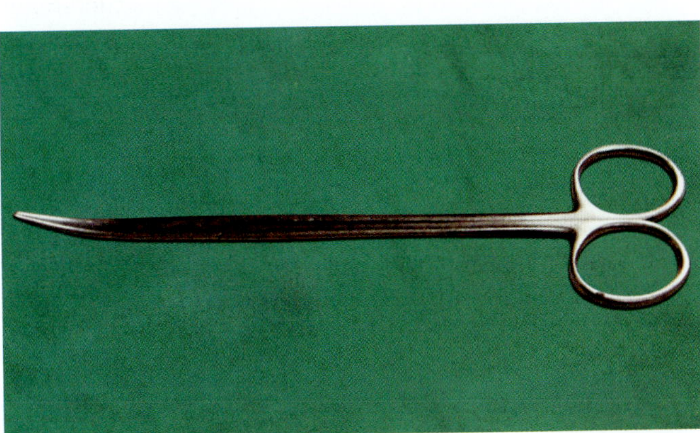

**Fig. 13.69:** Curved scissors

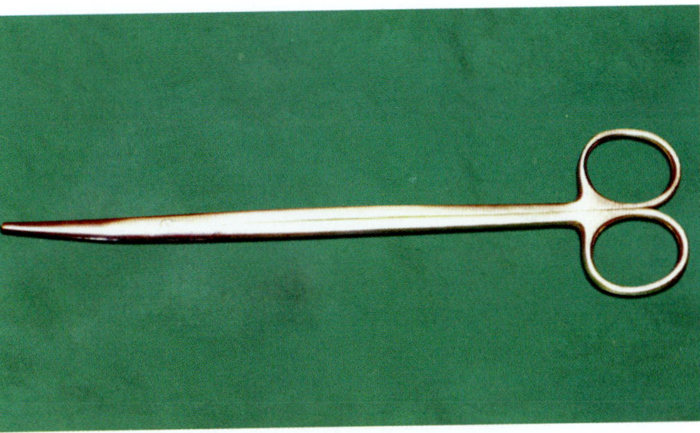

**Fig. 13.71:** Metzenbaum scissors

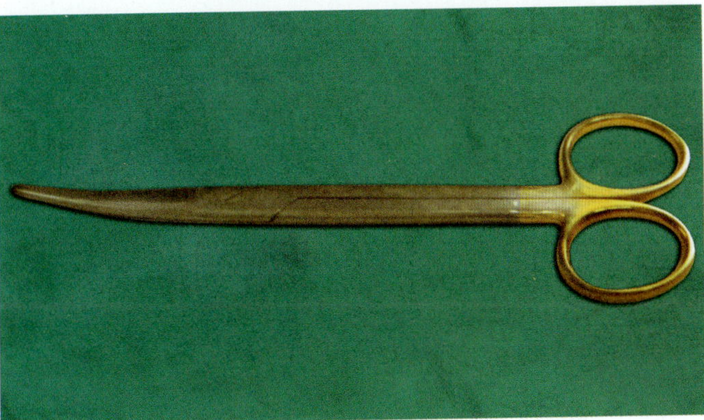

**Fig. 13.70:** Mayo's scissors

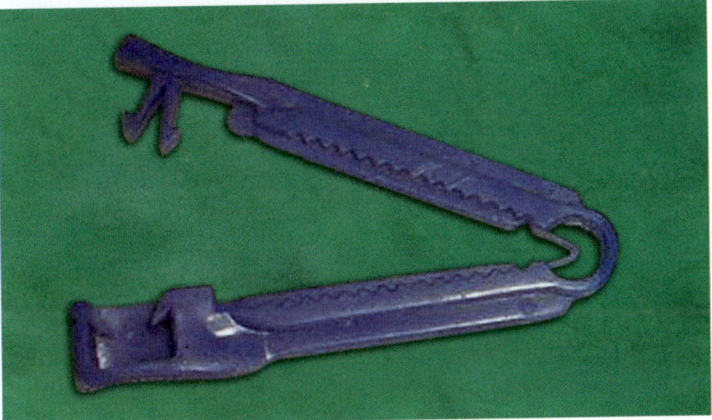

**Fig. 13.72:** Umbilical cord clamp

- Early cord clamping prevents the transfer of this extra blood to the fetus. This is done in the following cases:
    - Rh isoimmunization (to prevent antibody transfer from mother to baby)
    - Asphyxia
    - Preterm babies (to prevent hypervolemia)
    - Diabetic mother
    - Low birthweight babies.

## Bonney's Myomectomy Clamp (Fig. 13.73)

### DESCRIPTION

It is a specialized instrument designed by Victor Bonney for reducing intraoperative blood loss during various surgeries. It has three parts:

1. *Blades:* These are at an angle of 120° to the shaft. It has overlapping transverse bar dividing it into two compartments. Usually there is rubber tubing in anterior half of the compartment, which prevents trauma to the structures it holds.

2. *Shaft*

3. *Handle:* Handle has two pairs of finger grips. Distal finger grip is used for applying and removing the instrument. Proximal finger grip can open up the instrument wider in cases where the uterus is bulky.

### USES

To control bleeding during the following surgeries:
- Abdominal myomectomy
- Hysterotomy
- Metroplasty.
    Use has become less because myoma can be removed by latest methods.

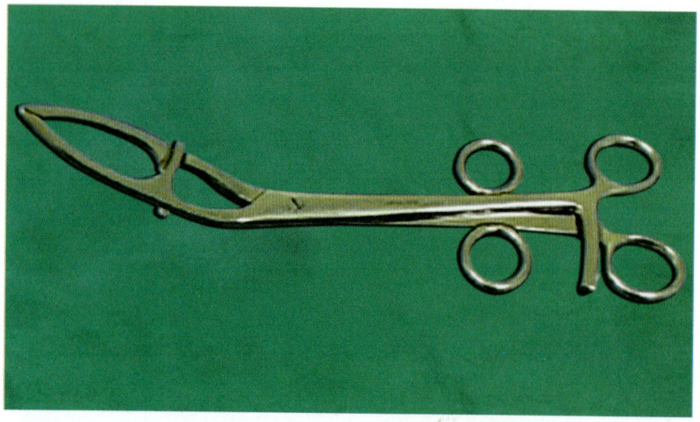

## Iris Scissors (Fig. 13.74)

### DESCRIPTION

They are small and delicate pair of scissors.

### USES

- Used for precise vaginal and vulvar surgery
- Used for delicate dissection.

## Sharp-Curved Mosquito Hemostat (Fig. 13.75)

### DESCRIPTION

This is a small variety of artery forceps.

### USES

- Used for holding delicate structures such as fascia and peritoneum

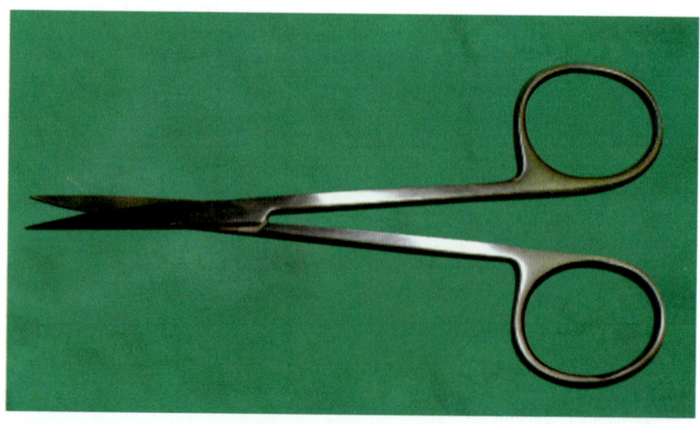

**Fig. 13.74:** Iris scissors

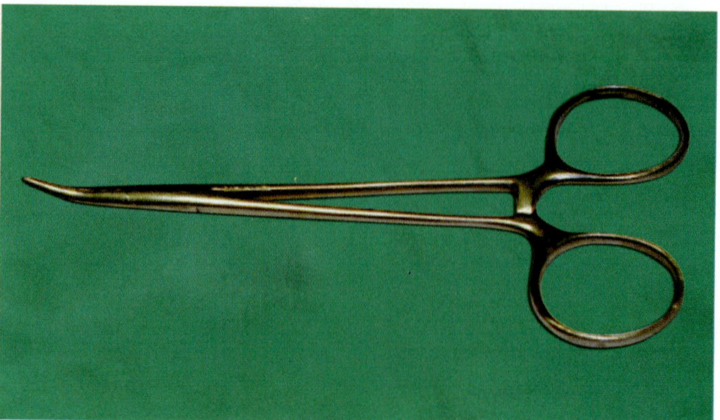

**Fig. 13.73:** Bonney's myomectomy clamp

**Fig. 13.75:** Sharp-curved mosquito hemostat

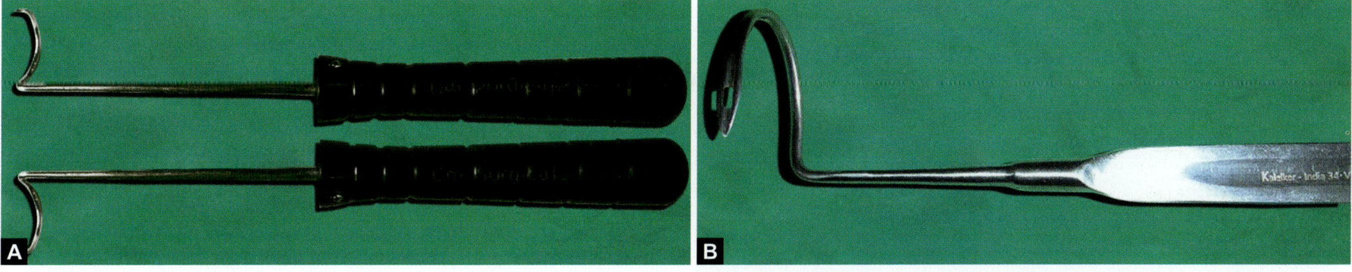

**Figs 13.76A and B:** (A) Shirodkar cervical encerclage needles of both the sides; (B) Left sided Shirodkar cervical encerclage needle

- Holding free ends of sutures in case of vulvar/vaginal surgery
- For opening up the cavities of small abscesses.

# Shirodkar Cervical Encerclage Needles (Figs 13.76A and B)

## DESCRIPTION

These are two Shirodkar cervical encerclage needles, one for the right side and other for the left side. Each sided needle is half circled and has an eye at tip. These two needles are mirror image of each other. They are 5 cm long. These needles are used for giving cervical cerclage, which is usually administered at 14 weeks of gestation or 2 weeks before the age of gestation at which the patient aborts.

## USE

- They are used for application of modified Shirodkar cerclage surgery for incompetent cervix. In this surgery, a cervical encircling nonabsorbable suture is passed around cervix at the level of internal os. This surgery helps in disturbing uterine polarity, thereby preventing early "taking up" of the lower segment.

# Intrauterine Insemination Cannula (Fig. 13.77)

It is a thin flexible catheter which is placed in uterine cavity for intrauterine insemination.

## USES

- This catheter is used for the purpose of artificial intrauterine insemination.

*Indications for Artificial Insemination of Husband's Semen*

- *Mild to moderate male subfertility:* Oligospermia, asthenospermia, teratospermia, oligoasthenoteratozoo-

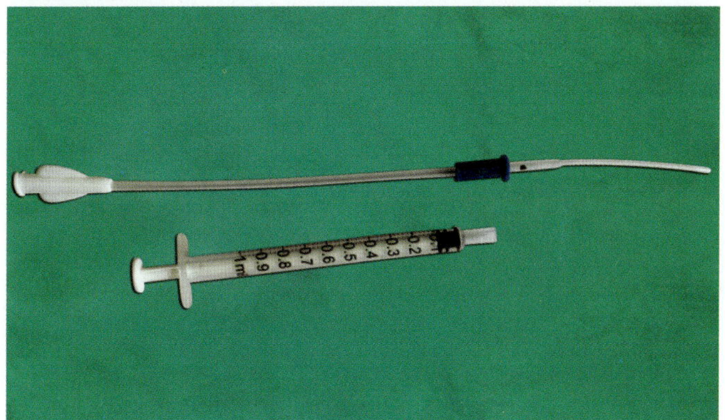

**Fig. 13.77:** Intrauterine insemination cannula

spermia, pyospermia, semen volume and liquefaction defects.
- Impotency
- Premature ejaculation, retrograde ejaculation
- Anatomical defects, i.e. hypospadias, vaginal and cervical defects.
- Unexplained infertility
- Cervical factor, i.e. hostile cervical mucus, antisperm antibodies in cervical mucus
- *Immunological factors:* Presence of antisperm antibodies
- *Endometriosis:* Mild or moderate
- Chronic anovulation
- HIV positive woman or man.

*Indications for Artificial Insemination of Donor's Semen*

Artificial insemination using donor's semen is performed for following indications:
- Azoospermia
- Immunological factor if not correctable
- Genetic disease in the husband.

# Electrosurgical Loop (Fig. 13.78)

This is a thin wire, semicircular electrode made of stainless steel or tungsten and is used for loop electrosurgical excision

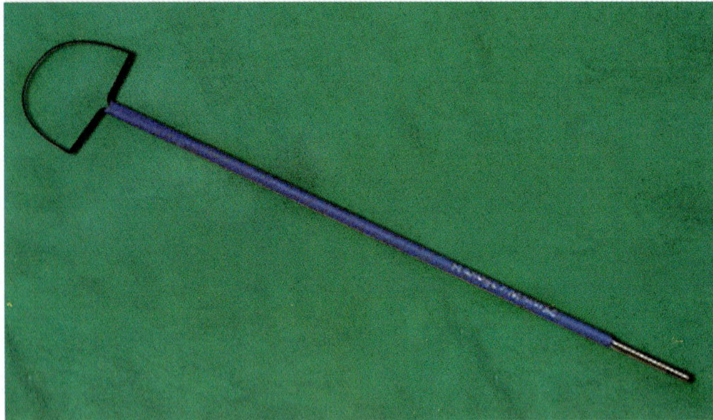

**Fig. 13.78:** Electrosurgical loop

procedure (LEEP). For this procedure, other equipment which are required include electrosurgical unit, wire loop electrode, insulated speculum and smoke evacuation system.

## USES

- Loop electrosurgical excision procedure
- Large loop excision of transformation zone (LLETZ).

# Cervical Punch Biopsy Forceps (Fig. 13.79)

## DESCRIPTION

The instrument has two blades. Smaller blade has sharp cutting edge and fits into larger blade. The two blades are used to punch out the tissue required for taking biopsy.

Tissue specimen is held between the two blades like a basket. Handle of the equipment is angulated to avoid obstruction of field of vision.

## USES

Cervical punch biopsy may be taken for the following indications:
- Recurrent cervicitis, cervical ulcers/growths and nonhealing erosions
- Postcoital bleeding per vaginum
- Abnormal Pap smear
- Abnormal finding on Schiller's test, i.e. iodine negative areas on colposcopy.

# Cryomachine (Fig. 13.80)

## DESCRIPTION

Cryomachine is an equipment used for performing cryosurgery/cryocautery/cryotherapy, which is an ablative method used for elimination of cervical intraepithelial lesion. The equipment comprises of a cryoprobe, and a refrigerating gas cylinder. Tip of the cryoprobe is made of silver or copper and is in contact with surface of cervix. Cryoprobe is attached with connecting tube to a cylinder of refrigerating gas, i.e. nitrous oxide cylinder with pressure gauge. The procedure of cryotherapy has been described in details in Chapter 10.

## USES

Cryocautery is performed in cases of cervical intraepithelial neoplasia (CIN) confirmed by colposcopy/cervical biopsy and there is no evidence of invasive cancer. The following conditions must be fulfilled:

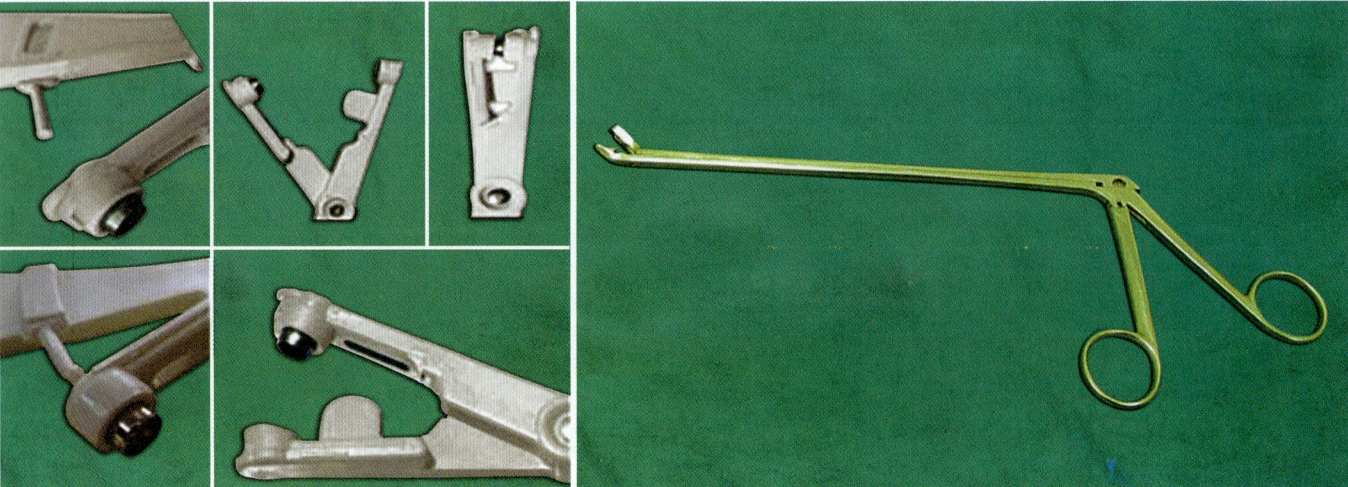

**Fig. 13.79:** Cervical punch biopsy forceps

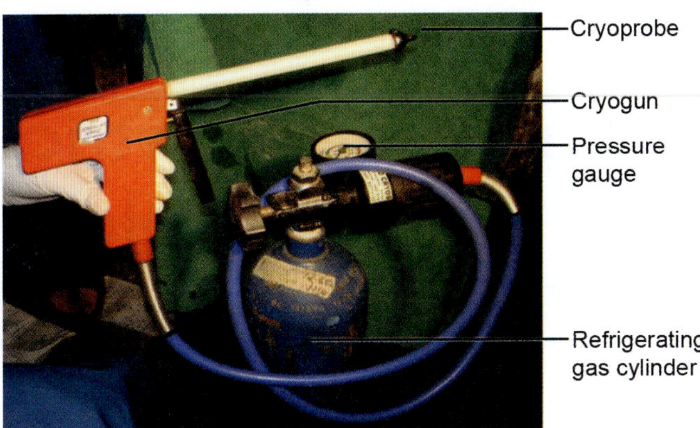



**Fig. 13.80:** Cryomachine

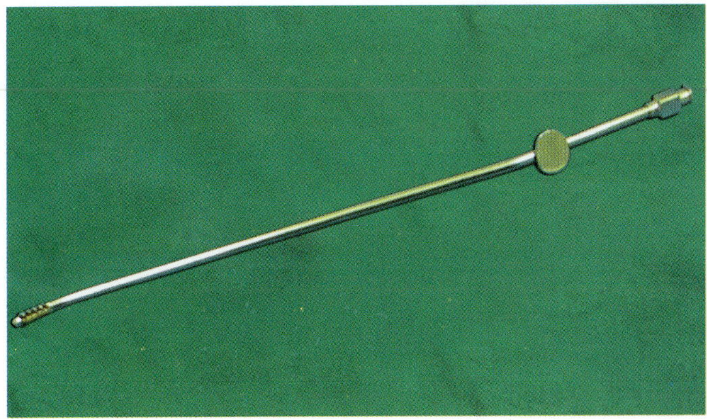

**Fig. 13.81:** Novak's endometrial biopsy curette

- The entire lesion is located in ectocervix with no extension in endocervix and vagina
- The lesion is visible in its entire extent and does not extend more than 2–3 mm into the endocervical canal
- The lesion should be adequately covered by the largest cryoprobe and lesion should extend less than 2 mm beyond the cryoprobe.

# Novak's Endometrial Biopsy Curette (Fig. 13.81)

## DESCRIPTION

Novak's endometrial biopsy curette is a long tubular instrument used for endometrial biopsy. This is a hollow and blunt tipped instrument. The tip has a whistle subterminally, which is notched and has a serrated cutting edge. The instrument is angulated about 5 cm from tip for easier introduction in the uterine cavity. The procedure of endometrial biopsy has been described in details in Chapter 10.

## USES

Endometrial biopsy may be performed for the following indications:
- Diagnosis of DUB
- *Diagnosis of corpus luteum insufficiency:* Biopsy is taken on D21–24
- *Diagnosis of anovulation:* Biopsy is taken on D21–28 and if cycles are irregular, biopsy is taken of DI
- *Diagnosis of tuberculosis:* Endometrial biopsy for diagnosis of tuberculosis is done in late premenstrual phase because tubercles are present in superficial endometrial layers and are shed during menstruation.

## FURTHER READINGS


1. Agarwal K. Instruments and Procedures in Obstetrics and Gynecology, 1st edition. New Delhi: Jaypee Brothers Medical Publishers; 2014.
2. Hibbard BM. (2000). The Obstetrician's Armamentarium: Historic Obstetric Instruments and Their Inventors (Norman OB/GYN Series, No. 4), 1st edition. Jeremy Norman Co; 2000.
3. Nemitz R. Surgical Instrumentation: An Interactive Approach, 2nd edition. St Louis, Missouri: Saunders; 2013.

# Specimens in Obstetrics and Gynecology



## Description of Specimen

### GROSS APPEARANCE OF THE SPECIMEN

While describing the specimen, the main organ must be firstly described. The description must be brief and oriented towards the likely pathology in question. The approximate size, shape and external surface of the organ, which is visualized, must be described. Size of the uterus must be described in terms of weeks of gestation, e.g. 8 or 10 weeks, etc. Other related organs (if present in the specimen) along with the main organ must also be briefly described. The student must never start the answer by mentioning the exact diagnosis, for example, if one is shown the specimen of fibroid uterus, one must never start answering by saying that this is a specimen of fibroid uterus. Instead, one must first describe the organ (uterus in this case) and then describe the presence of a tumorous growth. One can end the answer by giving the most preferential diagnosis.

### Cut Specimen or Not

In case of a cut-section of a specimen, the layers of the organ in concern must be described. For example, in case of cut-section of the uterus, various layers such as serosa, myometrium, endometrium and the endometrial cavity need to be described in that particular order.

### Diagnosis

The differential diagnosis and the most probable diagnosis (preferential diagnosis) must be given.

## Obstetric Specimens

### ANENCEPHALY

#### Gross Appearance

This is a specimen of fetus (male or female if the baby's sex can be identified), showing the following features (Fig. 14.1):
- There is deficient development of vault of skull and brain tissue but facial portion is normal
- Eyeballs are protruding
- Ears are lowest and the chest is bulging

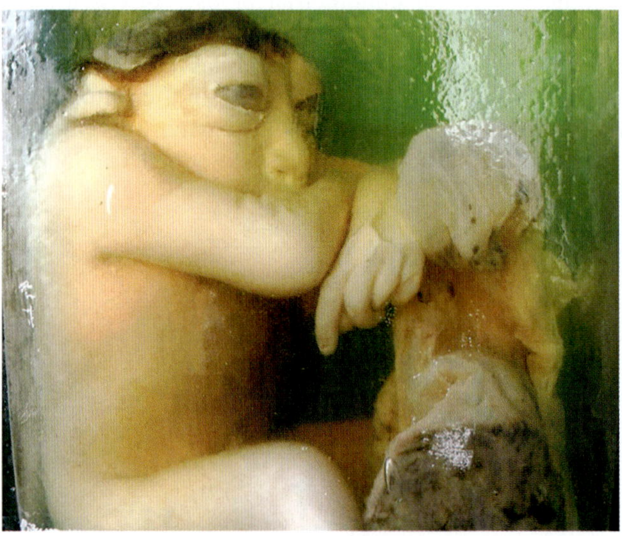

**Fig. 14.1:** Specimen of anencephaly

- Pituitary gland is absent
- There may be the presence of associated malformations such as hydrocephaly, clubfoot, etc. The fetal back must be particularly examined to detect presence of spinal cord anomalies such as spina bifida (Figs 14.2A and B), meningocele, myelocele, etc.

## Diagnosis

My preferential diagnosis would be a (male/female) fetus with anencephaly with or without spina bifida.

### Q. How is the diagnosis of anencephaly confirmed?

**Ans.** In early pregnancy, i.e. around 13 weeks of gestation, there is an increased level of alpha-fetoprotein in amniotic fluid and/or maternal serum.

### Ultrasound Findings

The ultrasound findings help in confirming the diagnosis. At about 10 weeks of gestation, there is absence of cranial vault and there may be presence of angiomatous brain tissue. Later in pregnancy, there may be an inability to measure the biparietal diameter. There may be the failure to identify the normal bony structure and brain tissue cephalad to the orbits.

### Clinical Examination

*Abdominal examination:* On abdominal examination, in the latter half of pregnancy, there may be difficulty in locating fetal head.

*Spring sign:* On vaginal examination in labor when the cervix is sufficiently dilated, if upon palpation of fetal head, it moves suddenly like a spring, this is suggestive of anencephaly. This occurs due to stimulation of fetal brain reflex centers.

### Q. What steps can be taken to prevent the occurrence of neural tube defects?

**Ans.** To prevent the occurrence of neural tube defects, supplementation with folic acid in the dosage of 4 mg daily must be started 1 month prior to conception.

### Q. How should a case of anencephaly be managed?

**Ans.** If the diagnosis of anencephaly has been confirmed before 20 weeks of gestation, pregnancy may be terminated after adequate counseling of the parents because this congenital anomaly is incompatible with extrauterine life. Prostaglandin E2 gel may be required in cases, which are refractory to stimulation by oxytocin. Shoulder dystocia can be managed by cleidotomy.

### Q. What complications can occur in cases of anencephaly during pregnancy?

**Ans.** During pregnancy, the following complications can occur: hydramnios, malpresentations (face and breech presentations), premature labor, tendency for postmaturity, etc.

During labor, complications such as shoulder dystocia and obstructed labor can occur. Shoulder dystocia can occur because a small head tries to escape through the incompletely dilated cervix.

### Q. What is the likely clinical presentation in such a patient?

**Ans.** There are no specific signs and symptoms in early pregnancy suggestive of anencephaly. Diagnosis is usually established with help of ultrasound examination. The woman may develop polyhydramnios later in pregnancy. The clinician should also enquire about any previous history of neural tube defects because there is 2% risk of recurrence of anencephaly in the subsequent pregnancy.

### Q. What are the most common types of neural tube defects which are encountered in the clinical practice?

**Ans.** The most common types of neural tube defects encountered in clinical practice include anencephaly and spina bifida.

## RUPTURED UTERUS

Figure 14.3 is a hysterectomy specimen of an enlarged uterus (recently delivered) showing a rent/tear with ragged margins in the fundal region suggestive of a uterine rupture in the fundal region.

Figure 14.4 is a hysterectomy specimen of the enlarged uterus (recently delivered) with a longitudinal rent extending just below the uterus up to the isthmus. This appears to be related to a previous longitudinal scar in the uterus as a result of classical cesarean section.

Figure 14.5 is a specimen of enlarged uterus (recently delivered) with a transverse rent in the lower segment of

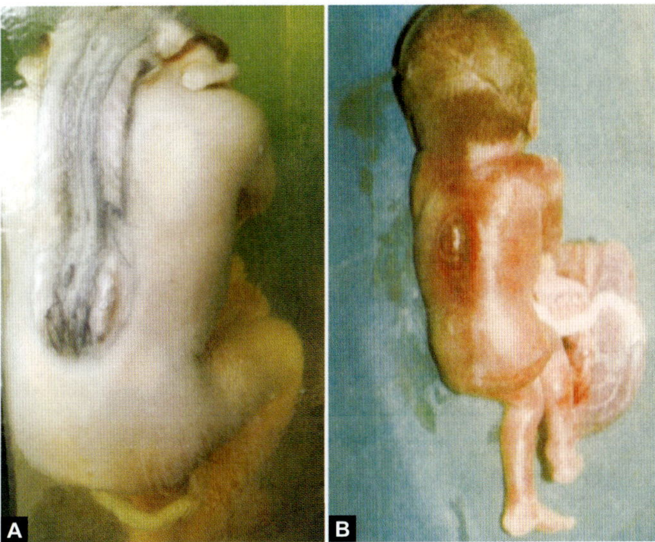
**Figs 14.2A and B:** Spina bifida

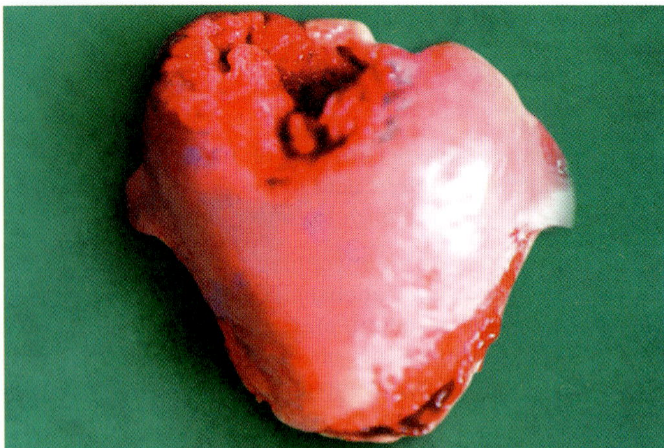

**Fig. 14.3:** Fundal rupture

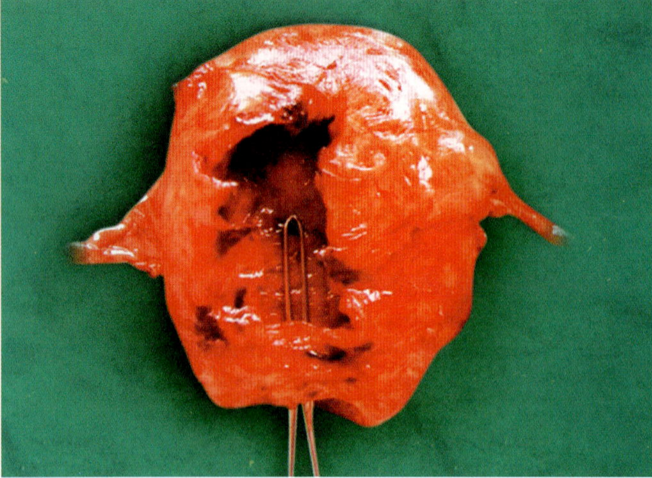

**Fig. 14.4:** Hysterectomy specimen of classical scar rupture

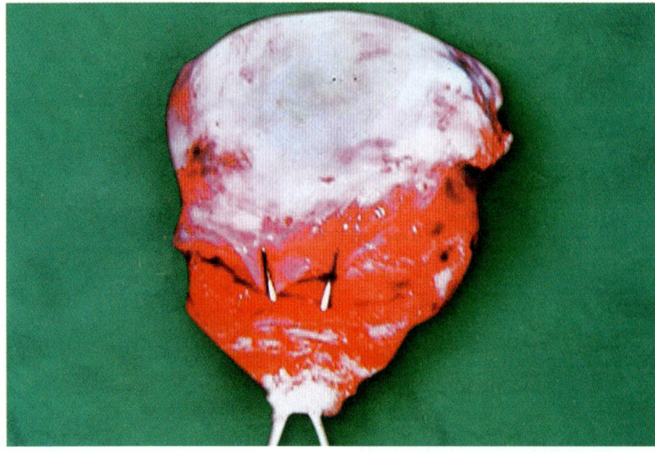

**Fig. 14.5:** Hysterectomy specimen of lower segment rupture

the uterus, about 5–6" in size. This is probably related to the rupture of a previous lower segment cesarean scar at the time of future vaginal delivery.

For clinical questions related to scar rupture as a result of previous cesarean delivery, kindly refer to Chapter 5.

## ECTOPIC PREGNANCY

Figures 14.6A and B are specimens showing a tube-like structure, which most likely appears to be a fallopian tube. No portion of the adjacent organs (either uterus or ovary) can be identified. This implies that only salpingectomy was performed for the pathology in the fallopian tube. There appears to be an oval-shaped structure at the distal end of the tube (identified by the fimbriae). It appears to be filled with clotted blood and whitish frond-like structures (probably chorionic villi). No gestational sac could be, however, identified. My preferential diagnosis in this case would be that of ectopic gestation for which a salpingectomy was performed.

### Q. What is the most common clinical presentation in cases of ectopic pregnancy?

**Ans.** The classical triad of symptoms of ruptured tubal pregnancy include amenorrhea followed by abdominal pain and vaginal bleeding. In case of a ruptured ectopic pregnancy, on general physical examination, there may be an evidence of hemodynamic instability (hypotension, collapse, signs and symptoms of shock). Low blood pressure could be related to significant amount of intraperitoneal bleeding. In severe cases, even shock may be present. Signs of peritoneal irritation (abdominal rigidity and guarding) may be also present. On bimanual examination, uterus appears bulky and there may be extreme tenderness upon palpation of fornices or movement of cervix. Uterine size does not correspond to the period of gestation. An adnexal mass may be palpated (with or without tenderness).

For other clinical questions related to ectopic pregnancy, kindly refer to Chapter 7.

## NORMAL PLACENTA

### Gross Appearance

Figures 14.7A and B show the specimen of placenta with an attached umbilical cord. Figure 14.7A shows maternal surface of placenta. Surface of placenta is grayish-brown in color studded with multiple cotyledons separated from each other by septa. The umbilical cord does not appear to be attached to this surface of the placenta.

Figure 14.7B shows the fetal surface of the placenta covered by thin smooth membranes (amnion and chorion). The umbilical cord appears to be arising from this surface of the placenta.

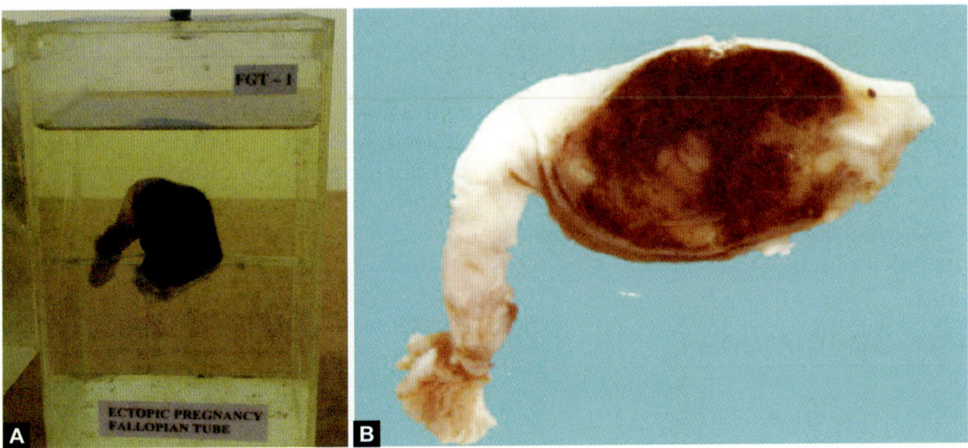

**Figs 14.6A and B:** Ectopic pregnancy

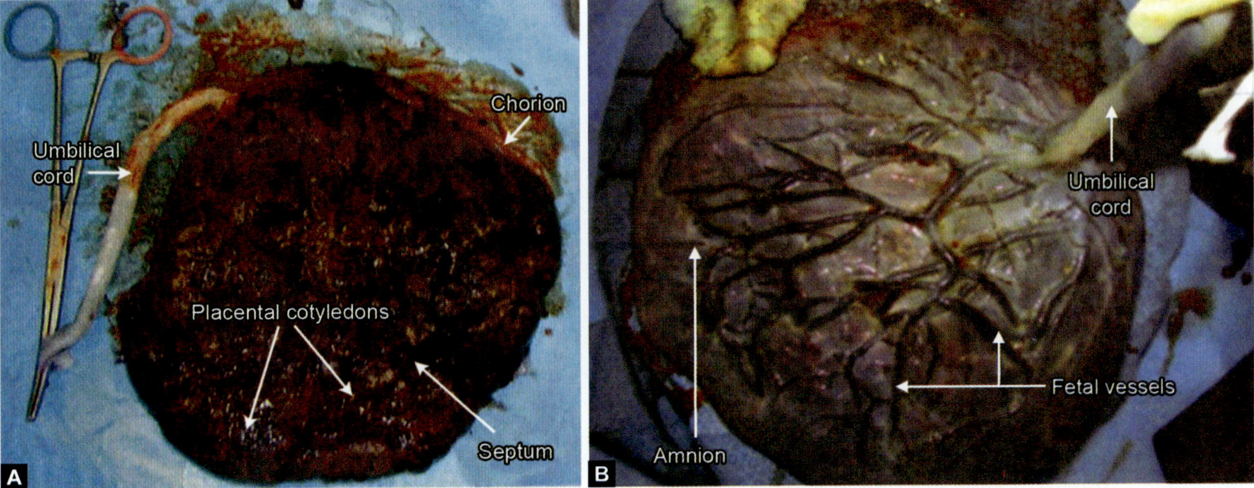



**Figs 14.7A and B:** (A) Maternal surface of placenta; (B) Fetal surface of placenta

**Q. What are the main functions of the placenta?**

**Ans.** The main functions of placenta are as follows:

- Transfer of nutrients and waste products
- Endocrine function: Production or metabolism of the hormones and enzymes necessary to maintain pregnancy
- Barrier function
- Immunological function.

## COUVELAIRE UTERUS

Figure 14.8 shows specimen of uterus removed at the time of hysterectomy. The uterus appears port wine in color probably as a result of intravasation of blood into the uterine musculature up to the level of serosa. The blood gets infiltrated between the bundles of muscle fibers. There can be effusions of blood beneath the tubal serosa, connective tissues of broad

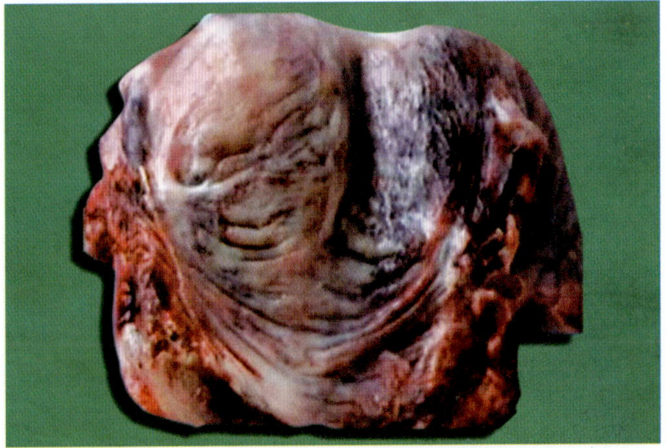

**Fig. 14.8:** Couvelaire uterus or uteroplacental apoplexy

ligaments, substances of the ovaries as well as free blood in the peritoneal cavity. These myometrial hemorrhages may interfere with uterine contractions to produce PPH. This condition has been found to be associated with severe forms of concealed placental abruption and is known as the Couvelaire uterus. However, Couvelaire uterus per se is not an indication for cesarean hysterectomy. In this case, cesarean hysterectomy was performed to save the patient's life due to severe uncontrollable PPH.

# Gynecological Specimens

## FIBROIDS

### Gross Appearance

This is a specimen of the uterus (probably removed by hysterectomy). The uterus is enlarged in size. The size of the uterus must be described in terms of weeks depending upon the type of specimen shown. There appears to be a nodular growth arising from endometrium/myometrium. These nodular growths are well-defined, showing a whorled appearance and surrounded by pseudocapsule. Whorled appearance and trabeculation may be due to the presence of fibrous tissue and muscle bundles. The fibroids vary in size from tiny, microscopic growths (seedling leiomyomas) to huge ones.

Uterine shape is distorted/not distorted by single/multiple nodular growth of varying sizes. The size, location and characteristics of the various fibroids present should then be described.

Figure 14.9 shows a cut specimen of uterus with a uniformly enlarged uterus having a size of 10–12 weeks of gestation. Cut-section shows presence of a large, single nodular growth, pinkish-white in color having a whorled appearance, about 10 cm in diameter arising within the myometrial fibers. My preferential diagnosis would be a single large intramural fibroid, having a diameter of 10 cm, arising in the uterine myometrium. The external surface of the uterus appears smooth.

Figure 14.10 shows a cut-section of the uterus with a centrally located smooth nodular growth suggestive of a submucous fibroid 8 × 6 cm in dimensions, having a smooth, uniform surface, centrally located within the uterine cavity.

Figure 14.11 shows a cut-section of the uterus with a large intramural nodular growth, having dimensions of 6 × 6 cm, suggestive of an interstitial fibroid.

Figure 14.12 is a cut-section of uterus showing multiple nodular growths arising within the uterine myometrium and one of them is a pedunculated growth having a diameter of 2 cm with the pedicle attached to the uterine serosa.

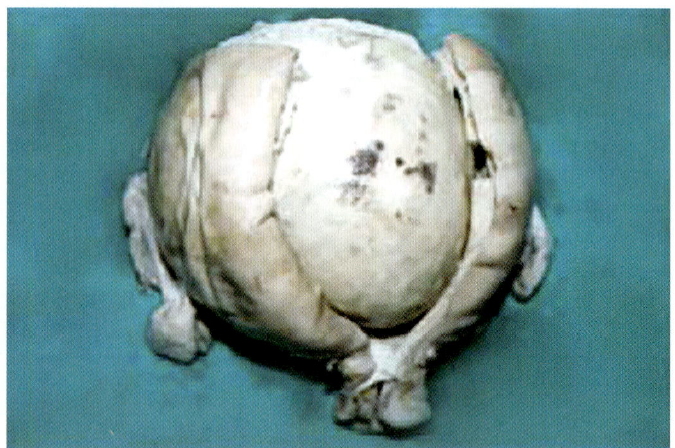

**Fig. 14.10:** Large submucous fibroid

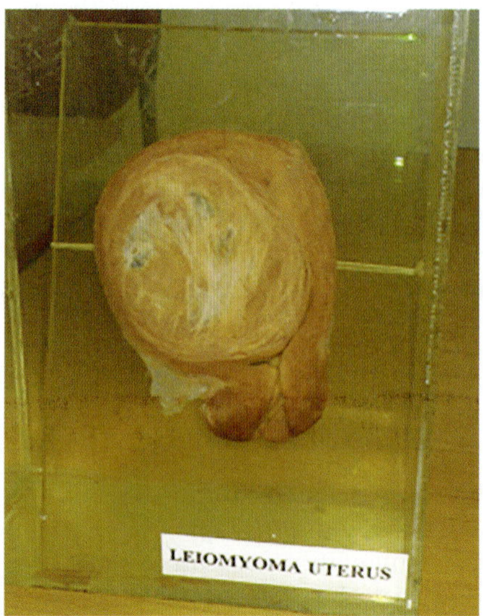


**Fig. 14.11:** Cut-section of the uterus showing a large interstitial fibroid

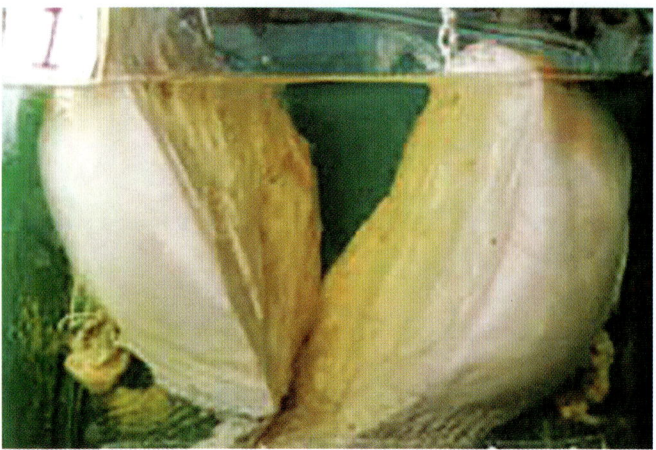

**Fig. 14.9:** Large intramural fibroid

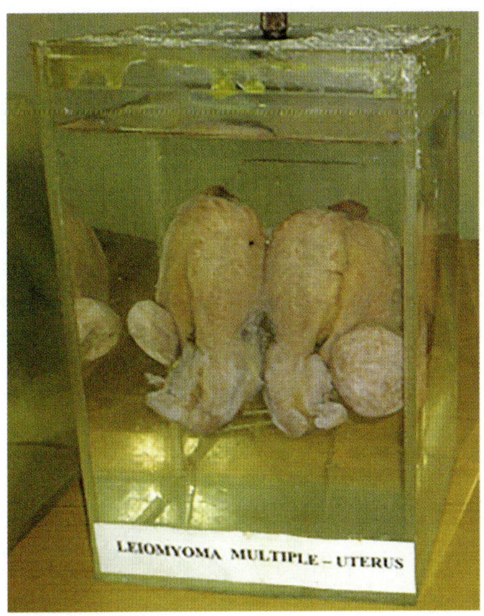

**Fig. 14.12:** Cut-section of uterus showing multiple fibroids

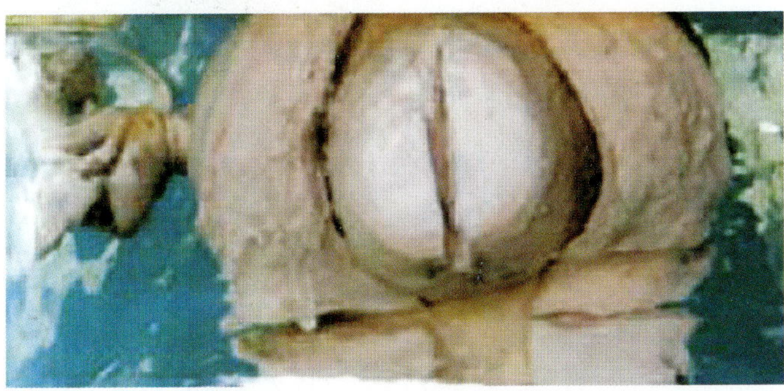

**Fig. 14.13:** Large submucous fibroid occupying the endometrial cavity

Figure 14.13 is a cut specimen of uterus showing large submucous fibroid size of $10 \times 6$ cm, with uterine cavity enlarged and myometrium thinned out.

### Q. What are the different types of fibroids?

**Ans.** Depending on their location, different types of fibroids may be classified as:

- Interstitial or intramural
- Subperitoneal or subserous
- Submucous.

For details related to other clinical questions, which may be asked in a specimen of fibroid uterus, kindly refer to Chapter 9.

## VESICULAR/HYDATIDIFORM MOLE

### Gross Appearance

This is a specimen showing a cluster of grayish/pinkish-brown colored, translucent vesicles/grape-like structures, which are connected to each other by strands of connective tissues. The vesicles may be of variable size, varying in diameter from 2 cm to 5 cm. The vesicles are filled with a clear fluid, rich in hCG.

The hydatidiform moles could be of two types: partial and complete mole. Difference between the two has been described in Chapter 9. On gross inspection, the complete mole does not show presence of any fetal/placental tissue (Fig. 14.14), whereas there might be presence of remnants of fetal/placental tissue in a case of partial mole (Fig. 14.15).

For details related to other clinical questions, which may be asked in a specimen of hydatidiform mole, kindly refer to Chapter 9.

## ENDOMETRIOSIS

Chocolate cyst of ovaries represents the most important manifestation of endometriosis.

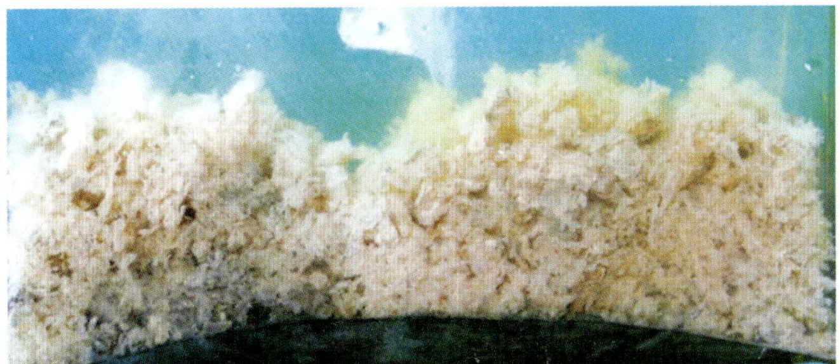

**Fig. 14.14:** Complete vesicular mole

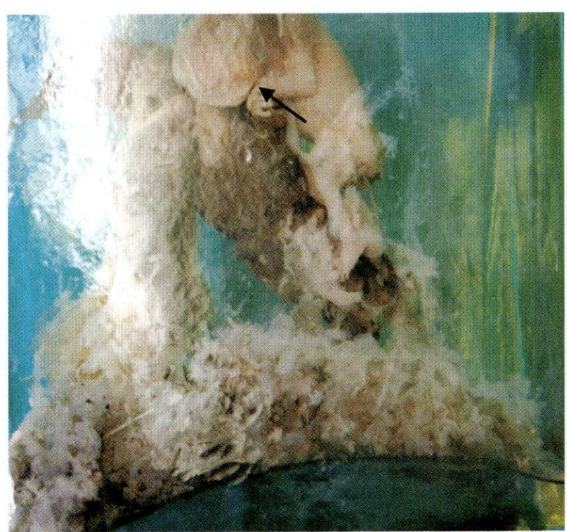

**Fig. 14.15:** Partial vesicular mole (The arrow indicates presence of fetal parts)

## Gross Appearance

Figure 14.16 is a specimen showing cut-section of the uterus with left ovary. Indication for hysterectomy was DUB in this case. Tunica albuginea, the outer covering of ovary appears to be thickened. Brownish-black vascular adhesions are also well marked on the undersurface of the ovary. The ovary shows presence of a cyst having dimensions of $5 \times 5$ cm. The inner surface of the cyst wall appears to contain areas of dark-brown tissue or liquid, suggestive of clotted blood. Figure 14.17 is a specimen showing ovaries of both the sides, each having a thin-walled, smooth cyst-like structure filled with dark-brown liquid-like material suggestive of clotted blood. My preferential diagnosis in this case would be chocolate cyst of ovary.

For details related to other clinical questions, which may be asked in a specimen of endometriosis, kindly refer to Chapter 9.

## ENDOMETRIAL CANCER

### Gross Appearance

Figures 14.18A and B are specimens showing cut-section of an enlarged uterus with cervix and bilateral adnexa. There is a fungating growth, which is localized in the upper part of uterine cavity close to fundus. Surface of the growth appears irregular with the areas of hemorrhage and necrosis.

For details related to other clinical questions, which may be asked in a specimen of endometrial cancer, kindly refer to Chapter 9.

## NEOPLASTIC GROWTHS OF OVARY

### Mucinous Cystadenoma of Ovary

Figure 14.19 is a specimen showing cut-section of an organ, which most likely appears to be the ovary, harboring a large

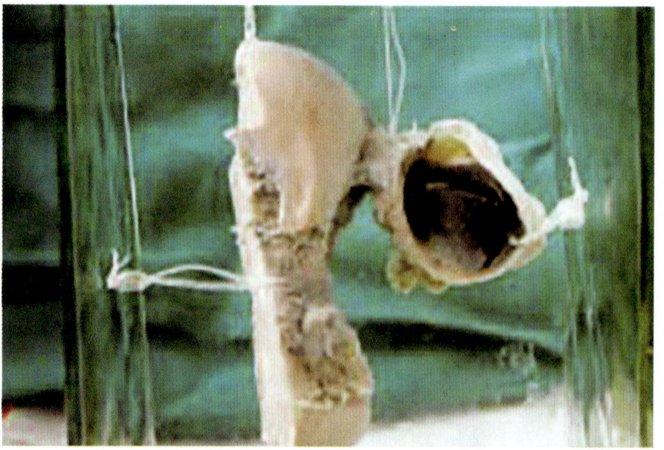

**Fig. 14.16:** Cut-section of uterus and ovary with dark colored clotted blood suggestive of chocolate cyst of ovary

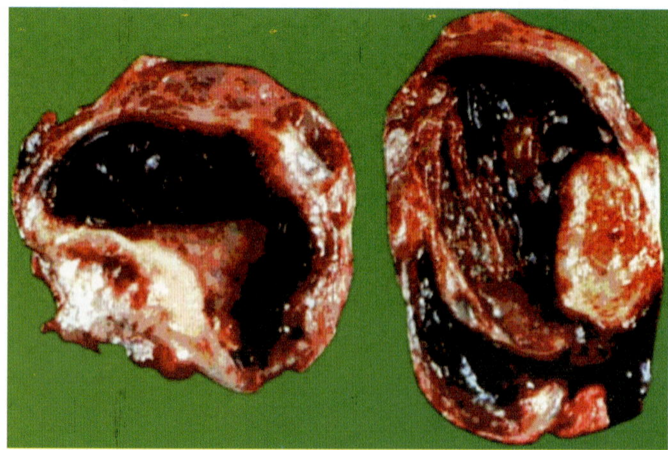

**Fig. 14.17:** Cut-section of both the ovaries, which show the presence of chocolate cyst

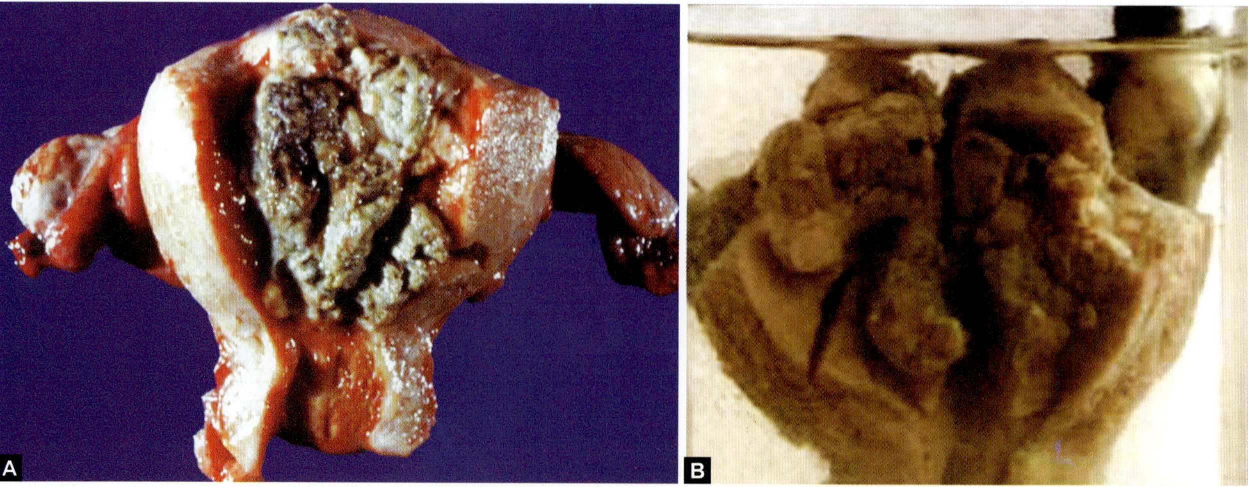


**Figs 14.18A and B:** Specimen showing endometrial carcinoma

mass having a diameter of 10–12 cm. There are presence of several septa within the mass, which give it a multiloculated appearance. Some of the loculi appear to be filled with a thick, viscid, straw-colored, mucin-like material. A few of the loculi appear to be empty probably because the fluid had been washed out at the time of mounting the specimen. There appear to be no solid areas of hemorrhage or necrosis inside the mass. My preferential diagnosis would be that of a mucinous cystadenoma. The diagnosis, however, needs to be confirmed on histopathological examination.

For details related to other clinical questions, which may be asked in a specimen of benign ovarian neoplasms, kindly refer to Chapter 9.

## Serous Cystadenoma of Ovary

Figure 14.20 is a specimen obtained after hysterectomy in which the uterus along with the bilateral adnexa had been removed. On the right side, there appears to be a large

cystic mass having diameter of about 8–10 cm arising from the left ovary. External surface of this cystic mass appears smooth and lobulated. The capsule appears thin, translucent, glistening and brownish-pink in appearance. There are no areas of hemorrhage, necrosis, papillae or adhesions on the external surface. A few dilated blood vessels can be seen on the surface of the mass. My preferential diagnosis would be a benign ovarian neoplasm, which in this case most likely is serous cystadenoma. A histological examination of the tissue is required to confirm the diagnosis.

Figure 14.21 is a specimen showing cut-section of an organ, which most likely appears to be ovary, harboring a cystic mass containing clear fluid-like substance. The cut-section shows presence of a few septae, which gives the tumor a multiloculated appearance. The loculi are of different sizes and appear to contain a thin, colorless, clear, serous fluid. There are no solid areas of hemorrhage or necrosis inside the tumor. My most preferential diagnosis in this case would be a serous cystadenoma. Sometimes, a long stretched, tubular structure may be present on the upper surface of the mass. This structure can be identified as fallopian tube due to the presence of fimbriae at its lateral end. This further helps in identifying the mass as having an ovarian origin. For details related to other clinical questions, which may be asked in a specimen of benign ovarian neoplasms uterus, kindly refer to Chapter 9.

Figure 14.22 is a cut specimen of an ovary, harboring a large tumor mass, having the dimensions of about 8 × 6 cm. The tumor has a smooth surface. There appears to be presence of heterogeneous material within the tumor. In the upper part, there is a presence of yellow cheesy substance, probably suggestive of sebaceous material. In the lower part of the tumor, there is presence of grayish-brown tissue. The origin of this tissue can be identified only on histopathological examination. My preferential diagnosis would be that of a (benign) dermoid cyst of the ovary, which needs to be confirmed on histopathological examination. No solid areas

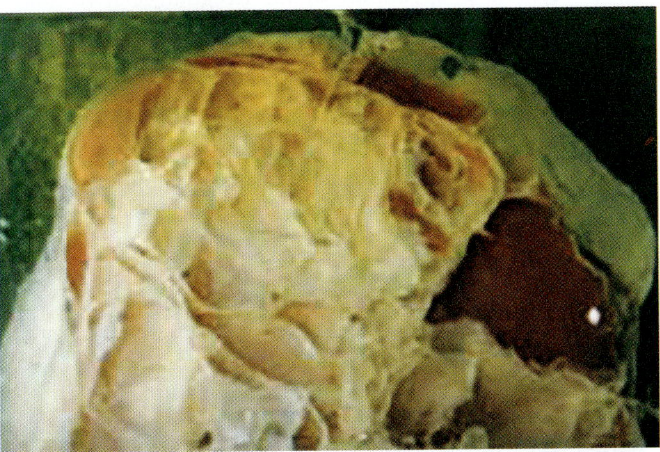

**Fig. 14.19:** Specimen showing mucinous cystadenoma of ovary

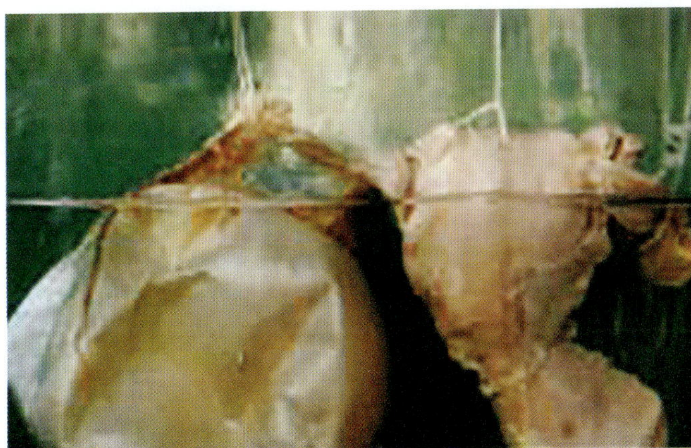

**Fig. 14.20:** Cut- section of ovary showing serous cystadenoma

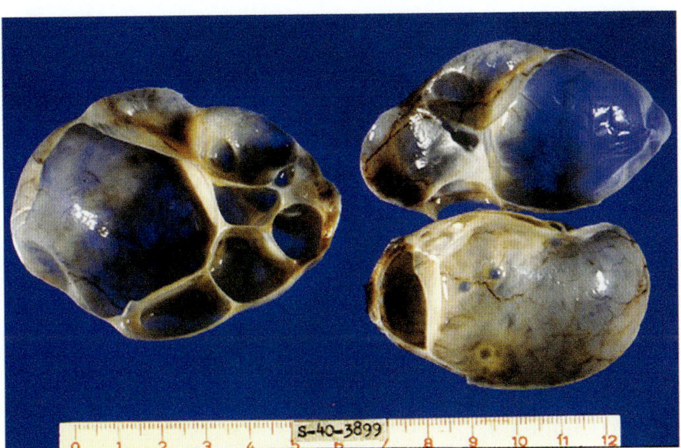

**Fig. 14.21:** Cut-section of ovary showing serous cystadenoma

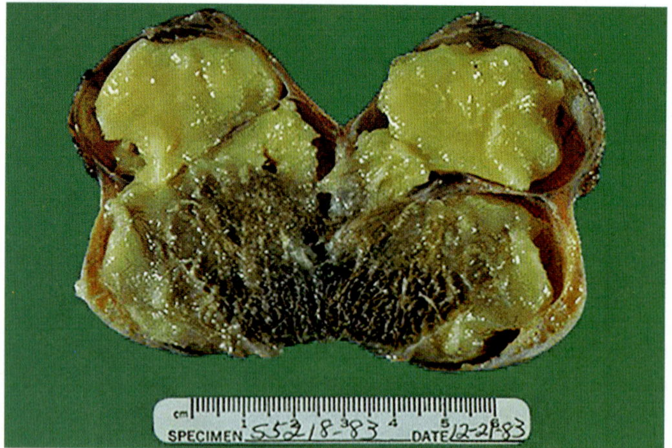

**Fig. 14.22:** Cut-section of ovary showing mature cystic teratoma

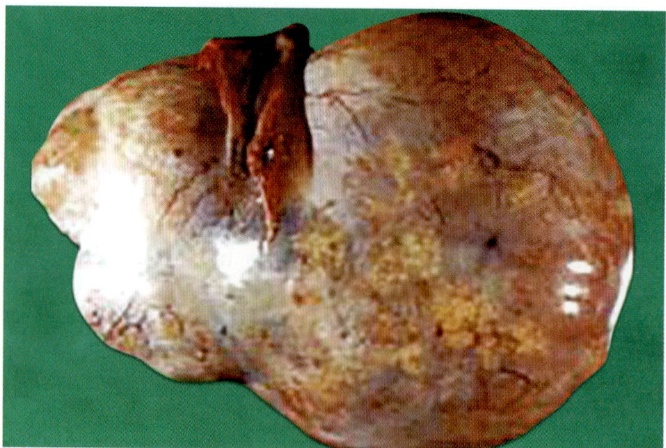

**Fig. 14.23:** Malignant ovarian tumor

or areas suggestive of hemorrhage or necrosis could be identified within the tumor. Sometimes, structures such as hair shaft, teeth, etc. can also be identified within the mass.

### Q. What is a teratoma?

**Ans.** Ovarian teratomas are a complex group of tumors that are subdivided into three major categories: (1) immature, (2) mature, and (3) monodermal and highly specialized. The majority of germ cell tumors are benign cystic teratomas, also known as dermoids.

*Immature teratomas:* Immature teratomas primarily contain immature tissues, most commonly of neuroectodermal origin. However, they may sometimes also contain varying quantities of mature tissue as well. Immature teratomas are essentially malignant.

*Mature teratomas:* Unlike the immature teratomas, the mature teratomas are exclusively composed of mature tissues. Mature teratomas could be either solid or cystic (dermoid cysts). In most cases, the tumor contains elements derived from all three germ layers. The dermoid cysts are benign ovarian masses, which may appear as masses having various sonographic appearances ranging from anechoic to echogenic due to variety of internal contents. The solid areas may be due to the presence of hair follicles in combination with the calcified elements within dermoid. These materials are responsible for producing echogenicity within the cyst. These cysts may contain hair, which because of its high echodensity may produce a typical acoustic shadow. Other types of tissues which may be present include teeth, bone, cartilage, thyroid tissues, bronchial tissues and sebaceous material.

For details related to other clinical questions, which may be asked in a specimen of benign ovarian neoplasms, kindly refer to Chapter 9.

## Ovarian Cancer

Figure 14.23 is a specimen of an irregular-shaped mass, appearing to arise from the ovary. The cut-section of the tumor cannot be seen so it is difficult to describe the contents of the mass. As seen from the external surface, the capsule of the mass appears to be smooth and glistening. Through it, tissues having varied consistency can be identified. There appear to be multiple solid areas within the mass. Areas of hemorrhage and necrosis can also probably be identified. Multiple blood vessels can also be seen traversing the surface of the ovary. From the various characteristics as described, the mass appears to be malignant in nature. However, this needs to be confirmed on histopathological examination. My preferential diagnosis would be that of a malignant ovarian tumor.

For details related to other clinical questions, which may be asked in a specimen of ovarian cancer, kindly refer to Chapter 9.

## HYDROSALPINX

Figure 14.24 is a hysterectomy specimen of uterus and cervix along with the right-sided adnexa. There appears to be retort-shaped, cystic mass, having dimensions of $10 \times 5$ cm arising from the right-sided tube. The walls of this mass appear to be thin and translucent having a smooth external surface. No adhesions can be seen on the external surface. The tubal fimbriae cannot be visualized because they are indrawn. My preferential diagnosis would be of a hydrosalpinx (moderate grade).

### Q. What is hydrosalpinx and how is it formed?

**Ans.** Hydrosalpinx is a cystic mass filled up with serous or clear fluid, commonly developing in the fallopian tubes as a result of distal tubal blockage. As the tubes get substantially

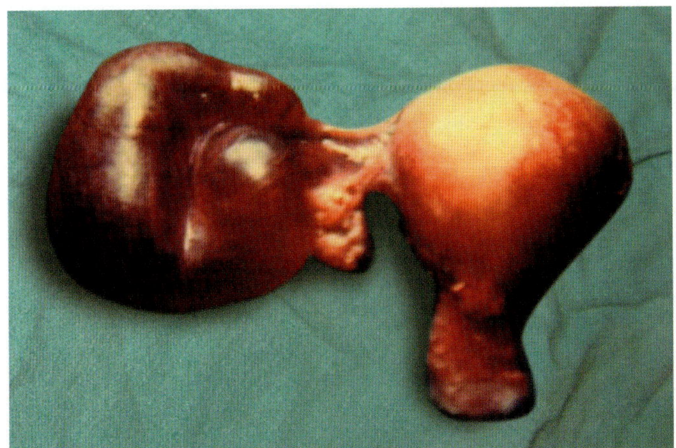

**Fig 14.24:** Specimen of hydrosalpinx

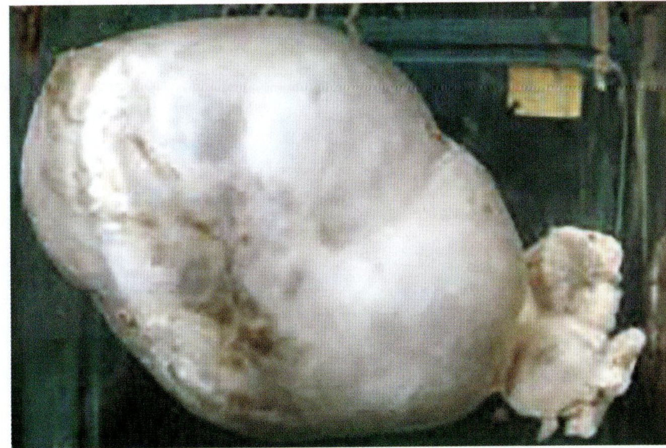

**Fig. 14.25:** Specimen showing ovary with multiple follicular cysts

distended, this results in the formation of a retort-shaped mass.

Hydrosalpinx commonly develops as a result of acute pelvic inflammatory disease. Infection causes obstruction of the cornual or fimbrial end openings of the tube. Inflammatory pus or exudate, which is formed initially, results in the formation of a mass, pyosalpinx. Gradually, over the period of time, this inflammatory exudate gets absorbed, leaving behind a clear fluid, which results in the formation of hydrosalpinx.

### Q. Why is hydrosalpinx retort shaped?

**Ans.** At the time of formation of hydrosalpinx, when the inflamed tube distends with pus or exudate, the thick mesenteric border of the ampullary portion of the tube restricts its stretching and enlargement, whereas the thin antimesentric portion readily expands. The thick isthmic portion of the tube is also resistant to expansion. All this results in the formation of a retort-shaped/sausage-shaped structure.

### Q. How is hydrosalpinx graded?

**Ans.** Hydrosalpinx is graded based on the maximum diameter of the tube. The grading is done as shown in Table 14.1.

| Table 14.1: Grading of hydrosalpinx | |
| --- | --- |
| *Grade* | *Diameter of the tube* |
| Mild | 0–2 cm |
| Moderate | 2–5 cm |
| Severe* | >5 cm |

*In severe hydrosalpinx, endosalpingeal mucosa (especially the cilia) is also irreparably damaged

## POLYCYSTIC OVARIES

### Gross Appearance

Figure 14.25 is a specimen showing an enlarged ovary having dimensions of 6 × 4 × 2 cm. Normal size of the ovary can be considered as 3 cm (length) × 2.5 cm (width) × 1 cm (thickness). In the above-described specimen, the ovarian capsule is thickened and pearly whitish-gray in color. From the external surface multiple small follicles, probably filled with clear fluid can be seen. My preferential diagnosis in this case would be that of polycystic ovary. Since the cut surface of the ovary is not seen, it is not possible to visualize small follicular fluid-filled cysts present at the periphery, which are commonly seen in a case of polycystic ovary.

For details related to other clinical questions, which may be asked in a specimen of polycystic ovary, kindly refer to Chapter 9.

## CARCINOMA CERVIX

Figure 14.26 is a specimen, showing cut-section of the uterus, cervix and bilateral adnexa. Vaginal cuff along with a part of parametrial tissue attached to the isthmus laterally can also be identified. A large fungating growth arising from the cervix can be observed. Areas of hemorrhage and necrosis can also be identified within this growth. Therefore, my preferential diagnosis in this case would be carcinoma cervix for which a Wertheim's hysterectomy was probably performed. It is not possible to give the exact staging just by seeing the specimen.

For details related to other clinical questions, which may be asked in a specimen of carcinoma cervix, kindly refer to Chapter 9.

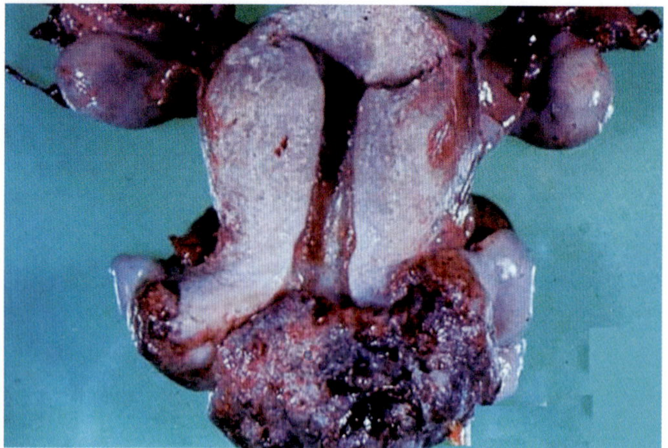

**Fig. 14.26:** Specimen of carcinoma of the cervix; the specimen was removed by Wertheim's operation; note that the cervix has been almost entirely eroded by the growth

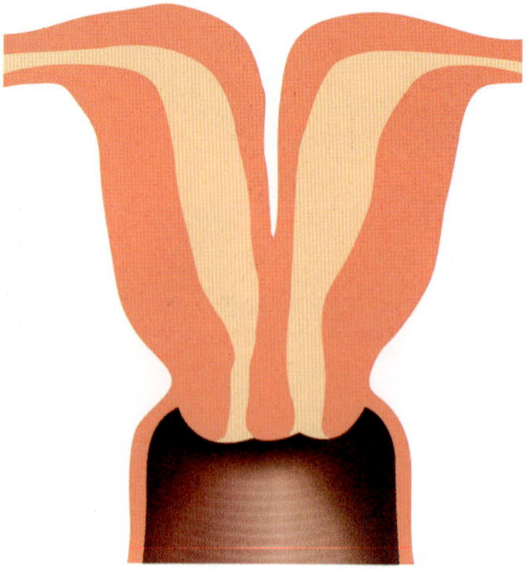

**Fig. 14.28:** Bicornuate uterus bicollis

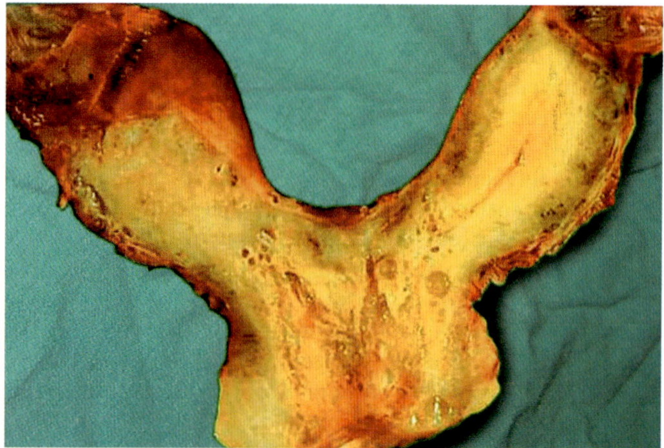

**Fig. 14.27:** Specimen showing cut-section of a bicornuate uterus with a single cervix

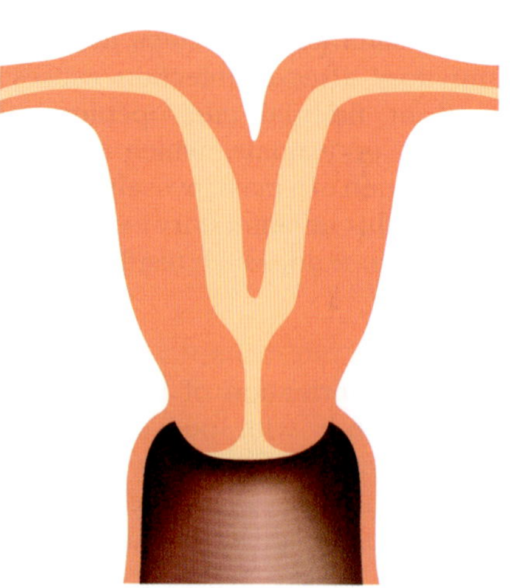

**Fig. 14.29:** Bicornuate uterus unicollis

## MÜLLERIAN DUCT ANOMALIES

Müllerian duct anomalies result due to defective fusion, canalization or absorption of the median septum of the female reproductive systems during embryonic development. Figure 14.27 shows cut specimen of the uterus, where the upper part has two horns, with each horn being connected to the single fallopian tube of the respective side. This gives the uterus a heart-shaped appearance. The pathology is related to the defective fusion of the upper parts of the Müllerian tubes. The fusion in the caudal parts occurs normally as a result of which the lower parts of the uterus and cervix are normal while the upper parts are bifurcated. My diagnosis in this case would be that of a bicornuate uterus, more specifically bicornuate uterus unicollis.

Bicornuate uterus could be of two types depending upon the involvement of the cervical canal. When the bifurcation of the central myometrium extends up to the external cervical os, there are likely to be two separate cervical canals. This condition is known as bicornuate uterus bicollis (Fig. 14.28). When the bifurcation of the central myometrium extends up to the internal cervical os, this results in a single cervical canal. This condition is known as bicornuate uterus unicollis (Fig. 14.29).

Figures 14.30A and B show a specimen where the uterus appears to be present as a paired organ. There are two uteri, two cervical canals and probably two vaginae. Each uterus has an ipsilateral fallopian tube facing the respective ovary. This condition is also known as uterus didelphys. This condition usually develops when the two Müllerian ducts fail to fuse

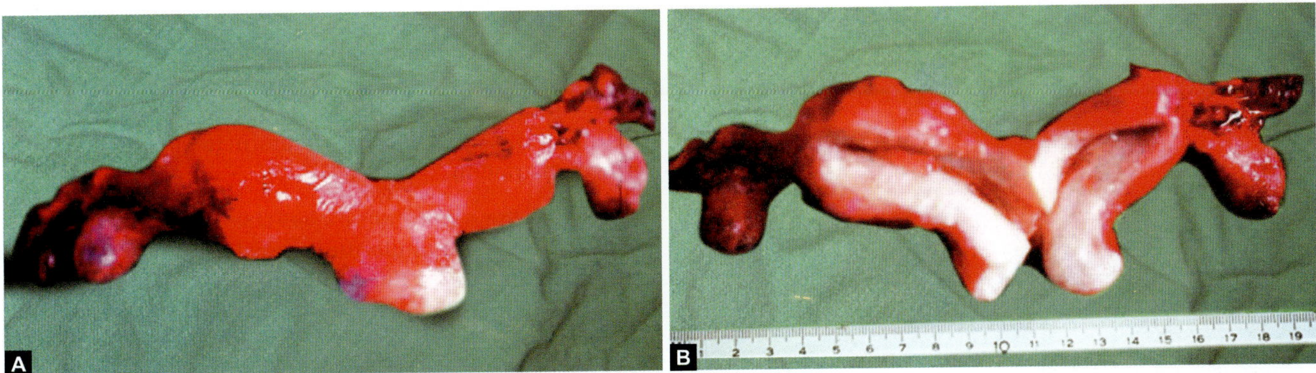

**Figs 14.30A and B:** Double uterus. (A) Uncut specimen; (B) Cut specimen

along the whole of their length, but develop normally and remain separate.

### Q. What management is required in cases of uterus didelphys?

**Ans.** Patients with uterus didelphys usually require no treatment. However, various uterine anomalies such as bicornuate uterus, septate uterus, etc. may be associated with reproductive abnormalities such as recurrent pregnancy loss, preterm births, malpresentation (breech, transverse presentation), etc. Since patients with uterus didelphys are usually left untreated, they may require special attention during pregnancy due to the high rate of pregnancy-related complications.

### Q. What treatment is required in cases of bicornuate uterus?

**Ans.** Metroplasty or unification of the two uterine horns in cases of bicornuate uterus is recommended only for those women who have experienced more than three recurrent spontaneous abortions, midtrimester losses or premature births, and in whom no other etiologic factor for pregnancy wastage has been identified. Strassman metroplasty is commonly performed in cases of bicornuate uterus.

### Q. What is a septate uterus?

**Ans.** Septate uterus is a uterine anomaly where the uterine cavity may be bifurcated due to presence of a septum, which extends downwards from the uterine fundus. The uterine septum usually results from incomplete resorption of the median septum after complete fusion of the Müllerian ducts has occurred. The septum could be of two types: partial and complete. The complete septum extends from the fundal area to the internal os and divides the endometrial cavity into two components. This anomaly is often associated with a longitudinal vaginal septum. The partial septum does not extend to the os and, therefore, may permit partial communication between the endometrial cavities. If there is presence of two separate cervices, this entity should be distinguished from the didelphys uterus because management of both the pathologies would be different.

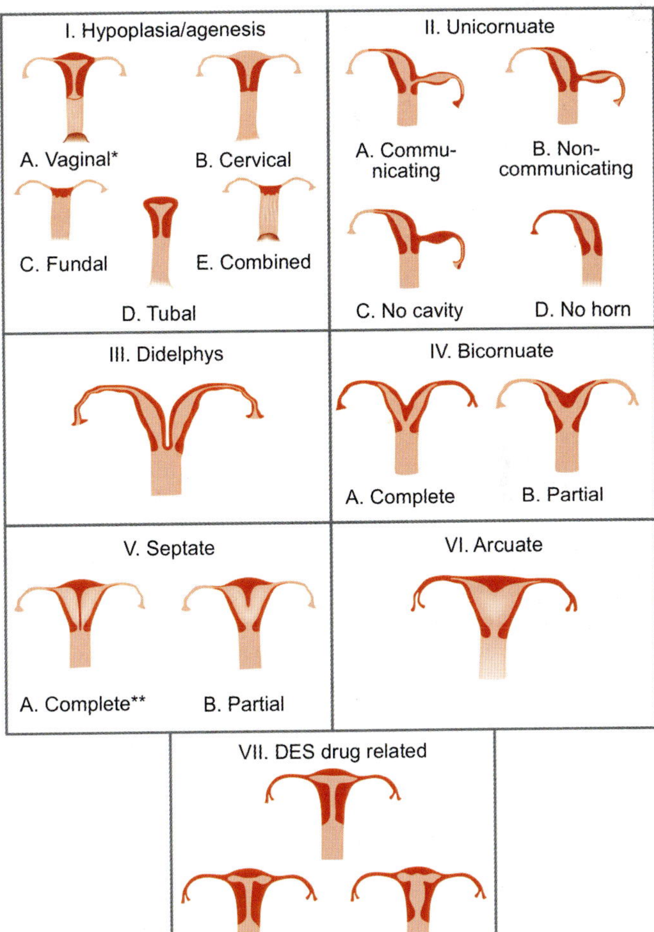


**Fig. 14.31:** Classification of the uterine anomalies by the American Society for Reproductive Medicine (1998). *Uterus may be normal or take a variety of abnormal forms. **May have two distinct cervices
*Source*: The American Fertility Society classifications of adnexal adhesions, distal tubal occlusion, tubal occlusion secondary to tubal ligation, tubal pregnancies, müllerian anomalies and intrauterine adhesions. Fertil Steril. 1988;49(6):944-55

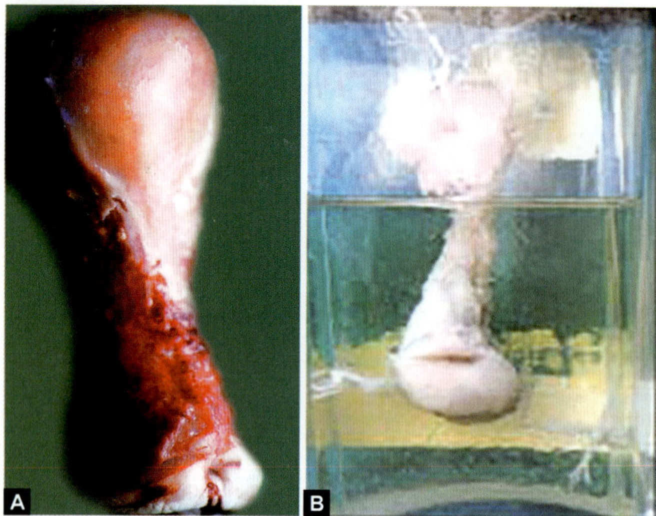

**Figs 14.32A and B:** Uterine prolapse with supravaginal elongation of cervix

A complete septum would be removed hysteroscopically while no surgical intervention would be recommended for the uterine didelphys.

### Q. How can one differentiate between bicornuate and septate uterus?

**Ans.** The diagnostic modalities, which are commonly used to establish a definitive diagnosis, include HSG, hysteroscopy and laparoscopy. Hysteroscopy helps in visualizing the interior of the uterine cavity and, therefore, identification of uterine septum. Laparoscopy helps in visualizing the external surface of the uterus, which may appear bifurcated in case of a bicornuate uterus. The external surface of the uterus may appear more or less normal in case of a septate uterus. Ultrasonography and MRI are also useful investigations for differentiating between the two anomalies.

### Q. What is arcuate uterus?

**Ans.** In an arcuate uterus, there is no actual septum in the region of fundus but instead of usual dome-shaped convexity of the fundus, there is shallow concave depression. The condition can cause abortion, preterm labor and intrauterine growth restriction.

### Q. How are the uterine anomalies classified?

**Ans.** Classification of uterine anomalies as described by the American Society for Reproductive Medicine is described in Figure 14.31.

## UTERINE PROLAPSE

### Supravaginal Elongation of Cervix

Figures 14.32A and B is a specimen of uterus and cervix removed by vaginal hysterectomy. No adnexa can be seen, so probably they were retained at the time of hysterectomy. Cervix appears to be elongated by approximately 5 cm. Normal length of cervix is about 2.5 cm, wherein the vaginal and supravaginal parts are equal in length. Elongation of the supravaginal part is commonly associated with uterine prolapse. Sometimes, this could also be due to congenital anomaly or chronic cervicitis. The elongation commonly occurs due to the straining of cervix as a result of the pull of cardinal ligaments to keep the cervix in position, whereas the weight of uterus makes it fall through the vaginal axis. Chronic interference of venous and lymphatic drainage also results in cervical elongation. My preferential diagnosis in this case is supravaginal elongation of cervix. The probable cause for this pathology can be gathered only if more information, particularly patient's history has been provided.

## FURTHER READING

1. Inamdar S, Khatri M. Color Atlas of Pathological Specimens & Instruments in Obstetrics & Gynecology, New Delhi, India: Jaypee Brothers Medical Publishers (P) Ltd; 2009.

**15**

CHAPTER

# Drugs in Obstetrics and Gynecology



# Atosiban

## Introduction

Atosiban is a peptide analog of oxytocin, acting as antagonist at the oxytocin receptors. In Europe and UK, it is available for inhibition of labor between 24 and 33 weeks of gestation, and may offer better benefit: risk ratio than other tocolytics. However, it is not yet approved for use in USA and India.

## Mechanism of Action

By acting as an antagonist at the oxytocin receptors, it may help in suppressing premature uterine contractions.

## Indications

- Tocolytic agent: Used as a tocolytic agent in cases of premature labor. This drug is available in Europe and UK for inhibition of labor between 24 and 33 weeks of gestation. However, it is not yet approved for use in USA and India.
- Recurrent implantation failure: It is also used for improving pregnancy outcome in cases of in vitro fertilization and embryo transfer (IVF-ET) with recurrent implantation failure.

## Route of Administration

Intravenous route.

## Dosage

An initial bolus dose of 6.75 mg is given intravenously over 1 minute. This is followed by a continuous IV infusion of 300 µg/minute for 3 hours. This is followed by an intravenous infusion of 100 µg/minute for a maximum of 45 hours. The maximum duration of treatment is 48 hours and the maximum dose to be administered is 330 mg.

## Contraindications

Atosiban is contraindicated in the following conditions:
- Pregnant women with gestational age below 24 or over 33 completed weeks
- Premature rupture of the membranes at more than 30 weeks of gestation
- Cases with intrauterine growth restriction
- Cases with abnormal fetal heart rate
- Antepartum uterine hemorrhage (placenta previa or abruptio placenta) requiring immediate delivery
- Eclampsia and severe preeclampsia requiring emergency delivery

- Intrauterine fetal death
- Suspected intrauterine infection
- Any other conditions in the mother, or fetus, where continuation of pregnancy is hazardous.

## Side Effects

Though it is less effective than β2 agonists regarding its tocolytic activity, it has been found to be associated with fewer cardiovascular and metabolic complications in comparison to β2 adrenergic agonists. It can cause minor side effects such as nausea, vomiting, arthralgia and chest pain.

# Bromocriptine

## Introduction

It is a synthetic ergot derivative (2-bromo-α-ergocryptine), acting as potent agonist on D2, but as partial agonist or antagonist on D1 receptors. It is also a weak α-adrenergic blocker but not an oxytocic.

## Mechanism of Action

Most of the actions of this drug are based on its activity on D2 receptors. It decreases the release of prolactin from the pituitary gland by activating dopaminergic receptors on lactotrope cells. Therefore, it acts as a strong antigalactopoietic drug. It also increases GH release in normal individuals.

## Indications

Bromocriptine is administered in the following conditions:
- Hyperprolactinemia due to microprolactinomas causing galactorrhea, amenorrhea and infertility in women. Bromocriptine and cabergoline are the first-line drugs for most cases. Bromocriptine should be stopped when pregnancy occurs, though no teratogenic effects have been yet reported.
- Hyperprolactinomas causing gynecomastia, impotence and sterility in men.
- Induction of ovulation: It can be used in combination with clomiphene citrate (CC) in patients with CC resistant anovulation.
- Suppression of lactation and breast engorgement in cases of neonatal death.
- Nongynecological disorders: Parkinsonism, type 2 diabetes mellitus, hepatic coma, acromegaly due to small pituitary tumors.

## Route of Administration

Oral route.

## Dosage

Bromocriptine should always be started at a low dose, 1.25 mg BD and then gradually increased till response occurs or until the side effects become limiting. Bromocriptine in the dosage of 2.5–10 mg/day proves to be useful in most cases.

## Contraindications

Bromocriptine is contraindicated in patients having following disorders:
- Mental disturbances
- Coronary diseases
- Peripheral vascular diseases
- Cerebrovascular diseases
- Hypertension
- Chronic heart diseases.

## Side Effects

The various side effects, which can occur with bromocriptine, are as follows:
- *Early:* These include nausea, vomiting, constipation, nasal stuffiness/blockage and conjunctival injection. Postural hypotension/syncope may occur at the initiation of therapy.
- *Late:* Behavioral alterations, mental confusion, hallucinations, abnormal movements, livedo reticularis.

# Cabergoline

## Introduction

It is a newer D2 agonist; more potent; more D2 selective and is longer acting (half-life > 60 hours) in comparison to bromocriptine.

## Indications

Some patients not tolerating or not responding to bromocriptine have been successfully treated with cabergoline. It is preferred for treatment of hyperprolactinemia and acromegaly.

## Route of Administration

Oral.

## Dosage

Cabergoline is administered in the dosage of 0.25 mg twice weekly. If required, it can be increased after every 4–8 weeks up to a maximum of 1 mg twice weekly.

## Contraindications

The drug is contraindicated in the following conditions:
- Patients with uncontrolled hypertension
- Known hypersensitivity to ergot derivatives.

## Side Effects

Incidence of complications such as nausea and vomiting are also lower with cabergoline in comparison to bromocriptine.

# Cerviprime Gel

Cerviprime gel and its insertion have been described in details in Chapter 6. Kindly refer to Chapter 6 for further details.

# Clomiphene Citrate

## Introduction

Clomiphene citrate is a nonsteroidal triphenylethylene derivative, acting as selective estrogen receptor modulator (SERM) having both estrogen antagonist and agonist effects.

## Mechanism of Action

Whether CC would act as an agonist or an antagonist depends upon the prevailing levels of endogenous estrogens in the body. If the levels of endogenous estrogens are too low, estrogen agonist properties of the drug are manifested. Otherwise in presence of normal levels of endogenous estrogens, antiestrogenic properties are exhibited. Clomiphene citrate is largely believed to exert its antiestrogen effect by competing with the estrogen receptors at the level of hypothalamus, pituitary and ovaries. By blocking the estrogen receptors within the hypothalamus, CC alleviates the negative feedback effect exerted by endogenous estrogens. As a result, the GnRH release gets normalized. Therefore, the secretion of FSH and LH is able to re-establish the normal process of ovulation and is capable of normalizing follicular recruitment, selection and development.

## Indications

- Women in whom the cause of infertility is anovulation or anovulatory disturbances
- Women with unexplained fertility problems
- Polycystic ovarian disease
- Anovulatory dysfunctional uterine bleeding
- Harvesting oocytes before an IVF cycle
- Oligospermia (in males).

## Route of Administration

Oral.

## Dosage

*Standard protocol:* The standard dose of CC is 50 mg PO once a day for 5 days, starting on the days 3–5 of the natural spontaneous menstrual cycle or after progestin-induced bleeding. In case there is no response with 50 mg dosage, it can be increased up to a dosage of 250 mg/day. The dosage is increased in the increments of 50 mg every 5 days. The response to CC is monitored using pelvic ultrasonography starting on the day 12 of the menstrual cycle. The follicle should develop to a diameter of 23–24 mm before a spontaneous LH surge occurs.

*Extended protocol:* Therapy with CC in the dosage varying between 50 and 250 mg/day is administered over 8–10 days. This protocol, however, can be associated with significant side effects and so it is not commonly used.

*Combination protocols:* These protocols are usually used in women who are resistant or refractory to standard treatment with CC. The following combinations can be offered to such women:
1. CC + hCG (5,000–10,000 IU).
2. CC + insulin sensitizing agents (e.g. metformin, 1,000–2,000 mg/day in divided doses).
3. CC + glucocorticoids (0.5 mg dexamethasone or 5 mg prednisolone daily at night).
4. Sequential CC with gonadotropins: CC is administered in the dosage of 50–100 mg/day on days 5–9 of the cycle. This is immediately followed by low dose of FSH (e.g. 75 IU/day) on days 9–12 of the cycles.

### Clomiphene Failure

This is defined as absence of pregnancy despite the occurrence of ovulation with CC. This could be related to causes such as abnormal cervical or endometrial environment, low fertilization/implantation rate, and deficient function of the corpus luteum (luteal dysfunction).

### Clomiphene Resistance

This is defined as absence of ovulation even after treatment with CC in the dosage of 100 mg/day for 5 days for three cycles.

## Contraindications

Clomiphene citrate is contraindicated in the following conditions:
- Ovarian cysts/tumors
- Ovarian failure
- Hepatic dysfunction
- Occurrence of visual disturbances
- Pregnancy
- Previous history of breast cancer (use is controversial).

### Side Effects

The main risk for the women who are being prescribed CC is that this drug may be associated with the risk of multiple pregnancies. Women undergoing treatment with CC should be offered ultrasound monitoring during at least the first cycle of treatment to ensure that they receive a dose that minimizes the risk of multiple pregnancy. Another important adverse effect associated with the use of this drug is the thickening of the cervical mucus under the antiestrogenic effect of CC. This may create an iatrogenic cervical factor, which may be responsible for producing infertility in a patient who has otherwise ovulated. Other adverse effects, which may be rarely associated with CC, include hot flushes (vasomotor flushes), scotomas, breast tenderness, nausea, dryness of the vagina, headache and ovarian hyperstimulation.

Anovulatory women with PCOS, having a BMI of more than 25 who have not responded to CC alone, should be offered metformin in combination with CC. Women who are prescribed metformin should be informed about the side effects, such as nausea, vomiting and other gastrointestinal disturbances, associated with its use.

# Cyproterone Acetate

### Introduction

Cyproterone acetate is a synthetic, steroidal antiandrogen drug, which also has additional progestogen-like properties.

### Mechanism of Action

Cyproterone inhibits LH release by its progestational activity. Lowering of serum testosterone occurs consequent to LH inhibition. This helps in supplementing the direct antiandrogenic action of cyproterone.

### Indications

- Precocious puberty in boys (prevention of pubertal changes).
- Inappropriate sexual behavior in men (suppression of libido and androgenic anabolism).
- Acne and hirsutism in women (usually in combination with an estrogen).
- Combined oral contraceptive pills: Due to its progestogenic effects, cyproterone acetate is a component of some combined oral contraceptive pills (e.g. Dianette and Diane): These pills may be especially useful in women with severe acne and hirsutism desiring contraception.
- Metastatic prostate carcinoma (efficacy of this drug is inferior to other forms of androgen deprivation).

### Route of Administration

Oral.

### Dosage

- In COCPs, cyproterone acetate (2 mg) is combined with 35 µg of ethinyl estradiol. This is taken for 21 days followed by 7 days of pill-free interval.
- For cases of hirsutism and hypersexuality, a dose of 25 mg BD is sufficient although dose up to 100 mg/day is permissible.
- For treatment of metastatic prostate cancer, dosage of up to 300 mg/day are sufficient.

### Contraindications

The drug is to be prescribed with caution in the following conditions:
- History of allergy or sensitivity to any of the ingredients in the medicine.
- Breastfeeding/pregnancy.
- History of jaundice, gallstones, porphyria, systemic lupus erythematosus, hereditary angioedema, chorea.
- Inflammatory bowel disease such as Crohn's disease or ulcerative colitis.
- History of hypertension, renal problems, a family history of hypertriglyceridemia, thromboembolic problems (e.g. heart attack, angina, stroke, deep vein thrombosis, pulmonary embolism, etc.), chloasma, depression, liver tumors, migraine or severe headache.
- Presence of risk factors for developing cervical cancer.
- Sickle cell anemia.
- Vaginal bleeding having unknown cause.
- Risk factors for developing breast cancer.

### Side Effects

Use of this drug in men can be associated with complications such as decreased libido, erectile dysfunction, inhibition of gonadal function, reduced sexual drive and reduced sperm production and volume of semen. This may be associated with fertility problems. Less commonly, the use of this drug can result in complications such as a feeling of lack of interest or lack of energy, breast enlargement, and/or tenderness, breathing difficulties, weight changes, depressed mood, feeling of restlessness, hot flushes, liver problems including jaundice, sweating, tiredness, etc. Rarely, it may result in complications such as benign breast lumps, galactorrhea, hypersensitivity reactions, etc.

# Danazol

### Introduction

Danazol, a synthetic androgen is the derivative of ethinyl testosterone, which has been shown to be highly effective drug for relieving the symptoms of endometriosis by inhibiting pituitary gonadotropins (FSH and LH).

## Mechanism of Action

By inhibiting the pituitary production of gonadotropins, danazol may result in the development of a relative hypoestrogenic state. Endometrial atrophy is the likely mechanism, which provides relief from pain due to endometriosis. Danazol acts by inhibiting the mid-cycle FSH and LH surges and preventing steroidogenesis in the corpus luteum.

## Indications

It is a highly effective drug for treatment of endometriosis.

## Route of Administration

Oral.

## Dosage

Danazol therapy is started when the patient is menstruating, usually on the 1st day of the menses. The initial dosage should be 800 mg/day, given in two divided oral doses, but this dosage can be titrated down as long as amenorrhea persists and pain symptoms are controlled. Patients with less severe symptoms may be given 200–400 mg/day, in two divided oral doses. Treatment is usually administered for 6 months in cases of endometriosis, but can be extended to 9 months in responsive patients with severe disease.

## Contraindications

Contraindications for the use of danazol include the following:
- Pregnant and lactating women
- Porphyrias
- Epileptic seizures
- Breast cancer
- Impaired renal/hepatic/cardiac function
- Undiagnosed abnormal uterine bleeding.

## Side Effects

The adverse effects caused by danazol are primarily related to estrogen deficiency and the androgenic effects. Estrogen deficiency can result in symptoms such as headache, flushing, sweating, atrophic vaginitis and breast atrophy. Androgenic effects associated with danazol include acne, edema, hirsutism, deepening of the voice and weight gain.

# Diazepam

## Introduction

Diazepam is the oldest and an all-purpose benzodiazepine derivative.

## Mechanism of Action

It is used as a sedative, hypnotic, anxiolytic, muscle relaxant, premedicant, anesthetic and an anticonvulsant agent.

## Indications

- Status epilepticus, eclampsia
- Preeclampsia
- Preoperative medication for surgeries such as D&C, medical termination of pregnancy, laparoscopy, etc.

## Route of Administration

Oral/intramuscular/intravenous.

## Dosage

*Lean regimen for eclampsia:* In this regime, loading dose of 10 mg, IV is administered over 2 minutes, followed by IV infusion of 40 mg in 500 mL normal saline for next 24 hours. This drug is nowadays not preferred as it causes lethargy and apnea of the newborn.

*Mild-to-moderate preeclampsia:* In these cases, diazepam is administered in the dosage of 10 mg every 6 to 8 hourly.

## Contraindications

Diazepam is contraindicated in the following disorders:
- Pregnant or lactating women
- Liver disorders
- Severe depression
- Psychosis
- Hypersensitivity or allergy to any drug in the benzodiazepine class
- Liver/renal disorders
- Acute narrow-angle glaucoma.

## Side Effects

*Maternal side effects:* Benzodiazepines are relatively safe drugs. Maternal side effects at hypnotic doses are dizziness, vertigo, ataxia, disorientation, amnesia, respiratory depression, hypotension, shock, prolongation of reaction time, resulting in impairment of psychomotor skills, etc. Therefore, the patients who have been given preanesthetic medication with diazepam should be instructed not to drive by themselves immediately after undergoing surgery. Some less commonly occurring complications include weakness, blurring of vision, dry mouth, urinary incontinence, etc. The dependence and hangover producing liability of diazepam is low.

*Fetal side effects:* This drug can cross the placental barrier resulting in side effects such as respiratory depression, apneic spells, hypotonia, hypotension, impaired temperature regulation, hyperbilirubinemia, neonatal sedation, increased incidence of teratogenicity (e.g. cleft lip, cleft palate, etc.).

# Drotaverine Hydrochloride

## Introduction

It is a highly effective antispasmodic agent, commonly used for relieving muscle spasms for various obstetric and gynecological indications.

## Mechanism of Action

Drotaverine hydrochloride is an isoquinolone derivative, which is a selective phosphodiesterase 4 inhibitor. Thereby, this drug increases the concentration of cAMP and cGMP resulting in the relaxation of smooth muscles. Simultaneously, the drug does not have any anticholinergic side effects.

## Indications

*Active management of labor:* This drug is only administered in cases where active labor has been established (i.e. cervix is more than 3–4 cm dilated). Forty milligrams (1 ampoule) of the drug is administered slowly via intramuscular or intravenous route after diluting it with 10 mL of saline. This is repeated after every 2–3 hours for a maximum of 3 doses. It is  likely to reduce the duration of active phase of labor by hastening cervical dilatation.

*Dysmenorrhea:* In cases of dysmenorrhea, this drug is administered in the dosage of 1 or 2 tablets (40–80 mg) three times a day for 3–5 days.

*Uterine cramps due to IUCD in situ:* One or two tablets are given three times a day.

*Preoperative medication:* It can be administered along with mefenamic acid at the time of paracervical block in cases of gynecological procedures such as hysteroscopy and endometrial biopsy.

*Nongynecological indications:* Treatment of nongynecological/obstetric causes of colicky pain (e.g. renal colic, abdominal colic, etc.), functional bowel disorders, etc.

## Route of Administration

Oral/intramuscular/intravenous/subcutaneous.

## Dosage

40–80 mg orally three times a day.

## Contraindications

The drug should be used with caution in the following conditions:
- Pregnancy and lactation
- Severe hepatic/renal/cardiac dysfunction
- Porphyria.

## Side Effects

No major side effects have been observed with this drug. It can be associated with minor side effects such as vertigo, nausea, and vomiting, dry mouth, etc. With high doses, hypotension may occur if the drug is administered in nonrecumbent position.

# GnRH Agonists

## Introduction

This is a synthetic peptide molecule which interacts with the GnRH receptors to elicit the biological response by stimulating the release of pituitary hormones FSH and LH. Since the physiological release of GnRH is in pulses, whereas these agonists act continuously, soon following the initial episode of stimulation, GnRH analogs produce a hypogonadotropic-hypogonadic state by inhibiting the secretion of gonadotropins by causing the downregulation of pituitary gland.

## Mechanism of Action

After an initial episode of stimulation, by eventually causing the downregulation of pituitary gland, GnRH agonists produce a hypogonadotropic-hypogonadic state. They also act by inhibiting the mid-cycle FSH and LH surge and preventing steroidogenesis in the corpus luteum. Spermatogenesis or ovulation comes to an end and testosterone or estradiol levels fall to the castration levels. Recovery usually occurs within 2 months of stopping treatment. Currently, goserelin and leuprolide acetate are the most commonly used GnRH agonists.

## Indications

- *Endometriosis:* Efficacy of GnRH agonists for providing pain relief is similar to that of danazol. Treatment is usually restricted to monthly injections for 6 months.
- *Estrogen-dependent disorders:* These include conditions such as menorrhagia, adenomyosis or uterine fibroids. GnRH agonists are effective in these cases by producing a hypoestrogenic state.
- *Precocious puberty:* GnRH agonists are useful in treating precocious puberty in both boys and girls.

- *Ovarian stimulation protocols:* In these cases, GnRH agonists produce a hypoestrogenic state by causing the downregulation of hypothalamo-pituitary axis. FSH is then administered followed by hCG to trigger ovulation.

## Route of Administration

Intramuscular/subcutaneous/intranasal/implants: Some GnRH agonist preparations are also available in the form of implants. The action of implants can last from 1 to 12 months. Injectable preparations are formulated for daily, monthly or quarterly use.

## Dosage

Leuprolide is used in the dosage of a single monthly 3.75 mg depot injection given intramuscularly. Goserelin, in a dosage of 3.6 mg, is administered subcutaneously every 28 days. The dose of goserelin is 3.6 mg SC q28d or 10.8 mg SC q12wk for 6 months. A nasal spray of nafarelin (synarel) is also available and is used in the dosage of 400 µg twice daily.

## Contraindications

- Pregnancy/lactation
- Hypersensitivity to the constituents of a GnRH preparation.

## Side Effects

Similar to danazol, use of GnRH agonists may result in hypoestrogenic side effects. Their use is specifically associated with the loss of trabecular bone density, which is restored by 2 years after cessation of therapy. Other prominent adverse effects include hot flushes, mood swings, breakthrough bleeding, reduced libido, depression, vaginal dryness, etc.

There has been much recent research regarding whether the simultaneous use of add-back therapy would be helpful in preventing osteoporosis and other hypoestrogenic symptoms associated with the use of GnRH agonists. Various agents which can be used as the add-back therapy include hormone replacement therapy preparations (a combination of conjugated estrogen 0.625 or 1.25 mg with norethindrone 5 mg/day), OCPs (containing ethinyl estradiol and desogestrel), progestins (norethindrone 5–10 mg/day), tibolone maleate, bisphosphonates, etc. Use of add-back therapy does seem to reduce some of the hypoestrogenic side effects associated with the use of GnRH agonists, thereby allowing longer duration of therapy with these agents.

Hypersensitivity reactions also have been sometimes reported. Ovarian hyperstimulation, resulting in polycystic ovary, lower abdominal pain, ovarian bleeding and shock can also occur in women who are administered GnRH agonists.

# GnRH Antagonists

## Introduction

The GnRH antagonists are the latest generation of drugs that block the secretion of pituitary gonadotropins without an initial flare-up effect. These are synthetic peptide molecules having a structure similar to GnRH agonists. However, they exert an antagonist effect on the hypothalamus. The advantages of GnRH antagonists over the long-acting GnRH agonists are as follows:

- GnRH antagonists produce a quick suppression of gonadotropin secretion by competitive antagonism. Therefore, they are usually started only from the 6th day of ovarian hyperstimulation.
- GnRH antagonists carry a lower risk of ovarian hyperstimulation syndrome in comparison to the GnRH agonists. However, the pregnancy rate may be similar or even lower in comparison to the GnRH agonists.
- They achieve more complete suppression of endogenous gonadotropin secretion.

## Mechanism of Action

These drugs bind to the GnRH receptors in the pituitary gland thereby blocking the release of LH and FSH. In women, administration of GnRH antagonists suppresses the release of estrogen, whereas in men it suppresses the release of testosterone. Various GnRH antagonists which are commonly used include cetrorelix, ganirelix, abarelix and degarelix.

When used for the induction of ovulation, the GnRH antagonists are administered as a single dose on the 6–8th day of the menstrual cycle. Use of GnRH antagonists has the advantage of blocking the LH surge at the periovulatory period; therefore, premature luteinization or spontaneous LH surge does not occur. As a result, the pituitary gland is not downregulated at the beginning of the menstrual cycle. Due to this, smaller amounts of gonadotropins are required to stimulate ovulation.

## Indications

### Women

- Ovarian stimulation protocols
- Endometriosis (for providing relief from pain)
- Uterine fibroids.

### Men

- Prostate cancer (advanced cases of prostate cancer): Use of GnRH antagonists results in a reduction in the size of tumor

- Benign prostatic hyperplasia (under investigation)
- Contraception (under investigation).

## Route of Administration

GnRH antagonists can be either administered by intramuscular injection (abarelix) or subcutaneous injection (cetrorelix, degarelix and ganirelix).

## Dosage

In cases of infertility, GnRH antagonists can be administered either as a single dosage protocol or as multiple dosage protocol. In a single dosage protocol, high dose of cetrorelix (3 mg) is administered in the follicular phase (day 8 or 9) of the stimulation cycle. In the multiple-dose protocol, the drug is administered daily from day 6th or 7th of gonadotropin stimulation including the day when hCG is administered.

## Contraindications

GnRH antagonists are contraindicated in the following situations:
- Undiagnosed vaginal bleeding (due to the suspicion of underlying cancer)
- Hypersensitivity or severe allergic reactions to the drug or its components
- Pregnant women
- Hepatic/renal insufficiency.

## Side Effects

It can result in side effects such as headache, nausea, weight gain and hot flushes. When used for cases of fertility treatment, it can result in side effects such as ovarian hyperstimulation and abdominal pain. Injection of this drug can result in injection site reactions, systemic allergic reactions, etc.

# Isoxsuprine

## Introduction

Isoxsuprine is a β2 adrenergic agonist causing relaxation of the smooth muscles of the uterus and the blood vessels.

## Mechanism of Action

The drug exerts β sympathomimetic and sympatholytic actions. The β actions are mediated through cAMP, which phosphorylates a number of intracellular cAMP-dependent protein kinases, thereby initiating a series of reactions, eventually reducing the frequency and intensity of uterine contractions. In higher doses, the drug exerts a direct papaverine-like antispasmodic and smooth muscle relaxant action on the muscles of corpus as well as cervix.

## Indications

- Acts as a tocolytic agent used for the treatment of preterm labor
- For producing uterine relaxation in cases of tetanic uterine contractions
- Cervical relaxation of rigid cervix.

## Route of Administration

Isoxsuprine can be administered through intramuscular/ intravenous or oral routes. Preparation of isoxsuprine hydrochloride (duvadilan) is available in the form of oral tablets, intramuscular and intravenous ampoules.

## Dosage

In cases of preterm labor, initially an IV infusion at the dose rate of 0.3–0.5 mg/minute is started by adding 40–60 mg of isoxsuprine in 500 mL of 5% glucose or normal saline. This is followed by 10–20 mg intramuscularly 6–8 hourly for 2 days and then oral isoxsuprine in the dosage of 20 mg TDS for an average of 14 days.

## Contraindications

- Pregnancy
- Bleeding disorders
- Glaucoma
- History of heart diseases (especially heart attack).

## Side Effects

Administration of isoxsuprine through intramuscular/intravenous route can result in side effects such as flushing, tachycardia, hypotension, etc. Administration through oral route can result in side effects such as nausea, stomach upset, flushing, giddiness, headache, etc. Rarely, severe allergic reactions (rashes, itching, swelling, difficulty in breathing, etc.) can also occur with this drug.

# Labetalol

## Introduction

Labetalol, the first adrenergic antagonist is a nonselective β-blocker, which also has vascular α1 receptor blocking capabilities. It has gained wide acceptance for use during pregnancy.

## Mechanism of Action

This drug produces its action by blocking both α and β receptors. It helps in lowering BP smoothly but rapidly, without causing tachycardia.

## Indications

Labetalol is used for the following indications:
- It is a moderately potent hypotensive agent used for the treatment of preeclampsia (pregnancy-induced hypertension)
- Acute or chronic hypertension associated with pheochromocytoma
- Clonidine withdrawal
- Essential hypertension.

## Route of Administration

- It can be administered via oral/intravenous route.
- Labetalol is available in the form of 100 mg, 200 mg and 300 mg tablets. Ampoules of labetalol are available containing 5 mg/mL of solution.

## Dosage

Labetalol is given as a 20 mg intravenous bolus, followed by 40 mg after 10 minutes. If the first dose is not effective, then 80 mg is administered every 10 minutes. Maximum total dose of 220 mg can be administered. It can also be administered in the form of a continuous infusion—250 mg of labetalol in 250 mL of normal saline, administered at the rate of 20 mg/hour (20 mL/minute). The onset of action of intravenous dosage is within 5–10 minutes. Orally, labetalol is administered in the dose of 100 mg 8-hourly, which may be increased to 800 mg/day.

## Contraindications

Labetalol is contraindicated in the following conditions:
- Asthma, airway obstructive disease
- Third-degree, second-degree heart block, or moderate-to-severe-first-degree heart block
- Congestive heart failure
- Bradycardia
- Hypotension
- Cardiogenic shock.

## Side Effects

This drug can produce side effects like flushing, headache, nausea and vomiting. It is contraindicated in women with asthma and first-degree heart block. Therefore, its use must be avoided in women with asthma or congestive heart failure. Due to a lower incidence of side effects like maternal hypotension, the use of labetalol now supplants that of hydralazine. When administered orally to women with chronic hypertension, it seems to be as safe and effective as methyldopa, although neonatal hypoglycemia can occur with higher doses.

# Letrozole

## Introduction

Aromatase inhibitors, such as letrozole and anastrozole, inhibit the action of the enzyme aromatase, which is responsible for the process of aromatization (conversion of androgens into estrogens). As a result, estrogen levels are dramatically reduced, releasing the hypothalamic-pituitary axis from its negative feedback.

## Mechanism of Action

It is an orally active nonsteroidal (type 2) compound that reversibly inhibits aromatization all over the body, including that within the breast cancer cells, resulting in nearly total estrogen deprivation.

## Indications

- *Early breast cancer:* Letrozole is a first-line drug for adjuvant therapy after mastectomy in postmenopausal women with positive estrogen receptors.
- *Advanced breast cancer:* Current guidelines recommend letrozole as first-line therapy because of longer time to disease progression and higher response rate obtained with this drug in comparison to tamoxifen.
- *In vitro fertilization:* Though the Food and Drug administration (FDA) has not approved the use of aromatase inhibitors for induction of ovulation in cases of PCOS, this off-label use is legal in some countries such as the US and UK. Its use as an ovulation inducing agent has been banned in India since 2011.

## Route of Administration

Oral.

## Dosage

It is prescribed in the daily dosage of 2.5 mg.

## Contraindications

- Premenopausal women
- Pregnancy/lactation.

## Side Effects

This drug can be associated with side effects such as hot flushes, nausea, diarrhea, dyspepsia, thinning of hair, etc. Joint pain is common and bone loss may be accelerated. However, this drug is not associated with an increased risk of endometrial hyperplasia, endometrial carcinoma, venous thromboembolism or deterioration of the lipid profile.

# Magnesium Sulfate

## Introduction

During pregnancy, magnesium sulfate is usually used in the patients with severe preeclampsia/eclampsia, once the decision for delivery has been made. The Magpie study (2002) has demonstrated that administration of magnesium sulfate to women with preeclampsia reduces the risk of an eclamptic seizure. It is also used in cases of preterm labor where it acts by providing fetal neuroprotection.

## Mechanism of Action

Magnesium sulfate is associated with cerebral vasodilatation and is a blocker of N-methyl-D-aspartate (NMDA) receptors in the brain, the pathway for anoxic cell damage. It acts as a tocolytic by competing with $Ca^{2+}$ ions for entry into myometrium through both voltage sensitive as well as ligand gated $Ca^{2+}$ channels.

## Indications

- *Prevention and treatment of seizures in preeclampsia and eclampsia:* In these cases, magnesium sulfate must be administered while awaiting delivery and in the immediate postpartum period for up to 24 hours following delivery or 24 hours after the last seizure, whichever is later. Magnesium sulfate is now also considered as an anticonvulsant of choice for treating eclampsia.
- *Prevention of preterm labor:* Administration of magnesium sulfate is likely to provide fetal neuroprotection in cases of anticipated early preterm delivery (less than 32 weeks of gestation). It is also likely to provide short-term prolongation of pregnancy (up to 48 hours), thereby allowing time for the administration of antenatal corticosteroids in pregnant women between 24 and 34 weeks of gestation, who are at risk of preterm delivery within 7 days. The US FDA (2013) has advised against use of magnesium sulfate injection for more than 5–7 days to stop preterm labor in pregnant women due to the concerns for fetal and neonatal bone demineralization and fractures associated with long-term in utero exposure to magnesium sulfate.

## Route of Administration

Intramuscular/intravenous.

## Dosage

*Preeclampsia and eclampsia:* A total dose of 14 g is administered in the form of loading and maintenance dose. The following regimens can be given: Zuspan, Sibai and Pritchard regimen (refer to Chapter 5 for details).

*Preterm labor:* In cases of preterm labor, magnesium sulfate is administered in as 4–6 g bolus dose (IV) for 20 minutes, then 2–3 g/hour.

## Contraindications

It is contraindicated in the following conditions:
- Maternal renal disease
- Reduced patellar reflexes in the mother.

## Side Effects

*Maternal:* Administration of magnesium sulfate may result in maternal side effects such as flushing, lethargy, muscle weakness, diplopia, etc. The therapeutic levels of magnesium range between 4 mEq/L and 7 mEq/L. In doses exceeding the therapeutic range, magnesium sulfate can result in certain toxic effects such as loss of patellar reflexes, followed by oliguria and ultimately resulting in cardiovascular and respiratory depression. Therefore, further dose of magnesium sulfate is adjusted based on the patient's reflexes, urinary output, respiratory rate, patient's clinical condition and serum magnesium levels. The aim should be to maintain magnesium concentration at 4 mEq/L. Toxicity to magnesium sulfate is a life-threatening emergency and the following steps must be taken immediately:
- Intubation and bag and mask ventilation must be done.
- External cardiac massage may also be required.
- 10 mL of 10% calcium gluconate must be slowly administered intravenously. This serves as an antidote for magnesium sulfate poisoning.

*Newborns:* Administration of magnesium sulfate may result in symptoms such as lethargy, hypotonia, demineralization, etc. in the newborn. There may be signs of magnesium toxicity (i.e. respiratory and/or neuromuscular depression) in the newborn, if the mother has received intravenous magnesium sulfate prior to delivery (especially if for a period of longer than 24 hours). Equipment for assisted ventilation as well as intravenous calcium should be immediately available for the first 24–48 hours after delivery.

# Metformin

## Introduction

Metformin belongs to the biguanide group of oral hypoglycemic agents.

## Mechanism of Action

Biguanides do not cause insulin release, but presence of insulin is vital for their action. Metformin lowers blood glucose by exerting the actions some of which are described next:
1. Suppression of hepatic gluconeogenesis and reduction of glucose output from liver. This is the major

action responsible for lowering of blood glucose in diabetics.

2. Enhances insulin-mediated glucose uptake and disposal in skeletal muscle and fat.
3. Overcoming insulin resistance exhibited by type 2 diabetics. This is manifested by following actions:
   - Increasing glycogen storage in skeletal muscles
   - Reduced lipogenesis in adipose tissue and enhanced fatty acid oxidation.
4. Interference with mitochondrial respiratory chain and promotion of peripheral glucose utilization through anaerobic glycolysis.

Metformin improves insulin sensitivity and decreases hepatic gluconeogenesis and, therefore, reduces hyperinsulinism, basal and stimulated LH levels, and free testosterone concentration. Consequently, the patient with PCOS becomes responsive to CC induced ovulation induction. Metformin is used as an insulin sensitizer. It helps in treating the root cause of PCOS and improves fertility by rectifying endocrine and metabolic functions. This results in spontaneous ovulation. It also helps in lowering the requirement of ovulation inducing drugs, thereby, resulting in better rates of implantation.

## Indications

- *Type 2 diabetes mellitus:* Metformin is now established as a first choice drug for all patients with type 2 diabetes mellitus, except when not tolerated or contraindicated.
- *Polycystic ovarian disease:* Metformin has been found to improve ovulation and fertility in some infertile women with polycystic ovary. Patients with PCOS, having a BMI more than 25 are often resistant to treatment with CC alone. These patients commonly have other problems, such as hyperinsulinism and hyperandrogenism, associated with acanthosis nigricans. This group is amenable to metformin treatment in combination with CC.

## Route of Administration

Oral.

## Dosage

In cases of PCOS, the initial dose of metformin is 500 mg PO once a day for 7 days, then 500 mg BID for another 7 days, and finally 500 mg TID for 3 months. Since patients can ovulate while on metformin treatment, pelvic ultrasonography is required for documentation of ovulation. In case ovulation does not occur with the use of metformin as a sole therapy, CC is started at the initial dose of 50 mg/day for 5 days.

## Contraindications

- Hypotension
- Heart failure

- Severe respiratory, hepatic and renal disease
- Alcoholics (due to an increased risk of lactic acidosis).

## Side Effects

Though side effects can commonly occur with metformin, they are not usually serious. Frequently occurring adverse effects of metformin include gastrointestinal intolerance, nausea, vomiting, abdominal cramps, anorexia, bloating, metallic taste, mild diarrhea and tiredness. Weight loss has also been observed. These side effects usually tend to subside with time. Metformin does not cause hypoglycemia except in overdose.

Lactic acidosis is a rare complication which can be further precipitated by alcohol ingestion. With high dose of metformin, vitamin B12 deficiency can also occur due to interference with its absorption.

# Methergine

## Introduction

Ergotamine is an alkaloid isolated from a fungus *Claviceps purpurea,* which commonly occurs in cereals like rye, wheat, etc. Methergine is methylergometrine maleate, a semisynthetic derivative of ergometrine/methergine is available in the form of 1 mL ampoules.

## Mechanism of Action

Both methylergonovine (methergine) and ergometrine cause generalized smooth muscle contraction. As a result, the upper and lower segments of the uterus contract tetanically and pass into a state of spasm without any relaxation in between.

## Indications

- Prophylaxis and treatment of severe atonic PPH
- Active management of third stage of labor
- Following LSCS/hysterectomy, to facilitate uterine contractions.

## Route of Administration

It can be administered through intramuscular/intravenous or oral routes. Ergometrine (ergonovine) is available in ampoules of 0.25 mg and 0.5 mg and tablets of 0.5 mg and 1 mg. Methergine is available in ampoules of 0.2 mg and tablets of 0.5 mg and 1 mg.

## Dosage

Methergine is administered in the dose of 0.2 mg intramuscularly or intravenously stat for controlling atonic PPH as well as following the delivery of anterior shoulder in cases of normal vaginal delivery (active management of third stage of labor). A typical dose of methylergonovine, 0.2 mg administered intramuscularly, may be repeated as required at intervals of 2–4 hours. The dose of ergometrine is 0.25 mg IM which can be repeated every 5 minutes up to a maximum dose of 1.25 mg. The onset of action on the uterus after oral administration is 15 minutes, after IM injection 5 minutes and after intravenous injection onset is almost immediate. It can be administered directly in the uterine muscle, if necessary. The total dose of ergometrine in 24 hours must not exceed 1,000 µg. Ergot alkaloids are sometimes used orally in a dose of 0.125 mg TDS for a maximum of 7 days to help in uterine involution in cases of secondary PPH.

## Contraindications

Ergometrine should be used with caution in the following cases:

- *Suspected multifetal pregnancy:* Administration of ergometrine with the delivery of the first baby can result in the entrapment of second baby due to tetanic contractions of the uterus.
- *Organic cardiac disease in the mother:* It may cause sudden sequestration of the uterine blood into the general circulation causing overloading of the right heart resulting in pulmonary edema.
- *Severe preeclampsia and eclampsia:* Injection of ergometrine in these cases can result in a sudden rise in blood pressure.
- *Rh-negative mothers:* Injection of ergometrine can result in fetomaternal hemorrhage.

## Side Effects

Since the stimulant action of ergometrine also involves the lower segment of the uterus along with the upper segment, this can occasionally result in the entrapment of the separated placenta. Its use can result in adverse effects such as vomiting, elevation of blood pressure and pain after birth requiring analgesia. It can inhibit lactation if higher doses are used for many days postpartum, as it inhibits prolactin release (dopaminergic action). Its prolonged use may lead to gangrene of the toes due to its vasoconstrictive effect. Rarely, it may cause chest pain due to acute coronary spasm.

# Methotrexate

## Introduction

Methotrexate is a folic acid analog, which is one of the oldest and highly efficacious antineoplastic drugs. Besides being used in the treatment of various neoplastic lesions, it is also used for treatment of several other nonmalignant conditions in the field of obstetrics and gynecology.

## Mechanism of Action

Once folic acid has entered the body cell, it is sequentially transformed to dihydrofolate and tetrahydrofolate with the help of the enzyme dihydrofolate reductase. Methotrexate acts by inhibiting this enzyme, dihydrofolate reductase, thereby blocking the conversion of dihydrofolic acid to tetrahydrofolic acid. This eventually results in the depletion of the nucleotide pool because tetrahydrofolic acid is an essential coenzyme required for one carbon transfer reactions in de novo purine and pyrimidine synthesis and amino acid interconversions. Folic acid is also required for the de novo synthesis of the nucleoside thymidine. Therefore, methotrexate inhibits the synthesis of DNA, RNA, thymidylates and proteins.

## Indications

### Uses in Obstetrics

It can be used for the following indications in cases of obstetrics:

- Treatment of nonmetastatic persistent trophoblastic disease
- Choriocarcinoma
- Medical treatment of unruptured ectopic pregnancy
- Medical abortion
- Conservative treatment of placenta accreta/retained placenta
- Nongynecological malignancies: Methotrexate is widely used for the treatment of various nongynecological malignancies such as non-Hodgkin lymphoma, breast, bladder, head and neck cancers, osteogenic sarcomas, maintaining remission in cases of leukemia, etc.
- Nongynecological/nonmalignant disorders: Methotrexate acts as a prominent immunosuppressing agent in cases of rheumatoid arthritis, psoriasis and many other autoimmune disorders.

## Route of Administration

Methotrexate can be administered systemically [intravenously (IV), intramuscularly (IM), or orally]. It can also be administered in the form of a direct local injection into the ectopic pregnancy sac.

## Dosage

### Hydatidiform Mole

*Nonmetastatic persistent trophoblastic disease*: Nonmetastatic disease can be treated with a single chemotherapeutic drug, most commonly, methotrexate. Methotrexate can be used alone or in combination with folinic acid (to overcome the adverse effects of methotrexate). Some commonly used regimens of methotrexate alone include:

- Methotrexate in the dosage of 0.4 mg/kg (maximum 25 mg) intravenously or intramuscularly daily for 5 days per treatment course.
- Weekly doses of 30–50 mg/m$^2$ of IM methotrexate has been found to be the most cost-effective, taking into consideration factors such as efficacy, toxicity and cost.
- 50 mg intramuscularly to be repeated every 48 hours for a total of four doses.

The regimen of methotrexate in combination with folic acid is as follows:

- Methotrexate in the dose of 1 mg/kg intramuscularly is given on days 1, 3, 5 and 7 along with calcium leucovorin rescue in dose of 0.1 mg/kg on days 2, 4, 6 and 8, 30 hours following injection of methotrexate.
- Courses are repeated every 14 days dependent on toxicity, i.e. first course on day 1; second course on day 15; third course on day 29 and so on. An adequate response to chemotherapy is defined as fall in the β-hCG levels by 1 log after a course of chemotherapy. If the response to 1 mg/kg dose is inadequate, the dose is increased to 1.5 mg/kg for each of the four treatment days. If even then, the response after two consecutive courses of methotrexate-folic acid is inadequate, the patient is considered resistant to methotrexate.

### Choriocarcinoma

*Low-risk metastatic gestational disease:* Low-risk metastatic disease is treated with single or multiple drug chemotherapy. Methotrexate is administered intramuscularly, alternating daily with folinic acid for 1 week followed by 6 days of rest.

*Moderate-risk metastatic gestational disease:* Moderate-risk patients (WHO score of 5–7) have been treated with multiagent chemotherapy. The most commonly used combination chemotherapy include: MAC based combination (methotrexate, dactinomycin, cyclophosphamide or chlorambucil) or EMA (etoposide, methotrexate and dactinomycin).

*High-risk metastatic gestational disease:* Women with high-risk GTN usually require combination chemotherapy (EMA CO).

### Medical Abortion

The FDA has approved the use of methotrexate for medical termination of pregnancy up to 49 days following the last menstrual period. The regimen comprising the use of methotrexate and misoprostol is discussed below.

Administration of methotrexate in the dose of 50 mg/m$^2$ IM on day 1, followed by the vaginal administration of misoprostol 800 µg vaginally, 3–7 days later. The dose of misoprostol can be repeated every 48 hours up to 3 doses until the pregnancy

is terminated. Efficacy of methotrexate in inducing medical termination of pregnancy reduces with an increase in the gestational age.

### Ectopic Pregnancy

On the day of treatment, methotrexate is injected in the dosage of 50 mg/m$^2$ of BSA (body surface area) via intramuscular route.

$$BSA = \sqrt{\frac{(\text{Height in cm} \times \text{Weight in kg})}{3,600}}$$

- The effect of methotrexate dosage can be estimated by measurement of the β-hCG levels (day 4), which serve as the baseline level against which subsequent levels are measured. Subsequently, the serum β-hCG levels are measured on day 7.
- If the β-hCG level has dropped by 15% or more since day 4, weekly hCG levels must be obtained until they have reached the negative level.
- If the weekly levels plateau or increase, a second course of methotrexate may be administered.
- Second dose of methotrexate may also be required if decline in β-hCG levels is less than 25% on day 7.
- If no drop has occurred by day 14, surgical therapy is indicated.

## Contraindications

- Pregnancy: Methotrexate should not be used in pregnant women with psoriasis or rheumatoid arthritis. For treatment of neoplasms in women, methotrexate must only be used if the potential benefits outweigh the risk to the fetus
- Lactation
- Alcoholism/history of liver diseases (chronic liver diseases, alcoholic liver diseases, etc.)
- Blood dyscrasias/hematological dysfunction (bone marrow hypoplasia, leukopenia, thrombocytopenia or significant anemia)
- Known hypersensitivity to methotrexate
- Active pulmonary disease
- Immunodeficiency disorders.

## Side Effects

Methotrexate can result in side effects such as nausea, vomiting, ulceration, alopecia, abdominal pain, temporary hair loss, swelling of feet and lower legs, back pain, cough or hoarseness, headache, shortness of breath, bone marrow depression, renal tubular necrosis and hepatotoxicity. It may cause birth defects in unborn babies if administered to pregnant women.

# Mifepristone

## Introduction

It is a synthetic, 19-norsteroid compound having potent antiprogestational and significant antiglucocorticoid, and antiandrogenic activities.

## Mechanism of Action

It acts as a progesterone receptor antagonist due to which it serves as an abortifacient in the early pregnancy. When administered during the follicular phase, its antiprogestin action results in decrease of the mid-cycle gonadotropin surge from pituitary gland. This causes slowing of follicular development and delay/failure of ovulation. If administered during the luteal phase, it prevents secretory changes by blocking the action of progesterone on the endometrium. Later in the cycle, it blocks progesterone support to the endometrium, liberating the release of prostaglandins (PGs) from it, thereby stimulating uterine contractions. Mifepristone also sensitizes the myometrium to PGs and induces menstruation. If implantation has occurred, mifepristone blocks decidualization, thereby causing dislodgement of the conceptus. If hCG production falls, secondary luteolysis occurs resulting in the reduction of endogenous progesterone secretion and cervical softening. All these effects eventually result in miscarriage.

Mifepristone also serves as a powerful antagonist agent at the glucocorticoid receptors.

## Indications

- *Termination of pregnancy*: For termination of pregnancy up to 7 weeks of gestation, 600 mg of mifepristone can be administered in the form of a single oral dose. This single dose regime is successful in nearly 60–85% cases. To improve the success rate, mifepristone can be followed up to 48 hours later by a single oral dose of 400 mg misoprostol. This combination regimen is associated with a success rate of greater than 90% and is the accepted nonsurgical method of early first trimester abortion.
- *Cervical ripening*: Mifepristone, in the dosage of 600 mg, administered 24–30 hours before attempting surgical abortion or induction of labor, helps in cervical softening and the facilitation of the procedure of surgical abortion.
- *Postcoital/emergency contraception:* Mifepristone in the dosage of 600 mg administered within 72 hours of intercourse interferes with implantation and is a highly effective method of emergency contraception.
- *Once-a-month contraceptive agent*: A single dose of 200 mg mifepristone administered 2 days after mid-cycle each month prevents conception on most occasions.
- *Induction of labor*: Mifepristone helps in blocking the relaxant action of progesterone on uterus, late in pregnancy, thereby promoting labor. It may also be administered in cases with intrauterine fetal death and to deliver abnormal fetuses.
- *Cushing's syndrome:* Mifepristone has palliative effect due to glucocorticoid receptor blocking property and may be used for inoperable cases of Cushing's syndrome.
- *Other uses:* Other proposed uses of mifepristone include endometriosis, uterine fibroids, certain breast cancers and meningioma.

## Route of Administration

It is most commonly administered via the oral route.

## Dosage

Dosage of mifepristone used for the termination of pregnancy has been described in the "indications".

## Contraindications

- Presence of IUCD
- Ectopic pregnancy
- Adrenal failure
- Hemorrhagic disorders
- Inherited porphyrias
- Intake of anticoagulants
- Long-term corticosteroid therapy.

## Side Effects

Side effects such as nausea, vomiting, diarrhea, weakness, dizziness, bleeding or cramping may commonly occur. Rarely, there may be symptoms of a serious allergic reaction, including rashes/itching/swelling (especially of the face/tongue/throat), severe dizziness, dyspnea, etc.

# Misoprostol

## Introduction

Misoprostol is a synthetic prostaglandin E1 analog (PGE1) that increases uterine tone and reduces postpartum bleeding. Though recently use of misoprostol for several obstetric indications has considerably increased, misoprostol has been approved by the US FDA for its use only in the prevention of NSAID induced gastric ulcers. Moreover, its use was contraindicated in pregnant women. However, since the past decade there has been an increase in off-label use of misoprostol for induction of labor. The manufacturer of misoprostol (Cytotec) Searle issued a warning letter in the year 2000 against the use of misoprostol in pregnant women. The drug was cited as being an abortifacient and associated with the risk of complications such as uterine rupture, maternal and fetal deaths. This had generated much controversy regarding the use of misoprostol for induction of labor.

## Mechanism of Action

It acts by stimulating uterine contractions and causing the cervix to ripen.

## Indications

Recently, misoprostol is being used for several obstetric indications, which are described next:

- *Induction of medical abortion:* Misoprostol for induction of medical abortion serves as a better alternative to surgical termination of pregnancy because it is cheaper, simpler, less invasive, does not require administration of anesthesia and is also free from complications associated with surgical methods (perforation, etc.). The ACOG now acclaims that there is substantial evidence regarding the use of misoprostol for induction of labor. However, labor induced with misoprostol must be closely monitored. The US FDA has still not given its approval for the use of this drug to induce labor.
- *Cervical priming before surgical abortion:* Use of misoprostol for cervical priming prior to suction evacuation is likely to facilitate this procedure.
- *Treatment of PPH:* Although misoprostol is widely used in the treatment of PPH, it is presently not approved by the US FDA for this indication. Misoprostol, however, is safe, inexpensive, stable at room temperature, has a long shelf life and is easily storable. Therefore, it has a high potential of usefulness in developing countries. Its administration also reduces the incidence of PPH in the home birth setting. There is evidence that misoprostol does not provide any additional benefits when used in combination with another uterotonic drug like oxytocin. Moreover, oxytocin is still the drug of choice for prevention of PPH as it is less expensive than misoprostol and is associated with fewer side effects.
- *Induction of labor:* Misoprostol is nowadays commonly being used for induction of labor at term and in cases of IUD. Though the US FDA has still not given its approval for the use of this drug to induce labor, the ACOG now acclaims that there is substantial evidence regarding the use of misoprostol for induction of labor. However, labor induced with misoprostol must be closely monitored.

## Route of Administration

Misoprostol can also be rapidly absorbed by the sublingual, vaginal and rectal routes.

## Dosage

- *Medical termination of pregnancy:* Misoprostol can be administered either as a single agent or as an adjuvant for medical induction of first trimester abortion.
  - Misoprostol as a single agent: Misoprostol in the dosage of 200–800 µg vaginally can be used alone for first trimester of pregnancy (up to the gestational age of 8–10 weeks).
  - Misoprostol in combination with mifepristone: Medical termination of pregnancy of up to 7 weeks has been achieved with high success rate by administering mifepristone (antiprogestin) 600 mg orally 2 days before a single oral dose of misoprostol 400 µg. It is now a valuable alternative to suction-evacuation. Uterine contractions are provoked and the conceptus is expelled within the next few hours. Intravaginal misoprostol is now favored by many as it produces fewer side effects. Sublingual route is also advocated by some experts.
  - Misoprostol in combination with methotrexate: Methotrexate administered along with misoprostol is also highly successful for inducing abortion in the first few weeks of pregnancy (8–9 weeks of gestation). Methotrexate is administered via intramuscular route in the dose of 50 mg/m$^2$ followed by vaginal misoprostol in the dosage varying between 500 µg and 800 µg.
- *Medical induction of second trimester abortion:* Misoprostol is administered vaginally in the dosage of 400 µg every 4 hourly until 20 weeks of gestation. Between 20 and 24 weeks of gestation, misoprostol is administered in the dosage of 200 µg vaginally every 6–12 hours.
- *Incomplete abortion/missed abortion:* Misoprostol has a role in cases of incomplete abortion, missed abortion and molar gestation. However, delayed and erratic action and incomplete abortion are complications associated with the use of misoprostol. Misoprostol is administered in the dosage of 400 µg vaginally (or orally) every 4 hourly for 3 doses.
- *Cervical priming before surgical abortion:* Misoprostol is administered in the dosage of 400–600 µg vaginally approximately 3–4 hours prior to first trimester pregnancy termination by suction evacuation.
- *Induction of labor in cases of intrauterine death:* Misoprostol can be used as an inducing agent in cases of second or third trimester intrauterine death. In cases of fetal death between 13 and 24 weeks, 200 µg of misoprostol is administered vaginally after every 3–4 hours. In cases of fetal death after 24 weeks of gestation, misoprostol is administered in the dosage of 100 µg every 6–12 hours or 50 µg every 4 hourly.

- *Induction of labor at term*: Misoprostol is a relatively new agent for prelabor cervical ripening and induction of labor. Misoprostol is administered in the dose of 25–50 µg through the vaginal route (instillation in the posterior fornix) every 3–4 hours. Misoprostol can also be administered via oral route in the dose of 200 µg, which has been found to be as effective as the vaginal route. However, the oral route is associated with a higher incidence of complications such as tachysystole and hyperstimulation.
- *Postpartum hemorrhage*: For controlling PPH, misoprostol can be administered sublingually, orally, vaginally and rectally. Doses range from 600 µg to 1,000 µg. The dose recommended by FIGO (2012) for prevention of PPH is a single dose of 600 µg misoprostol administered orally immediately after delivery of the newborn. For treatment of PPH, FIGO (2012) recommends a single dose of 800 µg misoprostol, to be administered sublingually immediately after PPH is diagnosed. This dose must be administered irrespective of the prophylactic measures which had been previously taken.
- *Prophylactic management of third stage of labor*: Prophylactic administration of misoprostol for active management of third stage of labor is 600 µg sublingually or vaginally. The vaginal route is more potent and side effects are also fewer in comparison to the sublingual route. However, the vaginal route could be inappropriate in patients with heavy bleeding. In such cases, 600 µg can be administered sublingually or 800–1,000 µg can be given rectally.

### Contraindications

- Presence of a uterine scar
- Hypersensitivity to the drug
- Pregnant women (for reducing the risk of NSAID induced gastric ulcers): Misoprostol is likely to increase the uterine tone and contractions in pregnancy, resulting in partial or complete abortions. Also, its use in early pregnancy is likely to be associated with birth defects.

### Side Effects

Misoprostol is effective in the treatment of various above described obstetric indications, but side effects such as diarrhea, fever, shivering, etc. may limit its use. Uterine cramps, vaginal bleeding, nausea, vomiting, headache, dyspepsia, flatulence, constipation and diarrhea are the common side effects. Misoprostol can commonly cause side effects such as maternal pyrexia and shivering. In rare cases, misoprostol can cause uterine tachyphylaxis, which can lead to uterine tetanus and the risk of uterine rupture.

# Oxytocin

### Introduction

Oxytocin is a nonapeptide, released by the posterior pituitary in the body. It is synthesized within the nerve cell bodies in supraoptic and paraventricular nuclei of hypothalamus. It is transported down the axon and stored in the nerve endings within the neurohypophysis. Stimuli such as coital activity, parturition, suckling, etc. help in the release of oxytocin molecule. The synthetic form of oxytocin (syntocinon or pitocin) used as a drug is a decapeptide.

### Mechanism of Action

*Uterus:* Oxytocin, which has uterotonic action, helps in increasing the force and frequency of uterine contractions. In the full-term gravid uterus, oxytocin causes physiological uterine contractions, i.e. the contraction of upper uterine segment and retraction of the lower segment. With low doses, full relaxation occurs in between the uterine contractions. Basal tone increases only with high doses of oxytocin. Nonpregnant uterus and that during early pregnancy is rather resistant to oxytocin; sensitivity increases progressively in the third trimester, with a sharp increase occurring near term. The sensitivity quickly falls during the puerperium.

Action of oxytocin on myometrium is related to the specific G-protein coupled oxytocin receptors, which mediate the response mainly by depolarization of muscle fibers and influx of $Ca^{2+}$ ions, through phosphoinositide hydrolysis as well as IP3-mediated intracellular release of $Ca^{2+}$ ions.

*Breasts*: In the breast tissues, oxytocin contracts the myoepithelial cells of mammary alveoli, thereby forcing the milk into the bigger milk sinusoids, resulting in the "milk ejection reflex". This reflex is initiated by suckling so that the ejected milk may be easily sucked by the infant.

### Mode of Administration

Being a peptide molecule, oxytocin is inactive orally and is most commonly administered by IV route, rarely by intranasal/intrabuccal spray. Oxytocin can also be administered by intramuscular/subcutaneous routes. However, these routes are not commonly used because the response through these routes may be erratic and the dose cannot be titrated to the response. Oxytocin is available in the form of ampoules of Pitocin (5 units/0.5 mL) and syntocinon (5 units/mL), where 1 IU of oxytocin is equal to 2 µg of pure hormone. In order to preserve their potency, synthetic oxytocin ampoules must be stored in a refrigerator.

(1 IU of oxytocin = 2 µg of pure hormone). The oxytocin ampoules need to be stored in a refrigerator at 2–6°C.

## Indications

### Postpartum Hemorrhage

Oxytocin (syntocinon) is an effective first-line treatment for PPH. Oxytocin 10–20 IU/500 mL of Ringer's lactate or normal saline may be administered by IV infusion for an immediate response, especially in hypertensive women in whom ergometrine is contraindicated. It is infused at a rate of 125 mL/hour (60 drops/minute) over 4 hours. As much as 500 mL can be infused over 10 minutes without complications. For a sustained effect, continuous infusion of oxytocin is usually preferred. In cases of circulatory collapse, 10 units may be administered intramyometrially. Oxytocin acts by forcefully contracting the uterine muscle, which compresses the blood vessels passing through its mesh work to arrest hemorrhage from the inner surface exposed by placental separation.

### Active Management of the Third Stage of Labor

It is used for the active management of third stage of labor. Oxytocin is recommended as the first-line drug in active management of third stage of labor due to its short half-life and good intensity of action. Also, its action can be quickly terminated and it does not cause contraction of the lower segment.

### Induction of Labor

It may be required to induce the labor in cases of postmaturity, preeclampsia, gestational diabetes, erythroblastosis, ruptured membranes or placental insufficiency.

*Oxytocin titration technique:* For this purpose, oxytocin is administered via slow IV infusion wherein 5 IU of oxytocin is diluted in 500 mL of glucose or normal saline solution (10 mIU/mL). Infusion is started at a low rate (1–2 mIU/minute) and progressively accelerated at an interval of 20–30 minutes according to response (1–2 mIU/minute). When the optimal response is achieved, i.e. there are about three uterine contractions in 10 minutes, with each uterine contraction being sustained for about 45 seconds; the particular oxytocin concentration which was being used is continued. The oxytocin infusion is described in terms of milliunits/minute. The oxytocin infusion rate can either be manually regulated by counting the number of drops per minute or the other option is to use an oxytocin infusion pump, which automatically controls the infusion rate. Before starting oxytocin infusion, the following prerequisites (Table 15.1) need to be confirmed:

*Continuous monitoring:* While inducing the patient with oxytocin infusion, uterine contractions, fetal heart rate and any other complications must be closely monitored after every 5–10 minutes. The drug is discontinued when the uterine contractions become strong enough. The oxytocin dose can be increased in the range of 1–32 mIU/minute. Majority of patients respond to the dose of 16 mIU/minute or less. This dose rate can be attained by adding 2 IU of oxytocin to 500 mL of Ringer's lactate solution, with a drop rate of 60 drops/minute (where 15 drops =1 mL). There is no upper limit to the permitted dose. If the uterus still remains inert at the oxytocin dosage of 100 mIU/minute, it may be wise to consider using prostaglandins for stimulation of the uterus. The accuracy and control of infusion can be greatly improved by using an oxytocin infusion pump. Table 15.2 shows the correlation between oxytocin dosage and drop rate per minute, while Table 15.3 shows ACOG guidelines for the administration of oxytocin.

### Uterine Inertia

In cases where the uterine contractions are not strong enough and labor is not progressing satisfactorily, uterine contractions can be augmented by intravenous administration of oxytocin. Oxytocin, however, must not be used for

**Table 15.1:** Prerequisites to be fulfilled before starting oxytocin infusion

- Fetus is in cephalic presentation
- Fetal lungs are adequately mature
- There is no cephalopelvic disproportion
- There is no placenta previa
- There is no fetal distress
- No uterine scar due to previous surgery

**Table 15.2:** Calculation of oxytocin dosage (delivered in mIU/ minute) and its correlation with drop rate per minute

| Units of oxytocin mixed in 500 mL of Ringer's lactate solution (1 unit = 1,000 milliunits) | Drops/minute (15 drops = 1 mL) | | |
|---|---|---|---|
| | 15 | 30 | 60 |
| 1 | 2 | 4 | 8 |
| 2 | 4 | 8 | 16 |
| 8 | 16 | 32 | 64 |

**Table 15.3:** ACOG guidelines (2011) for administration of oxytocin

| Regime | Starting dose (mIU/ minute) | Increase by (mIU/ minute) | Dosage interval (minutes) | Maximum dose (mIU/ minute) |
|---|---|---|---|---|
| Low dose | 0.5–2 | 1–2 | 15–40 | 20 |
| High dose | 6 | 1–6* | 15–40 | 42 |

*The incremental dose is decreased to 3 mIU in presence of recurrent hyperstimulation

accelerating the labor, which is progressing normally on its own. Before starting oxytocin infusion for strengthening the uterine contractions, all the prerequisites as described in Table 15.1 must be fulfilled. Oxytocin is the drug of choice for inducing and augmenting labor and is usually preferred over ergometrine/PGs for the following reasons:

- Intensity of oxytocin action can be controlled and be quickly terminated due to its short half-life and slow IV infusion.
- When used in low concentrations, oxytocin allows normal relaxation in between uterine contractions. Therefore, the fetal oxygenation is not compromised.
- Since the lower uterine segment is not contracted, fetal descent is not affected.
- Uterine contractions are consistently augmented.

### Breast Engorgement

Oxytocin is effective in cases where the breast engorgement occurs in the woman due to inefficient milk ejection reflex. Oxytocin is administered by an intranasal spray few minutes before suckling. It does not increase milk production, rather just causes milk ejection.

### Oxytocin Challenge Test

This test is performed to determine uteroplacental adequacy in cases of high-risk pregnancies. Oxytocin is administered via IV infusion at very low concentrations till uterine contractions are elicited every 3–4 minutes. Marked abnormalities in fetal heart rate, particularly late decelerations, indicate uteroplacental compromise. This test is rarely performed nowadays.

## Adverse Effects

- *Strong uterine contractions*: Injudicious use of oxytocin during labor can result in strong uterine contractions. This may force the fetal presenting part through incompletely dilated birth canal, resulting in harmful effects such as maternal and fetal soft tissue injury, rupture of uterus, fetal asphyxia and death.
- *Tachysystole/uterine hyperstimulation*: Injudicious use of oxytocin can result in continuous uterine contractions or strong uterine contractions. Tachysystole can be associated with a persistent pattern of more than five uterine contractions in 10 minutes, with each contraction lasting for 2 minutes (or more) or contractions of normal duration occurring within 1 minute of each other, there being no resting tone between contractions.
- *Maternal cardiovascular side effects*: Administration of oxytocin can cause certain side effects related to the cardiovascular system in the mother. These can include side effects such as increase in the heart rate, systemic venous return and cardiac output, cardiac arrhythmias, premature ventricular contractions, etc.
- *Water intoxication*: This occurs due to its antidiuretic hormone like action when administered in high doses (30–40 mIU/minute) along with IV fluids, especially in conditions such as preeclampsia and renal insufficiency. Water intoxication may manifest in the form of symptoms of hyponatremia such as confusion, coma, convulsions, congestive cardiac failure and death.
- *Hypotension*: Bolus intravenous injection should be avoided in patients with PPH where patient is hypovolemic or in patients with heart disease because of the risk of development of hypotension. Occasionally, oxytocin may also produce anginal pain.
- *Fetal side effects*: It can result in fetal side effects such as bradycardia, neonatal jaundice, low APGAR score, etc.

## Contraindications

### Absolute Contraindications

The administration of oxytocin is contraindicated in the following situations:

- Grand multipara (risk of uterine rupture)
- Vaginal delivery is contraindicated (e.g. obstructed labor)
- Evidence of intrapartum fetal distress
- Pregnant women with underlying cardiac disease (to avoid the occurrence of fluid overload)
- Previous history of anaphylactic shock.

### Relative Contraindications

- Previous uterine scar
- Vertex not fixed in the pelvis
- Unfavorable cervix
- Breech presentation
- Hydramnios
- Multiple pregnancy.

# Pethidine

## Introduction

Pethidine is a medicine which helps in providing relief against moderate-to-severe degree pain. It is a synthetic opioid analgesic drug (morphine-like), belonging to the phenylpiperidine class and acts by mimicking the effects of the body's endogenous endorphins. Though once commonly used at the time of labor and delivery, nowadays, its use is rarely employed in obstetric practice due to the availability of better treatment options.

## Mechanism of Action

Though chemically unrelated to morphine, it interacts with μ opioid receptors and its actions are blocked by naloxone. Dose to dose, it is one-tenth in analgesic potency in comparison to morphine. However, analgesic efficacy approaches near to morphine and is greater than codeine. It is equally sedative and euphoriant and has similar abuse potential in comparison to morphine.

## Indications

### Obstetric Indications

- An analgesic agent in preanesthetic medication.
- *Labor analgesia:* Pethidine must only be administered in cases of established labor. It is usually given when the cervix is fully dilated and delivery appears eminent in about half-an-hour's time. It should not be administered if the delivery is likely to occur in the next 4–5 hours because the metabolic products of pethidine may cause neonatal depression.
- *Eclampsia:* Pethidine can be administered in the dosage of 50–100 mg IM every 6 hours or it can be used in alteration with drugs like diazepam. Though rarely used nowadays, pethidine in combination with chlorpromazine and promethazine can be used as a part of Krishna Menon's lytic Cocktail regimen, which was previously used in cases of preeclampsia.
- Postoperative analgesia.
- Left ventricular failure and pulmonary edema.

### Nonobstetric/Gynecological Indications

- It may be used for the treatment of nongynecological/obstetric cause of pain such as biliary spasm, renal colic, pain due to diverticulosis, etc.

## Route of Administration

- *Oral route:* Tablets (available in the form of hydrochloride salts) or in the form of syrup.
- *Parenteral route:* Intramuscular/intravenous/subcutaneous routes.

## Dosage

- *Severe pain:* 25–100 mg, 4 hourly (IM/IV/SC)
- *Moderate pain:* 50–150 mg, 4 hourly (oral route)
- *Obstetric analgesia:* 50–100 mg (IM/SC) for a maximum dosage of 400 mg/24 hours
- *Preoperative medication:* 25–100 mg, 1 hour prior to the surgery (IM/SC route)
- *Postoperative pain relief:* 25–100 mg, every 2 to 3 hourly after surgery till required (SC/ IM).

## Contraindications

Pethidine is contraindicated in the following conditions:
- Asthma
- Epilepsy
- Pheochromocytoma
- Respiratory depression
- Status epilepticus
- Tetanus
- Liver diseases
- Hypersensitivity
- Raised intracranial pressure
- Renal diseases
- Supraventricular tachycardia
- Alcohol consumption
- Avoid use with drugs/foodstuffs where there is a possibility of serotonin syndrome.

## Side Effects

### Maternal Side Effects

*Common side effects:* These include side effects such as sedation, mental clouding, lethargy, vomiting (occasionally in recumbent patient), constipation, respiratory depression, blurring of vision, urinary retention, hypotension, etc. Some atropinic effects such as dry mouth, blurred vision, tachycardia, etc. can also occur.

*Idiosyncrasy and allergy:* Allergic reactions manifesting as urticaria, swelling of lips may occur infrequently. Anaphylactoid reaction is rare.

*Interaction with other drugs:* Serotonin syndrome may occur in patients receiving concomitant therapy with selective serotonin reuptake inhibitors or monoamine oxidase inhibitors (e.g., furazolidone, isocarboxazid, phenelzine, procarbazine, selegiline, tranylcypromine, etc.). This may result in symptoms such as agitation, delirium, headache, convulsions and/or hyperthermia.

### Neonatal Side Effects

*Apnea of the newborn:* This may occur when pethidine is administered to the mother during labor. Naloxone 10 μg/kg injected in the umbilical cord acts as the antidote of choice.

# Primiprost

## Introduction

This is an oral preparation of the prostaglandin E2, dinoprostone, commonly used for induction of labor. The gel formulation of this drug (commonly available in the form of cerviprime gel) has been described in details in Chapter 6.

### Mechanism of Action

The exact mechanism of action of dinoprostone is yet not clearly understood. It probably acts by stimulating the smooth muscles of myometrium and causing cervical ripening due to its collagenolytic property. The advantages of using primiprost over oxytocin for the induction of labor are as follows:

- It is a convenient and a noninvasive method for induction.
- Patient can remain ambulatory at the time of induction.
- It is associated with minimal side effects (e.g. uterine hyperstimulation).

### Indications

- Induction of labor (at or near term)
- Augmentation of labor.

### Route of Administration

- It is administered via oral route.
- It can also be sometimes administered via vaginal route.
- It is available in the form of a box containing four tablets, with each tablet containing 0.5 mg of synthetic dinoprostone.

### Dosage

In the beginning one tablet is administered orally. If there is no response, the dosage can be increased by administering 1 tablet at every 1–2 hours intervals until good uterine contractions have been established or a maximum of three additional tablets have been administered (a total of 4 tablets).

### Contraindications

Kindly refer to Chapter 6 for details related to contraindications for dinoprostone insertion.

### Side Effects

Use of primiprost can be associated with the following side effects:

- Hyperstimulation of uterus (rarely)
- Failure of induction of labor
- Gastrointestinal side effects: Nausea, vomiting, diarrhea.

# Prostodin

### Introduction

It is a synthetic prostaglandin PGF2α analog that predominantly acts on the myometrium. PGF2α enhance uterine contractility and cause vasoconstriction. Therefore, this prostaglandin is most commonly used for controlling PPH and for inducing uterine stimulation in cases of first and second trimester MTP.

### Mechanism of Action

Mechanism of action of prostodin has been described in the introduction.

### Indications

Prostodin is used for the following indications:

- Atonic PPH
- Medical termination of pregnancy (both first and second trimester).

### Route of Administration

One vial of 15-methyl prostaglandin F2α, or carboprost contains 2.5 mg/10 mL, i.e. 250 g/mL. Hemabate is carboprost tromethamine available as 250 µg/mL sterile solution suitable for intramuscular use. It is available in the form of 1 mL ampoules.

### Dosage

*Atonic PPH*: For prophylaxis of atonic PPH, 0.1–1 mL of carboprost tromethamine is administered IM at the birth of anterior shoulder or following the delivery of placenta. Presently, methylergometrine is preferred over carboprost for active management of third stage of labor due to its lower cost and fewer side effects in comparison with methylergometrine.

For treatment of atonic PPH, carboprost is usually administered intramuscularly in a dose of 0.25 mg; this dose can be repeated every 15–90 minutes for a total dose of 2 mg or a maximum of eight doses. In severe cases of PPH, carboprost can also be administered intramyometrially. Carboprost has been proven to control hemorrhage in up to 84–96% of patients. Its use will often obviate the requirement for surgical intervention in a case of atonic PPH. It has been shown that prostaglandins are not preferable over conventional uterotonics like oxytocin for the active management of third stage of labor and the prevention of PPH. However, if PPH occurs even after the administration of oxytocin, administration of parental prostaglandins serves as an effective form of treatment.

*Second trimester medical termination of pregnancy:* One ampoule of carboprost containing 250 µg of carboprost tromethamine is injected IM, following which it is repeated every 3 hourly until the patient aborts. A maximum of four injections are usually required.

*First trimester medical termination of pregnancy:* One ampoule of carboprost is administered half an hour prior to suction evacuation for facilitating cervical softening and dilatation.

## Contraindications

Carboprost should be used with caution in patients with asthma, hypertension, hepatic or renal diseases. It is contraindicated in patients with cardiovascular, renal, pulmonary or hepatic dysfunction.

## Side Effects

Some of the common side effects associated with the use of carboprost include nausea, vomiting, diarrhea, hypertension, headache, flushing, bronchoconstriction, pyrexia, etc. Some of the less common side effects include abdominal pain, flushing, shivering, headache, dizziness, hypotension, fever/chills, dyspnea, etc. Rarely, uterine hyperstimulation and rupture of uterus can also occur.

# Rhesus Anti-D Immunoglobulins

For detailed information related to rhesus anti-D immuno-globulins, kindly refer to Chapter 5.

# Ritodrine Hydrochloride

## Introduction

This is a tocolytic agent, which was the first drug to be approved by the US FDA for tocolysis.

## Mechanism of Action

It is a selective $\beta_2$ agonist, which causes relaxation of the uterine smooth muscles without causing excessive cardiac activity.

## Indications

- *Preterm labor:* Management of preterm labor in selected patients with period of gestation less than or equal to 20 weeks. Due to the tocolytic action of ritodrine hydrochloride, the clinician is able to delay the labor by few days, thereby allowing time to the fetus for attaining lung maturity.
- *Fetal distress:* This drug is used for cases of acute fetal distress due to uterine hyperstimulation at the time of labor.
- *Prevention of preterm labor after surgery:* Ritodrine hydro-chloride is used for preventing preterm labor in pregnant women who have to undergo surgery during their pregnancy (e.g. cardiac surgery).

## Route of Administration

- This drug can be administered by intravenous/oral routes.
- 5 mL ampoules are available containing 10 mg/mL of the drug; 10 mg tablets are available for oral use. Sustained release tablets of 40 mg are also available.

## Dosage

Three ampoules (50 mg/ampoule) of ritodrine hydrochloride (total of 150 mg) are added into 500 mL of compatible IV diluent (usually 5% dextrose and not saline) to make a solution of 0.3 mg/mL concentration. A controlled infusion device, having a microdrip chamber is used for administering IV infusions. Initial IV infusion is started at the rate of 0.1 mg/minute (0.33 mL/minute, 20 drops/minute). Based on the patient's clinical condition, this is gradually increased by 0.05 mg/minute (0.17 mL/minute, 10 drops/minute, every 10 minutes until the desired result is attained. The effective dosage usually ranges between 0.15 and 0.35 mg/minute (0.50 to 1.17 mL/minute, 30 to 70 drops/minute). This dose is continued for approximately 12–48 hours after the contractions cease. This is followed by maintenance therapy using oral preparation of ritodrine hydrochloride which is started 30–60 minutes before stopping the parenteral therapy. One tablet (10 mg orally is administered every 2 hourly for 24 hours; thereafter 1–2 tablets are administered every 4–6 hours or one slow release tablet (40 mg) can be administered three times a day. About 80–120 mg of ritodrine hydrochloride can be administered every day.

## Contraindications

Use of ritodrine hydrochloride is contraindicated in the following situations:
- Hypersensitivity to ritodrine or any of the components of the preparation
- Pregnancies less than 20 weeks of gestation
- Antepartum hemorrhage
- Eclampsia, severe preeclampsia, uncontrolled hypertension
- Intrauterine fetal death
- Chorioamnionitis
- Maternal cardiac disease, pulmonary hypertension
- Maternal hyperthyroidism
- Uncontrolled maternal diabetes mellitus.

## Side Effects

*Maternal Side Effects*

- *Gastrointestinal side effects:* Nausea, vomiting, constipation, diarrhea.
- *CNS:* Headache, weakness, tremor, nervousness, restlessness, emotional upset, anxiety, malaise, giddiness, tremors.
- *Cardiovascular side effects:* Flushing, tachycardia, increase in systolic BP, decrease in diastolic BP, palpitations, chest pain, supraventricular tachycardia, etc.
- *Respiratory:* Dyspnea, hyperventilation, postpartum pulmonary edema.
- *Hypersensitivity:* Anaphylactic shock, rash.
- *Other:* Erythema, transient elevation of blood glucose, hypokalemia.

*Fetal Side Effects*

Fetal tachycardia, hypotension, hypoglycemia, hypocalcemia, etc. in neonates (whose mothers were administered other β-adrenergic agonists).

# Tranexamic Acid

## Introduction

Tranexamic acid, an antifibrinolytic drug, is a competitive inhibitor of plasminogen activation, which prevents the conversion of plasminogen to plasmin, thereby preventing dissolution of the clot. It is a synthetic analog of the amino acid lysine and is used for the prevention of excessive blood loss related to several medical disorders.

## Mechanism of Action

Since tranexamic acid has a very high affinity for the lysine binding sites of plasminogen, it blocks these sites and prevents binding of activated plasminogen to the fibrin surface, thereby exerting its antifibrinolytic effect by preventing the conversion of fibrin to fibrin degradation products. Placental bleeding appears to result from structural weakness and vascular defects in uteroplacental blood vessels. Tranexamic acid retards this process by preventing clot lysis.

## Indications

*Gynecological Indications*

- Dysfunctional uterine bleeding
- *Menorrhagia:* It is used for controlling excessive blood loss related to uterine fibroids/ IUCD insertion, etc.
- *Prevention of bleeding after minor surgical procedures:* This drug can be used for controlling bleeding following the minor surgical gynecological procedures (e.g. cervical conization).

*Obstetric Indications*

- *Abruptio placentae:* It is used for the treatment of fibrinolytic stage of acute disseminated intravascular coagulation (especially related to abruptio placentae).
- *Postpartum hemorrhage:* Tranexamic acid is now also being considered for reducing excessive bleeding due to atonic PPH in combination with oxytocin infusion and/ or fundal massage. A large, international, randomized, placebo controlled trial (WOMAN trial) regarding the use of tranexamic acid for the management of primary PPH is currently underway. Once the results of this trial are published, the role of tranexamic acid in the treatment of PPH would become clearer.

*Nongynecological Indications*

- *Prevention/control of excessive bleeding:* It is used for prevention/treatment of excessive bleeding due to the use of fibrinolytic drugs, cardiac, liver, vascular, orthopedic surgery, tonsillectomy, prostatic surgery, tooth extraction in hemophiliacs, etc.
- Recurrent epistaxis, hyphema due to ocular trauma, bleeding due to peptic ulceration.
- Treatment of Von Willebrand's disease.

## Route of Administration

*Intravenous/oral:* It is available in 500 mg/5 mL ampoules for IV use and 250/500 mg oral tablets.

## Dosage

- *Treatment of menorrhagia and IUCD induced bleeding:* It is administered orally in the dosage of 0.5–1 g, repeated 3–4 times per day for 4–6 days.
- *Prevention of bleeding after surgery:* Tranexamic acid is administered in the dosage of 0.5–1.0 g intravenously 2–3 times daily after surgery. This is soon replaced by oral dosage, which is started 2–4 days following surgery.

## Contraindications

- Acquired defective color vision
- Patients with subarachnoid hemorrhage (danger of cerebral edema and cerebral infarction)
- Patients with active intravascular clotting
- Hypersensitivity to tranexamic acid
- Severe renal insufficiency/hematuria.

## Side Effects

Its side effects are nausea, vomiting, diarrhea, headache, giddiness, dizziness, fatigue, hypersensitivity reactions, potential risk of thrombosis, retinal degeneration (animal studies), visual disturbances (in postmarketing trials), thrombophlebitis of the injected vein and disturbances in color vision.

## FURTHER READINGS

1. Briggs GG, Freeman RK, Yaffe SJ. Drugs in Pregnancy and Lactation: A Reference Guide to Fetal and Neonatal Risk, 9th edition. Philadelphia; Lippincott Williams & Willkins: 2011.
2. Zatuchni GI, Slupik RI. Obstetrics and Gynecology Drug Handbook, 2nd edition. London: Mosby; 1996.

# SECTION 4

# Appendices

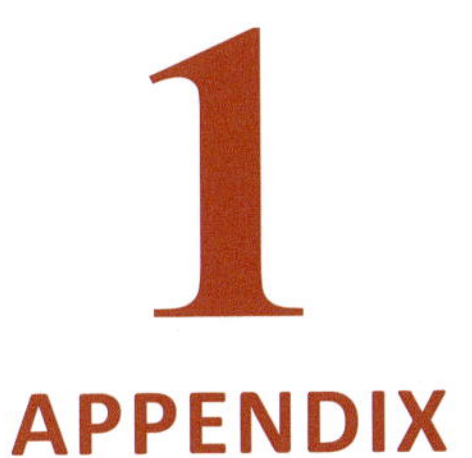



# Nutritional Values of the Common Food Stuffs

| S. No. | Food stuff | Calories (kCal) | Proteins (g) |
|---|---|---|---|
| | **Beverages** | | |
| 1. | 100 mL buffalo milk | 117 | 4 |
| 2. | 100 mL cow's milk | 67 | 3 |
| 3. | 1 cup buttermilk | 15 | 1 |
| 4. | 100 mL skimmed milk | 29 | 2 |
| 5. | 1 cup hot tea (without sugar) | 34 | 0.6 |
| 6. | 1 cup hot tea (with sugar) | 52 | 0.6 |
| 7. | 1 cup instant coffee | 149 | 1.0 |
| 8. | 1 glass lemonade | 107 | 0.3 |
| | **Breakfast** | | |
| 9. | 1 (250 mL) glass orange juice | 118 | 1 |
| 10. | 1 bowl cornflakes with milk | 291 | 9.8 |
| 11. | Bread (one slice) | 46 | 2.3 |
| 12. | 1 glucose biscuit | 15.9 | 0.2 |
| 13. | 1 boiled egg (small) | 57 | 4.64 |
| 14. | 1 omelette (of a small egg) | 77 | 5.38 |
| 15. | Semolina upma (1 bowl) | 147 | 2.3 |
| 16. | Vegetable upma | 192 | 4.4 |
| 17. | Semolina halwa (100 g) | 408 | 9.05 |
| 18. | Poha | 298 | 2.8 |
| | **Main Meals** | | |
| 19. | 100 g cooked vegetables | 125 | 2.3 |
| 20. | 100 mL dal (cooked lentils) | 108 | 8.3 |
| 21. | 100 g (boiled rice) | 111 | 2.2 |

| S. No. | Food stuff | Calories (kCal) | Proteins (g) |
|---|---|---|---|
| 22. | Plain chapati (phulka) without oil (35 g) | 85 | 3.0 |
| 23. | Plain paratha (50 g) | 150 | 4.0 |
| 24. | Puri (25 g) | 80 | 2.7 |
| 25. | 1 bowl curd (150 g) | 70 | 4.0 |
| 26. | Ice cream (1 cup vanilla, small) | 170 (vanilla) | 4.0 |
| | **Other Items** | | |
| 27. | Khichdi (150 g) | 182 | 7.0 |
| 28. | Pizza (small, with cheese) | 225 | 10.6 |
| 29. | Pav bhaji (one serving) | 118 | 3.3 |
| 30. | 100 g almond | 655 | 21.4 |
| 31. | 100 g cashew nuts | 596 | 18.22 |
| 32. | 100 g raisins | 150 | 2.4 |
| 33. | 100 g groundnuts | 567 | 15.0 |
| 34. | 100 g cheese | 348 | 24.0 |
| | **Fruits** | | |
| 35. | 1 banana (100 g) | 116 | 1.3 |
| 36. | 1 mango (200 g) | 160 | 0.8 |
| 37. | 1 apple (100 g) | 59 | 0.2 |
| | **Nonvegetarian food** | | |
| 38. | 100 g chicken breast | 298 | 33.0 |
| 39. | 100 g mutton | 279 | 36.0 |
| 40. | 100 g cod fish | 290 | 63.0 |

**APPENDIX**

# Reference Intervals: Biochemistry

Drugs (and other substances) may interfere with any chemical method as these effects may be method-dependent; it is difficult for the clinician to be aware of all possibilities. If in doubt, discuss with the lab.

| Substance | Specimen | Reference | Interval |
|---|---|---|---|
| Acid phosphatase (total) | S | 1–5 | IU/L |
| Acid phosphatase (prostatic) | S | 0–1 | IU/L |
| ACTH | P | < 80 | ng/L |
| Alanine aminotransferase (ALT) | P | 5–35 | IU/L |
| Albumin | P | 35–50 | g/L |
| Aldosterone | P | 100–500 | pmol/L |
| Alkaline phosphatase<br>  – Fetoprotein<br>  – Amylase | P<br>S<br>P | 30–300<br>< 10<br>0–180 (Somogyi) | pmol/L<br>kU/L<br>IU/dL |
| Angiotensin II | P | 5–35 | pmol/L |
| Antidiuretic hormone (ADH) | P | 0.9–4.6 | pmol/L |
| Aspartate transaminase (AST) | P | 5–35 | IU/L |
| Bicarbonate | P | 24–30 | mmol/L |
| Bilirubin | P | 3–17 | μmol (0.25–1.5 mg/100 mL) |
| Calcitonin | P | < 0.1 | μg/L |
| Calcium (ionized) | P | 1.0–1.25 | mmol/L |
| Calcium (total) | P | 2.12–2.65 | mmol/L |
| Chloride | P | 95–105 | mmol/L |
| Cholesterol | P | 3.9–7.8 | mmol/L |
| Very-low-density lipoprotein (VLDL) | P | 0.128–0.645 | mmol/L |
| low-density lipoprotein | P | 1.55–4.4 | mmol/L |
| high-density lipoprotein | P | 0.9–1.93 | mmol/L |
| Cortisol | P | Early morning (450–700)<br>Midnight (80–280) | nmol/L<br>nmol/L |
| Creatine kinase (CK) | P | Female (24–170)<br>Male (24–195) | IU/L<br>IU/L |
| Creatinine (related to lean body mass) | P | Female (0.5–1.1)<br>Male (0.6–1.2) | mg/dL |
| Ferritin | P | 12–200 | μg/L |
| Folate | S | 2.1 | μg/L |

(Contd ...)

*(Contd ...)*

| | | | |
|---|---|---|---|
| Follicle-stimulating hormone (FSH) | P/S | 2–8 | U/L (luteal) 18 |
| Gamma-glutamyl transpeptidase (GTT) | P | Male (11–50)<br>Female (7–33) | IU/L<br>IU/L |
| Glucose (fasting) | P | 3.5–5.5 | mmol/L |
| Glycated (glycosylate) hemoglobin | B | 5.8% | |
| Growth hormone | P | < 20 | mU/L |
| Iron | S | Male (14–31)<br>Female (11–30) | mmol/L |
| Lactate dehydrogenase (LDH) | P | 70–250 | IU/L |
| Luteinizing hormone (LH)<br>(Premenopausal) | P | 3–16 | U/L (luteal) |
| Magnesium | P | 0.75–1.05 | mmol/L |
| Osmolality | P | 278–305 | mosmol/1Kg |
| Parathyroid hormone (PTH) | P | < 0.8–8.5 | pmol/L |
| Phosphate (inorganic) | P | 0.8–1.45 | mmol/L |
| Potassium | P | 3.5–5.0 | mmol/L |
| Prolactin | P | Male (< 450)<br>Female (< 600) | U/L<br>U/L |
| Prostate-specific antigen | P | 0–4 | Nanograms/mL |
| Protein (total) | P | 60–80 | g/L |
| Red cell folate | B | 0.36–1.44 [160–140 (μg/L)] | μmol/L |
| Renin (erect/recumbent) | P | 2.8–4.5/1.1–2.7 | pmol/mL/h |
| Sodium | P | 133–145 | mmol/L |
| Thyroid-binding globulin (TBG) | P | 7–17 | mg/L |
| Thyroid-stimulating hormones (TSH)<br>NR widens with age<br>Thyroxine (T4)<br>Thyroxine (free) | P<br><br>P<br>P | 0.5–5.7<br><br>70–140<br>9–122 | mU/L<br><br>nmol/L<br>pmol/L |
| Total iron binding capacity | S | 54–75 | μmol/L |
| Triglyceride | P | 0.55–1.90 | mmol/L |
| Tri-iodothyronine (T3) | P | 2.5–6.7 | nmol/L |
| Urea | P | 1.2–6.7 | mmol/L |
| Urate | P | 6210–480<br>1150–390 | μmol/L<br>μmol/L |
| Vitamin B12 | S | 0.13–0.68 | Nmol/(< 150 ng/L) |

*Abbreviations:* P = plasma (heparin bottle); S = serum (clotted; no anticoagulant); B = whole blood (edetic acid-EDTA-bottle); IU = international unit

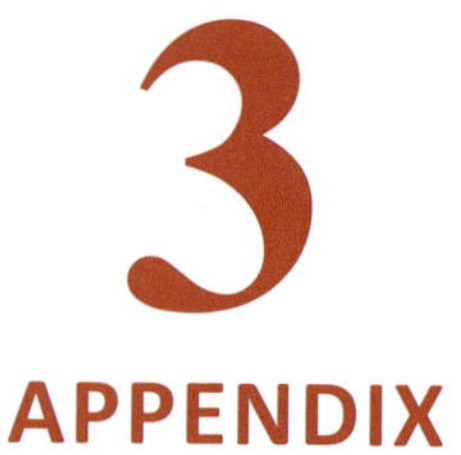



# Reference Intervals: Urine

| Substance | Reference | Interval |
|---|---|---|
| Cortisol (free) | < 280 | nmol/24h |
| Hydroxyindoleacetic acid | 16–73 | µmol/24h |
| Hydroxymethylmandelic acid (HMMA, VMA) | 16–48 | µmol/24h |
| Osmolality | 350–1,000 | mosmol/kg |
| 17-Oxogenic steroids | Male (28–30)<br>Female (21–66) | µmol/24h<br>µmol/24h |
| 17-Oxosteroids (neutral) | Male (17–76)<br>Female (14–59) | µmol/24h<br>µmol/24h |
| Phosphate (inorganic) | 15–50 | mmol/24h |
| Potassium | 14–120 | mmol/24h |
| Protein | < 150 | mg/24h |
| Sodium | 100–250 | mmol/24h |

# Reference Intervals: Hematology

| Measurements | Reference |
| --- | --- |
| White cell count (WCC) | $4.0–11.0 \times 10^9$/L |
| Red blood cell (RBC) count | Male ($4.5–6.5 \times 10^{12}$/L)<br>Female ($3.9–5.6 \times 10^{12}$/L) |
| Hemoglobin | Male (13.5–18.0 g/dL)<br>Female ($11.5 \times 16.0$ g/dL) |
| Packed red cell volume (PCV) or hematocrit | Male (0.4–0.54 L/L)<br>Female (0.37–0.47 L/L) |
| Mean cell volume (MCV) | 76–96 L |
| Mean cell hemoglobin (MCH) | 27–32 pg |
| Mean cell hemoglobin concentration (MCHC) | 30–36 g/dL |
| Neutrophils | $2.0–7.5 \times 10^9$/L; 40–75% WCC |
| Lymphocytes | $1.3–3.5 \times 10^9$/L; 20–45% WCC |
| Eosinophils | $0.04–0.44 \times 10^9$/L; 1–6% WCC |
| Basophils | $0.0–0.10 \times 10^9$/L; 0–1% WCC |
| Monocytes | $0.2–0.8 \times 10^9$/L; 2–10% WCC |
| Platelet count | $150.0–400.0 \times 10^9$/L |
| Reticulocyte count | Expressed as percentage when the RBC count is normal (0.8–2.0 %). Absolute value is used when the RBC count is not normal ($25–100 \times 10^9$/L) |
| Erythrocyte sedimentation rate | Depends on age |
| Prothrombin time (factors II, VII, X) | 10–14 seconds |
| Activated partial thromboplastin | 35–45 seconds |

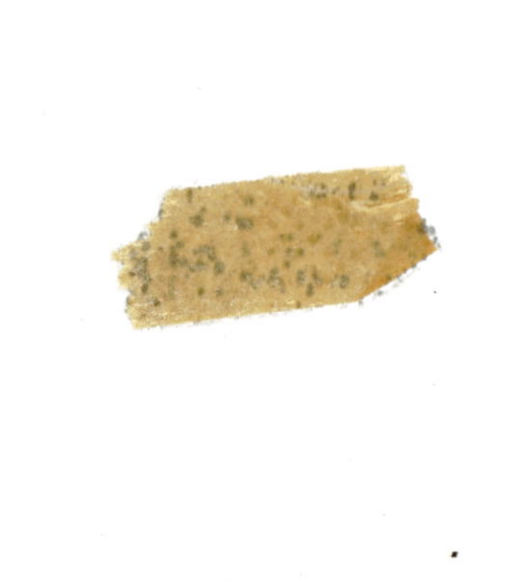